FAMILY MEDICAL ADVISER

AN A-Z GUIDE TO EVERYDAY AILMENTS, THEIR SYMPTOMS, CAUSES AND TREATMENT

FAMILY MEDICAL ADVISER

 PUBLISHED BY THE READER'S DIGEST ASSOCIATION LIMITED, LONDON

FAMILY MEDICAL ADVISER
was edited and designed by
The Reader's Digest Association Limited
London

Editor Joe Barling
Art Editor Mavis Henley

First edition
Copyright © 1983
The Reader's Digest Association Limited
Berkeley Square House
Berkeley Square
London WIX 6AB
Reprinted with amendments 1994

Typesetting
Jolly & Barber Limited, Rugby
Sprint Limited, Beckenham
Colour separations
Gilchrist Bros Limited, Leeds
Paper
C. Townsend Hook & Company Ltd.
Printing and binding
Usines Brepols, Turnhout, Belgium

® READER'S DIGEST, THE DIGEST and the
Pegasus logo are registered trademarks of
The Reader's Digest Association Inc.
of Pleasantville, New York, U.S.A.

Printed in Belgium

ISBN 0 276 00240 7

CONTENTS

CONTRIBUTORS

CONSULTANT EDITOR

Keith Hodgkin, BM, BCh, FRCGP, FRCP
Previously General Practitioner in
Redcar, Yorkshire, and
Professor and Chairman of
General Practice,
Memorial University, Newfoundland,
Canada
Visiting Professor in General Practice
Universities of Glasgow and Dundee;
Visiting Fellow
University of Western Australia

REVISIONS EDITORS

Dr James Cox, MB, BS, FRCGP, MICGP
General Practitioner in
Caldbeck, Cumbria

Dr Sheena Meredith, MB, BS, LRCP, MRCS
Medical Writer

EDITORIAL CONTRIBUTORS

Arnold E. Bender, BSc, PhD, FRSH, FIFST
Professor of Nutrition
Queen Elizabeth College
University of London

David A. Bender, BSc, PhD
Lecturer in Biochemistry
Courtauld Institute of Biochemistry
Middlesex Hospital Medical School
University of London

Dr George Birdwood, MA, MB, ChB, MIL

Professor James Calnan, FRCS, FRCP, DA, DTM & H, LDS, RCS, FCST
Professor of Plastic and Reconstructive
Surgery
University of London
at Hammersmith Hospital, London

Margaret E. Carter, SRN, SCM
Queen's Nurse

Dr Robert Catty, MB, BS, MRCGP
General Practitioner in Durham

Professor Geoffrey Chamberlain, RD, MD, FRCS, FRCOG
Department of Obstetrics and Gynaecology
St George's Hospital Medical School
London

Dr John Clarke, DSc, MD, MB, ChB

Dr Aubrey Colling, MD, FRCGP
General Practitioner in Stockton-on-Tees
Cleveland

Sarah Collins

Dr John Cormack, MD, FRCGP, DObst. RCOG
General Practitioner in Edinburgh

Ann Darnbrough,
Disability Consultant
to the Appropriate Health Resources
and Technologies Action Group

Dr Alan Maryon Davis, MB, BChir, MSc, MRCP, MFCM
Medical Officer
The Health Education Council, London

Dr Roland Freedman, MA, MB, BChir, FRCGP
General Practitioner in Gosforth,
Newcastle upon Tyne
Lecturer in Family Medicine
University of Newcastle upon Tyne

Dr John Fry, OBE, MD, FRCS, FRCGP
General Practitioner in Beckenham, Kent

Jean Gaffin, BSc(Econ), MSc
Child Accident Prevention Trust

Dr Max M. Glatt, DSc, MD, FRCP, FRCPsych, DPM
Alcoholism Teaching Clinic
University College Hospital, London

Dr Muir Gray, MD
Community Physician
The Radcliffe Infirmary, Oxford

Christina Gregory

Dr Mark Harries, MD, BS, MRCP, MRCS
Lecturer in Medicine
Guy's Hospital Medical School, London

Dr Frank Hull, MB, BS, FRCGP, DObst. RCOG
General Practitioner in Wellesbourne,
Warwick
Senior Lecturer in General Practice
University of Birmingham Medical School

Professor Bernard Isaacs, MD, FRCP(Glasgow & Edinburgh)
Department of Geriatric Medicine
University of Birmingham

Dr Sally Jobling, MRCS, LRCP, MRCGP, DObst.RCOG
General Practitioner in Oxford

Elizabeth MacKenzie Keeble

Professor J. D. E. Knox, MD, FRCP(Edinburgh), FRCGP
Department of General Practice
University of Dundee

Dr Douglas MacAdam, MA, MD, BChir, BD, FRCGP, FRACGP
Senior Lecturer in Community Practice
University of Western Australia

Dr Colin Mackenzie, MB, ChB, MRCGP
General Practitioner in Stockton-on-Tees
Cleveland

Mairi Mackenzie, BDS, LDS, DOrth, RCS
Department of Orthodontics
West Middlesex Hospital

Dr Nicola McClure, MB, BS, MRCS, LRCP
General Practitioner in London

Dr Harvey Marcovitch, MA, MB, BChir, MRCP, DObst.RCOG, DCH
Consultant Paediatrician
Horton General Hospital, Banbury

Marion Mathews

Dr Judith Millac, MB, BS, MRCS, LRCP, MRCGP, DObst.RCOG, DCH
General Practitioner in Leicester

Dr Kenneth Mourin, MA, MB, BChir,
MRCS, LRCP, DObst.RCOG, FRCGP
General Practitioner in Dereham, Norfolk

David Sutherland Muckle, MB,
BS(Dunelm), FRCS, MS, MD
Consultant Orthopaedic Surgeon
Medical Adviser FIFA

Dr Stuart Murray, PhD, MRCP(UK),
FRCP(Glasgow), FRCGP, DObst.RCOG
General Accident Senior Lecturer
Department of General Practice
University of Glasgow

Dr Frank Preston, VRD, MB, ChB, DA,
FFOM, FRAes
Director Medical and Safety Services
British Airways

Martin Raw, BA, MPhil
Department of Psychology
St George's Hospital Medical School
London

Dr Peter Roylance, RD, MB, ChB
Executive Medical Director, Medical
Operations, Merck, Sharp and Dohme,
New Jersey

John Talbot, MB, BS, FRCS, MRCS, LRCP
Consultant Ophthalmologist
Royal Hallamshire General Hospital
Sheffield

Janet Thrush, LCST

Ian Williams, BA, FITD, AEMT
Training Officer
British Red Cross

Jim Williams, MITD
British Red Cross

ARTISTS

Andrew Aloof

Keith Campbell

Jennifer Eachus

Nicholas Hall

Gordon Lawson

Malcolm McGregor

Howard Pemberton

Charles Pickard

Stephen Pointer

Bill Prosser

Charles Raymond

Edward Williams

PHOTOGRAPHER

Clive Arrowsmith

ADVISERS

Infant Feeding Sister Jane Armstrong
and the Parentcraft staff at
Queen Charlotte's Maternity Hospital
London

Dr Rosemarie A. Balliod
Department of Nephrology and
Transplantation
Royal Free Hospital, London

Anthea A. Blake
Nursing Officer, Neonatal Unit
University College Hospital, London

Alice Burns
Health Programmes Organiser
Women's National Cancer Control
Campaign, London

Professor Leslie Collier
Head of Department of Virology
London Hospital Medical College

Mr E. E. Douek, FRCS
Consultant Otologist
Guy's Hospital, London

David Griffin
Research Fellow
Department of Obstetrics and Gynaecology
King's College Hospital, London

Anne de J. Harvard
Great Ayton, Cleveland

Christopher R. Hayne
Physiotherapist specialising in Ergonomics
and Occupational Health

Dr A. M. Hewlett
Chairman, Intensive Therapy Unit
Northwick Park Hospital, Middlesex

Rosemary Hodgkin
Great Ayton, Cleveland

Alan Jones

Mr Alan Lynch
Orthodontist

Miss A. L. Lyness
Lecturer in Clinical Ophthalmology
Moorfields Eye Hospital, London

D. E. Maynard, MPhil, PhD
EEG Department
The London Hospital (Whitechapel)

Dr John K. Morgan
Kirkby-in-Cleveland

Dr P. F. Prior
St Bartholomew's Hospital, London

Carol Redvanly
PETT Program Project Administrator
Brookhaven National Laboratory, New York

Professor E. O. R. Reynolds
Professor of Neonatal Paediatrics
School of Medicine, University College, London

H. S. J. Siford, MBE
Consultant, Disability Training Centre
British School of Motoring Limited, London

Janet Silver
Principal Ophthalmic Optician
Moorfields Eye Hospital, London

Hugh Spencely. MA(Cantab), RIBA, MRTPI

Stephen Thorpe
Architect, Sudbury, Suffolk

David Ward, MD, MRCP
Cardiology Department
Brompton Hospital, London

HOW TO USE THIS BOOK

There are three ways to get at the information contained
in FAMILY MEDICAL ADVISER:

- by turning straight to an entry in the main A–Z section of the book;
- by using the Symptom Sorter;
- by looking up a key word in the index.

1. Using the main A–Z section
pages 56–537

If you know the name of the
ailment you wish to look up,
turn straight to it in the A–Z
section. There you will find a
description of the disorder
together with advice on how to
deal with it presented under the
following headings:

Symptoms
Duration
Causes
Complications
Treatment in the home
When to consult the doctor
What the doctor may do
Prevention
Outlook

2. Using the Symptom Sorter *pages 10–29*

In many cases, you may not know the name of the ailment, and so not know where to look. The symptoms, though, will be all too obvious—a cough, a high temperature, a sore throat, a rash, a headache, a back pain and so on.

When you see your doctor, with a medical complaint, the first thing he needs to know about is your symptoms.

By studying them he can go on to give a diagnosis of the complaint, and so prescribe the correct treatment.

The symptom sorter is organised like a consultation with your doctor.

Turn first to the symptom that is troubling you.

There you will be told how to interpret it and what immediate action, if any, to take. Each symptom entry lists the illnesses which may be causing the trouble and directs you to the appropriate entries in the main A–Z section of the book.

EMERGENCIES
Turn straight to the First Aid section *pages 538–612*

3. Using the Index
pages 613–623

Sometimes an ailment may have more than one name, making it difficult to track down in the A–Z section.

In that case, turn to the index at the back of the book.

Every illness mentioned in the book is listed under its alternative names.

The index also tells where in the book you can find specific items of medical information which do not have separate A–Z entries.

PART 1 SYMPTOM SORTER

A guide to understanding your symptoms and identifying their possible causes

ABDOMINAL PAIN

Pain in the abdomen is frequently a symptom of trivial disorder, but it may also point to a serious illness. It can arise from disorders of the DIGESTIVE SYSTEM (page 44), the URINARY SYSTEM (page 46), or, in women, the FEMALE GENITAL SYSTEM (page 48). For abdominal pain in children see also CHILD CARE page 155.
Immediate treatment
• Rest, taking fluids only.
When to consult the doctor
Immediately if:
• The pain is unchanged, or getting worse, after four hours.
• The sufferer is, or may be, pregnant.
• The pain is associated with vomiting, bleeding or abnormal periods.
As soon as possible if:
• The sufferer has had previous abdominal disorders such as DUODENAL ULCER, suspected APPENDICITIS or CHOLECYSTITIS.
• The pain is severe and interfering with sleep or the ability to work.
• The sufferer is elderly or very young (under six). In such cases even slight abdominal pain may have a serious underlying cause.
Possible causes
• Digestive disorders
Pain may be in the upper or lower abdomen, and associated with taking food, vomiting, nausea or diarrhoea.
Common causes: INDIGESTION; GASTROENTERITIS.
Less likely causes: APPENDICITIS; DUODENAL ULCER; GASTRIC ULCER; DIVERTICULAR DISEASE OF THE COLON; BOWEL OBSTRUCTION.
• Urinary disorders
Pain is felt in the lower abdomen, and also over the kidneys (in the back below the ribs) or in the genitalia. There may be blood in the water, frequent urination or burning pain on passing water.
Common causes: CYSTITIS.

Less likely causes: STONES IN THE URINARY TRACT; PYELONEPHRITIS.
• Disorders of the female genital system
Pain is usually in the lower abdomen and also in the lower back area. There may be abnormalities of periods, discharge, or abnormal bleeding from the vagina.
Common causes: PERIOD PROBLEMS; OVULATION SYNDROME; labour and childbirth (see PREGNANCY).
Less likely causes: Miscarriage (see ABORTION); ECTOPIC PREGNANCY; SALPINGITIS; ENDOMETRIOSIS.

AMNESIA

See SYMPTOM SORTER—MENTAL ACTIVITIES, FAILURE OF
See also page 71

ANKLE PROBLEMS

Pain and swelling are the symptoms most likely to affect the ankle. They often appear together, but not always. Symptoms usually follow a known injury or a chronic disease of which the sufferer is aware, such as GOUT or ARTHRITIS.
Immediate treatment
• Rest the affected ankle. Raise the foot.
• Take painkillers in recommended doses. *See* MEDICINES, 22.
When to consult the doctor
• If the ankle cannot bear the sufferer's weight.
• If the ankle appears deformed.
• If there is extensive purple bruising.
• If pain on weight-bearing persists after two days' rest.
• If the swelling is painless, affects both feet and is not caused by injury— especially if the sufferer is elderly.
Possible causes
• Pain

Common causes: SPRAIN; SYNOVITIS; some fevers.
Less likely causes: FRACTURE; ACHILLES TENDON RUPTURE; GOUT; RHEUMATOID ARTHRITIS; OSTEOARTHRITIS; RHEUMATIC FEVER.
• Swelling of both ankles
Common causes: Hot weather; prolonged standing; PREGNANCY; OBESITY.
Less likely causes: VARICOSE VEINS; HEART FAILURE; NEPHRITIS.

ANUS, PROBLEMS OF

Problems affecting the anus include bleeding, pain when passing a motion, swellings around the anus, and itching.
Immediate treatment
• Bathe the area, dry thoroughly and apply a soothing cream or lotion.
When to consult the doctor
• If there is bleeding from the anus, either with or after passing a motion.
• If passage of mucus or slime is noticed. This is often of no significance, but occasionally it may be a sign of serious disease.
• If irritation is persistent enough to cause embarrassment.
Possible causes
• Bleeding
Common causes: Babies and children— CONSTIPATION; ANAL FISSURE.
Adults—PILES; ANAL FISSURE.
Less likely causes: Babies—INTUSSUSCEPTION.
Adults—DIVERTICULAR DISEASE OF THE COLON; POLYPOSIS; cancer of the BOWEL; ULCERATIVE COLITIS.
• Pain when passing a motion
Common causes: PILES; ANAL FISSURE; CONSTIPATION; injury during labour.
Less likely causes: Internal PILES; RECTAL PROLAPSE (especially in babies).
• Irritation
See ANAL IRRITATION.

APATHY

A state of listlessness or fatigue in which the patient appears to have lost interest in the world about him. People may also refer to the symptom as malaise, tiredness, prostration and weakness. Apathy is a common symptom of many disorders both trivial and serious, but because it occurs frequently it is difficult to define, has many variations in meaning and is difficult to interpret. Only the presence of other symptoms, such as fever and loss of weight, make it possible to differentiate between many causes of both psychological and physical origin. If other symptoms are absent, relatively trivial causes are probably responsible.
Possible causes
Common causes: Monday morning feeling; hangover; FEVER; infection; ANXIETY; DEPRESSION; INSOMNIA; MYALGIC ENCEPHALOMYELITIS.
Less likely causes: ANAEMIA; MYXOEDEMA; serious mental diseases such as DEPRESSION and SCHIZOPHRENIA; many other chronic diseases and infections.

APPETITE, LOSS OF

A symptom of a wide variety of diseases. The medical name is anorexia. The significance of loss of appetite varies with the age of the patient.
When to consult the doctor
• If, in the case of babies, loss of appetite persists for more than 24 hours and the cause is not obvious.
• If, in the case of teenagers and adults, loss of appetite persists for more than seven days, earlier if there is also loss of weight, vomiting, diarrhoea, cough or abdominal pain.
• If an old person living alone is

involved—since loss of appetite in these circumstances can lead to malnutrition.

Possible causes
Loss of appetite is a side-effect of all fevers and many disorders of children. Many disorders are trivial, but a few may be serious. *See also* CHILD CARE *page 149.*
• Loss of appetite for less than seven days
This is a common symptom of minor infections and many trivial disorders, such as: MOTION SICKNESS, hangover, INDIGESTION, GASTROENTERITIS, COMMON COLD, TONSILLITIS, and other infections. Other symptoms usually make the cause clear.
• Loss of appetite for longer than seven days
Common causes: PREGNANCY; GASTROENTERITIS; alcohol and ALCOHOLISM.
Less likely causes: HEPATITIS; GLANDULAR FEVER; TUBERCULOSIS; ulcerative COLITIS; STOMACH and other CANCERS; RHEUMATOID ARTHRITIS; ANOREXIA NERVOSA; DEPRESSION; DRUG ABUSE; CIRRHOSIS OF THE LIVER.

ARM PROBLEMS

Problems with the arm such as pain, swelling or stiffness usually relate to the movement of joints or to parts of the arm. For example, pain may be greatest with shoulder movement, or tremors may be most obvious in the hand. Problems in the arm are dealt with in this Symptom Sorter under the part of the arm most affected.

Occasionally, after major breast operations, swelling and pain may affect the whole arm, this should be reported to the doctor.

BACK PAIN

However agonising, back pain is usually the result of some minor strain or injury. Only rarely does it have a serious cause. *See page 84*

BAD BREATH

Known medically as halitosis, it is usually due to poor care of the teeth and gums, sometimes to digestive disorders. Regular cleaning of teeth, combined with regular perborate mouth washes and advice from a dentist are essential for complete cure. Individuals especially liable to bad breath must avoid foods such as onions or garlic.
See TEETH.

BALANCE PROBLEMS

Problems with balance are often just the result of slight changes in posture or blood pressure, but occasionally they may be a symptom of more serious disease.
Immediate treatment
• Sit or lay the patient down until the difficulty has passed.
• Do not attempt to drive or carry on with your job.
When to consult the doctor
• If the dizziness persists for longer than 30 seconds or if it recurs.
• If it interferes with any activity, especially if this involves machinery or heights.
Possible causes
• Dizziness and lightheadedness
The sufferer has a sensation of unsteadiness which usually passes after a

minute or so.
Common causes: Standing up suddenly; FAINTING ATTACK; excess of alcohol; sleeping-pills; hot rooms.
Less likely causes: TRANSIENT ISCHAEMIC ATTACK; VERTEBRO-BASILAR INSUFFICIENCY.
• Vertigo
A spinning sensation identical to that felt after being spun several times on a rotary chair. The patient staggers to one side and is unable to stand up. *See* VERTIGO.
• Ataxia
Movements are clumsy, speech may be slurred, and walking may be unsteady.
Common causes: Excess of alcohol or other drugs; fatigue.
Less likely causes: STROKE; MULTIPLE SCLEROSIS; ST VITUS'S DANCE; BRAIN TUMOUR; TABES DORSALIS.

BEDWETTING

See CHILD CARE *page 159.*

BEHAVIOUR, ABNORMAL

Unusual or extreme behaviour may occur in adults or children (*see* CHILD CARE *page 159*). Such behaviour is disturbing to those in contact with the patient, and unfortunately it is often difficult to identify the cause.
ANXIETY, COMPULSIVE OBSESSIONAL BEHAVIOUR, DEPRESSION, HYSTERIA, PARANOIA, PHOBIA and SUICIDE all have entries in the A-Z section of this book and should be consulted directly.
Immediate treatment
• It is often necessary to report such behaviour to family or friends. Ensure that the patient is not a harm to himself or others.
When to consult the doctor
• If normal activity is being interfered

with, and if the patient could endanger others or himself.
Possible causes
• Agitated behaviour
The sufferer is unusually irritable, overactive, restless, anxious or shows great variations in mood.
Common causes: Extremes of worry; ALCOHOL; DRUG ABUSE.
Less likely causes: HYSTERIA, HYPOMANIA, DEPRESSION, SCHIZOPHRENIA, DIABETES; DRUG ABUSE; stimulants (*see* MEDICINES, 20).
• Aggressive behaviour
Aggressiveness and anger are normal adult reactions to any situation of insecurity, fear or worry. However, abnormal aggression and sudden swings of mood may be a symptom of disorder.
Common causes: Excess of alcohol; extreme fear or anger; ANXIETY; stimulants (*see* MEDICINES, 20); living alone for long periods.
Less likely causes: EPILEPSY; insulin overdose (DIABETES); head injury with concussion (POST-CONCUSSIONAL SYNDROME); HYPOMANIA; SCHIZOPHRENIA; BRAIN TUMOUR.
• Delusions and hallucinations
The sufferer is completely certain that unlikely events, voices heard or visions seen have actually happened. SCHIZOPHRENIA in its early stages is a likely cause.
• Guilt
Extreme feelings of guilt are not uncommon in perfectly normal individuals.
Common causes: DEATH AND BEREAVEMENT; any close involvement with a major catastrophe.
Less likely causes: DEPRESSION; PHOBIA.
• Irritability
A normal reaction to tension and worry. ANXIETY; PREMENSTRUAL TENSION; INSOMNIA and fatigue are common causes.
• Odd behaviour
Behaviour that is clearly abnormal or completely out of character may arise in certain disorders.
Common causes: Excess of alcohol; sedatives or stimulants (*see* MEDICINES, 17, 20).

Less likely causes: EPILEPSY; CONCUSSION; insulin overdose (DIABETES); HYPOMANIA.

• Paranoia or persecution complex
Abnormal feelings; delusions about being persecuted.
Common causes: Living alone, especially in old age.
Less likely causes: SCHIZOPHRENIA; PARANOIA.

See SYMPTOM SORTER—MENTAL ACTIVITIES, FAILURE OF

BLACKOUTS

See SYMPTOM SORTER— CONSCIOUSNESS, DISTURBANCES OF

BLEEDING

If bleeding is a result of injury *see* FIRST AID *page 564*. Other sites of bleeding include the nose (*see* NOSE-BLEED), moles and other skin blemishes (*see* SYMPTOM SORTER—SKIN ABNORMALITIES), and the vagina.

TENDENCY TO BLEED
Some individuals bleed and bruise more easily and for longer than others. This is rarely a cause for concern unless a NOSE-BLEED or bleeding after removal of teeth cannot be stopped: medical help may then be needed. Consult a doctor if the tendency develops.

UNEXPECTED BLEEDING FROM THE VAGINA
If your periods have stopped (amenorrhoea), are painful (dysmenorrhoea), heavy or irregular (menorrhagia and dysfunctional menstrual bleeding). *See* PERIOD PROBLEMS.

Unexpected bleeding (between periods, during pregnancy, after childbirth, during or after sexual intercourse or after the MENOPAUSE) should always be taken seriously although it may be harmless, as in the case of mid-point spotting which often arises when taking the contraceptive pill. In general, large losses require more immediate action than smaller ones.
Immediate treatment
• Bed-rest.
When to consult the doctor
Immediately if:
• You are or may be pregnant.
• You have just had a baby.
• Bleeding is associated with pain in the lower back.
As soon as possible if:
• The pain is severe or starts unexpectedly.
• Bleeding occurs after intercourse, or after the menopause.
• You are in any doubt about the origin of the blood.
Possible causes
Common causes: Spontaneous ABORTION; the Pill; the onset of childbirth, when there is a small flow of blood.
Less likely causes: ANTEPARTUM HAEMORRHAGE (during pregnancy); childbirth (post-partum haemorrhage); cancer of the UTERUS; CERVICAL CANCER; ECTOPIC PREGNANCY; uterine fibroids; dysfunctional menstrual bleeding (*see* PERIOD PROBLEMS).

See also SYMPTOM SORTER—BLOOD

BLINDNESS

Loss of sight may develop gradually or suddenly, and may affect one or both eyes, partially or completely. The cause may be serious.
Immediate treatment
• If loss of sight is sudden, rest in a chair with eyes closed until medical help is obtained.

When to consult the doctor
• As soon as possible.
Possible causes
• Sudden blindness in one or both eyes, complete or partial
Common causes: MIGRAINE (blindness passes off in ten to 20 minutes).
Less likely causes: CIRCULATION PROBLEMS IN THE EYE; DETACHED RETINA; ARTERITIS (temporal); GLAUCOMA (acute).
• Gradual onset of blindness in one or both eyes
Common causes: CATARACT; amblyopia (lazy eye).
Less likely causes: GLAUCOMA (chronic); IRITIS; DETACHED RETINA; CIRCULATION PROBLEMS IN THE EYE; DIABETES; inflammation of the retina.

BLISTERS

Causes of blisters include friction, allergy, burning, or various diseases.
See page 91

BLOOD

Blood may be seen in any bodily discharge or may appear as undiluted blood. It should always be reported to a doctor.

BLOOD IN THE MOTIONS
If the blood is from the large bowel or anus, it will be bright red and may be passed on its own or mixed with a motion. If the blood is from higher up in the digestive tract—from a gastric or duodenal ulcer—the motion may be black and tarry (not red) because of digestive action. This is called a melaena stool.
Immediate treatment
• Rest in bed and take sips of water.
When to consult the doctor
• Immediately if a black, tarry motion or

blood is passed.
Possible causes
Common causes: Severe NOSE-BLEED or taking iron or bismuth (black motion); PILES (red motion).
Less likely causes: DUODENAL or GASTRIC ULCER; CIRRHOSIS OF THE LIVER; STOMACH and BOWEL CANCER; ulcerative COLITIS; POLYPOSIS or DIVERTICULAR DISEASE OF THE COLON; SCHISTOSOMIASIS in some countries.
See SYMPTOM SORTER—MOTIONS, ABNORMAL.

BLOOD IN SEMEN
If blood appears in semen, consult the doctor.

BLOOD IN SPIT
If spit contains blood, or is tinged red or rusty, or if blood is coughed up (haemoptysis), disease in the lungs is suspected. Vomited blood probably arises from the digestive system.
Immediate treatment
• Complete bed-rest until the cause of the bleeding is identified.
When to consult the doctor
• As soon as possible.
Possible causes
• Frequently, full observation and investigation fail to reveal the cause or site of such bleeding.
Common causes: SINUSITIS (acute); NOSE-BLEED.
Less likely causes: PNEUMONIA; PULMONARY EMBOLISM; TUBERCULOSIS of lung; LUNG CANCER.

BLOOD IN THE URINE
Passing urine that is red or tinged with red (haematuria) indicates bleeding in the urinary system unless caused by dye of some kind. Sometimes, despite full investigation in hospital, no obvious cause is found.
When to consult the doctor
• If there is any red discoloration (even a faint tinge) of the urine that cannot be attributed to something eaten.
Possible causes
Common causes: Eating beetroot and foods

coloured by certain red dyes; CYSTITIS. *Less likely causes*: NEPHRITIS (acute); STONES IN THE URINARY TRACT; injury; kidney and bladder CANCER; SCHISTOSOMIASIS in some countries.

BLOOD IN VOMIT
Vomiting blood (haematemesis) usually indicates bleeding in the digestive system. Blood that is coughed up is more likely to be from the lungs.

If the blood is from the mouth or nose it is bright red. When bleeding is from the food pipe (oesophagus), stomach or duodenum, fresh red blood may be vomited up or just appear in the mouth. If the blood has remained in the stomach for an hour or so before it is brought up, it may be dark brown and look like coffee grounds.

Occasionally after an obvious NOSE-BLEED some blood may be subconsciously swallowed and then vomited up an hour or so later.

Immediate treatment
- Rest in bed without food or drink.
- Rinse mouth out with water.

When to consult the doctor
- Immediately, regardless of the quantity of blood, unless the bleeding is clearly due to a trivial cause such as a nose-bleed.

Possible causes
Common causes: Bleeding from the gums or mouth; NOSE-BLEED.
Less likely causes: DUODENAL or GASTRIC ULCER; OESOPHAGITIS; CIRRHOSIS OF THE LIVER; STOMACH and OESOPHAGUS CANCER.

See also SYMPTOM SORTER—BLEEDING

BOWEL PROBLEMS

Any change of an otherwise well-established bowel habit should be reported to the doctor.
See SYMPTOM SORTER—BLOOD
SYMPTOM SORTER—MOTIONS, ABNORMAL

SYMPTOM SORTER—DIARRHOEA
CONSTIPATION

BREAST PROBLEMS

Breasts vary naturally in shape, size and colour. Only if a change is noticed is there cause for concern. In a normal woman the nipples of one or both breasts may be inverted—turned in—and appear to be absent. Correction of this defect is simple and allows normal breast-feeding.

A doctor should be consulted before treatment for cosmetic reasons. *See* COSMETIC SURGERY.

When to consult the doctor
- As soon as possible if any lump is found.
- At once if there is pain related to breast-feeding because a BREAST ABSCESS may develop.
- If the nipples become cracked, painful and then inflamed during breast-feeding. *See page 372.*
- If there is puckering of the skin and discharge from the nipple.

Possible causes
- Lumps
Common causes: FIBROADENOMA OF THE BREAST; breast-feeding; BREAST ENGORGEMENT.
Less likely causes: BREAST CANCER; nodular MASTITIS; BREAST ABSCESS.

BREATHING DIFFICULTIES

There are three main types of breathing difficulty: noisy breathing, painful breathing and shortness of breath or breathlessness.

NOISY BREATHING
Noisy breathing is of two kinds: wheezy breathing, where the noise occurs on

breathing out, and hoarse or difficult breathing which is noisy on breathing in and out. It is often difficult to distinguish the two types of noisy breathing but they have different sets of causes.

Immediate treatment
- Rest in a pleasantly warm, airy room.
- Steam inhalations.

When to consult the doctor
As soon as possible if:
- A baby under six months is affected.
- A baby or toddler is restless or looks grey in colour.
- There is obvious difficulty or distress in getting breath—breathing may be rapid and the lower ribs may be drawn in with each breath.
- There is heart disease of any kind.
- There is any possibility of a FOREIGN BODY IN THE EAR, NOSE OR THROAT.

Possible causes
- Wheezy on breathing out
Common causes: COMMON COLD; RESPIRATORY INFECTION (acute). Toddlers and children are especially affected by this condition.
Less likely causes: ASTHMA; BRONCHIOLITIS and certain virus infections.
- Noisy breathing in and out
Common causes: CROUP; LARYNGITIS; RESPIRATORY INFECTION (acute upper).
Less likely causes: EPIGLOTTITIS; certain virus infections.

PAINFUL BREATHING
Breathing that is painful is called pleuritic respiration. It is a serious symptom and suggests disorder in the lungs, their lining (pleura), or in the bones, muscles or skin of the chest. The pain forces the sufferer to catch all breaths, which are therefore short and often rapid. A cough is often present as well.

Immediate treatment
- Rest.
- Take painkillers in recommended doses. *See* MEDICINES, 22.
- Apply local heat to the chest by means of a hot-water bottle.

When to consult the doctor
As soon as possible if:
- Pain is severe.

- There is breathlessness.
- There is fever or blood-stained spit.

Possible causes
Common causes: Chest injuries; FIBROSITIS (chest).
Less likely causes: FRACTURE; PLEURISY; PNEUMONIA; PNEUMOTHORAX; PULMONARY EMBOLISM.

SHORTNESS OF BREATH
Shortness of breath is of two types: type 1, air hunger, is when the sufferer feels that he cannot get enough air and takes large, deep, sighing breaths while the rate of breathing is unchanged or slowed. This symptom is well known to every adult and is usually a reaction to feeling oppressed either physically (a crowded or overheated room) or mentally (ANXIETY, taking a driving test). The reaction is quite normal and best ignored. Type 2, breathlessness, is when the sufferer is out of breath as if he had just run upstairs and the rate of breathing is increased. This type of breathlessness, if it occurs at rest or after unexpectedly small amounts of exertion, is a symptom of disorder of the RESPIRATORY SYSTEM *(page 42)* or the CIRCULATORY SYSTEM *(page 40)*. Breathlessness associated with increasing facial pallor may be a symptom of ANAEMIA, especially if there is unusual blood loss such as nose-bleeds or heavy periods.

Immediate treatment
- Sit in the position of greatest comfort.

When to consult the doctor
Immediately if:
- Onset of breathlessness is sudden, severe or associated with either chest pain or blood-stained spit.
As soon as possible if:
- Breathlessness occurs at rest.
- There are other symptoms such as a cough, swelling of ankles, fever, or previous loss of blood.
- Serious disease is known to be already present.

Possible causes
- Respiratory system
Breathlessness associated with a cough,

chest pain related to breathing, or a recent attack of pneumonia.
Common causes: Poor physical condition; OBESITY; SMOKING; ASTHMA.
Less likely causes: BRONCHITIS (chronic); EMPHYSEMA; LUNG CANCER; PNEUMONIA; BRONCHIECTASIS; TUBERCULOSIS; PULMONARY EMBOLISM.
• Circulatory system
Breathlessness occurs at night or on lying down, it may be accompanied by swelling of the ankles or chest pain not related to breathing.
Common causes: Poor physical condition; normal PREGNANCY; OBESITY.
Less likely causes: HEART FAILURE in all forms; CORONARY THROMBOSIS.

CATARRH

Nasal catarrh is a harmless but annoying symptom that may be difficult to cure. It is present for a few days in many infections of the nose and sinuses.
Immediate treatment
• Nose blowing and decongestive nasal drops (*see* MEDICINES, 41) may help at first, but drops themselves can cause catarrh if taken for longer than ten days.
When to consult the doctor
• If the blockage persists for longer than two to four weeks.
• If the discharge is blood-stained.
Possible causes
Common causes: COMMON COLD and other infections; SMOKING.
Less likely causes: SINUSITIS; NASAL POLYPS; RHINITIS (chronic and allergic).

CHEST PAIN

There are two main types of chest pain: pain which is clearly related to breathing (*see* SYMPTOM SORTER—BREATHING

DIFFICULTIES), and pain which is not related to breathing. Such pain may be unrelated to anything, or have a clear relationship to exertion or eating.
Chest pain brought on by exertion is usually 'crushing', may radiate to the neck, shoulders or arms, and passes off with rest. Such pain is usually a symptom of disorder of the heart and is sometimes called cardiac or anginal pain.
Immediate treatment
• Rest, and take half an aspirin.
• Take painkillers in recommended doses. *See* MEDICINES, 22.
• Apply heat to chest by means of hot-water bottle.
When to consult the doctor
Immediately if:
• Pain is severe.
• There is shock—pallor and sweating.
• A heart condition is suspected; either because the patient has already suffered a heart attack or because the pain fits the description of cardiac or anginal pain given above.
• The pain is not improved after an hour's rest.
Consult the doctor in most other cases of chest pain because even slight pain may have a serious cause.
Possible causes
• Cardiac-type chest pain
Common causes: ANGINA PECTORIS.
Less likely causes: CORONARY THROMBOSIS; ISCHAEMIC HEART DISEASE; MYOCARDITIS; severe ANAEMIA; THYROTOXICOSIS; other rare heart diseases.
• Chest pain related to eating or swallowing
Common causes: INDIGESTION.
Less likely causes: OESOPHAGITIS; DUODENAL ULCER.

COLD LIMBS OR BODY

Sensation of cold in the limbs, hands or feet is dealt with in this Symptom Sorter under the part of the body affected.

General feeling of cold, accompanied by shivering, is usually caused by cold weather, but may be a sign of raised temperature. *See* SYMPTOM SORTER—FEVER.
Occasionally coldness may be a sign of lowered temperature. *See* HYPOTHERMIA.

COLLAPSE

The term collapse is often used loosely and means different things to different people. Used by a doctor it refers to loss of consciousness.
See SYMPTOM SORTER—CONSCIOUSNESS, DISTURBANCES OF

CONCENTRATION, LOSS OF

See SYMPTOM SORTER—MENTAL ACTIVITIES, FAILURE OF

CONFUSION

See SYMPTOM SORTER—MENTAL ACTIVITIES, FAILURE OF
See also page 176

CONSCIOUSNESS, DISTURBANCES OF

Faints, dizzy turns, blackouts, fits, convulsions, breathholding attacks, TRANSIENT ISCHAEMIC ATTACKS and strokes are all terms often used by both doctors and lay people. They may mean different things to different people, but all

imply the same thing: that consciousness has been lost for a short time.
Temporary loss of consciousness is of two types. The first is unconsciousness caused by poor blood supply to the brain. All the well-known symptoms of a faint are present—extreme pallor, sweating, weak pulse and low blood pressure. The second is unconsciousness caused by loss of control by the brain. Other symptoms are twitching movements, tongue biting, noisy breathing, leaking of urine or motion. Pulse, colour and blood pressure stay normal. After an attack there may be drowsiness, odd behaviour, weakness of a limb or difficulties of speech.
Immediate treatment
• During a fit or faint, turn the patient half on his front so that his tongue comes forward and his airway is clear (unconscious position). Keep him as warm and still as possible—this applies in open or public places as well as in the home. Do not try to give food or drink. Call a doctor or ambulance. *See* FIRST AID *page 611.*
When to consult the doctor
• Immediately, if the symptom occurs. If the patient has recovered quickly and is in his own home, immediate advice over the telephone may be enough.
Possible causes
• Unconsciousness due to poor blood supply to the brain
Common causes: FAINTING ATTACK due to pregnancy, blood loss, excessive standing; old age.
Less likely causes: VERTEBRO-BASILAR INSUFFICIENCY; HEART BLOCK; breathholding attacks (*see* CHILD CARE *page 159*).
• Unconsciousness caused by loss of control by the brain
Common causes: Concussion (POST-CONCUSSIONAL SYNDROME); head injury.
Less likely causes: Fever fit (*see* CHILD CARE *page 154*); EPILEPSY; birth injury to brain; BRAIN TUMOUR; STROKE; TRANSIENT ISCHAEMIC ATTACK; SUBARACHNOID HAEMORRHAGE; MENINGITIS.

CONSTIPATION

Most constipation is caused by an unbalanced diet or lack of exercise. Only rarely is it a symptom of serious disease. Consult the doctor if there is abdominal pain or if a change in bowel habit persists for longer than two or three weeks.
See page 178
See also CHILD CARE *page 153*

CONVULSIONS

See SYMPTOM SORTER—CONSCIOUSNESS, DISTURBANCES OF

COUGH

A cough is a protective reflex which helps the body to rid the lungs of unwanted phlegm and inhaled foreign matter. Coughing has a wide variety of causes.
Immediate treatment
• Stay quiet in a warm room.
• Take soothing medicines if the cough interferes with sleep or appears to tire the sufferer. *See* MEDICINES, 16.
When to consult the doctor
• If there is blood in spit.
• If there is chest pain, shortness of breath or persistent fever.
• If the cough is getting worse or persists after two or three weeks.
• If there is a possibility of an inhaled foreign body. *See* FIRST AID *page 572*.
Possible causes
A cough that is hoarse or painful is usually a symptom of CROUP, LARYNGITIS or infection of the windpipe (trachea). In whooping cough the 'whoop' is always heard when the breath is drawn in after a

spasm of coughing.
The cause of a cough can be identified by the length of time it persists.
• Cough lasting less than ten days.
Common causes: Coughs; COMMON COLD; RESPIRATORY INFECTION (acute upper); MUCUS COLLECTION IN THE PHARYNX; INFLUENZA; many other viral respiratory infections.
Less likely causes: MEASLES; WHOOPING COUGH; PHARYNGITIS; LARYNGITIS; BRONCHIOLITIS; PNEUMONIA.
• Cough lasting more than ten days
Common causes: SMOKING; habit; ALLERGY.
Less likely causes: BRONCHITIS (chronic); BRONCHIECTASIS; ASTHMA; TUBERCULOSIS (lungs); LUNG CANCER.
See also CHILD CARE *page 154*

CYANOSIS

Blueness of skin usually seen in the face and hands of a person who is cold. If such blueness is seen in a person whose face and hands are warm it may be a symptom of serious heart or lung disease such as PNEUMONIA, HEART FAILURE or CONGENITAL HEART DISEASE, and should be reported to the doctor.
In babies and young children cyanosis should always be reported to the doctor.
Immediate treatment
• Put the patient in a warm room and if possible avoid applying heat directly to the cold part.
• If the patient is in the open, or exposed, attempt to keep the whole body warm, or at least prevent it from losing heat.

DEAFNESS

Deafness may develop in one or both ears at any age. There are two kinds of

deafness: conductive deafness affecting the middle ear; and nerve deafness affecting the inner ear.
Immediate treatment
• None. Deafness from serious causes rarely develops suddenly.
When to consult the doctor
• If deafness is suspected in a person of any age including babies.
• If ringing noises are heard in the ear (TINNITUS).
• If there is discharge or pain in the ear.
• If a child shows any deafness after an ear infection.
• In children deafness from 'glue ear' (chronic secretory OTITIS MEDIA), often develops after a simple ear infection. Be sure to take the child back to the doctor if further checks are requested.
Possible causes
Common causes: NOISE INJURY; EUSTACHIAN TUBE BLOCKAGE (after flying or diving); EAR WAX; OTITIS MEDIA.
Less likely causes: EAR INJURY; PERFORATED EAR-DRUM; OTOSCLEROSIS; congenital DEAFNESS; DEAFNESS of old age; MÉNIÈRE'S DISEASE.

DELUSIONS

See SYMPTOM SORTER—BEHAVIOUR, ABNORMAL

DEPRESSION

A state of low spirits felt by most people at some time in their lives, but which becomes an illness if prolonged or severe.
See page 193

DIARRHOEA

An extremely common symptom caused by a wide range of conditions.
Diarrhoea can be acute (lasting less than seven days), or chronic and recurrent. Acute diarrhoea is usually caused by food poisoning due to bacterial or viral infection. When associated with abdominal pain it may be due to harmless colic, but alternatively may be a symptom of more serious disease (*see* SYMPTOM SORTER—ABDOMINAL PAIN). In general, the causes of chronic diarrhoea are usually more serious than those of acute diarrhoea.
Babies under one year and frail, elderly patients are at special risk in any acute attack of diarrhoea because of the dangers from fluid loss. *See* CHILD CARE *page 153*.
Immediate treatment
• Bed-rest and frequent intake of fluids. Many cases will clear up with this treatment alone.
When to consult the doctor
• If the patient is a baby under one year or frail and elderly.
• If there is blood in the motions.
• If symptoms are exceptionally severe or persist for longer than three days.
• If others have been simultaneously affected.
• If you have recently returned from a foreign country.
• If you are residing in a country where the water supply is suspect or where TYPHOID, AMOEBIASIS, SCHISTOSOMIASIS, SPRUE or CHOLERA are known to occur.
Possible causes
Common causes: Diet; laxatives (*see* MEDICINES, 3); GASTROENTERITIS; mild DYSENTERY; irritable BOWEL.
Less likely causes: APPENDICITIS; COLITIS; DIVERTICULAR DISEASE OF THE COLON; BOWEL CANCER; COELIAC DISEASE; AMOEBIASIS; CYSTIC FIBROSIS; ILEITIS; GIARDIASIS.

DIZZINESS

See SYMPTOM SORTER—BALANCE PROBLEMS

DROWSINESS

There are rarely any serious causes of drowsiness. It is usually the result of fatigue or alcohol, or drugs such as tranquillisers, sedatives and hypnotics (*see* MEDICINES, 17); analgesics and narcotics (*see* MEDICINES, 22); and antihistamines (*see* MEDICINES, 14).
Very rarely drowsiness may be a symptom of NARCOLEPSY, HYPOTHERMIA, ENCEPHALITIS or other brain disorders.

EAR PROBLEMS

Problems affecting the ear include earache, discharge, noises in the ear (*see* TINNITUS), rash (*see* OTITIS EXTERNA) and EAR INJURY. *See also* SYMPTOM SORTER—DEAFNESS and *page 188.*

EARACHE AND DISCHARGE
Earache is a very common symptom in children under ten years. It usually indicates the presence of infection behind the ear-drum in the middle ear. The pain is caused by pus stretching the drum, and ceases if the pus perforates the drum—appearing at the ear-hole as discharge.
The condition settles rapidly with treatment in children. In adults it is less common but should be taken seriously because complications are more likely.
Immediate treatment
• Rest in a warm room.
• Take painkillers in recommended doses.
See MEDICINES, 22.

• Do not put drops into a discharging ear unless instructed by the doctor.
When to consult the doctor
• If a baby is in pain. A very young baby may not be able to indicate the site of pain (*see* CHILD CARE—CHILDHOOD ILLS *page 151*).
• If earache persists after four to eight hours' rest.
• If there is discharge.
• As soon as possible if pain develops in an ear that is already discharging.
• If ear problems develop after flying, diving or respiratory infections.
Possible causes
Common causes: OTITIS MEDIA (all types); EUSTACHIAN TUBE BLOCKAGE; boil (ABSCESS); FOREIGN BODY IN THE EAR.
Less likely cause: OTITIS MEDIA (chronic).

ELBOW PROBLEMS

Pain, stiffness and swelling are common problems affecting the elbow. It is also subject to those disorders affecting the joints in general (*see* SYMPTOM SORTER—JOINT PROBLEMS).
Immediate treatment
• Rest the elbow, put the arm in a sling.
When to consult the doctor
• If pain persists for longer than three to ten days.
• If other joints are affected.
• If there is fever.
Possible causes
Common causes: Sprain; PULLED ELBOW OF CHILDREN; FRACTURE and injury; TENNIS ELBOW.
Less likely causes: BURSITIS; ARTHRITIS of all kinds.

EYE PROBLEMS

Symptoms affecting the eyes should always be taken seriously and reported to the doctor early. The eye is a small, complicated and vital organ in which it is often difficult even for doctors to differentiate between trivial and serious disease.
Immediate treatment
• Chemicals and other foreign bodies in the eye can cause serious damage and must be washed from the eye at once. Open the affected eye, with a finger if necessary, and wash it under a running tap or in clean fresh water in a bowl. *See* FIRST AID *page 585.*
• For other symptoms, close the eye and ensure complete rest.
When to consult the doctor
• Immediately after undertaking emergency treatment in the case of injury.
• Immediately if there is sudden blindness, partial or complete, in one or both eyes.
As soon as possible if:
• A grey cloud or blurred area obscures the sight of one or both eyes.
• There is severe pain in the eyeball.
• The pupils of the two eyes are different in size (some eye drops may cause this).
• A double image is seen.
• Redness occurs in the white of the eye within $\frac{1}{10}$ in. (2·5 mm.) of the iris.
• Sudden pain strikes, or there is the possibility of a foreign body or welding flash.
Any eye symptom which develops slowly or persists for more than three to five days should be reported to the doctor.

EYE SYMPTOMS WHICH MAY HAVE SERIOUS CAUSES
Possible causes
• Pain and irritation in the eye
Common causes: CONJUNCTIVITIS; foreign body in the EYE; injury.
Less likely causes: CORNEAL ULCER; IRITIS;

acute GLAUCOMA.
• Redness of the eyeball
Common causes: CONJUNCTIVITIS; SUBCONJUNCTIVAL HAEMORRHAGE; foreign body in the EYE; injury.
Less likely causes: CORNEAL ULCER; IRITIS; acute GLAUCOMA.
• Spasm of the eyelid, dislike of bright light, and inability to open the eye
Common causes: Foreign body in the EYE; CONJUNCTIVITIS; injury.
Less likely causes: IRITIS; CORNEAL ULCER.
• Persistent (longer than three to five days) eye symptoms or visual disturbances
Common causes: REFRACTIVE ERRORS; FLOATERS; SQUINT; MIGRAINE.
Less likely causes: CATARACT; chronic GLAUCOMA; IRITIS; DIABETES; HYPERTENSION.

EYE SYMPTOMS WHICH RARELY HAVE SERIOUS CAUSES
Possible causes
• Sticky eyes
CONJUNCTIVITIS; BLEPHARITIS.
• Watering eyes
Blocked TEAR-DUCT; ECTROPION.
• Swollen and painful eyelids
STYES; ECTROPION; ALLERGY.
• Sore, red, scaly eyes
BLEPHARITIS.

FACIAL PROBLEMS

Changes in the face often reflect disorder elsewhere in the body. Even if the change is not a symptom of serious disease it may cause the sufferer distress and the doctor should be consulted.
Immediate treatment
• Depends on the nature of the underlying cause.
When to consult the doctor
As soon as possible if:
• There is severe pain.
• Pain, weakness or swelling starts suddenly.

• Any facial swelling, redness or infection associated with fever.
Possible causes
• Pain
Common causes: Toothache (*see* TEETH); boil (ABSCESS); STYE.
Less likely causes: SINUSITIS; TRIGEMINAL NEURALGIA; SHINGLES.
• Weakness, paralysis, drooping
Common causes: BELL'S PALSY.
Less likely causes: STROKE; brain disorders; MYASTHENIA GRAVIS; MUSCULAR DYSTROPHY.
• Lack of expression
Common causes: DEPRESSION.
Less likely causes: PARKINSON'S DISEASE; MYXOEDEMA.
• Swelling
Common causes: OBESITY; local inflammation from teeth; boil (ABSCESS); STYE; MUMPS; ALLERGY.
Less likely causes: SINUSITIS; GLANDULAR FEVER; corticosteroid treatment (*see* MEDICINES, 32, 37).
• Lumps
Common causes: SEBACEOUS CYST; boil (ABSCESS).
Less likely causes: SKIN CANCER.
• Blue
See SYMPTOM SORTER—CYANOSIS.
• Flushed, red or inflamed
Common causes: Blushing; heat; SUNBURN; fevers; boil (ABSCESS); STYE.
Less likely causes: CELLULITIS; ERYSIPELAS; ROSACEA; SCARLET FEVER and other rashes.
• Pallor
Common causes: FAINTING ATTACK; shock; blood loss; ANAEMIA (iron deficiency).
Less likely causes: Rarely ANAEMIA (pernicious); chronic diseases.
See SYMPTOM SORTER— CONSCIOUSNESS, DISTURBANCES OF.
• Yellow
See JAUNDICE.

FAINTING

See SYMPTOM SORTER— CONSCIOUSNESS, DISTURBANCES OF
See also page 250

FATIGUE

See SYMPTOM SORTER—APATHY

FEARS

See ANXIETY
PHOBIA

FEVER

Raised temperature, shivering, chills and feeling hot make up fever. It is a symptom, not, as a lay person might think, a specific illness such as scarlet fever or malaria. Fever is a very common symptom with a wide variety of causes.

When a patient has a fever it means that his body is fighting infection and that he needs rest and, where appropriate, anti-infective medicines (*see* MEDICINES, 25). A raised temperature is a sign that a child should be kept indoors, or an adult should stay off work.

Normal temperature for most individuals is 98.6°F (37°C). A few people have a normal level that is 1°F (0.5°C) either above or below this. Temperatures up to 104°F (40°C) often arise at the start of many childhood infections, *see* CHILD CARE *page 154*. In adults temperatures

usually rise to a lesser extent, but are physically more upsetting. In the elderly, serious infections can be present even though the temperature remains normal —a result of their reduced ability to fight infection.
Immediate treatment
• Rest in a warm (not hot) room.
• Take plenty of fluids.
• Take painkillers: adults—of the aspirin type; children—paracetamol. *See* MEDICINES, 22.
• Sponge the patient with tepid water if a temperature is over 102°F (39°C).
When to consult the doctor
• Immediately if a baby has a temperature over 104°F (40°C).
• If a baby under one year has a temperature.
• If fever persists for more than three days in an adult.
• If serious disease is suggested by other symptoms.
• If there is the possibility of contact with other infected individuals.
• If severe shivering, shaking and chattering of teeth occur with fever. This condition is called a rigor, and should be reported because it suggests PNEUMONIA, PYELONEPHRITIS or MALARIA.
Possible causes
These are recognised by the other symptoms present.

FITS

See SYMPTOM SORTER— CONSCIOUSNESS, DISTURBANCES OF

FLATULENCE

An annoying, harmless, very common symptom of indigestion which is caused by swallowing air or overfilling the

stomach. Only when associated with other symptoms is flatulence a useful pointer to disease.
See SYMPTOM SORTER—INDIGESTION WIND

FOOT PROBLEMS

Injury, excessive weight-bearing, wear and tear and disorders of the circulation affect the feet and toes causing discomfort and deformity.
Immediate treatment
• Rest the foot and avoid wearing uncomfortable shoes.
When to consult the doctor
• If pain, weakness, swelling or other symptoms persist for longer than seven days or if daily activities are interfered with.
Possible causes
• Rash or blisters
Common causes: Injury; friction.
Less likely causes: TINEA; ECZEMA (contact).
See SYMPTOM SORTER—SKIN ABNORMALITIES.
• Pain
Common causes: Sprains; injuries; BUNION; FLAT FOOT; METATARSALGIA; INGROWING TOE-NAIL.
Less likely causes: FRACTURE; GANGRENE; GOUT; OSTEOARTHRITIS; PLANTAR FASCIITIS.
• Weakness, paralysis
Common causes: None.
Less likely causes: SLIPPED DISC; STROKE; MULTIPLE SCLEROSIS.
• Itching
See also page 323.
• Feeling cold, white appearance
Common causes: Cold weather.
Less likely causes: RAYNAUD'S SYNDROME; MYXOEDEMA.
• Swelling (both feet)
Common causes: OBESITY; hot weather; prolonged standing.
Less likely causes: HEART FAILURE; NEPHRITIS; VARICOSE VEINS.

- Swelling (one foot)
Common causes: SPRAIN; injury.
Less likely causes: FRACTURE;
OSTEOARTHRITIS; RHEUMATOID ARTHRITIS;
GOUT.

FORGETFULNESS

See SYMPTOM SORTER—MENTAL
ACTIVITIES, FAILURE OF

GROIN SWELLING

A soft, painless swelling in the groin is a
symptom of a HERNIA. A harder lump or
swelling suggests an enlarged lymph
gland which may develop after a boil
(ABSCESS), GLANDULAR FEVER, or more
serious disease affecting lymph glands.
Immediate treatment
- Rest in the lying flat position.
When to consult the doctor
- Any swelling in the groin that recurs
or persists for longer than two or three
days should be reported to a doctor.

GROWTH

See SYMPTOM SORTER—SKIN ABNORMALITIES
for growths on the skin. Growth is also a
popular but ill-defined term for CANCER,
being a shortened form of the medical
term for cancer—'new growth' or
'neoplasm'.

GUM PROBLEMS

See TEETH

HAIR PROBLEMS

Problems with hair include BALDNESS,
DANDRUFF, LICE, PSORIASIS, and excessive
hair (HIRSUTISM). For cradle cap *see*
CHILD CARE *page 159*.
See also HAIR

HALLUCINATIONS

See SYMPTOM SORTER—BEHAVIOUR,
ABNORMAL

HAND, FINGERS AND WRIST

Problems affecting the hand, fingers and
wrist include pain, swelling, weakness,
tremor, rash and colour changes.
Immediate treatment
- Rest, warmth and painkillers in
recommended doses provide suitable early
treatment for most hand conditions. A
sling may be helpful.
When to consult the doctor
- If any symptom in the hand persists for
longer than two or three days, or earlier
if there is injury or severe pain.
Possible causes
- Pain
Common causes: Injuries; WHITLOW;
ABSCESS; SPRAIN; CHILBLAIN.
Less likely causes: POLYMYALGIA
RHEUMATICA; CARPAL TUNNEL SYNDROME;
OSTEOARTHRITIS; RHEUMATOID ARTHRITIS;
CERVICAL RIB SYNDROME; CERVICAL
SPONDYLOSIS.
- Deformity and swelling
Common causes: Injuries; SPRAIN;
FRACTURE (including Colles' fracture);
GANGLION; CHILBLAINS; ABSCESS;
RHEUMATOID ARTHRITIS; OSTEOARTHRITIS;
MALLET FINGER; DUPUYTREN'S CONTRACTURE.
- Weakness
Common causes: None.
Less likely causes: CARPAL TUNNEL
SYNDROME; CERVICAL RIB SYNDROME;
CERVICAL SPONDYLOSIS; STROKE; MOTOR
NEURONE DISEASE; MULTIPLE SCLEROSIS;
POLYNEUROPATHY.
- Tingling, pins and needles and
numbness
Common causes: Cold weather; CHILBLAINS.
Less likely causes: CARPAL TUNNEL
SYNDROME; CERVICAL RIB SYNDROME;
POLYNEUROPATHY.
- Tremor
Common causes: Alcohol.
Less likely causes: PARKINSON'S DISEASE;
THYROTOXICOSIS.
- Cold and white
Common causes: Mild RAYNAUD'S
SYNDROME; CHILBLAINS.
Less likely causes: Severe RAYNAUD'S
SYNDROME.
- Blue
See CYANOSIS.
- Rash (on the hands only)
Common causes: CHILBLAINS; SCABIES
(very itchy); injuries.
Less likely causes: ERYTHROMELALGIA;
ECZEMA (contact).
See SYMPTOM SORTER—RASH

HEADACHE

CHILDREN
See CHILD CARE *page 155*.

ADULTS
The most common form of headache
originates in the muscles of the scalp and
forehead after periods of concentration,
driving or ANXIETY. Aching is in the
forehead or over the top or back of the
head. This type of headache is worse at
the end of the day or with mental fatigue,
rarely lasts longer than an hour or so and
does not keep the sufferer awake. There is
no need to consult the doctor. Some
people suffer more from headaches than
others. *See* TENSION HEADACHE.
  Sometimes, however, a headache can
be caused by changes in the circulation
inside the skull.
Immediate treatment
- Rest in a darkened room.
- Take painkillers in recommended doses
(*see* MEDICINES, 22).
When to consult the doctor
Immediately if:
- Headache and drowsiness follow head
injury.
- Very severe headache starts suddenly.
As soon as possible if:
- There are other associated symptoms,
such as vomiting or visual disturbances.
- Headache is associated with stiffness of
the neck or back.
- If headache is aggravated by coughing,
or moving or lowering the head, and has
persisted for more than three days.
- If there is no satisfactory explanation
for a headache that is continuous or
getting worse after three days.
Possible causes
Common causes: Any raised temperature;
MIGRAINE; ANXIETY.
Less likely causes: SINUSITIS;
HYPERTENSION; POST-CONCUSSIONAL
SYNDROME; CLUSTER HEADACHE; BRAIN
TUMOUR; BRAIN ABSCESS; MENINGITIS;
SUBDURAL HAEMATOMA;
SUBARACHNOID HAEMORRHAGE.

HEARTBEAT DISORDERS

See SYMPTOM SORTER—PALPITATIONS

HEARTBURN

A hot sensation behind the breastbone coming on after meals. Heartburn occurs in most types of indigestion, but occasionally, if severe, it may be a symptom of DUODENAL ULCER.
See SYMPTOM SORTER—INDIGESTION
ACID REGURGITATION

HEEL PAIN

If injury is not the cause of the pain see PLANTAR FASCIITIS.

HIP PAIN

See SYMPTOM SORTER—LIMP

HOARSENESS

BABIES AND YOUNG CHILDREN
See SYMPTOM SORTER—BREATHING
DIFFICULTIES.

OLDER CHILDREN AND ADULTS
Immediate treatment
• Rest the voice.
• Use inhalations such as steam or

Friar's balsam.
• Take painkillers in recommended doses.
See MEDICINES, 22.
When to consult the doctor
• If hoarseness persists for more than 14 days.
Possible causes
Common causes: LARYNGITIS (acute).
Less likely causes: LARYNGITIS (chronic); growth in LARYNX.

INCONTINENCE

The inability to control the discharge of motions from the anus (faecal incontinence), or the involuntary passing of urine (urinary incontinence).

FAECAL INCONTINENCE IN CHILDREN
Faecal incontinence in children is usually a behaviour problem which follows fears and insecurities. Consult your doctor; such soiling may be difficult to cure.

FAECAL INCONTINENCE IN ADULTS
Immediate treatment
• See HOME NURSING.
When to consult the doctor
• This is an unpleasant symptom, and early advice from a nurse or doctor is usually indicated.
Possible causes
Common causes: Oily laxatives. See MEDICINES, 3.
Less likely causes: DEMENTIA; FAECAL IMPACTION.

URINARY INCONTINENCE IN CHILDREN AND ADULTS
See SYMPTOM SORTER—URINE AND
URINATION PROBLEMS.

INDIGESTION

Any minor discomfort coming on after meals tends to be called indigestion. Symptoms generally described as indigestion include a feeling of fullness in the stomach, discomfort in the upper abdomen, burping, HICCUPS, a hot feeling behind the breastbone (heartburn), regurgitation of water (waterbrash) and acid (see ACID REGURGITATION and FLATULENCE).
Sometimes symptoms of indigestion are caused by serious disease such as DUODENAL ULCER. More often the causes are trivial such as eating or drinking too much.
Immediate treatment
• Rest in a chair.
• Take antacids (see MEDICINES, 1), or half a teaspoon of bicarbonate of soda in a glass of water.
• Drink fluids in small amounts, no alcohol.
When to consult the doctor
• If the symptoms are persistent or getting progressively worse.
• If there is abdominal pain, cough, loss of appetite or loss of weight.
Possible causes
Common causes: Eating too much rich, fatty or fried foods, drinking too much alcohol.
Less likely causes: DUODENAL ULCER; GASTRIC ULCER; GASTRITIS; OESOPHAGITIS; CHOLECYSTITIS; GALLSTONES; ALCOHOLISM.

INSOMNIA

Difficulty getting to sleep, waking frequently in the night, or waking early can have a number of causes, but by far the most common is worry.
See page 320

IRRITABILITY

See SYMPTOM SORTER—BEHAVIOUR,
ABNORMAL

ITCHING

Itching is often associated with skin rash, see SYMPTOM SORTER—SKIN ABNORMALITIES.
See also page 323

JAUNDICE

Excess of yellow pigment in the body tissues, seen in the skin and whites of the eyes, is caused by a number of serious disorders. The doctor should be consulted as soon as jaundice is noticed.
See page 324

JAW PROBLEMS

Problems with the jaw include stiffness, pain and swelling, and should usually be reported to the doctor—or dentist, since often the teeth are involved.

JOINT PROBLEMS

An affected joint may be painful, hot and sometimes red, and swollen from fluid. Movements may be stiff, painful and limited. Problems in the joints are also dealt with in this Symptom Sorter under the part of the body affected.

Immediate treatment
- Rest the joint.
- Take painkillers in recommended doses. *See* MEDICINES, 22.
- Apply heat to the joint by means of a hot-water bottle or poultice.

When to consult the doctor
- If symptoms are severe, persist for longer than seven days, or if normal activities are prevented.

Possible causes
Joint disorders may be caused by injury (SPRAIN, BURSITIS, dislocation and FRACTURES), ageing with wear and tear (OSTEOARTHRITIS), or inflammation (RHEUMATOID ARTHRITIS, GOUT, RHEUMATIC FEVER, POLYMYALGIA RHEUMATICA).

In general, different diseases affect different joints. Osteoarthritis affects mainly the hips, knees and spine of the elderly. Rheumatoid arthritis affects mainly the hands, knees and feet of the middle-aged. Gout affects mainly the big toe and leg joints. Polymyalgia affects mainly the arms of the elderly.

KNEE PROBLEMS

Disorders of the knee joint, from whatever cause, usually start with pain which is made worse by movement; then stiffness develops, and the knee becomes hot and finally swollen.

Immediate treatment
- Rest and painkillers in recommended doses. *See* MEDICINES, 22.

When to consult the doctor
- If pain is severe.
- If symptoms persist for longer than four to seven days.
- If normal activities are prevented.

Possible causes
Common causes: Injury; SPRAIN; OSTEOARTHRITIS.
Less likely causes: Torn CARTILAGE; torn

LIGAMENT; RHEUMATOID ARTHRITIS; RHEUMATIC FEVER; GOUT.

LEG PROBLEMS

Many problems in the legs clearly originate in a particular joint, and are dealt with in this Symptom Sorter under the joint affected. Other, more general, problems are covered below.

Immediate treatment
- Keep the leg at rest in the position of greatest comfort. Most disorders in the legs need rest initially, and many will clear with rest alone.
- Take painkillers in recommended doses if necessary. *See* MEDICINES, 22.

When to consult the doctor
- If there is recent injury causing any deformity, or extensive bruising.
- If pain is severe or has not cleared up after three days' rest.
- If, in the absence of injury, symptoms are severe or getting worse, or if symptoms are persisting after three to seven days' rest.
- If symptoms have occurred before.

Possible causes
- Pain, aching, stiffness
Common causes: Injury; unaccustomed exercise; FIBROSITIS; SLIPPED DISC.
Less likely causes: Ruptured TENDON or muscle; FRACTURE; INTERMITTENT CLAUDICATION (pain in the calf); RHEUMATOID ARTHRITIS; OSTEOMYELITIS (acute); THROMBOPHLEBITIS.
- Swelling in one leg
Common causes: Injury, boils (ABSCESS).
Less likely causes: FRACTURE; VARICOSE VEINS; THROMBOPHLEBITIS; WHITE LEG.
- Swelling in both legs
Common causes: Prolonged standing; PREGNANCY; hot weather; OBESITY.
Less likely causes: VARICOSE VEINS; HEART FAILURE.
- Weakness
Common causes: Fatigue and unaccustomed use.

Less likely causes: SLIPPED DISC; STROKE; MULTIPLE SCLEROSIS; PARKINSON'S DISEASE; rare diseases affecting the nerves of the spinal cord.
- Numbness and tingling
Common causes: Compression of the sciatic nerve by the edge of a chair.
Less likely causes: SLIPPED DISC; STROKE; MULTIPLE SCLEROSIS; POLYNEUROPATHY.
- Redness, red lines
Redness or red lines from a wound, boil (ABSCESS) or CELLULITIS, are signs of a spread of infection. Rest the leg completely and consult the doctor.
- Redness with localised swelling and tenderness
Such a symptom indicates a local inflammation such as a boil (ABSCESS), CELLULITIS or uncommon allergic reactions.
- Red patch without swelling or tenderness
A red patch may be a symptom of PSORIASIS, ECZEMA (discoid or varicose), or ERYTHROMELALGIA.
See SYMPTOM SORTER—RASH
- Ulcers in the lower leg
Common causes: Injury; VARICOSE VEINS.
Less likely causes: WHITE LEG; GANGRENE; ARTERIAL THROMBOSIS; DIABETES.
See SYMPTOM SORTER—LIMP.

LIGHTHEADEDNESS

See SYMPTOM SORTER—BALANCE PROBLEMS

LIMP

LIMPING IN A CHILD
Although a limp in a child is often due to trivial causes, it may occasionally be a symptom of serious bone disease.

Immediate treatment
- Rest the affected leg.

When to consult the doctor
- If a limp has no obvious cause and persists after one to three days' rest.
- If there is severe pain in the affected leg.

Possible causes
Common causes: Injuries; cuts; BLISTER; SPRAIN; BRUISE.
Less likely causes: PERTHE'S DISEASE and other rare bone diseases; CONGENITAL DISLOCATION OF THE HIP; OSTEOMYELITIS.
See also CHILD CARE page 157.

LIMPING IN ADULTS
Immediate treatment
- Rest the affected leg.
- Take painkillers in recommended doses. *See* MEDICINES, 22.

When to consult the doctor
- If an elderly person has difficulty walking after a fall.
- If, after seven to 14 days' rest, pain is still causing a limp.
- If other joints are affected or if other symptoms suggest more widespread disease.

Possible causes
Common causes: Injuries; SPRAIN; excessive use; SLIPPED DISC.
Less likely causes: OSTEOARTHRITIS; RHEUMATOID ARTHRITIS; FRACTURE (neck of thigh bone).

LIPS

If the lips appear blue *see* SYMPTOM SORTER—CYANOSIS. The lips may also become cracked in cold weather (*see* CHAPPED LIPS) or subject to repeated COLD SORES. These disorders are harmless and, though annoying, heal quickly. Any ulcer or lump which persists for longer than two weeks should be reported to the doctor.
See CLEFT PALATE and HARE-LIP

Most lumps, bumps, cysts, moles and birthmarks are present at birth or appear and grow slowly. They generally range in diameter from $\frac{1}{5}$-4 in. (5-100 mm.).
Immediate treatment
- None.

When to consult the doctor
As soon as possible if:
- Any lump is found in the breast.
- Any bleeding occurs.
- The abnormality increases in size, spreads or there are changes in the surrounding skin.
- Other similar abnormalities appear.
- An open sore or ulcer develops.
- If the abnormality affects appearance or daily living.

Possible causes
Identification of the abnormality is made by colour.
- Deep red, purple or blue raised areas
Common causes: CHERRY SPOTS; MONGOLIAN SPOTS.
Less likely causes: PORT-WINE STAIN; STRAWBERRY NAEVUS; SPIDER NAEVUS.
- Brown raised areas
Common causes: SEBORRHOEIC WARTS; PIGMENTED NAEVUS; benign MELANOMA.
Less likely causes: Malignant melanoma (*see* SKIN CANCER); KERATOSIS.
- Raised areas the colour of normal skin, inflamed red or with pus
Common causes: Boil (ABSCESS); SEBACEOUS CYSTS (soft lumps); KELOID (found in scars only); SKIN TAGS; ACNE.
Less likely causes: SKIN CANCER (hard lumps, or pearl-like rodent ulcer on the face); MOLLUSCUM CONTAGIOSUM.
- Coloured marks or stains, not raised
Common causes: FRECKLES; CHLOASMA (brown marks appearing during pregnancy); VITILIGO (white marks); STRETCH MARKS (marks like scars); MONGOLIAN SPOTS (blue marks).
Less likely causes: PORT-WINE STAIN.

See also SYMPTOM SORTER—PENIS

See SYMPTOM SORTER—MENTAL ACTIVITIES, FAILURE OF

See SYMPTOM SORTER—PERIOD PROBLEMS
See also page 403

Some failure of mental powers is almost universal after the age of 50. It is usually minimal and best ignored. However, obvious failure may be caused by disorder of some kind and occasionally, as in DEMENTIA, the failure may be extreme. There may be lack of concentration, confusion and loss of memory.

LACK OF CONCENTRATION
Most people suffer lack of concentration at some time especially those involved with figures, reading and writing. Sufferers may exaggerate the importance of its effects to explain other deficiencies. Worry, tension, ANXIETY and HYPERACTIVITY in children are common causes.

CONFUSION
Minor or short-lived degrees of confusion are very common. They may follow drinking alcohol, sudden awakening, mental fatigue, lack of sleep and the use of sedatives. Temporary confusion may follow head injuries, concussion (*see* POST-CONCUSSIONAL SYNDROME) and EPILEPSY. Any of these disorders should be reported to the doctor.

Permanent or long, continued states of confusion may have a serious cause and should always be reported by others if the sufferer is too confused to do so himself.

LOSS OF MEMORY
The medical name for loss of memory is amnesia. Failure of memory for recent events, recent dates and recent names becomes increasingly apparent to many people after the age of 50. Although annoying, this symptom rarely interferes with normal activities. It is best dealt with by the use of simple memory aids, such as writing down important matters. *See* AMNESIA.
Immediate treatment
- Usually no treatment is effective in reversing memory loss.

When to consult the doctor
- If symptoms interfere with normal activities.

Possible causes
Common causes: Worry; alcohol; sedatives and tranquillisers (*see* MEDICINES, 17); ANXIETY; OLD AGE.
Less likely causes: HYSTERIA; concussion (POST-CONCUSSIONAL SYNDROME); ALCOHOLISM; EPILEPSY; ATHEROMA; STROKE; DEMENTIA; very rarely BRAIN TUMOUR.

See SYMPTOM SORTER—LUMPS

Abnormalities of the motions (also called stools or faeces) include variations in colour, shape and consistency.

BLOOD IN MOTIONS
See SYMPTOM SORTER—BLOOD.

BLACK, TARRY MOTIONS
Unless caused by taking bismuth or iron medicines, black, tarry motions are a symptom of bleeding in the digestive system. *See* SYMPTOM SORTER—BLOOD.

PALE, CLAY-COLOURED MOTIONS
If associated with the passage of dark urine, pale, clay-coloured motions may be a symptom of JAUNDICE. This type of motion is common and rarely abnormal in babies.

PALE, BULKY, OFFENSIVE MOTIONS
Offensive-smelling, pale, bulky motions are a symptom of GIARDIASIS, or, less commonly, COELIAC DISEASE, CYSTIC FIBROSIS or SPRUE.

LOOSE, RUNNY MOTIONS
See SYMPTOM SORTER—DIARRHOEA.

MUCUS OR SLIME PASSED
Persistent passage of mucus or slime should be reported to the doctor because it is occasionally a symptom of COLITIS or BOWEL CANCER.

WORMS
When passed in the motions worms are white. THREADWORMS are threadlike, less than $\frac{1}{2}$ in. (13 mm.) long, and moving. ROUNDWORMS are the size and shape of an earthworm. TAPEWORMS are rectangular or cylindrical segments $\frac{2}{5}$-$\frac{4}{5}$ in. (10-20 mm.) long which do not move. A few segments are passed with each motion.

PAINFUL MOTIONS
In babies and children, pain on passing a motion usually indicates an ANAL FISSURE.
In adults anal fissure is often the cause, but painful motions are also a symptom of internal PILES. Severe attacks of diarrhoea may also cause a spasm of anal discomfort (tenesmus).

MOUTH AND TONGUE PROBLEMS

Pain, soreness, rashes and ulcers are all common in the mouth and on the tongue.

Immediate treatment
- Use mouthwashes and lozenges. *See* MEDICINES, 42.
- Take painkillers in recommended doses. *See* MEDICINES, 22.
- Follow a fluid diet.

When to consult the doctor
- If discomfort prevents eating for more than two days.
- If rashes, bleeding or ulcers are present in the mouth.
- If the tongue is sore and ulcerated for more than 14 days.
- If there is any swelling of face, jaw, gums or mouth.

Possible causes
- Pain and soreness

Common causes: THRUSH; MOUTH ULCERS (aphthous); MUMPS; dental problems (*see* TEETH); STOMATITIS.
Less likely causes: ANAEMIA (iron deficiency or pernicious anaemia); tongue CANCER.
- Rashes and ulcers

Common causes: THRUSH; MOUTH ULCERS; STOMATITIS; MEASLES; dental problems (*see* TEETH).
Less likely causes: Tongue CANCER; LICHEN PLANUS.

See also page 509

MUSCLE PROBLEMS

Problems with the muscles are dealt with in this Symptom Sorter under the part of the body affected.

NAIL ABNORMALITIES

Acute pain with pus under the nail is a symptom of acute PARONYCHIA. Deformities of the nails may follow chronic PARONYCHIA, PSORIASIS, injuries to the nail bed or old age. Brittle nails are caused by excessive submersion of the nails in water, or periods of ill health. Rarely, clubbing of the nails may be noted in patients with chronic heart or lung disease.

Deformities of the toe-nails are common in the elderly, and although they are harmless a chiropodist should be consulted.
See INGROWING TOE-NAIL

NAUSEA

A very common symptom associated with many disorders. Diagnosis of its cause requires other symptoms to be taken into account.

Immediate treatment
- Rest.
- Antacids (*see* MEDICINES, 1), anti-emetics and antihistamines (*see* MEDICINES, 21) may help.
- Take sips of water.

When to consult the doctor
- If nausea is severe and followed by vomiting.
- If pregnancy or other symptoms such as abdominal pain suggest the need for advice.

Possible causes
Common causes: Eating or drinking too much; sudden changes of posture; PREGNANCY; MOTION SICKNESS; MIGRAINE; most fevers; GASTRITIS; GASTROENTERITIS.
Less likely causes: Many disorders of the digestive tract and many chronic disorders.

NECK PAIN

A stiff neck that starts suddenly and is painful to move and twist is common in both adults and children. Often there are no other symptoms, and with rest the pain settles in one or two days. FIBROSITIS is a possible cause. CERVICAL SPONDYLOSIS may cause prolonged or repeated attacks.

A special form of stiff neck sometimes occurs in association with certain acute bacterial or viral infections. There is clearly fever, the back of the neck is stiff and the sufferer is unable to bend his head forward, either to touch the knees with his nose or push his chin on to his chest. This combination of symptoms should be reported to a doctor immediately to exclude the possibility of MENINGITIS.

NOSE PROBLEMS

Common problems with the nose are bleeding, deformity, blocking and colour change.

Possible causes
- Bleeding from the nose
See NOSE-BLEED.
- Deformity or swelling
The usual causes of deformity or swelling are injury, especially during boxing (nose FRACTURE), or rhinophyma (ROSACEA).
- Blocked nose
See COMMON COLD.
- Persistent blocked nose
Common causes: COMMON COLD; enlarged ADENOID (in children); RHINITIS (allergic).
Less likely causes: DEVIATION OF NASAL SEPTUM; NASAL POLYPS; RHINITIS (chronic); SINUSITIS.
- Blue nose
See SYMPTOM SORTER—CYANOSIS.
- Red nose
Common causes: Frequent blowing; COMMON COLD; boil (ABSCESS).
Less likely causes: Drinking too much; ROSACEA.

NUMBNESS

Cold or sitting in an awkward position can cause temporary numbness. Persistent numbness should be reported to the doctor, especially if it is associated with an inability to feel pain and heat, and loss of touch sensation. Rarely, the condition may be a symptom of disorder of the nerves which supply the limbs.

Sometimes numbness develops in limbs following sudden or gradual interference with circulation to the limb as in RAYNAUD'S SYNDROME, BUERGER'S DISEASE and ARTERIAL THROMBOSIS.

Immediate treatment
- Keep the limb warm in the position of greatest comfort.

When to consult the doctor
- If there is persistent numbness and no other symptoms.
- If numbness is associated with severe pain or colour changes in the limb. If such changes are not related to cold and are of sudden onset, consult the doctor immediately.

PAIN

Pain is dealt with in this Symptom Sorter under the part of the body affected.
See also page 398

PALPITATIONS

Healthy people are normally unaware of their heart beating except after exercise or while experiencing fear or ANXIETY. In other circumstances awareness of the heart beating (palpitations) may sometimes be a sign of heart disease.
Immediate treatment
• None.
When to consult the doctor
• If palpitations persist over several hours.
• If there are other symptoms associated with the palpitations.
Possible causes
Common causes: Exercise; fear; some drugs; ANXIETY.
Less likely causes: EXTRASYSTOLES; PAROXYSMAL TACHYCARDIA; more serious disorders of rhythm such as ATRIAL FIBRILLATION and ATRIAL FLUTTER; THYROTOXICOSIS.

PALLOR

See SYMPTOM SORTER—FACIAL PROBLEMS

PARALYSIS

Medically, paralysis means muscle weakness which varies greatly in its extent and severity. It is not, as a lay person might believe, a complete inability to move. Weakness is dealt with in this Symptom Sorter under the part of the body affected.
See also page 400

PENIS, FORESKIN AND URETHRA

Disorders affecting the penis are pain, discharge, rashes and itching, ulcers and nodules, and deformities.

PAIN
Usually felt at the tip of the penis during urination, pain may be a symptom of disorder within the penis and in other parts of the body.
Immediate treatment
• Take painkillers in recommended doses. *See* MEDICINES, 22.
• Avoid intercourse.
When to consult the doctor
• If there is any pain in the penis.
• As soon as possible if there is also discharge or the possibility of SEXUALLY TRANSMITTED DISEASE.
Possible causes
Common causes: CYSTITIS; COLD SORES; URETHRITIS; GONORRHOEA.
Less likely causes: BALANITIS; REITER'S DISEASE.
See SYMPTOM SORTER—URINE AND URINATION PROBLEMS.

DISCHARGE
Immediate treatment
• None, avoid intercourse.
When to consult the doctor
• As soon as possible if discharge is noticed, especially if there is a possibility of SEXUALLY TRANSMITTED DISEASE.
Possible causes
Common causes: URETHRITIS; GONORRHOEA.
Less likely causes: BALANITIS; REITER'S DISEASE.

RASHES AND ITCHING
Immediate treatment
• None, avoid intercourse.
When to consult the doctor
• If the symptoms occur, especially if there is a possibility of venereal disease.
Possible causes
Common causes: SCABIES; THRUSH; VENEREAL DISEASE; HERPES SIMPLEX.

Less likely causes: Generalised rashes affecting the whole body. *See* SYMPTOM SORTER—RASH.

ULCERS AND NODULES (LUMPS)
In adults any nodule or ulcer should be regarded as evidence of sexually transmitted or serious disease unless the doctor has proved otherwise.
Immediate treatment
• None, avoid intercourse.
When to consult the doctor
• As soon as possible if there are any ulcers or nodules on the penis.
Possible causes
Common causes: WARTS (anogenital) which are usually sexually transmitted.
Less likely causes: SEXUALLY TRANSMITTED DISEASES.
In babies small, harmless ulcers may arise on the penis and cause pain as part of nappy rash (*see* CHILD CARE *page 158*).

DEFORMITIES
Infection of the foreskin (BALANITIS) or retraction of a tight foreskin, especially in toddlers and children, may cause a sudden swelling of the tip of the penis (PHIMOSIS). Immediate treatment is needed. The outlook then is excellent.

PERIOD PROBLEMS

Disorders of menstruation include irregularity, emotional upset, puffiness, and migraine. The other main problems, pain, absence, flooding, change of pattern and bleeding after the menopause, are covered on *page 403*.

IRREGULAR PERIODS
Many normal women suffer from periods which are irregular in time or amount of loss. Irregularity is often annoying for the sufferer but is not a sign of infertility. Consult the doctor if pregnancy is desired but has not been achieved, or if mis-carriage or the menopause are possible.

DEPRESSION, WEEPINESS, IRRITABILITY AND TENSION
See PREMENSTRUAL TENSION.

PUFFINESS OF FACE AND HANDS, AND MIGRAINE
Normal alterations in body fluids during the menstrual cycle cause many annoying but harmless symptoms. *See* PREMENSTRUAL TENSION.

UNEXPECTED BLEEDING FROM THE VAGINA
See SYMPTOM SORTER—BLEEDING.

PHOBIA

A condition in which intense anxiety and abnormal fear are triggered off by specific situations, such as open spaces and heights, or by specific objects, such as spiders and snakes.
See page 408

PIMPLES AND PUSTULES

See SYMPTOM SORTER—SKIN ABNORMALITIES

PULSE, RAPID

Accurate taking of the pulse requires constant practice and may be difficult even then. A rapid or weak pulse is often associated with fear, fever, shock, blood loss, or simple exercise. Occasionally, a rapid or irregular pulse that occurs while at rest may be a symptom of serious heart disorder. The doctor should be consulted if this is considered to be a possibility.

For most people the normal resting

pulse rate is about 70. A rate of 20-30 above, at rest, is usually considered to be abnormal.

See SYMPTOM SORTER—PALPITATIONS

Rashes tend to change their character or distribution from day to day. Most rashes represent the body's reaction to physical or allergic irritation. After severe sunburn, for example, the skin first becomes red, then itching nettlerash or pimples may follow. Blisters develop if exposure to the sun is continued, and finally the rash heals with scaling or crusts.

Because rashes vary so greatly with each stage, identification depends less on the appearance of the rash than on the area of the body that it affects and the other symptoms, such as fever or cough, which are present.

There are three main kinds of rash.

RASHES WHICH AFFECT THE WHOLE BODY AND ARE ASSOCIATED WITH GENERAL SYMPTOMS SUCH AS FEVER OR COUGH
This type of rash is usually a symptom of an infection and children are mainly affected.
Immediate treatment
• Rest.
• Take fluids.
• Take painkillers in the recommended doses.
See MEDICINES, 22.
When to consult the doctor
• If the general symptoms are severe.
• If contacts may be at risk. A pregnant woman, for example, should avoid contact with GERMAN MEASLES.
Possible causes
Common causes: GERMAN MEASLES; MEASLES; CHICKENPOX; SCARLET FEVER.
Less likely causes: GLANDULAR FEVER; TYPHOID; SYPHILIS (adults only).

RASHES WHICH AFFECT THE WHOLE BODY WITHOUT ASSOCIATED GENERAL SYMPTOMS
Such rashes are frequently due to allergies, are often itchy, are more likely to affect adults, and may appear as scaling, nettlerash or fine red pimples.
Immediate treatment
• Stop whatever might be causing the rash.
When to consult the doctor
• If the cause of the rash seems to be a drug prescribed by the doctor, or a substance used at work.
• If the rash is severe or persistent.
Possible causes
Common causes: SUNBURN; DRUG RASH; ECZEMA; SCABIES (the rash is very itchy); irritants and chemicals.
Less likely causes: PSORIASIS; PITYRIASIS; PRICKLY HEAT; ICHTHYOSIS (present from birth).

RASHES WHICH AFFECT ONE PART OF THE BODY ONLY
The part of the body affected usually indicates the likely cause.
Immediate treatment
• Depends on the cause.
When to consult the doctor
• If the rash spreads or persists for more than seven days.
Possible causes
Common causes: IMPETIGO, COLD SORES and ROSACEA affecting the face; CANDIDIASIS affecting the breasts or groin.
Less likely causes: Discoid and varicose ECZEMA affecting the legs; TINEA affecting the groin; ATHLETE'S FOOT; contact ECZEMA; SHINGLES (accompanied by pain).

Most people in normal health have times when the scalp itches or appears to be flaking, or hair seems to be falling out at an alarming rate. These problems are usually caused by dryness of the scalp or the natural variation in rate of hair loss. However, when these symptoms persist or are severe the scalp may be affected by some disease.

ITCHING
Scalp irritation may be caused by LICE, but can also arise in other local skin disorders that produce scurf such as DANDRUFF, PSORIASIS or ECZEMA.

SCALING
Common scaling disorders include DANDRUFF, ECZEMA and PSORIASIS. In babies scaling is often caused by cradle cap (*see* CHILD CARE *page 159*).

HAIR LOSS
See BALDNESS.

LUMPS
After scalp injury, especially in children, large lumps may suddenly appear in the scalp. The lumps, which are really bruises, usually disappear without treatment in two to ten days. Persistent soft lumps are usually caused by SEBACEOUS CYSTS.

See SYMPTOM SORTER—BLOOD

Although shaking (tremor) may affect the head and legs, it is most obvious in the hands and fingers.
See SYMPTOM SORTER—HAND, FINGERS AND WRIST

See SYMPTOM SORTER—FEVER

Pain felt in the shoulder when moving the arm is usually related to injury, less often more general disorders are responsible.
Immediate treatment
• Rest.
• Keep the shoulder still.
• Take painkillers in recommended doses.
See MEDICINES, 22.
When to consult the doctor
• As soon as possible if injury, deformity and shoulder pain suggest either a fracture or a dislocation of the shoulder.
• If pain persists following previous injury.
• If there is no injury, but pain with movement persists for longer than two or three weeks.
Possible causes
Common causes: Injury; SPRAIN; FIBROSITIS.
Less likely causes: FRACTURE or dislocation from injury; FROZEN SHOULDER; ROTATOR CUFF LESION; CERVICAL RIB SYNDROME; SHOULDER HAND SYNDROME; OSTEOARTHRITIS; RHEUMATOID ARTHRITIS.

There are two main groups of skin disorders: those which involve lumps, bumps, cysts, moles, birthmarks and other abnormalities that remain relatively unchanged for long periods (*see* SYMPTOM SORTER—LUMPS); and those which involve rashes that tend to change in size and character from day to day (see SYMPTOM SORTER—RASH). Other skin abnormalities include changes in texture and colour, and itching.

BLISTERS
See page 91.

CRACKING
Cracks in the skin occur at the start of many skin disorders such as CHAPPED LIPS or ECZEMA.

CRUSTING
Healing of a skin disorder such as IMPETIGO or ECZEMA is usually recognised by crusting, often associated with slight irritation.

DRY SKIN
See SKIN.

GREASY SKIN OR BLACKHEADS
See ACNE
SEBORRHOEA
SKIN.

SEVERE ITCHING
Immediate treatment
• Avoid scratching if possible. Calamine lotion or painkillers in recommended doses (see MEDICINES, 22) may help.
When to consult the doctor
• If itching is severe.
Possible causes
Common causes: SCABIES; ECZEMA.
Less likely causes: LICHEN PLANUS.
See also page 323.

LUMP
See SYMPTOM SORTER—LUMPS.

RASH
See SYMPTOM SORTER—RASH.

ROUGHNESS OR THICKENING
When eczema or another abnormality is healing, roughening or thickening of the skin may occur. Sometimes it follows prolonged itching or scratching.
See CALLUSES and ITCHING (neurodermatitis).

ULCER
Any open sore or ulcer that fails to heal after two or three weeks should be reported to a doctor.

YELLOW SKIN
See JAUNDICE.

BLUE SKIN
See CYANOSIS.

PALE SKIN
See ANAEMIA.

SLEEPLESSNESS

See INSOMNIA
For sleep problems in children see CHILD CARE page 157.

SPEECH PROBLEMS

If a child is affected see page 479.
Sudden difficulty with speech in an adult, when there may be slurring or inability to find the right words, may be a symptom of STROKE, TRANSIENT ISCHAEMIC ATTACK, too much to drink, or drugs (see DRUG ABUSE; MEDICINES).
Nasal speech suggests defects or blockage of the nasal airway. This may happen with the COMMON COLD, enlarged ADENOID and CLEFT PALATE. Less likely causes are NASAL POLYP and DEVIATION OF NASAL SEPTUM.

SPINE, ABNORMAL CURVATURE OF

The spine may be affected by a number of disorders, most of these cause BACK PAIN.

A few cause deformities and abnormalities without pain. These disorders lead to increased curvature of the spine backwards at chest level (hunchback or KYPHOSIS), forwards at waist level (LORDOSIS) or abnormal curvature sideways at any level (SCOLIOSIS). Any of these abnormalities may be seen at any age in children or young adults. They may be painless, and in children aged 12 and over can easily be overlooked by parents and teachers.
Immediate treatment
• None.
When to consult the doctor
• As soon as possible if any curvature is of recent onset, is associated with pain or appears to be getting rapidly worse.
Possible causes
Common causes: Slight increases in curvature which are not a sign of disease. Some growing children may be slightly 'round shouldered'.
Less likely causes: OSTEOCHONDRITIS; OSTEOMALACIA; rarely, congenital defects of the spine or tuberculosis of the spine.

SPOTS

See SYMPTOM SORTER—SKIN ABNORMALITIES

STIFFNESS

Stiffness is dealt with in this Symptom Sorter under the part of the body affected.

STOMACH PAIN

See SYMPTOM SORTER—ABDOMINAL PAIN

SWALLOWING DIFFICULTIES

A sensation of catarrh at the back of the throat (MUCUS COLLECTION IN THE PHARYNX) or of a lump in the THROAT is known to most people. Persistent inability to swallow or sensation that food is sticking behind the breastbone should be reported to a doctor if it is present for more than seven to 14 days, because it may be a symptom of severe ANAEMIA, OESOPHAGITIS, or cancer of the OESOPHAGUS.

SWEATING

The body cools itself by sweating. Healthy individuals may vary greatly in the amount that they sweat. Unexpected sweating may be caused by exercise, extremes of heat, fear or severe pain as well as fever. It is also a symptom of insulin overdose. Every diabetic (see DIABETES) should be aware of this fact. Sweating is sometimes excessive at the MENOPAUSE and in THYROTOXICOSIS.

SWELLING

Swelling is dealt with in this Symptom Sorter under the part of the body affected.

TEMPERATURE, RAISED

See SYMPTOM SORTER—FEVER

See TENSION HEADACHE
ANXIETY
PREMENSTRUAL TENSION

TESTICLES AND SCROTUM, PROBLEMS OF

Disorders of the testicles and scrotum include the absence of one, or both, of the testicles, and pain, swelling or deformity.

ABSENCE OF TESTICLES
The doctor usually checks presence of the testicles at birth. If one, or both, is missing then the boy may require treatment at about five years. See TESTICLES, UNDESCENDED.

PAIN, SWELLINGS OR DEFORMITIES OF TESTICLES OR SCROTUM
Immediate treatment
• Bed-rest.
• Support the testicles.
• Take painkillers in recommended doses. See MEDICINES, 22.
When to consult the doctor
• As soon as possible if the pain is acute or associated with swelling.
• If there is swelling without pain.
Possible causes
Common causes: HERNIA.
Less likely causes: ORCHITIS; HYDROCELE; torsion of TESTICLES; TUMOUR OF THE MALE GENITAL SYSTEM.

THIRST

Excessive thirst which persists for longer than 24-48 hours should always be reported to the doctor, especially in

children. The cause is probably fever, but DIABETES is a possibility.

THROAT, SORE

The exact cause of this extremely common symptom can only be identified as other symptoms develop.
Immediate treatment
• Rest.
• Take soothing throat lozenges and painkillers in recommended doses. See MEDICINES, 42, 22.
When to consult the doctor
It is rarely necessary to call in the doctor for a sore throat, unless the patient is either very young or very old, or the doctor has indicated that the patient may be at risk.
Possible causes
Common causes: COMMON COLD; PHARYNGITIS; TONSILLITIS; INFLUENZA and other similar viruses.
Less likely causes: GLANDULAR FEVER; QUINSY.
See also THROAT, LUMP IN.

TIREDNESS

See SYMPTOM SORTER—APATHY

TOOTHACHE

Pain in the teeth is usually a symptom of dental decay, gingivitis or other dental disorder, but it may also be caused by disorders such as SINUSITIS and NEURALGIA. If toothache is severe or persistent, consult your dentist.
See TEETH

TREMOR

Shaking (tremor) can affect the head and legs but is most common in the hands and fingers. See SYMPTOM SORTER—HAND, FINGERS AND WRIST; PARKINSON'S DISEASE; THYROTOXICOSIS

UNCONSCIOUSNESS

See SYMPTOM SORTER—
CONSCIOUSNESS, DISTURBANCES OF

UNSTEADINESS

See SYMPTOM SORTER—BALANCE PROBLEMS

URINE AND URINATION PROBLEMS

Common disorders of urination are pain, frequent urination, lack of control, failure to urinate and abnormalities of urine.

PAINFUL URINATION
Pain during urination, known medically as dysuria, may range from mild discomfort to a sensation of severe burning.
Immediate treatment
• Drink plenty of fluids.
• Rest if the pain is severe.
• Take painkillers in recommended doses (see MEDICINES, 22).
When to consult the doctor
• If pain is severe or has no obvious trivial cause, or if there is a possibility of pregnancy or SEXUALLY TRANSMITTED DISEASE.

Possible causes
Common causes: CYSTITIS; intercourse.
Less likely causes: SEXUALLY TRANSMITTED DISEASE; PYELONEPHRITIS; STONES IN THE URINARY TRACT; PROSTATITIS; enlarged PROSTATE GLAND.

FREQUENT URINATION
This annoying symptom (called *frequency* by doctors) is sometimes of trivial origin and occasionally has a serious cause.
Immediate treatment
• None.
When to consult the doctor
• If frequency is associated with pain or blood in the urine.
• If SEXUALLY TRANSMITTED DISEASE is possible.
• If it is necessary to urinate many times at night (nocturia). In older men this is a symptom of enlarged PROSTATE GLAND.
Possible causes
Common causes: Normal menstruation; excessive fluid intake; PREGNANCY; diuretics (see MEDICINES, 6); CYSTITIS.
Less likely causes: SEXUALLY TRANSMITTED DISEASE; DIABETES; PYELONEPHRITIS; enlarged PROSTATE GLAND.

INCONTINENCE IN CHILDREN
In babies and children incontinence—lack of control over urination—is normal as late as five years. See CHILD CARE page 159.

INCONTINENCE IN ADULTS
In adults mild incontinence is common. Women who have had children may experience a harmless loss of urine after coughing or laughing (stress incontinence). Men with enlarged prostates may dribble urine after urinating.
Immediate treatment
• Depends on the cause.
When to consult the doctor
• If lack of control is causing offence or interfering with normal life.
Possible causes
Common causes: PREGNANCY; childbirth; UTERINE PROLAPSE; old age; enlarged PROSTATE GLAND.
Less likely causes: MULTIPLE SCLEROSIS; spinal injury and other nervous disorders.

FAILURE TO URINATE

Consult the doctor immediately if failure to urinate lasts longer than 15-20 hours.

ABNORMALITIES OF URINE

• Red urine may be caused by food or bleeding. *See* SYMPTOM SORTER—BLOOD IN THE URINE.
• Dark urine is a symptom of jaundice (*see* JAUNDICE).
• Blue or green urine is usually caused by proprietary medicines. Offensive or fishy-smelling urine is sometimes a symptom of infection, so is cloudy, warm urine, but a deposit or cloud that develops after urine has cooled is normal.

VAGINA AND VULVA, PROBLEMS OF

Disorders of the vagina and vulva may cause discharge, itching or painful intercourse, and swellings or sores.

DISCHARGE

Vaginal discharge is not always abnormal. Heavy vaginal discharge called leucorrhoea, or 'the whites', may cause distress but is not necessarily a sign of disease. However, a discharge that is yellow, stained with blood, painful or offensive is a symptom of infection.
Immediate treatment
• Normal hygiene.
When to consult the doctor
• If a discharge is offensive, yellow, brown, red or frothy.
• If a discharge is associated with frequent or painful urination.
• If intercourse is painful.
• If there is a possibility of SEXUALLY TRANSMITTED DISEASE.
Possible causes
Common causes: Normal leucorrhoea; chemical irritants, for example disinfectants or deodorants; foreign body or retained TAMPON; VAGINITIS (thrush and trichomonal vaginitis).
Less likely causes: SEXUALLY TRANSMITTED

DISEASE; atrophic VAGINITIS; CANCER of the vulva, UTERUS or vagina.

ITCHING OR PAINFUL INTERCOURSE

Itching in the vagina or pain on intercourse are usually symptoms of infection. Causes are the same as Discharge, above. Painful intercourse may also be a sign of lack of lubrication in the vagina (*see* SEX PROBLEMS). For itching of the vulva *see* ITCHING.

SWELLINGS AND SORES

Soft swellings commonly follow overstretching during childbirth and are called cystocele and rectocele. Other swellings or sores may have serious causes.
Immediate treatment
• Normal hygiene.
When to consult the doctor
• As soon as possible if any swelling of the vagina or vulva is noticed.
Possible causes
Common causes: Cystocele and rectocele; PROLAPSE of the uterus; WARTS.
Less likely causes: BARTHOLIN'S CYST AND ABSCESS; CANCER of the vulva or vagina; SYPHILIS.

VOICE PROBLEMS

See SYMPTOM SORTER—HOARSENESS LARYNGITIS

VOMITING

A common symptom with many causes.

CHILDREN
See CHILD CARE *page 153.*

ADULTS
Immediate treatment
• Rest in bed or a chair.

• Take sips of water only.
When to consult the doctor
• If there is abdominal pain, or blood or what looks like coffee grounds in the vomit.
• If vomit contains food eaten more than four hours previously.
• If vomiting continues over four hours.
• If there is also severe diarrhoea or muscle cramps.
Possible causes
Common causes: Eating or drinking too much alcohol; MOTION SICKNESS; GASTRITIS; GASTROENTERITIS; PREGNANCY; fevers.
Less likely causes: PYLORIC STENOSIS; GASTRIC ULCER; DUODENAL ULCER; STOMACH CANCER.

WEAKNESS

Weakness is dealt with in this Symptom Sorter under the part of the body affected.
See SYMPTOM SORTER—APATHY for general fatigue.

WEIGHT LOSS

Loss of weight, that is not the result of a deliberate attempt to slim, should always be taken seriously, especially if other symptoms suggest the possibility of serious disease.
Immediate treatment
• Take milk or milky drinks and eat nourishing food if possible.
When to consult the doctor
• If there is progressive weight loss over four weeks.
• If loss of weight is associated with other symptoms such as persistent cough, vomiting, diarrhoea or absent periods.
Possible causes
Common causes: Dieting; acute fever or operation; chronic ALCOHOLISM; old age and loneliness.

Less likely causes: Chronic GASTRITIS; DEPRESSION; ANOREXIA NERVOSA; STOMACH CANCER; chronic infections such as TUBERCULOSIS and COLITIS.

WHEEZING

See SYMPTOM SORTER—BREATHING DIFFICULTIES

WIND

See SYMPTOM SORTER—INDIGESTION
See also page 527

WORMS

See SYMPTOM SORTER—MOTIONS, ABNORMAL

YAWNING

A common, harmless symptom of drowsiness about which sufferers occasionally become self-conscious and anxious.
See SYMPTOM SORTER—DROWSINESS ANXIETY

YELLOW EYES OR SKIN

See SYMPTOM SORTER—JAUNDICE
See also page 324

PART 2 THE SYSTEMS OF THE BODY

A guide to the functions of the different parts of the human body

INFECTIOUS DISEASES

An infection occurs when harmful organisms—known as pathogens—invade the body. These organisms include viruses, bacteria, protozoa, rickettsiae, fungi and worms. All can be passed from one person to another by various routes. Droplets containing organisms expelled during coughing and sneezing may be breathed in. Organisms are spread by direct contact during kissing or sexual intercourse, or by contact or transfusion with infected blood or body fluids. Animals may be intermediate hosts for the organisms: for example, mosquitoes convey the malaria protozoa plasmodium, and parrots may transmit the bacteria which cause psittacosis. Harmful organisms lie in contaminated food and drink or the soil, and may enter the body through the mouth or an open wound. Organisms may also be passed from an infected mother to her baby during the period of pregnancy or during birth.

THE INCUBATION PERIOD
Once harmful organisms enter the body they begin to reproduce, but it takes some time for them to become numerous enough to cause symptoms. The time that elapses between the organism entering the body and the appearance of symptoms is known as the incubation period, and it may last from a few hours in the case of cholera, to five months in certain forms of hepatitis, or longer.

When a person is attacked by an infectious disease his body develops antibodies to combat the infection. These antibodies remain after the infection has been cured, conferring natural immunity against the same organism.

Artificial immunity to infectious diseases can be given by stimulating the body to produce antibodies. Vaccines consist of a substance which causes the immune system to react to a specific disease without producing the disease itself.

Vaccines do not exist for all infections, but some of the most severe ones can be controlled this way.

TREATMENT
The success of medical treatment for infectious diseases depends on the organism responsible. Antibiotics, such as penicillin, eliminate bacteria. Bacterial infections include diphtheria, gonorrhoea, forms of pneumonia, scarlet fever, whooping cough, syphilis, tuberculosis and typhoid.

Infections caused by protozoa (malaria, for example) and fungi (athlete's foot and thrush, for example) are also usually treatable with drugs. However, few drugs, including antibiotics, seem to affect viral infections. These include chickenpox, hepatitis, colds and influenza, measles, mumps, rabies, and poliomyelitis.

HIGH-RISK GROUPS
- People living in or travelling in countries where infectious diseases are widespread.
- Babies under three months.
- The family of someone suffering from an infectious disease.
- Adults who catch childhood diseases may get them more severely.
- Pregnant mothers should not be in contact with German measles.
- The old and the ill can lose their immunity to many infections.

MAIN SYMPTOMS OF INFECTIOUS DISEASE
The following symptoms all have entries in the SYMPTOM SORTER.
- Diarrhoea.
- Fever.
- Headache.
- Rash.

EMERGENCIES
- If diphtheria is suspected.
- If bitten by any mammal abroad, or in a known rabies-infested area.

HOW TO HELP PREVENT INFECTIOUS DISEASE
- Make sure your child has all the vaccinations your doctor recommends.
- Before you go abroad check whether there are any widespread infectious diseases there and consult your doctor.
- Avoid unsterilised water, ice-creams and uncooked foods in countries where infectious disease is widespread.

Infectious diseases

Each of the disorders listed here has its own entry in the book. There it is described in detail and you are told what to do about it.

AIDS	MENINGITIS
AMOEBIASIS	MUMPS
ATHLETE'S FOOT	PARATYPHOID
BLACKWATER FEVER	PNEUMONIA
BORNHOLM DISEASE	POLIOMYELITIS
	PSITTACOSIS
BRUCELLOSIS	Q FEVER
CAT-SCRATCH FEVER	RABIES
CHICKENPOX	ROCKY MOUNTAIN SPOTTED FEVER
CHLAMYDIA INFECTIONS	ROUNDWORMS
CHOLERA	SANDFLY FEVER
COLD SORES	SCARLET FEVER
COMMON COLD	SCHISTOSOMIASIS
CYTOMEGALO-VIRUS INFECTION	SHINGLES
	SLEEPING SICKNESS
DENGUE FEVER	SMALLPOX
DIPHTHERIA	SYPHILIS
ERYSIPELAS	TETANUS
GERMAN MEASLES	THREADWORMS
	THRUSH
GLANDULAR FEVER	TOXIC SHOCK SYNDROME
GONORRHOEA	TOXOCARIASIS
HEPATITIS	TOXOPLASMOSIS
HISTOPLASMOSIS	TUBERCULOSIS
HYDATID CYST	TULARAEMIA
INFLUENZA	TYPHOID FEVER
LEGIONNAIRE'S DISEASE	TYPHUS
	WHIPWORM
LEISHMANIASIS	WHOOPING COUGH
LEPTOSPIROSIS	YAWS
MALARIA	YELLOW FEVER
MEASLES	

THE MENTAL SYSTEM

The mental system controls the personality, behaviour and feelings rather than the physical functions of the human body such as digestion or circulation. That is not to say, though, that there may not be physical causes of some mental illnesses just as there are some physical remedies —drugs acting on the brain, for example.

All of us are troubled at some time—a few of us a lot of the time—by mental symptoms which might be considered abnormal. This does not necessarily mean that we are ill. A doctor makes his diagnosis on the basis of the combination and severity of the symptoms shown.

In mental illness changes in behaviour may be the first sign that something is wrong. During childhood we learn to fit in with a pattern of behaviour decided by the society in which we live. A wide range of physical and emotional behaviour is accepted. Each individual has his personal pattern of behaviour, and it is when this pattern changes so drastically that the sufferer finds it difficult to take his place in society that he may need medical help.

The mentally ill are all too often rejected by the communities in which they live. Because we often do not understand mental illness we fear it. It is difficult to treat mental illness the same way as physical illness, but manic depression is no more the 'fault' of the sufferer than a broken leg. A sufferer needs help, sympathy and understanding from his family and friends, rejection may only make his illness worse.

DISORDERS OF THE MENTAL SYSTEM
There are three main groups of mental disorders: neuroses, psychoses and mental deficiency.

Neuroses are illnesses in which normal thoughts or feelings are exaggerated to such a degree that they interfere with the sufferer's everyday life. The severity of the neuroses varies widely from patient to patient. The sufferer is always aware of his disorder and its effects. Neuroses account for nearly two-thirds of all mental illness in Britain, and anxiety is by far the commonest form. Other neuroses include hysteria, phobia and depression.

The psychoses cause the major mental problems and it is psychotics who may be popularly termed mad. A sufferer from a psychosis is out of touch with reality and cannot function in society. The illness is apparent to outsiders, but the psychotic himself may not realise that he is ill and is unlikely to seek treatment. In some cases psychotics may require compulsory admission to hospital. Psychoses include manic depression, recurrent severe depression, and the various forms of schizophrenia. There is some evidence that psychoses may be associated with chemical changes in the brain.

Mental deficiency, or retardation, is a general name for a group of conditions in which the sufferer is in some way mentally handicapped. The many different causes include infection of the baby in the womb, brain damage at birth, and genetic abnormalities as in Down's syndrome. Mental deficiency is usually diagnosed in childhood, and unlike neuroses and psychoses it is generally permanent.

HIGH-RISK GROUPS
Some people appear to be especially vulnerable to mental illness because of their heredity, background or surroundings. Large low-income families, unemployment, lack of a close friend or confidant, single parent families, prolonged serious illness and alcoholism are just some of the factors that seem to play a part in mental illness. Extreme stress, loneliness or times of marked change of life-style such as marriage or retirement may also contribute to mental illness.

SYMPTOMS OF MENTAL DISORDER
Patterns of abnormal behaviour, such as apathy or irritability, which might be a symptom of mental illness are dealt with in the SYMPTOM SORTER. Some conditions, such as anxiety or depression, also have entries in the A–Z section of the book.

EMERGENCIES
True emergencies do not often occur in mental illness. Only when life is threatened should urgent action be taken. This may be necessary when a depressed patient threatens, or has attempted, to commit suicide, or when a psychotic patient threatens to harm himself or others. In these cases the doctor, and occasionally the social services or the police, will have the patient compulsorily admitted to hospital.

HOW TO HELP PREVENT MENTAL PROBLEMS
• Try to lead a healthy life. Eat and drink in moderation, take regular exercise and get enough sleep.
• Try to have interests outside yourself to counter boredom and loneliness.
• Try to avoid stress. Attempt to sort out problems quickly instead of worrying about them. Take a regular holiday and weekend breaks.
• Do not take any drugs that have not been prescribed by a doctor.

Disorders of the mental system

Each of the disorders listed here has its own entry in the book. There it is described in detail and you are told what to do about it.

ANOREXIA NERVOSA	DEPRESSION
	HYPERACTIVITY
ANXIETY	HYPOMANIA
AUTISM	HYSTERIA
BULIMIA NERVOSA	MANIC DEPRESSION
COMPULSIVE OBSESSIONAL BEHAVIOUR	NEUROSIS
	PHOBIA
	SCHIZOPHRENIA
CONFUSION	SUICIDE

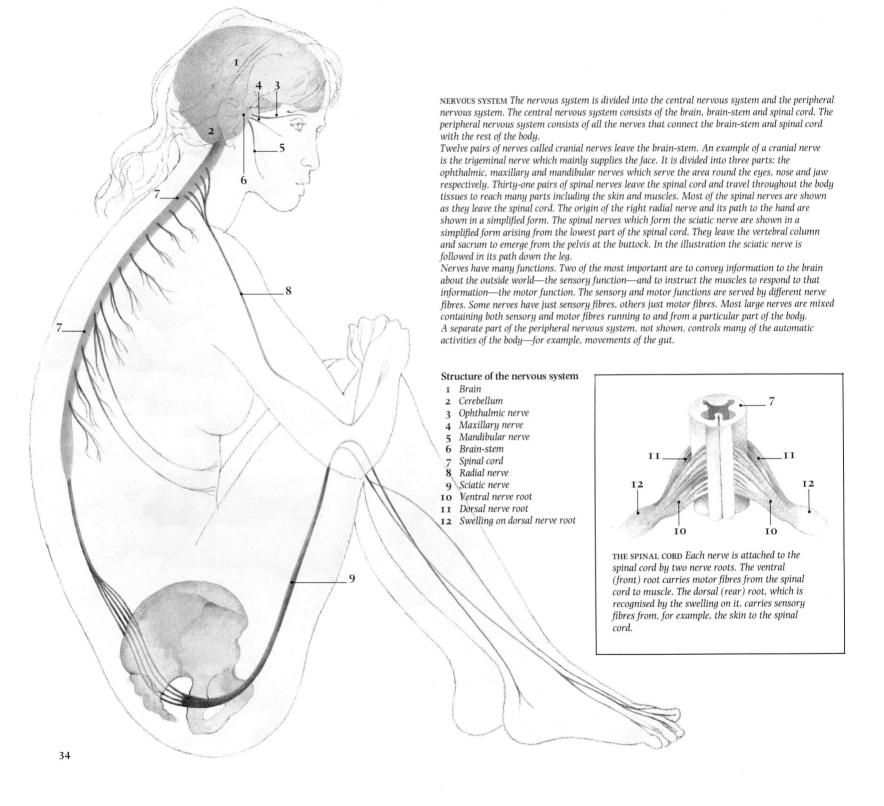

NERVOUS SYSTEM *The nervous system is divided into the central nervous system and the peripheral nervous system. The central nervous system consists of the brain, brain-stem and spinal cord. The peripheral nervous system consists of all the nerves that connect the brain-stem and spinal cord with the rest of the body.*

Twelve pairs of nerves called cranial nerves leave the brain-stem. An example of a cranial nerve is the trigeminal nerve which mainly supplies the face. It is divided into three parts: the ophthalmic, maxillary and mandibular nerves which serve the area round the eyes, nose and jaw respectively. Thirty-one pairs of spinal nerves leave the spinal cord and travel throughout the body tissues to reach many parts including the skin and muscles. Most of the spinal nerves are shown as they leave the spinal cord. The origin of the right radial nerve and its path to the hand are shown in a simplified form. The spinal nerves which form the sciatic nerve are shown in a simplified form arising from the lowest part of the spinal cord. They leave the vertebral column and sacrum to emerge from the pelvis at the buttock. In the illustration the sciatic nerve is followed in its path down the leg.

Nerves have many functions. Two of the most important are to convey information to the brain about the outside world—the sensory function—and to instruct the muscles to respond to that information—the motor function. The sensory and motor functions are served by different nerve fibres. Some nerves have just sensory fibres, others just motor fibres. Most large nerves are mixed containing both sensory and motor fibres running to and from a particular part of the body.

A separate part of the peripheral nervous system, not shown, controls many of the automatic activities of the body—for example, movements of the gut.

Structure of the nervous system

1 *Brain*
2 *Cerebellum*
3 *Ophthalmic nerve*
4 *Maxillary nerve*
5 *Mandibular nerve*
6 *Brain-stem*
7 *Spinal cord*
8 *Radial nerve*
9 *Sciatic nerve*
10 *Ventral nerve root*
11 *Dorsal nerve root*
12 *Swelling on dorsal nerve root*

THE SPINAL CORD *Each nerve is attached to the spinal cord by two nerve roots. The ventral (front) root carries motor fibres from the spinal cord to muscle. The dorsal (rear) root, which is recognised by the swelling on it, carries sensory fibres from, for example, the skin to the spinal cord.*

THE NERVOUS SYSTEM

The nervous system consists of the brain and the nerves that connect it with every part of the body. All the nerves—except the cranial nerves—leave the brain along the spinal cord, a solid bundle of nerves running along a canal in the spine. Individual nerves branch off from the spinal cord through the gaps between the spinal vertebrae to connect with all the muscles in the body.

Two particular groups of nerves—the sympathetic nerves and the parasympathetic nerves—control such body functions as breathing, heartbeat, stomach activity, erection, ejaculation, sweating, blood pressure and the circulation of blood to the limbs. The sympathetic nerves oppose the parasympathetic nerves and so maintain the fine adjustment of these functions. For instance, sympathetic nerves speed up heartbeats and parasympathetic nerves slow them down; sympathetic nerves enlarge the eye pupils and para-sympathetic nerves make them smaller.

Each individual nerve is made up of a chain of nerve cells (neurones) with long branches that are protected by a sheath of myelin—a complex material which, if damaged, disrupts the workings of the nerves involved and causes such disorders as multiple sclerosis. The branches transmit messages from the brain to the body as fast as 328 ft (100 m.) a second. The sensory nerves send signals about such physical sensations as pain, touch, heat and cold; and the motor nerves then instruct the body to react in an appropriate manner—for example, by contracting muscles to move a limb away from a flame.

In general, the left side of the brain controls the right side of the body, and the right side of the brain controls the left side of the body.

DISORDERS OF THE NERVOUS SYSTEM

Changes in the motor nerves, which control the muscles, can cause many of the disorders that affect the nervous system. Increase in motor activity, for example, due to causes such as epilepsy, head injury or meningitis, can lead to convulsions. Reduced motor activity leads to muscle weakness or paralysis.

The intensity of these and other disorders depends upon the patient's general physical and mental condition and upon the root cause.

Two of the most common disorders are fainting, in which the blood supply to the brain is abruptly, if briefly, reduced—and tension headache.

Another frequently encountered disorder is neuralgia, a severe stabbing pain—often in the face—which usually extends along the length of a nerve.

Other disorders include: multiple sclerosis, a chronic disease affecting areas of the brain and spinal cord; Parkinson's disease, in which the muscles twitch; and spina bifida, a congenital defect of the spine.

HIGH-RISK GROUPS

● There are no specific groups of people who, because of their work or life styles, run a high risk of developing a disorder of the nervous system. However, those who have already suffered from such an illness should look out for any signs that it may be about to recur and report them to their doctor.

● Epilepsy, muscular dystrophy and some forms of ataxia tend to run in certain families.

MAIN SYMPTOMS OF NERVOUS DISORDER

The following symptoms all have entries in the SYMPTOM SORTER.

● Collapse.
● Convulsions.
● Headache.
● Tremor.
● Unconsciousness.
● Vertigo.

EMERGENCIES

● An epileptic seizure in someone aged 30 or over, who is not known to suffer from epilepsy, may indicate a brain tumour.

● Severe headache, stiff and painful neck or back, vomiting and high temperature—which may be signs of meningitis.

● Dizzy spells, vertigo or unconsciousness when tilting the neck can indicate stroke, transient ischaemic attack or vertebro-basilar insufficiency, in which the flow of blood to the base of the brain is impeded. There may also be double vision and weakness of a limb.

Disorders of the nervous system

Each of the disorders listed here has its own entry in the book. There it is described in detail and you are told what to do about it.

BELL'S PALSY	NARCOLEPSY
BRAIN ABSCESS	NEURALGIA
BRAIN TUMOUR	NEURO-FIBROMATOSIS
CATAPLEXY	
CERVICAL RIB SYNDROME	NOCTURNAL MYOCLONUS
CLUSTER HEADACHE	PARKINSON'S DISEASE
DELERIUM TREMENS	POLY-NEUROPATHY
DEMENTIA	ST VITUS'S DANCE
ENCEPHALITIS	SPINA BIFIDA
EPILEPSY	STROKE
EXTRADURAL HAEMATOMA	SUBARACHNOID HAEMORRHAGE
FALLS	SUBDURAL HAEMATOMA
GUILLAIN-BARRÉ SYNDROME	TABES DORSALIS
HYDROCEPHALUS	TENSION HEADACHE
MIGRAINE	TIC
MOTOR NEURONE DISEASE	TRIGEMINAL NEURALGIA
MULTIPLE SCLEROSIS	VERTEBRO BASILAR INSUFFICIENCY
MUSCULAR DYSTROPHY	VERTIGO
MYASTHENIA GRAVIS	

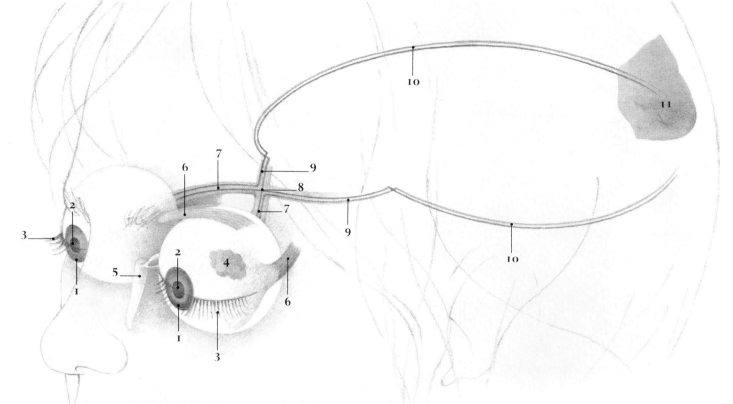

Structure of the eye

1 Iris
2 Pupil
3 Eyelash
4 Lacrimal gland
5 Nasolacrimal duct
6 Eye muscles
7 Optic nerves
8 Optic chiasma
9 Optic tracts
10 Optic radiations
11 Right visual cortex
12 Conjunctiva
13 Cornea
14 Aqueous humor
15 Lens
16 Ciliary body
17 Vitreous humor
18 Sclera
19 Choroid
20 Retina
21 Macula lutea
22 Blind spot

EYE *Light entering an eye passes through the transparent cornea on the front of the eye before reaching the lens. Between the cornea and the lens is a space filled with watery fluid, the aqueous humor. The opening, or pupil, in the iris (the coloured part of the eye) grows larger when there is little light and smaller when there is much light so allowing the correct amount of light to fall on to the retina. Light is focused on to the retina by the lens. The major part of the inside of the eye consists of the vitreous humor which partly gives shape to the eyeball.*

The retina contains special cells (receptors), which convert light waves into nerve impulses. The impulses pass to other cells in the retina before leaving the eye to travel along the optic nerve to the optic chiasma.

Each side of the brain has a specialised part (visual cortex) for interpreting information from the eyes. Each visual cortex receives some information from both eyes. At the optic chiasma information from the left eye, for example, is distributed, some continuing to the left side of the brain along the left optic tract and radiation, some crossing over to the right side. The same process happens with information from the right eye.

The eyeball is moved by small muscles which surround it. The lacrimal gland produces tear fluid which constantly moistens the cornea and is drained through the nasolacrimal duct into the nasal cavity.

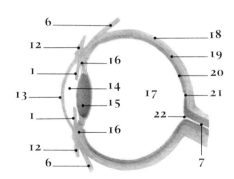

SECTION OF THE EYE *Lining the eyelids and the white of the eye is a membrane, the conjunctiva. The outermost of the three main layers of the eyeball is formed by the sclera, the white of the eye, and the cornea. The middle layer consists of the choroid, iris and ciliary body. Part of the ciliary body adjusts the shape of the lens to focus the eye. The choroid contains pigment and blood vessels. The inner, light-sensitive layer, is the retina. The optic nerve leaves the eyeball at the blind spot. The macula lutea is the point of most acute vision.*

THE EYE

The parts of the eye include the eyelids, conjunctiva, cornea, sclera, pupil, the iris, lens, aqueous humor, vitreous humor, retina, choroid and optic nerves.

The eyelids act as protective shutters for the eyeball and like the visible part of the eye itself, are lined by the conjunctiva, a thin membrane filled with blood vessels. Behind the conjunctiva lies the cornea (the 'window' through which light enters) and the sclera, or white of the eye.

The amount of light entering the eye is controlled by the pupil, a hole in the centre of the iris. The light is then focused by the lens—a firm, transparent, convex body behind the iris. The space between the cornea and the lens is bathed by a watery fluid called the aqueous humor.

Light passes from the lens through the vitreous humor, a transparent, jelly-like substance that forms the bulk of the eyeball. From there, the light is focused on to the retina, a light-sensitive sheet of nerve cells and fibres lining the interior of the eyeball. Between the retina and the sclera is the choroid, a layer of blood vessels that nourishes the retina.

The optic nerve, behind the retina, transmits the light signals to the brain, which interprets them, and we see.

DISORDERS OF THE EYE

By far the most common disorder that a doctor will have to deal with is a foreign body in the eye. Foreign bodies include dust, eyelashes and small insects. All cause pain and, sometimes, swelling.

The second most common disorder is conjunctivitis, in which the conjunctiva covering the white of the eye is red and swollen and has a discharge.

Third in order of occurrence are refractive errors, in which the light rays are not focused on the retina due to a fault, or faults, in the refractive process—or because the eyeball is affected by astigmatism (whereby the image of an object is distorted) or by long-sightedness or short-sightedness.

Styes—hard, pus-filled cysts at the base of the eyelid—are also fairly common.

Other less frequent disorders include: blepharitis, an inflammation of the eyelids; cataract, an opacity in the lens of the eye which causes blurred vision; squint, in which the eyes are abnormally aligned; subconjunctival haemorrhage, a gathering of bright red blood on the surface of the white of the eye; and floaters, a sensation of black streaks floating in the field of vision, caused by blood leaking into the eyeball.

HIGH-RISK GROUPS

- Children who squint. If a child is suspected of having a squint at any age after six months, he should be taken to a doctor. Without treatment, the affected eye could malfunction and go blind.
- Metal workers using high-speed drills and workers using oxyacetylene torches. If these workers fail to wear goggles they are liable to suffer an eye injury.
- People whose parents, brothers or sisters have glaucoma. These people are at risk of developing glaucoma, in which abnormally high pressure in the eye causes loss of vision. Regular eye check-ups can ensure early detection.
- Diabetics. Failure by diabetics to control their disease properly can lead to poor eyesight.

MAIN SYMPTOMS OF DISORDER OF THE EYE

The following symptoms are dealt with in the SYMPTOM SORTER under EYE PROBLEMS.
- Blindness and other visual difficulties.
- Eyelid problems.
- Pain in the eye.
- Red eye.

EMERGENCIES

- Foreign body that cannot easily be removed from the eye.
- Chemical burns caused by caustic acid or alkali. The eye should be washed immediately under a tap or with plain water. *See* FIRST AID *pages 585–6.*
- 'Arc eye', a very painful condition caused by exposure to ultra-violet light—usually from an oxyacetylene flame.
- Sudden and severe pain or loss of vision.

HOW TO HELP PREVENT EYE PROBLEMS

- Wear spectacles if they are prescribed for you. It is almost impossible to rectify faulty eyesight without using spectacles or contact lenses.
- Do not cover a sore or red eye with a pad or patch unless advised to by a doctor. Otherwise infection may occur.
- Do not use drops, ointments or solutions unless prescribed for you by a chemist or doctor, they could harm the eyes.
- Wear goggles when working with a high-speed drill, oxyacetylene torch or chisel. This applies as much to DIY enthusiasts working around the house or doing their own car repairs as it does to people in industry.
- Do not read or do close work in poor light, especially if you are elderly.

Disorders of the eye

Each of the disorders listed here has its own entry in the book. There it is described in detail and you are told what to do about it.

BLEPHARITIS	INTURNED
CATARACT	EYELASHES
CIRCULATION	IRITIS
PROBLEMS IN	MACULAR
THE EYE	DEGENERATION,
COLOUR	SENILE
BLINDNESS	MEIBOMIAN CYST
CONJUNCTIVITIS	NIGHT BLINDNESS
CORNEAL ULCERS	OPTIC NEURITIS
DETACHED RETINA	REFRACTIVE
ECTROPION AND	ERRORS
ENTROPION	SQUINT
EPISCLERITIS	STYES
EYE, FOREIGN	SUBCONJUNCTIVAL
BODY IN	HAEMORRHAGE
FLOATERS	TEAR-DUCT,
GLAUCOMA	BLOCKED

EAR *Sound-waves enter the external ear which consists of the pinna (ear flap) and the external canal. About 1 in. (25 mm.) from the opening of the external canal the sound-waves meet the tympanic membrane (ear-drum). On the other side of the ear-drum is the middle ear, a small cavity containing air, which is within a bone deeply placed in the skull behind the eye socket. The Eustachian tube links the middle ear with the nasopharynx which is behind the nasal cavity and helps to regulate air pressure within the middle ear. Sound-waves are conveyed via the ear-drum to the internal ear by the auditory ossicles. There is a chain of three small bones called malleus, incus and stapes because their shape resembles a hammer, an anvil and stirrup. The internal ear consists of a complicated series of fluid-filled spaces and twisting canals to which another descriptive name, the labyrinth, is given. Three semicircular canals and the vestibule are concerned with maintaining balance. Another part of the internal ear—called the cochlea because it looks like a shell—receives sound-waves from the middle ear and converts them into nerve impulses which pass to the brain.*

Structure of the ear

1	Pinna	8	Incus (separated from stapes to show parts of the inner ear)
2	External canal		
3	Middle ear	9	Stapes
4	Inner ear	10	Vestibule
5	Eustachian tube	11	Cochlea
6	Tympanic membrane (ear-drum)	12	Semicircular canals
7	Malleus	13	Auditory nerve

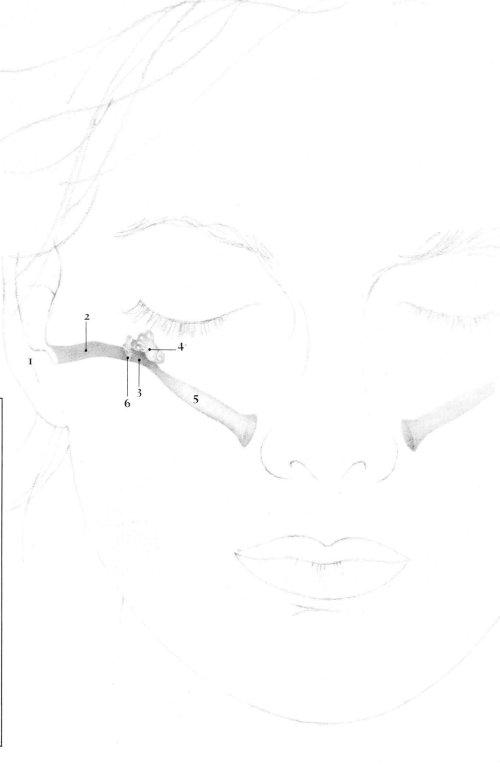

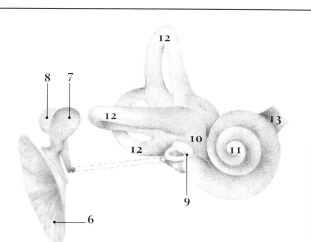

PATH OF SOUND *Sound-waves cause the ear-drum to vibrate. Vibrations from the ear-drum are picked up by the malleus, attached to the inside of the ear-drum, and then passed in turn to the incus and the stapes. The stapes fits into the vestibule of the internal ear where its vibrations are passed on to the fluid in the cochlea, and specialised cells in the cochlea convert the sound-waves into nerve impulses which are passed along the auditory nerve to the brain.*

THE EAR

The ear is made up of three parts—the outer ear, the middle ear and the internal ear. The outer ear, the part we can see, consists of the pinna (the ear flap) and the ear canal. The middle ear contains the ear-drum, the auditory ossicles, and the Eustachian tube. The inner ear contains the cochlea and the balance mechanism.

The ear flap plays a part in collecting sounds and directing them along the ear canal to the ear-drum. Sounds, which are small fluctuations in air pressure, vibrate the drum. For the drum to be sensitive to sound, the air in the middle ear must be at the same pressure as the air in the outer ear and this pressure is equalised by the Eustachian tube, which connects the ear with the back of the throat. Sometimes the air can be felt passing up or down the Eustachian tube, especially when going uphill or when flying or diving. The 'popping' sensation sometimes felt on these occasions is a result of uneven pressures being equalised.

The ear is protected from infection by wax, which is continuously produced by small glands in the outer ear. Tiny hairs, called cilia, move the wax outwards and that is why soft, moist wax comes out of the ear. The wax is meant to be there and no attempt should be made to remove it.

Besides being the organ of hearing, the ear also contains the organ of balance. This lies within the inner ear and consists of three connected semicircular canals containing a fluid called endolymph. When the head moves, the fluid in the canals presses on receptors which carry signals to the brain.

DISORDERS OF THE EAR
Almost everyone loses some degree of hearing as they get older, constant exposure to loud noises may make hearing loss more severe. Partial or complete deafness may be congenital (present from birth) or caused by disease. Sometimes deafness results from failure in the mechanism that conducts sound to the middle ear (it may be as simple as a lump of wax in the ear canal) or there may be failure to transmit sound-waves to the brain (nerve deafness).

The ear is a common site of infection, this causes earache, and may sometimes be dangerous. Infection may develop in the outer ear canal causing a condition known as otitis externa. Infection in the middle ear is called otitis media. In severe cases infection in the middle ear may spread to the mastoid area causing mastoiditis, or the build up of pus in the middle ear may cause perforated ear-drum if it is not released. However, antibiotics (see MEDICINES, 25) usually cure the infection rapidly. A perforated ear-drum may also be caused by injury.

Some people experience various noises in the ear (tinnitus) which may be a symptom of a number of diseases or have no identifiable cause at all.

Because the ear also plays a part in regulating balance, disorders of the semicircular canals may cause dizziness. One such disorder is Ménière's disease.

HIGH-RISK GROUPS
- Children. About one in 10,000 children is born deaf. The deafness, known as congenital deafness, may be partial, one sided, or total. In most cases the cause is unknown, but German measles in the first 13 weeks of pregnancy, some other diseases, and certain drugs taken by pregnant women can all be responsible. Children are also more liable than others to attacks of otitis media and to mastoiditis. Most cases of foreign bodies in the ear involve children.
- Swimmers and divers. Water in the ear can cause otitis externa.
- The elderly. Deafness of old age begins in some people at the age of fifty.
- People working in foundries or other noisy places may suffer noise injury.

MAIN SYMPTOMS OF DISORDERS OF THE EAR
The following symptoms all have entries in the SYMPTOM SORTER.
- Deafness.
- Dizziness.
- Ear problems, particularly earache, discharge or bleeding from the ear and noises in the ear.

EMERGENCIES
- Discharge or bleeding from the ear.
- Pain due to foreign body in the ear.
- Persistent earache.
- Sudden deafness.

HOW TO HELP PREVENT EAR DISORDERS
- Consult a doctor if deafness in a child or adult persists for more than two weeks.
- Wear ear protectors if working in noisy conditions.
- Do not wear a hearing aid without first asking your doctor if you need one.
- Do not try to remove ear wax: you could push it into the ear canal and damage the ear-drum.
- Do not let a child play with small things that it could push into its ears.
- Do not try to remove foreign bodies from the ear. Consult your doctor.

Disorders of the ear

Each of the disorders listed here has its own entry in the book. There it is described in detail and you are told what to do about it.

DEAFNESS	MOTION SICKNESS
EAR INJURY	NOISE INJURY
EAR WAX	OTITIS MEDIA
EUSTACHIAN TUBE,	OTITIS EXTERNA
BLOCKAGE OF	OTOSCLEROSIS
FOREIGN BODY IN	PERFORATED
THE EAR	EAR-DRUM
LABYRINTHITIS	TINNITUS
MASTOIDITIS	
MÉNIÈRE'S	
DISEASE	

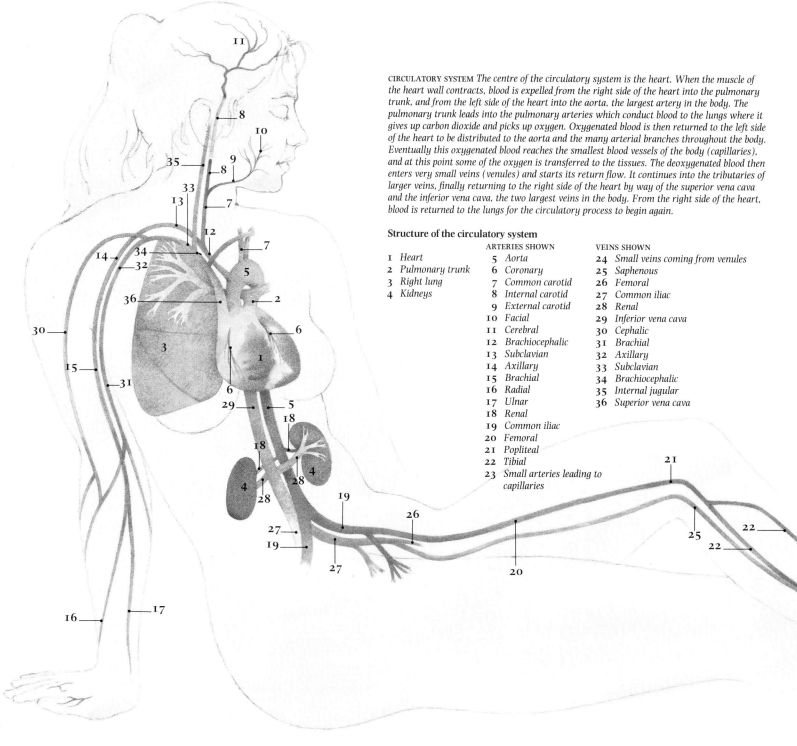

CIRCULATORY SYSTEM *The centre of the circulatory system is the heart. When the muscle of the heart wall contracts, blood is expelled from the right side of the heart into the pulmonary trunk, and from the left side of the heart into the aorta, the largest artery in the body. The pulmonary trunk leads into the pulmonary arteries which conduct blood to the lungs where it gives up carbon dioxide and picks up oxygen. Oxygenated blood is then returned to the left side of the heart to be distributed to the aorta and the many arterial branches throughout the body. Eventually this oxygenated blood reaches the smallest blood vessels of the body (capillaries), and at this point some of the oxygen is transferred to the tissues. The deoxygenated blood then enters very small veins (venules) and starts its return flow. It continues into the tributaries of larger veins, finally returning to the right side of the heart by way of the superior vena cava and the inferior vena cava, the two largest veins in the body. From the right side of the heart, blood is returned to the lungs for the circulatory process to begin again.*

Structure of the circulatory system

ARTERIES SHOWN		VEINS SHOWN
1 *Heart*	5 *Aorta*	24 *Small veins coming from venules*
2 *Pulmonary trunk*	6 *Coronary*	25 *Saphenous*
3 *Right lung*	7 *Common carotid*	26 *Femoral*
4 *Kidneys*	8 *Internal carotid*	27 *Common iliac*
	9 *External carotid*	28 *Renal*
	10 *Facial*	29 *Inferior vena cava*
	11 *Cerebral*	30 *Cephalic*
	12 *Brachiocephalic*	31 *Brachial*
	13 *Subclavian*	32 *Axillary*
	14 *Axillary*	33 *Subclavian*
	15 *Brachial*	34 *Brachiocephalic*
	16 *Radial*	35 *Internal jugular*
	17 *Ulnar*	36 *Superior vena cava*
	18 *Renal*	
	19 *Common iliac*	
	20 *Femoral*	
	21 *Popliteal*	
	22 *Tibial*	
	23 *Small arteries leading to capillaries*	

THE CIRCULATORY SYSTEM

The circulatory system comprises the heart, arteries and veins through which blood is carried to and from the organs and tissues of the body. In the high-pressure system of arteries blood is pumped from the heart through large arteries, which branch into smaller ones (arterioles) to a set of very fine, thin-walled capillaries. At this stage gaseous and chemical exchange occurs between the blood and tissue fluid outside the capillaries. Oxygen and other nutrients are supplied and carbon dioxide and other waste products are returned to the circulation. Capillary blood then enters small veins (venules) and returns to the heart in the low-pressure system of veins.

To maintain a satisfactory flow of blood to vital organs such as the brain and kidneys a certain level of pressure is required. This level is regulated by pressure receptors in the arteries and by chemical control of the blood which adjusts the heart rate and degree of contraction of the arteries.

DISORDERS OF THE CIRCULATORY SYSTEM

The most common problems of the heart and circulation are caused by atheroma—degenerative changes in the walls of the arteries, which restrict the flow of blood. If atheroma occurs in the heart or brain it can lead to strokes or heart attacks when there is complete blockage of blood flow; or angina, dizziness, disturbances of vision and collapse when the blockage is partial.

Severe atheroma in the leg arteries may reduce the circulation to such an extent that gangrene develops in the feet.

The heart valves can become infected by bacteria and viruses in the blood-stream, leading to obstruction of the blood flow.

In some conditions the mechanism controlling rhythm may be disturbed and the heart may beat very fast and/or irregularly. This may be due to a congenital abnormality or, in adults, a deterioration in the nerves controlling the heartbeat or in their blood supply.

Heart rate and rhythm are also very sensitive to the chemical state of the blood, for example, the concentration of oxygen, carbon dioxide, calcium, sodium and potassium.

General diseases and infections can affect the heart muscle. The heart and circulation also respond to emotional changes, such as anxiety and fear.

HIGH-RISK GROUPS

• Babies. Exposure to certain drugs and diseases, especially GERMAN MEASLES, during pregnancy, can be related to congenital abnormalities of the heart in babies.
• Smokers. Smoking is known to have harmful effects on arteries, both within the heart and in the general circulation.
• The middle-aged and elderly. The heart may be affected by disease elsewhere in the body. Serious lung disease, such as chronic bronchitis and obstructive airways disease, strains the heart.
• People with high blood CHOLESTEROL.

MAIN SYMPTOMS OF DISORDER OF THE HEART AND CIRCULATORY SYSTEM

The following symptoms all have entries in the SYMPTOM SORTER.
• Breathing difficulties, particularly shortness of breath.
• Chest pain.
• Cold limbs.
• Collapse or fainting.
• Cyanosis (blueness of skin).
• Fatigue.
• Heartbeat disorders such as jumping, thumping, jerking, or missing a beat.
• Swelling of the ankles.

EMERGENCIES

Professional care is vital in emergencies of the heart and circulation, but first aid can be applied until help arrives.
• Seat people who are short of breath or in pain.
• Lie unconscious patients who are breathing on their sides.
• Apply immediate heart massage and artificial respiration to patients who are unconscious and not breathing. See FIRST AID *pages 552–7.*

HOW TO HELP PREVENT CIRCULATION PROBLEMS

• Keep to your ideal weight (*see page 525*).
• Take plenty of exercise.
• Eat sensibly. See NUTRITION.
• Do not smoke. Smoking affects the arteries and harms babies whose mothers smoke during pregnancy.

Disorders of the circulatory system

Each of the disorders listed here has its own entry in the book. There it is described in detail and you are told what to do about it.

ACROCYANOSIS	ERYTHRO-MELALGIA
ANEURYSM	
ANGINA	EXTRASYSTOLES
PECTORIS	GANGRENE
AORTIC	HEART BLOCK
INCOMPETENCE	HEART FAILURE
AORTIC VALVE	HYPERTENSION
STENOSIS	LYMPHOEDEMA
ARTERIAL	MITRAL
THROMBOSIS	INCOMPETENCE
ARTERITIS	MITRAL STENOSIS
ATHEROMA	MYOCARDITIS
ATRIAL	PAROXYSMAL
FIBRILLATION	TACHYCARDIA
ATRIAL FLUTTER	PERICARDITIS
BUERGER'S	PULMONARY
DISEASE	EMBOLISM
CARDIO-	RAYNAUD'S
MYOPATHY	DISEASE
CLAUDICATION,	RHEUMATIC
INTERMITTENT	FEVER
COARCTATION OF	THROMBO-
THE AORTA	PHLEBITIS
CONGENITAL	VARICOSE ULCER
HEART DISEASE	VARICOSE VEINS
CORONARY	VENTRICULAR
THROMBOSIS	FIBRILLATION
COR PULMONALE	
ENDOCARDITIS	

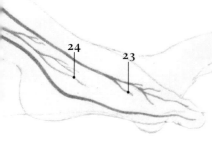

24   23

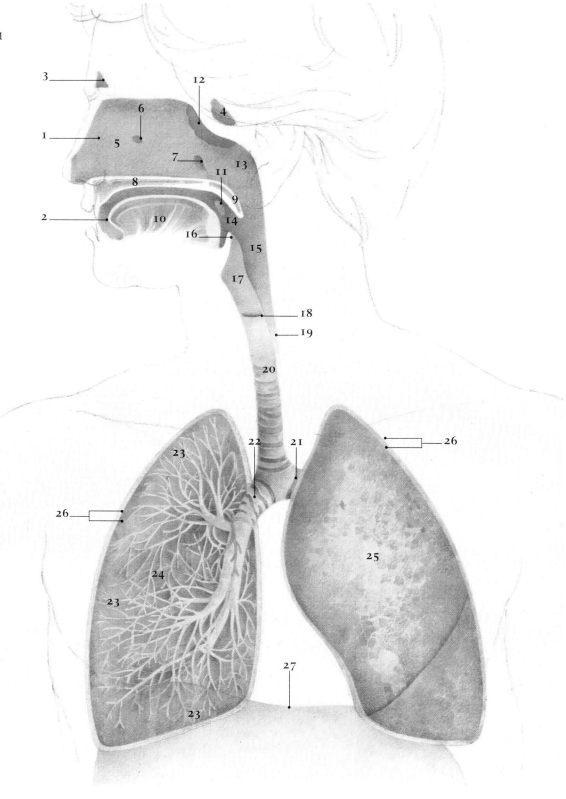

RESPIRATORY SYSTEM *Air enters the upper part of the respiratory system through the nose where it is moistened and warmed by the linings of the two nasal cavities. Foreign particles—dust and bacteria—in the air stick to the mucus on the walls of the cavities purifying the air. Small channels lead off from each nasal cavity to the nasal sinuses. If the nose is blocked, air enters through the mouth. At the back of the mouth lie the tonsils, and behind the nasal cavities lie the adenoids. Both tonsils and adenoids are part of the immune system involved with producing antibodies against infection. Also behind the nasal cavities are openings to the Eustachian tubes which connect with the middle ears.*

Purified air passes through the pharynx (throat) and descends into the larynx, past the epiglottis—a small flap which is one of several mechanisms that help to prevent food entering the windpipe. The vocal cords lie in the larynx and sounds can be produced as air passes over them. From the larynx the air passes into the trachea (windpipe) which is connected to each lung by a tube called a bronchus. Each bronchus subdivides many times and some of these smaller tubes are called bronchioles. Beyond the bronchioles the tubes get smaller still and finally the air enters tiny, thin-walled sacs called alveoli. In these sacs oxygen is transferred from the air to the red blood cells in the small blood vessels of the lung; and carbon dioxide is given up.

Moist membranes called pleura surround the lungs and allow them to move freely so that they can function properly. During breathing, the diaphragm, below the lungs, contracts. This increases the space in the chest and so allows the lungs to expand.

Structure of the respiratory system

1	Nose	14	Oropharynx
2	Mouth	15	Laryngeal pharynx
3	Frontal sinus	16	Epiglottis
4	Sphenoidal sinus	17	Larynx
5	Nasal cavity	18	Vocal cords
6	Opening of the	19	Oesophagus
	maxillary sinus	20	Trachea
7	Opening of the	21	Left bronchus
	Eustachian tube	22	Right bronchus
8	Hard palate	23	Bronchiole
9	Soft palate	24	Right lung
10	Tongue	25	Left lung
11	Tonsils	26	Pleura
12	Adenoids	27	Upper limit of the
13	Nasopharynx		diaphragm

THE RESPIRATORY SYSTEM

The respiratory system consists of all the organs of the body contributing to breathing. It includes the nose, mouth, upper throat, larynx, trachea and bronchi, which are all air passages. These lead to the lungs, where oxygen is passed into the blood and carbon dioxide is given off.

The air passages not only route air to the lungs, but they filter it. This is why colds, runny noses and sore throats are so common. The nose and throat trap infection, and localise it before it can reach the lungs and develop into serious disease such as pneumonia.

DISORDERS OF THE RESPIRATORY SYSTEM

More than 25 per cent of all conditions reported to the doctor occur in the respiratory system, and for every case reported three or four more never appear in the surgery.

About 200 different organisms, either viruses or bacteria, can attack the respiratory system, and attempts at identification are usually impractical or impossible. Because of this difficulty doctors tend to label respiratory disorders with the name of the area affected. This practice gives rise to names such as tonsillitis—inflammation of the tonsils; bronchitis—inflammation of the bronchial tubes; and many other 'itises'. The vast majority of infections get better with simple treatment in one to five days. However, it is all the more important to consider the possibility of serious disease if symptoms do not begin to improve within five days.

The respiratory system is particularly susceptible to allergy, because it provides the easiest access to the body for allergic substances. If an allergic reaction blocks the nose, breathing through the mouth means that the filtering effect of the nasal passages is bypassed. Allergic substances pass straight into the trachea and then the lungs, causing catarrh, breathlessness, asthma and other disorders.

Benign or malignant tumours of the mouth, throat or the voice-box are rare. Lung cancer is more common, accounting for 6 per cent of all deaths in Britain. It is 15 times more common among cigarette smokers than among non-smokers.

HIGH-RISK GROUPS
- Babies under six months.
- Children under three, particularly if there are other symptoms such as fever, reluctance to take food, or a seizure.
- Frail, elderly people. This group is particularly vulnerable to acute bronchitis or pneumonia.
- People with a history of chest disease such as chronic bronchitis or asthma.
- Any individual suffering from chronic ill-health from other causes.
- Those who smoke.

MAIN SYMPTOMS OF THE RESPIRATORY SYSTEM
The following symptoms all have entries in the SYMPTOM SORTER.
- Blood in spit.
- Breathing difficulties.
- Catarrh.
- Chest pain made worse by breathing.
- Cough.
- Hoarseness.
- Sore throat.

EMERGENCIES
- Choking, see FIRST AID *pages 572–4.* Do not attempt to remove a foreign body from the throat yourself unless the patient is choking. Consult the doctor immediately. Do not put fingers in the throat or try to make the patient vomit.
- A young child with a feverish illness having difficulty breathing which is not relieved by inhaling steam.
- Severe asthma attack, especially in a child.

HOW TO HELP PREVENT AND TREAT RESPIRATORY PROBLEMS
- Do not smoke.
- Keep elderly people warm in winter and when they are ill to prevent hypothermia.
- Keep cool a patient with a feverish respiratory infection, particularly if the patient is a child. Keep the room at a comfortable temperature (59–64°F, 15–18°C); remove nightclothes and roll down bedclothes; give extra drinks and paracetamol in the recommended dosage. *See* MEDICINES, 22.
- Do not participate in sport or heavy work too soon after a respiratory illness. This may cause infection to descend to the lungs, or heart-rhythm disturbances.
- Do not use nose drops or sprays to clear a stuffy nose unless they have been prescribed by a doctor.
- Do not give small children peanuts, beads or other small objects to eat or play with; they may choke on them.

Disorders of the respiratory system

Each of the disorders listed here has its own entry in the book. There it is described in detail and you are told what to do about it.

ADENOID, ENLARGED	HYPER-VENTILATION
ASTHMA	LARYNGITIS
BRONCHIECTASIS	LARYNX
BRONCHIOLITIS	GROWTH IN
BRONCHITIS	LUNG CANCER
CLEFT PALATE	MUCUS
AND HARE-LIP	COLLECTION
COMMON COLD	IN THE
CROUP	PHARYNX
DEVIATION OF	NASAL POLYP
THE NASAL	NOSE-BLEED
SEPTUM	PHARYNGITIS
DIPHTHERIA	PLEURISY
EMPHYSEMA	PNEUMONIA
EPIGLOTTITIS	PNEUMOTHORAX
FOREIGN BODY	QUINSY
IN THE EAR,	RESPIRATORY
NOSE OR	INFECTION
THROAT	RHINITIS
GLANDULAR	SINUSITIS
FEVER	TONSILLITIS
	THROAT, LUMP IN

DIGESTIVE SYSTEM *The easiest way to understand the digestive system is to follow the route taken by food once it is in the mouth. Each mouthful that is swallowed is usually called a bolus, and may be dry, liquid or a mixture of both. The food is chewed by the teeth and then the bolus, especially if dry, is acted on by saliva which contributes fluid and enzymes for the first stage of digestion. Saliva is produced by glands—the sublingual glands (under the tongue), the parotid glands (on the side of the face), and submandibular glands (under the lower jaw). Many other very small saliva-producing glands line the cheeks. From the mouth the food passes with little or no change through the pharynx (throat) and oesophagus (gullet) to the stomach. In the stomach the food is acted upon by acid and more enzymes from the stomach lining and is turned into a semi-fluid mass known as chyme, which is released into the first part of the small intestine—the duodenum. In the duodenum more enzymes from the pancreas, and bile from the liver, break down the food further. The gall-bladder acts as a small reservoir for bile which passes into the duodenum via the bile duct behind the pancreas. From the duodenum, the mixture passes into the next part of the small intestine, the jejunum, and then into the ileum. It is in these two parts of the intestine that most of the nutrients in the food are absorbed into blood in veins which will carry them to the liver for further digestion. The liver also receives blood from other abdominal organs, for example the spleen, which lies partly behind and to the left of the stomach. The remaining mixture, which has had all the nutrients removed, moves on into the colon via the ileocaecal junction, which lies above the appendix, and progresses through the caecum, and the ascending, descending, transverse and sigmoid colons. As it passes through these parts of the digestive system it is progressively dehydrated before being passed out of the body via the rectum and anal canal.*

Structure of the digestive system

1	Teeth	14	Duodenum
2	Mouth	15	Jejunum
3	Sublingual gland	16	Ileum
4	Parotid gland	17	Ileocaecal junction
5	Submandibular gland	18	Caecum
6	Pharynx	19	Appendix
7	Oesophagus	20	Ascending colon
8	Stomach	21	Transverse colon
9	Spleen	22	Descending colon
10	Liver	23	Sigmoid colon
11	Bile duct	24	Rectum
12	Gall-bladder	25	Anal canal
13	Pancreas		

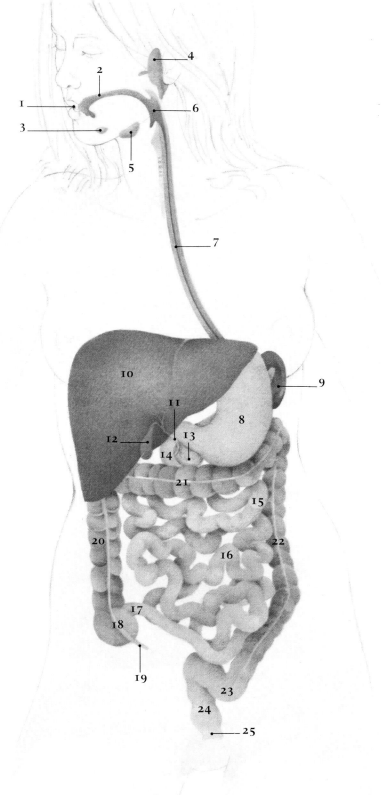

The digestive system consists of the digestive tract (alimentary canal) which forms a continuous passage from the mouth to the anus, together with the pancreas, liver and gall-bladder.

In the digestive tract food is broken down so that the sugars, fats, proteins, minerals, vitamins and water that it contains may be absorbed into the blood-stream to fuel the body.

The motion which passes out at the anus consists of all the waste, unusable elements of food—mainly cellulose—and the bacteria which help the breakdown of food in the intestines. However, even though some elements of food do not nourish the body, they do play an important part in digestion. The roughage, or fibre, in food helps to carry away wastes and may even help to protect against diverticular disease and cancer of the colon and rectum. *See* NUTRITION.

THE DIGESTIVE SYSTEM

DISORDERS OF THE DIGESTIVE SYSTEM
The digestive tract is extremely tolerant of the wide variety of substances that pass through it, but it reacts strongly against infected foods, poisons and other irritants. These may cause vomiting or diarrhoea. Many minor disorders of the digestive tract, including indigestion, gastritis, food poisoning and gallstones, follow eating the wrong things. Many serious diseases are caused, or persist, because the digestive process prevents the healing of small injuries and infections. Duodenal, oesophageal or gastric ulcers and pancreatitis are examples.

However, most diseases of the digestive tract are caused by several different factors acting at once. Thus, heredity, diet, infection, immune processes and mechanical blockage may all play different parts in causing a single disorder.

HIGH-RISK GROUPS
• Babies and elderly people risk dehydration from gastroenteritis.
• Duodenal ulcer and polyposis often run in families.
• Obese women risk gallstones.

• Adults under stress are predisposed to duodenal ulcer and possibly colitis.

MAIN SYMPTOMS OF DIGESTIVE DISORDERS
The following symptoms have entries in the SYMPTOM SORTER.
• Abdominal pain.
• Loss of appetite.
• Blood in vomit or the motions.
• Constipation.
• Diarrhoea.
• Indigestion.
• Vomiting or nausea.
• Weight loss.
• Yellow skin or eyes.

EMERGENCIES
• Vomiting large amounts of blood, or blood in the motions.
• Prolonged or severe vomiting especially with abdominal pain and diarrhoea.
• Prolonged or severe diarrhoea especially with vomiting or bleeding.
• Severe abdominal pain when the patient's condition is deteriorating.
• Tenderness and pain in a hernia which cannot be pushed back.
• Rapid deterioration in a baby or elderly person with diarrhoea or vomiting.

HOW TO HELP PREVENT DIGESTIVE PROBLEMS
• Eat plenty of high-roughage food such as fresh vegetables, meat, wholemeal bread and bran.
• Eat regular, frequent meals. Do not bolt food.
• Tell your children about the dangers of eating poisonous plants and drinking from strange bottles.
• Do not eat creamy foods, processed meat or fish, which have been left more than eight hours at room temperature 65–70°F (18–21°C).
• Do not just warm up cooked meat once it has gone cold. Either eat it cold or heat it through thoroughly.
• Do not strain too hard over motions to relieve constipation, or encourage children to do so during toilet training.
• Do not become overweight.

Disorders of the digestive system

Each of the disorders listed here has its own entry in the book. There it is described in detail and you are told what to do about it.

ACHALASIA OF THE CARDIA	HICCUPS
ACID REGURGITATION	ILEITIS, REGIONAL
ANAL FISSURE	JAUNDICE
ANAL IRRITATION	MESENTERIC ADENITIS
APPENDICITIS, ACUTE	MOUTH ULCERS
BOWEL, CANCER OF	OBESITY
BOWEL, IRRITABLE	OESOPHAGITIS
CIRRHOSIS OF THE LIVER	OESOPHAGUS, CANCER OF
COELIAC DISEASE	OESOPHAGUS, STRICTURE OF
COLITIS, ULCERATIVE	PANCREATITIS
COLON, INACTIVE	PERITONITIS
CONSTIPATION	PILES
CYSTIC FIBROSIS	POLYPOSIS OF COLON
DIVERTICULAR DISEASE OF THE COLON	PROCTITIS
DUODENAL ULCER	PYLORIC STENOSIS
DYSENTERY	RECTAL PROLAPSE
FAECAL IMPACTION	SALIVARY GLANDS— INFECTIONS, STONES AND TUMOURS
FISTULA IN ANO	STEATORRHOEA
GALLSTONES	STOMACH, CANCER OF
GASTRIC ULCER	TAPEWORM
GASTRITIS	THREADWORMS
GASTROENTERITIS	TONGUE PROBLEMS
GIARDIASIS	
HERNIA	

URINARY SYSTEM *Urine is produced in two kidneys. Each kidney contains about a million glomeruli—small clusters of tiny blood vessels (capillaries) which filter the blood. The filtrate (the solution filtered out of the blood) passes through many tubules within the kidney. The function of these tubules is to reabsorb a lot of water from the filtrate and to alter its chemical composition until a correct chemical balance is achieved to suit the requirements of the body. When the remaining filtrate leaves the kidney to enter the expanded upper part of the ureter in the abdominal cavity, it has been greatly reduced in volume and this remaining solution, containing waste products, is called urine.*

The ureters descend from each kidney into the pelvis and connect with the back of the urinary bladder. The bladder lies between the pubic symphysis and the womb in the female, and between the pubic symphysis and the rectum in the male. Urine can be temporarily stored in the bladder but eventually it is released via the urethra. In the female the urethra is very short and lies just in front of the vagina. In contrast, the male urethra is much longer and in the early part of its course is surrounded by the prostate gland before it enters the penis. The male urethra serves a dual function in that it conveys either urine or ejaculatory fluid.

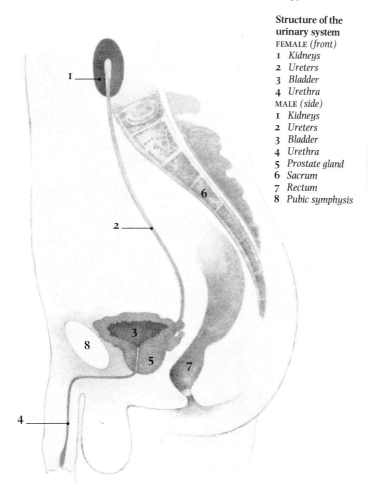

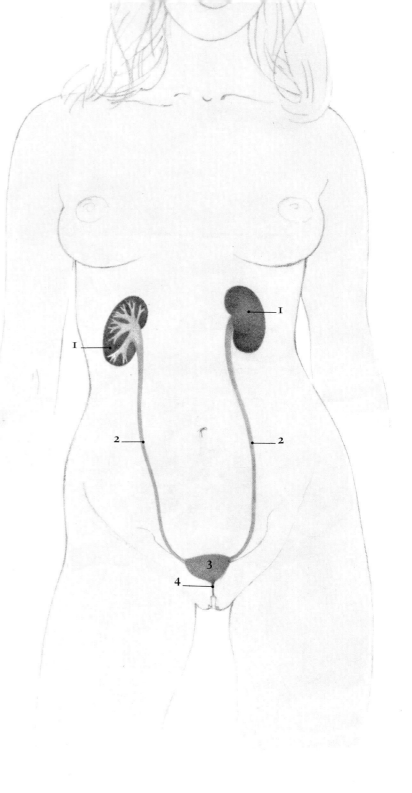

Structure of the urinary system
FEMALE *(front)*
1 *Kidneys*
2 *Ureters*
3 *Bladder*
4 *Urethra*
MALE *(side)*
1 *Kidneys*
2 *Ureters*
3 *Bladder*
4 *Urethra*
5 *Prostate gland*
6 *Sacrum*
7 *Rectum*
8 *Pubic symphysis*

THE URINARY SYSTEM

The urinary system consists of the kidneys, ureters, bladder and urethra. The function of the kidneys is to keep the blood healthy by filtering off unwanted material and keeping the water, salts and acids in the blood at a constant level. All the body's blood passes through the kidneys many times each day and is thus kept constantly purified. Neither kidney does nearly as much work as it is capable of performing, and the body can, if need be, function efficiently on only one kidney. Solution containing waste (urine) passes from the kidneys through the ureters to the bladder and then out through the urethra. About $2\frac{1}{2}$ pints (1.4 litres) of urine are passed every 24 hours.

DISORDERS OF THE URINARY SYSTEM

About 6 per cent of all conditions reported to the doctor are disorders of the urinary system. In most cases the disorder is due to an infection in or near the bladder, and in all but a small percentage of infections a bacterium called *Escherichia coli* is responsible. The germ usually lives in the bowel, from which it gains entry to the bladder via the urethra. This passage is much shorter in the female than in the male and therefore the bacteria have less distance to travel to reach the bladder—which is one reason why women are much more prone than men to cystitis (inflammation of the bladder).

If the natural flow of urine is impaired by the narrowing of the urethra (such as occurs with an enlarged prostate gland), urine in the bladder can become stagnant. If an infection is present, germs will multiply rapidly in the stagnant urine, often making the infection chronic (persistent) or recurrent.

Most bladder infections are not severe and some will clear up on their own. Occasionally, however, infection may spread to the kidneys and cause pyelonephritis, inflammation of part of the kidneys. Treatment with antibiotics is required for these disorders.

Inflammation of the glomeruli in the kidneys, nephritis, is not due to infection but to a process called autoimmune disease: the body produces antibodies that attack its own tissue.

There is a large group of very rare conditions, called by doctors nephrosis and nephrotic syndrome, in which there is swelling of body tissue. Causes include diabetes mellitus, and poisoning from certain drugs such as aspirin.

Kidney diseases form only a fraction of a percentage of urinary tract disorders, but are important because they can lead to kidney failure and victims may require dialysis or kidney transplants.

Tumours of the urinary tract are most common in the bladder. Stones—hard masses of mineral salts—can form in the kidney or the bladder and are the result either of an infection or a blood abnormality, such as gout.

The bladder is regulated by nervous control. This can be disturbed following damage to the brain, the spine or the nerves leading to the bladder.

HIGH-RISK GROUPS

- Babies and young children. There may be few symptoms of urinary infection—perhaps pallor, a failure to put on weight and wetting the bed or pants after being dry—but developing kidneys are especially susceptible to damage, so a doctor must be told as soon as infection is suspected.
- Newly married and pregnant women. Infection of the urinary tract tends not to be serious but a doctor should be consulted in the event of back pain and raised temperature.
- Industrial workers. A higher than average incidence of bladder cancer occurs in people who have worked in the chemical, dyestuff or rubber industries.
- People with high blood pressure or diabetes.
- Immigrants. Tuberculosis of the urinary system is more common than usual in immigrants from India and Pakistan.
- The elderly. Incontinence (inability to retain urine) is one of the most common problems of old age. Enlargement of the prostate gland is common among elderly men and causes other urinary problems, including incontinence.

MAIN SYMPTOMS OF DISORDER OF THE URINARY SYSTEM

The following all have entries in the SYMPTOM SORTER.
- Back pain and pain that spreads from the lower back down to the penis or scrotum.
- Swelling of face, legs and arms.
- Urination problems especially burning pain related to urination, frequent passage of urine, or blood or discoloration of urine.

EMERGENCIES
- Inability to pass urine.
- Blood in urine.
- Severe pain in the lower back beneath the ribs.

HOW TO HELP PREVENT URINARY PROBLEMS
- Keep the genitals and surrounding area clean. Women must be especially careful to wipe from front to back after defecating to avoid infecting the bladder with *Escherichia coli*.
- Drink plenty of fluids, especially in hot weather.
- Do not exceed the recommended dose of paracetamol and other painkillers. Excess dosage can damage the kidneys.

Disorders of the urinary system

Each of the disorders listed here has its own entry in the book. There it is described in detail and you are told what to do about it.

FEMALE GENITAL SYSTEM *The female genital system is designed to produce eggs (ova) and receive sperm, and also to nurture the embryo if fertilisation occurs.*
Each month an egg is produced in one or other of the two ovaries of a woman of childbearing age. The egg is carried from the ovary to the womb (or uterus) by the Fallopian (or uterine) tube.
Sperm enter the system via the vagina during sexual intercourse. Around the entrance to the vagina are folds of fat-filled skin called labia. At the front, between the labia, lies the clitoris. During first intercourse the small membrane guarding the entrance to the vagina—the hymen —is stretched. Sperm travel up the vagina, through the opening of the neck of the womb (cervix) into the womb and from there to the Fallopian tube. It is in the outer third of the Fallopian tube that fertilisation takes place. The fertilised egg travels along the Fallopian tube to the womb where it becomes implanted in the wall of the womb. If an egg is not fertilised by a sperm, it is shed during the next menstrual period.
In the non-pregnant adult female the womb lies in the pelvis behind and partly on top of the bladder. During pregnancy the womb enlarges as a result of the growth of its wall and contents and eventually can be felt almost as high as the level of the diaphragm.
The breasts also enlarge during pregnancy, partly because of an increase in glandular tissue within them. After the birth of the child milk is produced by the glandular tissue in the breasts and conducted to the tip of the nipple by milk ducts.

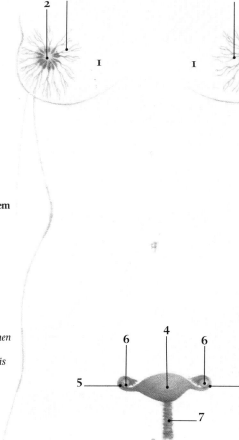

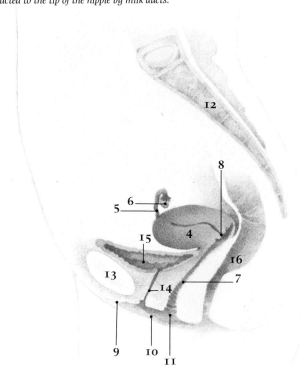

Structure of the female genital system

I	Breasts
2	Nipples
3	Milk ducts
4	Womb
5	Fallopian tubes
6	Ovaries
7	Vagina
8	Cervix
9	Clitoris
10	Labium
11	Position of hymen
12	Sacrum
13	Pubic symphysis
14	Urethra
15	Bladder
16	Rectum

THE FEMALE GENITAL SYSTEM

The female genital system consists of the parts of the female body concerned with reproduction; these include the ovaries, Fallopian tubes, uterus, vagina, vulva, breasts and nipples.

Two months before a girl is born her ovaries contain a total of 7 million cells, their number drops to about 1 million at birth. At puberty about 300,000 cells remain, each of which could develop into a follicle which produces hormones and an egg. Because the period between the start of menstruation and the menopause is about 30–40 years and since normally only one egg is produced each month, the number of cells which actually turn into eggs is about 400, the rest degenerate.

The hormone oestrogen is chiefly responsible for the development of the female genital organs at puberty, the breasts, uterus, vagina and the rest of the genital tract enlarge, fat is distributed to form feminine curves and hair grows under the arms and in the pubic region.

DISORDERS OF THE FEMALE GENITAL SYSTEM

Difficulties with menstrual periods, such as pain, irregularity and heavy bleeding, are very common disorders of the female genital system. The normal pattern of menstruation varies greatly: some women have brief, light periods at short intervals; other women have longer, heavier periods. The doctor should be consulted if the normal pattern changes.

The vagina is a common site of infection. Many infections clear up spontaneously without the need to consult the doctor, but $2\frac{1}{2}$ per cent of consultations in general practice are due to vaginal infection.

After the menopause the vaginal walls and vulva shrink and become dry. This can cause soreness and sometimes even infection. In the vulva there may be abnormal skin changes.

The Fallopian tubes are also a site of infection, usually spread from the uterus or vagina. Infection of the pelvic area is sometimes known as pelvic inflammatory disease or salpingitis.

The egg-producing follicles in the ovary can become cysts—swellings filled with fluid. These swellings may remain unnoticed unless an operation is carried out for something else, occasionally they grow very large. They may cause pain. Very rarely the cysts are cancerous.

Many women experience tenderness and lumpiness of the breast before a period. Sometimes there is an isolated lump which is soft and tender. Unfortunately, cancer of the breast starts as a small lump in the breast and so all lumps should be reported to the doctor as soon as they are discovered.

HIGH-RISK GROUPS
- Women over 40 are more likely to develop breast cancer.
- Women over 50 are more likely to develop cancer of the body of the uterus.
- Women who are sexually active are more likely to develop cervical cancer.
- Women who are overweight are more likely to develop prolapse.

MAIN SYMPTOMS OF FEMALE GENITAL DISORDER
The following symptoms all have entries in the SYMPTOM SORTER.
- Abdominal pain.
- Problems of the vagina and vulva.
- Period problems (*see also page 403*).

EMERGENCIES
- Severe, lower abdominal pain and collapse in early pregnancy.
- Bleeding in the second half of pregnancy.
- Severe bleeding after childbirth.

HOW TO HELP PREVENT FEMALE GENITAL PROBLEMS
- Examine your breasts every month. Report any changes in appearance or lumps. *See* BREAST CANCER.
- Have regular cervical smear tests, at least one every three years.
- Do not wear tight panty girdles, tight jeans, nylon tights, or use vaginal deodorants if you are prone to thrush. The Pill may also increase the likelihood of your getting thrush.
- Wipe from front to back after a bowel motion.
- Do not forget to remove your last tampon at the end of your period.
- If you are breast-feeding, keep your nipples soft and supple by regular use of a lubricant such as olive oil.
- Do not let the baby suck on the end of the nipple, make sure he is properly fixed to the areola.

Disorders of the female genital system

Each of the disorders listed here has its own entry in the book. There it is described in detail and you are told what to do about it.

ANTEPARTUM HAEMORRHAGE	OVARIAN CYST
BARTHOLIN'S CYST AND ABSCESS	OVULATION SYNDROME
BREAST ABSCESS	PREMENSTRUAL TENSION
BREAST ENGORGEMENT	SALPINGITIS
CERVICAL CANCER	SEXUALLY TRANSMITTED DISEASES
CERVICAL EROSION	TAMPON, RETAINED
CERVICAL SMEAR	THRUSH
D & C	UTERUS, CANCER OF
ECTOPIC PREGNANCY	UTERUS, PROLAPSE OF
ENDOMETRIOSIS	UTERUS, RETROVERSION OF
FIBROADENOMA OF THE BREAST	VULVA, CANCER OF
FIBROIDS, UTERINE	VAGINITIS AND VULVITIS
GENITAL HERPES	WARTS, ANOGENITAL
MASTITIS, NODULAR	
MENOPAUSE	
NIPPLE, CRACKED	

MALE GENITAL SYSTEM *Sperm are produced in the two testes which are contained within the scrotum. Each testis releases its sperm through a series of small channels to a tube called the vas deferens, a cord-like structure at the top of the scrotum. The vas deferens on each side passes through a canal in the abdominal wall to enter the abdominal cavity and then travels towards an area behind the bladder where two small glands—the seminal vesicles—lie. On either side a duct from the seminal vesicle joins the terminal part of the vas deferens. This combination of vas deferens and seminal vesicle duct is called the ejaculatory duct. The two ejaculatory ducts enter the part of the urethra lying within the prostate gland immediately below the bladder.*

During intercourse sperm are delivered into the vagina from the urethra within the penis. The volume of ejaculate (or semen) is increased by fluid from the seminal vesicles and prostate gland.

Structure of the male genital system

1 *Bladder*
2 *Penis*
3 *Testis*
4 *Scrotum*
5 *Urethra*
6 *Vas deferens*
7 *Prostate gland*
8 *Seminal vesicles*
9 *Sacrum*
10 *Pubic symphysis*
11 *Rectum*

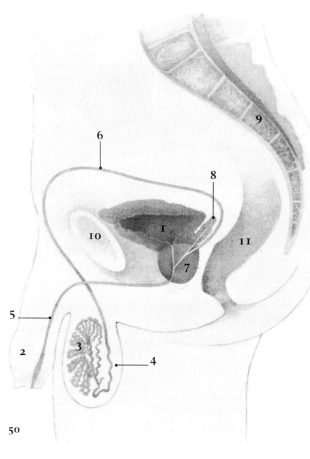

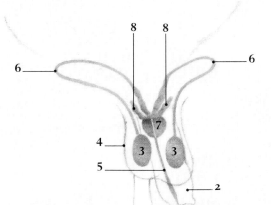

THE MALE GENITAL SYSTEM

The male genital system consists of the urethra, prostate gland, testes, scrotum, vasa deferentia, seminal vesicles and penis.

Sperm are produced in the testes or testicles, two oval-shaped organs which are enclosed in a pouch of skin called the scrotum behind the penis. The testes are protected by several layers of muscle and fibre.

On each side a tube called the vas deferens conveys sperm from the testes to the seminal vesicle, a gland which produces most of the fluid that combines with sperm to make semen.

The prostate gland lies at the base of the bladder and surrounds the top part of the urethra. During ejaculation it secretes a fluid that becomes part of the semen.

The urethra is a tube about 8 in. (200 mm.) long leading from the bladder to the tip of the penis. It passes sperm from the testicles and urine from the bladder out of the body.

The penis is the organ through which the greater part of the urethra passes. It is composed of sponge-like tissue which normally hangs limp, but when the tissue is distended with blood the penis becomes rigid and erect. The enlarged end of the penis is known as the glans. It is covered by the foreskin (prepuce), unless this has been removed by circumcision.

DISORDERS OF THE MALE GENITAL SYSTEM

Most disorders of the male genital system affect the external organs and different conditions occur at different ages. They should all receive medical attention.

Boys may have problems with a tight foreskin and infection between the foreskin and glans.

In men, discharge from the penis is nearly always due to a sexually transmitted disease, particularly gonorrhoea. Lice which occur in the pubic hair are usually transmitted sexually too. Blood in the semen may be caused by sexual overactivity, but occasionally may be the result of serious disorders such as tuberculosis.

Swelling of the testes, with or without pain, may be due to bacterial or virus infection, orchitis or occasionally cancer.

Itching of the penis is most often caused by an allergy to a contraceptive or an item of clothing.

After the age of 60 enlargement of the prostate gland becomes increasingly common. The enlargement tends to strangle the urethra, causing difficulty in urination and retention of urine.

Older men can also suffer from an infection of the glans, and soreness or itching is a common symptom of diabetes. Sores on the penis may be due to sexually transmitted diseases or they may indicate cancer. In any event they should be reported to a doctor.

A skin rash on the genitals and surrounding area can occur at any age and can be due to napkin rash, eczema, intertrigo, pubic lice, or ringworm.

HIGH-RISK GROUPS
• People who are promiscuous. The risk of sexually transmitted disease and perhaps of cancer of the penis may be reduced by wearing a sheath.
• Males with undescended TESTICLE are at increased risk of testicular torsion and testicular cancer.

MAIN SYMPTOMS OF DISORDERS OF THE MALE GENITAL SYSTEM
The following symptoms all have entries in the SYMPTOM SORTER.
• Problems of penis, foreskin and urethra including pain and swelling.
• Problems with urination such as pain while urinating and failure to urinate.
• Problems of testicles and scrotum such as pain and swelling.

EMERGENCIES
• Torsion, or twisting, of the testicles. This is more common among teenagers and young adults but can also occur in infants.
• Painful swollen penis (in males above the age of three or four), with the foreskin stuck in the retracted position behind the glans.

HOW TO HELP PREVENT GENITAL DISORDERS
• Keep the foreskin clean by drawing it back daily and washing underneath with soap and warm water.
• Use a sheath to reduce the risk of contracting sexually transmitted disease, including AIDS.
• Seek medical advice if you have any concern about male genital symptoms, particularly if you have several sexual partners.
• Carry out self-examination of the scrotum, in order to detect testicular tumours. Every month, after a shower or bath, gently but thoroughly feel all around the surface of each testicle within the scrotum. Report any unusual lumps or bumps to your doctor.
• Do not use force to draw back a little boy's foreskin to clean it. If smegma (a white, cheese-like substance exuded by the foreskin) collects around the base of the child's glans this is nothing to worry about. It will go away in due course.

Disorders of the male genital system

Each of the disorders listed here has its own entry in the book. There it is described in detail and you are told what to do about it.

BALANITIS	SYPHILIS
CRAB LICE	TESTICLES,
GONORRHOEA	UNDESCENDED
HYDROCELE	TORSION OF THE
INTERTRIGO	TESTICLES
ORCHITIS	TUMOURS OF THE
PHIMOSIS	MALE GENITAL
PROSTATITIS	SYSTEM
PROSTATE GLAND,	VARICOCELE
ENLARGED	WARTS,
SEXUALLY	ANOGENITAL
TRANSMITTED	
DISEASE	

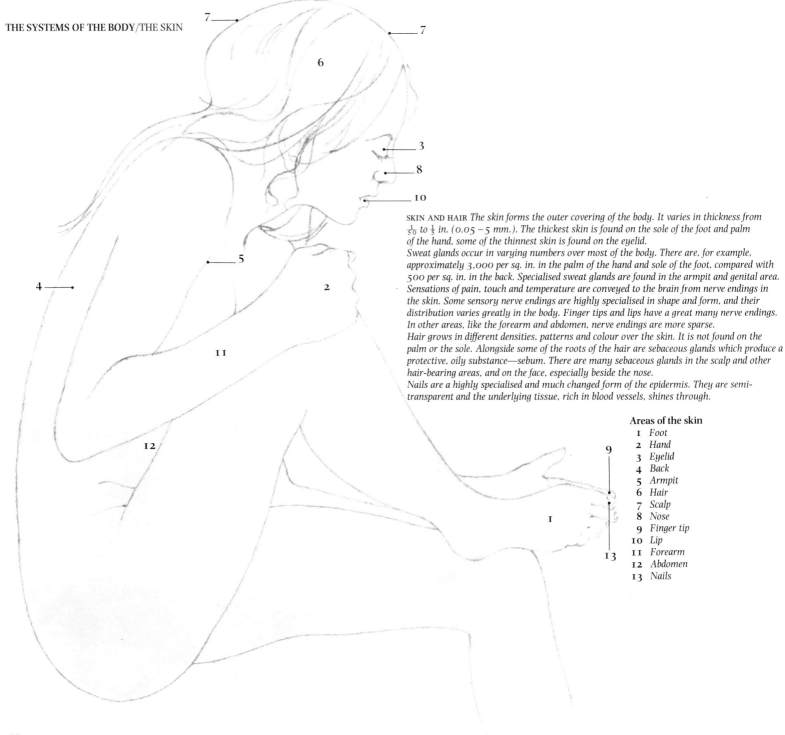

SKIN AND HAIR *The skin forms the outer covering of the body. It varies in thickness from $\frac{1}{50}$ to $\frac{1}{5}$ in. (0.05 − 5 mm.). The thickest skin is found on the sole of the foot and palm of the hand, some of the thinnest skin is found on the eyelid.*

Sweat glands occur in varying numbers over most of the body. There are, for example, approximately 3,000 per sq. in. in the palm of the hand and sole of the foot, compared with 500 per sq. in. in the back. Specialised sweat glands are found in the armpit and genital area.

Sensations of pain, touch and temperature are conveyed to the brain from nerve endings in the skin. Some sensory nerve endings are highly specialised in shape and form, and their distribution varies greatly in the body. Finger tips and lips have a great many nerve endings. In other areas, like the forearm and abdomen, nerve endings are more sparse.

Hair grows in different densities, patterns and colour over the skin. It is not found on the palm or the sole. Alongside some of the roots of the hair are sebaceous glands which produce a protective, oily substance—sebum. There are many sebaceous glands in the scalp and other hair-bearing areas, and on the face, especially beside the nose.

Nails are a highly specialised and much changed form of the epidermis. They are semi-transparent and the underlying tissue, rich in blood vessels, shines through.

Areas of the skin

1 Foot
2 Hand
3 Eyelid
4 Back
5 Armpit
6 Hair
7 Scalp
8 Nose
9 Finger tip
10 Lip
11 Forearm
12 Abdomen
13 Nails

THE SKIN

The skin is a strong elastic covering that encloses the body and protects it from damage by injury or infection. An average man is covered by approximately 18 sq. ft (1.7 sq. m.) of skin which weighs about 9 lb. (4.1 kg.). The skin is made of an outer layer of cells (epidermis), an underlying part containing blood vessels (dermis), and a deeper subcutaneous layer (from cutis—the medical name for skin).

In the deeper parts of the dermis are hair follicles, from which hair grows. It varies in thickness from about $\frac{1}{5000}$ in. (0.005 mm.) in the fine 'lanugo' hair covering a fetus, to $\frac{1}{125}$ in. (0.2 mm.) in beard hair. It varies in length from $\frac{1}{25}$ in. (1 mm.) or less, to 5 ft (1.5 m.) in extreme instances.

DISORDERS OF THE SKIN

It is a special feature of the skin that while serving many vitally important functions it also plays a major role in appearance. Like the internal systems of the body it may be subject to serious disease, but unlike the internal systems, relatively minor disorders, such as acne, dandruff or psoriasis, cause distress to the sufferer out of all proportion to their effect on his or her physical well-being.

The tendency to certain skin disorders seems to be inherited; psoriasis, ichthyosis and some forms of eczema are examples.

Contact with certain substances may produce a reaction in the skin (contact eczema) and the skin may also show other symptoms, including itching, blistering or rash—which are signs of diseases such as measles, or of allergies.

The skin is a site of infection. Two of the most common virus infections are cold sores and warts. Impetigo is a common bacterial infection and common fungal infections include thrush and athlete's foot.

Growths on the skin are usually benign, but in rare cases they may be cancerous. Any new growth or change in a mole or its surrounding skin should always be reported to the doctor since most skin cancers are curable if treated early.

The most common form of balding (alopecia) is male pattern balding which seems to run in families. Unfortunately there is very little that can be done to remedy it. Occasionally women may also lose hair, but in most cases this is only temporary. Increased growth of hair (hirsutism), which can distress women, is sometimes due to a hormonal abnormality but usually no cause can be found.

HIGH-RISK GROUPS

• Blood relatives of people suffering from allergies are more likely than average to have similar troubles.

• People with fair skin and fair hair. These people, particularly red-heads, are very sensitive to sunlight.

• People exposed to chemicals. Housewives using detergents or workers with mineral oils, dyes and chemicals. *See* OCCUPATIONAL HAZARDS.

MAIN SYMPTOMS OF SKIN DISORDER

The following symptoms all have entries in the SYMPTOM SORTER.

• Lumps.
• Rash.
• Skin abnormalities.
• Itching (*see also page 323*).

EMERGENCIES

• Acute urticaria. If there is swelling of the tongue or throat a doctor should be seen as soon as possible.

• Burns and scalds. Remove watches, rings and tight clothing. Hold the burnt area under cold running water for at least ten minutes. Cover with a clean, non-fluffy dressing; never apply ointments or fats.

HOW TO HELP PREVENT SKIN PROBLEMS

• Wear gloves when handling detergents, oils or chemicals.

• Wash thoroughly after handling chemicals even if gloves have been worn.

• Do not use towels or face-cloths which have been used by others.

• Cover fair skin in sunlight with a broad-brimmed hat and cotton sleeves.

• Do not sunbathe for hours at a time on the first day of a holiday.

Disorders of the skin

Each of the disorders listed here has its own entry in the book. There it is described in detail and you are told what to do about it.

ABSCESS	ORF
ACNE VULGARIS	PARONYCHIA
BALDNESS	PEMPHIGOID
BARBER'S RASH	PEMPHIGUS
BLISTER	PHOTO-SENSITIVITY
BODY ODOUR	PIGMENTED NAEVUS
BRUISES	PITYRIASIS
CELLULITIS	PORT-WINE STAIN
CHAPPED LIPS	PRICKLY HEAT
CHERRY SPOTS	PSORIASIS
CHLOASMA	RINGWORM
COLD SORES	ROSACEA
CORN	SCABIES
DANDRUFF	SEBACEOUS CYST
DRUG RASH	SEBORRHOEA
ECZEMA	SEBORRHOEIC WARTS
GENITAL HERPES	SHINGLES
HAIRY PIGMENTED NAEVUS	SKIN CANCER
HIRSUTISM	SKIN TAGS
ICHTHYOSIS	SPIDER NAEVUS
IMPETIGO	STEROID SKIN CHANGES
INSECT BITES AND STINGS	STRAWBERRY NAEVUS
ITCHING	STRETCH MARKS
KELOID	SUNBURN
KERATOSIS, SENILE	SWEATING, EXCESSIVE
LENTIGO	TATTOO
LEPROSY	THRUSH
LICE	URTICARIA
LICHEN PLANUS	VITILIGO
MELANOMA	WARTS
MILIA	WHITLOW
MOLLOSCUM CONTAGIOSUM	
MONGOLIAN SPOTS	
MYXOEDEMA	

SKELETAL SYSTEM *There are 206 major bones in the human body. In a living person bones are pliable structures consisting of proteins impregnated with mineral substances. This combination gives properties of resistance to compression, tension and a certain amount of elasticity. Bones change dramatically in shape and size with age and it is growth of bones that determines a person's adult height. Here most of the individual bones of the skeleton are shown. Bones are interconnected by means of joints, and there is great variation in the shape and mobility of joints to suit their particular functions. For example, the joints in the adult skull are usually fused together so that the bones of the skull form a solid casing to protect the brain. In the limbs where a great deal of mobility is required, the bones are separated by joint cavities. Movable joints are supported by ligaments and are moved and partly supported by muscles. The vertebral column, or spine, surrounds and protects the spinal cord. The spinal nerves emerge from small holes in the sides of the vertebral column. Intervertebral discs lie between the individual vertebrae. The largest discs are in the lumbar region.*

Structure of the skeleton

1   Skull
2   Mandible
3   Cervical vertebrae
4   Clavicle
5   Scapula
6   Humerus
7   Ulna
8   Radius
9   Carpals
10 Metacarpals
11 Phalanges
12 Ribs
13 Sternum
14 Thoracic vertebrae
15 Lumbar vertebrae
16 Ilium
17 Sacrum
18 Coccyx
19 Femur
20 Tibia
21 Fibula
22 Tarsals
23 Metatarsals
24 Phalanges
25 Lumbar discs
26 Deltoid muscle

THE SKELETAL SYSTEM

Together, the bones of the human skeleton support the rest of the body, and give it the shape we all recognise. They also protect the vital organs and act as levers enabling movement to take place. Less obviously, they manufacture blood and store and distribute essential minerals—calcium in particular. There are four types of bone, classified by shape—long, short, flat and irregular.

Long bones each consist of a shaft with a knob at each end. The shaft is a thick-walled tube of dense bone filled with yellow marrow, while the ends are made of spongy bone covered by a thin layer of dense bone. Leg, arm and rib bones are typical long bones.

Short bones are box-like structures made of spongy bone enclosed in a thin crust of denser bone. They are formed in places such as the ankle and wrist where strength is required along with a capacity for limited movement.

Flat bones have similar construction to that of short bones. Examples are the shoulder-blades and the skull bones.

Any bones which do not fit into the other three categories are called irregular bones. They include the bones of the face and the spinal column.

Spongy bone contains red marrow which produces blood cells. In children, the shafts of long bones also contain this marrow; but in adults it is replaced by yellow marrow which produces blood cells only when the body is under stress.

The bones are connected by joints, which fall into three categories: immovable, slightly movable and freely movable. Immovable joints hold the bones tightly together with tough fibrous tissue, as in the skull. Slightly movable joints hold the bones together by a disc of cartilage, as in the spine. Freely movable joints hold the bones together by a fibrous capsule containing a lubricating fluid, as in the elbows and knees.

SOME DISORDERS OF THE SKELETAL SYSTEM
Aches, pains and stiffness in the bones and joints are a relatively common symptom in adult patients. Each year some 20 million people in the United Kingdom suffer from a skeletal disorder involving the loss of 40 million working days a year.

Among adults, some 5 million people suffer from osteoarthritis, in which the cartilage linings between the bones of the joint are worn away. Back pain alone is the next most common disorder, followed by rheumatism, a general term for any pain affecting the muscles and joints.

HIGH-RISK GROUPS
• Hospital nurses. More than 220,000 nurses in Britain suffer from back pain each year—caused by bending over or lifting bedridden patients. This can be eliminated by bending correctly. *See* BACK PAIN and HOME NURSING.
• People in their mid-60s and upwards. Rheumatic disorders affect at least 40 per cent of men and women aged 65. Left untreated the disorders can cripple.
• Coal-miners, building workers and the like are prone to injuries which can lead to rheumatic disorders.

MAIN SYMPTOMS OF DISORDER OF THE SKELETAL SYSTEM
The following symptoms all have entries in the SYMPTOM SORTER under the part of the body affected.
• Pain.
• Stiffness.
• Swelling.

EMERGENCIES
If any of the following symptoms occur, a doctor should be consulted without delay.
• Bruising, swelling or deformity of a bone, following injury, which may mean that it is fractured. *See* FIRST AID *page 588*.
• Joint pain.
• Pain in the lower back radiating into the buttock, thigh and leg can be a sign of sciatica—which, in turn, may indicate a more serious back disorder.
• Neck and shoulder pain.
• Acute pains in the limbs or joints of a growing child may indicate infection such as osteomyelitis.

HOW TO HELP PREVENT SKELETAL PROBLEMS
• When lifting or carrying, follow the advice given on *pages 86–87*.
• Always wear seat-belts in a car and a crash-helmet on a motor-cycle. Wear a lightweight helmet when riding a bicycle.
• Always wear well-fitting, low shoes.

Disorders of the skeletal system

Each of the disorders listed here has its own entry in the book. There it is described in detail and you are told what to do about it.

ACHILLES	OSTEOARTHRITIS
TENDON RUPTURE	OSTEO-
ANKYLOSING	CHONDRITIS
SPONDYLITIS	OSTEOMALACIA
BUNION	OSTEOMYELITIS
BURSITIS	OSTEOPOROSIS
CALLUS	PAGET'S DISEASE
CARPAL TUNNEL	OF THE BONE
SYNDROME	PERTHES'
CARTILAGE,	DISEASE
TORN	PLANTAR
CERVICAL	FASCIITIS AND
SPONDYLOSIS	CALCANEAL SPUR
COCCYDYNIA	POLYMYALGIA
CONGENITAL	RHEUMATICA
DISLOCATION	RHEUMATOID
OF THE HIP	ARTHRITIS
DUPUYTREN'S	ROTATOR CUFF
CONTRACTURE	LESION
FIBROSITIS	SPRAIN
FLAT FEET	SYNOVITIS
FOOT STRAIN	SLIPPED DISC
FRACTURES	SLIPPED
FROZEN	FEMORAL
SHOULDER	EPIPHYSIS
GANGLION	TENNIS ELBOW
INGROWING	TENOSYNOVITIS
TOE-NAIL	TORN LIGAMENT
MALLET FINGER	WHIPLASH
METATARSALGIA	

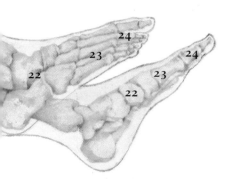

PART 3   A-Z OF HEALTH PROBLEMS

A guide to maintaining health and coping with common disorders and diseases

ABDOMINAL PAIN

Abdominal pain, in all its forms and in all ages, may frequently be a symptom of trivial disorder, but also has many serious causes which often require careful medical observation.

See SYMPTOM SORTER—ABDOMINAL PAIN

ABORTION

In the minds of many people, the word abortion is limited to the artificial termination of pregnancy, whether carried out legally by a doctor when it is known as a therapeutic abortion, or illegally—the so-called backstreet abortion. To doctors, however, the word simply means the expulsion or removal of a fetus before the 24th week of pregnancy—for whatever reason. There is no medical distinction between an artificial abortion, legal or illegal, and a spontaneous abortion (miscarriage). The vast majority of abortions are spontaneous.

SPONTANEOUS ABORTION
There are no precise numbers for pregnancies that fail, but medical research has shown that probably about one-third of all pregnancies abort spontaneously within four weeks of conception. In many cases the woman never knows that she has been pregnant, for the abortion occurs about four weeks after her last menstrual period and so passes unrecognised. In other cases abortion may occur a week or so later and she just thinks that she has a late period.

Spontaneous abortions may be nature's way of terminating a pregnancy that is in some way likely to be unsatisfactory.

Symptoms
- In the early stages of spontaneous abortion, the commonest symptom is loss of blood from the vagina. This may be bright red if it is fresh, or brown if the blood has been retained in the vagina for some hours. If the embryo has not been dislodged it is, at this stage, a *threatened abortion* and the pregnancy may still be saved. If the condition becomes worse, pain may come and go at regular intervals like small labour pains. This is a sign that the threatened abortion may become *inevitable* if the embryo is dislodged. The bleeding may also increase at this stage.

Treatment in the home
- Any woman in early pregnancy who has any spotting

of red or brown blood, or pains like period pains, should rest. It is not necessary to go to bed.

When to consult the doctor
- As soon as any unusual bleeding or pain is noticed.

What the doctor may do
- At first, he may decide to wait and to be informed if the condition progresses to heavier bleeding or painful contractions of the uterus.
- Send the woman to hospital if she passes from the threatening abortion stage to the inevitable stage.
- First priority for the doctor or hospital is to stop the woman losing too much blood and to help her to regain her health for any future pregnancy.
- In hospital the woman may have an evacuation of the uterus, under anaesthetic, to remove any placenta or membrane left behind.

Prevention
- Once a woman has become aware that she is pregnant, she should avoid unnecessary fatigue and vigorous sporting activities, especially if there is a risk of injury.
- It is sensible to avoid sexual intercourse during the times when periods would normally be due.
- If the woman's blood group is rhesus negative, the doctor will give her an injection to prevent problems in future pregnancies.

INCOMPLETE ABORTION
Some women experience a slight loss of blood during the first three months of pregnancy, which is not necessarily related to any abnormality. Spotting may occur during the times when periods would normally be due. Such a loss has, however, to be treated as a possible abortion.

MISSED ABORTION
If the embryo dies but is not expelled from the uterus, the acute bleeding may well stop for a time. However, when bleeding starts again some days or even weeks later, the remains in the uterus must be removed to give the woman a better chance of starting another pregnancy.

SEPTIC ABORTION
Sometimes after an incomplete abortion, the remains inside the uterus become infected. This is very dangerous. Not only is the woman's health at risk, but so, too, is her chance of future pregnancy. The infection may spread from the uterus to the Fallopian tubes and block them, so stopping contact between future eggs and sperm.

Symptoms
- Nausea.
- Headache.
- Pain in the lower stomach.
- Pus may be discharged from the vagina.

When to consult the doctor
- Immediately, if any raised temperature occurs in association with discharge from the vagina.

What the doctor may do
- He will examine the woman and send her to hospital if he suspects septic abortion.
- In hospital, treatment will consist of antibiotics, intravenous fluids and probably evacuation of the uterus under general anaesthetic when the woman is well enough.

HABITUAL ABORTION
Although spontaneous abortion is common, if a woman miscarries three times in a row, her condition is known as habitual abortion. It is wise for her to go into a hospital gynaecological department to see if the problem is caused by something which can be corrected.

Causes
- The commonest cause is an abnormality in each of the embryos. This results in a fetus which is so abnormal that nature does not allow it to develop into a baby.
- A deficiency of the hormone progesterone.
- A structural abnormality of the uterus, which can be seen on a special X-ray.
- The cervix or neck of the uterus being incompetent—that is to say, unable to support the developing fetus safely inside.

What the doctor may do
- Arrange for the woman to be examined at a hospital gynaecological department. To check for progesterone deficiency there may be tests on the woman's blood. If the deficiency is confirmed it can be made good by an injection of the hormone early in pregnancy.
- Insert a stitch around the neck of the womb to prevent it from opening too early in pregnancy.

THERAPEUTIC ABORTION
In many countries of the Western world, a pregnancy can legally be terminated in its early stages if doctors advise that its continuation would seriously affect the health of the mother. The exact position varies from one country to another and from year to year.

Legal grounds for abortion
In the United Kingdom, the commonest situation is when two doctors recommend termination of pregnancy because in their opinion the health or life of the mother may be jeopardised.

In practice, this means that a wide range of physical and psychological disorders can be considered as grounds for a legal abortion. One doctor, usually the patient's family doctor, can send the woman to a consultant gynaecologist if he considers she needs an abortion. If the gynaecologist agrees, he will perform the operation. In all, about 160,000 (1991) legal abortions take place each year in England. The vast majority of these are in the first few weeks when the operation is straightforward and the risk small. Unless an abnormality has been found, doctors rarely consider abortion after the 16th week, because of the extra medical risks involved.

The most common reasons for an abortion are psychological problems; the risk of an existing condition, such as raised blood pressure, becoming worse; or a serious risk of abnormality to the baby. For example, the pregnant woman may have been exposed to German measles, which can cause her child to be born with mental abnormalities. The mother may have had tests taken which show that she is carrying a baby with Down's syndrome (mongolism).

In addition, termination of pregnancy is allowed in Great Britain if its continuation would adversely affect the health of the other children in the family. This reason is not often used, but it is one of the few times that a medical act of such a serious nature as the stopping of a life can be taken on the grounds of improving the quality of life of other members of the family.

A woman should consider the following two guidelines carefully before taking any decisions about having an abortion:

Firstly, she should discuss the physical and psychological reasons for wanting a termination both with those involved—her partner and, perhaps, her parents and friends—and with an understanding doctor, probably her family doctor. If, for any reason, her family doctor is unable to give advice, she should discuss the matter with the doctor at the local family planning clinic.

Secondly, she should consider the long-term reactions of herself and her partner, if she is considered to be legally eligible for termination. Such feelings may involve both guilt and depression.

What the doctor may do

The exact method used to carry out a therapeutic abortion depends upon the stage of pregnancy that has been reached.

If a woman is in the first 12 weeks of pregnancy, the uterus may be evacuated under anaesthesia through the vagina. The neck of the womb is gently dilated and a small tube is passed into the uterus. By making a vacuum through this, the contents of the uterus are sucked out.

For most women this is not a major operation. It usually requires no more than an overnight stay in the hospital or clinic. The woman bleeds for a few days afterwards, though probably less than during a normal menstrual period. It is wise to consider future contraceptive pre-

cautions at the same time, to make sure that the woman does not become pregnant again by mistake. *See* FAMILY PLANNING.

If the woman has passed 12 weeks of pregnancy, it is difficult to remove the embryo through the neck of the womb and so one of two methods may be used. Some doctors remove the fetus through the stomach wall by performing a mini Caesarean section, to open the uterus. The woman stays in hospital for about ten days after this, and there is a small scar on the uterus which should be drawn to the doctor's attention in future pregnancies.

Many gynaecologists, however, now try to terminate at any stage of pregnancy by making the uterus contract so as to expel its own contents. This can be done by using doses of hormones called prostaglandins.

These are the same hormones that the woman would produce later in pregnancy to cause her to go into normal labour. These hormones can be given by mouth, pessary or a small injection into the uterine cavity or into the vagina. Either way they work by causing the uterus to contract and a mini labour occurs some hours later. Sometimes the labour is not complete and a small operation may be required to remove remaining fragments of membrane and placenta retained in the uterus.

After-effects of a therapeutic abortion

Most women who decide to have an abortion and go through it willingly have no serious physical after-effects. Termination carried out in hospital does not affect future pregnancies or make them harder to achieve. There are risks of infection and bleeding but these are diminished by consulting doctors in hospital who perform the operation.

The women who are sure that they want an abortion usually have no psychological regrets. But there are some women who undergo an abortion while having grave doubts about it, and they may have problems, such as guilt and depression afterwards. It is this group that doctors worry about most when they have to decide to end the pregnancy in the first instance.

ABSCESS

An abscess is a local pocket of infection. In the skin, where it often starts around a hair follicle, it is known as a boil. The follicle and surrounding cells in the skin are killed by bacteria and form pus. The pocket of pus increases. The boil comes to a head, or increases. The pus then bursts through the skin and escapes.

A carbuncle is a collection of boils. It develops when more than one hair follicle becomes infected. The pocket of pus may be extensive and spread below the skin before pointing in two or more heads and bursting.

Hairy sites and areas of friction are most likely sites for abscesses. These include nostrils, armpits, back of the neck and between the legs and buttocks.

Symptoms

• Painful swelling in the infected area. The amount of pain will depend on the position of the swelling, for instance a small boil on the nose is painful only if pressed, or if it becomes large.

• At first the area is tender, inflamed and swollen. Later the boil points with a yellow centre before bursting.

• Infection from an abscess may spread into the bloodstream making the person feel ill, and run a fever.

• Most boils burst within a week of starting, but if the infection goes very deep, it may take two weeks for the pus to come to the surface of the skin.

Causes

• Boils and carbuncles are most often due to infection by bacteria.

• A person with low resistance due to excessive tiredness, poor nutrition, diabetes mellitus or a blood disorder is more likely to develop abscesses.

Treatment in the home

• Rest the infected part, and move it as little as possible. This allows the body's defences to work, and reduces the chance of internal spread.

• Local heat and magnesium sulphate poultices will help bring a boil or carbuncle to a 'head'.

• Do not apply creams or antiseptics to the skin, they will not help cure an abscess because no penetration takes place.

• When the boil bursts, frequent changes of the soiled dressing are important. A clean, dry dressing is all that is needed.

• Take paracetamol or aspirin to relieve the pain.

• Use disinfectant in the bathwater, following the manufacturer's instructions.

• Boils tend to spread between members of a household. Sufferers should use their own towels and if possible scald underwear and handkerchiefs while the boil is discharging.

When to consult the doctor

• If the boil is very painful.

• If the inflammation around the boil spreads without coming to a head.

• If the boil does not discharge pus, although a head has developed.

• If a person has many boils at the same time, or a sequence of infections.

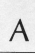

What the doctor may do
• Lance, or cut into the abscess to release the pressure and ease the pain.
• Take swabs from the nose and skin, as well as from the boil, to discover the type of bacteria.
• Give antibiotics by mouth, or injection, to stop the spread of infection. *See* MEDICINES, 25, 43.
• Test the urine to exclude diabetes.
• Test the blood to find out if any other diseases are reducing resistance to infection.
• Prescribe antibiotic ointments for the nose, to treat germs that may remain there as a source of further infection.

Prevention
• Attention to diet, rest and relaxation will assist the body's protection against infection.
• Strict hygiene while the abscess is discharging will reduce the chance of infection spreading.
• Control of diabetes, or any other disorder.
• Treat other members of the family.

Outlook
• Abscesses will heal completely if the person is generally fit.
• If an abscess does not heal, some other cause than a boil should be suspected.

See SKIN *page 52*
DIGESTIVE SYSTEM *page 44*

ACHALASIA OF THE CARDIA

A rare disease in which the muscles of the oesophagus (gullet) fail to work properly. Normally, when food is swallowed, these muscles automatically set up a wavelike movement to the oesophagus that pushes the food down towards the stomach. The sphincter (muscle ring) at the lower end of the oesophagus relaxes and lets the food through. In achalasia, the oesophageal muscles and sphincter do not respond to a swallow, and so food and saliva are retained in the oesophagus, which becomes swollen.

Symptoms
• Difficulty in swallowing both liquids and solids; initially intermittent, later continuous.
• Food is felt to stick behind the breastbone.
• Chest pain, ranging from mild to severe.

• Regurgitation of undigested food and saliva.
• Food and saliva may be breathed into the lungs, especially when the patient is lying in bed. This causes coughing, breathlessness and chest infections.

Causes
• Not known.

Complications
• PNEUMONIA, BRONCHIECTASIS.
• Higher incidence than normal of OESOPHAGEAL CANCER.

Treatment in the home
• Eat small meals sitting up.
• Take frequent drinks in small quantities.

When to consult the doctor
• If any of the above symptoms persist for longer than a week.

What the doctor may do
• Check to exclude more serious causes of symptoms.
• Send the patient to a consultant surgeon who may order tests including barium swallow X-rays and internal examination with an endoscope—an instrument with a light which can be passed down the throat into the oesophagus.
• Treatment may require an operation to cut or stretch the muscles of the lower oesophagus sphincter in order to allow food to pass into the stomach.

Prevention
• None is possible.

Outlook
• Reasonably good with treatment.

See DIGESTIVE SYSTEM *page 44*

ACHILLES TENDON RUPTURE

The Achilles tendon is the tendon which attaches the calf muscles of the leg to the back of the ankle. When a rupture occurs it is always complete: the tendon snaps in two.

Symptoms
• A sudden severe pain at the back of the ankle, often as if it has been struck by a blow.
• Tenderness at the site of the rupture.
• An inability to stand on tip-toe with the affected foot.
• Walking is possible but only with a limp, and the patient will not be able to run.

Duration
• With treatment, the rupture will take from about six to eight weeks to heal.

Causes
• The rupture occurs most often in early middle age after some sudden activity, such as the first game of squash or tennis of the season.

Treatment in the home
• None is advised.

When to consult the doctor
• Immediately the condition is suspected or the symptoms occur.

What the doctor may do
• He will send the patient to the nearest hospital emergency department.
• At the hospital the lower leg may be X-rayed to make sure the symptoms are not the result of a fracture.
• If the rupture is diagnosed early, the lower leg will be immobilised in plaster for six to eight weeks, and a shoe with a raised heel or a heel set into the plaster will need to be worn for a further two to six weeks.
• If diagnosis is delayed, treatment will depend on age. A young adult may have the snapped tendon sewn together, then a plaster applied.

Prevention
• Avoid sudden, strenuous activity after a long period of only moderate exercise.

Outlook
• If the condition is not treated, the separate parts of the tendon will unite spontaneously but, in doing so, will make the tendon longer. This can leave the patient either with a limp or without a spring in his step.
• If treatment is carried out early, the foot will return to normal in about ten weeks.
• If treatment is delayed, recovery takes longer.

See SKELETAL SYSTEM *page 54*

ACID REGURGITATION

A condition in which the contents of the stomach flow back into the oesophagus and cause inflammation.

Symptoms
• A burning sensation behind the breastbone, which may spread up to the back of the mouth as wind is brought up, giving a taste of acid and food.

Duration
• The symptoms persist unless treated.

Causes
- Lax muscles at the lower end of the oesophagus (food pipe) where it joins the stomach. They allow acid to flow back up from the stomach.
- Overindulgence in food or drink.
- Wearing tight corsets and belts.
- Bending down or lying flat tends to force food from the stomach backwards into the oesophagus, with consequent aggravation of symptoms.

Complications
- Peptic or reflux OESOPHAGITIS. The lining of the oesophagus becomes inflamed and then ulcerated by the action of stomach juices.
- Stricture (narrowing) of the oesophagus.
- Bleeding, usually a slow loss, resulting in ANAEMIA.

Treatment in the home
- Do not wear tight clothes or corsets, and avoid bending forward. Try to bend only at the knees.
- Eat small, frequent meals and sit upright while eating so that your oesophagus stays vertical.
- Avoid being overweight.
- Take milky drinks and antacids which coat the lower end of the oesophagus. *See* MEDICINES, 1.

What the doctor may do
- Prescribe antacids or drugs to reduce acid. If the symptoms persist he may send you to hospital for a barium swallow X-ray or ENDOSCOPY.

Prevention
- Avoid overeating, overdrinking and being overweight.
- Do not wear tight clothes.

See DIGESTIVE SYSTEM *page 44*

ACNE VULGARIS

The most common of all skin conditions, acne affects the face, shoulders, back and chest. A sebaceous gland, which supplies sebum to lubricate the skin, becomes blocked at its opening on the surface and the contents become infected and inflame the surrounding skin. In mild cases there may be only blackheads and small pimples, but in more severe cases these may fill with pus or turn into cysts. Acne usually occurs around puberty and can cause great distress at an age when personal appearance is very important.

Symptoms
- Blackheads and small pimples erupt on the face, shoulders, back or chest.

- The pimples fill with pus.
- Inflamed, painful cysts deep in the skin occur in severe acne. On healing, these often leave scarring and pitting which cause permanent unsightly appearance.

Duration
- The number of spots and pimples vary from week to week; in women they often increase just before a menstrual period.
- Usually the infection clears by the early twenties.

Causes
- Blockage of sebaceous glands in the skin, which may then become infected.
- Heredity, hormones and skin hygiene may contribute.
- Some industrial chemicals produce or worsen acne.

Complications
- Scarring.
- Loss of confidence.

Treatment in the home
- Wash regularly with medicated soap or detergent lotion and hot water. This will help by removing layers of oil which block the skin pores, and also by disinfecting the skin.
- Proprietary acne lotions and drying creams will often help, but the instructions on the container must be followed. *See* MEDICINES, 43.
- Sunbathing and ultraviolet lamps often help to improve acne. Take care to build up exposure gradually to avoid burning and the risk of skin cancers.
- Eat sensibly. It is not true that particular foods such as chocolate or chips cause acne, but a healthy diet with plenty of fresh fruit and vegetables will improve the general skin condition.

When to consult the doctor
- If the condition is not getting any better despite the recommended home treatment.
- If any of the proprietary lotions causes a skin reaction.
- If there are cysts. These, if left untreated, will leave scars.

What the doctor may do
- Prescribe abrasive treatments to apply to the skin. These help to lessen the severity of an acne attack and to minimise scarring.
- Prescribe antibiotic creams or a special vitamin A preparation (tretinoin) to use on the skin.
- Advise about diet, careful sunbathing or use of ultraviolet lamps.
- Prescribe antibiotics to be taken by mouth. These need to be taken for at least three months, and sometimes for much longer.
- For women, prescribe a special hormone combination (Dianette) which helps to counter acne and HIRSUTISM. (It also acts as an oral contraceptive.)

- In severe cases, refer the patient to a skin specialist for treatment with isotretinoin, a vitamin A preparation taken by mouth, available only in hospital.

Prevention
- Acne cannot be prevented, only controlled.
- Scarring can be prevented by early medical treatment of severe acne.

Outlook
- At whatever age acne starts, it is unlikely to go on getting worse indefinitely. Sooner or later it will improve.

See SKIN *page 52*

Do's and don'ts if you have acne

☐ *Do* wash with detergent lotion or medicated soap, and do use proprietary lotions and drying creams.

☐ *Do* sunbathe or use an ultraviolet lamp—with care.

☐ *Do* keep to a balanced diet.

☐ *Do* consult your doctor.

☐ *Don't* wear your hair in a fringe. Hair falling on to your forehead or face can increase the number of spots. Wash your hair regularly and keep it reasonably short or tied back.

☐ *Don't* use oily or greasy cosmetics to hide your spots. If you have to use cosmetics choose non-greasy ones. Ask your chemist's advice.

☐ *Don't* squeeze or pick at acne spots. They will become larger and inflamed, and scarring is more likely. Single, large, unsightly blackheads may be removed with a blackhead extractor after first washing the skin.

☐ *Don't* become impatient if the spots do not clear up immediately. Treatment may take weeks or months to work.

ACOUSTIC NEUROMA

A rare growth on the acoustic nerve of hearing and balance. The growth is not malignant, but it slowly grows inside the skull and causes pressure on the nerve and surrounding brain. It is this pressure that causes problems.

Symptoms
- Slowly increasing deafness often associated with 'singing', in one ear.
- Clumsiness and unsteadiness in walking.
- Dizziness, which is not usually severe.
- In more advanced cases, there may be pain on the side of the face, weakness and headache.

Duration
- Symptoms may gradually increase over a period of from two to ten years.

Causes
- It is not known what causes the growth.

Complications
- Removal of the growth always makes the affected ear deaf.

When to consult the doctor
- If there is gradually increasing deafness in one ear, especially if there is clumsiness and unsteadiness in walking and dizziness.

What the doctor may do
- Examine the ears with an auriscope (an instrument with a magnifying lens and a light).
- Test the degree to which the patient's hearing is impaired with a tuning fork.
- Examine the eyes for nystagmus (a horizontal flickering of the eyes).
- Arrange further examination and tests such as a CAT scan by an ear, nose and throat specialist or a neurologist, who will be able to confirm the presence of a growth.
- If the diagnosis is confirmed, the specialist will arrange for an operation to remove the growth.

Prevention
- It is not known how to prevent an acoustic neuroma from forming.

Outlook
- Although hearing will not be restored in the affected ear, early removal of the tumour has good results; though it may leave weakness of the muscles of one side of the face. The danger of removal increases as the tumour slowly grows bigger.

See EAR *page 38*

ACROCYANOSIS

A harmless but persistent deficiency in the circulation of the extremities (hands, fingers, feet and toes) of young women.

Symptoms
- There is no pain, but the fingers and hands are always cold and blue.

Duration
- A persistent complaint, but as the patient gets older the symptoms abate.

Causes
- The blood vessels of the hands and feet are unusually sensitive to cold. The reason for this sensitivity is unknown.

Treatment in the home
- Keep the fingers and hands warm.

When to consult the doctor
- If the condition persists and worries you.

What the doctor may do
- Make sure it is nothing more serious.

Prevention
- Protect hands from cold.

Outlook
- Good, though the condition will persist for several years.

See CIRCULATORY SYSTEM *page 40*

ACROMEGALY
A disease in which the skin thickens and the hands, feet and face, particularly the lower jaw, enlarge. It is the result of over-production of growth hormone by the pituitary gland, which lies in the brain. A benign (non-cancerous) tumour of the gland causes the excess production.

Treatment consists of destroying the tumour by radiotherapy or by removal of the gland. Acromegaly occurs after the age at which normal growth stops; excessive production of growth hormone in children produces a different condition, GIGANTISM.

ACROPARAESTHESIA
An intense prickling or tingling sensation in the extremities of the body, the fingers or the toes. The feeling may be caused by pressure on a nerve, as for example when it is experienced after sleeping in an uncomfortable position.

More rarely, it may be a sign of a trapped nerve, as in CARPAL TUNNEL SYNDROME, a disease of the nervous system, or a disorder of the circulatory system such as RAYNAUD'S SYNDROME. Acroparaesthesia is more common in women than men, and is thought to be associated with the chemical changes in the female body caused by menstruation.

ACUPUNCTURE

A method of attempting to treat illness or to anaesthetise part of the body by putting the tips of silver alloy or stainless-steel needles into certain areas of the patient's skin and then often vibrating them. The technique was first described by Chinese writers 4,500 years ago. Today it is practised by about a million therapists in China, and it is being used increasingly, often in conjunction with orthodox medicine, in North America, Western Europe, Japan, Russia and elsewhere.

Acupuncturists claim that the technique can alleviate or cure many physical and mental ailments. They include migraine, ulcers and digestive troubles, lumbago, arthritis, fibrositis, neuritis, sciatica, rheumatism, dermatitis, eczema, asthma, bronchitis, depression and anxiety.

Acupuncture has also been used to reduce the unpleasant symptoms of withdrawal from drugs like heroin, and may help in stopping smoking, but it is less effective for alcoholism.

Acupuncture is not suitable for conditions like appendicitis which need an urgent operation, nor for serious illnesses like meningitis or injuries like broken bones. It may not work for everyone.

DOES IT WORK?
Some doctors remain sceptical of acupuncture and say that any results achieved are as a result of suggestion. However, acupuncture has been used successfully to treat animals, and they are unlikely to respond to suggestion.

Recent research has shown that in humans, acupuncture applied to certain points—though not all—stimulates production of morphine-like chemicals in the body. These substances, called endorphins, are produced naturally in response to injury and during childbirth.

As a result of this finding, acupuncture is gaining increased acceptance from orthodox medicine, and many Western doctors now boast acupuncture training as a helpful addition to their medical skills. Most of them, however, prefer mechanical and biological explanations of the technique's successes to the Eastern philosophy underlying traditional Chinese acupuncture.

HOW IT WORKS
The needles used for acupuncture are long and thin. They may look alarming when in place, but they should not hurt unless the muscles are very tense – all that the patient usually feels is a warm tingling sensation. Usually no more than four or five needles are used, sometimes only one. They may be inserted for a short time or left in for as long as 20 minutes, and patients return for repeat treatments as necessary. All reputable practitioners use sterile needles, so there is no risk of infection.

In acupuncture, disease is seen as a disturbance of the whole person: mind, body and soul. Practitioners ask about your general health, lifestyle, feelings and habits as well as specific symptoms.

THE CHINESE PHILOSOPHY
Traditional Chinese medicine holds that health and happiness depend on the normal flow of life energy, called Chi, present throughout the universe. When our Chi is in harmony, there is perfect balance between the two universal forces, Yin and Yang, which represent opposite poles such as female/male, passive/active, cold/hot. If we are ill or upset, these forces are in a state of imbalance.

According to traditional acupuncture philosophy, life energy flows through the body in a series of 26 meridians representing different bodily systems. On each meridian lie five major points relating to the symbolic elements—earth, wood, water, metal and fire—and many minor points, making a total of more than 1,000 over the whole body.

Internal, external and emotional factors may create imbalances of the forces flowing along the meridians, and one disrupted meridian may in turn affect others. Acupuncture, by applying needles or other stimulation to the appropriate points, can restore healthy balance to the life forces and eliminate the causes of illness.

VARIATIONS ON ACUPUNCTURE
Needles are the easiest and most effective method of acupuncture, but there are traditional variations and modern developments based on the same principles.
Moxibustion applies heat to the points by burning a wad of the herb moxa, either attached to the end of a pre-inserted acupuncture needle or simply held near to the skin points.
Shiatsu or *acupressure* uses massage rather than needles.

As well as pressure by fingers, buttons or studs may be pressed over a particular point. Wrist bands with a tiny button to stimulate a point on the wrist are now widely available to alleviate motion sickness. Stimulation of the same point has been used in hospitals to help morning sickness in pregnancy, and nausea and vomiting during drug treatment for cancer.
Ear acupuncture, developed in France, uses either needles or studs designed to stay in place for a few weeks at a time. These are popular as an aid to dieting or stopping smoking: when massaged they cut down cravings for food or cigarettes.
Electroacupuncture may use a tiny electric current passed down needles, or simply stimulate the skin over acupuncture points without needles. Hand-held devices are now available for self-treatment.

See SMOKING

ADDISON'S DISEASE

A very rare disorder in which the body becomes incapable of reacting to physical stresses because the adrenal glands, the glands which control the metabolism of salts, cease to work.

Symptoms often come on gradually and may be difficult to recognise, but if early symptoms are neglected the first apparent symptom may be sudden collapse.
Symptoms
- Increasing weakness and tiredness leading to complete exhaustion.
- Loss of appetite, nausea and abdominal pains.
- Faintness on standing, caused by low blood pressure.
- Darkening of the skin, accentuated by sunlight.
- Dark patches inside the mouth.
- Collapse after minor physical stresses such as slight infections or injuries.
Duration
- The condition is permanent and drug treatment must continue indefinitely.
Causes
- Destruction of the outer layers of the adrenal glands by autoimmune processes, that is, the body's own defences somehow react against the gland's tissue.
- Very rarely, tuberculous infection is responsible.
Complications
- Failure of the circulation from low blood pressure.
- Severe infection—such as PNEUMONIA.

Treatment in the home
- None is advisable until the condition has been diagnosed.
- Once the condition has been diagnosed and stabilised, close collaboration between patient and doctor is required to manage the disorder.
- Sufferers must learn how to regulate the dosage of the drugs they take.
When to consult the doctor
- As soon as any of the above symptoms occur.
- Once management of the condition has begun, the doctor should be consulted if there are any unusual symptoms or problems.
What the doctor may do
- Arrange for blood tests to confirm the diagnosis.
- Refer the patient to a hospital specialist.
- The specialist will probably admit the patient to hospital for further tests to show the levels of salt and extent of steroid hormone deficiency.
- If Addison's disease is confirmed, special steroid tablets will be prescribed to replace the gland's own hormones.
See MEDICINES, 32.
Outlook
- Addison's disease is readily controlled with tablets that replace the hormones produced by the adrenal glands, and with treatment the outlook is good.
- If undiagnosed and untreated, the condition can cause eventual circulatory collapse and death.

ADENITIS
Inflammation of any glands. The term usually refers to lymph glands, especially those in the neck, armpit and groin, which are the most commonly affected.

ADENOID, ENLARGED

The adenoid is a single pad of lymphoid tissue (the tissue that helps to protect the body from infection) lying at the back of the nose close to the point where it joins the mouth cavity. It is small at birth, but begins growing at about the age of three. It reaches maximum size at about the age of eight, and by puberty no longer causes obstruction. Enlargement of the adenoid may block the opening of the Eustachian tube (the tube that connects the middle ear to the throat) into the nose, resulting in OTITIS MEDIA. The adenoid may also obstruct the flow of air from the nose to the throat, forcing the child to breathe through the mouth. The flow of air through the mouth then causes the tonsils to become larger.

Symptoms
- Breathing through the mouth.
- Blocked nose, and nasal speech.
- Snoring, and disturbed sleep.

Duration
- May be short-term, up to a few months.
- In some children, mouth breathing becomes persistent. If untreated, complications may be life-long.

Causes
- Recurring or long-standing infection of the adenoid.

Complications
- Recurrent ear infections may cause deafness.
- Recurrent throat, sinus and lung infections.
- The face may take on permanent adenoidal features—gaping mouth, prominent incisor teeth, narrow nose and a high arched palate ('adenoidal facies').
- Impaired learning capacity, and in very severe cases, mental retardation.

Treatment in the home
- There is no home remedy for enlarged adenoids.
- Offer supportive treatment during throat, ear or chest infections.

When to consult the doctor
- If the child has severe earache, throat or chest infections or recurrent episodes of mouth breathing.
- If mouth breathing lasts for more than a month.

What the doctor may do
- Examine the ears and mouth.
- Test to see how well the child can breathe through one nostril at a time.
- Test the hearing.
- Send the child to an ear, nose and throat specialist.
- The specialist may decide that an operation is necessary to remove the adenoid and possibly the tonsils at the same time. Recovery is usually rapid.

Outlook
- From the age of eight, the adenoid decreases in size and both the risk of complications and symptoms decrease. The specialist's decision to operate on it depends on reaching a balance between symptoms and age of the patient.

See RESPIRATORY SYSTEM *page 42*

ADHESION

Fibrous tissue that joins together two normally unconnected surfaces within the body. It can be caused by inflammation of the affected area or by abnormal healing of a wound, ulcer or surgical cut.

ADRENALINE

A hormone produced by the adrenal glands. Whenever a person faces an emergency or feels anger, shock, fear or some other strong emotion, adrenaline is passed rapidly into the bloodstream to speed up the heart rate and breathing, to make the muscles work faster and longer than usual and so to prepare the body for action. Injections of adrenaline are used to treat bronchial ASTHMA, a severe ALLERGY, and other conditions.

AIDS

Acquired Immune Deficiency Syndrome is an infection which causes the body's defences against other infections and certain cancers to be severely diminished. Because the disease was only recognised in 1981 it is difficult to predict the long-term effects of the virus, but it seems that most, if not all, of those infected will develop AIDS, which may take many years to appear.

Symptoms
- Early symptoms may be vague and ill-defined. They include weight loss, fever, diarrhoea, oral THRUSH, and HERPES infections. Not all sufferers of early symptoms will go on to develop the full-blown illness.
- If the disease progresses to full-blown AIDS the patient may develop infections such as pneumonia or meningitis, cancers such as Kaposi's sarcoma (a skin cancer) or lymphoma (cancer of the LYMPH system) and he may become demented because of the effect of the virus on the brain.

Incubation period
- Not everyone exposed to the virus, even by sexual or blood contact, becomes infected.
- There is a four to twelve-week 'latent' period between exposure to the virus and development of a positive blood test. The affected individual is, however, infectious during this time.
- Although an infected person may never go on to develop AIDS, he is likely to be permanently infectious to others.

Causes
- AIDS is caused by the human immunodeficiency virus (HIV).
- It is transmitted by blood or semen, for example by hypodermic needles and syringes shared by drug addicts, by means of sexual intercourse, especially anal intercourse among homosexuals, and from mother to baby during pregnancy.
- As far as is known, the virus is not transmitted by

touch or other non-sexual contact.
- There is no risk to a blood donor in the U.K.

Treatment
- There is no effective cure.
- The progress of AIDS can be slowed by the anti-viral drugs AZT and acyclovir.

Prevention
- The safest course is to have only a single, faithful sexual partner.
- Avoidance of sexual intercourse or intimate kissing with anyone who might be infected.
- Avoidance of rectal sex or any act that might cause bleeding.
- Using a condom reduces the risk of AIDS (as well as other sexually transmitted diseases).
- Drug users should avoid injecting, or at least avoid sharing equipment.
- Those at risk from AIDS should not be blood donors.
- At present there is no vaccine against AIDS.
- Those at risk can have their blood tested for HIV antibodies and, if possible, counselled accordingly.

Outlook
- For an individual who develops AIDS, the likelihood of death within a year is very high.
- For the community, until an effective vaccine or treatment is available, the number of cases is likely to increase rapidly.

ALCOHOLISM

People like to believe they can handle alcohol. A pint or two at lunchtime; wine with a meal and a liqueur after it; the occasional modest drink with colleagues or friends. Kept to these limits, alcohol will do few people any serious harm. It helps to reduce tension and puts people more socially at ease.

But after a time some social drinkers find that they cannot call a halt. They start drinking heavily because of the psychological relief it gives them—the temporary feeling of physical well-being it bestows—or they find that without consuming alcohol they feel permanently below par.

Heavy drinkers, whether they consume alcohol steadily or go on 'sprees' punctuated by periods of abstinence, are in danger of developing health and social problems and eventually of becoming dependent on alcohol. The danger zone is entered when the individual does not know—or does not care—when to say 'no' to himself, or to those with whom he is drinking.

Later the individual drinks in secret, hides his bottles at home and refuses to discuss his problem with anyone. By this time he is probably a true dependent.

Whatever pattern he adopts, he is either physically or psychologically dependent upon drink. Without it, he is unable to face up to life with its stresses, problems and challenges.

Physical dependence can be seen only when the drinker's supply of alcohol is suddenly stopped or reduced dramatically. This is followed by various withdrawal symptoms, including fits resembling those of EPILEPSY and the hallucinations and shakings of DELIRIUM TREMENS.

Psychological dependence may reveal itself when someone who is otherwise intelligent and rational insists upon drinking heavily—in spite of appreciating that alcohol is a drug which is doing him grave and possibly lasting harm.

TYPES OF ALCOHOLISM

There are no direct figures for the number of sufferers from alcoholism in the United Kingdom, but all the related figures—consumption of alcohol; convictions for drunkenness; convictions for drunken driving; admissions to hospital with alcoholism; and deaths from alcohol-related diseases such as cirrhosis of the liver—have been steadily rising since 1948, when the number of problem drinkers in Britain was first estimated. There are several possible causes for this spread in alcoholism. The wider social acceptance of heavy drinking; greater prosperity, particularly among women and young people; and the more general sale of alcohol in supermarkets and grocers' shops, as well as in off-licences and wine merchants.

As a result of these factors, sufferers from alcoholism—of either sex—can come from almost any age bracket, occupational group, or social category.

Patterns of alcoholism vary widely. The American social scientist Professor E. M. Jellinek, who pioneered the modern scientific approach to the problem, described five types of alcoholism. Two or more of them may be found in the same individual at the same time, and there is no such person as a 'typical' alcoholic.

Type 1 (Alpha alcoholism) The drinker has a deep-seated psychological problem—such as depression or anxiety—and he drinks excessively to try to overcome it.

Type 2 (Beta alcoholism) The drinker is not necessarily dependent on alcohol, but his continual drinking leads to physical or mental deterioration—producing, for example, CIRRHOSIS OF THE LIVER, polyneuritis, or DEMENTIA. Publicans are particularly prone to this type of alcoholism.

Type 3 (Gamma alcoholism) The characteristic feature is that the drinker can go for long periods without touching alcohol. However, once he starts to drink socially, he finds it difficult or impossible to stop, and the 'one or two' he may have set as his limit turn into many. In addition, his periods of abstinence gradually get fewer and shorter. That pattern of going 'on the wagon' and then having 'binges' is most commonly found among British and North American problem drinkers, possibly because in Britain and the USA there is more shame attached to heavy drinking than in wine-drinking countries.

Type 4 (Delta alcoholism) The drinker is never really drunk, but keeps on topping up with alcohol in relatively small quantities throughout the day and cannot break the habit. That pattern is more common in wine-drinking countries such as France, with its liberal licensing laws.

Type 5 (Epsilon alcoholism) Formerly known as dipsomania. This type afflicts the drinker who only takes alcohol periodically. His craving is not satisfied until he loses control of himself and he may finally pass out. The Epsilon drinker is sober most of the time, unlike the Gamma drinker who is drunk most of the time.

ALCOHOLISM AS A DISEASE

Despite the dangers of all five types, Jellinek regards only Gamma and Delta alcoholism as being addictive and involving physical dependence. He also considers Gamma and Delta alcoholism to be diseases because of the physical changes that occur in the drinkers' cell metabolisms, or chemical processes.

One of the quickest and easiest ways of determining whether someone is, or is about to become, alcohol-dependent is the *CAGE* test—so called from the initials of its key words. It was introduced in 1974 by the American Psychiatric Association and consists of four questions:
1. Does the drinker ever feel he should *Cut* down on his drinking?
2. Does he ever get *Annoyed* when people criticise his drinking?
3. Does he ever feel bad or *Guilty* about his drinking?
4. Does he ever have an *Eye-opening* drink first thing in the morning in order to steady his nerves or to ease a hangover?

If the drinker answers yes to all of the questions—or even just to number 4—then there is a strong likelihood that he is dependent on alcohol. If he answers yes to just one or two then he should watch his drinking.

HIGH-RISK GROUPS

To identify those people who are at most risk of becoming addicted, medical experts examine three vital aspects of the individual's background. They are: his underlying psychological and physical make-up; the environments in which he lives, works and seeks his entertainment; and the physical effects of drink upon his system.

Surveys carried out since the beginning of the century show that certain occupations have a high alcoholic risk due to the stresses and strains associated with them. In England and Wales the Registrar-General's office periodically issues occupation mortality rates from cirrhosis of the liver, which is commonly caused by prolonged and heavy drinking

The statistics show that people working in the drink trade are most at risk. That is largely because they can easily obtain alcohol at work, and because they may feel the need to drink with their customers to promote business.

Doctors, journalists, sailors, retired army officers, travelling salesmen and people working in hot, dusty environments have long had high alcoholism rates. That is particularly true in Britain and America, where clinical observations of problem drinkers—seen in and outside hospital—have been made for the past 40 years.

Apart from such 'occupational drinkers', there is likely to be a high proportion of problem drinkers among the accident prone; motorists who frequently drive when under the influence of drink; people with suicidal tendencies; those, mainly women, who habitually take more tranquillisers or sedatives than their doctors have prescribed for them, and the sons and daughters of people with a drink problem.

THE NEW DRINKERS

Forty years ago in Britain, problem drinkers were usually male and aged 40 or over. But that pattern no longer applies. The proportion of men to women who are addicted to drink has changed from about four to one in the 1950s to less than two to one.

The women most likely to become dependent on alcohol include those who go out to work and then suffer from an identity conflict, in which they are unsure whether they are truly fitted to be career women, or whether they would gain more satisfaction from solely being wives and mothers. Bored, lonely, middle-aged housewives whose children have grown up and left home, whose husbands are preoccupied with their jobs, and who have no careers of their own are equally at hazard.

Problem drinking is not restricted to adults, married or otherwise. The increase in alcoholism among teenagers and schoolchildren, inferred from the rise in convictions for drunkenness and consumption of alcohol, is one of the most alarming social trends of recent years. Partly, it may be due to the greater affluence of young people, but some sociologists believe that advertisements in which drinking hard liquor is equated with sophistication or manliness also play a part.

WHAT ALCOHOLISM CAN DO

Potential or actual alcoholism can affect four areas of people's lives: mental; physical; professional; and domestic and social.

Mental depression The most common mental ailments are anxiety, tension and depression. These may be caused by drink itself, by financial worries, by feelings of guilt or insecurity, or by a combination of all three. However, anxiety, tension and depression may themselves have been the cause of the alcoholism: it is often difficult to identify the root of the problem.

In 10 per cent of sufferers, more serious complaints develop with the advance of alcoholism. The drinker may develop phobias, start hearing things and seeing things, and show signs of schizophrenia—delusions and hallucinations—marked disturbances of thinking and contact with reality. Some sufferers develop Korsakoff's syndrome—named after the 19th-century Russian neurologist Sergei Korsakoff—in which the drinker suffers marked loss of memory which he unwittingly tries to disguise by relating stories of non-existent experiences.

Alcoholic dementia may occur. This is an irreversible intellectual deterioration in which the drinker shows loss of memory, comprehension and judgment similar to senile dementia.

If the drinker is deprived of alcohol he suffers the withdrawal syndrome—hallucinations, tremors, seizures and, worst of all, delirium tremens. The main features of this are restlessness, confusion, distortion of sense of time and place, and also frightening and vivid visual hallucinations.

Physical degeneration The central nervous system and the liver are the parts of the body most frequently damaged by alcohol. The nervous system can be affected by polyneuritis (inflammation of the nerves), and at a later stage dropfoot—when the muscles of the front foot cannot support the toes which drop below the level of the heel, so that the sufferer looks as though he is walking on a feather mattress. The patient may also be stricken by Wernicke's encephalopathy—named after the German neurologist Karl Wernicke—in which he is confused, unsteady on his feet and has weakness in some eye muscles.

Problems at work After a while, many problem drinkers find that they cannot do their work as well as they could before, or that they are absent more frequently to recover from their drinking. As a result, they may lose their jobs, and drink even more to compensate.

Misery at home The alcoholism of one member of a family can affect all the others. The husbands or wives and the children of drinkers often suffer from anxiety and depression, and there may be physical effects, too.

HAS HE A DRINK PROBLEM?
The four stages in the development of alcoholism

Stage 1: The pre-alcoholism phase

Anyone who answers 'yes' to any of these questions—particularly question 4—should control his drinking habits, as they could lead to serious problems later.

1 Does he drink to feel at ease on social occasions?
2 Does he drink to forget worry or anxiety?
3 Does he feel more efficient or confident in his work when he is drinking?
4 Does he need to drink more than he used to in the past to obtain the same effect?

Stage 2: The warning phase

The answer 'yes' to one or more questions shows that the drinker is well on the road to alcoholism. He should cut down his intake sharply. Most people can manage to do that without outside help at this stage.

5 After a period of drinking during which he was not obviously drunk, does he find it difficult to remember things he said or did?
6 Does he drink surreptitiously or secretly?
7 If he thinks there will not be enough to drink at a party, does he 'top up' with alcohol beforehand?
8 Does he arrange appointments so that they do not interfere with the opening hours of public houses?
9 Does he gulp his drink?
10 Does he look for work in jobs which provide easy access to alcohol?
11 Does he occasionally or frequently drive after he has had several drinks?

Although most problem drinkers strive to be good marriage partners and parents, they may, in drunkenness, go from vocal abuse to actual physical violence against members of their families. Some suffer from paranoid jealousy, in which the drinker is mistakenly convinced of his partner's infidelity and may become violent in attempting to justify his suspicions.

In addition to mental and physical injuries, the family may also be faced with financial hardship because the drinker has lost his job, or because he or she squanders money on alcohol. Sexual problems such as impotence and frigidity are also common.

The constant need for money to pay for their liquor drives many sufferers to crime, and the depressive effects of excessive drink lead others to take, or attempt to take, their own lives.

Stage 3: The crucial phase

Every 'yes' is a red warning light, indicating that the drinker must cut down drastically, or in certain cases stop drinking altogether. He may need encouragement to do so from his family or friends, or to seek medical advice. He is not necessarily yet a fully fledged victim of alcoholism but he will be unless he changes his habits immediately.

12 Does he continue drinking after previously deciding to have 'just one or two'?
13 Does he frequently suffer from hangovers?
14 Does the idea of 'a hair of the dog' as a remedy for a hangover appeal to him?
15 Does he suffer from morning shakes?
16 Does he have a drink first thing in the morning?
17 Does he neglect his meals because of his drinking?
18 Does he feel guilty about his drinking?
19 Does he prefer to drink alone?
20 Does he lose time from work because of drinking?
21 Does his drinking harm his family in any way?
22 Does he need to drink at a definite time each day?
23 Does he need to 'top up' with a drink every few hours?
24 Does he carry drink with him, for example, in his car or brief-case?
25 Does his drinking make him irritable?
26 Has he become jealous of his wife since he started heavy drinking?
27 Does his drinking cause physical symptoms, such as stomach pains?

28 Does drinking make him restless, or prevent him from sleeping?
29 Does he need a drink to be able to sleep?
30 Does he lose self-control after drinking?
31 Does he show less initiative, ambition, concentration or efficiency than previously?
32 Has his sexual desire decreased?
33 Is he particularly moody?
34 Has he become more isolated and lost friends?
35 Have his wife and children had to change their way of life—for example, by not going out, or not inviting guests—because of his drinking?
36 Has drinking made him harder to get on with, or otherwise changed his personality?
37 Does he tend to drink in places where he hopes he will not meet friends or acquaintances, or with people of a different background to his own?
38 Does drinking affect his peace of mind?
39 Does he feel resentful, self-pitying or that everyone is treating him unfairly?
40 Is drinking jeopardising his job or damaging his reputation?

Stage 4: The chronic phase

The answer 'yes' to any one of the first three questions means that there is a strong likelihood that the drinker is dependent on alcohol. The answer 'yes' to any one of the last five questions means that he is dependent on it. He needs help *now* or he may do himself irreversible mental or physical harm.

41 Has he ever seriously considered suicide when drinking?
42 Does he feel incapable of coping with life, whether or not he has been drinking?
43 Does he suffer from any of the following conditions, all of which (in the absence of any other cause) are complications of heavy drinking? Vomiting blood; passing blood in the stools; severe abdominal pains; unsteadiness of gait when not drinking; pain in the calves; epileptic-like fits; hallucinations (delirium tremens, or 'DTs'); severe tremors or sweating at night.
44 Does he go on alcoholic 'binges', drinking for several days in succession?
45 Does he get obviously drunk on much less than in the past?
46 Is he unable to take any action unless he has fortified himself with a drink beforehand?
47 Does he feel unable to give up drinking, even though he has been warned it is going to kill him?
48 Does he return to uncontrolled, excessive drinking again and again, even though he has tried to cut it down or give it up altogether?

BRAIN DAMAGE

The CT—Computerised Tomography—X-ray technique enables an arc of sensors to probe deep into the body. It has revealed that the brains of heavy drinkers can be affected at an early stage of their affliction—and that organic changes such as widening of the brain's ventricles, or cavities, may take place. So far, however, the significance of these changes is not fully understood. The changes in the nervous system are largely caused by vitamin B deficiency, and can to some extent be reversed by taking vitamin pills or by injections.

PHYSICAL DAMAGE

In contrast, liver damage is mostly due to the poisonous action of the alcohol itself. There are three such types of liver disease:

1. **Alcoholic fatty liver.** This occurs in most problem drinkers and is reversible if the patient stops drinking and follows a planned diet.
2. **Alcoholic hepatitis** (inflammation of the liver). This may be reversible, or it may worsen and lead to cirrhosis.
3. **Alcoholic cirrhosis** (replacement of liver cells by fatty tissue). This is irreversible, although with abstinence it may not progress.

OTHER PHYSICAL DISORDERS

There may also be other physical disorders. GASTRITIS (inflammation of the stomach lining) is widespread and many problem drinkers have a history of GASTRIC ULCER and may have undergone a partial GASTRECTOMY. CARDIO-MYOPATHY (heart-muscle disease), ANAEMIA (reduction of the number of red blood cells) and PANCREATITIS (inflammation of the pancreas) also occur.

Some types of CANCER are more often found in problem drinkers than in other people, perhaps because they are also often heavy smokers—for example, in cases of cancer of the mouth, larynx, pharynx or oesophagus.

Sufferers from alcoholism tend to bleed easily. The number of platelets in their blood is reduced and their blood does not coagulate as quickly as normal. Cirrhosis may lead to varicose veins, in the oesophagus and the rectum, which may burst and thereby cause vomiting of blood or bleeding piles. This adds to the hazards when the sufferer has to undergo surgery; and even after a successful operation, recovery may be complicated by withdrawal symptoms.

HOW MUCH ALCOHOL IS SAFE?

People vary widely in the amount of alcohol they can drink without damaging their health. This partly depends on their size—large bodies can absorb more than tiny ones. And women seen to tolerate alcohol less well than men, and are generally smaller too, so for them the 'safe' levels are lower still.

The risk increases with the amount consumed regularly. One 'unit' contains about 8 grams of alcohol: it is equivalent to half a pint of beer, one glass of wine or a single measure of spirits.

	Men	Women	
Sensible drinking	Up to 21	Up to 14	units/week
Moderate risk	22–49	15–36	units/week
Definitely harmful	50 or more	36 or more	units/week

DRINK AND YOUNG PEOPLE

Today, when no more than 5 per cent of men and 15 per cent of women in Britain are teetotal, most youngsters are, sooner or later, faced with the question: 'Shall I start to drink or not?'

Some experts believe it is safer to give children small amounts of drink—possibly diluted with water—with their meals at home, than to allow them to start drinking without any parental guidance. However, this approach is no guarantee against heavy drinking later.

Parents who nag, scold or preach at their children about the 'evils' of alcohol run the risk of making them drink out of defiance. The example of the father's and

---

Some don'ts about drinking

There are 'don'ts' which apply to everyone who drinks, and which are largely dictated by common sense. For instance:

☐ *Don't* drink at all before driving a car.

☐ *Don't* drink for medical reasons such as anxiety, depression or to combat stress.

☐ *Don't* drink alone.

☐ *Don't* drink early in the morning.

☐ *Don't* drink on an empty stomach.

☐ *Don't* fall into the habit of taking alcohol as an aid to sleep. This can easily lead to dependence.

☐ *Don't* mix alcohol with any other drug, especially tranquillisers.

☐ *Don't* gulp alcohol. Sip slowly.

☐ *Don't* drink to alleviate loneliness.

---

mother's own moderate drinking habits is far more important than any verbal warning.

Teachers, parents and anyone in charge of young people should know about the dangers of heavy drinking, and be able to discuss them unemotionally with the youngsters at the right opportunity.

WHERE HELP CAN BE OBTAINED

Advice and help for the problem drinker and—equally important—for his family are available from a wide variety of organisations. To find the best one for a particular case, it may be necessary to try several. Often the task has to be shared among various organisations and individuals.

NON-SPECIALIST SOURCES

The family doctor In the majority of cases, the family doctor—working perhaps in liaison with a community

nurse and social worker—can give advice and practical help.

The Church Frequently, the sufferer feels unable to discuss his illness with a doctor or health worker or social worker. In some cases an understanding clergyman or priest may be able to persuade the drinker to seek medical advice.

The Samaritans Initial advice and assistance is available from the local branch of The Samaritans, which is a voluntary organisation. Their number is in the local telephone directory.

SPECIALIST ORGANISATIONS

Alcohol Concern, 275 Grays Inn Road, London WC1X 8QF (071-833 3471). Alcohol Concern, a voluntary organisation, has information and advice centres throughout the United Kingdom. The centres provide specially trained counsellors, and are referred to in cases where residential care or treatment is necessary.

The addresses and telephone numbers of the numerous local centres in England, Wales and the Channel Islands can be obtained from the London headquarters or from local town halls.

The equivalent bodies in Scotland and Northern Ireland are the *Scottish Council on Alcoholism,* 137-145 Sauchiehall Street, Glasgow G2 3EW (041-333 9677), and the *Northern Ireland Council on Alcohol,* 40 Elmwood Avenue, Belfast BT9 6AZ (0232 664434).

Alcoholics Anonymous, General Service Office, PO Box 1, Stonebow House, Stonebow, York YO1 2NJ (0904-644026), is an organisation that helps anyone who drinks abnormally and who wants to stop. As its name implies, it offers the drinker anonymity, as only first names are used. He will be befriended by other sufferers from alcoholism who have stopped drinking and with whom he can identify, as they have undergone similar experiences to his own.

AA holds closed meetings for sufferers only, and open meetings which the members' families and friends can attend.

Information about groups throughout the UK—including times and places of meeting—can be obtained from AA's General Service Office.

Al-Anon Family Groups UK and Eire, 61 Great Dover Street, London SE1 4YF (071-403 0888). A similar organisation to Alcoholics Anonymous, it helps the families of problem drinkers. Group meetings are held regularly and information about them can be obtained from the London headquarters.

Alateen is an organisation which helps the teenage children of problem drinkers. Contact is made through Al-Anon in London.

Medical Council on Alcoholism, 1 St Andrew's Place, London NW1 4LB (Tel. 071-487 4445). A voluntary body which informs doctors about the problems of alcoholism.
Regional Alcoholic Units, The National Health Service runs about 25 such units in England and Wales and a number in Scotland. Their aim is the rehabilitation of sufferers, and they provide specialised in-patient and out-patient services, home visiting services, and sometimes special hostels and day centres.

They often work closely with AA, using group-therapy methods. Treatment usually starts with detoxification (cleansing the system of alcoholic poison). A few units have their own detoxification centres and some independent centres are run by voluntary groups—which also organise most of the special hostels. Drugs designed to deter sufferers from drinking may also be used.

Information about the units can be obtained from the Medical Council on Alcoholism (see above). Details about local facilities are also available from local social service departments and area health authorities. They may include community and social work services, and day and residential care at homes and hostels.

TYPES OF TREATMENT AVAILABLE
There is no miracle drug and no miracle cure for alcoholism. Because of the various factors involved in the illness, treatment is usually based on a combination of techniques. The three main ones are:
1. Psychological treatment This consists of examining and discussing the drinker's problem, either through individual counselling or group therapy. Behaviour therapy is also used in which an attempt is made to improve a person's drinking behaviour.
2. Social treatment This aims to help the drinker to readjust to society and to resume a useful role in it. He is helped in his return to family life, and housing difficulties are also dealt with. He can also join in self-help groups run by AA.
3. Drug treatment This is sometimes used in addition to the other two treatments, especially during the first stage of detoxification—when vitamins and possibly anticonvulsants (to guard against fits) may be given. Tranquillisers can be dangerous in chronic alcoholism; when tranquillisers are taken with alcohol the effects of both are increased.

The only other long-term drugs in common use are those which, when combined with alcohol, produce highly unpleasant effects such as headache, vomiting and breathing difficulties, and which act as a deterrent to drink. There are two proprietary brands available: Antabuse (disulfiram) and Abstem (CCC). These deterrents are available only on prescription, and have largely taken the place of the emetics previously used in alcohol aversion treatment.

CONCLUSION
The aim of any treatment is to restore the drinker and his family to a healthy, contented and satisfying way of life. Most medical experts believe that this can be brought about only by total abstinence, as an alcoholic is never completely 'cured'—he is only resisting the temptation to drink.

That is also the view of Alcoholics Anonymous. But there is a minority which considers that certain people dependent on alcohol can learn—through behaviour therapy—to become 'controlled' drinkers.

The outlook for the majority of sufferers is much more optimistic than most people—including many doctors—believe.

Those drinkers who sincerely want to end their addiction or dependence can do so—provided they seek and accept qualified help. All the specialist organisations will give a sympathetic and understanding hearing to all who approach them and provide assistance and treatment where required.

Alcoholism is no longer regarded as a crime or a disgrace. It is a disease that can often be cured and in most cases checked. There is no longer any reason—or any excuse—for people with a drink problem to suffer in shame and silence.

ALEXANDER TECHNIQUE
A method of improving an individual's posture and movement, based on the idea that there are 'correct' and 'incorrect' methods of standing, sitting and moving—which may vary according to the person. Use of the correct method, which mainly involves keeping the neck and spine straight, is said to benefit physical and mental health. The technique is not an exercise programme, but requires practice and experiment with the guidance of a tutor. Nothing in the technique conflicts with orthodox medical opinion, and it has the respect, though not the unqualified approval, of physicians.

ALKALI
A substance that neutralises an acid. Alkalis in the body help to ensure that the blood and the digestive juices from the liver and pancreas are kept slightly alkaline. The main body alkali is sodium bicarbonate, formed from sodium in the diet and carbon dioxide.

ALKALOSIS
A disorder caused by a considerable rise of alkali in the blood and in other body fluids. It can be caused by prolonged vomiting, which passes hydrochloric acid out of the system; by taking too much sodium bicarbonate to treat indigestion; or by abnormally deep breathing that results in an excessive loss of carbon dioxide. Symptoms include tingling skin, muscle weakness and cramp. When vomiting is the cause, a transfusion of a saline solution may be needed.

ALLERGY

A wide variety of apparently unrelated ailments—including ASTHMA, HAY FEVER, ECZEMA and URTICARIA (nettle-rash)—are all due to allergies. If you have an allergy, your body is sensitive to—and therefore reacts to—one or more of the vegetable and animal substances to which most people are exposed in everyday life. Substances which cause the body to react are called antigens. They include pollen, animal hair, house dust mites, and foods such as shellfish and eggs.

When antigens invade the body of an allergic person, it defends itself by producing antibodies—proteins designed to neutralise the antigens. It is the subsequent reaction between antibody and antigen inside the body which is responsible for producing the sufferer's allergic ailments.

HOW THE ENEMY PENETRATES
Antigens act by penetrating the body. They dissolve in water, rendering vulnerable any part of the body that is not waterproof. The body is protected on the outside by the skin—a waterproof layer antigens that cannot penetrate unless it is broken, as it is by a disease such as dermatitis.

But the body has several openings, and it is here that an antigen makes its entry. The lungs provide by far the easiest access. As we breathe, they take in particles of vegetable or animal matter from about 350 cu. ft of air every 24 hours. This vast volume of antigen-laden air is distributed over the entire surface area of the lungs' air sacs which, if opened out, would be the size of a football pitch. Some antigens, too, get into the body through the intestines, in what we eat and drink.

THE BODY'S DEFENCES
The body is armed with defences to combat invaders, such as bacteria and viruses, which cause harm. The first

line of defence is the production of a protein antibody called globulin, which circulates in the blood. Globulin is made in bone marrow in response to invasion by foreign material.

Scientists have identified five classes of globulin; the one which reacts with antigens to cause allergies is known as IgE. People who make a lot of IgE antibody tend to have allergic reactions more readily than those who do not. They develop blisters and itching of the skin when their doctor pricks it during tests for allergies; and they also have a tendency to develop eczema.

The more IgE antibody in the blood, the greater the likelihood of eczema; and it may be that people with eczema have skin which is readily penetrated by antigens, and so make a lot of antibody in response. Eczema sufferers comprise between 15 and 25 per cent of Britain's population. The condition runs in families, and is most common in childhood, becoming less severe as the sufferer grows older.

WHAT HAPPENS IN AN ALLERGIC REACTION?

Scattered throughout the tissue lining the surface of the body—skin, nose, eyes, ears, lips, mouth, lungs and intestines—are millions of single cells called mast cells, which act as 'factories' for the manufacture and storage of chemicals. One of these chemicals is histamine—the 'trigger' of the allergic reaction. The IgE antibody is stuck around the surface of the mast cells, waiting for the appropriate antigens to penetrate the body in order to do their work.

When antigen enters the body and comes into contact with the IgE, a chemical reaction between antigens and antibody begins within the cells. As a result, enough energy is generated to release the histamine in the cells into the surrounding tissues. Here the histamine accumulates in clefts called receptors. Once the receptors are filled, they trigger off more chemical reactions, a process that culminates in symptoms of allergy. All of this takes between 30 seconds and two minutes.

WHAT ARE THE SYMPTOMS?

The exact symptoms of allergy depend on where the antigen enters the body, on how many mast cells release their histamine, and on the amount of histamine discharged at one time.

In the skin The release of histamine into the skin produces irritation and itching. Within a minute or so the histamine distends the little blood vessels near the surface, causing the skin to redden. The blood vessels most heavily saturated with histamine begin to leak and allow plasma—the clear fluid in which blood corpuscles are suspended—to seep out into the surrounding tissues,

where it is trapped beneath the skin. This raises a rash of little white bumps rather like gnat bites. They are called weals or hives—giving this allergic ailment its name of hives, or urticaria.

Although eczema is an allergy symptom that appears on the skin, it is not known to be caused by the release of histamine into the skin—in fact, none of the mechanism that produces the symptoms of eczema is as yet understood. It cannot, therefore, be prevented; though it can be treated.

In the eyes Mast cells line the delicate membranes of the eyes and eyelids. Antigen arriving here causes irritation and streaming—the ailment called conjunctivitis. On occasion the membranes may be so swollen that the eyes are completely closed. Tears run into the nose and cause stuffiness and snuffles.

In the nose Mast cells line the entire nose cavity. The release of histamine here brings immediate irritation, which causes continual sneezing. The mucous cells of the nose are stimulated by the irritation and begin to produce mucus. This condition is rhinitis. Once the nose is blocked, the sufferer begins to breathe through the mouth. The filtering effect of the nose is bypassed, and antigen is inhaled straight down into the lungs.

When allergic symptoms occur in eyes and nose together, the combination is called hay-fever. This is produced by grass pollen—it is nothing to do with allergy to hay; nor is it a fever.

In the lungs The bronchial tubes through which we breathe are lined with mast cells. They are also lined with muscle, and the release of histamine from the mast cells causes an asthma attack to develop.

The muscle contracts and the bronchial tubes narrow, reducing the amount of air getting in and out. It is normal for the bronchial tubes to widen slightly when we breathe in, and narrow a little when we breathe out; but the picture changes under the influence of histamines. The bigger bronchial tubes do not change in diameter very much because they are held open by rigid bands of cartilage, but the smaller tubes contract a great deal, and it becomes harder to breathe out than in. As air is forced in and out, it makes a characteristic whistling or wheezing sound.

Not only is the flow of air in the small tubes obstructed, but the smallest tubes of all shut down completely. As a result the level of oxygen in the blood falls, and the victim becomes breathless.

Histamine irritates mucous cells in the lungs in the same way as it does those in the nose. The cells stream mucus, which becomes sticky and contributes to blocking the smaller bronchial tubes.

The asthma attack starts as tightness in the chest with

breathlessness, then progresses to more severe breathlessness. Because it is more difficult to breathe out than in, air gets trapped in the lungs, and the chest is blown up like a balloon. When monitoring an asthma attack, a hospital doctor may measure the diameter of the patient's chest with a tape. If the chest is getting smaller, this is a good sign, but if the circumference is increasing, the attack is worsening.

In the intestine Mast cells line the intestine throughout its length. The release of histamine from these cells may be caused by allergies to food, such as shellfish. The discharged histamine makes the intestinal muscle contract, resulting in stomach pain and profuse diarrhoea. Frequently a rash breaks out somewhere on the body, presumably because the antigen in the food is absorbed into the blood and is carried simultaneously to the mast cells of the skin.

Anaphylactic shock When antigen is injected into the bloodstream, as happens with a bee or wasp sting, it spreads rapidly to large numbers of mast cells all over the body; and this results in the simultaneous discharge of very large quantities of histamine.

The resulting symptoms—a condition called anaphylactic shock—are explosive and dramatic. Within a minute or two, weals develop all over the skin. Because the tissue around the face is soft, it can swell easily; and the tissue around the eyes may become so puffy that within five minutes or so the eyes may close completely. The lips swell up, and the throat feels thick, due to swelling of tissue around the tongue and mouth. The wholesale inflammation of the skin causes a massive drop in blood pressure, so that the victim develops a rapid heartbeat, and may actually faint. Asthmatic people may find their asthma getting worse during such an attack.

HOW ALLERGIES ARE TREATED

What can I do? The best treatment is to avoid the cause, and this may be a relatively simple matter if the cause is known. For example, an allergy which is proved to be due to cat fur improves six to eight weeks after the cat has been removed and sufficient time has elapsed to ensure that all the fur has been collected by vacuuming or other cleaning.

But some antigens are more difficult to avoid. Allergy to house dust is due to the droppings of house mites—microscopic insects which live as parasites in bedding, armchairs and sofas, feeding on the skin scales that fall from the human body day and night. People spend about one-third of their lives in bed. Tossing and turning abraids the skin, which then collects in the feathers of pillows and duvets, the bed covering or the hair of the mattress.

Furthermore, mites like warmth and moisture, so a bed provides an endless supply of food in a pleasantly temperate climate.

To make life as difficult as possible for house mites, use Terylene pillows and duvets, which do not retain skin fragments as effectively as feathers; and put a plastic cover over the mattress. The food source can be reduced by vacuuming the bedding each day. Some sprays are now available which help to kill off the mites.

What can the doctor do? For certain allergies your doctor may recommend a course of desensitisation injections, which can reduce your sensitiveness to antigens. Extracts of the antigens themselves are injected. Graded injections of increasing concentration are usually administered every one to two weeks over a period of about ten weeks.

Unfortunately, desensitisation injections can produce anaphylactic shock (see page 70) which may be fatal. Treatment is only carried out if the allergy is severe and resuscitation facilities are immediately available. Reactions can occur up to two hours later, so patients are kept under observation.

Because of the risks involved, desensitisation against grass pollens and house dust mites are not usually recommended. Your doctor may prescribe a steroid inhaler or nose spray. Steroids reduce inflammation and swelling of the air passages. They do not work immediately and must be taken regularly to have any effect.

Your doctor may also prescribe antiallergy drugs, which forestall or treat the symptoms. Hay fever frequently improves with antihistamines—drugs that block the damaging effect of histamine by occupying the histamine receptors. However, most antihistamines make the sufferer drowsy, especially if taken with alcohol, and this may have serious implications for motorists.

Antihistamines are ineffective against asthma; but some skin rashes do respond to them, and itching may be relieved within half an hour of taking a single tablet.

REVOLUTIONARY DRUG
The treatment of respiratory allergy has been revolutionised with the introduction of sodium cromoglycate, which prevents the mast cell from discharging its histamine. It can be dropped as a solution into the eyes, or inhaled through the mouth as a powder, or sprayed up the nose as an aerosol. Sodium cromoglycate is helpful only if taken before symptoms have developed, and it needs to be taken regularly to forestall them. So, too, does another preparation for puffing up the nose—a spray containing cortisone, a HORMONE that works by reducing the inflammation caused by allergies.

Nose drops containing isoprenaline may be given. They constrict the blood vessels and widen the bronchial tubes.

They give immediate but short-lived relief of asthma symptoms; in the long run they become habit-forming, and should be used sparingly.

Bronchodilator drugs also give immediate relief to asthmatics, by widening the bronchial tubes. They are not habit-forming, and are puffed or sprayed up the nose or into the mouth. The use of such inhalants may bring instant relief to asthma sufferers.

Do's and don'ts about allergies

☐ *Do* make a note of when you come into contact with something to which you may be allergic, and of your reaction to it. Such records can be a better means of diagnosis than medical tests.

☐ *Do* look for a pattern in your suspected allergy. Asthma in spring, but not during the rest of the year, may indicate an allergy to grass pollen. A rash around the waist may be caused by the elastic in the waistband. One on the wrist could be an allergy to nickel in a watch strap.

☐ *Do* make every effort, once you know you are allergic to something, to avoid it. For instance, if you have a food allergy, check the list of ingredients in packaged foodstuffs.

☐ *Do* remember, if you are a new mother and have asthma or eczema, that your baby may also be allergic. Protect him from the antigens in cow's milk by breast-feeding for the first six months if you can.

☐ *Don't* expect instant results once you have eliminated things to which you may be allergic. Animal fur, for instance, may remain in the house for several months after the animal has gone.

☐ *Don't* assume that you are allergic to penicillin if you develop a rash while being treated with it. Check with your doctor, because the spots may be due to the bacterium causing the illness.

Bronchodilators such as aminophylline are taken as tablets, but they can have side-effects such as trembling of the limbs and insomnia, and they take half an hour or so to begin working. But they may remain effective for a long period—a full night's respite, for instance—whereas the effects of inhalants last only two or three hours.

ALOPECIA
The medical term for baldness or loss of hair. Mostly it occurs on the head, but other parts of the body may occasionally be affected. The condition is usually inherited, but it may be caused by disease or drugs.
See BALDNESS

ALZHEIMER'S DISEASE
This is the commonest form of pre-senile DEMENTIA, a progressive decline in mental faculties which may begin as early as age 45. The brain shrinks, its nerve fibres become tangled, and deposits of a protein called amyloid are found in various brain sites. Its exact cause is unknown, but it has been linked with heredity, virus infections and intake of aluminium.

AMBLYOPIA
One type of reduction in the sharpness of vision. In most cases it is not caused by any disease of the eye but is either hereditary or the result of an uncorrected SQUINT in childhood. In some cases, however, it is due to damage to the optic nerve that has been caused by excessive use of alcohol or tobacco, poor diet or certain drugs.

AMNESIA
Loss of memory, either partial or total, that is so pronounced as to cause worry or problems for the sufferer. It can be caused by a head injury, and indicates the presence of concussion, *see* FIRST AID; by the patient's emotional state such as HYSTERIA; or by a number of illnesses including ALCOHOLISM, MENINGITIS, SYPHILIS, BRAIN TUMOUR and EPILEPSY. In retrograde amnesia, the victim loses his or her memory for events that happened before some injury or emotional shock; in anterograde amnesia, the loss of memory is for events that happened afterwards.

In many cases of amnesia, the patient's memory returns with the passing of time or with the clearing up of the underlying condition. But if the cause is emotional disturbance, this could mean that the mind subconsciously wishes to 'erase' some occurrence that is too distressing to contemplate; and psychiatric help is needed.

AMNION

The membranous sac which encloses the fetus in the womb. Inside the sac the fetus floats in, and is cushioned by, a liquid called amniotic fluid. The bursting of the amnion and release of the fluid usually signals the beginning of childbirth. When there is a risk that a fetus may be suffering from SPINA BIFIDA, DOWN'S SYNDROME, a RHESUS FACTOR problem or one of certain other abnormalities, a sample of amniotic fluid is withdrawn from the womb through a hollow needle (amniocentesis). The cells of the fetus in the fluid are then examined for evidence of the abnormality.

AMOEBIASIS

A parasitic disease found world-wide, but more commonly in tropical countries. The infection is spread by food or water which has been contaminated by flies carrying the germ from human faeces. Travellers to the tropics, especially areas where amoebic dysentery is common, should avoid water, unless they know it has been purified, and fruit and vegetables from sources where contaminated water may have been used to wash them. Iodine-releasing tablets added to the water will kill the amoebae, but they cannot be destroyed simply by boiling water or adding chlorine to it.

Symptoms
- Diarrhoea. This may be profuse with blood and mucus (amoebic dysentery), or less severe and intermittent.
- Abdominal cramps.
- If the infection spreads to the liver it will produce an abscess which can be felt by the doctor, and the patient will suffer fever, sweats and weight loss.
- Sometimes there are no symptoms, but the patient is carrying the disease and will excrete germs in his faeces.

Duration
- Infections may persist indefinitely if not treated.

Causes
- A parasite called *Entamoeba hystolytica* which attacks the intestines.

Treatment
- In severe cases bed-rest and replacement of lost fluids are essential.

When to consult the doctor
- If there is a severe or prolonged attack of DYSENTERY, particularly if the patient is in an area where amoebic dysentery is known to occur.

What the doctor may do
- Check stools for amoebae or their cysts.
- Prescribe an antiamoebic drug. *See* MEDICINES, 28.

See INFECTIOUS DISEASES *page 32*

AMPUTATION

The removal by a surgeon of a diseased part of a limb or organ of the body. An amputation is normally performed to prevent the spread of infection or cancer from diseased to healthy tissues, or to remove a structure that cannot carry out its usual function in order that an artificial substitute or prosthesis may be fitted.

AMYLOID DISEASE

A disorder in which an abnormal wax-like protein called amyloid invades the tissue of internal organs. The disease sometimes occurs as a complication of prolonged infections, such as TUBERCULOSIS, prolonged inflammatory illnesses, such as RHEUMATOID ARTHRITIS, or certain other disorders, including HODGKIN'S DISEASE. In other cases, amyloid disease occurs in isolation. The organs most commonly affected are the spleen, liver and kidneys. When the disorder is secondary to some underlying illness, treatment consists of controlling that illness.

ANAEMIA

A reduction in the quantity of oxygen-carrying haemoglobin in the blood. Anaemia is the most common of all the blood diseases and occurs in various forms—iron deficiency, pernicious, sickle cell and megaloblastic.

Symptoms
- Tiredness.
- Shortness of breath.
- Dizziness.
- Disturbed vision.
- Headache and insomnia.
- Palpitation.
- Pallor of skin.
- Loss of appetite and indigestion.
- Swelling of the ankles in severe cases.
- Chest pain in older patients.

Each form of anaemia may have one or two additional symptoms which are specific to it. These are listed below under the relevant form.

IRON DEFICIENCY ANAEMIA

The most common form of anaemia. It is caused by a lack of the iron in the body necessary for the production of haemoglobin. The condition is aggravated by pregnancy, heavy periods or any blood loss. Premature babies are very liable.

Symptoms
- Sore tongue and inflammation on the side of the mouth.
- Dry, brittle nails.

Duration
- The condition persists until treated.

Causes
- Loss of blood due to heavy periods or tooth extraction, for example.
- A diet deficient in iron.
- Diseases of the bowel in which absorption of iron is prevented.
- Many chronic infections which interfere with blood formation.
- Diseases such as GASTRIC ULCER, CANCERS and PILES in which there is hidden blood loss.
- RHEUMATOID ARTHRITIS and MYXOEDEMA.
- Several diseases of the blood in which the red blood cells are destroyed.

Complications
- In severe cases, OEDEMA and HEART FAILURE.

Treatment in the home
- Eat more foods containing iron, such as meat and pulses.

When to consult the doctor
- If the symptoms described develop.

What the doctor may do
- Examine the patient.
- Take a blood sample for testing.
- If the diagnosis is confirmed, prescribe a course of iron tablets or, occasionally, iron injections.
- Treat any underlying cause.

Prevention
- Ensure that the diet contains enough iron.
- Report any excessive loss of blood to the doctor so that it can be treated before anaemia develops.
- During pregnancy and heavy periods, women should seek medical advice and take iron tablets conscientiously.

Outlook
- Excellent. The condition should be cured within six months of treatment. If the underlying cause is diagnosed and treated, anaemia is much less likely to recur.

PERNICIOUS ANAEMIA

A form of anaemia which develops when the bone marrow lacks vitamin B12 or other substances needed for the proper formation of blood. The condition is commoner in people with blood group A than in those with blood group O.

Symptoms
- The tongue is sore, smooth and inflamed in places.
- Persistent diarrhoea.
- Tingling in the fingers and toes.
- In severe cases, the facial skin may assume a lemon-yellow tint.

Duration
- The condition persists until treated.

Causes
- Failure of the stomach to produce an enzyme—the intrinsic factor—which is needed for the absorption of vitamin B12 from food.
- This failure results from autoimmunity, certain drugs or follows removal of the stomach (GASTRECTOMY).

Complications
- With early treatment these are few. They may include heart failure, degeneration of the spinal cord and cancer of stomach.

Treatment in the home
- None.

When to consult the doctor
- Immediately the symptoms described develop.

What the doctor may do
- Take a blood sample for testing.
- Refer the patient to hospital for further examination, which may include testing the stomach or a sample of bone marrow.
- If the diagnosis is confirmed, prescribe a course of vitamin B12 injections.

Prevention
- The only types of pernicious anaemia which can be prevented are those which have an underlying cause, such as a gastrectomy, or prolonged treatment with an antiepileptic drug.

Outlook
- Good. After the initial course of treatment, injections must be given indefinitely to stop recurrence.

SICKLE-CELL ANAEMIA
An inherited condition found almost exclusively in black people. Symptoms start in childhood. Both sexes are affected equally.

Symptoms
- Slight yellow discoloration of the skin and eyeballs.
- Feverishness, weakness and anaemia, especially after strenuous physical exercise.
- Anything causing deep or rapid breathing may result in a crisis when the symptoms are particularly severe.
- Blood clots may occur anywhere in the body.

Duration
- The condition is chronic, persisting throughout a patient's life.

Causes
- An abnormal haemoglobin present in the blood. Haemoglobin is the red pigment in the blood which carries oxygen from the lungs to the tissues. If, because of exertion or respiratory infection, the amount of oxygen in the blood is reduced, the abnormal haemoglobin causes the blood cells to deform into a sickle shape. These cells are then destroyed by the body's immune system, causing anaemia.

Complications
- Ulcers and local infections may occur in bones, kidneys and other organs.

Treatment in the home
- None.

When to consult the doctor
- If any symptoms of the illness are noticed.

What the doctor may do
- Take blood tests to find out whether abnormalities are present.
- Arrange for the patient to have regular blood transfusions if sickle-cell anaemia is diagnosed. This is the only form of treatment available.

Prevention
- There is no way of preventing the disease, but avoiding strenuous physical activity may reduce the risk of severe crises occurring.

Outlook
- Complications arising from the anaemia may result in death at any age, but many sufferers survive beyond middle age.

MEGALOBLASTIC (FOLATE DEFICIENT) ANAEMIA
A form of anaemia similar to pernicious anaemia. It develops if the diet is deficient in folic acid, which is present in liver and vegetables. Pregnant women and the elderly are particularly vulnerable. The symptoms are similar to those of pernicious anaemia. The treatment is to give folic acid tablets. This is why such tablets are given often as a preventative to those who may be at risk.

ANAESTHESIA
Loss of sensation in part or all of the body. This may occur as the result of injury to or disease of a nerve, as happens in LEPROSY, but the term is generally used to describe the deliberate medical removal of sensitivity to pain by means of an anaesthetic drug administered by injection or inhalation so that surgery can be performed.

ANAL FISSURE

Split in the lining of the anal canal. The split is often difficult to heal because it is held open by muscular spasm caused by the pain of inflammation.

Symptoms
- Pain during and after passing a motion.
- Blood on the paper after wiping the anus.

Causes
- Usually passing a hard motion.

Treatment in the home
- Soaking in a bath of hot water or holding a hot, wet sponge against the anus may help to relieve muscular spasm and pain.
- Before or after opening bowels apply a painkilling ointment to the fissure with the finger.
- Eat plenty of fruit and take either bran, a bulk laxative, or a lubricant laxative. *See* MEDICINES, 3.

What the doctor may do
- Examine you to confirm the diagnosis and make sure there are no other reasons for the pain and bleeding.
- In severe cases send you to a surgeon for an operation to either cut out the fissure or stretch the anus.

See DIGESTIVE SYSTEM *page 44*

ANAL IRRITATION

Chronic itching around the anus, known medically as pruritis ani. The moist skin becomes inflamed and soggy. The more the sufferer scratches, the worse the irritation becomes.

Causes
- Most cases have no obvious cause.
- Irritating soap, powders and ointments.
- Rough clothes.
- Poor anal hygiene.
- Complaints such as PILES (haemorrhoids), and ANAL FISSURES.
- Infections caused by THREADWORMS or THRUSH.
- Disorders which cause itching, such as DIABETES mellitus or JAUNDICE.

Treatment in the home
- Do not scratch. Wear gloves in bed to stop scratching while asleep.

- Keep the skin around the anus clean and dry and use only a bland talcum powder, such as baby powder.

When to consult the doctor
- If the itching persists.

What the doctor may do
- Prescribe a steroid cream to apply to the affected area around the anus.
- Take a swab or examine stools to check for THREAD-WORMS or FUNGUS INFECTION.
- Take urine and blood samples to check for DIABETES or JAUNDICE.

See DIGESTIVE SYSTEM *page 44*

ANDROGENS

Male sex hormones whose function is to produce secondary sexual characteristics after puberty—for example, facial hair and a deep voice. Most androgens, including the principal one, testosterone, are produced in the testicles; others are formed in the adrenal glands, on top of the kidneys.

Small amounts of androgens are also produced in women's ovaries and adrenal glands; when production is excessive it causes VIRILISM. If the sexual development of an adolescent boy is retarded, he may be given injections of natural or synthetic androgens. These are also used to treat breast cancer in women.

ANENCEPHALY

A rare abnormality in which the major part of the brain of a fetus fails to develop. The bones at the back of the head are also partly or completely missing. Death occurs at birth. The abnormality tends to run in families. A pregnant woman from such a family can have early tests carried out on the fetus and, if these indicate anencephaly, she can have the pregnancy terminated.

ANEURYSM

Local swelling of an artery, like a blow-out on an inner tube, which can develop if the artery is diseased or weakened, especially when the blood pressure is high. The artery most commonly affected is the aorta (the main artery of the chest and abdomen), but small congenital aneurysms (those that are there at birth) can occur in otherwise healthy arteries supplying the brain. *See*

SUBARACHNOID HAEMORRHAGE. Rupture is the most serious risk of an aneurysm. Sometimes a rupture is incomplete and between the inner and outer layers of the arterial wall.

Symptoms
- Many aneurysms have no symptoms, especially those in the abdomen, and are found only by chance on routine examination or X-ray.
- Those which develop in the chest are more likely to press on surrounding tissues and to interfere with the proper function of the heart, causing chest pain and shortness of breath.

Duration
- *See* ATHEROMA.

Causes
- The most common cause is atheroma (degenerative change) of the wall of the artery.
- Untreated SYPHILIS (now rare) occasionally causes an aneurysm of the aorta many years after the original infection.
- The cause of congenital aneurysm is not known.

When to consult the doctor
- As soon as the condition is suspected.

What the doctor may do
- If an aneurysm is causing symptoms, the doctor will investigate to see whether it can safely be removed by surgery. An aneurysm without symptoms is often not treated.
- If the aneurysm ruptures, emergency surgery is required immediately.

Prevention
- *See* ATHEROMA.

Outlook
- Aneurysms in the chest which cause symptoms are serious, and without surgery they may be fatal.
- Those elsewhere may remain for many years without causing serious trouble, but when pain or pressure symptoms develop, the risk of rupture has to be balanced carefully against the risks of removal by surgery.

See CIRCULATORY SYSTEM *page 40*

ANGINA PECTORIS

Attacks of choking or throttling pain across the upper part of the chest, due to reduction of the blood flow through the coronary arteries which supply the heart muscle. It occurs in spasms and is usually brought on by exertion

and relieved by rest. Although atheroma of the coronary arteries is the most common cause, other diseases, such as anaemia, may produce the same type of pain.

Symptoms
- The pain usually begins across the upper part of the front of the chest and can spread to the jaw and down the left arm, and sometimes the right also.
- The pain can be described as tight, heavy, constricting or crushing, and sometimes numbing or burning. It is never throbbing or knife-like.
- The pain usually lasts a few minutes, and is precipitated by exertion or a meal and passes off with rest.

Duration
- Once angina develops, the attacks usually recur. With treatment the frequency of attacks can be reduced and may cease completely.
- Occasionally, despite treatment, attacks become increasingly frequent.

Causes
- Exertion, such as walking—especially against the wind or up an incline.
- Cold weather.
- Emotion, which can be brought on by an argument, shock, violence or excitement on television.
- Heavy meals.

Complications
- A clot may form and block the coronary artery and cause CORONARY THROMBOSIS.

Treatment in the home
- Sit down and rest. If you are walking in the street, stand still. The pain should be relieved within a few minutes.
- Reduce emotional stress if possible. Attacks brought on by emotion are sometimes difficult to relieve.
- Do not continue exercise or activity. Angina is not likely to work off without rest. Further activity during an attack may be harmful.

When to consult the doctor
- If the pain is not relieved within ten to 15 minutes, or if you have never had angina before.

What the doctor may do
- The doctor will need to find out the cause of the angina and to assess its severity. If it is mild, no treatment will be needed, but if it is serious then various medical treatments are available. *See* MEDICINES, 8.
- If it is not responding to medical treatment, the diseased artery can be surgically bypassed by a vein graft, or opened up by inflating a tiny balloon in the artery (angioplasty).

Prevention
- Avoid conditions which produce the pain—for instance exertion, especially after heavy meals in cold or windy weather. Your doctor may prescribe tablets which

you can safely take before exertion to prevent the onset of pain.

• For long-term prevention, do not smoke. Keep your weight down to an ideal level (*see* WEIGHT). Increase physical activity, but avoid precipitating an attack of angina by using your tablets if necessary. Physical conditioning by exercise often reduces the severity of angina. But be guided by your doctor.

Outlook

• The outlook for angina sufferers depends on the underlying cause. Even when the coronary arteries are diseased, reduction of weight and stopping smoking may relieve the angina completely, and may also improve the condition of the arteries.

See CIRCULATORY SYSTEM *page 40*

ANGIONEUROTIC OEDEMA

A form of urticaria or nettlerash. Tongue, throat, lips and face may become swollen. Very rarely the swelling is so severe that immediate treatment with an injection of adrenaline is necessary. The cause is usually a bee sting, a food or a drug.

See ALLERGY

ANKLE

The symptoms most likely to affect the ankle joint are pain and swelling. The joint is a common site for injuries such as sprains, strains and fractures and is also subject to the disorders and diseases that affect the other joints of the body.

See SYMPTOM SORTER—ANKLE PROBLEMS

ANKYLOSING SPONDYLITIS

A disease of the joints affecting mainly young men in their twenties and thirties. It usually affects the spine, causing joints to fuse by an unusual process of bone formation.

Symptoms

• Onset of symptoms is gradual over a period of months or years.

• Repeated attacks of backache in a healthy, fit person (aged 20-35).

• Early morning back pain and stiffness. This can radiate down one or both legs.

• Increasing stiffness of the whole spine which may be revealed if the sufferer tries to bend down and touch his toes.

• Tenderness over the hip joints.

• Chest expansion may be limited.

• Spinal joints are the main ones involved, but in some cases the shoulder, hips and knees may be affected.

Duration

• Slowly progressive for many years.

Causes

• No definite cause has been isolated, but the condition sometimes runs in families.

Complications

• In the long term, regional ILEITIS, ulcerative COLITIS, and certain heart defects may develop.

• IRITIS (inflammation of the eye) can occur in 25 per cent of cases.

• Long-term disease can cause the spine to become rigid, and this in turn leads to KYPHOSIS (curvature of the spine) which with neck distortion can result in a crippling handicap.

Treatment in the home

• None possible, except under medical direction.

When to consult the doctor

• Immediately the disease is suspected.

What the doctor may do

• He may X-ray the lower part of the back and carry out a blood test to confirm the diagnosis. If the diagnosis is confirmed, referral to hospital is usual.

• Painkillers and anti-inflammatory drugs will be prescribed to relieve the symptoms and slow down the progress of the disease. *See* MEDICINES, 22, 37.

• Physiotherapy will also be arranged to strengthen the spinal muscles and mobilise the joints.

• If the pain persists despite treatment with drugs, and the condition is getting worse, then radiotherapy may be tried. In early cases the results are excellent, with the disease process being apparently arrested. More advanced cases with fixed deformity can also benefit from radiotherapy.

• Not all specialists favour radiotherapy because it involves a risk of leukaemia, in about three cases in 1,000.

Prevention

• Where there is a family history of the disease, tests can assist in early diagnosis, allowing early active treatment.

Outlook

• For cases which are treated by anti-inflammatory drugs and radiotherapy in the early stages, the outlook is good. For cases in the more advanced stages a combina-

tion of these measures can often restore the patient to a reasonable level of activity.

See SKELETAL SYSTEM *page 54*

ANOREXIA NERVOSA

A disorder in which the individual refuses food because of an unnatural fear of putting on weight. It mainly affects adolescent girls in affluent Western communities, although occasionally older married women may be affected. One patient in 15 is male. Anorexia nervosa is becoming increasingly common—a recent survey in Scotland showed that three people in 200,000 suffer from it. The condition is distressing for the sufferer's family and friends, because they cannot understand her subconscious self-deception regarding the need for food. The sufferer convinces herself that she is too fat, that she has not lost weight and that she does not need either treatment or food. She is unlikely to listen to advice from family or friends about the need for food, so they should be prepared to seek medical help on the patient's behalf. Treatment is essential and although most cases recover, occasional fatalities do occur.

Symptoms

• Failure to eat for long periods.

• Loss of weight. This may be considerable and obvious to everyone except the sufferer.

• Vomiting occurs. The patient's changed attitude towards food leads to vomiting being self-induced, often concealed by the patient.

• Menstrual periods stop.

• Sexual desire may be lost.

• Reluctance to undress in front of others, probably because of a subconscious desire to conceal weight loss.

Duration

• From a few months to three or four years.

Causes

• The causes are uncertain, but the condition has many features of PHOBIAS and COMPULSIVE OBSESSIONAL BEHAVIOUR.

• Disturbances in secretion of sex hormones may occur.

• Strained family relationships and emotional upsets are extremely common, but it is often not clear if these have preceded or followed the onset of symptoms.

Complications

• Severe loss of weight, anaemia, infertility, brittle bones and loss of sexual desire are common.

- Very occasionally death can occur.

Treatment in the home
- None is advised until medical advice has been sought.

When to consult the doctor
- As soon as the condition is suspected.

What the doctor may do
- Get the sufferer to accept the need for medical help. This is usually the first and most difficult step in the treatment.
- Confirm the diagnosis.
- Refer the sufferer to a psychiatrist, if she is willing to go. Often, she will accept treatment only from her family doctor.
- Agree a target weight to be achieved with the patient.
- Ensure, if necessary by admission to hospital, that food is being eaten, that vomiting is not concealed or being self-induced in private, and that the weight target is being achieved.

Prevention
- None known.

Outlook
- In about 80 per cent of cases response to treatment is good. About 20 per cent are unaffected by treatment and the symptoms may continue for several years.

See MENTAL SYSTEM *page 33*

ANOXIA
An insufficient supply of oxygen to the tissues of the body. In 'anaemic anoxia', the reduction in the supply of oxygen to the tissues is caused by deficiencies in the constituents of blood—there may be a shortage of red, oxygen-carrying, blood cells, or a fault in the chemical make-up of haemoglobin.

Sometimes anoxia is said to be 'stagnant', in which case it is the result of general or localised slowing (stagnation) of circulating blood. Stagnant anoxia may be caused by problems such as HEART FAILURE, shock, the blockage of a blood vessel in THROMBOSIS, or a spasm of the muscular wall of a blood vessel.

Deficiencies in the respiratory system may also cause anoxia, and in this case the condition is known as 'anoxic anoxia'. Sufferers from chronic BRONCHITIS, for example, often have a degree of anoxia because the amount of lung tissue available for the exchange of oxygen and carbon dioxide during breathing is reduced. Anoxic anoxia may also be caused by an asthmatic attack, where the airways are constricted, or by weakness or disease of the muscles that are used in breathing. More rarely, the condition may be a result of a reduced oxygen content of the air that is breathed, as at high altitudes.

ANTEPARTUM HAEMORRHAGE

Any bleeding from the vagina that occurs during pregnancy. It may well be symptomatic of a condition that is serious for mother and baby, and a doctor should be summoned right away.

Symptoms
- Any blood loss during pregnancy. The loss may be heavy and contain clots.

Duration
- How long the bleeding lasts will vary from case to case.

Causes
- If the haemorrhage occurs during the first three months of pregnancy, it is usually due to a threatened miscarriage (*see* ABORTION) which is common, or a complete miscarriage.
- Otherwise, it is usually due to PLACENTA PRAEVIA, or detachment of afterbirth.
- Detachment of the afterbirth from the wall of the uterus (womb) due to toxaemia of pregnancy.

Treatment in the home
- Rest in bed until the doctor arrives.
- Keep any blood clots that have been passed so that the doctor can examine them.

When to consult the doctor
- Summon the doctor as soon as any bleeding occurs.

What the doctor may do
- Treatment depends on the cause and severity of the bleeding. Often the mother is immediately admitted to hospital. In some cases bed-rest is all that is needed.

Prevention
- All unnecessary strenuous activity should be avoided during pregnancy. If a woman is in doubt about any activity she should discuss it with her doctor or midwife. Sexual intercourse can safely be continued during pregnancy unless the woman has a history of miscarriage or antepartum haemorrhage, in which case she should discuss the matter with her doctor.

Outlook
- The outlook for mother and baby depends on the cause, but is usually good provided a doctor is consulted immediately any bleeding occurs.
- Occasionally antepartum haemorrhage ends in premature labour or a still birth.

See FEMALE GENITAL SYSTEM *page 48*

ANTHRAX
A disease of farm animals that can be passed on to man. It attacks either the skin, producing deep ulcers, or the lungs, causing PNEUMONIA and, in untreated cases, eventual death. Any outbreak of the disease is brought under strict control in most countries, and anthrax in man is extremely rare.

ANTHROPOSOPHICAL MEDICINE
A philosophical theory, developed in the late 19th century, that tries to make man aware of his spiritual reality.

Anthroposophy—the name comes from two Greek words meaning 'mankind' and 'wisdom'—maintains that man has four dimensions: his physical body; his creative and imaginative capacity; his emotions and drives; and his sense of himself as an individual.

Anthroposophists reason that, in attempting to treat illness, all four dimensions should be taken into account. In their view, an anthroposophical physician should therefore have not only an orthodox medical training, but an ability to relate the physical condition of the patient to his other three dimensions.

One logical extension of this philosophy is that a 'good' physician is naturally an anthroposophist, whether he has formally studied anthroposophy or not.

ANUS
The opening at the lower end of the digestive canal through which motions are discharged. The anus is a muscular sphincter (valve) which allows control over the opening and closing of the bowels. Bleeding from the anus should always be referred to a doctor. Other problems include pain, irritation, discharge and swelling.
See SYMPTOM SORTER—ANUS PROBLEMS

ANXIETY

A state of uncertainty, worry or fear that is not only perfectly normal but is usually also a necessary part of performing any difficult task well. There are four main factors which determine when anxiety becomes a medical problem.

1. If the symptoms of anxiety are unpleasant the sufferer will want them relieved, or present them to the doctor as evidence of a serious physical disease.

2. We are usually worried by the symptoms of anxiety only because we are unable to link them with their cause. Thus, we may accept feelings of nausea or an attack of diarrhoea before a driving test or an important interview—because we see the link between the symptoms and the cause. On the other hand, we may report the same symptoms to the doctor if the cause is more distant and less easily defined, for example, a long-term but understandable anxiety about a child, money or a job. This inability to link symptoms and cause often makes us feel, quite wrongly, that we are imagining our symptoms.

3. Doctors are only beginning to understand how anxiety about everyday life can cause the physical symptoms described below. These symptoms are not imagined, but are like rocks that only show up when the tide goes out. Through the action of chemical compounds found in the brain, fatigue, boredom, ill health and worry can lower the 'tide level' of our consciousness and expose the physical symptoms of anxiety, including pain. If, for example, someone at work dies from a sudden heart attack, several anxious workmates might, unknown to each other, report unexplained palpitations, chest pains or discomfort to their doctors. Similar complaints might come from a hard-pressed housewife who has been looking after an old mother with a weak heart.

4. Anxiety and lack of understanding of the symptoms—including the fear that they are imagined—may add to a person's worries about a specific challenge in his life. The result is a vicious circle where worry about the cause of symptoms, in turn, aggravates them. Sometimes the person will realise this, and label himself a 'chronic worrier'.

All these factors confuse the way in which all of us, including medical personnel, present symptoms to the doctor.

Symptoms
- Listlessness, weakness and fatigue.
- Headaches and head pressures.
- Tenseness, nervousness and irritability.
- Depression, usually at night.
- Unexplained pains in any part of the body, but particularly in the chest, abdomen and back.
- Dizzy spells.
- Deep sighing breaths.
- Panic, or palpitations.
- Nausea, vomiting, diarrhoea and frequent passing of urine.
- Insomnia.

Duration
- The symptoms tend to come and go as long as the person has cause to be anxious—but they do not usually get progressively worse in either frequency or severity.

Causes
- There are as many causes as there are challenges which affect people. Conflicts—especially of loyalty—are particularly able to produce the symptoms of anxiety. Both doctors and patients tend to describe these challenges and conflicts loosely as 'stress'.

Complications
- Some people are especially liable to develop symptoms of anxiety over many years—the so-called chronic anxiety.

Treatment in the home
- Anyone helping to deal with long-standing anxiety symptoms in a friend or relative has the difficult task of encouraging the sufferer to undertake a maximum of productive activity and a minimum of introspection. Being over-sympathetic, on the one hand, or telling the sufferer, on the other, to pull himself together or that his symptoms are imagined, is liable to aggravate the condition, rather than improve it.

When to consult the doctor
- Symptoms which could be due to anxiety are best reported to the doctor as soon as possible—for two reasons. Firstly, they may be caused by a serious disease and not by anxiety at all. Secondly, if a doctor can reassure you early on about the cause of the symptoms, it will help to prevent the vicious circle of chronic anxiety from developing.

What the doctor may do
- Find out your medical history, and examine you in order to exclude the possibility of serious disease.
- Explore those areas of your life which involve challenge, conflict and worry. These may include sexual and family relationships, finance and jobs.
- Discuss conflicting challenges. This often helps individuals to put their worries into perspective.
- Explain the nature and causes of the symptoms of anxiety. This may help the individual to see wider problems. If this is done with understanding, the symptoms may gradually disappear.
- Prescribe a tranquilliser or beta-blocker to help break the vicious circle of worry. These drugs should never be seen as a long-term solution, however.
See MEDICINES, 17, 22.
- Send the sufferer to a psychiatrist, if the condition is extreme and is persistently preventing the sufferer from functioning normally or forming proper relationships.

Prevention
- Anxiety helps most of us to face the challenges of life successfully. Usually, all that we need to do is to recognise it and to manage our reactions to it. Perhaps the best prevention is the full enjoyment of relationships with our family and friends.

Outlook
- In a few people, the vicious circle of chronic anxiety may persist for years. The majority, however, eventually come to terms with their symptoms and manage to live relatively normal lives as they develop rewarding relationships.

See MENTAL SYSTEM *page 33*

AORTIC INCOMPETENCE

The aortic valve lies at the exit of the main pumping chamber (ventricle) and should close after each heart-beat, preventing the backflow of blood into the heart. When diseased, the valve becomes thickened and does not close adequately; blood leaks backwards and causes pressure in the heart. As well as being incompetent, the valve may be narrowed (stenosed). *See* AORTIC VALVE STENOSIS.

Symptoms
- In mild cases there are no symptoms, and the condition goes undetected.
- Shortness of breath occurs when there is a large blood leakage.

Causes
- RHEUMATIC FEVER as a child.
- Sclerosis, or hardening of the valve.
- Infection.
- Congenital abnormalities of the heart.

Treatment in the home
- Avoid exertion causing shortness of breath.

When to consult the doctor
- If undue breathlessness occurs.

What the doctor may do
- Try to treat the breathlessness with drugs.
- The diseased valve may be surgically replaced, depending upon the patient's age and general health.

Prevention
- None.

Outlook
- A slight blood leakage makes little difference to the quality and length of life of the sufferer. A larger leak may lead to heart failure, but this may be controlled by drugs. Surgical replacement of the diseased valve improves the outlook considerably, but the operation is not without risk.

See CIRCULATORY SYSTEM *page 40*

AORTIC VALVE STENOSIS

A disease of the heart valves. The aortic valve, which consists of three cusps (valve flaps), normally opens with each heartbeat to let the blood flow forward to the body. When diseased, the cusps become thick, hard and often fused. The opening is stenosed (narrowed) and obstructs the forward flow of blood, especially to the brain and coronary arteries. As well as being narrowed, the valve may be incompetent. *See* AORTIC INCOMPETENCE. Some people are born with the stenosis, it may follow infections in young people or it may develop as a result of hardening of arteries.

Symptoms
- ANGINA PECTORIS (pain across the upper part of the chest related to exertion).
- Shortness of breath.
- Dizziness, especially when standing up from a sitting or lying position.
- Fainting on exertion.

Duration
- Symptoms persist unless the condition can be treated.

Causes
- RHEUMATIC FEVER in early life, which sometimes may go unrecognised. The valves are inflamed and the three cusps become fused and rigid as years go by.
- Sclerosis (hardening) of the valves, which occurs in older people.
- The cause of congenital aortic stenosis is not known.

Treatment in the home
- Avoid too much exertion, and take care when standing suddenly from a sitting or lying position.
- Avoid becoming overweight, smoking and drinking.

When to consult the doctor
- If you get angina, shortness of breath, dizziness or fainting.
- If you know that you have aortic stenosis and there is a change in your symptoms—for example, worsening of angina or increasing shortness of breath.

What the doctor may do
- Send you for X-rays, an ECG and other tests to assess the severity of the stenosis.
- Surgery may be necessary, but if the strain on the heart is not great, then a regular check-up may be all that is required.
- Prescribe antibiotics before surgery or tooth extraction, if you have a wound or sore throat, to prevent infection and further damage to the valve.

See MEDICINES, 25.

Prevention
- *See* RHEUMATIC FEVER.

Outlook
- Stenosis discovered by chance and causing few symptoms may change very little over the years.
- Severe stenosis may lead to heart failure and shortened life expectancy. Surgery involving valve replacement, or splitting the valve in the young, may improve the outlook.

See CIRCULATORY SYSTEM *page 40*

APATHY

A state of listlessness or fatigue in which the patient appears to have lost all interest in the world about him. Apathy can manifest itself in both acute and long-standing diseases which may have either physical or psychological origin.

See SYMPTOM SORTER—APATHY

APGAR SCORE

A method of estimating the degree of asphyxia, or oxygen shortage, in a newborn baby. A score of 2, 1 or 0 is given to each of the following: the baby's colour (2 if he is pink all over, 0 if he is completely blue), type of breathing, heart rate, muscle activity and response to a stimulus in the nose. A score of 4 or less out of the maximum possible of 10 is a sign of severe asphyxia.

APOPLEXY

An alternative term for stroke—a sudden serious illness resulting from damage to the BRAIN. It may be caused by a blood clot or a haemorrhage affecting the arteries of the brain.

See STROKE

APPENDICITIS

Inflammation of the appendix (a 3-4 in. (75-100 mm.) long blind tube arising from the beginning of the large intestine). There are two kinds of appendicitis: acute, which strikes suddenly and usually requires immediate hospital admission for an operation to remove the appendix, and chronic, which may continue for months before an operation is necessary.

ACUTE APPENDICITIS
Symptoms
- These may develop over four to 48 hours.
- The first sign is usually pain that comes and goes. At first it may be felt near the navel or sometimes only in the lower right side of the abdomen.
- After a few hours there is severe constant aching in the lower right side of the abdomen, which is tender to pressure. The pain is worse on moving and may interfere with sleep.
- The patient feels sick and may vomit. There is often constipation, but sometimes the bowels may be loose or normal.
- Food and drink are usually refused.
- It may hurt to walk around or to pass urine.
- There may have been a previous similar attack of pain that subsided.
- The breath may be foul smelling.
- The temperature usually rises moderately—up to 102°F (39°C). In children, higher temperatures may be noted.

Duration
- An immediate operation is usually needed, after which patients are discharged from hospital within one or two weeks and can go back to work after three weeks.
- Sometimes the pain will stop after a few hours. But patients should never delay seeking medical help if appendicitis is suspected.

Causes
- The open end of the appendix becomes blocked by kinking, swelling inside the walls, or by a hard mass of faecal material, and infection flares up into an abscess.

Complications
- The abscess may burst, spreading the inflammation all over the abdominal cavity and causing PERITONITIS.
- Sometimes the appendix bursts and the spread of inflammation is localised to the appendix area—this is an appendix abscess.

Treatment in the home
- Let the patient lie still with a hot-water bottle to ease the discomfort.
- Do not give food or drinks—the mouth can be rinsed out with sips of water only.
- Do not give any painkilling tablets, laxatives, or any other medicines.

When to consult the doctor
- If pain has persisted for more than four hours. But call the doctor earlier if the pain gets worse, becomes continuous, or keeps the patient awake. Diagnosis of acute appendicitis is always difficult, because the symptoms are so variable, so an immediate medical opinion is essential—especially in children and the elderly.

What the doctor may do
- Send the patient to hospital immediately for observation or surgery if acute appendicitis is suspected.
- Occasionally, if the diagnosis is in doubt or the pain has cleared, the doctor may decide to observe the patient at home.

Prevention
- None.

Outlook
- With early observation, leading to early diagnosis and treatment, the outlook is excellent.
- Recurrent attacks of acute appendicitis arise if the appendix is not removed.

CHRONIC APPENDICITIS
A condition in which the patient feels bouts of vague discomfort in the right lower abdomen, often for some months, although acute appendicitis rarely develops. Often an operation is performed to see if there are other reasons for the discomfort, but rarely are any found. The appendix is usually removed and in most cases the symptoms disappear.

See DIGESTIVE SYSTEM *page 44*

APPETITE, LOSS OF
A symptom of a wide variety of diseases. The medical name for loss of appetite is anorexia. In children, especially babies, consult the doctor early. *See* CHILD CARE. In adults and teenagers loss of appetite, if it persists, may be a symptom of serious disease.
See SYMPTOM SORTER—APPETITE LOSS

ARM
Problems in the arm almost always involve the shoulder, elbow or wrist joints, or the hand, and they include pain, swelling and stiffness.
See SYMPTOM SORTER—ARM PROBLEMS

ARTERIAL THROMBOSIS

Clotting of blood in a short segment of an artery which obstructs the normal flow of the blood. The arteries of the heart, brain and leg are the most commonly affected, but any artery can be involved, *see* CORONARY THROMBOSIS. For arterial thrombosis of the leg, *see* intermittent CLAUDICATION.

Symptoms
- Sudden onset of pain, usually in a limb, when at rest.
- The affected limb is colder and paler than the other.

Causes
- Usually ATHEROMA. This is a degenerative condition which begins in early adult life and causes increasing symptoms with age.

Complications
- Even with treatment there is a high risk of gangrene of the leg, requiring amputation, and of death.

Treatment in the home
- None. Consult the doctor at once.

What the doctor may do
- Arrange urgent admission to hospital. It may be possible to remove the clot by drugs or surgery.

Prevention
- Do not smoke.
- Do not overeat and avoid being overweight. *See* ATHEROMA.

Outlook
- Prospects have improved considerably, but even if the clot can be safely removed the artery may remain diseased and may need grafting.

See CIRCULATORY SYSTEM *page 40*

ARTERITIS

Inflammation of an artery. Arteritis may occur in small arteries, such as in the fingers, or larger arteries, such as the temporal artery on the side of the head.

Symptoms
- Pain in the region of the artery.
- An artery near the surface of the body will be tender.

Duration
- The symptoms are usually relieved quickly with proper treatment, but treatment may need to be continued for months or even longer to maintain relief.

Causes
- Usually unknown.
- Sometimes arteritis is associated with other diseases. For example, RHEUMATOID ARTHRITIS.

Complications
- If untreated the artery may become thrombosed.

When to consult the doctor
- If there is pain with tenderness in a particular area that persists for longer than 12 hours and has no obvious cause.

What the doctor may do
- Look for the underlying cause of inflammation and treat with anti-inflammatory drugs. *See* MEDICINES, 37.

Outlook
- With treatment, the outlook for arteritis is good.

See CIRCULATORY SYSTEM *page 40*

ARTHRITIS
A general term for inflammation of a joint. Acute arthritis is rare and may follow injury or bacterial infection—(septic) arthritis. Chronic arthritis usually results from RHEUMATOID ARTHRITIS or the wear and tear of ageing—OSTEOARTHRITIS.

ASBESTOSIS
A lung disease caused by inhaling minute particles of asbestos fibre. It usually affects only people working in the asbestos industry.

See OCCUPATIONAL HAZARDS

ASCITES
An abnormal build up of fluid in the abdominal cavity. The abdomen swells and becomes tense and uncomfortable. There may be shortness of breath, regurgitation of food, and loss of appetite. Ascites may occur in diseases of the heart, liver, lungs or kidneys.

See DIGESTIVE SYSTEM *page 44*

ASPERGILLOSIS
A fungus infection of the lungs and airways caught from dead leaves, compost heaps, hay, and other decaying vegetation. It causes asthma and recurring chest infections, and can be diagnosed by skin or blood tests. If caught by a patient already ill with a serious malady such as leukaemia, it can be fatal.

ASPERMIA
Also called 'azoospermia'. Semen ejaculated by the male contains no sperm. If sperm numbers are low, the condition is known as 'oligospermia'. The cause may be a failure of the seminiferous tubules that form sperm, as in ORCHITIS, or a blockage of the ducts that carry the sperm.

See also INFERTILITY

Living with asthma

With properly prescribed medical treatment, and by following a few simple self-help hints, most people suffering from asthma can lead a normal or near-normal life.

☐ First, get to know your limitations and do not be afraid to admit them. If something bothers you, such as cigarette smoke, say so.

☐ Keep a diary about your asthma. Jot down when you get attacks and what brings them on. This can help you and your doctor understand the value of various types of treatment.

☐ Keep regular hours and get as much sleep as you need. You should avoid emotional and physical stress.

☐ Do not behave like an invalid, or allow your child to become one. Take as much exercise as you can cope with physically. Swimming is particularly helpful as it teaches breathing control—and usually swimming pools are free from dust and pollen.

☐ On the other hand, do not try to pretend the asthma does not exist, as you may overlook a build-up to severe illness.

☐ Always carry prescribed medication with you. You will feel more confident and be less likely to get an attack if you know you have an inhaler or tablets in your pocket or handbag.

☐ Avoid irritants where you can. Dust the bedroom regularly, and avoid woollen blankets, feather pillows or eiderdowns, and keep the mattress covered. Vacuum the room and mattress daily.

☐ Do not acquire furry or feathered pets if you have an asthmatic child. Fish are fine.

ASTHMA

Asthma involves breathing difficulties caused by narrowing of the airways. During a classic asthma attack, sufferers have a marked wheeze and visibly struggle for breath—often very alarming for onlookers as well as for the patients themselves.

Note that wheezy breathing in babies and young children is common, and although understandably worrying, does not necessarily mean they have asthma or are liable to develop it.

Asthma attacks occur when air-flow is partly obstructed: the bronchial passages of the lungs are narrowed by inflammation, mucus, or constriction of the muscles surrounding the air tubes (bronchospasm). In between attacks, breathing may be normal.

In susceptible people, attacks may be triggered by external factors (extrinsic asthma)—this is the usual pattern when asthma begins in childhood or adolescence. Sometimes attacks are due to internal factors, often unknown (intrinsic asthma)—this pattern is more likely when asthma appears in later life (late-onset asthma). This type of asthma is often much more disabling, and tends to be associated with recurring chest infections. In older people, symptoms of asthma may be confused with those of heart disease or bronchitis.

Asthma tends to run in families, and in children is often associated with ECZEMA and allergic RHINITIS. Typically a child develops eczema first, then this improves and asthma worsens. Fortunately, 75 per cent of sufferers improve during puberty; only a minority continue to have severe symptoms in adult life.

Symptoms
• Coughing, wheezing and difficulty in breathing. The main difficulty (and wheeze) is related to breathing out and not in.
• Cough with sputum may be the only symptom, particularly in children who tend to cough at night.
• Fast pulse (more than 90 beats per minute).
• Drawing in of the lower ribs on breathing in. This is especially obvious in babies and young children.

Causes
• Respiratory infections.
• ALLERGY to various substances, including the house dust mite, animal fur, feathers, pollens and foods.
• Night-time attacks in children are often due to pets, feather pillows, or house dust mites in bedding.
• Occupational exposure, as to chemicals or fumes.
• Exercise, or anxiety or other emotions.

• Some drugs, particularly aspirin and beta-blockers.

Treatment in the home
• Both a child with asthma and the family must learn to adjust to the long-term problems of recurrent asthma.
• The child must be encouraged to lead as full and normal a life as possible, yet at the same time be helped and supported to do this by parents and doctors who understand how modern drugs can be used to prevent and control attacks.

When to consult the doctor
• Mild and transient wheezy breathing occurring for the first time in a child should be reported to the doctor.
• If the wheezing causes distress.
• If there is cyanosis.
• If there is indrawing of the chest on breathing in.
• If the pulse-rate is fast (more than 90 beats per minute).
• If the wheezing continues for several days.
• In adults the doctor should be consulted if any of the above symptoms cause distress or anxiety, or in the event of a sudden severe attack.

What the doctor may do
• Assess the severity of the asthma by tests of lung function, and often teach the patient to monitor breathing capacity at home with a peak flow meter.
• Prescribe drugs to help prevent attacks and/or to treat acute attacks. Bronchodilator drugs act by relaxing the muscles around the air tubes, and steroids reduce swelling and inflammation in the air passages. Both can be taken by inhaler.
• Assess allergies, advise on means of reducing exposure and prescribe anti-allergy drugs.
• Prescribe antibiotics for respiratory infections.
• Send the patient to hospital for specialist assessment, or for admission during a severe attack.

Prevention
• Asthma cannot be prevented, but the likelihood of an attack can be reduced by taking certain precautions:
• Do not smoke.
• Keep out of dusty, smoky surroundings.
• Medicines such as cromoglycate, if taken regularly as prescribed by the doctor, may prevent asthma attacks.
See RESPIRATORY SYSTEM page 42
ALLERGY

ATAXIA
Ataxia is a symptom of many different diseases affecting the brain and spinal cord. The patient moves clumsily, and frequently loses his balance. Ataxia is treated according to its cause.
See NERVOUS SYSTEM page 34

ATHEROMA

A degeneration of the walls of the arteries. The condition is also known as atherosclerosis and arteriosclerosis. Fatty deposits develop on the artery walls, which then harden, making the arteries rigid (sclerosis). The deposits enlarge into plaques (raised circular areas), which together with the sclerosis lead to narrowing of the artery.

Atheroma begins in early adult life and increases with age. If a crack or fissure forms in a fatty plaque, a blood clot may develop inside the artery. This is an ARTERIAL THROMBOSIS, which may break away, leading to CORONARY THROMBOSIS or STROKE.

Atheroma causes no symptoms until it reaches the stage when the narrowing of an artery interferes with the circulation of the blood. Symptoms then depend on the part of the body affected.

Symptoms caused by narrowing of the artery

When the heart is affected:
• Chest pain on exertion, which is relieved by rest. *See* ANGINA.

When the brain is affected:
• Temporary disturbances of balance, vision, speech and use of limbs. *See* TRANSIENT ISCHAEMIC ATTACKS.

When the legs are affected:
• Pain in the calves when walking, which is relieved by rest. *See intermittent* CLAUDICATION.

Symptoms caused by blocking of the artery

When the heart is affected:
• Sudden onset of severe and persistent pains in the chest.

• The pain may occur during rest. *See* CORONARY THROMBOSIS.

When the brain is affected:
• Weakness, or loss of use, in arms and legs.
• Speech difficulties.
• Sometimes unconsciousness. *See* STROKE.

When the legs are affected:
• Usually sudden onset of severe pain in the affected limb, which goes cold and turns pale. *See* ARTERIAL THROMBOSIS.

Causes

The cause is still uncertain, but:
• There is a hereditary tendency.
• The risk is much greater among men than women, and increases in women after the menopause, suggesting a hormonal link.
• High blood-cholesterol levels increase the risk.

Do's and don'ts about atheroma

FOR THE OVERWEIGHT

☐ *Do* keep a strict record of everything that is eaten and drunk for seven days (only water is non-fattening).

☐ *Do* include in your diet reasonable amounts of wholemeal bread (two to four slices a day), potatoes (not cooked in fat), fruit and vegetables.

☐ *Always* eat other foods in moderation.

☐ *Don't* eat sugar, confectionery, puddings, biscuits, cakes, ice-cream or other sweet foods.

☐ *Don't* eat foods cooked in fat—use corn oil or maize oil instead.

☐ *Don't* drink alcohol or sweetened drinks.

☐ If you *must* eat something sweet, try eating a few grapes, raisins or dates, which are all rich in natural sugar.

Most people will lose weight on this diet. Those who do not should see their doctor.

FOR THOSE OF IDEAL WEIGHT

☐ *Do*, wherever possible, eat meat from animals that have fed free range (for example, wild rabbits, hares, pigeons and fish).

☐ *Do* eat plenty of potatoes, wholemeal flour, beans, peas and lentils—these provide the same amount of protein as moderate quantities of meat.

☐ *Do* include some of the following in the diet: fish, liver, kidneys, brain, green vegetables, nuts, berries.

☐ *Don't* eat more than modest amounts of meat from chickens, cows, sheep, pigs and other animals reared by man: even the lean meat of these contains a large amount of fat.

☐ *Don't* eat foods cooked in fat—use corn oil or maize oil instead.

☐ *Don't* eat food cooked with white flour, including white bread. Instead, eat wholegrain bread, oats, unpolished rice—and food cooked with wholemeal flour.

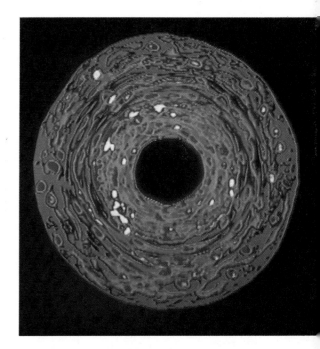

HARDENED ARTERY *The mainly red outer ring in this ultrasound scan represents the normal thickness of the artery wall. The inner circle of white-flecked purple is made up of fatty deposits which have narrowed the channel through which the blood flows.*

When to consult the doctor
- If any of the described symptoms occur.
- If there is doubt about whether exercise to help prevent atheroma can be taken.

What the doctor may do
- He will examine you to discover which artery is causing symptoms and whether it is narrowed or completely blocked.
- Perform examinations, blood tests and X-rays to assess the severity of atheroma in other arteries.
- If an artery is completely blocked, an operation may be necessary to remove the blocked portion or bypass it with part of a healthy vessel from elsewhere in the body.
- Arteries other than those treated are likely to be diseased, though they may not yet be causing symptoms. To prevent their condition worsening, the doctor will suggest the general preventive measures which are described below.
- He may test the blood in order to estimate the level of fats it contains.

Prevention
- Stop smoking. This is the most important of all preventive measures.
- Exercise regularly—at least twice a week, and hard enough to leave you out of breath and quicken your pulse. If exercise is resumed in middle age after years of inactivity, there should be a gradual build-up to strenuous activity and you should consult your doctor first.
- Some doctors believe that very low doses of aspirin—half a tablet or less every other day—help to prevent heart attacks.
- Avoid excess alcohol consumption. Small amounts may, however, have beneficial effects on blood lipids.
- Avoid overeating. Part of any excess food that is eaten is deposited as fat in the arteries. *See* WEIGHT.
- Keep to a good diet by following the recommendations on page 81.

Outlook
- The prospects for those with a specific disorder caused by atheroma, *see* **Symptoms**, page 81, are given in the entry on that disorder.

See CIRCULATORY SYSTEM *page 40*

ATHETOSIS
A rare condition of the nervous system in which the patient is unable to keep any group of muscles in one position. Particularly affected are those of the fingers, toes and tongue.
See NERVOUS SYSTEM *page 34*

ATHLETE'S FOOT

A fungus infection which is most marked between the toes and on the soles of the feet. It is known medically as tinea pedis and is a form of RINGWORM. Athlete's foot is rare in young children but becomes common in adolescents and young men who use public changing-rooms.

Symptoms
- Itching, sometimes intense, between the toes and on the soles and sides of the feet.
- The skin, especially between the fourth and little toes, becomes soggy, flaking and peeling with cracks between the skin creases.
- Small blisters and rashes occur around the toes and soles.
- The skin on the soles and heels may become covered with white scales; the underlying skin is bright red with inflammation.

Duration
- The condition persists until treated.

Causes
- Fungus infections.
- Damp, sweaty skin encourages infection.

Treatment in the home
- Wash the feet frequently and dry carefully between the toes.
- Change socks and footwear daily or more often, especially if the feet are sweaty.
- Use antifungal proprietary foot powders and creams daily. These are obtainable without prescription from a chemist.

When to consult the doctor
- If the diagnosis is uncertain. Types of ECZEMA or PSORIASIS of the foot can be confused with athlete's foot.
- If the condition does not get better after using proprietary remedies.
- If there is pain or swelling, and inflammation spreading towards the ankle. These are symptoms of bacterial infection.

What the doctor may do
- Examine a scraping from the skin of the foot under a microscope.
- Prescribe antifungal creams and antibiotics to treat bacterial infection. *See* MEDICINES, 26.
- Occasionally prescribe antifungal drugs to be taken by mouth.

Prevention
- Wear rubber or wooden sandals in public places like gymnasiums, changing-rooms and swimming-pools. The fungus infection is spread by people going barefoot.
- Keep the feet cool by wearing sandals as much as possible, and change sweaty socks and shoes after activity, periods of standing or after work.
- Use antifungal foot powders, otherwise shoes and socks will cause reinfection.

Outlook
- Treatment will clear up the skin on the foot but recurrence is likely because of reinfection from footwear and floors, and the difficulty of clearing infection from the nails. Inadequate drying between the toes and sweaty feet also increase the chance of recurrence.

See SKIN *page 52*

ATOPIC
A term used to describe an ALLERGY which produces a reaction away from the point of contact with the allergy-causing substance. For example, an allergy to certain foods can cause a skin rash.

ATRIAL FIBRILLATION

An irregular beating of the heart. The atrium is the chamber of the heart from which rhythmical contractions spread to the rest of the heart. In atrial fibrillation the contractions lose their rhythm and the heart beats irregularly. Atrial fibrillation may occur in sudden intermittent attacks, but more usually it persists once it has developed. Older people are most affected.

Symptoms
- Palpitations.
- Shortness of breath.
- Vague feeling of tiredness or being unwell.
- Sometimes there are no symptoms.

Duration
- Intermittent attacks may last minutes or hours, and they may recur over many years before becoming established.
- Persistent atrial fibrillation lasts for ever, without treatment.

Causes
- Very often no underlying cause can be found.
- Congenital deformity of the heart.
- THYROTOXICOSIS.

Complications
- Heart failure with congestion of lungs and swelling of

ankles. This will cause shortness of breath, palpitations or an irregular pulse.

- PULMONARY EMBOLISM is a frequent condition.

Treatment in the home
- Sit down and rest.

When to consult the doctor
- As soon as possible, if an irregularity of the heart rhythm is suspected.

What the doctor may do
- If the heart is still beating irregularly at the time of examination the doctor will usually be able to diagnose atrial fibrillation, which he will often confirm by an ECG, a tracing of the heart rhythm.
- If the attack has stopped, he will be unable to say for certain what caused it, and will look for an underlying cause.
- He may prescribe treatment to help the heart beat more slowly and efficiently, or send you to hospital for electric-shock treatment to the heart to stop the irregularity.
- As there is a danger of blood clots developing in the heart, anticoagulant drugs may be prescribed. In this case it will then be necessary for the patient to have regular blood checks. See MEDICINES, 10.

Prevention
- Little is known about preventing atrial fibrillation.

Outlook
- With medical treatment, atrial fibrillation can continue indefinitely without ill effect.

See CIRCULATORY SYSTEM *page 40*

ATRIAL FLUTTER

An uncommon disturbance of the normal heart rhythm in which heart-muscle contractions are stimulated at a very fast regular rate. Only a proportion of stimulations cause contractions of the heart muscle. The ratio of stimulations to contractions may be two to one or every three or four to one.

Atrial flutter is linked with degenerative heart conditions, and is consequently seen most frequently in older people.

Symptoms
- The onset of symptoms is sudden.
- Awareness of rapid heartbeat.
- Breathlessness.
- Chest pain on exertion (ANGINA PECTORIS).

Duration
- Though atrial flutter may occur in spells, it usually continues until treated.

Causes
- Myocardial infarction—the death of part of a heart muscle. See CORONARY THROMBOSIS.
- Congenital abnormalities of the heart.
- ISCHAEMIC HEART DISEASE, in which the blood supply is restricted.
- RHEUMATIC FEVER, which is characterised by scarring and inflammation of the heart.

Treatment in the home
- Remain at rest in bed or a chair until seen by a doctor.

When to consult the doctor
- If you are aware of a disturbance in the heartbeat.
- If there is undue breathlessness, or chest pain. See ANGINA PECTORIS.

What the doctor may do
- Try to slow the heartbeat if it is too fast, by pressure on one of the two carotid arteries in the neck.
- Arrange for an ECG, to reveal the nature of the disturbance.
- Send the patient to hospital for treatment by drugs, or electric shock to the heart to convert the abnormal rhythm to normal. See MEDICINES, 5.

Prevention
- This depends on the disease causing the condition. See Causes, above.

Outlook
- When an attack has stopped, drugs may be given to prevent another attack.
- Long-term outlook will be related to the disease causing the condition.

See CIRCULATORY SYSTEM *page 40*

AUTISM

The cause of this rare childhood condition, which affects boys more than girls, is unknown. From the age of a few months the autistic child does not appear to be able to relate to others but prefers to live in a world of his own, causing great distress to his parents. He resents change, and his games tend to be simple and repetitive.

Autistic children are not physically handicapped. Most of them are mentally retarded, however, and few grow up to lead a normal life.

The certain diagnosis of autism is difficult and often requires prolonged co-operation between parents and paediatricians. The parental burden of an autistic child may be considerable and once a certain diagnosis has been made, parents are advised to discuss their present and future problems fully with their family doctor and paediatrician; also parents are strongly advised to contact the *National Autistic Society*, 276 Willesden Lane, London NW2 5RB (Tel. 081-451 1114), or *The Scottish Society for Autistic Children*, 24D Barony Street, Edinburgh EH3 6NY (031-557 0474).

AUTOIMMUNE DISEASE
A disorder characterised by a fault in the body's defence system. Normally the body produces antibodies only to fight invading germs and other harmful substances. In an autoimmune disease it creates antibodies that attack its own tissues. Known autoimmune diseases include disseminated lupus erythematosus. Disorders suspected of belonging to the category include RHEUMATOID ARTHRITIS and pernicious ANAEMIA.

AUTOSUGGESTION
A technique used in psychiatry. The patient is told to keep repeating to himself a favourable idea of himself until eventually, convinced of its truth, he finds his mental state or behaviour improved.

AYURVEDA
'Knowledge of life'—the literal translation of ayurveda—is a system of sacred medicine within the Hindu religion. It was developed in India more than 2,000 years ago, and is still widely practised there. Although ayurveda uses physical treatments—for example, specially prepared medicines, controlled diets and blood-letting—it is largely based upon the rituals and metaphysical concepts of Hinduism, and it therefore appears unscientific to most Westerners.

BACH FLOWER REMEDIES
A system of treatments akin to HOMEOPATHY and HERBALISM, which uses curative properties claimed to exist in certain plants. The remedies themselves are prepared by submersing the plants in pure spring water and allowing them to stand in the sun for a few hours. The water is then diluted and given to the patient in small doses. Practitioners of the system maintain that the process transfers a 'life force' from the plant to the patient, and alleviates mental and physical disorders.

BACK PAIN

Each year in Britain about 26 million days are lost from work because of back pain. Indeed, most people probably suffer back pain at some time in their lives, but in very few cases is it a symptom of serious disease. Back pain, however agonising, is usually the result of some minor strain or injury, and nearly 75 per cent of the sufferers recover within a week and nearly 90 per cent of the remainder within a month.

The lower spine is very mobile and can bend forwards, backwards, sideways and also rotate, and most cases of back pain are due to a minor upset in these movements. Pain can also come from the muscles round the spine,

Structure of the lower back

1	First lumbar vertebra	4	Fourth lumbar vertebra	7	Coccyx
2	Second lumbar vertebra	5	Fifth lumbar vertebra	8	Sacroiliac joint
3	Third lumbar vertebra	6	Sacrum	9	Hip bone

which control the movement between the adjacent vertebrae and help the spine to bend and straighten.

This type of mechanically caused back pain is usually made worse by activity—even coughing. It is eased by rest and the patient recovers with little treatment. Mechanical back pain tends to run in families and affect certain types of individuals. In addition there is usually an obvious cause, such as unaccustomed heavy manual work, like digging the garden or moving furniture. These occasional heavy tasks should be undertaken with caution. It helps, too, to take a reasonable amount of moderate exercise each week, particularly walking and swimming. However, any sudden or unusual form of exercise should be avoided. *See* EXERCISE.

In the majority of cases treatment consists of rest, the application of heat to the affected area and the taking of painkilling drugs, such as aspirin. Muscle-relaxing drugs,

prescribed by a doctor, may also be helpful. Heat can be provided by a hot-water bottle or an electric pad. Many people obtain relief by sleeping on a firm base—either by placing the mattress on the floor or by putting a hard board under the mattress.

If back pain lasts for more than two or three days, a doctor should be consulted. Even so, countless sufferers from back pain gain little from conventional treatment and seek the help of osteopaths, masseurs and other non-medical practitioners. Sometimes these treatments give relief, and not all doctors are opposed to them. But a doctor would normally advise a spinal X-ray before any form of treatment by manipulation.

HIGH-RISK CATEGORIES
The elderly The older you are, the more likely you are to suffer back pain as joints and muscles lose their supple-

ness. The elderly are at special risk for OSTEOPOROSIS (weakening of the bones).
Previous sufferers More than half of all patients with slipped discs, seen by doctors, have had earlier attacks.
Manual workers People like miners and construction workers, who have to lift, carry and bend; typists who have to operate their machines at arm's length; and housewives making beds and carrying babies (especially lifting out of a cot) run a high risk of back trouble.
The obese The spines of overweight people often cannot support the extra stress of the abnormal loads put on them.
Tall people There is evidence that people above average height suffer more back trouble than other people.

See SKELETAL SYSTEM *page 54*
CARING FOR YOUR BACK *see over*

THE CAUSES OF BACK PAIN *Since man's remote ancestors learned to stand upright, the human race has had to contend with back pain. Several million years of evolution have not, apparently, fully adapted a spine originally designed for four-legged locomotion to our present two-legged stance. Consequently, additional stress is put on the spine—especially in the neck and lower back where the vertebrae are not supported by the rib cage. Back pain occurs most frequently and most severely in the lower back, where strained muscles and ligaments are the commonest cause. The spine is supported by a complex web of ligaments and muscles. It is never still—even breathing causes it to move as the rib cage expands and contracts—and every muscular effort, however slight, involves the spine. This is why many people stricken by back pain cannot relate its onset to any specific activity. However, unaccustomed tasks such as digging or heavy lifting are the likeliest causes. Similar activities are often responsible for a disc prolapse (slipped disc), particularly from middle age onwards. Overweight people and pregnant women are also liable to strain the sacroiliac joint, which lies between the sacrum and the ilium (hip bone), as they bend the spine backwards to compensate for more weight in front.*

Causes of back pain

Apart from sprains and minor injuries, each of the causes listed below has its own entry where you are told what to do about it.

☐ **Lower back**	☐ **Upper back**
(*common cause*)	(*common cause*)
FIBROSITIS	FIBROSITIS
KIDNEY TROUBLE	Sprains and minor injuries
MUSCLE STRAIN	
See FIRST AID *page 607*	
OSTEOARTHRITIS	☐ **Upper back**
Sprains and minor back injuries leading to SCIATICA and SLIPPED DISC	(*less-likely cause*)
	DUODENAL ULCER
	HEART DISEASE
	OSTEOCHONDRITIS
	PLEURISY
	PNEUMONIA
☐ **Lower back**	SCOLIOSIS
(*less-likely cause*)	SHINGLES
ANKYLOSING SPONDYLITIS	TUBERCULOSIS OF THE SPINE
CANCER	
COCCYDINIA	
OSTEOPOROSIS	
RHEUMATOID ARTHRITIS	

CARING FOR YOUR BACK
A self-help programme to prevent and ease back pain

The best way to avoid back trouble is to adopt a good, natural posture at all times. This means that you should neither slouch nor hold yourself rigidly erect. Women should wear flat-heeled shoes for shopping and household duties. People already suffering from back pain should never sleep on their stomachs.

Here are some examples of the wrong and right ways of holding your spine.

SLEEPING

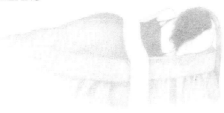

WRONG *A soft bed does not support the spine and can cause pain. Even so, many people use a 'comfortable' mattress that sags in the middle.*

RIGHT *It is essential to have a firm bed to support the spine. If you do have a soft bed, place a firm board under the mattress. Some people find it most comfortable to lie with their knees bent, and their legs partly drawn up.*

WORKING IN THE GARDEN

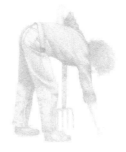

WRONG *Do not bend from the hips with straight legs to pick out weeds. This action, not digging itself, is the commonest cause of backache in the garden.*

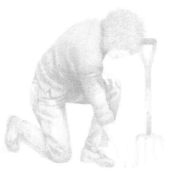

RIGHT *Do go down on one— or both knees—as close to the weeds as possible to save stretching. This applies to picking up any object, not just sorting weeds in the garden.*

SITTING AND DRIVING

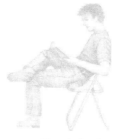

WRONG *Do not slouch or slump when seated, and do not hunch when driving or reading. Although slouching may feel more comfortable, it puts great strain on the back.*

RIGHT *Choose chairs which support the small of your back— and avoid those that are too soft or bucket-shaped. Adopt an upright position and hold the book up and away from your knees.*

LIFTING FURNITURE

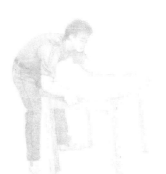

WRONG *Do not try to lift a heavy, household object—such as a table— by yourself.*

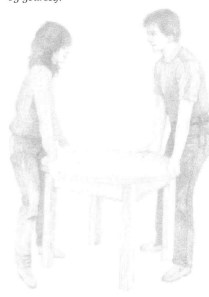

RIGHT *Find someone to help you. Bend your knees and keep your back naturally straight.*

LIFTING AN AWKWARD OBJECT

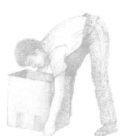

WRONG *Never stoop when lifting an object such as a tea-chest or packing-case. Lifting and handling in the wrong way are common causes of back pain.*

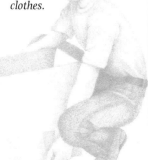

RIGHT *Squat by the object to be lifted. Keep your feet about 12 in. (300 mm.) apart. Keep close to the load and pull it into your body while carrying. Wear loose clothes.*

LIFTING A TYPEWRITER

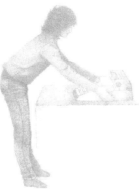

WRONG *Do not stoop to pick up a typewriter—and do not lift it with the keys towards you.*

RIGHT *Bend your knees and turn the machine so that the back, heavy end, is facing you.*

CARRYING HEAVY LOADS

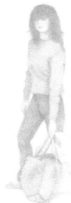

WRONG *If you have a heavy load when out shopping do not put all your purchases into one large shopping-bag—to be carried in one hand. To do so makes you lop-sided and puts strain on the spine.*

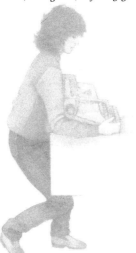

RIGHT *Carry two evenly loaded shopping-bags, one in each hand, so that you are well balanced. Do not overtire yourself and rest if necessary, putting the shopping-bags down on the ground.*

BAD BREATH
Known medically as halitosis, this common, harmless though trying disorder is usually due to poor care of the teeth and gums, or to digestive disorders. Regular cleaning of teeth, combined with regular perborate mouth washes and advice from a dentist are essential for complete cure. Individuals especially liable to bad breath must avoid foods such as onions, spicy foods or garlic.
See TEETH, CARE OF

BALANCE
Dizziness or problems with balance or staying upright often follow slight changes in posture or blood pressure. Marked disturbances may be a symptom of more serious disease.
See SYMPTOM SORTER—BALANCE PROBLEMS

BALANITIS

Inflammation between the tip of the penis glans and the foreskin.
Symptoms
• The foreskin swells and there is a discharge of pus from under the foreskin.
• There may be pain or a burning sensation in the penis when urine is passed.
Duration
• The inflammation may last for several days or weeks if not treated.
Causes
• Some cases are caused by a failure to keep the foreskin clean.
• In children with a long or irretractable foreskin, dirt or fibres of clothing may be trapped between the foreskin and glans.
• Occasionally, DIABETES may be the cause.
Treatment in the home
• Bathe the affected area.
• Avoid intercourse.
When to consult the doctor
• If the symptoms described occur.
What the doctor may do
• Ask for a urine sample and enquire about recent sexual activities. This is to exclude a sexually transmitted disease as the cause of the balanitis.
• Give advice about cleaning the penis.

- Prescribe antibiotics. *See* MEDICINES, 25.
Prevention
- Unless balanitis is caused by diabetes, good hygiene is all that is needed to prevent it in adults. It may be difficult to prevent in children with a long or irretractable foreskin.
Outlook
- Non-diabetic balanitis always clears up with treatment, but circumcision may be needed to prevent recurrence of the condition.

See MALE GENITAL SYSTEM *page 50*

BALDNESS

Loss of hair, known medically as alopecia. The most common form of baldness is 'male-pattern baldness'. This is hereditary and not caused by wearing hats, or washing and brushing the hair too much. Hair begins to thin at the temples and the crown, and thinning may show itself before the teens are over. Very rarely is all hair lost. Even in severe cases there is usually a fringe of hair left. Women sometimes start to lose their hair after the menopause, but not as severely as men.

Patches of baldness (alopecia areata) often develop between the ages of 12 and 40. In the majority of cases the hair grows back again. Thinning of hair may follow two or three months after severe illness or childbirth. Some drugs can cause loss of hair, especially anticancer drugs, and so can certain diseases such as SHINGLES, PSORIASIS and RINGWORM if they affect the scalp. Scarring causes permanent loss of hair.

Increased hair loss is natural at different times of the year, and in women is seldom an advance warning of baldness. Transient loss of hair and changes in hair texture may be noticed with menstruation, pregnancy and many general disorders.
Symptoms
- Hair loss: either generalised thinning or patchy.
Duration
- Male baldness progresses with age and cannot be reversed.
- Alopecia areata usually clears up within six to 12 months.
- Thinning of hair following illness, pregnancy or stopping the Pill rarely lasts more than six months.
- Hair lost because of drugs will grow again when the drugs are no longer taken.

- Hair will never grow again on skin that is scarred.
Causes
- It is unknown why certain conditions lead to hair loss and why some men are bald at the age of 25 and others still have a fine head of hair at 80.
Treatment in the home
- Nothing can be done to reverse male-pattern baldness, but if baldness is causing distress the possibility of a wig should be considered.
When to consult the doctor
- If patches of total hair loss develop.
- If loss of hair occurs at the same time as other symptoms of body upsets.
- If there is great fear of going bald.
What the doctor may do
- Examine the scalp with a magnifying glass.
- Examine the patient for other disorders or ask for a specialist's opinion.
- Prescribe steroid creams, or sometimes Minoxidil. *See* MEDICINES, 32.
- Occasionally advise surgical transplantation of hair follicles.
Prevention
- Baldness cannot be prevented.
Outlook
- Usually only baldness from scarring and hereditary baldness are permanent. In all other instances the hair usually grows again.

See HAIR CARE

BARBER'S RASH

An infectious rash, known medically as sycosis barbae or folliculitis, which affects the areas where facial hair grows on men.
Symptoms
- There is redness and swelling in the hair follicles (the tiny indentations out of which each hair grows).
- Shaving becomes difficult and painful, and the affected skin area is unsightly.
- In severe cases, the hair follicles contain pus which may seep out to form crusts on the face.
Duration
- Without treatment, the infection may continue for several weeks.
Causes
- Bacteria, which may be picked up from dirty towels or

unhygienic shaving equipment. The infection, once contracted, spreads from one follicle to another.
Complications
- None.
Treatment in the home
- Wash the face regularly with hot soapy water.
- If possible, stop shaving until the condition clears up. Otherwise, sterilise your shaving kit in an antiseptic solution after use. An electric shaver may be more comfortable to use than a blade.
When to consult the doctor
- If the home treatment described fails to cure the condition after three or four days.
What the doctor may do
- Prescribe an antibiotic. *See* MEDICINES, 25.
Prevention
- Practise careful hygiene in general. In particular, do not use dirty towels or other people's shaving equipment.
Outlook
- The condition usually responds very quickly to treatment, leaving no harmful after-effects.

See SKIN *page 52*

BARIUM SULPHATE
A thick white fluid that is passed into the digestive tract when it needs to be X-rayed. Barium sulphate is opaque to X-rays and so any abnormalities of the tract, such as an ulcer or growth, are shown up on the X-ray film.

For a barium swallow (to examine the gullet) or a barium meal (to investigate the stomach and/or upper intestine) the patient drinks the fluid; in a barium enema (to examine the rectum or lower intestine), it is pumped up the rectum.

BARTHOLIN'S CYST AND ABSCESS

Bartholin's glands are two lubricating glands at the back of the vulva, the external female genitals. In rare cases they become swollen and cysts form. A cyst may become infected and a painful abscess then develops.
Symptoms
- Swelling of the vulva, usually on one side.
- The swelling becomes painful and tender if there is an infection within the cyst.

- The cyst may enlarge and interfere with intercourse.
Duration
- Cysts and abscesses persist until treated.
Causes
- A blockage of one of Bartholin's glands causes a cyst. Infection of a cyst causes an abscess.
Treatment in the home
- If the swelling is painless and not interfering with sexual intercourse, immediate treatment is not necessary.
- To relieve pain, take painkillers in recommended doses.
When to consult the doctor
- Immediately, if the swelling is painful. If it is not, an appointment can be made at any time.
What the doctor may do
- Prescribe a course of antibiotics. *See* MEDICINES, 25.
- Send the patient to a gynaecologist. If an abscess is present, the gynaecologist will drain it. He may also remove the cyst.
Prevention
- There is no way of preventing the disorder.
Outlook
- Treatment usually clears up the problem.

See FEMALE GENITAL SYSTEM *page 48*

BASAL METABOLIC RATE
This is the rate of expenditure of energy by the body in a resting and fasting state; that is, the energy needed to keep the body just 'ticking over', before the needs of digestion or exercise are taken into consideration. It determines the tendency of a person to lay down fat stores in the body, and is a balance between efficient use of calories from food and expenditure of stored energy reserves. BMR is thus important in determining body weight and in the tendency to obesity, as well as in dictating the precise calorific requirements of a person in particular circumstances.

Exactly what determines an individual's BMR is unknown. Undoubtedly it is affected by heredity, by the person's age and sex, by the amount and distribution of body fat, and by thyroid hormones. The levels of food intake and activity also play a role. Women have a lower BMR than men of the same height, fatty tissue contributes less to the BMR than muscular tissue, and the BMR declines with age.

BATES METHOD
A technique intended to improve defective vision, devised by an American eye specialist. The patient is taught to relax his eyes by covering them, when closed, with the palms of the hands, and there are special exercises involving movements of the eyes or the whole head and controlled blinking.

BATTERED BABIES   *See* CHILD ABUSE

BAZIN'S DISEASE
Blue, cold, symmetrical areas of deep ulceration surrounded by raised nodules on the shins. It is also called 'erythema induratum'. It is a rare but important condition because it usually signifies active TUBERCULOSIS, and may sometimes be the only sign of the disease. It occurs most often in young women.

BCG (Bacillus-Calmette-Guerin)
The vaccination against TUBERCULOSIS, prepared from bovine tubercle bacilli of cattle.

BEDBUG
A bloodsucking insect that lives in furniture and floors by day and emerges at night. Its bite causes an itching sore which can be relieved by calamine lotion but which may become infected. Bedbugs are now rare in the West; if they are discovered, the infested room should be sprayed thoroughly with an insecticide.

BEDSORES
Painful places where the skin cracks and weeps, caused by irritation and continuous pressure on the body. Also known as pressure sores, bedsores usually occur on the buttocks, heels and elbows of bedridden patients.

See HOME NURSING

BED-WETTING
Most children become dry at night between the ages of two and three. However, about 10 per cent still wet the bed at the age of five and a smaller percentage continue to do so, on and off, for some years afterwards. Most cases have cleared up by the age of eight, but bed-wetting can occasionally extend into adulthood, when it is more likely to occur if the person has drunk too much alcohol. The most common cause is that the nervous system, which controls the working of the bladder, is slow to mature. But it may be that a child who is a heavy sleeper may fail to wake up when the bladder needs emptying, or emotional problems—for example, parents quarrelling, the arrival of a new baby or fear of the dark—may be responsible. Rarely, CYSTITIS or PYELITIS is the cause. The problem runs in families, and boys are more affected than girls.

See CHILD CARE

BEHAVIOUR, ABNORMAL
Unusual or extreme behaviour may arise in adults and occasionally in children (*see* CHILD CARE). It is often difficult to determine the exact cause.

See SYMPTOM SORTER—BEHAVIOUR, ABNORMAL, IN ADULTS

BEHCET'S SYNDROME
An inflammatory disease with oral or genital ulcers, and changes in the eyes, skin and nervous system, often accompanied by arthritis, skin disease, gastrointestinal upsets, fever and weight loss. It is common among Mediterranean peoples. Its cause is unknown and treatment uncertain, although giving steroids may help to alleviate the symptoms.

BELL'S PALSY

Inflammation of the facial nerve causing one side of the face to droop. It affects less than one person in 1,000 each year, but can occur at any age.
Symptoms
- Sudden paralysis of one side of the face, including weakness of the muscles of the forehead and eyebrows. The patient is unable to close the affected eyelids. The eye may roll up under the paralysed lid from time to time to moisten and protect it.
- The corner of the mouth on the affected side droops. The skin creases flatten out and the eye will not close properly. Food collects between the teeth and lips, and saliva may dribble from the corner of the mouth.
- There is no paralysis elsewhere in the body.
- The sense of taste on the affected side of the tongue may be impaired.
- There may be some pain or discomfort around the ear.
Duration
- Eighty per cent of patients recover within a few weeks.

Causes
• The cause of the inflammation of the facial nerve is usually unknown. In rare cases, the weakness can be caused by SHINGLES.

Complications
• Damage to the cornea of the eye.
• Permanent facial paralysis.

Treatment in the home
• Gently close the affected eye with a finger from time to time, to prevent it from becoming too dry. Do not rub the eye.

When to consult the doctor
• Within 24 hours, to confirm the diagnosis.

What the doctor may do
• Prescribe a course of steroid tablets or injections, although the effectiveness of this treatment has not yet been proven. See MEDICINES, 32.
• Arrange for testing and physiotherapy for the affected facial muscles.

Prevention
• None known.

Outlook
• Recovery is usually complete after a period of weeks.
• Occasionally muscle power on the affected side of the face does not return completely and the patient is left with some permanent weakness.

See NERVOUS SYSTEM *page 34*

BENIGN TUMOUR
A non-cancerous growth of tissue—that is, one that does not invade surrounding tissue and spread to other parts of the body. Examples of benign tumours are FIBROIDS in the womb and PAPILLOMAS in the nose.

BERYLLIOSIS
A lung disease caused by inhaling dust or fumes containing beryllium, a metal which with its compounds is used in a variety of industries, including electronics and ceramics. Sudden attacks are characterised by breathlessness at rest and coughing. They are usually short-lived and clear up of their own accord. When the disease is gradual in onset and persistent, the main symptom is breathlessness on exertion. In many cases this chronic form responds to treatment with steroid drugs, but occasionally it proves fatal.

BILHARZIASIS
A tropical disease caused by Schistosoma worms which live in the blood vessels of the bladder or intestines of human beings and animals.
See SCHISTOSOMIASIS

BILIOUS ATTACK
Strictly, biliousness describes the condition in which bile is brought up into the mouth from the stomach, but it is commonly used to describe any form of nausea or vomiting.
See ACID REGURGITATION

BIOCHEMICS
A system of medicine devised in the 19th century, in which it is believed that 12 inorganic salts—all of which are present in the human body—are essential to life and health. The system's founder reasoned that a shortage of one or more of these salts could cause a wide range of illnesses, from biliousness to sciatica, and that doses of them could therefore produce a cure.

Preparations based on the original formulae are sold throughout the world. Practitioners of the system claim to have found many more essential salts than the original 12.

The theory behind biochemics is similar to that of HOMEOPATHY, but not all homeopaths approve of the system. Orthodox doctors believe that self-treatment with the salts is not harmful, provided that the sufferer seeks qualified medical help if the symptoms persist for more than a few days.

BIOFEEDBACK

A technique in which a patient, using scientific measuring devices, can monitor bodily responses of which he would otherwise be unaware—for example, various brain rhythms, skin tension and muscle tension—and is encouraged to try to control them through relaxation or breathing exercises, or through disciplines such as YOGA.

Since the 1960s, doctors have been experimenting with biofeedback to treat MIGRAINE, INSOMNIA, circulatory ailments and psychiatric disorders, as well as to assist in childbirth.

The results suggest that biofeedback can be successful, although there are doubts about how long the benefits may last in conditions such as ANXIETY.

From a medical viewpoint, biofeedback has great appeal if it can be used to treat ailments, such as high blood pressure, which are both common and normally combated by drugs that may have unpleasant side-effects.

The American pioneer of biofeedback techniques demonstrated from 1958 onwards that people can control the 'alpha rhythms' produced by the brain and normally associated with feelings of relaxation and wellbeing.

He developed a machine which made a sound in response to alpha rhythms emitted by the operator, and found that the users could be 'trained' to increase or reduce the alpha-rhythm levels of their brains.

Many 'biofeedback machines' are now marketed commercially. Some—such as the EEG, which is widely employed in hospitals to record brain impulses—should be used only after qualified instruction or when a doctor has ruled out the presence of a serious ailment. But those that measure the resistance of the skin, as determined by the amount of perspiration present, are held to be harmless and may help in counteracting tension.

With all biofeedback equipment, the ultimate aim is to condition the patient so that the pattern it induces becomes ingrained, and the equipment itself eventually becomes unnecessary.

BIOPSY
A process in which a small piece of tissue is taken from an organ or structure of the body and examined microscopically in order to detect the presence of abnormal or diseased cells. The sample of tissue is most commonly taken by means of a hollow needle that is passed into the organ under a local anaesthetic. A biopsy may confirm or assist in the diagnosis of many diseases, but is specially important in the early detection of cancer.

BIORHYTHMS
Human behaviour is influenced by various biological cycles within the body that affect a person's moods and energy levels. Some, called circadian rhythms, from the Latin words meaning 'about a day', recur roughly every 24 hours—sleeping and wakefulness, fluctuations in body temperature and changes in the heart rate. See TRAVEL AND HOLIDAYS.

Other cycles—for example, in the pattern of waves emitted by the brain—recur much more frequently. See BIOFEEDBACK.

Therapists who have studied the 'biological clocks' within the human body believe that their knowledge can help in predicting variations in behaviour and bodily responses, and in medical treatment. Although the practical work carried out in this area of medicine has been limited, some of the results obtained suggest that it could eventually have important applications in, for example, establishing the best time of day at which drugs should be administered.

BLACK EYE

Bruising and swelling of the skin around the eye. Because of the many blood vessels and the transparency of the skin, a blow usually causes a worse bruise here than it would elsewhere.
See BRUISE

BLACKHEAD

A plug of hardened, fatty material formed in a skin pore—the outlet of a sebaceous gland—and known medically as a comedo.
See ACNE

BLACKWATER FEVER

A serious complication of malignant tertian MALARIA, in which the red blood cells are destroyed. The disease gets its name from the colour of the patient's urine which turns dark.
Symptoms
• Jaundice.
• Black or very dark urine.
• There may be severe kidney failure.
Duration
• A day or two if the attack is mild.
Causes
• The exact cause is unknown, but blackwater fever may be due to the quinine used in treating malaria since it occurs in people taking the drug.
Treatment
• Absolute rest and careful nursing are essential to ensure recovery.
• If there is kidney failure, the patient may need treatment with a kidney machine.
• Plenty of alkaline fluids should be given, and the patient may need an intravenous drip of glucose and sometimes bicarbonate of soda.
• A blood transfusion may be necessary.
• Treatment with quinine should be stopped.

See INFECTIOUS DISEASES *page 32*

BLASTOMYCOSIS

A rare, infectious disease which has two distinct forms, each caused by a different fungus. North American blastomycosis, which occurs in the USA and Africa, mainly involves the lungs but sometimes spreads to other organs, the bones and the skin. South American blastomycosis is a disease of Central and South America. It can affect the skin, lymph nodes, internal organs or all three.

BLEEDING

Any unexpected or excessive bleeding may have serious implications. Bleeding at any time during pregnancy should be reported immediately to the doctor.
See SYMPTOM SORTER—BLEEDING and BLOOD

BLEPHARITIS

An irritation and inflammation of the margins of the eyelids, usually affecting both eyes.
Symptoms
• The margins of the eyelids become red, and little crusts develop. The eyelids feel gritty and irritated.
Duration
• Even with treatment blepharitis can last for weeks or even years.
Causes
• The cause of blepharitis is not precisely known, but it is commonly associated with dandruff of the scalp and is itself a form of dandruff.
Treatment in the home
• Bathing the eyelids in a solution of tepid water and salt (1 teaspoon of salt to 1 pint of water) will clear any crusts which begin to form. Vaseline applied to the eyelids at night is helpful.
• As the condition is often associated with dandruff, washing the hair once or twice a week with a medicated shampoo (containing a tar derivative or selenium) may help to prevent the blepharitis from becoming chronic.
When to consult the doctor
• If the redness and irritation persist for more than a few days.
What the doctor may do
• The doctor will examine the eyelids with a magnifying glass.
• If blepharitis is confirmed he will probably prescribe an ointment to be massaged into the eyelid margins. He

will also advise on the treatment of dandruff of the scalp.
Prevention
• The prevention of blepharitis really lies in the prevention of dandruff, by weekly washing of the hair and using special shampoos if dandruff begins to become a problem.
Outlook
• Although blepharitis can last a long time, it is not dangerous and will not affect the eyesight.

See EYE *page 36*

BLINDNESS

Loss of sight may occur in a variety of diseases. Particular diseases affect different age groups and have different prospects for cure.
See SYMPTOM SORTER—BLINDNESS

BLISTER

A blister is a swelling formed by an accumulation of clear fluid under the skin. The fluid usually consists of serum, which is the watery component of blood. Most blisters occur singly, on an area injured by heat, sunburn, irritant substances, or friction. A blister may also result from an insect bite.

Where multiple blisters are present without external injury they may result from an infection. *See* COLD SORES (herpes simplex), SHINGLES (herpes zoster), CHICKENPOX and IMPETIGO. Multiple blisters may also indicate serious disease.

BLISTERS CAUSED BY INJURY
Symptoms
• A blister resulting from heat, skin irritants or friction usually forms within an hour of the injury occurring. A bubble of colourless fluid appears beneath the skin. It may grow in size after the irritation has stopped, and may burst if there is continued friction.
• A blister often forms after the pain of the injury has ceased. It may be painless itself, unless it bursts. In this case, a lower level of skin or raw tissue is exposed and becomes sensitive to the air. Dirt or other irritants may get in, forming an inflamed sore.
Duration
• A blister formed under the epidermis (the outer layer of skin) heals within a week. If the lower level of skin is broken or infected, healing takes longer.

Causes
- Touching any hot object, such as a stove or iron.
- Friction. For example, badly fitting shoes may raise blisters on the feet, and unaccustomed heavy manual work may produce blisters on the hand.
- Exposure to skin irritants, such as certain detergents and metals.

Complications
- If a blister bursts there is risk of infection. The blister may form an open, inflamed sore, or ULCER.

Treatment in the home
- Avoid any further friction which may cause the blister to burst.
- Do not burst the blister deliberately, unless the taut skin is causing acute discomfort. Opening the sore increases the chances of infection.
- If a blister does break, expose it to the air as much as possible in hygienic surroundings. Keep it covered with a bandage, however, where there are obvious risks of dirt getting in.

When to consult the doctor
- If a blister becomes infected, with a swollen, tender or red inflamed area spreading around it.
- If blisters occur without any obvious cause of injury.

What the doctor may do
- Prescribe antibiotics if a blister has become infected. See MEDICINES, 25.
- If blisters occur without any obvious reason, the doctor may take blood tests or remove some fluid from the blisters to check for evidence of an infection or skin disorder. He may also administer a local anaesthetic and remove a piece of skin for examination.

Prevention
- Take care when working with heat: when cooking or ironing, for example.
- Wear protective gloves for any heavy manual work to which you are not accustomed.
- Avoid badly fitting shoes, and break in new shoes with only short periods of wear. Put on thick socks to prevent chafing on a long walk.
- Initial periods of exposure to sun or ultra-violet lamps should be very short (only a few minutes) and should be increased very gradually.

Outlook
- Most blisters form only under the outer layer of skin, and heal completely with or without treatment. Occasionally, a severe blister may affect the whole thickness of the skin. It will also heal completely, but may scar.

BLISTERS FROM SKIN DISORDERS
Skin disorders which may cause blisters include ECZEMA, erythema multiforme (a rare but harmless skin disease), PEMPHIGUS and SHINGLES. The shape and distribution of the blisters vary according to the disorder. However, they are generally multiple, unlike the isolated blisters caused by burns, irritants or friction.

Symptoms
- Eczema often produces multiple blisters. They may be vesicles (small blisters) which itch and do not burst, or bullae (large, watery blisters). When vesicles affect mainly the palms and soles, the condition is known as cheiropompholyx. Occasionally, a bulla may occupy the whole of a palm or sole.
- Erythema multiforme produces many types of skin rash, including blisters and sores on the hands, lips, mouth and genitals.
- Pemphigus is a condition which produces large blisters or bullae in babies or middle-aged and elderly people.

Duration
- See under the separate entries for the disorders mentioned above.

Causes
- See under the disorders mentioned above.

Complications
- If any blister bursts it becomes susceptible to infection. An open sore, or ulcer, may form.

Treatment in the home
- Unexplained blisters cannot be properly treated until their cause is identified through medical tests. Avoid home cures; they may cause bacterial infection of the blistered area.
- To reduce the risk of infection, avoid friction which may cause blisters to burst. Wash blistered areas carefully with hot, soapy water.

When to consult the doctor
- If any blisters are found on the body without any obvious cause (such as a burn or chafing).

What the doctor may do
- Take blood and a sample of blister fluid if there is no obvious cause. Further treatment will depend on the cause (see under the disorders mentioned above).
- Recommend a skin cream, and prescribe sedatives to relieve itching and discomfort.

Prevention
- Some forms of eczema are due to allergic causes. Once the cause of the allergy is identified, prevention by avoidance or protection is often possible.

Outlook
- This depends on the nature of the disorder causing the blisters to form. In most cases, medical treatment will ease the symptoms even where no complete cure is available.

See SKIN *page 52*

BLOOD

Every cell in the body is linked by the flow of blood. As it circulates, it acts as both a transport system—carrying oxygen, vitamins and nutrients to the body's tissues—and as a defence mechanism, fighting infection. If the circulation stops, death occurs within minutes.

Blood is made up of cells floating in a pale yellowish liquid called plasma. Many specialised cells and chemicals are suspended, or floating, in the liquid while others are dissolved. If a test tube full of blood is left standing for a time, the plasma floats to the top, leaving the solid structures deposited at the bottom.

BLOOD'S COMPONENTS AND FUNCTION
Every chemical and structure in the blood has a specific function. The red blood cells, or erythrocytes, which are produced in the bone marrow, carry oxygen around the body. They contain haemoglobin, a chemical which makes blood red and takes up oxygen from the lungs and forms a compound in the blood called oxyhaemoglobin. As the blood passes through the tissues of the body, it releases the oxygen into individual cells to help generate energy. Carbon dioxide—a waste product of the chemical reaction which releases energy—is then absorbed into the blood and carried back to the lungs where it is exhaled. The heat given off during these reactions warms the blood as it circulates and is spread throughout the body, maintaining the temperature.

There are about 500 red blood cells to every white blood cell. The white blood cells, or leucocytes, form part of the body's defence mechanism. They come in five different types, most of which are produced in the bone marrow. Each type has a different function. Some engulf and digest bacteria and foreign bodies; others contain chemicals such as heparin, which prevents blood coagulation, and histamine, which responds to allergens in conditions such as hay fever and ASTHMA, and causes allergic reactions. Another type of leucocyte—the eosinophil—produces an antihistamine which, by inhibiting some of the effects of the histamine in the body, controls allergic reactions.

The blood also protects the body by its ability to clot and seal off wounds. Every cubic millimetre of blood contains about 250,000 tiny particles, or platelets. When any blood vessel is ruptured, the platelets clump together at the site of the injury. They then interact with chemicals in the plasma known as clotting factors. As a result of a series of chemical reactions, the blood is converted from a liquid to a solid state. If the blood lacks any of these clotting factors, as in the condition called haemophilia, it clots very slowly and the patient may experience prolonged bleeding after an injury.

As well as carrying oxygen and spreading heat, sealing wounds and fighting infection, the blood transports nutrients to every cell in the body. Foods are broken down by the digestive system and carried in the blood—fats as tiny globules, proteins in the form of amino acids, carbohydrates in the form of glucose, and vitamins. These provide the raw materials for the release of energy and the building and maintenance of the tissues. At the same time, the blood transports hormones—chemical messengers produced by the endocrine glands; these control many bodily functions.

After a serious accident, or during an operation, it may be necessary to give a patient a limited blood transfusion, in order to restore and maintain the volume of blood circulating in the body, which on average is about 9 pints (just over 5 litres). The body can naturally make up the loss of 1 pint but a larger loss requires emergency action. In certain diseases of the blood, such as haemolytic disease of the newborn, it may be necessary to perform an 'exchange' transfusion and change the patient's blood completely.

Transfusions direct from a donor to a recipient are performed rarely. This is because people belong to a variety of different blood groups, some of which are mutually incompatible.

Human blood is not all the same. It subdivides into four main groups which do not always mix with one another —a vital factor when blood transfusion is necessary.

The four main groups are: A, B, AB or O.

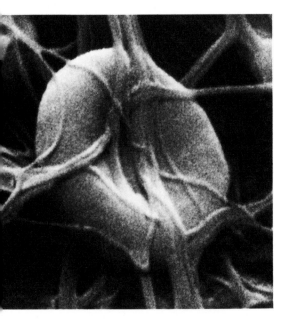

HOW BLOOD CLOTS *The blood protects the body by its ability to seal off open wounds. This is a dual process, first tiny cells called platelets clump together at the site of the injury, then red cells bind into clots. In this scanning electron micrograph, a single red blood cell—enlarged many thousands of times—is shown in the process of being drawn into a clot. The strands surrounding the blood cell, and which enmesh it in a clot, are made of material called fibrin which solidifies out of protein in the blood in reaction to injury. Fibrin first binds the red blood cells together in a jelly-like substance. Further chemical reactions take place which eliminate most of the liquid from the jelly, leaving it as a solid seal over the wound.*

Symptoms of blood diseases

Each of the possible causes listed after the symptoms below has its own entry. There it is described in detail and you are told what to do about it.

☐ **Abdominal pain**
Possible cause: sickle-cell ANAEMIA

☐ **Chest pain**
Possible cause: ANAEMIA (iron deficiency)

☐ **Diarrhoea**
Possible cause: ANAEMIA (pernicious)

☐ **Dizziness**
Possible cause: ANAEMIA (iron deficiency, pernicious or megaloblastic), GLANDULAR FEVER
Other possible cause: LYMPHOMA, HODGKIN'S DISEASE, LEUKAEMIA (acute or chronic), sickle-cell ANAEMIA

☐ **Headache, insomnia, disturbed vision**
Possible cause: ANAEMIA (iron deficiency, pernicious or megaloblastic)

☐ **Loss of appetite, indigestion**
Common cause: ANAEMIA (iron deficiency)
Other possible cause: LYMPHOMA, HODGKIN'S DISEASE, LEUKAEMIA (acute or chronic), sickle-cell ANAEMIA

☐ **Muscle pain, high temperature**
Common cause: GLANDULAR FEVER

☐ **Pallor**
Common cause: ANAEMIA

☐ **Shortage of breath on exertion**
Common cause: ANAEMIA (iron deficiency, pernicious or megaloblastic)

☐ **Sore throat**
Common cause: GLANDULAR FEVER

☐ **Sore tongue**
Common cause: ANAEMIA (iron deficiency, pernicious or megaloblastic)
Other possible cause: LEUKAEMIA (acute or chronic)

☐ **Swelling of the ankles**
Possible cause: ANAEMIA (iron deficiency)

☐ **Swelling of the glands** (lymph node enlargement)
Common cause: GLANDULAR FEVER
Other possible cause: LYMPHOMA, HODGKIN'S DISEASE, LEUKAEMIA (acute or chronic)

☐ **Tiredness**
Common cause: ANAEMIA (iron deficiency, pernicious or megaloblastic), GLANDULAR FEVER
Other possible cause: LYMPHOMA, HODGKIN'S DISEASE, LEUKAEMIA (acute or chronic), sickle-cell ANAEMIA

Forty-six per cent of people in the West are blood group O, 42 per cent group A, 9 per cent group B and 3 per cent group AB. The definition of these groups is based on the presence or absence of two chemicals, or agglutinogens, A and B. Blood group O contains neither agglutinogen.

Blood in group A contains antibodies, or agglutinates, which, if mixed, will react against the agglutinogens of blood group B. The mixture will then clot. As a result, group A blood clots if given in transfusion to a group B recipient and vice versa.

Blood group O is known as the 'universal donor blood' because it can be given in limited quantities to any recipient; blood group AB is called the 'universal recipient' because it can accept limited blood transfusions from any other group.

The following table shows which blood groups can be used in transfusion for each of the four groups:

Donor's blood group	Blood group of people from whom donor can receive blood	Blood group of people to whom donor can give blood
A	A, O	A, AB
B	B, O	B, AB
AB	A, B, AB, O	AB
O	O	A, B, AB, O

This system of classification is only one, though the most important, of many other blood group systems—among them the Rhesus system. Like the main A, B, AB and O system, the Rhesus system is based on the presence or absence of a group of agglutinogens—the RHESUS (Rh) FACTOR. Eighty-five per cent of the population has the Rhesus factor and are termed Rh-positive; the other 15 per cent lack the factor and are termed Rh-negative. Since the two groups are incompatible, they can cause reactions during blood transfusions and haemolytic disease of the new-born. All blood has therefore to be tested and matched before transfusion.

Blood for transfusion is usually stored under its different groups in blood banks. In Britain, it is given by donors through the National Blood Transfusion Service. Giving blood does not hurt and does not harm the donor. Each donor gives 500 ml (less than a pint) of blood at a time and usually gives blood three times a year. If you wish to give blood, you can find the address of the Blood Transfusion Service in your local telephone directory.

There are several hundred different blood tests. Each has been developed to test one of the many functions of the blood. For example, a measure of haemoglobin level gives information about the blood's oxygen-carrying capability while blood urea levels give information about the body's capacity to remove waste products.

BLOOD PRESSURE

A term used to mean high blood pressure—known medically as hypertension—but in fact covering pressure of blood in the blood vessels whether high or low.
See HYPERTENSION

BLOOD SYMPTOMS

Any blood in the stools, spit or urine may have serious implications.
See SYMPTOM SORTER—BLOOD and BLEEDING

BLUE BABY

A baby with blue-tinged lips and skin (cyanosis), the result of a certain type of heart disorder present from birth. Some of the baby's blood passes from one side of the heart to the other for immediate recirculation instead of first passing through the lungs to receive oxygen (which gives blood its red colour). Blue babies often have enlarged (clubbed) fingertips. They tire easily and develop slowly. The defective heart can often be corrected by surgery.
See CONGENITAL HEART DISEASE

BODY ODOUR

Body odour is normal. Every individual has a distinctive odour which is recognised by animals with a keen sense of smell. It becomes a problem only if it becomes offensive. Perspiration is the main cause. The body secretes moisture constantly through sweat glands all over its surface. The sweat itself is virtually odourless and normally evaporates quickly. Offensive smells result, not from the perspiration but from the bacteria which live on it. They accumulate especially in areas where sweat cannot evaporate freely: in the armpits, the groin and around the feet. Bathing or showering frequently is the most effective remedy.

BOIL

An example of an abscess within the skin, a boil is a raised, tender, pus-filled area on the skin caused by local bacterial infection.
See ABSCESS

BORNHOLM DISEASE

A painful virus infection that may occur in epidemic form and which mainly affects children and young adults. It gets its name from Bornholm, a Danish island in the Baltic Sea where it was first identified. It is also known as devil's grip, epidemic myalgia and pleurodynia.
Symptoms
• Sudden attacks of severe pain in the upper abdomen or chest.
• Rapid shallow breathing, with increased pain on deep breathing, laughing or yawning.
• High temperature.
• Profuse sweating.
• There may be a slight cough, but there will be no vomiting.
Incubation period
• Three to five days.
Duration
• Three to seven days.
Causes
• A virus, spread by direct contact, especially coughing and sneezing.
Complications
• As with many virus diseases, infections of the pleura, lungs, heart, brain or liver occasionally occur.
Treatment in the home
• Rest.
• Take painkilling tablets in doses recommended on the container. *See* MEDICINES, 22.
• Hold a hot-water bottle (wrapped so as to prevent burning the skin) against the most painful area to ease the pain.
When to consult the doctor
• Immediately, if there is severe chest pain or abdominal pain.
What the doctor may do
• Examine the patient to make sure he is not suffering from another illness with similar symptoms, such as pneumonia or appendicitis.
• Prescribe stronger painkillers once the diagnosis is certain.
Prevention
• Avoid contact with affected individuals.
Outlook
• Recovery is complete within a few days.
• Relapses may occur soon after apparent recovery.

See INFECTIOUS DISEASES *page 32*

BOTULISM

A serious bacterial form of food poisoning. Usual symptoms are double vision, difficulty in swallowing and extreme weakness. In about one-third of cases there may be either vomiting or diarrhoea. About 10-20 per cent of all infections are fatal within 24 hours. Botulism is extremely rare and most outbreaks result from eating food that has either been canned at home or inadequately canned. Food should never be eaten from damaged cans or from cans that are blown—that is with the ends blown outwards like the back of a spoon.

BOWEL, CANCER OF

Cancer of the colon and rectum. About 65 per cent of cases occur low down in the bowel, in the rectum and pelvic colon. Some 20 per cent occur in the transverse and descending colon (that part lying across the upper abdomen and down the left side); and the remaining 15 per cent occur on the right side, in the caecum and ascending colon. The growths may be flat or warty with surface ulceration and bleeding, or ring-like round the gut, causing constriction.

Symptoms
• Passing dark red blood, especially if mixed with the motions. Mucus or slime may be passed as well.
• Change of bowel habit: there may be constipation, a frequent urge to empty the bowels, or diarrhoea. There may be faecal incontinence as well, sometimes with painful anal spasms.
• Abdominal pain which may be a generalised ache, or localised in the left lower abdomen with feelings of distension. A severe, intermittent sharp pain may be felt if the growth is constricting the bowel.
• Unexplained anaemia, loss of weight, loss of appetite and a general feeling of ill health.

Causes
• Cancers may arise in polyps. See POLYPOSIS OF THE COLON.
• Studies comparing different countries suggest that diet may be related to cancer. The low-fibre diets of Western countries are particularly suspect.

Complications
• BOWEL OBSTRUCTION.
• Perforation and PERITONITIS.
• Spread of growth to stomach, liver and bladder.

Treatment in the home
• None advised. Seek medical advice.

When to consult the doctor
• If there is any change of bowel habits—such as constipation or diarrhoea, or the passage of blood, mucus or slime—that persists for more than 14 days. This particularly applies to people aged 35 or over.
• In the great majority of cases the changes are likely to stem from a non-malignant bowel condition (PILES may cause rectal bleeding, for example).

What the doctor may do
• Perform a rectal examination to try to determine the cause of the symptoms. He may insert a proctoscope, a short tube, to look at the bowel wall.
• Arrange for an X-ray and special investigations in hospital.
• If cancer is diagnosed, surgery is the usual form of treatment.

Prevention
• High fibre diet.

Outlook
• Good with early treatment.

See DIGESTIVE SYSTEM *page 44*

BOWEL, IRRITABLE

A disorder of bowel action, usually starting before the age of 30. It is also known as spastic colon.

Symptoms
• Some people have urgent, painless diarrhoea during or after meals, or immediately on getting up in the mornings. Other people have colicky or continuous aching pain over the lower colon (in the lower left abdomen), with periodic constipation or diarrhoea, sometimes alternately.
• Passing mucus with the stool is common.
• Tiredness, lack of concentration, anxiety and depression may occur.

Duration
• Individual episodes may last from days to months.
• Episodes may come and go for years.

Causes
• Stress, tension, anxiety or mild depression causes the bowel to react by overactivity of the muscles of the lower colon.

Treatment in the home
• Remember that it is stress, often self-imposed, that causes the symptoms, so relax and try to avoid stressful situations.

• Occupy yourself with alternative activities, especially physical exercise.
• Try bland bulk-building agents in recommended doses, or bran—1 tablespoon three times daily.

When to consult the doctor
• If you have troublesome or persistent symptoms.
• If depression or anxiety is marked.

What the doctor may do
• Give advice about diet and exercise.
• Prescribe drugs to reduce overactivity of the bowel muscle.
• Treat any anxiety or depression.
• If he has any doubt about the diagnosis, he will send you for X-rays and stool investigations.

Prevention
• Take plenty of exercise.
• Avoid stressful situations that are known to cause symptoms.

Outlook
• The tendency is usually lifelong.

See DIGESTIVE SYSTEM *page 44*

BOWEL OBSTRUCTION

A serious condition in which the bowel is blocked. The obstruction may be a mechanical one, for instance, a hernia, a twisted gut or cancer of the bowel; or it may be due to a condition known as ileus, when the natural wave-like movements of the bowel that push the food on are stopped by PERITONITIS, or following surgery.
See SYMPTOM SORTER—ABDOMINAL PAIN

BOW LEGS

Outward curving of one or both legs leaving a gap between the knees, known medically as genu varum. Many children show bow legs when they are learning to walk, but almost always grow out of them.
See CHILD CARE

BRADYCARDIA

An adult heart rate of less than 60 beats a minute. The normal rate is 60–90 beats, the average being 72–78. Bradycardia is naturally present in many athletes and other healthy, vigorous people. However, it can be caused by HEART BLOCK or JAUNDICE and may also occur during convalescence after an infectious disease—for example, INFLUENZA or PNEUMONIA. Except in cases of heart block, the rate returns to normal as the patient recovers from the disease.

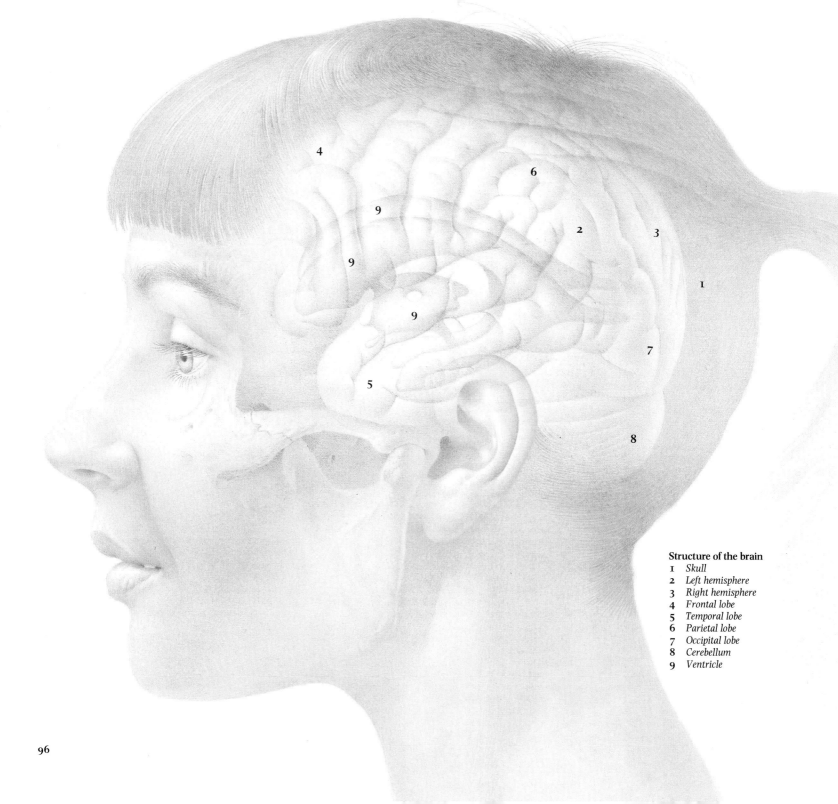

Structure of the brain
1 *Skull*
2 *Left hemisphere*
3 *Right hemisphere*
4 *Frontal lobe*
5 *Temporal lobe*
6 *Parietal lobe*
7 *Occipital lobe*
8 *Cerebellum*
9 *Ventricle*

BRAIN

LOOKING AT THE BRAIN *Inside the rigid casing formed by the bones of the skull, the brain floats in cerebrospinal fluid, which both nourishes it and cushions it against shock. The cerebrospinal fluid is contained between the layers of a protective membrane called the meninges. Seen through the skull, the most obvious feature of the brain is the grey, wrinkled, walnut-like mass of the cerebrum. This divides into two hemispheres, each of which consists of four main areas—the frontal, temporal, parietal and occipital lobes, which are divided from one another by deep grooves. The frontal lobes play a part in the control of our thought processes and emotions, the others control our senses—hearing, smell, touch and sight. At the base of the brain, just above the spinal cord, is the cerebellum, which controls balance and co-ordination. Lying at the centre of the brain are four interconnecting chambers called ventricles which secrete and store cerebrospinal fluid. On average, the brain weighs 3 lb. (1.4 kg.) in a man and 2 lb. 12 oz. (1.25 kg.) in a woman. The difference in weight appears to relate to the difference in body size between the sexes.*

The brain is the command centre of the human body and the home of the mind. Without the individual being aware of most of its activity, it co-ordinates and controls all the body's functions. It is often compared with a computer, but the largest and most sophisticated computer conceivable has only a fraction of the brain's capacity. There are about as many cells in the human brain, at least 100,000,000,000, as there are stars in the Milky Way galaxy—yet they are all housed in the skull, a container little more than the size of a quart pot.

Control of the physical activity of the body is exercised through a complex network of nerves which link all parts of the body to the brain. One set of nerves, the sensory nerves, sends signals to the brain registering sensations such as sight, smell, touch, taste. The brain acts upon this information by sending signals back down another set of nerves, the motor nerves. The signals passing to and from the brain are transmitted along the nerves by electrical impulses. Within the brain, signals between cells are passed by chemicals that carry messages from output to input terminals connected to each cell.

Anatomists divide the brain into three main parts—the hindbrain, the midbrain and the forebrain or cerebrum. Each of these is further subdivided, with each subdivision having its own specialist function.

The hindbrain, located at the base of the skull, consists of part of the brain stem (the pons and medulla oblongata) and the cerebellum. The brain stem is the connecting link with the spinal cord along which all signals to and from the brain must pass. It also controls the main automatic functions of the body, including heartbeat, breathing and consciousness. The cerebellum controls balance.

The midbrain is the small part of the brain stem that joins the hindbrain to the forebrain.

The cerebrum, the largest and most highly developed part of the brain, consists of two hemispheres which look very like the mirror-image halves of a walnut kernel. This wrinkled outer material—the so-called grey matter—is where the brain cells of the cerebrum are concentrated. In general the left hemisphere controls the right side of the body and vice versa. Deep grooves divide each hemisphere into four lobes. The temporal (side) lobes control hearing and smell. The parietal (top) lobes control touch, with precisely defined areas responsible for particular parts of the body—a single fingertip, the face, an ear lobe and so on. All aspects of vision are processed by the occipital (rear) lobes, while the frontal lobes are concerned with thought, emotion and the 'higher' mental functions associated with intelligence.

Every year, new techniques are developed which give further insight into the workings of the brain. Sophisticated machines such as the PET, NMR and CAT scanners can detect activity which appears to relate to mental processes. But, for the most part, those functions of the brain which relate to intelligence, memory, learning and personality remain hidden. For one thing, they seem to involve more than one area of the brain, and to depend on the complex circuits which connect those 100,000,000,000 cells one with another.

Brain disorder

Disorder within the complex and delicate structure of the brain arises from seven main causes:

□ **Defects at or before birth**
(such as DOWN'S SYNDROME and MENTAL SUBNORMALITY).
See NERVOUS SYSTEM *page 34*

□ **Electrical disturbance**
(such as MIGRAINE and EPILEPSY).
See NERVOUS SYSTEM *page 34*

□ **Infection**
(such as MENINGITIS and ENCEPHALITIS).
See INFECTIOUS DISEASES *page 32*

□ **Injury**
(such as CONCUSSION).
See FIRST AID *page 574*

□ **Interruption of blood supply**
(such as STROKE).
See NERVOUS SYSTEM *page 34*

□ **Tumour**
See BRAIN TUMOUR

□ **Mental disorders**
(such as SCHIZOPHRENIA and DEPRESSION).
See MENTAL SYSTEM *page 33*

BRAIN ABSCESS

An area of infection (like a boil) within the brain. The abscess forms a capsule around itself. Brain abscesses are rare.

Symptoms
- Headache, which is worse on lying down and in the mornings.
- Vomiting.
- Confusion, depression or irritability.
- Usually the temperature is raised at some stage.
- Neurological symptoms may develop (for example, there may be muscle weakness, loss of balance or partial loss of vision), depending on the position of the abscess within the brain.
- Fits.
- Symptoms are similar to those of BRAIN TUMOUR, but can usually be distinguished from it because in an abscess symptoms develop more quickly—in one to six weeks— and because there is evidence of infection (or injury) elsewhere in the body.

Duration
- Until treated.

Causes
- Fifty per cent of cases follow an attack of acute OTITIS MEDIA (an ear infection), or occur in patients with chronic otitis media or sinusitis. The infection spreads through the skull to the brain.
- Patients with certain types of congenital heart disease are more at risk.
- Infection can spread to the brain, via the bloodstream, from infection elsewhere in the body, for example from BRONCHIECTASIS.

EXPLORING THE MYSTERIES OF THE BRAIN
Mapping the functions of the brain by measuring changes in cerebral blood flow

The varying rate of blood flow in the brain relates to how hard each part of the brain is working. The pictures here show flow patterns in the left side of the brain for different activities, composed by a computer from scans taken from a number of normal subjects.

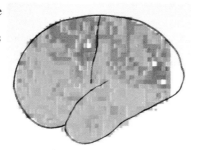

LOOKING AT A MOVING OBJECT

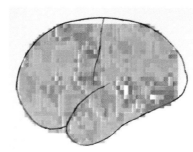

READING ALOUD

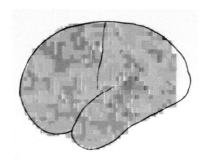

LISTENING TO WORDS

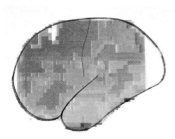

RESTING The subject is lying down with eyes closed. In all the pictures, green is average activity, orange and red more than average, and blue less than average.

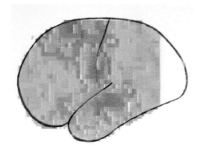

AUTOMATIC SPEECH: COUNTING

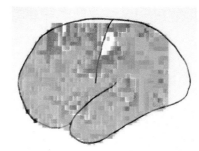

NAMING OBJECTS BY TOUCH

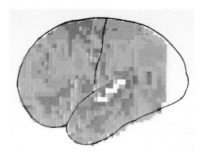

LISTENING TO MUSIC

Complications
- Permanent brain damage may occur.

Treatment in the home
- None is advised. If the condition is suspected, seek medical advice.

When to consult the doctor
- If the above symptoms occur.

What the doctor may do
- Examine the nervous system, and particularly the eye. Signs of pressure on the optic disc, seen through an ophthalmoscope, may be a clue to an abscess.
- Arrange tests in hospital. These may include brain scans and sampling of the fluid around the spinal cord (lumbar puncture).
- If an abscess is confirmed, give treatment by a course of antibiotic injections. *See* MEDICINES, 25.
- Send the patient for surgery if necessary to remove or drain the abscess.

Outlook
- Although fortunately rare, brain abscess is a serious disease. Even with modern treatment a complete cure cannot be guaranteed, and 30 per cent of survivors have lasting after-effects, such as muscle weakness, loss of balance, impaired speech or loss of vision.

See NERVOUS SYSTEM *page 34*

BRAIN TUMOUR

Because the brain is confined within the skull, which cannot expand, a growing tumour increases the pressure within the skull. Symptoms of brain tumours may result from a direct effect of the tumour on the nerves of the brain, or from the increase in pressure within the skull. They will depend upon which part of the brain is affected. Brain tumours do not spread to other parts of the body as do malignant cancers that develop elsewhere. Doctors often refer to brain tumours as 'expanding' lesions of the brain.

Symptoms
- An epileptic seizure in a person over the age of 30 may be the first symptom.
- Muscle weakness or lack of co-ordination.
- Personality changes.
- Increasing drowsiness.
- Loss of balance or loss of part of the field of vision.
- Headache and vomiting may indicate increasing pressure. The headache is worse when coughing or lying down, and may be particularly severe in the mornings.
- Tumours in children may affect the cerebellum—the area of the brain controlling co-ordination. The child will then become increasingly unsteady on his feet and have flickering eyes. Headache and the feeling of increased pressure within the skull often develop slowly in children because their skulls are slightly 'elastic'.

Duration
- Extremely variable. Many brain tumours are slow growing and their development is difficult to recognise.
- Most take from one to six months to develop, some may take several years.

Causes
- Brain tumours may arise from the nerves of the brain itself, when they are called gliomas.
- Tumours may arise from the meninges (the lining between the brain and skull, or spinal cord and vertebrae). These are usually called meningiomas.
- Cancers elsewhere in the body (particularly in the lung, breast, kidney, ovary or colon) may spread to produce a tumour or tumours in the brain. These are called 'secondary' tumours.

Complications
- Permanent brain damage.

Treatment in the home
- None.

When to consult the doctor
- If any of the above symptoms occur, or if you have headaches, and fear you may have a brain tumour.

What the doctor may do
- Check for abnormal reflexes, numbness and muscle weakness.
- An examination of the nervous system, particularly looking at the back of the eyes with an ophthalmoscope, may reveal signs of a tumour.
- Arrange skull and chest X-rays.
- More sophisticated tests such as an EEG, NMR scan or CAT scan may be advised if there is evidence of a tumour.
- Some, but not all tumours, can be removed by an operation. Some 'secondary' tumours (for example, from the kidney) may diminish or even disappear if the primary tumour is removed.

Outlook
- The outlook depends upon the type of tumour. Some can be completely removed and cause no further problems, others may be much more serious and produce rapid deterioration.
- Early diagnosis and surgery when possible, to remove the tumour, reduces the extent of local damage to the brain and nerves.

See NERVOUS SYSTEM *page 34*

BREAST
The breasts may become painful or red, or lumps may form in them. Any abnormalities, deformities or lumps should always be reported to the doctor.
See SYMPTOM SORTER—BREAST ABNORMALITIES

BREAST ABSCESS

An abscess caused by infection entering the breast through a CRACKED NIPPLE, which is usually due to breast-feeding. If the abscess is not treated, it will spread and become more painful. The condition is not common.

Symptoms
- Gradually increasing pain in the breast, eventually becoming severe.
- Part of the breast becomes tender and hard.
- The skin over the tender area may be red.
- Fever.

Duration
- With treatment, usually two to ten days.

Causes
- Bacteria entering the breast through a cracked nipple.

Treatment in the home
- Make sure the breast is well supported.
- Take painkillers in recommended doses. *See* MEDICINES, 22.

When to consult the doctor
- If there is pain or tenderness of the breast.

What the doctor may do
- Advise a woman who is breast-feeding about whether or not to continue doing so and about expressing her milk.
- Prescribe antibiotics. *See* MEDICINES, 25.
- If, as often happens, antibiotics fail to heal the abscess, minor surgery will be needed. With the patient under a general anaesthetic, a small incision (which leaves behind a barely visible scar) is made in the breast to drain off pus. Breast-feeding may then be stopped.

Prevention
- Treat cracked nipples as described in the entry on them.
- Keep the breasts clean by bathing them regularly.

Outlook
- Treatment usually clears up the abscess, but occasionally it will recur.

See FEMALE GENITAL SYSTEM *page 48*

BREAST CANCER

A malignant growth of the breast, responsible for one-fifth of all deaths from cancer in women. Women of menopausal age are particularly liable, but breast cancer is not uncommon in women under 35 years. Women who have had children are less likely to be affected than those who have not. Women with a family history of breast cancer, especially in a mother or sister, are at higher risk.

Symptoms
- A painless, usually hard lump in the breast.
- Bleeding from the nipple.
- Puckering of the skin or drawing in of the nipple.
- Ulceration on the surface of the breast.

Duration
- Death may occur within two years if the condition is not treated.

Causes
- Possibly associated with use of oral contraceptives.

Treatment in the home
- None is possible.

When to consult the doctor
- Immediately any lump in the breast is noticed.

What the doctor may do
- Send the patient to a specialist for assessment. This may involve a special breast X-ray (mammography), ultrasound scan, withdrawing fluid from a cyst with a needle, or a BIOPSY. Most breast lumps are *not* cancerous. Treatment may be by surgery or radiotherapy, or both. Nowadays removal of the whole breast (mastectomy) is rarely necessary. Most early cancers can be treated by removal of the lump alone (lumpectomy).

Prevention
- Woman aged 50 to 64 should have regular mammography X-rays of the breasts to detect early cancer. (For others, the risk of X-rays outweigh the benefit of routine mammography.)
- Regular self-examination of the breasts is reassuring, though it does not necessarily reduce risk.

Outlook
- With early treatment the outlook is good. Pregnancy should be considered only after consultation with the patient's doctor or surgeon.
- Conservation of the breast is usually possible. If mastectomy is necessary, reconstructive surgery may be carried out at the time or later. Modern artificial breasts (prostheses) are outwardly undetectable.

See FEMALE GENITAL SYSTEM *page 48*

SELF-EXAMINATION OF THE BREASTS
The early detection of possible warning signs

To check for possible signs of cancer you should become aware of your breasts, especially in everyday activities such as bathing, showering and dressing. You may spot an irregularity—from a difference in the size or shape of the breasts to over-prominent veins. Most irregularities are unlikely to mean that cancer is present, but to make absolutely sure, you should show any findings to your doctor.

LOOKING FOR POSSIBLE SIGNS

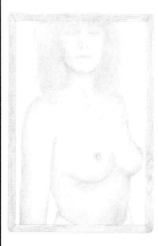

1 *Undress to the waist and stand in front of a mirror. Note the size and shape of each breast and note any existing irregularities. If you have not already done so, report these to your doctor. In future examinations look for any unusual changes or differences—such as swelling or discoloration of either breast.*

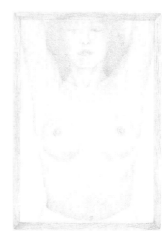

3 *Briefly stretch your arms above your head. Again, this will emphasise any difference between your breasts that has occurred during the month. You should also look for any unusual rash on the breasts or nipples and any unusually prominent veins over either breast.*

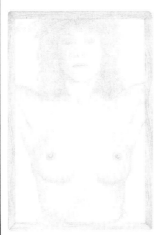

2 *Place your hands lightly on top of your head. This will emphasise any difference in size or shape between your breasts. Then concentrate on the nipples, looking for any excessive upward or outward thrust of either nipple. Look for any sign of bleeding or weeping from either nipple.*

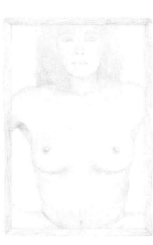

4 *Place your hands firmly on your hips and push inwards. Look at your breasts carefully while you continue pressing. This action will emphasise any puckering of the skin—or any turning in on itself of either nipple. Make sure to look at the undersides of your breasts for puckering, lifting up each breast to do so.*

FEELING FOR POSSIBLE SIGNS

When feeling for lumps or nodules you should lie on a firm surface with your head on a pillow. Place a folded towel under the shoulder on the side you are going to examine first— slightly raising it. Feel with the flat of the pads of the middle three fingers, keeping the fingers straight. Each time you feel, press the breast tissue gently but firmly towards the chest wall.

1 *Start to feel near the nipple, keeping your other arm by your side.*

2 *Move your fingers out over the breast, with a spiral motion.*

3 *Feel the bottom of the breast.*

4 *Feel the outside of the breast.*

5 *Place your other arm above your head and repeat the examination of the entire breast.*

6 *Thoroughly feel the part of the breast that extends towards the armpit.*

BREAST ENGORGEMENT

An uncomfortable filling of the breasts with milk three or fours days after the birth of a baby. Nearly all mothers experience the condition. Occasionally the breasts become so engorged that the baby is unable to suck from the nipple properly.

Symptoms
• The breasts feel tender and hard.

Treatment in the home or maternity unit
• Express a small amount of milk from the breast with the fingers, by gently squeezing the breast around the areola (the brown or pink skin surrounding the nipple). The midwife will show you how to do this.

When to consult the doctor or midwife
• If the engorged breast causes difficulties when feeding the baby.

What the doctor or midwife may do
• Examine the breasts, watch the baby feeding, show the mother how to encourage the baby to suck properly and advise on how to express milk.

Prevention
• Prevention is not possible.

See FEMALE GENITAL SYSTEM *page 48*

BREATHING DIFFICULTIES
There are three main types of breathing difficulty—shortness of breath, painful breathing and noisy breathing. Each difficulty may be a symptom of disease.
See SYMPTOM SORTER—BREATHING DIFFICULTIES

BREATHING EXERCISES
Control of the breathing to promote physical and mental wellbeing has been practised since ancient times, and forms, for example, part of the discipline of YOGA. Various modern therapists have devised their own breathing exercises, and breath control is widely used in the treatment of speech impediments and some stress-related conditions.

BRONCHIECTASIS

An increase in size of the bronchi and bronchioles—the airways of the lungs. The condition may be congenital (present at birth) but is more commonly the by-product of a disease or infection—in BRONCHITIS, for example, the area of lung tissue is reduced and the bronchi become weakened and widen as a result.

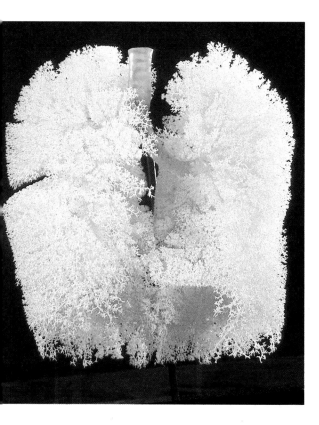

TREELIKE LUNG *The lung resembles a tree, of which the yellow trachea (windpipe) is the trunk. This trunk divides into the branches of the main bronchi, which in turn sub-divide into the twig-like bronchioles. These continue to branch until they end in clusters of minute air sacs called alveoli, which give up oxygen to tiny blood vessels and absorb carbon dioxide from them.*

Any infection in which the amount of air that reaches the lungs is reduced is likely to cause bronchiectasis—WHOOPING COUGH, PNEUMONIA, TUBERCULOSIS, as well as bronchitis are all associated with the condition. Sometimes the direct cause of the reduction of air is physical. A growth may impinge on the airway, or more commonly the airway may become blocked by a foreign body such as an inhaled peanut.

Commonly the infection of the bronchi in bronchiectasis leads to the formation of infected pus in airways and a severe cough. The bacterial infection is normally treated by antibiotics, and the pus drained through physiotherapy.

See RESPIRATORY SYSTEM *page 42*

BRONCHIOLITIS

Inflammation of the bronchioles (small air-tubes). It is an illness affecting babies under 18 months, mostly in winter. The air-tubes become filled with mucus and pus cells causing the baby to be seriously ill.

Symptoms
• The illness starts with a cough or cold; this infection then spreads down to the small air-tubes deep in the lungs.
• Shortness of breath with rapid breathing, sometimes with a wheeze, develops in a few hours.
• The baby's breathing gets more rapid and difficult, and the lower ribs and upper abdomen are sucked in with each breath taken.
• Restlessness and irritability.
• Difficulty with feeding. The baby may not even want liquids.
• The baby may look pale or even have a bluish tinge (cyanosis).

Duration
• One or two weeks.

Causes
• Many different viruses are capable of causing this serious infection in babies. Most such infections remain as a simple cold. In only a few cases does the virus spread to cause bronchiolitis.

Treatment in the home
• Keep the room temperature even. Do not let the bedroom become cold at night.
• Give frequent small feeds—liquids only if the baby refuses solids.

When to consult the doctor
- As soon as any of the above symptoms occur in any baby under 12 months.
- If there is indrawing of the ribs or rapid, noisy breathing in older babies and toddlers.

What the doctor may do
- Unless the illness is mild, he will send the child to hospital where specialist nursing and oxygen, if necessary, are available.

Outlook
- Good with full early care.

See RESPIRATORY SYSTEM *page 42*

BRONCHITIS

Inflammation of the larger air passages (bronchi) leading to the lung. There are two categories: acute and chronic.

ACUTE BRONCHITIS
Symptoms
- Wheezy breathing.
- Persistent cough.
- Phlegm which may contain pus giving it a yellow or greenish tinge.
- General upset, loss of appetite, headache, fever.

Duration
- Usually seven to 21 days. The condition is mild and self-limiting in otherwise healthy adults.

Causes
- A number of different germs, viruses and bacteria, which invade the lining of the tubes leading to the lungs and set up inflammation. The lining swells, narrowing the tubes, and the condition is made worse by the outpouring of mucus (phlegm) and other secretions. The irritation causes the cough, and the poisons cause the general upset.
- Acute bronchitis is often encountered as part of MEASLES.

Complications
- Bronchitis is more serious in babies and in the elderly because there is a greater risk of PNEUMONIA.

Treatment in the home
- Stay in bed for two or three days in a warm atmosphere (day and night).
- Take plenty of hot drinks and painkillers in recommended doses. *See* MEDICINES. 22.

When to consult the doctor
- If the illness is severe, or if the breathing becomes laboured or associated with pain in the chest.
- If the patient is elderly or a baby.

What the doctor may do
- Advise limitation of physical activity. This decreases the possibility of the infection being drawn down into the lungs and causing pneumonia.
- Prescribe antibiotics if there is a risk of pneumonia.
- Prescribe cough medicine. *See* MEDICINES, 16, 25.

Prevention
- Avoid smoking and smoky atmospheres.
- Those at special risk, such as the elderly or small babies, should not sleep in cold bedrooms and should avoid contact with people with colds or chest infections.

Outlook
- Acute bronchitis usually leaves no after-effects.

CHRONIC BRONCHITIS
This is characterised by a disorder of the lining of the bronchi. The normal mechanism that keeps the tubes clear and free from obstruction is destroyed. The tubes become narrowed. The disease is usually slowly progressive leading to destruction of the delicate air sacs of which the lungs are composed. Many of the remaining air sacs become distended (EMPHYSEMA) to fill the destroyed areas. This stops them functioning and oxygenating the blood. These changes cause obstruction to the flow of blood through the lungs, put a strain on the circulation and may lead to heart failure. It is still a common condition causing a great deal of suffering and death in the United Kingdom. It mainly strikes those over 40, men more than women, particularly those in dusty jobs.

Symptoms
- Chronic cough with spit, usually white and frothy.
- Wheezy breathing.
- Increasing breathlessness, at first experienced with mild exertion, and becoming more and more marked until it is present even at rest.
- A series of attacks of acute bronchitis.
- A general feeling of illness and ill-defined chest pain.

Causes
The causes are not fully understood, but among readily identifiable factors are:
- Air pollution, particularly by sulphur dioxide in waste gases produced by industry and where open fires are used in the home.
- Smoking increases the risk of infection and the damage done by it.

Complications
- EMPHYSEMA, HEART FAILURE, PNEUMONIA.

Treatment in the home
- Rest in a warm room.
- Avoid moving from a hot to a cold atmosphere.

When to consult the doctor
- If there is a persistent cough over a period of two or three weeks.
- If there is recurrence of a winter cough.

What the doctor may do
- Prescribe medicines to help the cough, and steam inhalations or antibiotics. *See* MEDICINES, 16, 25.

Prevention
- Keep away from smoky or dusty environments.
- Do not smoke.

Outlook
- Once the process has started it cannot be stopped, but stopping smoking slows it down.

See RESPIRATORY SYSTEM *page 42*

BRUCELLOSIS

This is chiefly a disease of cattle, pigs and goats, which is sometimes caught by humans. The disease is not very common in Britain where the type found affects cows only. It is caused by a bacterium called *Brucella abortus*, which often causes the infected cow to abort. It is also known as undulant or abortus fever. Brucellosis can be caught by people, such as farmers or vets, who are in contact with infected animals when they are calving or having a miscarriage, or by people working in slaughterhouses. It can also be caught by drinking milk straight from an infected cow without the milk first being pasteurised or sterilised. It is not likely to be caught by anyone else.

Symptoms
- Fever in recurring attacks.
- Headache.
- Sweating.
- Fatigue, weakness and lassitude.
- Joint pains.

Incubation period
- Seven to 21 days.

Duration
- Usually six weeks or longer without treatment.

Causes
- Bacteria.

Complications
- Not usually any, but very rarely the infection may affect the testes, lungs or heart.

Treatment in the home
- None.

When to consult the doctor
- If any of the symptoms appear in someone who is in contact with cattle or goats.

What the doctor may do
- Take blood tests to confirm the diagnosis.
- Prescribe a prolonged course of antibiotic tablets.
- Give a short course of injections. *See* MEDICINES, 25.

Prevention
- This depends upon eliminating the infection from cattle. Female calves can be immunised against brucellosis, but there is no necessity for human beings to be immunised.
- Farmers are obliged by law to slaughter infected cattle.
- Do not drink milk until it is pasteurised or sterilised.

Outlook
- With treatment, health should return completely to normal within a few weeks.
- Without treatment the infection may recur over many years and the affected person may feel unwell, weak and depressed over a long period of time.

See INFECTIOUS DISEASES *page 32*

BRUISE

A bruise is a discoloration in or below skin tissue. It generally results from an accidental injury. Blood leaks from damaged blood vessels, seeping into the surrounding body tissues. Some people bruise more easily than others, depending on the health of their circulation and blood vessels.

Symptoms
- The discoloration is often blue, purple or black, but fading to yellow with the passing of time.
- There may be some swelling on the site of the bruise.
- The bruise may be painful or painless. Discomfort tends to be greater if the bruise lies directly above a bone, because the congested tissues are more tightly stretched.

Duration
- Bruises fade as the blood is absorbed back into the circulation. A small bruise tends to disappear after two or three days; a more extensive one after two or three weeks. Bruises on the back of the hand due to senile purpura may last for over a month.

Causes
- A bruise is normally produced by a blow, or sharp pressure, to a part of the body. Blood spreads from damaged vessels beyond the site of the initial injury. It tends to seep downwards, responding to gravity. For

example, a bruise on the ankle may produce discoloration around the toes. A bruise on the eyebrow may result in a black eye.
- Certain blood disorders produce multiple bruises without any external cause of injury.
- In the elderly, the skin and body tissues tend to lose their elasticity and small blood vessels burst easily in the skin, this condition is called purpura.

Complications
- If a bruise is opened by a cut or scratch, there is some danger of infection entering and an ulcer forming.

Treatment in the home
- An ice pack applied immediately after the injury will help to reduce the bruising.
- Once a bruise has formed, there is little that can be done to speed its healing.

When to consult the doctor
- If pain is severe, or if there is difficulty in moving the affected part of the body 24 hours after the injury.
- If bruises occur without an external injury to account for them.

What the doctor may do
- Recommend X-rays; a severe bruise may be accompanied by damage to a bone or ligament, requiring treatment.
- Take blood tests to check for evidence of a blood disorder. Treatment will depend on the disorder in question.

Prevention
- Take all normal precautions to avoid accidents. Take particular care with elderly people to ensure that falls do not result from minor household hazards such as loose carpet edges, trailing flexes and so on. *See* SAFETY IN THE HOME.

Outlook
- All bruises can be expected to heal completely, unless some other illness is present.

See SKIN *page 52*

BUERGER'S DISEASE

Severe and progressive obliteration of the small arteries, mainly in the legs and feet, though the hands and arms are often involved. It is seen mainly in men under the age of 40 who are heavy smokers. Sections of the arteries and veins become inflamed and blocked. New blood channels develop, but the condition recurs at intervals over several years.

Symptoms
- Pain in the feet and legs which may occur at rest as well as on exertion.
- Cold feet, which may be discoloured, red or blue.
- Numbness of the feet.
- Burning, pins and needles of the feet.
- Discoloration of the feet and toes.
- Recurring bouts of inflammation and pain in leg veins (THROMBOPHLEBITIS).

Duration
- The symptoms will persist and will become worse without treatment.

Causes
- The exact cause is unknown, though the disease is almost always linked with heavy SMOKING.

Complications
- GANGRENE, which would involve amputation.

Treatment in the home
- Stop smoking.
- Reduce weight to normal.
- Take particular care of your feet. Cut toenails regularly and carefully, and wear well-fitting shoes.

When to consult the doctor
- If there are any of the above symptoms, suggesting poor circulation of the feet and legs.
- For those with established disease, when there is any sudden change in circulation, or if the skin produces ulcers, or shows discoloration.

What the doctor may do
- Arrange for an assessment of the circulation by ultrasound and X-rays.
- Give general advice, such as stop smoking.
- If gangrene has developed, or is beginning, he will suggest surgery to try to improve the circulation by cutting the nerves controlling the arteries. This is known as sympathectomy. Amputation may be necessary.

Prevention
- Stop smoking, as this is the only known factor influencing the disease.

Outlook
- Without treatment the outlook is poor. Ulcers on the toes and feet may occur, and lead eventually to gangrene that requires amputation. If smoking is abandoned, treatment usually improves the condition considerably.

See CIRCULATORY SYSTEM *page 40*
SMOKING

BULIMIA NERVOSA
Unlike ANOREXIA NERVOSA, which is characterised by self-imposed starvation, sufferers from bulimia nervosa eat

large amounts of often unhealthy food in 'binges', while at the same time wanting to be thinner. Bulimia mainly affects young women, who may be obese or of normal weight, but who tend to have low self-esteem. To compensate for a binge, the sufferer may make herself vomit, exercise intensively, abuse laxatives or starve herself.

Nutritional and psychological treatments take time but they are often helpful, particularly if the family is involved.

BUNION

A harmless swelling of the joint of the big toe. It is particularly common in middle-aged women and usually affects both feet.

Symptoms
• The joint gradually swells and the skin over it becomes hard, red and tender.
• Pressure from a shoe makes the bunion more painful.
• The big toe becomes displaced towards the other toes of the foot.

Duration
• A bunion will be permanent unless treated.

Causes
• Almost always badly fitting shoes. The feet of children, teenagers and young adults are especially at risk from such shoes because the bones of their feet are more easily deformed than those of adults, and they feel less pain from the displacement.

Treatment in the home
• Wear loose-fitting shoes and protect the bunion with felt pads, obtainable from a chemist.

When to consult the doctor
• If self-treatment fails to ease the discomfort.
• If the bunion becomes more inflamed and painful.

What the doctor may do
• Refer the patient to a hospital for an operation.
• Organise treatment by a chiropodist.

Prevention
• Always wear well-fitting shoes. This is especially important in the case of young people.
• If any swelling or inflammation begins to appear on the big-toe joint, protect it immediately with felt pads, then take extra care that shoes fit well.

Outlook
• Self-treatment, surgery or chiropody will nearly always considerably relieve or clear up the trouble.

See SKELETAL SYSTEM *page* 54

BURSITIS

A bursa is a sac containing a small amount of lubricating fluid that reduces friction where skin, a muscle or a tendon moves over bone. In bursitis, the bursa becomes inflamed and excess fluid forms in the sac and interferes with lubrication. The disorder commonly affects the kneecap (when it is known as housemaid's knee) and the elbow (student's elbow).

Symptoms
• Swelling of the affected area. It may be tender and hot.

Duration
• From a few days to many months.

Causes
• Housemaid's knee is due to excessive kneeling.
• Student's elbow is caused by keeping the elbow bent for long periods. In middle-aged people it may occur in conjunction with gout.

Treatment in the home
• Use the affected joint as little as possible. In some cases the bursitis will disappear of its own accord.

When to consult the doctor
• If the swelling persists for more than two weeks or gets bigger.
• If the bursa becomes painful, hot to the touch or interferes with activity.

What the doctor may do
• Anaesthetise the affected area and remove the excess fluid from the bursa through a fine needle.
• Inject hydrocortisone into the emptied sac in order to reduce the risk of recurrence.
• Prescribe antibiotics, in the case of infection.
• Refer the patient to a hospital, to have the bursa removed. This is a minor operation that requires only a local anaesthetic.

Prevention
• If possible, avoid activities which involve prolonged pressure on knees and elbows.
• If prolonged kneeling is unavoidable, kneel on a foam-rubber mat to reduce pressure on the knees.

Outlook
• The results of treatment are generally good.

See SKELETAL SYSTEM *page* 54

CAESAREAN SECTION
An operation, performed under an anaesthetic, to deliver a baby through the mother's abdominal wall. The abdomen and uterus are cut open and the baby eased out. A caesarean section is used when a vaginal delivery would be harmful to the baby.
See PREGNANCY

CALCIFICATION
1. The normal formation of bones from calcium phosphate.
2. Abnormal deposits of calcium salts in tissue. Calcification in joints is painful and may require surgery. In blood vessels it can cause ATHEROMA.

CALLUS

When abnormal pressure, or friction, is continually exerted on an area of skin, the skin thickens to form a callus, or callosity. The most common site is the sole of the foot, beneath a prominent bone. In nearly all cases there is an existing disorder of the foot: for example, the toes do not take their proper share of the weight borne by the foot, or the foot is turned inwards when walking.

Symptoms
• The skin of the affected area becomes hard, thick, slightly raised and insensitive.

Duration
• The callus remains for as long as the pressure continues to be exerted.

Causes
• Pressure from badly fitting shoes.

Treatment in the home
• Wear well-fitting shoes. Padding in a shoe may help to reduce pressure and pain.

When to consult the doctor
• If the calluses are causing considerable discomfort.

What the doctor may do
• Refer the patient for possible treatment of any underlying disorder of the foot.
• Refer the patient to a chiropodist who will pare away some of the thickened skin.
• Advise the patient on any means of prevention.

Prevention
• Wear well-fitting shoes, especially when young.

Outlook
• Calluses almost always clear up when properly fitting shoes are worn.

See SKELETAL SYSTEM *page* 54

CANCER

Cancer is not a single disease. It is a process that can affect any organ of the body, and each one will have different symptoms and different prospects for recovery.

Cancer is a disorder of cell growth in a part of the body.

Early warning check list

The following signs can indicate the presence of cancer at an early stage. If you notice any of these symptoms see your doctor at once, as early diagnosis increases the chance of successful treatment.

☐ Coughing up blood.

☐ Passing of blood in the urine.

☐ Passing of blood in the motions.

☐ Persisting changes in bowel habits—either constipation or loose motions.

☐ Blood-stained discharge from the vagina.

☐ Vaginal bleeding between periods, after intercourse or after menopause.

☐ Persistent cough or hoarseness.

☐ Lump in a breast.

☐ Lumps in the neck.

☐ Any change in a mole, or non-healing sores (ulcers) on the skin — especially the face and hands, which are more exposed to the sun.

☐ Unexplained persistent tiredness.

☐ Unexplained loss of weight.

☐ Unexplained indigestion.

The human body is made up of billions of microscopic cells, each with special roles and duties. Normally, each is orderly in growth and reproduction, but in cancer, cells in a part of the body become uncontrolled. They multiply rapidly and look different from normal cells under a microscope. Because of their growth they form a swelling which may become ulcerated.

Normal cells know their place in the body and remain within the limits of the organ of which they form a part. But cancer cells know no such bounds. They invade adjacent tissues and destroy them.

This excessive growth is not only in nearby tissues. Some cancer cells penetrate the blood and lymph vessels and spread to more distant organs, such as the lungs, liver, bones and lymph glands—where they establish new cancer colonies. This moving and 'settling' process is called metastasis (the transference of disease from a primary to a secondary part of the body), and the distant colonies are called metastases.

With such hectic, disordered and uncontrolled cell activity the body's energies are misused and wasted. If this continues unchecked, it will use up all of the body's reserves and result in death. But modern treatment can cure more than 30 per cent of all cancers.

WHO IS LIKELY TO GET CANCER?

Although cancers can occur at any age, the disease tends to become more likely as people grow older. From 40 onwards, the likelihood of getting cancer increases considerably. In any year only three people in every 1,000 develop the disease at 40; nine people in every 1,000 at 60; and 18 people in every 1,000 at 80.

The reason why ageing cells are more likely to become cancerous is not yet clear—although current research into the problem could provide the solution in the foreseeable future.

The areas of research include: the irritation of cells by smoking; harmful chemical reactions from certain foods; the lack of dietary fibre; the over-exposure of the skin to sun—especially in hot climates; and adverse reactions from industrial work with such materials as rubber and asbestos.

But despite this tendency to affect mainly the middle-aged and elderly, certain cancers such as leukaemia (cancer of the blood) and cancer of the brain and bone occasionally develop in children.

Cancer affects men and women almost equally, although certain organs are likely to be more affected in each sex. For example, breast cancers occur predominantly in women and lung cancers in men, who tend to smoke more than women—and who generally start smoking at an earlier age.

In Western countries such as Britain and America, one in four deaths will be from cancer, while two in four will be from heart disease and strokes, and one in four from other diseases.

Although the exact nature and causes of all cancers are still uncertain, there are clues pointing towards the causes of special cancers.

Family tendencies Despite popular belief, cancer does *not* run in families and is *not* an inherited disease. However, there are predispositions which tend to run in families and which can bring on cancer. For example, in some families there is a tendency to a rare form of bowel polyps which can turn cancerous, and which needs to be surgically treated as early as possible. There is also an incidence of lung cancer in families which smoke heavily.

High-risk occupations These occupations—which include some chemical industries and mining in poor safety conditions—predispose people to skin, bladder and lung cancers. *See* OCCUPATIONAL HAZARDS.

Chemical causes It is likely, but as yet unproven, that certain chemical properties in food, water or air can irritate some body cells and make them cancerous. The suspected dangers lie in the excessive consumption of alcohol; eating raw foods contaminated by as yet unspecified substances; the possible radioactive and chemical contamination of drinking water; and air pollution in factories or at home—which is more likely to occur in cities than in the country.

Cigarette smoking The medical world now agrees that there is a definite link between cigarette smoking and lung cancer. It is likely that the inhaled smoke from thousands of cigarettes over a period of 20–30 years in some susceptible people will irritate the cells of bronchial tubes enough for them to turn cancerous. *See* SMOKING.

Infections In some cases, infections can cause cancers in animals. Some children in Central Africa suffer from a neck cancer caused by a virus, and there may be other cancer-causing viruses responsible for some forms of LEUKAEMIA and for cancer of the neck of the womb (cervix). However, cancer is *not* infectious.

Moles and warts Most moles and warts are harmless. But some may change their shape and colour and become cancerous.

TERMS USED BY DOCTORS

As cancer is not a single disease, different terms are used in describing it. *Neoplasm* means a 'new growth' of useless cells. *Tumour* is a similar term, meaning a lumpy collection of tissue cells large enough to be seen or felt. *Malignancy* refers to the chaotic cell growth, the invasion and destruction of nearby tissues and the distant metastatic spread. Tumours and neoplasms are referred to as malignant (cancerous) or benign (non-cancerous). However, some benign tumours may later turn malignant and they are sometimes removed as a precautionary measure.

Some cancers are labelled by the cells that are involved. The group of cancers arising from the cells lining tubes, such as the gut or bronchi, or from the glands, is called *carcinoma*. And the group of cancers arising from the fibrous tissue in muscles, ligaments and bones is called *sarcoma*.

THE ORGANS MOST LIKELY TO BE AFFECTED
Of the organs of the body most affected by cancer, the stomach and bowels account for 24 per cent of the total. They are followed by the lungs (16 per cent), breast (15 per cent), bladder, kidneys and prostate gland (13 per cent), skin (9 per cent) and female organs such as the ovaries and the body and neck of the uterus (9 per cent). Other sites and types account for the remaining 14 per cent.

Today, the incidence of cancer is increasing in several organs of the body—the lungs, bowel, prostate gland, pancreas, breast, ovary and bladder.

However, the incidence is decreasing in some other organs—the stomach, mouth, lip, tongue and the neck of the womb. So far, there is no medical explanation for these changes.

SYMPTOMS AND SITES
The tell-tale symptoms of cancer depend on their primary site—and upon the effects they produce both in nearby tissues and in other, more distant, parts of the body.

A cancer will begin to produce local symptoms only when it has grown large enough to interfere with the working of an organ. These may include a troublesome and persistent cough; unaccustomed indigestion; constipation or diarrhoea; abdominal pain, and pain or difficulty in urinating. Blood or a mucous-like discharge in the faeces or urine may occur if bowel or bladder cancer has grown large enough to become ulcerated on the surface. In cases where a cancer is near the surface—as on the skin, breast or other organs—it may be felt as an obvious lump, which may later ulcerate.

Women should examine their breasts for lumps at least once a month. See BREAST CANCER.

In the earliest stages, cancer has no general symptoms; but later there may be symptoms such as loss of appetite, loss of weight and an apparently undue amount of tiredness.

Other symptoms may include pain (which is not usually an early symptom), jaundice, extreme changes of mood and mental attitude, and epileptic-type fits.

HOW CANCER IS DETECTED AND EXAMINED
Although there is no reliable medical check-up test that will reveal all cancers in their earliest stages, regular check-ups can still be of positive value. A doctor can examine any breast lumps and have them diagnosed. X-rays can be taken of the breasts and lungs to determine if they are cancerous. A check can be made on microscopic specks of blood in faeces. Urine and sputum samples can be analysed to see if cancer is present. And a cervical smear—taken every three years, or more regularly if advised—can ascertain the presence or otherwise of cancer at the neck of the womb.

When suspicions are aroused, a search is made for the site of the possible cancer. If a cancer is located, a portion of it is removed for a BIOPSY, an examination of living tissues—in this case for cancer cells. X-rays are taken of possibly affected organs; computers are used for diagnosis and analysis; and radioactive drugs and dyes show up any cancerous growths—provided they are large enough to be visible.

AVAILABLE FORMS OF TREATMENT
The aim of medical treatment is to remove or destroy the primary site of a cancer before it spreads to other sites—which are sometimes called secondary deposits as well as metastases.

Because the exact nature and causes of cancer are unknown, there is no single group of effective drugs that can be used against it—as, for example, antibiotics in the treatment of infection. Treatments for cancer are still rather crude in their attacks on the growths. The treatments are:

Surgical removal This involves cutting out the growth at the primary site, together with any adjacent tissues and local lymph gland to which the growth may have spread. This is possible, for example, with the breast, bowel, lungs, kidneys, testes, womb, ovary, bones and skin.

The surgeon can see and feel the bulky tumour; but he cannot tell how far the microscopic cancer cells may have spread. He can only hope to remove the growth before any large-scale spreading occurs, and then to kill off any few remaining cells by radiotherapy or chemotherapy. The results of surgery are generally good.

Radiotherapy X-rays and other forms of radioactivity are used to destroy cancer cells and leave normal cells undamaged. The treatment is based on the fact that abnormal and rapidly growing cancer cells are susceptible to low levels of radioactivity, and normal, more stable cells are not.

In some extensive cases of skin or breast cancer, radiotherapy may be the only practical treatment. It may also be used as a follow-up to surgery or chemotherapy.

The treatment requires precise calculations and expertise in the use of the potentially dangerous radiotherapy machines.

Chemotherapy There are certain drugs that destroy cancer cells without damaging normal cells. They are called cytotoxics (poisonous to cells). Excessive dosages, however, will also destroy normal cells and kill the patient, and so the drugs—which are taken in capsule form by mouth or by injection or drips—must be employed with great care.

Cytotoxics have been dramatically successful in curing cancers such as HODGKIN'S DISEASE (which mainly affects the lymph nodes and spleen), some forms of LEUKAEMIA, and certain rare cancers of the male and female genitals. Even when a complete cure has not been possible, they have been helpful in relieving pain and other distressing symptoms.

Unorthodox treatments There are also a number of unorthodox techniques including homeopathy (in which a disease is treated with minute doses of drugs that, in a healthy person, would produce symptoms similar to those of the disease); naturopathy (in which no drugs at all are used and cures are based upon diet and exercise); and faith-healing (in which illnesses are cured by the power of suggestion). People sometimes turn to fringe medicine when all other hope has been extinguished. Despite occasional reports of 'miracle cures', the non-traditional treatments are not repeatable for other cases, and their success has not been proved by scientifically organised trials.

On rare occasions, the body overcomes and destroys cancer without medical help. Most doctors have experienced such an inexplicable phenomenon at least once in their careers, and it reinforces the growing view that cancer—though still a deadly affliction—is not the 'unbeatable opponent' it was once thought to be.

Whatever the treatment used, it works best if given at the earliest possible stage—before any extensive spreading has taken place. This emphasises the importance of having regular check-ups and screenings—and so catching any cancers in their early stages.

Check-ups can be done for cancer of the lungs, breast, bowel, cervix, testes, skin, bladder and blood (leukaemia). Regular tests are also made for the possibility of cancerous cells in the urine and phlegm. Anyone who smokes should have a chest X-ray if he develops persistent chest symptoms.

THE INCREASE IN CURES
Today, with advancing medical knowledge and skill, cancer no longer means an inevitable death sentence. One in every three cancers results in the patient being

alive five years or more after treatment (the current definition of a cure). A growing degree of optimism is justified.

Some cancers are more curable and controllable than others. In the United Kingdom those with the highest success rates are:

Skin cancers: a nine in ten chance of cure;
Womb cancers: almost a one in two chance of cure;
Bladder cancers: just under one in two chance of cure;
Breast cancer: a one in three chance of cure;
Blood cancers: (such as leukaemia and Hodgkin's disease): a one in three chance of cure;
Prostate cancers: a one in four chance of cure;
Bowel cancers: a one in four chance of cure.

In 1981 doctors with the Imperial Cancer Research Fund in London announced improvements in the treatment of several kinds of cancer—especially those affecting children. The new treatments, together with better drug therapy, mean that 75 per cent of children with leukaemia now survive—compared with only 10 per cent ten years ago. However, several cancers—of the lung, brain, bone, stomach, pancreas, gall-bladder and kidneys—still have very low success rates and the research for possible cures continues.

CARE OF TERMINAL PATIENTS
Even though many people with cancer die, much can be done to make the final stages as peaceful and comfortable as possible. Drugs and skilled nursing can control symptoms such as pain, vomiting, incontinence, sleep difficulties and bowel problems.

A positive approach is now taken with terminal patients. They are encouraged to lead as normal a life as possible for as long as possible, and some patients are able to spend their last days at home. They are cared for by a doctor, nurse, home help and social workers—and they receive the comfort and support of their family and friends. But if such care is not possible, hospitals and hospices—nursing homes with special skills in caring for terminal cases—will take charge of the patients.

PREVENTION OF CANCER
Prevention of cancer is very much in the hands of the individual. There are certain 'do's and don'ts' which can be practised and which could greatly lessen the chances of contracting the disease in its various forms.

For instance, giving up smoking will reduce the risk of lung cancer. A high-fibre diet will supply plenty of roughage and so decrease the likelihood of cancer of the bowel. (In fact, some experts believe 'bland' foods such as dairy products can actually encourage cancer.)

Everyone should be on the look-out for any symptoms

—from unexplained loss of weight to enlarging moles— that could indicate cancer. Any such symptoms should immediately be reported to a doctor, and the golden rule is: if in doubt, find out.

See also BOWEL CANCER
BREAST CANCER
CERVICAL CANCER
LUNG CANCER
PANCREAS, CANCER OF
SKIN CANCER
STOMACH CANCER

CARBUNCLE
A cluster of boils that most commonly occurs on the back of the neck. A carbuncle is a more serious disorder than a single boil.
See ABSCESS

CARDIOMYOPATHY

A group of disorders of the heart muscle which leads to progressive weakness of the heart, disturbance of rhythm and eventual heart failure. The coronary arteries are usually normal. People of all ages, including children, may be affected.
Symptoms
• Shortness of breath.
• Cough.
• Angina.
Duration
• Cardiomyopathy is a progressive disease, usually lasting some years.
Causes
• The cause of cardiomyopathy is not usually known, though some types have a hereditary basis, and some are associated with other diseases.
• Alcohol.
When to consult the doctor
• If there is unexplained shortness of breath, a cough, or if physical exertion brings on ANGINA.
What the doctor may do
• The doctor will treat the symptoms with a variety of drugs. He will also send you for special tests to determine the precise nature of the disorder. These may include giving an anaesthetic to take a specimen of heart muscle for microscopic examination.

• A heart operation may sometimes be necessary to alleviate symptoms.
Prevention
• When there is a family history of heart-muscle disease or when there is an abnormality known to have a hereditary basis, the risks should be understood by those contemplating parenthood.
Outlook
• Once symptoms have developed, the disease is likely to be well advanced, but with treatment it may be controlled for many years. The outlook depends on the type of cardiomyopathy.

See CIRCULATORY SYSTEM *page 40*

CARPAL TUNNEL SYNDROME

A condition in which one of the nerves leading from the wrist to the hand is compressed as it passes through the carpal tunnel, a space in the wrist through which tendons that flex the fingers also pass. The pressure causes pain and loss of some use of the hand. Severe cases can lead to wasting and weakness of the small muscles at the base of the thumb. The disorder mainly affects middle-aged and elderly women, especially those who use their fingers a lot, such as typists, housewives or pianists.
Symptoms
• Pain, tingling and numbness in the thumb, index finger and middle finger of the affected hand. The pain tends to be worse at night or when very warm.
• Pain and tingling may spread up the forearm.
• Clumsiness when attempting fine work, such as sewing.
Duration
• Symptoms may get progressively worse over a period of weeks, months or years.
• The disorder lasts until a minor operation is carried out to cure it.
Causes
• A gradual thickening of the tendons that pass through the carpal tunnel. The thickened tendons press on the nerve.
• Reduction of the space in the tunnel as the result of other conditions, including OSTEOARTHRITIS of the wrist, MYXOEDEMA, RHEUMATOID ARTHRITIS and PREGNANCY.

Treatment in the home
- Try to avoid movements that cause pain.
- Pain at night can be relieved by hanging the arm out of the bed.

When to consult the doctor
- As soon as symptoms develop.

What the doctor may do
- Prescribe painkilling tablets. *See* MEDICINES, 22.
- Inject cortisone into the wrist. *See* MEDICINES, 32.
- Examine the hands and, if he suspects carpal tunnel syndrome, refer the patient to a hospital. There a simple operation will relieve the pressure on the nerve.

Prevention
- None.

Outlook
- Good. The result of the operation is generally satisfactory.

See SKELETAL SYSTEM *page 54*

CAR SICKNESS

Nausea and vomiting suffered by many people when travelling by car. The movement of the car causes an upset between what the person's eyes see and what his balance mechanism feels, and so signals from eye and ear do not agree.

See MOTION SICKNESS

CARTILAGE, TORN

A knee injury in which a sudden twisting movement tears one of the cartilages—two firm, elastic shock absorbers that lie between the ends of the bones in the knee joint. The tear is commonly sustained by sportsmen, particularly footballers and people who work in a squatting position—for example, miners.

Symptoms
- Pain in the knee following an abrupt twist of the joint.
- Swelling of the knee.
- Sometimes locking of the knee so that it cannot straighten fully.

Causes
- Twisting of the knee when the joint is bent and the lower leg is fixed firmly on the ground.

Duration
- Unless the torn cartilage is removed, the knee is susceptible to further disabling injuries.

Treatment in the home
- Keep weight off the affected knee.

When to consult the doctor
- Immediately symptoms develop.

What the doctor may do
- Advise resting the knee.
- Refer the patient to hospital for an operation to remove the torn cartilage.

Outlook
- The knee generally recovers satisfactorily, but a sportsman's ability may be affected.
- Ten to 20 years after the injury OSTEOARTHRITIS may develop in the knee.

See SKELETAL SYSTEM *page 54*

CATAPLEXY

A sudden collapse of posture provoked by excitement.

Symptoms
- The head slumps forward, the jaw drops and the knees buckle. The patient may fall to the ground, but remains conscious throughout.

Duration
- Attacks may last up to two minutes.

Causes
- An attack may be provoked by any strong emotion, such as gaiety, sadness or anger. A disturbance occurs in the part of the brain which controls the muscles. The condition occurs most often in people who suffer from NARCOLEPSY.

Complications
- None, unless an accident should occur as a result of the collapse.

Treatment in the home
- None advised.

When to consult the doctor
- If an attack occurs.

What the doctor may do
- Arrange hospital tests to check diagnosis.
- Prescribe drugs to reduce the frequency of attacks.

Outlook
- Cataplexy is a minor disorder. There is no complete cure. A sufferer usually experiences his or her first attacks during adolescence, and they are likely to persist throughout life.

See NERVOUS SYSTEM *page 34*

CATARACT

A painless misting of the lens of the eye. Cataract often affects both eyes, though usually one more than the other. Most people over the age of 65 have some degree of cataract, but in the majority of cases it causes little or no inconvenience.

Symptoms
- The vision, especially distant vision, becomes hazy or foggy, usually in one eye more than the other. Close work, such as reading or sewing, is usually at first little affected.

Duration
- Cataracts will last until they are surgically removed. They cannot be cured by drops, tablets or spectacles and they will not disappear naturally. Some develop so slowly that they cause little visual difficulty until the patient reaches the age of 80 or 90. Others develop steadily but slowly, and a few, for no known reason, get rapidly worse over a period of a few months.

Causes
- The commonest cause is advancing years. The blood supply which nourishes the lens becomes less efficient and the lens loses its transparency and becomes opaque.
- Other causes of cataract are diabetes and, rarely, the secondary effects of some eye diseases, for example iritis, glaucoma or detached retina.

Treatment in the home
- There are no simple treatments for cataract other than surgery, and this is better carried out late than early. This is because while it is possible to retain useful and comfortable vision even if one eye has a lens which is quite blind with cataract, it is uncomfortable and difficult to use the two eyes together when one has a lens in and the other does not. The time for treatment comes when the vision in the better eye deteriorates to the extent that normal activities and enjoyment are interfered with.

When to consult the doctor
- If you have any difficulty in seeing.

What the doctor may do
- Test your vision by asking you to look with each eye in turn at a card with lines of letters or figures of different sizes, to find out how small a line of print you can read with each eye, with or without spectacles. Examine your eyes with an ophthalmoscope.
- If you have cataracts but the vision with one eye is still quite good, the doctor may say that nothing needs to be done and ask you to return if you notice the vision in the 'good' eye getting worse, or arrange a check in six

months or a year. He may refer you to an eye specialist, who may also advise you to wait, or return from time to time to review the situation.

• If the vision in the better eye is bad enough to interfere with your way of life, the eye specialist will probably suggest an operation to remove the cataract. An artificial lens may be implanted at the same time, or special spectacles or contact lenses may be worn after the operation.

Prevention

• Generally, cataracts cannot be prevented, but if diabetic patients allow their diabetes to get out of control they may hasten the development of eye complications.

Outlook

• Although cataracts usually occur as you get older, only 15 patients out of every 1,000 over the age of 75 need to see a doctor about them, and only a few of these need an operation. When an operation is performed the results are generally excellent.

See EYE *page 36*

CATARRH

A widely used general term referring to the discharge of mucus, usually from the nasal sinuses, and the air passages in the nose and throat.

See SYMPTOM SORTER—CATARRH

CATHETER

A thin flexible tube that can be inserted into the opening of an organ, most commonly the bladder and the heart. A catheter is introduced into the bladder to enable urine to be passed when a disorder prevents this. A heart catheter is inserted into an artery or vein in the leg or arm and then passed up into the heart. There it records the heart's blood pressure and can withdraw blood for analysis.

CAT-SCRATCH FEVER

A rare disease affecting all the systems of the body. It may follow superficial damage to the skin from a cat bite or a scratch from a cat or a thorn.

Symptoms

• A few days after the scratch a small blister containing pus develops on the site of the injury.

• Between two to six weeks after the injury the site becomes painful and swollen.

• Lymph glands that drain the site of the injury may become inflamed and swollen with pus, sometimes with serious abscesses.

• There may be a slight increase in temperature, with headaches, chills, tiredness and a general feeling of ill health.

• Sometimes a rash appears on the hands and feet.

Duration

• The disease can last from two weeks to several months. If serious abscesses develop in the lymph glands, a long period of convalescence may be necessary.

Causes

• Cat-scratch fever is thought to be caused by a specific virus.

Treatment in the home

• Follow normal home treatment for a fever—rest in bed, a light diet and large quantities of fluid.

When to consult the doctor

• If a pus-filled blister develops on the site of the injury and becomes painful and swollen.

What the doctor may do

• As cat-scratch fever is not a condition that can normally be diagnosed by the family doctor, he will send the patient to hospital for tests.

• At the hospital, the doctor may take a sample of tissue from the blister for examination under a microscope in the laboratory.

• It may become necessary to drain any abscesses that form in the lymph glands.

Outlook

• Cat-scratch fever usually clears up spontaneously, within four weeks.

See INFECTIOUS DISEASES *page 32*

CAULIFLOWER EAR

An enlarged and deformed ear-flap caused by injury. Boxers and rugby players are particularly prone to the injury. Although damage to the flap itself may be severe, hearing will not be lost.

See EAR INJURY

CAUSALGIA

Intense, continuing, burning pain—often in a limb. It usually follows injury, but persists after the injury has healed, because of damage to a nerve. The pain is felt in the area supplied by the nerve, which is not necessarily the site of the injury.

See NERVOUS SYSTEM *page 34*

PHANTOM LIMB PAIN

CAUTERISE

To destroy diseased or damaged tissue by applying to it extreme heat or cold, a corrosive substance or the intense light of a laser beam. Commonly used to remove warts and small growths.

CELL

The basic unit of all living creatures. A man's body contains about 100 million million cells, each of which is only about a few hundred-thousandths of an inch across. A human cell is enclosed by thin tissue called a membrane. Cytoplasm forms the bulk of the interior. It is a thick liquid made up of proteins, carbohydrates, salts, fats and water. At its centre is the nucleus, which contains DNA (deoxyribonucleic acid). DNA enables the cell to reproduce itself—generally by splitting in two—and in sex cells is responsible for a person passing on characteristics to his or her children. Together, cytoplasm and the nucleus are known as protoplasm. The day-to-day functions of the cell are to absorb oxygen and nutrients from the blood and to pass into the blood carbon dioxide and other waste products.

CELLULITIS

Spreading inflammation of the skin and subcutaneous tissues. Diabetics are particularly vulnerable to the condition.

Symptoms

• The skin is hot, red, tender and shiny because of the swelling.

• Blisters may appear on the inflamed skin.

• Red lines of inflammation, LYMPHANGITIS, may be seen from the cellulitis to the nearest lymph glands, for example, up the leg or the arm.

• The nearest lymph glands may be swollen and tender.

• The person may soon feel feverish and ill.

Causes

• The most common cause is bacterial infection. The infection gets into the skin through a cut or an invisible skin puncture and spreads rapidly.

• Poison from an insect bite.

• Chemical poisoning.

Complications

• Boils and carbuncles may develop. Very occasionally the infection may spread into the blood or bones.

Treatment in the home
• Rest the affected area and keep it higher than the rest of the body. This reduces the spread of infection.
When to consult the doctor
• As it is not easy to distinguish cellulitis caused by infection from that due to other causes, it is always advisable to seek medical advice.
What the doctor may do
• Exclude other more serious diseases.
• Give antibiotic injections or tablets, which should quickly control the condition if it is caused by bacterial infection. *See* MEDICINES, 25.
Prevention
• There is no easy way to avoid accidental infection, but cellulitis is more likely to occur in dirty conditions.
Outlook
• The sooner treatment is started the quicker will be the recovery.
• As the infection settles, the dry skin may peel from the area which was most inflamed.
• There will be no scarring.

See SKIN *page 52*

CEPHALHAEMATOMA
A swelling on the head of a baby due to a collection of blood beneath the membrane covering the skull. A cephalhaematoma most commonly occurs on the scalp of a newborn baby as the result of pressure on the skull during labour. In older babies a blow can cause the swelling. In all cases it disappears without treatment in a few weeks.

CEREBRAL PALSY
The term cerebral palsy indicates a permanent disorder of the brain, usually present from birth, characterised by reduced muscle control and by muscle spasms (hence the old name 'spastic'), sometimes accompanied by lowered intelligence. The condition occurs with varying degrees of severity.

With support and encouragement from family, friends and teachers, exceptional successes can be achieved. For instance, many sufferers have completed university education.

Despite their problems, cerebral palsy sufferers can live enjoyable and fulfilling lives, as can those who are caring for them.

The term is occasionally used to describe the paralysis that follows any STROKE.
See NERVOUS SYSTEM *page 34*

CERVICAL CANCER

A malignant growth in the neck of the uterus (womb). Its incidence has increased in recent years, especially in younger women. It is linked with the human papilloma virus, which is transmitted by sexual intercourse and also causes genital warts.
Symptoms
• Bleeding between periods.
• Bleeding after sexual intercourse.
• Bleeding after the menopause.
• Brown or bad-smelling vaginal discharge
Duration
• Until the condition is treated.
Causes
• Probably an infection with human papilloma virus.
• Cervical cancer is linked with sexual intercourse—it does not occur in nuns.
• Risk increases with number of sexual partners, and with number of partners that each male partner has had.
• Smoking, and possibly the Pill, may increase risk.
Complications
• Cancer may spread from the cervix to other organs.
Treatment in the home
• None is possible.
When to consult the doctor
• Immediately there is any unexpected vaginal bleeding or discharge, whether before or after the menopause.
What the doctor may do
• Carry out an internal vaginal examination and take a CERVICAL SMEAR.
• Arrange an examination by a gynaecologist, who is usually able to destroy abnormal cells by laser, freezing, or minor surgery.
• In advanced cases, HYSTERECTOMY or radiotherapy will be necessary.
Prevention
• Avoid promiscuity and promiscuous sexual partners.
• Use a condom or diaphragm (cap).
• Regular smear tests every three years, or annually for those with genital warts.
Outlook
• Before cancer develops, cells in the cervix are in a pre-cancerous state which can last for several years. These cells can be detected with a cervical smear test and if treated at this stage the prospect is very good. Once cancer has developed sufficiently to cause symptoms, the chances of complete cure are reduced—hence the importance of regular cervical smear tests.

CERVICAL EROSION

An alteration in the outer covering of the cervix, the neck of the uterus (womb); it changes from its normal pink, smooth condition to a red, graze-like one that often oozes a slight discharge. The condition is very common, particularly in women who have had children, it is harmless and never leads to cancer.
Symptoms
• Many women have no symptoms; the erosion is only discovered after routine internal examinations.
• In others there is a yellow, green or occasionally brown discharge from the vagina, and occasionally low back pain.
When to consult the doctor
• If you have the symptoms described.
What the doctor may do
• Carry out an internal pelvic examination and take a CERVICAL SMEAR to exclude the possibility of CERVICAL CANCER.
• Cauterise the area of erosion. This is a painless and quick procedure.
Prevention
• There are no means of preventing the condition.
Outlook
• In most cases the affected area returns to normal naturally, in others cauterisation heals the area.

See FEMALE GENITAL SYSTEM *page 48*

CERVICAL RIB SYNDROME

Some people are born with an extra rib positioned above the normal ribcage, at the base of the neck. It is known as a cervical rib and generally causes no problem of any kind.

In a few cases, however, the rib may press on the nerves in the neck and produce an aching pain down the inside of the arm. This is likely to happen when heavy weights are carried in the hand or when the sufferer is tired. A slight numbness or weakness may also develop in the hand itself. An effect may also be felt in the eye; the lid may droop and the pupil become smaller.

If you notice such symptoms, report them to your doctor. He may recommend X-rays to find out whether a cervical rib is present, though in most cases the symptoms will have resulted from some other cause such as CERVICAL SPONDYLOSIS or CARPAL TUNNEL SYNDROME.

Pains in the arm may also result from a nerve getting trapped by a neck muscle.

However, if the syndrome is confirmed and symptoms are severe, the doctor may recommend that the cervical rib be removed by surgery. The operation usually results in a complete cure.

See NERVOUS SYSTEM *page 34*

CERVICAL SMEAR

A test to detect pre-cancerous cells in the tissue of the cervix of the uterus (the neck of the womb). Pre-cancerous cells are cells that if left untreated might become cancerous later. The test, which is performed either at a doctor's surgery or at a family planning clinic, takes only seconds and is almost always painless. A minute specimen of tissue is taken from the cervix for examination. If the test is positive—that is, if the cells are pre-cancerous— the doctor will send the patient to a gynaecologist.

Every woman should have regular cervical smears from the time she starts to have sexual intercourse until she is at least 65 years old. The doctor will say how often they should be carried out.

Cervical smears do not rule out cancer of the body of the uterus (*see* UTERUS, CANCER OF), and a recent negative smear should never make a woman hesitate to consult her doctor about unexpected vaginal bleeding or discharge—which may be symptoms of cancer of the uterus.

See FEMALE GENITAL SYSTEM *page 48*

CERVICAL SPONDYLOSIS

A disorder that causes pain in, and restricted movement of, the neck region of the spinal column. Cervical spondylosis mainly affects those over 40. It is sometimes accompanied by a SLIPPED DISC in the neck.
Symptoms
• Pain in the back of the neck or in the region of the shoulder-blade. This is often worse in certain positions,

for example, lying in bed with the head raised by several pillows.
• There may also be pain, tingling and numbness in a finger or hand.
Duration
• Treatment usually gets rid of symptoms within two or three months.
Causes
• Increasing age causes irreversible degeneration of the joints of the spine. Then injury or certain other factors— such as having the head raised too high in bed—can bring on the condition.
Complications
• Turning the head or looking up may occasionally slow up the blood supply to the brain causing dizziness or a brief blackout.
Treatment in the home
• Take painkillers in recommended doses to relieve the pain. *See* MEDICINES, 22.
When to consult the doctor
• If the pain in the neck or shoulder is not relieved by taking painkillers.
• If there is any pain, numbness or weakness in a finger or hand.
• If any temporary dizziness or blackout results from turning the head or looking up, such as when decorating a ceiling.
What the doctor may do
• Question the patient to discover whether injury or any factor such as a new car or new furniture has caused a change in posture.
• After examining the neck and testing reflexes and sensation in the upper arm, arrange X-rays.
• In mild cases he will prescribe pain-relieving drugs for the pain and possibly also arrange for the patient to have physiotherapy.
• In more severe cases, prescribe a special close-fitting collar to keep the neck in a fixed position.
Prevention
• Avoid postures that strain the neck and upper back.
Outlook
• About four-fifths of cases clear up permanently; in others the disorder recurs within two years.

See SKELETAL SYSTEM *page 54*

CHAGAS' DISEASE
A disease of poor communities in Mexico and South America, caused by a trypanosome—one of a group of parasites that also causes SLEEPING SICKNESS. In children Chagas' disease is often fatal. In adults it causes

long-standing damage to the heart and only rarely affects the brain. Unlike sleeping sickness there are no effective drugs against infection from this particular trypanosome.

CHALAZION
Swelling of an oil-secreting gland in the eyelid caused by blockage of the gland. It is slightly disfiguring and uncomfortable, but not painful. A hot compress applied for a quarter of an hour three times a day will help a chalazion to disappear. If there is no improvement after several weeks, a doctor should be consulted. Some cases require a minor operation to remove the gland.
See MEIBOMIAN CYST

CHANCRE
A painless ulcer that is the first symptom of SYPHILIS. In most cases it develops on the genitals, but it may also occur on the anus, lips, tongue or fingers.

CHANGE OF LIFE
Another name for the menopause, the period in a woman's life when menstruation begins to come to an end. In most women it begins between the ages of 45 and 55 and lasts from six months to three years.
See MENOPAUSE

CHAPPED LIPS

Sore, inflamed, roughened and cracked lips. The problem is usually caused by wind and cold, and can be cured by using lip salve.

Sometimes, the condition is confused with the swollen, painful red patches of COLD SORES. In other cases there may be a persistent crack at the corner of the mouth or a sore with a growth that is usually a WART, or ulcer, but may very occasionally be a cancer. When the lips are swollen, bright red and raw where they meet, the condition is called CHEILOSIS. This is usually caused by a vitamin B deficiency, or other nutritional disorder, especially when linked with sore eyes, and ridges of grey-white skin that radiate from the corners of the mouth (angular stomatitis). If chapped lips persist, and cause discomfort, it is sensible to consult the doctor.

See SKIN *page 52*

CHEILOSIS
Cracking and scaling of the lips and corners of the mouth. It is believed to be caused by a deficiency of B-group vitamins, which are found in meat, fish, dairy products and vegetables. High doses of the vitamins often improve the condition.

CHEMOTHERAPY
Control of treatment of disease by chemical substances. The term may be used to describe both anti-infective and anticancer agents.

CHERRY SPOTS

Bright red or purple papules (pimples) which appear on the chest and trunk in later life. They are usually about $\frac{1}{8}$ in. (3 mm.) across and consist of tiny blood vessels. Other names for the condition are cherry angioma and Campbell de Morgan spots. They are harmless, give no pain, and in spite of some people's fears do not turn into cancer.
Symptoms
• The spots cause no trouble unless injured, when they bleed easily.
Causes
• It is not known what causes cherry spots.
Treatment in the home
• There is nothing to be done in the way of home treatment.
When to consult the doctor
• If you are over-anxious about the spots.
What the doctor may do
• Reassure the patient that the condition is harmless.
Outlook
• With age the spots may become more numerous, but individual spots do not get bigger.

See SKIN *page 52*

CHEST PAIN
There are two types of chest pain—pain which is related to breathing and pain which is not. Either type may be a symptom of serious disease.
See SYMPTOM SORTER—CHEST PAIN

CHEYNE-STOKES BREATHING
Alternating periods of slow, shallow, quiet breathing and fast, deep, loud breathing. At the end of a shallow period, breathing may stop altogether for a while. The symptom occurs during severe HEART FAILURE, usually when the sufferer is in a coma.

CHICKENPOX

A common contagious disease caused by the virus *Varicella zoster*, which also causes SHINGLES (herpes zoster). Chickenpox, which is known medically as varicella, is mainly a disease of childhood, but it occasionally affects adults. It occurs in epidemics every two or three years and quickly spreads in schools or wherever children are together. One attack of chickenpox usually ensures immunity to the disease (which means that the sufferer cannot get it again), but the virus can lie dormant and cause shingles in later life. Some children develop immunity simply by being in contact with it and without developing characteristic symptoms.
Symptoms
• A highly irritating rash which starts on the body and spreads to the arms, legs, face and head. The rash begins as raised pink spots which rapidly change to watery blisters. These then burst or shrivel up and crust over to form scabs.
• The spots appear in crops over about four days, so that all stages of the rash may be on the body at the same time.
• Slightly raised temperature.
• The patient, especially an adult, may feel quite ill for a day or two.
Incubation period
• Twelve to 14 days.
Duration
• Scabs form on the blisters after about five days and gradually disappear over the next two weeks.
• The patient is infectious (that is, can pass the disease on to others) from about four days before the rash appears until all the blisters have formed scabs.
Causes
• A virus, spread by close contact with an infected person.
Complications
• The blisters may become infected, that is, inflamed and full of pus.
• Pneumonia is a rare but serious complication, more common in adults.
Treatment in the home
• Most cases of chickenpox do not require medical attention, and can be adequately treated at home.
• Keep the rash clean and dry.
• Have a quick shower each day and pat the skin dry.
• Apply calamine lotion to the rash twice daily to ease the itching.
• Do not pick the spots, or they will scar and leave little pock-marks.
• Drink plenty of liquids—it does not matter if the patient does not want to eat while he feels ill.
• Rest.
• Take paracetamol to help reduce fever and discomfort. Avoid aspirin. *See* MEDICINES, 22.
• In general, there is no need to isolate an infected child from other children. But try to avoid spreading the infection to babies under six months and to women in late pregnancy. If a mother has the disease within a few days of giving birth, the baby may have chickenpox and be quite ill.
• Chickenpox during early pregnancy is very unlikely to affect the unborn child.
• Elderly people should avoid close contact because they may contract SHINGLES.
When to consult the doctor
• If the child has a high fever, is vomiting or coughing excessively.
• If the eyes themselves (not simply the eyelids) are affected.
• If the spots become inflamed.
What the doctor may do
• Prescribe antibiotic medicines if the skin, lungs or ears have become infected. *See* MEDICINES, 25.
• Prescribe acyclovir, an anti-viral drug, in severe cases or if the child also suffers from other illnesses.
Prevention
• There is no immunisation against chickenpox. The only prevention is to avoid contact with an infected person, but it is usually better not to try to protect a child from catching the disease.
• People on drugs (such as steroids) that suppress natural immunity may be given an injection of antibodies to boost their defences, if they have been in contact with chickenpox.
Outlook
• Recovery is complete. The spots do not form scars unless they are picked or become infected.
• Rarely, chickenpox is fatal.

See INFECTIOUS DISEASES *page 32*

CHILBLAINS

Sore, reddish-blue swellings, usually on the toes or fingers, due to exposure to cold. Chilblains give a burning sensation and may be intensely itchy and painful, but they usually clear within two to three weeks if there is no further exposure to cold. They have become much less common with the advent of central heating.

Sometimes chilblains may be a sign of poor blood flow to the extremities, and occasionally they occur elsewhere on the body, such as on the buttocks in those working outdoors in tight jeans.

See SKIN *page 52*

CHILD ABUSE

At least one in every 100 children born is, at one time or another, physically abused, sexually molested or severely neglected. Parents are responsible for most cases of child abuse. Sexual abuse most often involves female children and male relatives, usually the father or stepfather. Physical and sexual abuse often co-exist. About 10 per cent of maltreated children are killed or suffer permanent brain damage. In addition, about one in ten of school-age children living in Western cities undergoes extremes of neglect, ill-treatment and distress, without actual physical abuse.

PARENTS WITH PROBLEMS

Parents who abuse their children are usually young and have housing, financial or marital problems. Often the mother has had an unhappy pregnancy or delivery and was separated from her baby soon after the birth. Fathers are often rigid authoritarians and relatively uninvolved in the child's upbringing. Above all, most of these parents have had an emotionally unhappy, physically violent, sexually abusive or excessively strict upbringing themselves. However, child abuse can also take place when none of these problems is present.

Any parents who are fearful that they might injure their child should immediately either seek help from a sympathetic friend or relative or telephone their health visitor or family doctor, a minister of religion or NSPCC officer, a local paediatrician, a local authority social worker or the local Samaritans or Helpline.

An elaborate system involving social and medical workers has been devised to try to halt child abuse once it has started and to help the parents involved. In some cases it is decided that for the child's sake it is best for the parents and child to be separated, temporarily or perhaps even permanently.

HOW YOU CAN HELP

If you suspect that a child in your neighbourhood is being abused by its parents, you should discuss your suspicions in *confidence* with a responsible person—such as an NSPCC officer, a child welfare officer or your local doctor. For legal reasons, you should *never* discuss your unproven suspicions with your friends, neighbours or the parents themselves.

See CHILD CARE *page 116*

CHILD CARE

A special section on child care gives advice on child-rearing from birth to the age of five.

See CHILD CARE *page 116*

CHIROPRACTIC

A system of manipulating the body joints, particularly those of the spine, to treat pains in or injuries to bones, joints and muscles, as well as some nervous or stress-related conditions. It is in many ways similar to OSTEO-PATHY, although its manipulation is more vigorous.

Chiropractic is widely recognised in North America, New Zealand and Western Australia. In the United Kingdom, it is not available on the National Health Service, but since 1977 doctors have been allowed to refer patients to chiropractors.

CHLAMYDIA INFECTIONS

Chlamydia are small bacteria responsible for a variety of infections. Diagnosis of chlamydia infections can be difficult, but they respond to antibiotics. Diseases caused by chlamydia include:

- TRACHOMA, the commonest treatable cause of blindness.
- Infant PNEUMONIA.
- Non-specific URETHRITIS, a sexually transmitted disease more common than GONORRHOEA and on the increase.
- SALPINGITIS, infection of the female Fallopian tubes that may result in sterility.
- Epididymitis, infection of the epididymis (the tube next to the testicles).
- LYMPHOGRANULOMA venereum, a sexually transmitted disease that causes swelling of the lymph glands in the groin of both men and women.
- REITER'S DISEASE (ARTHRITIS, CONJUNCTIVITIS and urethritis occurring together).
- PSITTACOSIS, a form of pneumonia caught from birds.

See INFECTIOUS DISEASES *page 32*

CHLOASMA

A darkening of the skin of the face in women. It can occur during pregnancy or while taking the oral contraceptive pill.

Symptoms
- Darkening of the skin of the face.
- The distribution of the increased pigment is mask-like, being greatest over the cheek-bones, bridge of the nose and around the mouth.
- A patchy pigmentation may be caused by a perfume.

Duration
- The condition is usually, but not always, temporary and disappears three or four months after childbirth or after stopping the oral contraceptive, or ceasing to use the offending perfume.

Causes
- Hormones stimulating melanin (dark pigment) in the skin are increased during pregnancy and use of the oral contraceptive pill.
- Oil of bergamot in perfumes makes pigment cells respond vigorously to sunlight.

Treatment in the home
- The condition is a temporary one and the brown marks can be covered by make-up.

When to consult the doctor
- If pigmentation occurs without an apparent cause, or is causing worry.

What the doctor may do
- Make sure the pigment is not due to other uncommon general medical disorders.

Prevention
- Avoid perfumes and cosmetics which cause the pigmentation.
- Stop taking the contraceptive pill.

Outlook
- It is rare for chloasma to persist.

See SKIN *page 52*

CHOLECYSTITIS

Inflammation of the gall-bladder. Prolonged, or chronic, inflammation can lead to stones forming in the gall-bladder.

See GALLSTONES

CHOLERA

An acute infectious disease that can occur in epidemic form throughout the world, but not in Britain. It is caused by a germ called *Vibrio cholerae*, which is found in the faeces of patients and carriers. Cholera is transmitted by contaminated water and flies, and spreads rapidly when sanitation is poor. A natural disaster, such as an earthquake or flood may result in an epidemic.

Symptoms
• Watery diarrhoea. This is painless, but very severe.
• Vomiting, which is often effortless and without nausea.
• The loss of fluid produces rapid weight loss and muscle cramps.

Incubation period
• Six to 48 hours.

Duration
• Two to seven days.

Causes
• Bacteria in water and uncooked food, especially fruit and vegetables that have been contaminated by carriers.

Treatment in the home
• If immediate medical help is not available, keep the patient at complete rest.
• Give plenty of glucose water and iced drinks such as lemon and barley-water.

When to consult the doctor
• Immediately, if cholera is suspected.

What the doctor may do
• Arrange for an intravenous saline drip to replace lost fluid. Once the fluid is replaced, recovery is rapid.
• Prescribe antibiotic injections or tablets, although this is less important than replacing fluid lost through diarrhoea. *See* MEDICINES, 25.

Prevention
• Cholera immunisation is available, but offers poor protection against the disease and often itself causes mild symptoms. Very few countries now ask travellers to provide proof of immunisation and many doctors are reluctant to give it.
• In countries where cholera occurs, all water should be boiled and food, especially fruit and vegetables, should always be well cooked.
• Careful personal hygiene and good sanitation.

Outlook
• With adequate treatment, to replace the large amounts of fluid lost from the bowel, recovery is complete and there is little chance of the patient dying from the disease.
• When epidemics occur suddenly, such as after a flood or earthquake, hospitals cannot always cope with the number of patients needing treatment.

See INFECTIOUS DISEASES *page 32*

CHOLESTEROL

A fat-like substance present in the body and in many foods. It is essential to many body processes, although its exact role is not fully understood. High cholesterol levels play some role in ATHEROMA and CORONARY THROMBOSIS, but to what extent the risks can be altered by diet remains undetermined.

See NUTRITION

CHROMOSOMES

Minute threadlike bodies present in the nucleus of each CELL in the body. Each chromosome consists of a string of genes, which determine an individual's characteristics—such as colouring, height, blood group and any inherited disorder. Human cells each contain 46 chromosomes, 23 inherited from the father, 23 from the mother.

See DOWN'S SYNDROME
HEREDITY

CHRONIC FATIGUE SYNDROME

See MYALGIC ENCEPHALOMYELITIS

CIRCULATION PROBLEMS IN THE EYE

The vision can be affected by haemorrhages or clots that block the blood vessels of the retina. High blood pressure or diabetes increases the risk of this happening.

Symptoms
• Blockage of the circulation to the eye can cause sudden painless loss of vision in one eye. If sudden blindness is total, it is probable that an artery has been blocked. If a vein is blocked, loss of vision may be only partial.
• If the circulation supplying the central retina becomes inefficient, or if there is bleeding in this area, the patient will gradually find it increasingly difficult to read or knit, or do fine work.
• Small, symptomless haemorrhages may also occur in people with high blood pressure or DIABETES.

Duration
• The speed and extent of recovery depend on the size and area of the damage to the retina. A degree of recovery of sight may occur over a period of a few weeks or months.

Causes
• The small haemorrhages which can occur with diabetes or high blood pressure are part of the general strain on the circulation which these conditions can cause. Blood-vessel blockages are usually caused by small clots which may form in arteries affected by ATHEROMA ('furring up'), or in veins crossed by small hardened arteries.

When to consult the doctor
• If you have any loss of vision, especially sudden loss of vision, seek medical help immediately.

What the doctor may do
• The doctor is likely to test your eyesight by means of an eye chart, test your field of vision and look in your eyes with an ophthalmoscope. He will also probably check the blood pressure and test the urine for sugar.
• If the vision has been lost suddenly, the doctor will almost certainly arrange emergency admission to an eye hospital.
• When a retinal artery is blocked, high doses of steroids (cortisone) may be needed to save the sight of the second eye. If a vein has been affected, tests and sometimes treatment will be needed to prevent the development of chronic GLAUCOMA. *See* MEDICINES, 39.

Prevention
• Do not smoke. There is evidence that hardening of the arteries, the underlying cause of most circulatory problems in the eye, may be associated with heavy cigarette smoking.
• If you suffer from high blood pressure or diabetes (other underlying causes) it is vital to continue under medical supervision.

Outlook
• Even if the sight of the affected eye cannot be saved, or can be only partially restored, it is quite possible to adapt well to sight with one eye only.
• If the central vision is affected, reading may become impossible although the patient will not go blind and will be able to see his way to get about, and do most tasks not requiring fine vision.

See EYE *page 36*

Child care

HOW TO ENJOY YOUR BABY—AND COPE WITH THE DAY-TO-DAY PROBLEMS OF MOTHERHOOD

From the day of your baby's birth, he already has certain abilities and instinctive reactions. But he has a lot to discover, and in his early years the gaps are made good by what he learns from his family—most of all, his mother. He learns with all his senses, but particularly by imitation and experience.

Watching a baby's body and mind grow is one of the delights of being a parent. At first the baby struggles to recognise the world around him by looking and listening. Then he reaches out to it: as his arms and legs grow strong, he begins to explore. Increasingly during his second and third years his personality reveals itself in the way he tries to control his world with his newly discovered skills.

As well as deriving pleasure from their baby, parents also encounter worries about health and development. The following pages tell you what to expect from normal children, how to cope with common problems and illnesses, and how to get the best out of yourself and your children.

1. FIRST DAYS

Getting to know your baby

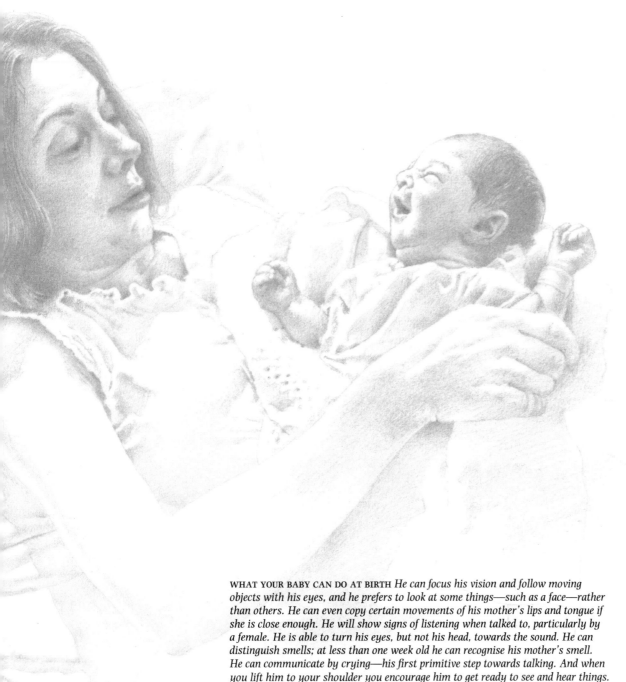

After a normal delivery of a baby the midwife removes the mucus from his nose and mouth, dries him with a towel, clamps the end of his umbilical cord and attaches a name tag to his wrist or ankle. In some cases the mother is given the baby to hold briefly before the midwife does those things; in others, she has to

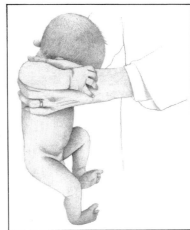

WHAT YOUR BABY CAN DO AT BIRTH *He can focus his vision and follow moving objects with his eyes, and he prefers to look at some things—such as a face—rather than others. He can even copy certain movements of his mother's lips and tongue if she is close enough. He will show signs of listening when talked to, particularly by a female. He is able to turn his eyes, but not his head, towards the sound. He can distinguish smells; at less than one week old he can recognise his mother's smell. He can communicate by crying—his first primitive step towards talking. And when you lift him to your shoulder you encourage him to get ready to see and hear things.*

'REFLEX ACTIONS' *A newborn baby will make walking steps if you hold him upright on a firm surface. He will also grip your fingers so tightly that you can lift him up. These are not deliberate actions but caused by an automatic reflex action (like blinking when something comes near your eye).*

wait until afterwards. If the midwife thinks the baby feels cold, she may suggest that before he is given to the mother he is put in a crib warmed by an electric blanket.

You may need some stitches in your vagina—particularly if delivery has been by forceps—and while these are being put in, the baby will probably be in a crib at your side.

Or you may have had a general anaesthetic, perhaps for a CAESAREAN SECTION, and will then probably not regain consciousness and see your baby until you have been moved to the maternity ward.

If you have decided to breast-feed (*see page 128*), the midwife may suggest letting the baby try to feed as soon as he is handed over to you.

WHAT HAPPENS IF A BABY DOES NOT BREATHE WHEN HE IS BORN?
A baby who does not start to breathe when the midwife removes the mucus from his nose and mouth is taken to a neonatal resuscitation trolley. There a doctor gives oxygen to the baby with a face mask while listening with a stethoscope to make sure the heart is beating rapidly

enough. The doctor may help oxygen to enter the baby's lungs by squeezing on a rubber bag attached to the mask. In the rare event that the baby fails to start breathing within a minute or two, the doctor or a midwife will insert a plastic tube through the baby's nose or mouth into his windpipe and pass oxygen directly into his lungs.

How to pick up a baby

A newborn baby may seem very delicate, but so long as you take care not to frighten him, and lift him gently but confidently, there is nothing to worry about.
Always take care to support his head; he will not be able to support it by himself until he is at least three months old. If his head is not supported he is likely to protest.

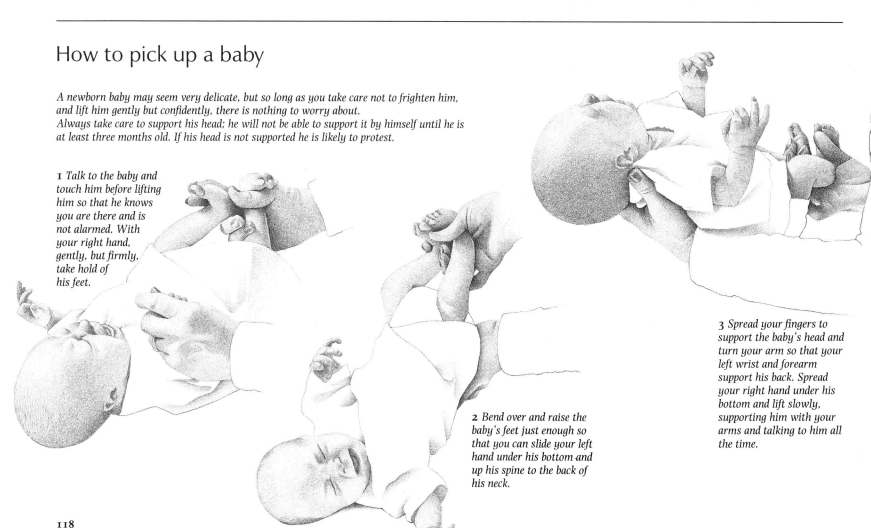

1 *Talk to the baby and touch him before lifting him so that he knows you are there and is not alarmed. With your right hand, gently, but firmly, take hold of his feet.*

2 *Bend over and raise the baby's feet just enough so that you can slide your left hand under his bottom and up his spine to the back of his neck.*

3 *Spread your fingers to support the baby's head and turn your arm so that your left wrist and forearm support his back. Spread your right hand under his bottom and lift slowly, supporting him with your arms and talking to him all the time.*

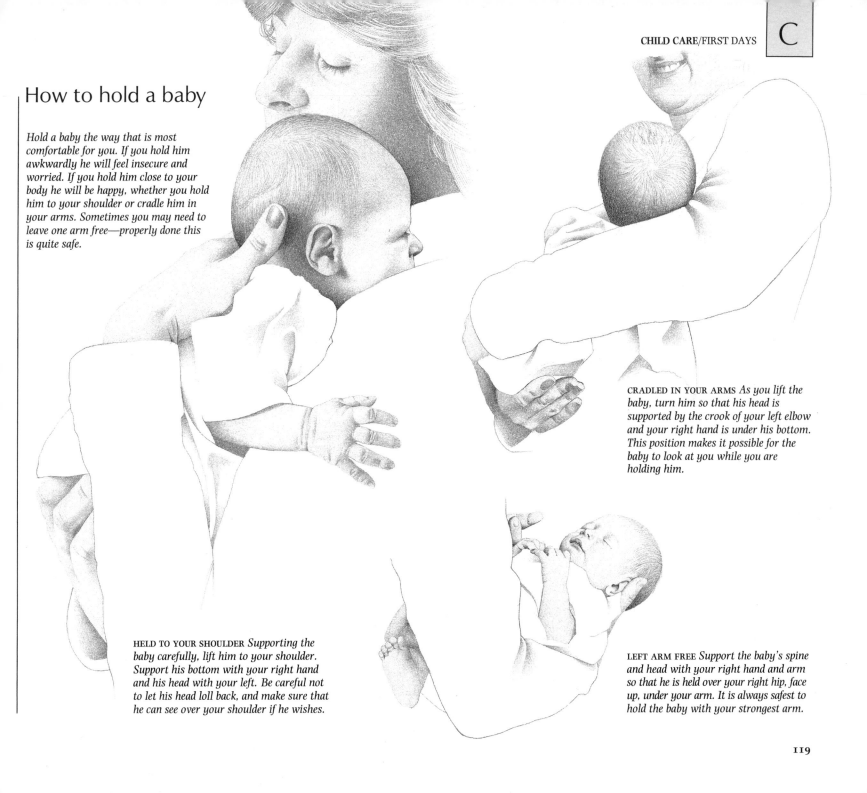

How to hold a baby

*Hold a baby the way that is most
comfortable for you. If you hold him
awkwardly he will feel insecure and
worried. If you hold him close to your
body he will be happy, whether you hold
him to your shoulder or cradle him in
your arms. Sometimes you may need to
leave one arm free—properly done this
is quite safe.*

CRADLED IN YOUR ARMS *As you lift the
baby, turn him so that his head is
supported by the crook of your left elbow
and your right hand is under his bottom.
This position makes it possible for the
baby to look at you while you are
holding him.*

HELD TO YOUR SHOULDER *Supporting the
baby carefully, lift him to your shoulder.
Support his bottom with your right hand
and his head with your left. Be careful not
to let his head loll back, and make sure that
he can see over your shoulder if he wishes.*

LEFT ARM FREE *Support the baby's spine
and head with your right hand and arm
so that he is held over your right hip, face
up, under your arm. It is always safest to
hold the baby with your strongest arm.*

CHECKING THAT THE BABY IS NORMAL

The first question most mothers ask after delivery is not whether the baby is a boy or a girl (the midwife usually announces this right away) but whether it is normal. It needs only a quick examination by the midwife—when she removes the mucus from the baby's mouth and dries him—to reassure you that all is well. But naturally, a minor abnormality, such as a small birthmark or an odd-shaped finger, may not be noticed.

If you are worried about any aspect of your baby's appearance in the first few days, tell the midwife or doctor. At some time during the first week a complete physical examination of your baby will be carried out.

NORMAL BIRTH WEIGHT

Birth weight is regulated by many things: whether the baby is a boy or a girl, whether it was born on time; how tall you and your partner are; what race you belong to; and whether you smoke (the babies of non-smokers tend to be heavier than those of smokers).

Most European babies born in the 40th week weigh between $5\frac{1}{2}$ lb. (2.5 kg.) and $9\frac{1}{4}$ lb. (4.2 kg.). Girls weighing less than $5\frac{1}{2}$ lb. and boys weighing less than $6\frac{1}{2}$ lb. (2.9 kg.) are called small-for-dates (SFD), or light-for-dates (LFD). The figures differ if the baby is born earlier or

How to lay down and wrap up a baby

Talk to the baby to reassure him as you lay him down—he may be upset at leaving the comfort of your arms. Put him down slowly, because a sudden move might frighten him. If you are going to wrap him up, spread the shawl diagonally in front of you and turn down the top corner ready to lie the baby on it.

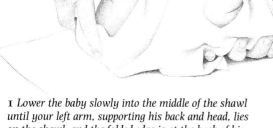

1 *Lower the baby slowly into the middle of the shawl until your left arm, supporting his back and head, lies on the shawl, and the folded edge is at the back of his head. Gently slide your hands from under his body.*

2 *Fold one side of the shawl down and across the baby's body, leaving his arms free if you are going to lie him on his front. If you are going to feed the baby or lie him on his side, wrap his arms inside the shawl.*

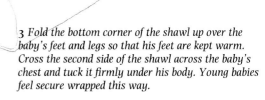

3 *Fold the bottom corner of the shawl up over the baby's feet and legs so that his feet are kept warm. Cross the second side of the shawl across the baby's chest and tuck it firmly under his body. Young babies feel secure wrapped this way.*

later than the 40th week.

If a baby is small-for-dates, this may mean that he will always have a slender build, but it can also mean that he is going to be of normal size and is small only because he has not grown well in the womb, possibly because the placenta has not kept him properly nourished. If this is so, he may have nourished himself with his own stores of food and because of this, may be short of food, particularly sugar, during his first day or two. The doctors may recommend extra feeds of milk or sugar-water, especially if you intend to breast-feed, and will take regular blood samples from him to check that his level of blood glucose is satisfactory.

LEARNING BABY CARE
A nurse in the maternity ward will show you how to hold, dress and undress the baby and when to pick him up. When a baby is held, the back of his head should be supported with one hand or against the body, since he cannot hold up his head by himself for more than one or two seconds. But do not worry if his head does flop occasionally, it is more likely to alarm than harm him.

The nurse will also show you how to bath the baby. The water should be comfortably warm when tested with your elbow. The baby is lowered gently into the water, with his shoulders and the back of his head supported by one hand and arm and with just his face showing

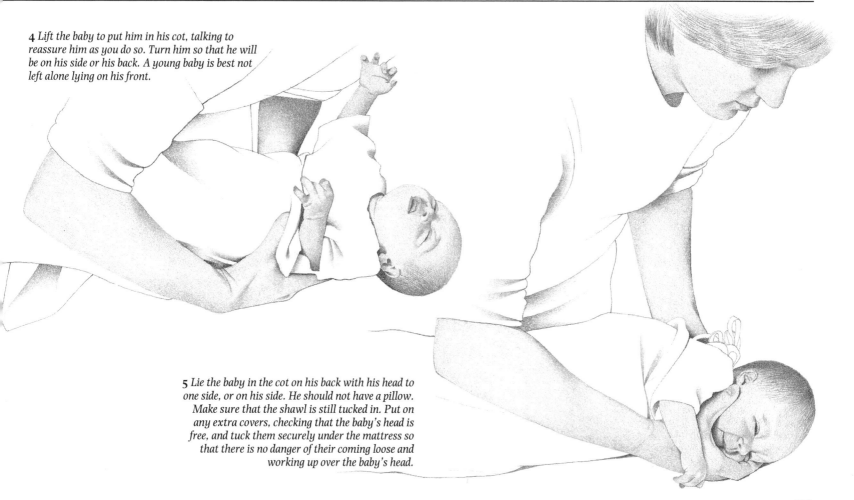

4 *Lift the baby to put him in his cot, talking to reassure him as you do so. Turn him so that he will be on his side or his back. A young baby is best not left alone lying on his front.*

5 *Lie the baby in the cot on his back with his head to one side, or on his side. He should not have a pillow. Make sure that the shawl is still tucked in. Put on any extra covers, checking that the baby's head is free, and tuck them securely under the mattress so that there is no danger of their coming loose and working up over the baby's head.*

above water. Use baby soap.

If your baby cries, go to him. He may be in an uncomfortable position, feel hungry or thirsty or have a pain. On the other hand, he may simply be passing urine. It is quite normal for him to cry when he does this. Doctors have studied the differences between young babies who are picked up as soon as they cry and those who are not. Those used to being picked up cry less often and for a shorter time. So at this age there is little danger of spoiling the baby.

When putting the baby down in his cot, the risk of cot death (sudden infant death) can be reduced if the baby is not placed on his front when he is laid down to sleep. There is no evidence that placing healthy babies on their backs brings an increased risk of death from choking or vomiting; and some experts point out that a baby on his back can see more of the world, which is good for his learning.

CIRCUMCISION

Should my son be circumcised?
Only if your religious beliefs demand that this be carried out. There is no good evidence that circumcision is a good thing. It is a painful operation and, rarely, there may be complications such as bleeding.

The foreskin cannot be drawn back at birth, indeed often not until the age of four or five. It should not be fiddled with. Ignore advice to draw it back forcibly; this can cause damage which, oddly enough, might mean that circumcision eventually becomes necessary at a later age.

Topping and tailing

There is no need to bath a new baby every day provided you 'top and tail' him instead. Have ready warm water and plenty of cotton wool, mild soap or baby lotion, any cream you use and a clean nappy. Spread a clean towel on a flat surface. Take off the baby's clothes, but not his nappy, and lie him on the towel.

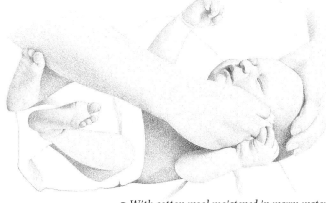

1 *With cotton wool moistened in warm water gently clean one side of the baby's face. Wipe around the eye first. Do not bathe the eye, tears do that. Then clean from the nose out to the ear. Do not probe inside the nose.*

2 *With a second swab wipe the other side of the baby's face. Using a clean swab for each side reduces the risk of spreading infection from one eye to the other.*

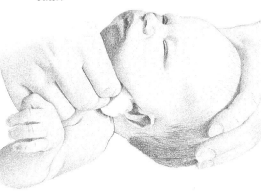

3 *With a third swab clean the baby's ears and neck. Do not wash inside the baby's ears. Clean only the outside, especially the area behind the ears.*

4 *Carefully dry the baby's face with cotton wool. Pay special attention to all the creases. If not dried thoroughly they may become inflamed. Clean and dry the baby's hands and under his arms. Put on his upper clothes so that he does not get cold.*

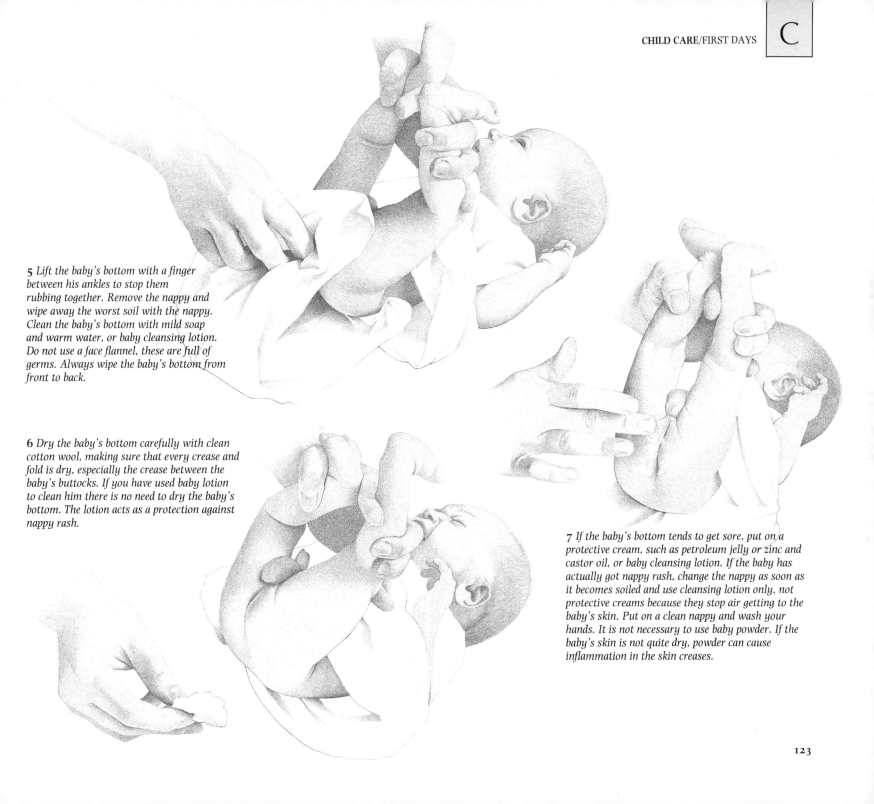

5 *Lift the baby's bottom with a finger between his ankles to stop them rubbing together. Remove the nappy and wipe away the worst soil with the nappy. Clean the baby's bottom with mild soap and warm water, or baby cleansing lotion. Do not use a face flannel, these are full of germs. Always wipe the baby's bottom from front to back.*

6 *Dry the baby's bottom carefully with clean cotton wool, making sure that every crease and fold is dry, especially the crease between the baby's buttocks. If you have used baby lotion to clean him there is no need to dry the baby's bottom. The lotion acts as a protection against nappy rash.*

7 *If the baby's bottom tends to get sore, put on a protective cream, such as petroleum jelly or zinc and castor oil, or baby cleansing lotion. If the baby has actually got nappy rash, change the nappy as soon as it becomes soiled and use cleansing lotion only, not protective creams because they stop air getting to the baby's skin. Put on a clean nappy and wash your hands. It is not necessary to use baby powder. If the baby's skin is not quite dry, powder can cause inflammation in the skin creases.*

Bathing a baby

Bath the baby in a warm room. Wash your hands, then collect everything you need where you can reach it easily as you bath the baby. Have ready clean cotton wool, baby soap or a proprietary cleansing solution, a large towel or towelling apron to put on your knee and another towel to wrap the baby in, a clean nappy, any cream you use, and a baby bath. Put about 3 in. (75 mm.) of water in the bath, pouring cold water in first—especially if the bath is a metal one—and then hot. Test the temperature with your elbow or the inside of your wrist. The water should feel neither hot nor cold. If you are using a solution, add it to the water following the manufacturer's instructions. Lift the baby on to your knee. Undress him, leaving his nappy on, and wrap him in a towel.

1 Before you put the baby in the bath, hold him under your left arm and wash his face with cotton wool and warm water from the bath. Use separate swabs for each side of his face and his ears and neck. Use more cotton wool to dry his face. Soap his head and rinse it, or wash it with solution from the bath. Pat his head dry with a towel. Take off his nappy, then wash his bottom carefully with cotton wool and soap, or cotton wool dipped in the solution. Wipe from front to back. Soap the baby's chest, arms and legs, then turn him over and soap his back. Soap him quickly so that he does not get cold. When the baby is older he can be soaped in the bath. If you are using solution you do not need to soap him. Dry your hands.

2 To put the baby in the bath, hold his left arm with your left hand and support his head with your left forearm. Hold his legs with your right hand—put a finger between his ankles to stop them rubbing together. Lower him into the water, talking gently to him. Do not remove your right hand until he is used to the feel of the water, especially if this is his first bath.

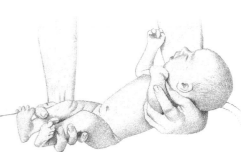

5 Lift the baby out of the bath, holding him as you did when putting him in. He is wet and slippery so take care. Wrap him in a dry towel.

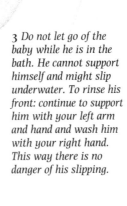

3 Do not let go of the baby while he is in the bath. He cannot support himself and might slip underwater. To rinse his front: continue to support him with your left arm and hand and wash him with your right hand. This way there is no danger of his slipping.

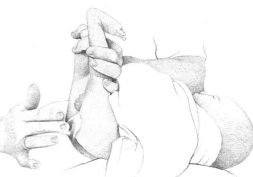

6 Pat dry the baby's bottom, paying special attention to the creases. Apply petroleum jelly, zinc and castor oil or lotion. Put on his nappy.

4 To rinse the baby's back: change hands and hold his left arm with your right hand so that he is leaning on to your wrist. Do not leave him in the water longer than is necessary to see that he is properly rinsed, or he will get cold.

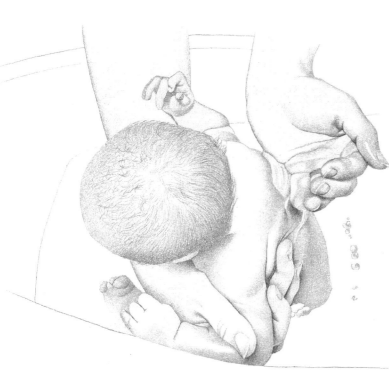

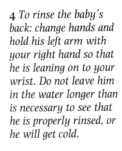

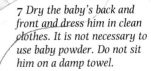

7 Dry the baby's back and front and dress him in clean clothes. It is not necessary to use baby powder. Do not sit him on a damp towel.

THE BOND BETWEEN MOTHER AND BABY

If newborn animals of certain species are taken from their mothers at birth and returned a day later, the mother may reject or even attack them. These newborn animals will follow and stay close to whichever creature looked after them in their first hours —even if a substitute mother was a completely different type of animal— and a bond is set up between the two.

Bonding also takes place between human babies and parents. However, there is disagreement about how soon after birth it happens, how easily it is disrupted by separation, and how much damage is done to the child by interference with the bonding process. Certainly some mothers who are unable to be close to their babies for the first few days or weeks have great problems with their feelings towards them for long afterwards. On the other hand, many mothers who have been separated from their children for the same amount of time become as loving as any other parent.

It is obviously a good thing if mothers and fathers can be with their babies as much as possible in the days after birth. In recognition of this, at some hospitals the baby is placed at the side (not the end) of his mother's bed, where she can see him and reach out to him and where he can be aware of her. Sleep is also important to the mother, so at night it is reasonable to keep the baby in a nursery within earshot, yet not so close that the mother wakes at every little snuffle.

Some mothers worry because when the baby is born they do not feel the affection that they thought they would. This may be because they are feeling so tired, sore or confused that all they want is sleep. Whatever the reason, the feeling is common and will nearly always pass as the days and weeks go by.

CONFLICTS

How will my husband feel?

If many mothers have confused feelings about their new baby it is hardly surprising that fathers may react in all sorts of ways—some quite unexpected. Of course he may be proud and excited; he may be delighted to have been able to be with you during the baby's birth. He could also be irritated, or even angry, particularly if he was unhappy about the pregnancy, or if you have, or are likely to have, major money or housing problems resulting from the baby's arrival.

Many men find it difficult to develop a close attachment to a newborn baby; it may seem to them that their partner is so totally involved with the baby that there is little room for them, so there can be feelings of jealousy or rejection. In the vast majority of cases this passes, and as the baby gets older, his father tends to take a greater interest and be more closely involved.

Some couples feel that bottle-feeding helps cement this relationship since it is an activity the man can share in from an early stage.

If you find that the arrival of a new baby seems to have provoked or worsened a bad relationship with your partner and you cannot easily solve the problem by talking together, seek the advice of your doctor or health visitor. Alternatively, you can contact a marriage guidance counsellor.

WHY THE BABY HAS A BLOOD TEST

In Britain, all babies have a small blood sample taken six or seven days after birth. The sample is usually taken by pricking the side of the baby's heel and letting two or three drops of blood fall on to specially prepared blotting-paper. The blood is then tested to ensure that the baby does not have a rare condition involving protein metabolism called phenylketonuria, which, if untreated, would eventually damage the brain and the liver. The treatment, which is highly successful, consists of adjusting the baby's diet.

In many hospitals a test is also performed for thyroid-gland insufficiency which can cause mental backwardness (cretinism), but which is completely preventable when it is detected early and the correct hormone treatment can be given.

Some babies also have other blood tests, for various reasons. Jaundiced babies may have a check on their blood level of bilirubin—the blood pigment responsible for yellow staining of the skin in jaundice. A baby suspected of being anaemic will probably have his blood tested. Blood glucose is checked in any baby who is unusually small or whose mother has diabetes. Certain blood chemicals may be checked in unusually nervous babies.

If your baby has an additional blood sample taken, do not hesitate to ask the midwife or doctor for the reason and the result.

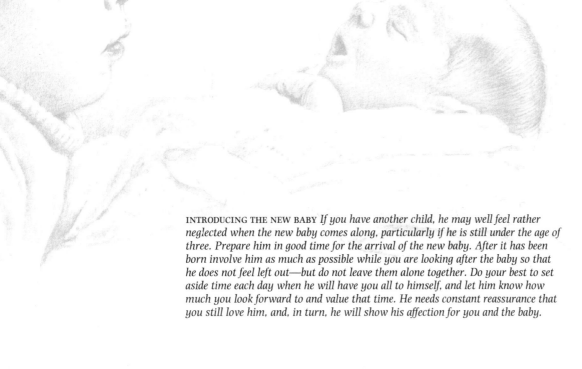

2. FIRST WEEKS

Meeting your baby's needs

When you return home with your baby, you and your husband will be involved straight away in feeding, changing nappies, bathing and ensuring that the baby is comfortable. But you will also want to resume living your own lives, and that partly involves getting back to your normal shape.

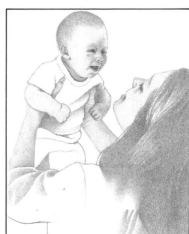

INTRODUCING THE NEW BABY *If you have another child, he may well feel rather neglected when the new baby comes along, particularly if he is still under the age of three. Prepare him in good time for the arrival of the new baby. After it has been born involve him as much as possible while you are looking after the baby so that he does not feel left out—but do not leave them alone together. Do your best to set aside time each day when he will have you all to himself, and let him know how much you look forward to and value that time. He needs constant reassurance that you still love him, and, in turn, he will show his affection for you and the baby.*

PICKING UP YOUR BABY *If your baby is crying, do not hesitate to pick him up and comfort him. There is no danger of your spoiling him. If he looks alert and ready to play, pick him up as much as you want, but do not keep picking him up when he seems ready for sleep or content just to gaze around.*

Breast-feeding versus bottle-feeding

BREAST MILK

Protein, fat and carbohydrate content
Ideally suited to the baby's intestine, so most is absorbed.

Minerals content
Ideally suited to the baby.

Concentration of contents
The strength of the milk is naturally regulated. It decreases when the baby has had enough, and he then stops feeding.

Nourishment
Ideal. However, some mothers produce too little milk and the baby fails to gain weight.

Protection against infections
Natural antibodies in the milk protect the baby against infections, particularly intestinal and respiratory infections.

Protection against other illnesses
Possibly provides some protection against eczema and asthma.

Contamination of milk
Not possible, unless there is a breast abscess.

Convenience
No equipment needed. Fewer dirty nappies, because the motions are smaller and fewer. You can feed the baby any time, anywhere. At night, particularly easier than bottle-feeding. However, only you can feed the baby; your partner or others cannot do it if you feel tired or ill (unless you collect and store breast milk in the freezer to be given with sterilised bottle-feeding equipment).

Supply
May diminish if you are tired, ill or miserable.

Baby's feelings
Probably enjoys the close contact with you.

Your feelings
You may feel very close and loving. You may get real pleasure.

Your health
A few women get cracked nipples or a breast abscess. Suckling also provokes the mother to produce a hormone which helps to shrink the uterus down to its normal size.

Your shape
Your breasts may end up larger, smaller or the same.

ARTIFICIAL MILK

Protein, fat and carbohydrate content
Less well absorbed by the intestine but, in practice, this is probably of little importance.

Minerals content
In the past, some babies have had fits because of too much phosphate and have suffered brain damage from too much sodium. This is now very rare and completely avoidable by feeding the correct amount, diluted the correct way.

Concentration of contents
The strength is constant. All you have to decide is how much to give.

Nourishment
It is easier to overfeed a baby with artificial milk and make him overweight.

Protection against infections
Provides no protection.

Protection against other illnesses
Not only provides no protection but in seven in 1,000 babies can cause diarrhoea, skin rashes or chesty illnesses.

Contamination
Unless bottles are cleaned and sterilised regularly, particularly in hot climates, bacteria can colonise the milk powder and cause gastro-enteritis in the baby.

Convenience
You need considerable equipment. This has to be regularly sterilised. Dirty nappies are more frequent and more unpleasant. The advantage of the method is that your partner or others can feed the baby when necessary.

Supply
Always available. Unaffected by your tiredness, illness or emotional distress.

Baby's feelings
Bottle-feeding a baby held close to you and in a loving way may well be as satisfying to him as breast-feeding.

Your feelings
You can obtain considerable enjoyment from bottle-feeding, and your husband can share this with you in a way that is not possible if you breast-feed.

Your shape
Unaffected.

BREAST-FEEDING, BOTTLE-FEEDING

It is only during this century that safe artificial baby milks have become available and have presented an alternative to the traditional method of breast-feeding. These artificial milks are made by adding water to dried cow's milk powder (or soya powder) supplemented with vegetable oils, iron and vitamins and fed to the baby from a bottle. Both methods of feeding have their advantages and disadvantages, and the table (*left*) shows these.

As can be seen from the table, most babies are better off being breast-fed than bottle-fed. Breast milk provides more balanced nourishment for the baby and greater protection of his health. Illnesses due to intestinal and respiratory infections are considerably lower in breast-fed babies than in bottle-fed ones. However, thousands of millions of babies have been bottle-fed without problems.

STARTING TO BREAST-FEED

Some women find breast-feeding in front of other members of the family embarrassing, perhaps because we are all too much exposed to breasts as sexual objects rather than as means of feeding babies. If you prefer privacy you can always find another room such as a bedroom, where you can concentrate on feeding your baby.

For the first 48–72 hours you will produce only a little milk (called colostrum). This is particularly good for the baby because it contains antibodies against infection, and he will need nothing else provided he is not premature, small-for-dates (*see page 120*), or ill.

A baby does not actually suck milk out of the nipple—with his gums, he squeezes the areola (the dark area of skin around the nipple) so that milk squirts out of the nipple into his mouth. If he is allowed to suck too hard at your nipple, it may become sore. Your midwife will show you how to position him at the breast to stop that happening.

DEMANDS

How often should I feed my baby?
The most natural method of breast-feeding is to give the baby milk whenever he demands it. During the first week or two, a baby may demand a feed up to a dozen times a day. Most babies then settle down to demanding a feed every three or four hours, but a few retain this early pattern of seeming to want virtually constant feeding. In time you will find that he establishes his own feeding pattern, and you can omit feeds during the night.

At night, keep the baby in a crib beside you. You will find that when he cries you can feed him almost without waking him up. Premature babies may be prescribed iron for the first few months. Some doctors recommend giving the baby fluoride drops to protect his developing teeth.

There are no rules about how long the baby should feed—let the baby decide. Make sure that he feeds from both breasts before he is full, otherwise one breast will become engorged.

WHEN A BABY GETS TOO LITTLE MILK
If you are an experienced mother you will know whether your baby is getting the right amount of milk. If the baby is your first, note the following points. If he is lively, alert and contented he is probably getting the right amount. If he is not putting on weight he may not be getting enough milk. Have his weight checked. This can be done at the welfare clinic, health centre, doctor's surgery, or by a health visitor at home.

An underfed breast-fed baby does not necessarily cry with hunger. Often he is quiet and uninterested in the world around him.

If your milk supply decreases or fails for any reason, consult your doctor, health visitor or midwife. You may be advised to make up for a decreased supply of breast milk with feeds of artificial milk. (Feeds given to top-up a breast-feed are known as complementary; those given in place of a breast-feed are called supplementary.)

However, giving artificial feeds may make the problem of decreased breast milk worse, since your body works on the principle that the more breast milk the baby takes, the more is produced, consequently the more artificial milk he gets, the less breast milk he takes and the less you will make.

Ninety-five per cent of women are able to breast-feed successfully. If you have any problems, consult your midwife or health visitor, talk to other mothers with experience of breast-feeding, or contact a branch of the National Childbirth Trust or La Leche League if there is one in your area.

RESTRICTIONS

What are the medical reasons for not breast-feeding?
Women who suffer from certain illnesses or are being treated with certain drugs should not breast-feed. If in doubt, consult your doctor on both points before starting to breast-feed. He will give you all the advice and reassurance that you need.

Stop breast-feeding temporarily if you have cracked nipples, and express the milk from your breasts until the nipples are healed. If breast-feeding becomes painful, seek immediate treatment.

If you begin breast-feeding but have to stop for any reason, do not be disappointed. The first days or weeks are the most important.

Feeding twins and triplets

☐ It is perfectly possible to breast-feed twins. Time rather than the quantity of milk is the likely problem (wet-nurses used to breast-feed as many as six babies, but it was a full-time occupation).

☐ It is even possible to feed them simultaneously by holding one under each arm carefully propped with cushions. If you want to try this, ask your health visitor to help you work out the best method. This may not work, especially if the babies wriggle or if they feed at a very different pace. In this case feed them one at a time but each from a different breast.

☐ Demand-feeding is difficult, because if they have different patterns you will get little rest. Wake one to feed him immediately after feeding the other.

☐ If you are bottle-feeding, you will find it virtually impossible to hold two bottles and two babies simultaneously. Propping up a bottle while one baby feeds can be dangerous or can introduce a lot of air which can produce wind. Unless you have help, demand-feeding is inadvisable, as you will find that the babies will take up much of your time.

☐ With both breast and bottle-feeding, one baby can be given a dummy while waiting for the other to finish.

☐ One in 7,000 pregnancies results in triplets. Feeding them without extra help is not impossible but certainly exhausting. Bottle-feeding is likely to be a little easier as your partner could share the work involved in preparing bottles.

Breast-feeding

Both mother and baby should be comfortable while feeding. Clothes that open down the front make it easier to bare your breasts. Sit on a comfortable low chair with your feet flat on the floor and with your back properly supported. If necessary put a pillow behind your back, or beneath the baby on your lap to adjust to an upright position that is comfortable both for yourself and the baby.

1 *Cradle the baby so that his mouth is level with the nipple. Support his head with your elbow or forearm. Gently stroke his cheek nearest the nipple. This lets him know that the breast is near.*

2 *The baby will turn his head towards the breast, purse his lips and touch the nipple. He will then take the nipple and areola in his mouth and start sucking. Do not let the baby suck on the end of the nipple. He will get no milk because his sucking closes the openings in the nipple, and you will get sore nipples. Make sure that the nipple and areola are both in his mouth.*

3 *If the baby seems to have difficulty in 'latching on', hold the breast between finger and forefinger at the edge of the areola. Gently press and guide the nipple into his mouth. It may be necessary to press nearer to the nipple if the nipples are very flat. If the breast is too swollen for the baby to grasp the nipple it sometimes helps to express a little milk before putting him to the breast.*

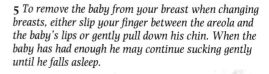

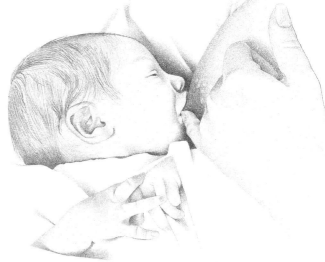

5 *To remove the baby from your breast when changing breasts, either slip your finger between the areola and the baby's lips or gently pull down his chin. When the baby has had enough he may continue sucking gently until he falls asleep.*

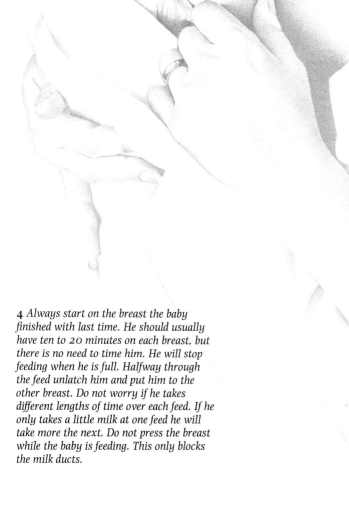

4 *Always start on the breast the baby finished with last time. He should usually have ten to 20 minutes on each breast, but there is no need to time him. He will stop feeding when he is full. Halfway through the feed unlatch him and put him to the other breast. Do not worry if he takes different lengths of time over each feed. If he only takes a little milk at one feed he will take more the next. Do not press the breast while the baby is feeding. This only blocks the milk ducts.*

Hand-expressing milk

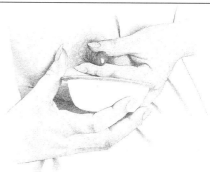

You may sometimes need to express your milk by hand. Place the index finger and thumb on the areola, and gently squeeze and push back towards the breastbone in the same movement. Do not squeeze the nipple.

Bottle-feeding

Sit in a low chair with your feet flat on the floor. Make sure your back is well supported, use a pillow if necessary. Cradle the baby in your arms so that his mouth is higher than his stomach and you can comfortably hold the bottle to his mouth. Hold the baby close to you. Do not give him the bottle propped up so that he can feed himself. He might choke, and he will be deprived of the comfort that a breast-fed baby gets from being cuddled by his mother.

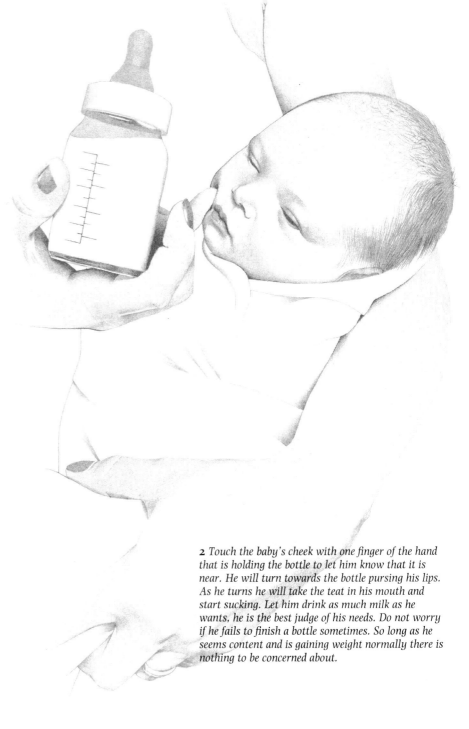

1 *Cold milk does not harm a baby and is safer than milk which is too warm, but the baby will prefer it at body temperature. Put the bottle of milk in a jug of hot water and leave it for five minutes. Test the temperature on your forearm. The milk should feel neither hot nor cold.*

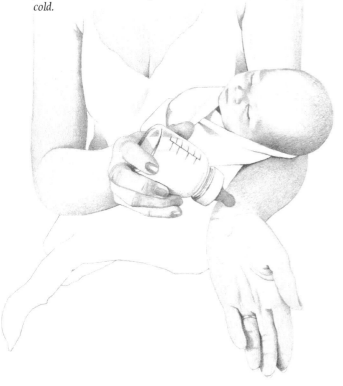

2 *Touch the baby's cheek with one finger of the hand that is holding the bottle to let him know that it is near. He will turn towards the bottle pursing his lips. As he turns he will take the teat in his mouth and start sucking. Let him drink as much milk as he wants, he is the best judge of his needs. Do not worry if he fails to finish a bottle sometimes. So long as he seems content and is gaining weight normally there is nothing to be concerned about.*

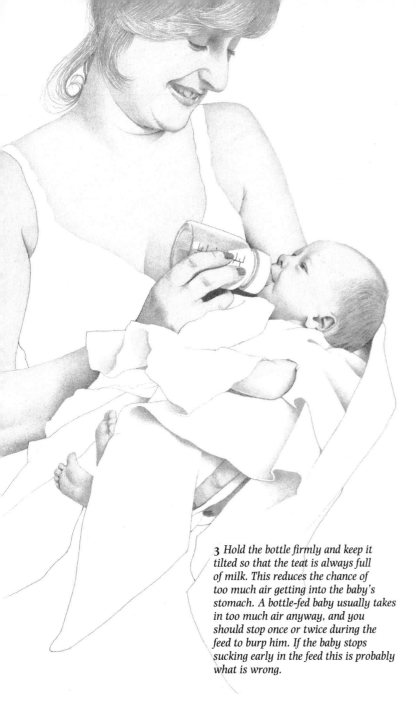

3 Hold the bottle firmly and keep it tilted so that the teat is always full of milk. This reduces the chance of too much air getting into the baby's stomach. A bottle-fed baby usually takes in too much air anyway, and you should stop once or twice during the feed to burp him. If the baby stops sucking early in the feed this is probably what is wrong.

BOTTLE-FEEDING

To bottle-feed a baby you will need: 2 feeding bottles, 4 teats, 2 bottle caps, 1 bottle brush, 1 sterilising container, 1 bottle of sterilising agent, tins or packets of milk powder, 1 measuring spoon (supplied with milk powders).

To make a bottle-feed, add dried cow's milk powder (which you buy from a chemist) to cooled boiled water. There is little to choose between different brands of powder, so it is sensible to buy the cheapest, but talk it over with the health visitor or doctor if you have any doubts. If you or your husband has asthma or eczema, your doctor may advise you to buy a soya-based powder. This contains no cow's milk, which may cause asthma or eczema in some babies.

It is vital that feeding equipment is sterile. In their first few months babies have very poorly developed ways of resisting infection, so it is important to keep bacteria and viruses away from them as much as possible.

When preparing bottles, your hands and all utensils should be clean. Bottles, caps and teats should be stored in a sterilising solution such as Milton, which should be changed according to the instructions on the bottle label.

Even Milton is not foolproof if there are deposits of dried milk in the bottle or teat, so straight after feeding wash them and scrub off any material clinging to the surface.

CALCULATING HOW MUCH MILK TO GIVE

Every 24 hours the baby requires about 2–3 oz. (60–90 ml.) of milk for every pound he weighs. The exact amount depends on the individual baby but is not necessarily related to his size: if he is small-for-dates (*see page 120*) he may have an enormous appetite, if large-for-dates a surprisingly small one. Feeds should be given about every four hours (though, as with breast-fed babies, the schedule need not be rigid). Very small or premature babies may need three-hourly feeds at first.

Do not worry if your baby refuses to finish a bottle or if he sleeps through the night without wanting a feed. The best guide to whether he is getting enough milk is his weight gain and degree of contentment. If you suspect he is taking the wrong amount, consult your health visitor, midwife or doctor.

DUMMIES

Should I give the baby a dummy?
If the choice is between an angry crying baby and a contented one with a dummy, give him a dummy. But remember it may be difficult to remove it. On the other hand, babies not allowed dummies may become thumb or finger suckers, and this is an even harder habit to break.

BRINGING UP THE BABY'S WIND

All babies—breast or bottle-fed—swallow air. In the case of bottle-fed babies you can lessen air swallowing by holding the bottle as shown. Once air has been swallowed it floats on top of the milk in the stomach. So, if you tilt the baby as shown, the air will escape up his food-pipe. Patting or rubbing his back may comfort the baby but is not essential. Wind him once in mid-feed and once afterwards. If nothing comes up, do not carry on for longer than a minute or two. If you keep interrupting the baby's feed he will cry and swallow even more air. Some babies are difficult to wind, but there is no foolproof method. *See* COLIC.

CHANGING NAPPIES
Babies will produce wet nappies at every feed and these will need to be changed. But the frequency with which they produce stools varies from baby to baby. Some do it after every feed, others (particularly breast-fed babies) as little as once a day.

Babies fed only on milk should pass soft stools with a porridge-like consistency. If your baby passes watery, frequent stools, this is not normal and you should consult your doctor. The colour of normal stools may vary from yellow to green, but the variation is rarely of medical significance.

NAPPY CHOICE

Disposable or terry-towel nappies?
This is a matter for you to decide. Terry-towel nappies, which you wash and use again and again, are only marginally cheaper than disposable nappies, but they are ecologically friendly. Not all disposable nappies can be flushed down the lavatory; this is especially so if you live in the country and have a septic tank. Some babies get nappy rash more readily with terry-towel nappies, others get the rash with disposable ones.

Changing nappies/Kite method

The kite nappy is suitable for either a boy or a girl, and since its length can be adjusted to the baby's size, it can be used for all ages. Have ready two closed nappy pins. Place the nappy diagonally in front of you on a flat surface.

Folding a kite

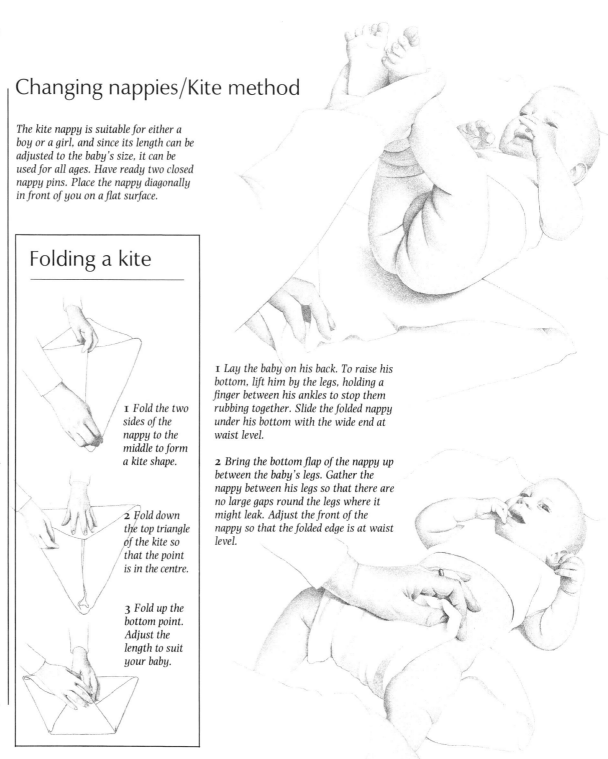

1 Fold the two sides of the nappy to the middle to form a kite shape.

2 Fold down the top triangle of the kite so that the point is in the centre.

3 Fold up the bottom point. Adjust the length to suit your baby.

1 Lay the baby on his back. To raise his bottom, lift him by the legs, holding a finger between his ankles to stop them rubbing together. Slide the folded nappy under his bottom with the wide end at waist level.

2 Bring the bottom flap of the nappy up between the baby's legs. Gather the nappy between his legs so that there are no large gaps round the legs where it might leak. Adjust the front of the nappy so that the folded edge is at waist level.

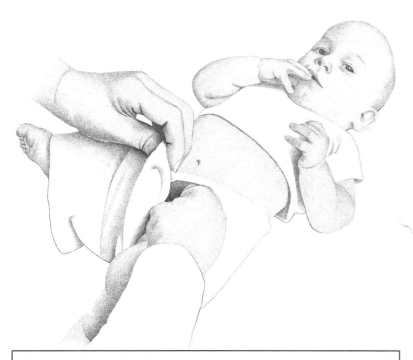

3 *Lift the right back corner of the nappy, bring it round to the baby's front, and tuck it under the front flap. Pin the corners together with a nappy pin and repeat the operation with the left corner.*

Using plastic tie-on pants

Plastic pants will prevent leakage, but should be left off whenever convenient since they trap urine close to the skin, which may lead to nappy rash. They may be held in place with elastic, poppers or ties.

1 *Lay the baby on his back on the plastic. Tie the two top ties across his front. Turn him over and tie the other two at his back.*

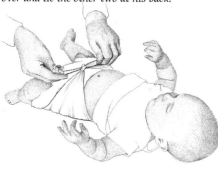

2 *Tuck in the edges round the legs where leaks may occur. This method of tying is more secure than tying at the sides.*

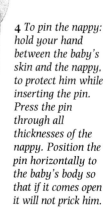

4 *To pin the nappy: hold your hand between the baby's skin and the nappy, to protect him while inserting the pin. Press the pin through all thicknesses of the nappy. Position the pin horizontally to the baby's body so that if it comes open it will not prick him.*

WASHING NAPPIES

Terry-towel nappies should be cleaned by removing solid waste with warm water, then washing the nappies in a washing-machine or in hot water, using soap powder (not an enzyme or biological detergent). Then soak them thoroughly in a solution of a sterilising agent specially manufactured for the purpose. Rinse the nappies in clean water and dry them.

USING PLASTIC PANTS

After you have removed the baby's nappy, clean his bottom carefully with cotton wool soaked in warm water. Use baby soap if he is very soiled. Pat him dry, then gently rub into the skin a barrier cream, which you can obtain from a chemist. Remove plastic pants whenever convenient, since they trap urine close to the skin and if this happens too often nappy rash will result. Plastic pants can be cleaned in warm water, soaked in a sterilising solution and hung up to dry—preferably outside.

Throw away the pants when they become hard, otherwise they will chafe his skin.

BATHING THE BABY

By the end of the day many babies are fairly smelly, so try to give the baby a bath every evening—though regular topping and tailing will serve the same purpose. Use only baby soap to wash him; other soaps and bubble baths could irritate his skin. And make sure you keep the soap out of his eyes.

When bathing the baby, do not touch what remains of the umbilical cord. If you leave it alone, it will come away sooner.

Changing nappies/Chinese method

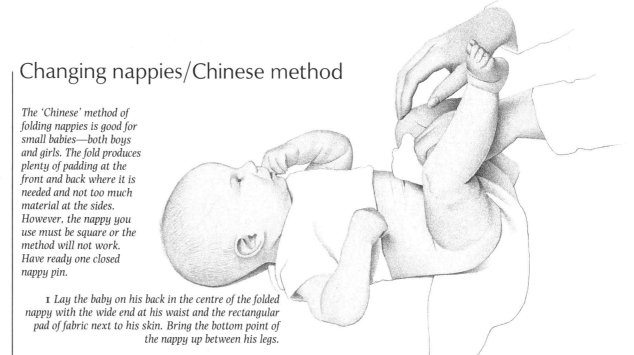

The 'Chinese' method of folding nappies is good for small babies—both boys and girls. The fold produces plenty of padding at the front and back where it is needed and not too much material at the sides. However, the nappy you use must be square or the method will not work. Have ready one closed nappy pin.

I Lay the baby on his back in the centre of the folded nappy with the wide end at his waist and the rectangular pad of fabric next to his skin. Bring the bottom point of the nappy up between his legs.

Folding a Chinese nappy

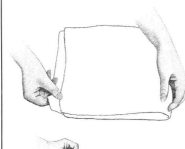

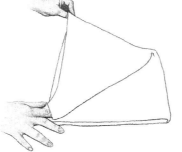

I Fold the nappy in half and then in half again to form a square. Place the square in front of you so that the edge of the second fold is on your left and the open corner is at the bottom to your right.

2 With your left hand, take hold of the top layer at the bottom right-hand corner. Holding down the under layers, pull the corner across to the left to form an overlapping triangle.

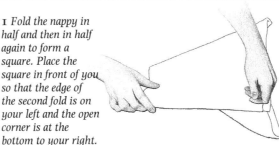

3 Turn the nappy over, top to bottom, so that the square is to your right. Fold over the right-hand third of the square. Do not disturb the triangle underneath.

4 Make a second lengthwise fold in the square so that there is now a thick rectangular pad of fabric lying in the middle of the triangle running from top to bottom.

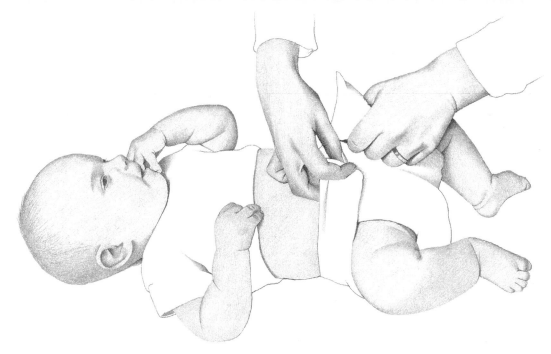

CLOTHING THE BABY

During pregnancy you should buy the following clothes for the baby:

All-in-one stretch garments,	4
Vests, preferably with ties at one side,	5
Nappies (the better quality last longer),	24
Nappy liners,	1 box
Plastic pants,	6
Bibs,	6
Sun hat,	1

A knitted bonnet, bootees and mittens are useful in winter, but coats and jumpers are not usually necessary for you to buy, nor are dresses, rompers and nightwear, since these are the items that are often bought or made as gifts.

If money is short, study the notice boards in the antenatal clinic and infant welfare clinic: second-hand clothes are often available. They can also be obtained at toddler clubs and parent groups, and your health visitor may well know of other places. You should not feel ashamed of buying second-hand clothes. There will not be time for them to become shabby, since babies grow out of their clothes so quickly.

2 *Hold the front flap in place with your left hand. Position your fingers so that the layer next to the baby's skin is left free. Bring the two side corners of the nappy across the baby's body so that they cross in the middle.*

3 *Protect the baby's body with the hand holding the flap as you insert the nappy pin. Fasten together the two side corners and the top layers of the pad, making sure that the pin is horizontal to the baby's body. Do not pin through the layer of fabric next to his skin.*

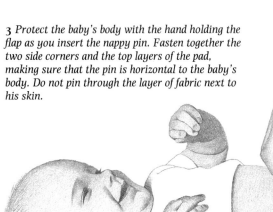

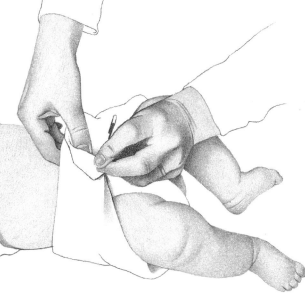

CORRECT CLOTHING

How warm does the baby need to be? In Britain overdressing a baby is more common than underdressing him. If he is red-faced and sweating, take off a layer of clothing. But if his bedroom gets very cold at night he will need clothing that covers his hands and feet.

THE BABY'S SLEEP

You will soon come to recognise the behaviour that shows your baby is ready to sleep—often a baby behaves as though he is uncomfortable. If the baby is lively, then, whatever the time of day, he is not yet ready for his sleep.

Many mothers are happy to use a carry-cot which can be used as a pram during the day. You will need a couple of flannelette sheets and two or three cellular blankets for use in the cot.

A pillow is unnecessary and can even be dangerous. A plastic sheet is useful to cover the mattress (and you will need a second plastic sheet for the pram mattress).

Do not allow the room to become too cold at night; but do not allow the baby to overheat by putting on too many clothes or blankets. Provide background heating at a minimum temperature of 55°F (13°C). But if the baby was premature and still weighs less than 6 lb. (2.7 kg.) this temperature may be too low—ask your doctor or health visitor for advice about this.

Do not put your baby to sleep face down.

COMFORTER

Should I let my child have a comforter?
When tired or unhappy, most young children turn to a comforter—a soft toy, blanket or even nappy that they fondle or cuddle—or suck their fingers. This behaviour is entirely natural and should not be stopped or mocked.

Dressing a baby

Lay the baby on a changing mat on the floor, in a cot, or hold him on your knee. Do not dress him on a table or bed where he might roll off on to the floor.

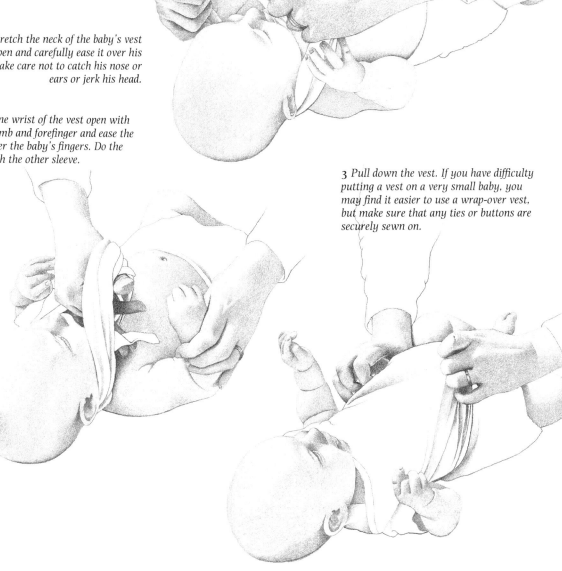

1 Stretch the neck of the baby's vest wide open and carefully ease it over his head. Take care not to catch his nose or ears or jerk his head.

2 Hold one wrist of the vest open with your thumb and forefinger and ease the sleeve over the baby's fingers. Do the same with the other sleeve.

3 Pull down the vest. If you have difficulty putting a vest on a very small baby, you may find it easier to use a wrap-over vest, but make sure that any ties or buttons are securely sewn on.

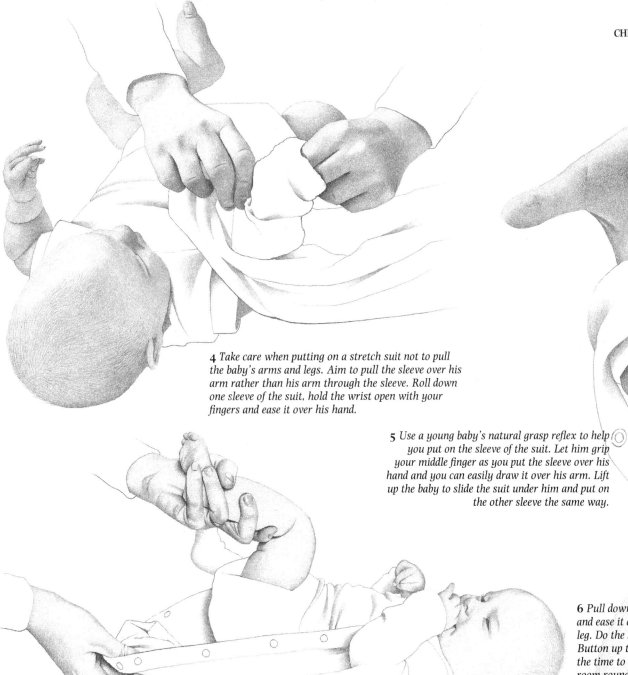

4 *Take care when putting on a stretch suit not to pull the baby's arms and legs. Aim to pull the sleeve over his arm rather than his arm through the sleeve. Roll down one sleeve of the suit, hold the wrist open with your fingers and ease it over his hand.*

5 *Use a young baby's natural grasp reflex to help you put on the sleeve of the suit. Let him grip your middle finger as you put the sleeve over his hand and you can easily draw it over his arm. Lift up the baby to slide the suit under him and put on the other sleeve the same way.*

6 *Pull down the suit, roll down one leg, and ease it on to the baby's foot and up his leg. Do the same with the other leg. Button up the front of the suit. This is the time to check that there is plenty of room round the baby's feet. If not, get a new suit, there may be harmful pressure on his feet and legs.*

MOVING THE BABY TO A FULL-SIZED COT

By the time your baby is able to sit up, a crib or carry-cot will no longer be safe for him to sleep in. You will need a full-size cot with a safety catch, preferably carrying the British Standards kite mark.

If you buy a second-hand cot which you intend to repaint, buy lead-free paint (it is called paint for toys and playthings).

You will need a cot mattress, plastic sheet, flannelette under-blanket, sheet and cellular blankets or infant's sleeping bag.

Cot bumpers are usually unnecessary unless your baby has a habit of banging his head against the bars (*see page 160*).

NIGHT NOISES

Is restlessness normal during sleep?
Yes. Most babies grunt, snort, sigh, whimper and kick when asleep. If the noise disturbs the sleep of you or your partner too much, put the baby in an adjoining room, from which you can hear him cry if he is in distress.

When you feel confident to do so, and if you have room, let him have his own room permanently.

TAKING THE BABY OUTSIDE

A new luxury pram is expensive and eventually becomes a white elephant. Many parents are happy simply with a carry-cot in a transporter, but do ensure that it has adequate safety attachments to prevent the cot falling out of the transporter when you take it down steps or if you stop suddenly.

When the baby is outside, it is a sensible precaution to fix a cat net to the pram, whether or not you keep a cat yourself. Both dogs and cats can carry diseases that infect children, so do not allow them to lick the baby or lie with him.

LOVE-MAKING

When can I make love again?
As soon as you want to, but you may not be interested in sex for a few weeks after the baby is born. You may be sore for a week or two. If the soreness still exists when you have your post-natal examination, tell the doctor. He may suggest using a lubricant jelly. If your sex life is still affected after one or two months, you can discuss it with your doctor.

Will breast-feeding stop me getting pregnant?
No.

If my periods have not returned, am I safe from pregnancy?
No.

OBTAINING HELP IN THE FIRST WEEKS

During your first few weeks with the new baby there will not seem to be enough hours in the day, and you will probably appreciate any help you can get. If you do not have a relative or friend who can help, ask your health visitor or the local social services department about the possibility of obtaining a home help.

If your mother is helping out, she may tend to spoil the baby. If you are happy to go along with her way of

doing things, there will be no problems. If not, then you should make it clear early on that your baby will be brought up your way.

FOOD AND DRINK

Do I have to 'eat for two' if I am breast-feeding?
No. But your appetite will increase a little and you will need to drink more.

GETTING BACK YOUR NORMAL SHAPE

You do not suddenly return to your normal shape immediately after your baby is born, but, provided you do not overeat, you should do so fairly soon. A greater problem than weight is the stretched muscles of your abdomen, which may make you more flabby there. The muscles will become firmer with time, but this natural process can be speeded up by regular exercises (*see page 248*).

POST-NATAL DEPRESSION

Nearly all women feel tearful, helpless or even frightened for a day or two after delivery. With a few mothers this reaction is more severe and lasts longer; it is known as post-natal depression. The mother becomes confused and cannot cope with her baby's needs, and she may also feel shaky, exhausted or generally ill. If you suffer post-natal depression, and relatives or friends are unable to help, talk to your doctor or health visitor. You may find that discussing how you feel is helpful, or you may even need treatment with anti-depressant tablets.

3. FIRST MONTHS

Helping your baby's development

When considering whether your baby is growing fast enough, there are two points to remember. Firstly, babies do not put on the same amount of weight each day. Rather, the line of their weight progress resembles a flight of steps, sometimes showing no gain for a few days, then leaping ahead. Secondly, some babies

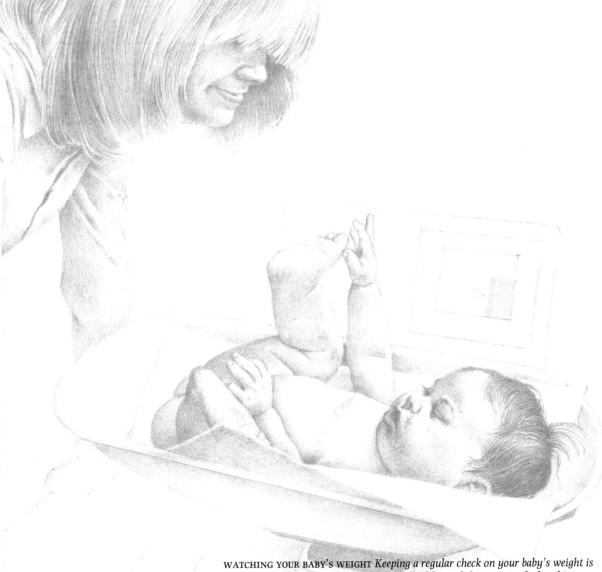

WATCHING YOUR BABY'S WEIGHT *Keeping a regular check on your baby's weight is an easy way of making certain that he is healthy and that you are feeding him adequately. There are various rules-of-thumb about how much weight should be gained in the first few months: a well-known one is 'an ounce a day except on Sundays'. However, beware of rules: each baby is unique and may follow a slightly different growth pattern. Rely on your health visitor or clinic nurse to guide you. Keep the clinic's weight book in your handbag; if your baby ever needs to be seen by a doctor the information in it may be helpful in discovering what is wrong.*

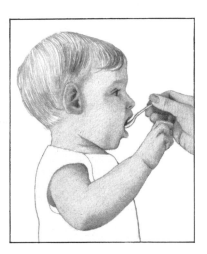

SPOON-FEEDING *Making a mess is all part of learning to cope. Let your baby use a spoon on his own and try out his newly discovered skills and he will learn much more quickly. However, feeding him with a spoon can be an enjoyable game and makes much less mess if you are in a hurry.*

start off heavy for their age, then put on only a little weight and become lighter for their age over a period of about three months. Others do the opposite. Although both these patterns are generally harmless, it is wise to consult your doctor if your baby follows either.

For the first six weeks have your baby weighed once a week; then fortnightly until three months; and after that once a month.

Do not be tempted to weigh the baby too often, since you may be needlessly worried by a succession of days when the baby gains no weight.

APPETITE

When do I increase the baby's feeds?
Firstly, if he seems hungry. Secondly, to keep his daily intake at about $2\frac{1}{2}$ oz. to every pound of his weight, or 150 ml. for every kilogram. If you offer a little more than this, you will soon know when he needs more.

INTRODUCING THE BABY TO SOLID FOOD
Babies will grow normally, and stay healthy, on milk alone for a year or more. But once a baby has teeth it is reasonable to offer solids, and once he can lift things to his mouth, let him practise with a rusk or biscuit. Solids in the early months can be harmful—by making the baby over-weight. A good compromise is to start solids some time between four and six months. However, babies who vomit their milk, and certain other babies, may need to go on to solids earlier. Let your health visitor or doctor guide you on the matter.

Introduce one solid at a time—then you will know if any particular food disagrees with the baby. Try cereals first. Then fruit, eggs, bread, butter, root vegetables, cheese, meat and fish. Most manufactured baby foods, which are sold in tins or jars, provide adequate nutrition. But it is worth looking at the list of ingredients. Foods with a lot of cereal, milk powder or lactose may be too fattening. All foods that you prepare yourself must be sieved or liquidised to break down large particles on which a baby could choke.

At a feed, offer solids first, then milk. As the baby takes more solids, he will want less milk. When fully weaned from the breast or bottle, he may require less than a pint daily. A few babies refuse milk once they have gone on to solids; this is not nutritionally harmful.

From about six months, the baby can drink ordinary bottled cow's milk. From that age also, there is no need to continue sterilising feeding vessels. Simply keep them as clean as possible.

MILK TEETH

Should I leave a bottle in the baby's bed?
No. Milk contains 7 per cent sugar, and sugar reacts with bacteria in the mouth to break down tooth enamel. At night, when the baby sleeps after each feed he takes, there is no longer, as there is in the day, a free flow of saliva and activity by the mouth to prevent the teeth being bathed in milk for long periods. So the baby's teeth are prone to decay.

DEVELOPMENT OF SKILLS

This table shows the ages by which nearly all babies have achieved various skills.

NOTE If your baby was premature, count his age from the day he should have been born.
Bear in mind that the table is only a guide and that some babies develop in an unusual way. For example, some stand before they can sit, and 'bottom-shufflers' may not walk until they are two or more. However, if you are worried about your baby's development in any of the skills listed, consult your doctor or health visitor, who will give the baby various tests to perform.
The doctor or health visitor will not regard the baby's performance of each test as a pass or failure. Instead, they look at the performances as a whole and observe how your baby behaves generally. And it may well be that even if your baby is very late in developing certain skills they will be able to reassure you that there is nothing fundamentally wrong.

MUSCULAR DEVELOPMENT

☐ **Can keep head steady when you sit him down**
Early 6 weeks *Average* 10 weeks
Late (but normal) 17 weeks

☐ **Rolls over**
Early 2 months *Average* 10 weeks
Late (but normal) 17 weeks

☐ **Bears some weight on legs**
Early 3 months *Average* $4\frac{1}{2}$ months
Late (but normal) $7\frac{1}{2}$ months

☐ **Sits without support**
Early 5 months *Average* $5\frac{1}{2}$ months
Late (but normal) 8 months

☐ **Can rise to sitting position unaided**
Early 6 months *Average* $7\frac{1}{2}$ months
Late (but normal) 11 months

☐ **Stands holding on to support**
Early 5 months *Average* $5\frac{1}{2}$ months
Late (but normal) 10 months

☐ **Walks round furniture**
Early $7\frac{1}{2}$ months
Average 9 months
Late (but normal) 13 months

☐ **Walks without support**
Early 11 months
Average 12 months
Late (but normal) 14 months

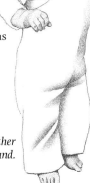

SUPPORT *Mother helps him to stand.*

SIGHT AND CO-ORDINATION OF EYES AND HANDS

□ **Can follow object from one side of vision to other (180 degrees)**
Early 7 weeks *Average* 2 months
Late (but normal) 4 months

□ **Gets hands together**
Early 5 weeks *Average* 2 months
Late (but normal) 3½ months

□ **Reaches for object**
Early 2½ months *Average* 3 months
Late (but normal) 5 months

□ **Grasps rattle**
Early 2½ months *Average* 3½ months
Late (but normal) 4 months

□ **Takes and holds two bricks**
Early 5 months *Average* 6 months
Late (but normal) 7½ months

□ **Bangs bricks together**
Early 7 months *Average* 8½ months
Late (but normal) 12 months

□ **Neat finger-thumb grip (of a raisin)**
Early 9 months *Average* 10½ months
Late (but normal) 14 months

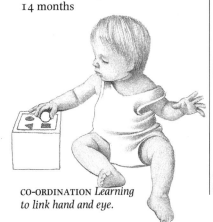

CO-ORDINATION *Learning to link hand and eye.*

SPEECH AND HEARING

□ **Laughs**
Early 6 weeks *Average* 7 weeks
Late (but normal) 3½ months

□ **Turns towards a voice**
Early 3½ months *Average* 5½ months
Late (but normal) 8½ months

□ **Imitates adult speech sounds**
Early 5½ months *Average* 7 months
Late (but normal) 11½ months

□ **Says 'Mama', 'Dada', indiscriminately**
Early 5½ months *Average* 7 months
Late (but normal) 10 months

□ **Says 'Mama', or 'Dada' to right person**
Early 9 months
Average 10 months
Late (but normal) 13 months

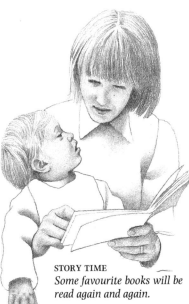

STORY TIME
Some favourite books will be read again and again.

RESPONSE AND PLAY

□ **Smiles in response to person**
Early Within days of birth
Average 5 weeks
Late (but normal) 7½ weeks

□ **Smiles spontaneously**
Early 6 weeks *Average* 8 weeks
Late (but normal) 5 months

□ **Feeds himself a rusk**
Early 4½ months *Average* 5½ months
Late (but normal) 8 months

□ **Plays peek-a-boo**
Early 6 months *Average* 6½ months
Late (but normal) 9½ months

□ **Plays pat-a-cake**
Early 7 months *Average* 9½ months
Late (but normal) 13 months

□ **Reacts shyly to strangers**
Early 5½ months
Average 9½ months
Late (but normal) 10 months

□ **Plays ball**
Early 10 months
Average 11½ months
Late (but normal) 16 months

□ **Indicates wants without crying**
Early 10½ months
Average 12½ months
Late (but normal) 14½ months

EXPERIMENT *Your baby feels shape and texture with his mouth.*

When you must turn to the doctor

Certain problems *must* be referred to the doctor. These are set out in the table below.

Problem	When to consult the doctor
□ No interest in surroundings	Immediately
□ No sign of seeing things	Immediately
□ No sign of hearing things	Immediately
□ Head not held up when lying on stomach	4 months old
□ Makes hardly any sounds	5 months old
□ Squint	6 months old
□ Not reaching out for toys	7 months old
□ Not sitting	9 months old
□ Not turning to voice	9 months old
□ Not taking weight on feet	12 months old

HELPING IN THE BABY'S DEVELOPMENT

Some aspects of development cannot be hurried—you cannot help the baby to walk earlier if his nerves and muscles have not developed enough for him to walk. Other aspects can be helped, however. The more you read to the baby, show him things, talk to him and play games with him, the more you encourage him to talk and the brighter he is likely to be.

WALKING

Should the baby have a baby-walker or bouncer?
These may provide the baby with fun but they will not help him to walk more quickly. And if he is a 'bottom-shuffler' (a baby who likes to move in a sitting position and will not take weight on his feet), a baby-walker may actually further retard his walking.

WHEN A BABY'S TEETH APPEAR

The following table shows when the average baby's teeth arrive. But bear in mind that babies differ considerably in their stages of development.

Lower central incisors
5 to 10 months

Upper incisors
8 to 12 months

Lower lateral incisors
12 to 14 months

First molars
12 to 14 months

Canines
16 to 22 months

Second molars
24 to 30 months

Teething problems upset most children to some extent. But it is very rare for them to be severe. Most mothers believe teething causes irritability, red cheeks, nappy rash, diarrhoea and fever. Most doctors do *not* believe that teething causes the last three. Indeed, diarrhoea and fever can be dangerous in a child and should never be blamed on teething— the cause may be something more

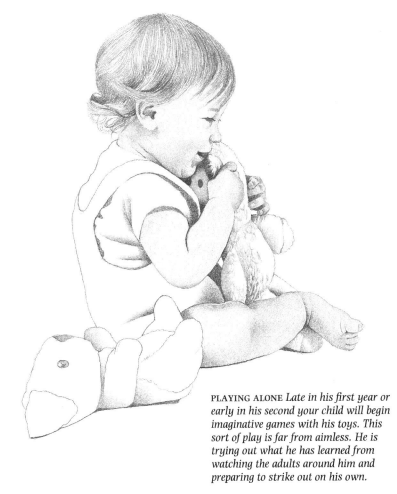

serious. It is a mistake to connect nappy rash with teething as the cause is quite different.

Teething never causes fits.

If your baby is uncomfortable and irritable when teething consult your doctor. He may prescribe a mild painkiller.

PLAYING ALONE *Late in his first year or early in his second your child will begin imaginative games with his toys. This sort of play is far from aimless. He is trying out what he has learned from watching the adults around him and preparing to strike out on his own.*

TOOTH CARE

How can I safeguard my child's teeth?
Good teeth are inherited. If yours or your partner's are of poor quality (as opposed to good teeth that have been allowed to decay), your child's will need special protection. To safeguard a baby's teeth, keep him off sweet foods as much as possible, and, since milk contains sugar, do not give him a bottle except at feeding times.

Teeth that have not yet developed can be protected by giving the baby fluoride if you do not live in an area where the tapwater is already fluoridated. Ask your doctor or dentist about this.

IMMUNISATION

During his first year the child should have the following immunisations:
Two months Diphtheria, tetanus, whooping-cough and HiB (haemophilus influenza, an important cause of MENINGITIS and EPIGLOTTITIS in children). At the same time, polio vaccine is given in the form of drops. Each of these immunisations is the first of a course of three given during the first year.
Three months The second combined diphtheria, tetanus and whooping-cough vaccination. The second HiB injection and polio vaccine drops.

Four months The third combined diphtheria, tetanus and whooping-cough vaccination. The third HiB injection and polio vaccine drops.

After the first year:

12 to 18 months Measles, mumps and rubella (MMR) vaccination.

Four to five years Diphtheria and tetanus. Polio vaccine drops.

10 to 14 years BCG vaccination against tuberculosis (if skin test is negative).

Thirteen years—for girls only German measles (rubella) vaccination.

Fifteen years, or on leaving school Tetanus vaccination and polio vaccine drops.

Any immunisation should be done when a child is well (though something like a persistently runny nose is not an illness).

A child who has suffered brain damage or who is prone to epileptic fits, or who has a close relative with epilepsy, should not be automatically immunised. Inform the doctor of the family history first, so that he can decide if immunisation is safe. If a child has any kind of allergy—for example, to penicillin, to hen's eggs—or if he has a disease such as leukaemia or Hodgkin's disease, or if he is on any kind of drugs, be sure to inform the doctor before vaccination. A child who has had a severe reaction to a vaccine should not have it repeated.

Your doctor will guide you in all these matters.

The ill-effects of vaccines on young children are much less common than most people think. The misconception may arise from the fact that during a child's first year he will probably have a few disorders, and that, by

the law of averages, one of these at least may well coincide with the time of an immunisation. Diphtheria, tetanus and polio vaccines are extremely safe. The first two sometimes cause swelling around the point of injection. Polio vaccine is

said to cause polio about once in every million doses. But polio is such a terrible disease that the slight risk is worth the protection provided for so many children.

There is a very rare possibility of an unimmunised parent developing

polio when a child is given the vaccine. Ideally, parents who have not previously had it should take the vaccine at the same time as the child.

Whooping-cough vaccine has had much publicity, because of rare cases

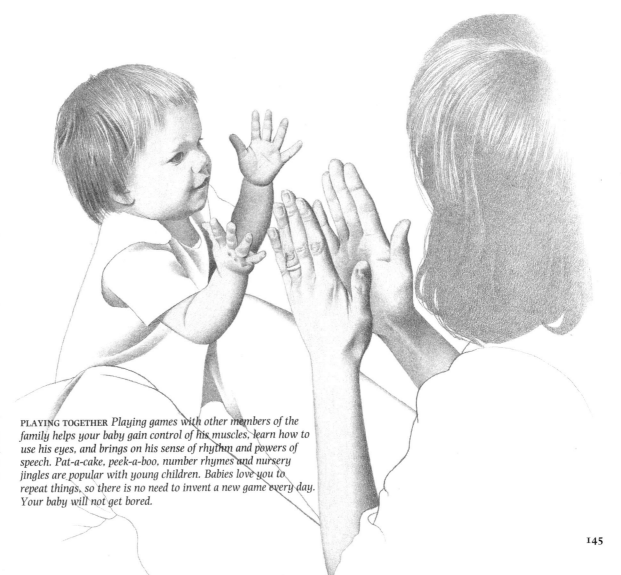

PLAYING TOGETHER *Playing games with other members of the family helps your baby gain control of his muscles, learn how to use his eyes, and brings on his sense of rhythm and powers of speech. Pat-a-cake, peek-a-boo, number rhymes and nursery jingles are popular with young children. Babies love you to repeat things, so there is no need to invent a new game every day. Your baby will not get bored.*

in which it has caused some degree of brain damage. The fact is that whooping cough is an unpleasant illness which, though usually harmless, is responsible for many more infant deaths than the vaccine is. By immunisation the number of deaths from whooping cough can be greatly reduced. Of children immunised against the disease, between one in 46,000 and one in 100,000 is estimated to have suffered brain damage. This incidence is much lower than the spontaneous risk of SUDDEN INFANT DEATH, PNEUMONIA and accidental death. In view of this and the risks of whooping cough, medical authorities still recommend that whooping-cough vaccine be given, provided the baby does not have any problems listed on page 145.

If you are in doubt about the matter, talk it over with your doctor.

HOW TO PREVENT ACCIDENTS
Young children are extremely curious and like exploring and putting interesting-looking objects in their mouth. Unless you take the necessary precautionary measures therefore, a child is likely to have an accident.

Once he is crawling, remove all dangerous objects from within his reach; go round each room on all fours yourself to see what is accessible.

Make sure the garage and garden shed are locked.

Do not store furniture polish, paint-stripper, bleach or any aerosol can where the child can reach them.

Put a gate at the top and bottom of any stairs.

Once the child can climb, keep upstairs windows locked.

Never have a fire alight without a guard around the entire fireplace.

Do not leave a child unattended in a room with a lighted paraffin heater.

Do not let the temperature of your hot water rise above 125°F (52°C).

Do not leave polythene bags lying around.

Do not use pots and pans that tip easily, when in use on a stove. Or if you already have these, buy pan guards to prevent them from tipping.

Lock away all medicines and tablets.

Make sure that the child cannot open the garden gate.

If the child is to travel in the family car, fit a safety harness.

Be careful not to say 'No' to a child when it is not really necessary: if he is always hearing the word, he will come to ignore it.

Do's and don'ts in your child's first year

There are several guidelines you can follow to keep your child healthy.

☐ *Do* give him more variety than rusks, biscuits, bread and sweets so that he does not get fat.

☐ *Do* encourage him to eat fruit and vegetables (puréed at first) as soon as he is eating solid foods.

☐ *Do* brush his teeth right from the start with a fluoride toothpaste, and give him fluoride tablets or drops to strengthen tooth enamel, unless you live in an area where the water is already fluoridated. Ask your dentist for advice.

☐ *Do* things with him so that he does not become bored.

☐ *Do* try to take him out with you every day, so that he gets regular fresh air.

☐ *Do* make sure that all your fires have proper guards, and avoid hanging tablecloths that can be pulled.

☐ *Don't* encourage him to develop a sweet tooth.

☐ *Don't* pacify him with sweets, if he is unhappy or irritable.

☐ *Don't* spend money on vitamins, except any your doctor may recommend.

☐ *Don't* smoke. Children who breathe in smoke from parents' cigarettes suffer more colds and chest infections than children of non-smokers.

☐ *Don't* let him get at medicines, tablets, household cleaners or other poisonous agents, bare electric wires or dog or cat droppings.

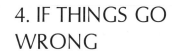

4. IF THINGS GO WRONG

Using the Health Service

As soon as possible after your baby is born you should register him as a patient with a general practitioner. If you fail to do this the baby is not entitled to National Health Service treatment, other than in an emergency (when any NHS doctor in

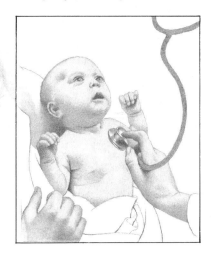

GAMES IN THE SURGERY *Your family doctor is not there just to treat illness. For example, your doctor may wish to test your baby's abilities and development from time to time. Most of the tests have been turned into games, such as checking for a squint by using a puppet for the baby's eyes to follow. Hearing, too, can be tested by persuading an infant to point to various toys when their names are whispered. If you are ever worried about aspects of your child's development, consult your family doctor, health visitor or clinic doctor. They will soon tell if anything is wrong with your baby, and give reassurance in the case of groundless fears.*

SEEING THE DOCTOR *Most things concerning children seem to go at a rapid pace. Illnesses are no exception. These frequently start suddenly and develop rapidly. Knowing this, your doctor will try to see you promptly. Happily, as your doctor knows, most childhood ills clear up quickly.*

the area where you are staying is obliged to provide treatment).

If you wish to visit the surgery of a GP who has an appointments system, the receptionist may ask you how urgent the problem is. Usually a baby will receive priority, but it would be unfair to other patients for you to insist on an immediate appointment for a minor complaint of long standing. If you think the receptionist is unreasonable in delaying an appointment, you can insist on speaking to the doctor. But remember that your reason for insisting should be valid. *See* DOCTOR.

Home visits by the doctor should rarely be necessary, particularly if you have a car or are very near the surgery. However, if you think your child is too ill to be taken to the doctor, try to phone before 10 a.m. for a visit. That is when most doctors plan their rounds.

At night, your phone call may be re-routed to another GP or a deputising service. If the phone rings for a long time, do not hang up. The re-connection may take some time.

Children in hospital

Each year one in every 15 children is admitted to hospital. For small children unused to separation from home and family a stay in hospital can be very upsetting. If the admission is an emergency and the child too young to understand an explanation, it is easy to imagine how terrified he might feel—even without any painful or unpleasant medical procedures taking place. Children from nine months to six years are most affected, some being more disturbed than others.

Avoiding distress
Much distress can be avoided if a parent, or other relative, remains with the child throughout the stay. Most hospitals arrange this routinely, and a polite but firm request to the ward sister will usually be met, even in those wards without special facilities for mothers.

If you cannot stay, it is best to be absolutely honest with the child. Do not pretend you are coming back when you are not.

Always leave behind something familiar belonging to you when you go. Try to have someone visit once or even more every day—a day can feel like half a lifetime to an infant. Tell the nurse any special words he uses or habits he has. If you get the chance, prepare your child for admission by talking about hospitals, playing nurse and doctor games, reading a book about a child going to hospital—and visiting the ward by arrangement with the sister.

Effect of separation
When children come home from hospital, their behaviour often changes. They may be clinging, not wanting to be left alone for a moment; children who were previously dry may now wet the bed; they may wake at night or refuse to sleep, develop headaches or stomach pains. All of this is a normal reaction to separation and will pass in time. Not all children react this way, but it is common enough to mean that unnecessary operations or hospital admission should be avoided if at all possible.

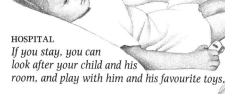

HOSPITAL
If you stay, you can look after your child and his room, and play with him and his favourite toys.

HOSPITAL SERVICES
If your child has an accident and you think he may need stitches, might have broken a bone or may have been knocked unconscious, go straight to the accident and emergency department of the nearest hospital. If he is suddenly taken seriously ill, do the same. But do not go because you want a second opinion or think your own doctor's treatment is not working.

WHEN TO CALL AN AMBULANCE
If a child has been in a road accident and has been unconscious, or you fear a broken limb.

If he is bleeding seriously or is unconscious.

If he is taken suddenly very ill and you do not have a car.
Note: if you do have a car and someone to go with you, this may be much quicker than waiting for an ambulance.

SEEING A SPECIALIST
You cannot walk into a specialist's consulting rooms without an appointment. Only your GP can arrange for you to see a specialist, except in a few inner-city areas where hospital paediatric departments have walk-in clinics. Officially, specialists are there to give an opinion to your GP rather than directly to you.

If your doctor thinks a second opinion is unnecessary he is almost

When to seek help urgently
(CHILD LESS THAN ONE YEAR OLD)

Take your child to the doctor at once if:

☐ He is not fully conscious or is unnaturally drowsy.

☐ He has had a fever fit *(see page 154)*.

☐ He becomes and stays very pale.

☐ He is blue around the lips or face—either all the time or intermittently.

☐ He has difficulty breathing or is wheezing badly.

☐ He suddenly develops a rash that looks like bleeding under the skin.

☐ You are frightened you might ill-treat him.

☐ *If in doubt, telephone your doctor. If he is unavailable, take your child to the nearest hospital accident and emergency department.*

Ask your doctor for a home visit if:

☐ Any of the above happens out of surgery hours.

☐ The child has a combination of two or more of the following: high fever, irritability or drowsiness, an altered type of cry, diarrhoea, vomiting, dry mouth and tongue, sunken eyes or a rash.

☐ He is unwell and you think he has an infectious illness such as MEASLES or CHICKENPOX.

☐ His breathing is noisy *(see CROUP)*.

Other reasons to call for help
(CHILD LESS THAN ONE YEAR OLD)

Ask for a surgery appointment the same day if there is:

☐ Less-severe wheezing, noisy or altered breathing.

☐ Diarrhoea and/or vomiting for more than six hours.

☐ Sudden development of excessive crying.

☐ Refusal to feed or sudden difficulty with feeding.

☐ Earache.

☐ Any fever in a child under six months.

☐ Fever for more than 24 hours in an older child.

☐ A stomach pain which is constant or worsening for longer than four hours.

☐ A headache which is constant for more than an hour or two.

Ask for an appointment within a day or two if you are worried about:

☐ Sore throat.

☐ Cough or cold, without difficulty in breathing.

☐ Headache which comes and goes.

☐ Minor amounts of diarrhoea and/or vomiting.

☐ Unexplained rashes without obvious fever.

Ask for a routine appointment or talk to your health visitor if:

☐ You are worried about the child's weight.

☐ He is a poor eater—but there has been no sudden change.

☐ You are worried about his sleeping.

☐ He has colic.

☐ He is constipated.

☐ He brings up some of his feeds.

☐ He has a sticky eye.

☐ He has a nappy rash.

☐ He is often miserable.

☐ You are unhappy or depressed and find him difficult to handle.

certainly right. But if he sees you are unhappy about this he will probably arrange one for you anyway. Remember, you have every right to ask for a second opinion. *See* DOCTOR.

THE ROLE OF THE HEALTH VISITOR

All health visitors are trained nurses and are experienced in midwifery. They are there to guide you with any problems you have looking after your child. They may be of help to you if you feel under stress and can put you in touch with other mothers, and help assess your child's sight, hearing and general development. The health visitor runs the child health clinic. She is told as soon as a baby is born and will call on you in the first few weeks and invite you to the clinic.

THE CHILD HEALTH CLINIC

At this clinic, sometimes called a child development clinic, you will be seen by either a health visitor or a doctor, who will examine your baby from time to time to see if he is developing as expected. Any questions you have about your child can be dealt with. When tiny, he will be weighed and measured on each visit. You will have the opportunity to meet other local mothers. You can buy powdered baby milk at some clinics. But the clinic doctor cannot normally prescribe medicines for you, unless he is also your GP. If the clinic is run by your own doctor it is a good place for him to get to know you better, and to help out with any family problems. After your first visit you will be told how often to attend.

PAEDIATRICIAN

He is a specialist in child health. One may possibly visit you in the maternity ward and you should feel free to ask him any questions you wish. Once you are home you can see him only by appointment through your GP, unless he has made a special arrangement with you about direct contact.

MIDWIFE OR SPECIAL CARE BABY UNIT STAFF

If your baby was in the special care baby unit and you got to know the staff well, you might want to talk to them about any problems in the first few weeks after going home. But if you think your baby is ill, contact your doctor.

For the first few days after birth, your midwife is available for advice. Again, she cannot help with a sick baby: contact your doctor.

SOCIAL WORKER

Social workers do not have training in child health. However, if your major worries are about housing, money or the state of your marriage you can request help from your social services department.

MOTHER AND BABY SUPPORT GROUP

This may offer a telephone number you can ring to talk at any time to another mother. It may have a place where mothers with babies can meet, and it can sometimes offer practical help. There may be one in your area. Look for notices in clinics, surgeries and libraries or ask your health visitor. Sometimes your local National Housewives' Register or similar groups will help.

PARENTLINE

Numerous local groups run a confidential, anonymous telephone service, along the lines of the Samaritans, for parents of children of any age. There is no connection with 'the authorities' (for example, health visitors, local authority social workers) unless the caller requests this kind of help. Many parents have praised its effectiveness in providing a link with another human being when everything is getting too much. Some local groups also run mother-toddler groups or provide a befriending service. They can be contacted through *Parentline*, Westbury House, 57 Hart Road, Thundersley, Essex SS7 3PD (Tel. 0268 757077).

NSPCC OFFICER

If you fear that caring for your baby is getting you down so much that you could lose your temper enough to hurt him, seek help straight away. Try your doctor or health visitor, or even the sister on the children's ward of your local hospital.

You could also try your local NSPCC Officer. He does not wear a uniform, does not deal just with 'cruelty', will respect your confidence and is trained in helping parents in difficulty with their children.

OTHER MOTHERS

They can often be your best source of help. If you do not know many people where you live, you can meet other mothers at the child health clinic, or at a play group, or through the local branch of the National Childbirth Trust or National Housewives' Register. Your health visitor can put you in touch with any local group of this sort.

If you are not too shy, try simply talking to other mothers you meet in the street, or in the park.

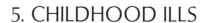

5. CHILDHOOD ILLS

Coping with common symptoms

The following pages list the common symptoms of childhood illness under the headings: The off-colour child; Problems of growth; Sleep problems; Skin problems: Behavioural problems.

Childhood disease

Other diseases of childhood are described in the main A–Z section. They include:

ADENOIDS	EPILEPSY
APPENDICITIS	FLAT FEET
ARTHRITIS	GERMAN
ASTHMA	MEASLES
BOILS	HAY FEVER
BRONCHIOLITIS	HERNIA
BRONCHITIS	IMPETIGO
CHICKENPOX	LICE
COELIAC	MEASLES
DISEASE	MUMPS
CONGENITAL	POLIOMYELITIS
DISLOCATION	PYLORIC
OF THE HIP	STENOSIS
CONJUNCTIVITIS	SCARLET FEVER
CROUP	URTICARIA
CYSTIC	WHOOPING
FIBROSIS	COUGH
DIPHTHERIA	

COPING WITH ILLNESS *Protection gained before birth or from breast milk lasts six months or so. After that most infants suffer several minor illnesses each year, the worst times being just after starting playgroup, nursery or primary school. Most illnesses need little more than extra comfort and extra love; the important thing is to recognise the difference between a child who is simply off colour and one who is really ill. This section aims to help you make that distinction, and to guide you on what you can do yourself and when you should seek medical advice.*

Causes of crying in a baby

Cause	**Hunger**
Clue	Some hours since feed, or last feed not very large
Remedy	Offer a feed

Cause	**Thirst**
Clue	Hot weather. Baby feverish or sweating
Remedy	Offer water

Cause	**Passing urine**
Clue	A sudden shriek
Remedy	Change nappy

Cause	**Discomfort**
Clue	Nappy rash, eczema, wet nappy, cold fingers and toes
Remedy	Treat or remove discomfort

Cause	**Colic**
Clue	Restless, draws up legs, sudden cry, then relaxes. Passes a lot of wind
Remedy	Carry baby over shoulder. Rock him in cradle. Take him for a drive. Check hole in teat if bottle-fed. Consult doctor or health visitor

Cause	**Loneliness and boredom**
Clue	Cries when he is alone, stops when you come in
Remedy	Keep him with you. Prop him up so that he can see you or other members of the family

Cause	**Habit**
Clue	Usually cries at night. Stops when you come in
Remedy	See SLEEP PROBLEMS (*page 157*)

Cause	**Teething**
Clue	May cause crying but less often than most people think
Remedy	Look for some other cause first. Consult a doctor if severe

Cause	**Tiredness**
Clue	Has missed a nap. A particular sort of moaning cry
Remedy	Try to get the baby to settle to sleep

Cause	**Personality**
Clue	No other cause found
Remedy	Consult doctor if worried

Cause	**Illness**
Clue	Off feeds. Feverish. Signs of cold. Pulls at ear. Vomiting, diarrhoea. Pain is suggested if crying is severe, fails to stop when baby is picked up and comforted, or is accompanied by pale skin or drawing up of legs
Remedy	Consult doctor

THE OFF-COLOUR CHILD

When a child is 'off-colour', 'poorly', or 'sickening for something' there will usually be a minor cause which will clear up in a day or two. Very occasionally the cause may be more serious.

The following descriptions of symptoms will help you to decide whether to take a child to the doctor.

CRYING

The normal baby generally cries only when he is hungry, angry, lonely, uncomfortable or in pain, and crying will stop when you solve his problem. At two weeks the average baby cries for two hours daily. Many babies cry in the evenings from about one month to three months, probably due to colic (*see this page*). One in five babies of about one year old cry or scream when put to bed.

It takes time to learn what the different sorts of crying mean. The only way to find out is by seeing what stops the baby crying. There are some babies, however, who cry for no obvious reason (see chart).

Treatment in the home

• Consult the chart and see if you find a remedy.

• If you are feeling jumpy and nervous yourself, realise that this can affect the baby.

• Find some way to keep calm.

• Be sure to get enough rest, perhaps by persuading your partner or asking relatives, friends or neighbours to help out. Your rest should come before housework or entertaining.

• If you feel desperate, seek the help of one of the people or organisations on page 150.

When to consult the doctor

• If the baby looks ill, has a fever, will not feed, appears to be in pain, or has any of the important symptoms listed on page 149.

• If you feel near the end of your tether.

What the doctor may do

• Check for ill-health and treat it.

• Give intestinal relaxant medicines for colic.

• Prescribe a sedative if essential.

• Help you by listening to your problems.

• Put you in touch with some person or agency who can take some of the load from you.

• Admit the baby to hospital for observation if all else fails, or if serious causes cannot be ruled out.

COLIC

Colic is probably due to the bowel not working properly, simply because it has not yet learned to do so. Instead of a smooth wave of contraction pushing food through, bubbles of air and gas become trapped between constrictions in the bowel and this is painful. For an unknown reason, colic is most common in the evenings from about five until ten, and generally stops when the baby is over three months.

Treatment in the home

• If you are bottle-feeding, check that the hole in the teat is the right size and that you are holding the bottle correctly (*see pages 132–3*).

• If you have just started feeding the baby solids, stop in case he is allergic to one or other of them.

• Do not add solids or change his

milk (a very few babies who are allergic to cow's milk do well on soya-bean milk, however).

• Try cuddling or rocking him, pushing him in his pram or even taking him for a drive.

When to consult the doctor

• If these simple measures fail and you think the baby is distressed; or you are exhausted or angry, so are in danger of exercising faulty judgment.

• If there are any other associated symptoms such as vomiting, diarrhoea or blood in the motions obtain a doctor's advice immediately.

What the doctor may do

• In severe cases, prescribe a sedative or, very rarely, arrange a short hospital stay.

OTHER FEEDING PROBLEMS

If the baby's weight gain is right (*see page 141*) then he is probably getting enough food, even if the total is less than 2½ oz. per pound of weight, or 150 ml. for every kilogram.

• If he fails to gain weight, check the amount of food taken. If this seems correct, check for other possible reasons, such as hunger, unusual vomiting or diarrhoea. If there are no other symptoms, wait until you have weighed the baby the following week.

When to consult the doctor

• If you think the baby is ill.

• If failure to gain weight continues.

• If other symptoms are also present.

• If you are approaching the end of your tether.

What the doctor may do

• Try to discover the cause.

• Suggest a diet change—but only if this is absolutely necessary.

• Arrange for frequent checks by the

health visitor.

• Treat any colic or other causes.

• Help you with your feelings of distress (*see page 169*).

VOMITING

A baby's vomiting can be one of three types:

Small amounts Many babies bring up a little curdled milk with winding. This is normal and nothing to worry about.

Moderate amounts Frequent small vomits throughout the day may be due to hiatus HERNIA, a congenitally short foodpipe or ACHALASIA.

Large amounts Vomits consisting of most or all of a feed coming out with great force may be due to PYLORIC STENOSIS (the most common cause), a urinary or other serious infection, or one of many other rarer abnormalities.

Treatment in the home

• If the baby is vomiting in moderation, sit him up in a baby chair after feeds and do not wind him too vigorously.

• Add a thickening agent such as Nestargel to his feed, remembering to enlarge the hole in the teat. Your health visitor can guide you.

When to consult the doctor

• If he is not gaining weight.

• If vomiting is associated with other symptoms such as diarrhoea, evidence of pain or fever.

• If large quantities of feed are vomited, consult your doctor at once.

What the doctor may do

• Make a diagnosis from your story, from examining the baby and the baby's urine, if it is obtainable.

• For moderate vomiting, he may prescribe medicines which might help a little; but usually the problem

gets better by itself as the months go by.

• If vomiting is severe, he will send the baby to hospital. Pyloric stenosis is treated by a simple operation.

CONSTIPATION IN BABIES AND TODDLERS

If the stools become hard and dry, are painful and difficult to pass, the child is constipated. Some mothers worry if the child does not empty his bowels each day, but they can easily tell if the child is constipated by the consistency of the stool. If it is soft, the child is not constipated—even if he only empties his bowels every few days.

A breast-fed baby is unlikely to become constipated as his mother's milk is perfectly balanced food. He may only need to empty his bowels infrequently because the milk is mostly absorbed and produces little waste matter. But it is quite normal if he has frequent bowel movements. A bottle-fed baby may become constipated if his feeds do not give him enough fluid, or sugar. An older baby on solid foods or a toddler on a normal diet may become constipated if they do not get enough fibre and fruit to eat. Also, toddlers and older children may become constipated if they do not respond to the urge to empty their bowels because they are involved in a game. Or they may deliberately refuse if toilet training has been allowed to become a battle.

Diseases in which the bowel is obstructed are very rare. *See also* main entry on CONSTIPATION.

Treatment in the home

• To prevent constipation in a baby, try giving more fluid such as water or fruit juices.

• Check that he is not underfed, then add a little sugar to each feed, until his stools are normal and soft, and then stop adding the extra sugar.

• In a toddler or older child, make sure he has plenty of roughage in his diet: add fruit and bran.

When to consult the doctor

• If passing a stool is painful or the stool is blood-stained. This may mean that the baby has an ANAL FISSURE— a split in the skin of the anus.

• If he has stomach pain or vomiting.

• If he begins to soil after he has been trained.

• If you think he needs a laxative (do not give a laxative unless the doctor prescribes it).

What the doctor may do

• Send the baby to hospital if he has a distended stomach and is vomiting, as there may be a genuine obstruction.

• Suggest diet changes or prescribe a laxative. Some children have chronic constipation and will need this daily, sometimes for months. In the worst cases the child will have to go to hospital to have the anus stretched under anaesthetic.

DIARRHOEA IN BABIES AND TODDLERS

Loose, runny or smelly stools in babies can be due to infection, either in the bowel or elsewhere in the body, an inability to absorb sugar in the feed—or the use of laxatives or other medicines such as antibiotics.

In older children it may be due to being seriously constipated, in which case the liquid contents of the upper bowel trickle around the hard stools and keep the lower bowel wide open. Allergies to certain foods, infection or even worry can also cause diarrhoea. *See also* GASTROENTERITIS.

Treatment in the home
• Check that there is nothing irritating in his diet—or yours if you are breast-feeding. Highly spiced food, peppers, curries, onions, tomatoes and rhubarb may provoke diarrhoea in some children.
• Stop feeding all milk (including breast milk) and solids to a baby. Let him drink plenty of orange or apple juice (not squash), Lucozade or a cola drink with the fizz removed by adding a little sugar. Best of all is a drink made with Dioralyte (sodium chloride and glucose), obtainable from your doctor or chemist. Feed him small amounts of the drink frequently—up to every two hours.
• When the diarrhoea stops, reintroduce breast milk, or bottle milk diluted with three times as much water. Gradually increase the strength over two or three days.
• With toddlers, go straight from clear fluids to solid foods that do not contain milk.
• Diarrhoea may be infectious. Other children can be protected if you wash your hands thoroughly after handling or changing the affected child; and if you wash him separately from the others. You should boil terry-towelling nappies.

When to consult the doctor
• If the baby is under six months and diarrhoea has lasted more than half a day.
• If he looks dehydrated with a dry mouth and sunken eyes and fontanelle (the soft spot on the head), or his skin loses its springiness and there are fewer wet nappies.
• If diarrhoea is associated with other symptoms such as vomiting, evidence of pain, failure to gain weight, or blood in the motions.
• If he has a temperature, looks ill, floppy or unnaturally sleepy.
• If he is well but the diarrhoea does not clear up.

What the doctor may do
• Change the baby's diet. In particular he may prescribe a special baby milk which contains no milk-sugar (lactose) or cane sugar (sucrose).
• Arrange to have a stool tested to check his diagnosis or to look for a germ causing GASTROENTERITIS.
• Prescribe a medicine such as kaolin or codeine which slows down bowel activity; but these medicines are less important than stopping milk.
• In severe diarrhoea, or if loose stools continue for a long time, he may refer you to a paediatrician.

COUGHS AND COLDS
The average toddler has about six coughs or colds each year—and while a few lucky children scarcely ever have a cold, others seem to have one constantly.

If your child seems to have a constant sniffly nose or is always coughing he may have an allergic condition such as ASTHMA or HAY FEVER. *See also* COMMON COLD.

Treatment in the home
• Keep him at home as quiet as possible. The object is to prevent minor infections from spreading down to the deeper parts of the lung.
• Treat a high temperature headache or sore throat with paracetamol (*not* aspirin) in recommended doses.
• Make sure he has plenty to drink. but there is no need to worry if he will not eat.

When to consult the doctor
• If he has earache.
• If a cough does not get better after three or four days.
• If the cough is in long spasms, since this may be whooping cough.
• If a cough is associated with other symptoms such as a wheeze, a whoop, vomiting or pain.
• If he (or you) is exhausted from lack of sleep.
• If there have been previous recurrent chest infections, or if chronic illness such as ASTHMA, DIABETES, COELIAC DISEASE or CYSTIC FIBROSIS renders the child vulnerable.

What the doctor may do
• Examine him to find out if there is infection in his throat, ears, air-tubes or lungs.
• Treat any underlying cause of infection. This may be in the ears (OTITIS MEDIA), the throat (TONSILLITIS or CROUP), or the lungs (BRONCHITIS or BRONCHIOLITIS).
• Cough medicines are not very effective, and doctors often suggest that the best treatment is a mild sedative in the form of paracetamol, or a medicine containing an antihistamine.
• Antibiotics are likely to be prescribed if the doctor considers that an infection is caused by bacteria, if there is a risk of infection later by bacteria, if the child has suffered from previous bacterial infections, or if the child for any reason needs protection from such infections. Antibiotics are not effective against simple virus infections.

HIGH TEMPERATURE
The body's normal temperature is 98.4°F (37°C), if taken with a thermometer in the mouth. The temperature in the armpit may be 1°F (0.5°C) lower.

However, not everybody has the same level of normal temperature, so that one of 99°F (37.3°C) need not be regarded as abnormal.

Temperature can rise for other reasons than illness, and these include strenuous physical exercise, crying or just swallowing a hot drink.

You can always tell if a child is ill without knowing his temperature.

If your child has had a FEVER FIT in the past it may be reassuring to check his temperature every four hours during the day while he is ill, so that you know when he is getting hot and can reduce his fever.

If a child is feverish, undress him, remove blankets from his bed and keep the room pleasantly warm— about 68°F (20°C), to avoid fever fits.

FEVER FITS
Seizures occurring in children during a feverish illness; also known as febrile convulsions.

Symptoms
• During a feverish illness the child suddenly goes 'vacant'. He goes stiff for a few seconds then begins to rhythmically twitch or shake his arms and legs.
• The symptoms can be extremely frightening for parents (and others), who may fear that the child is dead or dying. In fact recovery is rapid and complete.
• The seizure is followed by drowsiness or sleep.

Duration
• Ninety per cent of fever fits last less than 15 minutes.
• They usually occur between the ages of six months and five years.

• As many as 4 per cent of children (one in 25) have one at some time.
• Of all children who have had a fever fit, roughly one in three will have one more and one in ten will have more than one further seizure.

Causes
• Almost all cases occur when the body temperature is raised during an illness, particularly the virus infections such as pharyngitis, measles, mumps and chickenpox.

Treatment in the home
• Stay calm. The child will come out of the seizure on his own.
• Lay him on his side and make sure there is nothing outside his mouth blocking his airway.
• Do not attempt to prise open his jaws, or restrain the automatic movements.
• Cool him down by removing clothes, cooling the room and sponging with tepid water.

When to consult the doctor
• If this is the first seizure, call the doctor or an ambulance. If the seizure is over, contact the doctor or take the child to the hospital.

What the doctor may do
• If the seizure is prolonged he may give an injection of an anticonvulsant drug.
• Some children, particularly those under 18 months, will need a lumbar puncture examination of the fluid around the spinal cord to make sure that they are not suffering from meningitis.
• He will advise about keeping the child cool in the event of future feverish illnesses, to reduce the risk of further seizures.
• He may prescribe anticonvulsant medicine, or medicine to take at the start of a feverish illness. In many

cases no prescription is necessary.

Prevention
• Do not allow a child with a feverish illness to become too hot. Cool him down and give extra drinks. Do not 'wrap him up'. If a child is feverish he will recover more quickly, feel comfortable and be less likely to have a seizure if you can reduce his temperature.
• Remove his clothes.
• Open the windows.
• Do not overheat the room.
• Sponge him with tepid water if he is still feverish.
• Paracetamol in recommended doses will help to reduce the temperature.

Outlook
• Recovery from a fever fit is usually rapid and complete.
• Inevitably, because some adults are epileptic, some children who have fever fits will go on to develop epilepsy. Most will not. Those children at higher risk of developing epilepsy are those who: have a family history of epilepsy; have prolonged seizures (longer than 15 minutes); have 'focal features' (signs that one part of the brain in particular is affected).
• The doctor may well prescribe anticonvulsant medication to be taken regularly by children in these categories.

ABDOMINAL PAIN
Abdominal pain is not uncommon in children of all ages. The main problem is that although the majority of cases are of little significance, a certain number are due to acute appendicitis which if left untreated for long may have serious consequences.

When to consult the doctor
The following points about abdominal pain in children indicate that there might be a serious cause for your child's pain.
• If the pain has persisted for longer than four hours despite rest in bed on fluids only.
• If the pain is severe or getting worse, or has become continuous after being intermittent.
• If the pain has wakened or kept the child awake.
• If the pain is associated with vomiting, loose motions, or blood in the motions.
• If there is anything at all abnormal about the urine.
• If there have been previous attacks of which the cause has been uncertain.
• If for any reason you are worried about the possibility of acute APPENDICITIS.

In many instances of abdominal pain you will clearly need to consult your doctor to ensure that there is no serious cause for your child's pain. In most cases, no serious cause will be found. You will, however, find that by consulting your doctor and excluding serious causes you will be helped to treat other causes, such as school phobia, with knowledge and confidence.

HEADACHE
Headache is a common symptom in children as well as adults. As many as one in seven children have frequent headaches, but in only a few is there a serious cause.

Children under four rarely complain of headache. They may find it difficult to describe it.

Headaches in older children are of

two types:
Type 1 *Single headaches lasting a few hours*
The headache comes on without warning, is continuous for a few hours and the child is ill in other ways, being listless, hot, and off food.

Causes
• These headaches are almost always due to an infection and are associated with a high temperature. In children between four and ten years they are common. The headache is usually the first sign that the child is ill. High temperature and other symptoms develop over the next day or so. The infection may turn out to be general (measles, chickenpox, influenza), respiratory (pharyngitis, laryngitis, bronchitis), in the urine (cystitis, pyelitis), in the bowel (gastro-enteritis), or very rarely in the brain (meningitis, encephalitis).

Treatment in the home
• Confirm that the child has a temperature.
• Put the child to bed and give him fluids and paracetamol.
• The headache will not entirely disappear, but in an hour or so it will cease to bother the child and will in most cases be overshadowed by other developing symptoms.
• As other symptoms develop, consider (and treat) the likely cause. *See* SYMPTOM SORTER.

When to consult the doctor
• If other symptoms develop which indicate the need for medical treatment.
• If the headache is severe, especially if it fails to respond to paracetamol after two or three hours, or if it is associated with unusual symptoms such as a faint, fit or stiffness in the back, legs or back of the neck (an early or immediate medical opinion

is indicated).

What the doctor will do
• Check and treat the possible cause of infection.

Type 2 *Intermittent headaches passing off in an hour*
The headache disappears in an hour or so only to return one or two days or weeks later. Often (but not always) no other symptoms occur. This may pose a problem for parents (and doctors) because the absence of other symptoms may raise doubts about the 'genuineness' of the headache.

Causes
• Behavioural causes are common. Such headaches may genuinely follow a child's worry about school—perhaps a fear of bullying or of a teacher. Sometimes a headache may be reported when none exists to obtain sympathy, or as an excuse to avoid something unpleasant.
• Simply hunger, fatigue or boredom.
• Travel and MOTION SICKNESS.
• MIGRAINE and related conditions. The typical symptoms of migraine may not develop until the child is older or has suffered intermittent attacks of headache and nausea for several years (the so-called 'sick headache').
• Serious causes of headache, such as BRAIN TUMOUR, are rare. They can cause intermittent, progressively worsening attacks of headache, but in children the symptom of headache usually develops late or is overshadowed by other symptoms.
• Eyestrain and sinusitis, although often considered as causes of childhood headaches, are rarely found to be responsible.

Treatment in the home
• Check the temperature to exclude infectious causes (see **Type 1**).

• Show sympathy, not worry.
• Ask about worries at school or elsewhere, and try to allay them.
• Offer paracetamol if distressed.
• Find out unobtrusively if there are symptoms such as nausea, which might suggest MIGRAINE.
• Encourage the child to lead as normal a life as possible.

When to consult the doctor
• If the headache attacks are becoming worse or more frequent, especially if they stop the child from doing things he enjoys.
• If the headache attacks are associated with events suggesting migraine.
• If the headache attacks are associated with other symptoms such as faints, head injury or abdominal pain.

What the doctor may do
• Check the cause. Even when the cause is trivial this may be difficult and involve investigation in hospital or an EEG (ELECTROENCEPHALOGRAM).
• Treat the cause.

FOOD ALLERGIES
Some children are clearly allergic to certain foods, such as strawberries. A few babies are allergic to cow's milk.

Symptoms
Some or all of the following:
• Blotchy rash.
• Swollen mouth and tongue.
• Mild temperature.
• Blood-stained diarrhoea.
• Stomach pain.

Duration
• A few hours in mild cases; daily symptoms in the most severe.

Treatment in the home
• Experiment with suspect food by removing it totally. If the child improves, try him on it again to see

if his symptoms return. Repeat this two or three times to be absolutely sure. Do not remove milk from a baby with diarrhoea.

When to consult the doctor
• If excluding the suspect food fails.
• If you think the child needs a substitute (for example, in the case of cow's milk).

What the doctor may do
• If milk is the problem, he may prescribe 'non-allergic' milk substitutes made from soya beans.
• Prescribe medicines.

Prevention
• Avoid foods responsible, checking ingredients of packets or cans.

DRUG REACTIONS
Children are sometimes allergic to certain medicines which are seen by the body's defence as foreign material.

Symptoms
• Rash.
• Vomiting.
• Diarrhoea.
• Joint pains.
• Nettlerash (hives).

Duration
• A few hours to several days.

Treatment in the home
• None advised.

When to consult the doctor
• If you suspect that the symptoms are due to a medicine or drug that has been prescribed.

What the doctor may do
• Advise whether it is safer to stop the drug or continue.
• Prescribe antihistamine which will combat the allergy.

Prevention
• If a drug reaction has occurred once, always remind your doctor or chemist whenever you are given a

prescription or medicine in future.

Serious problems of growth in children are rare. The most common is obesity which can usually be dealt with at home, possibly with some advice from the doctor.

THE FAT CHILD
Generally, a child is considered to be obese if he weighs 20 per cent more than the right weight for his height.

The causes are complex; partly it may be inherited, partly the condition may be due to overfeeding in the early weeks. Only very rarely indeed has it anything to do with an abnormality of the thyroid, adrenal or pituitary gland. *See* OBESITY.

Treatment in the home
• Do not give your child snacks between meals.
• Do not give him food as a reward, to keep him quiet, or make him happy.
• Do not give him high carbohydrate food, such as cakes, biscuits and white bread. Instead, offer fruit, vegetables or wholemeal bread.
• Encourage older children to take plenty of exercise.

When to consult the doctor
• If the measures above do not help or if you would like regular, accurate weighing. Your health visitor is a good first person to contact.

What the doctor may do
• Help you to understand about diet.
• Arrange for the child to be weighed regularly and offer encouragement.

SHORT STATURE

There is no clear dividing line between children who are naturally small and those who are small because of some physical abnormality. Among children referred to a specialist because of concern about their lack of height, fewer than one in ten turns out to be abnormal.

Causes
- Parents or family are short.
- Child was very small at birth: 3–4 lb. (1–2 kg.).
- Delayed growth. Some small children, their weight correct for height, reach puberty late and go on growing longer than other people to reach a normal size eventually.
- Chronic ill-health.
- Rare glandular or genetic abnormalities.

Treatment in the home
- If you are worried, there is a simple formula for working out average height for children between 2 and 12: Age in years $\times 2\frac{1}{2} + 30$ in., or age in years $\times 6 + 77$ cm.

When to consult the doctor
- If you are concerned about your child's size.

What the doctor may do
- Check child's size against charts.
- Arrange X-rays and blood and urine tests, or refer you to a paediatrician.
- Enquire about your relationship with your child (children need love as well as food to grow).

BOW LEGS

Toddlers frequently have a bow-legged appearance which is quite normal and in most cases improves with time.

Causes
- The thigh bones are a little outwardly rotated in the hip sockets.
- Rarely RICKETS is responsible. Asian and other dark-skinned communities who live in temperate climates, low in sunlight, are at risk from rickets.

Treatment in the home
- None.

When to consult the doctor
- Not usually necessary; but do so if you are anxious or if the deformity is severe or increasing, or if the child has other symptoms such as bone pain, fits, severe chest infection.

What the doctor may do
- Offer you reassurance.
- Take blood tests to rule out rickets.

Outlook
- Rickets is treated with vitamin D.
- The remainder improve with time, without treatment.

KNOCK-KNEES

The child's knees appear too close together. The condition usually corrects itself of its own accord, but occasionally requires treatment.

Duration
- Many infants between 18 months and three years may look knock-kneed for several months.

Causes
- The thigh bones are a little inwardly rotated in the hip joint.

Treatment in the home
- None.

When to consult the doctor
- If the child is still knock-kneed by the age of seven.
- If, in a younger child, the gap between the inner side of the ankles is more than 3 in. (75 mm.) when the child stands knees together.
- If one knee is normal and the other faces in.

What the doctor may do
- Refer you to an orthopaedic surgeon, to decide whether there is an abnormality of the knee joint or leg bones which could require splinting or an operation. This is rare.

LIMPING

Limping in a child may be due to trivial injuries or infections, such as a cut, blister, boil, bruise or sprain. In all such cases the child will point to a painful area in which the cause will be obvious. If, however, a limp in a child persists for longer than one or two days in the absence of an obvious cause a doctor's opinion should be obtained.

Causes
- Any injury to lower limbs—usually obvious.
- Muscle cramps and stiffness following excessive exercise.
- Attention seeking—rarely maintained for long by a child.
- Infection or injury of hip or other limb joints (*see* ARTHRITIS, PERTHES' DISEASE and SLIPPED FEMORAL EPIPHYSIS). None of these conditions is common.
- Inflammation of spine and limb bones (OSTEOMYELITIS)—not common.
- Causes present since birth (CONGENITAL DISLOCATION OF HIP; weakness of limb muscles).
- Often the limp disappears before an obvious cause is identified.

Treatment in the home
- If the limp is obviously due to an injury or sprain and is not too severe, await natural recovery.
- Look for any sore place on the foot, or for a tight shoe.

When to consult the doctor
- If there is no evidence of any injury or sprain.
- If the child has limped for more than two days.
- If pain, but no injury, has been present for more than a day.
- Redness, swelling or tenderness of a joint or over a bone.

What the doctor may do
- Examine the child carefully.
- Request an X-ray.
- Seek a specialist's opinion.

SLEEP PROBLEMS

Babies, like adults, vary in the amount of sleep they need. The average hours of sleep each day are:
First weeks, 14 to 18 hours
Early months, 12 to 16 hours
One year, 10 to 13 hours
Three years, 9 to 12 hours
Seven years, 8 to 11 hours
Unfortunately for parents, there are some babies and infants who do not need much sleep, and others who do not develop a regular pattern of sleeping and waking.

It is normal for babies to wake for a night feed. Some drop this as early as six weeks, others not for several months.

By 18 months, six out of ten babies sleep through the night. A few wake occasionally, while nearly a quarter wake at least once on most nights.

WAKEFULNESS

Some babies have problems about sleeping and no one knows the reason. It seems little to do with the sex of the child, whether he was breast or bottle-fed, whether he was overactive by day, or whether or not he was picked up or taken into his parents' bed.

Treatment in the home
• To help a baby to go to sleep in the early weeks, keep him relaxed and soothed after each feed. Change his nappy gently and put him to bed.
• With an older baby, try not to let him get too excited or overtired when it is near bedtime, so that he learns to relax.
• If he wakes and cries in the night, let him cry for a few minutes before you go to him as he may go to sleep again. He may need to be lifted out and held for a few minutes, before settling to sleep. Try singing a lullaby to him. Or you may decide to take him to bed with you and cuddle him, though this may start a habit that can be difficult to break.
• If he frequently wakes, you may have to put up with it and try to make up your sleep during the day, while your baby sleeps.
• If a toddler refuses to go to sleep he may just not be ready, or he may be one of those who need little sleep. Try to tire him out in the day.
• Many toddlers wake in the night. Possibly a few can be cured by being hard-hearted and ignoring them, but not many.
• Try changing the normal routine of bath or bedtime. Try leaving a light on near his room.
• Cuddle him, and read him a story.
• Check that fear of the dark, or noise, or some physical cause such as itching or a blocked nose is not the problem if a baby who normally sleeps well changes his habit.

When to consult the doctor
• If you are exhausted, unable to cope, depressed or getting angry with the baby.

What the doctor may do
• He may suggest temporary use of a mild sedative for the baby.
• In really bad cases, if you are at the end of your tether with a very young baby, he may arrange for the child to spend a few days in a children's ward while you recover.

SLEEP-WALKING
Many children walk in their sleep. It is not a condition to cause you worry.
Causes
• Sometimes a sign of anxiety.
Treatment in the home
• A sleep-walking child should be gently guided back to bed without waking, but no harm will be done if the child is wakened.
When to consult the doctor
• Not necessary.

NIGHT TERRORS
Small children sometimes wake suddenly, apparently in great fear. They may scream, sob or talk incoherently; often they stare blankly into space.
Symptoms
• Screaming, sobbing or talking incoherently during the night.
Causes
• Largely unknown. Sometimes night terrors are sparked off by a sudden fright, shock or fever.
• Anxiety about separation from parents.
• Very rarely, a form of EPILEPSY, but other signs of this condition would usually be present.
Treatment in the home
• Keep calm.
• Comfort the child, reassure him if the cause is known.
• Waking a 'dreaming' child is not

harmful or dangerous.
When to consult the doctor
• If attacks are so frequent that the child loses sleep.
• If there are unusual symptoms such as headache, vomiting or twitching of arms or legs during an attack.
What the doctor may do
• Probably nothing more than satisfy himself of the diagnosis.
• Prescribe a sedative.
• Rarely, order an EEG (ELECTRO-ENCEPHALOGRAM).
Prevention
• None.
Outlook
• The child usually grows out of the habit eventually.

SKIN PROBLEMS

Babies rarely have a perfect skin. Newborn babies usually have patchy blue or lobster red areas which come and go during the first few days, and it is not unusual for jaundice to stain the skin yellow. In many babies, numerous spots that look like nettlerash, or bites, come and go all over the body in the first week. These are harmless.

On the baby's face little white spots called milia (millet seeds) can be caused by swelling of the glands which lubricate the skin. They disappear after a few days. By the second week, raised white dots, pinhead size, form on the cheeks, because of blockage of sweat glands. These dots may stay for several weeks.

Red areas frequently develop when

the baby sweats or where his skin rubs against clothes. All these spots are harmless and do not need treatment.

NAPPY RASH
A chafing of the surface layer of the skin caused by contact with ammonia, a chemical produced from urine by bacteria which normally live on moist skin. In addition, the baby may develop a skin allergy (eczema) which makes the rash worse. Sometimes, particularly if the skin is broken, there may be areas infected with bacteria or with the fungus *Monilia* (also called candida or THRUSH).
Treatment in the home
• Change the baby as frequently as possible—after every feed, if he seems wet and uncomfortable at other times, and at least once during the night. Use nappy liners to draw the urine away from contact with the skin.
• Leave his bottom bare for as often and as long as possible.
• Use plastic pants as infrequently as you can and rinse them often.
• Try terry-towel nappies instead of disposable (or vice versa).
• Wash and rinse nappies thoroughly. Use soap powder, not detergent, and while awaiting washing, keep them soaking in an antiseptic solution such as Napisan.
• Use a barrier cream such as zinc and castor oil, or cod-liver oil ointment, each time he is changed.
When to consult the doctor
• When these measures fail to work.
What the doctor may do
• Check for infection, either just by examining the rash or by swabbing its surface with a cotton-wool bud

which is then sent to a laboratory for testing. He will treat infection with a cream containing an antiseptic, antibiotic or antifungal agent.
- Prescribe a stronger barrier cream.
- Advise using a cream containing a steroid hormone. These creams are very effective, especially if there is any eczema present, but using a too strong variety for too long can damage the skin permanently. They should be used only under a doctor's close supervision.
- Never use a cream on your baby that has been prescribed for somebody else. It may contain a steroid and this could be dangerous.

ECZEMA
A baby suffering from eczema will have areas of reddened skin, which erupt into blisters which may weep and then crust over. Eventually the skin may become dry and thickened. Eczema is very itchy. Any part of the baby's body may be affected, although it is often seen spreading up from the nappy area or on the face. In older infants it may be confined to the inside of the elbows, backs of knees and wrists.

Although for some children, eczema comes and goes for many years, there are types which get better after a few months. *See also* main entry on ECZEMA.

Treatment in the home
- If there is nappy rash, treat as on page 158.
- If the rash started within a few days or weeks of taking a medicine, check with your doctor if the medicine could be a cause.
- Avoid soap. Wash the baby only when essential, by using emulsifying ointment instead of soap.

- Choose cotton clothes, and avoid woollen or nylon clothes next to the skin.
- Very occasionally a baby with eczema is allergic to cow's milk. Try cutting out milk from his diet for a few weeks.
- Keep the baby's nails short, so that he cannot scratch himself.
- Keep his room as dust-free as possible.
- Wash clothes with soap powder, rather than detergent, and rinse well.

When to consult the doctor
- If these measures fail.

What the doctor may do
- Firstly, he cannot 'cure' eczema, and you may have to settle for something less than a perfect skin.
- He may prescribe a steroid cream or ointment, and you should bear in mind that the use of too strong a variety for too long may cause permanent damage to the skin. A potent steroid suitable for the body may be unsuitable for the face where a weak preparation is safer.
- In chronic eczema, simple protective pastes may be used and sometimes these are in the form of medicated bandages which can be put on arms and legs at night.
- A sedative which also reduces itching may help him to sleep at night and stop his scratching.
- Suggest various diets.

CRADLE CAP
Many babies develop a harmless, scaly, brownish-coloured rash on the scalp which flakes like dandruff.

Treatment in the home
- Shampoo his head at least twice a week, gently rubbing away the scales. Take care to keep the lather out of the baby's eyes.

- If this is unhelpful, your doctor can prescribe special lotions and shampoos which are usually successful.

FLEA BITES
Fleas from cats and dogs frequently bite children, often because the fleas live in carpets on which babies and toddlers are playing.

Symptoms
- Usually a group of raised, itchy, pink spots on an arm or leg lasting three or four days; but a bite may be single and occur anywhere on the body.

Causes
- Cuddling animals.
- Contact of bare skin with rugs and carpets in which fleas live.

Treatment in the home
- Dust animal with flea powder.
- Dust all carpets with flea powder and then vacuum.

Prevention
- Fit a flea collar to your pet.

BEHAVIOURAL PROBLEMS IN YOUNG CHILDREN

Many children suffer from one or more behavioural problems in their early years. Usually there is some underlying emotional reason and the child grows out of the phase without medical help.

BED-WETTING
Wetting the bed regularly is unusual after the age of five, although one in seven normal children may still be wetting at this age.

Symptoms
- A wet bed—but occasionally a child may try to cover up by hiding pyjamas and sheets.

Duration
- Of those still wet at five, 15 per cent become dry each year. One in 100 18 year olds still has the problem.

Causes
- Frequently there is no certain cause—possibly an immaturity of the nerves controlling the bladder.
- Anxiety, particularly over house moves, parental arguments, separation—such as a stay in hospital.
- Too severe an attempt at pot training.
- Trying to train too early.
- Excessive punishment.
- Urinary infection.

Treatment in the home
- Do not try to train a child until he shows signs of being ready, such as calling attention to his need or even asking for a pot.
- Never use punishment to aid toilet-training.
- If a child wets, you will make it worse by shaming or criticising him.
- Always praise dry beds in such children.
- Offer small prizes—but not luxurious or expensive bribes.

When to consult the doctor
- At any age if you find that you or your partner are getting extremely upset or if you think your child is unnaturally anxious or unhappy. Otherwise at five or six years.

What the doctor may do
- Test the urine to check there is no infection.
- Show you how to use a nightly calendar with 'stars' for dry beds.
- Supply a buzzer alarm system.

- Prescribe a drug which may lessen wetting.
- Seek specialist help in difficult cases.

BREATH-HOLDING ATTACKS

Some children are able to hold their breath until they go blue, or faint, or—in the most severe cases—have a brief fit or convulsion. Occurs mainly in children aged 18 months to five years.

Causes
- Nearly always anger or frustration.

Complications
- None likely.

Treatment in the home
- Lay the child on his side and wait for him to recover.
- If unconscious, administer a single, non-painful slap.

When to consult the doctor
- If you are not sure whether the child is holding his breath or is having a fit.

What the doctor may do
- Make sure the diagnosis of breath-holding is correct and there is no suggestion of EPILEPSY.

Outlook
- The condition is frightening for the parent but harmless to the child, and disappears at age four or five.

HEAD BANGING AND ROCKING

A few infants and toddlers rock back and forth in their cot at night, and sometimes rhythmically knock their forehead or back of the head on the bars, headboard or wall.

Causes
- Anxiety caused by some upset in the family, but often there is no known cause.
- Sometimes the child finds the rhythmic movement pleasurable.

Treatment in the home
- Pad the bars or headboard.

When to consult the doctor
- If the habit shows no sign of stopping and it disturbs your sleep or worries you unduly.
- If the child is injuring himself.

What the doctor may do
- Ask you what might be upsetting your baby.
- Advise you to discourage the habit by paying no attention to it.
- If the problem is severe, prescribe a sedative.
- Refer you to a paediatrician, psychologist or child psychiatrist.

TANTRUMS

Almost inevitable between the ages of about two and four. The child is enraged, will not listen to any sort of reason, and may fling himself around or hurl toys.

Causes
- The child has reached an age where he begins to have strong ideas about what he wants to do, but is often unable to do it, or is prevented. The result is sudden outbursts of uncontrolled temper, during which the child is not capable of responding logically.

Treatment in the home
- There is no point in trying to reason, argue or punish.
- Keep as calm as possible, if necessary leaving the room.
- Tantrums in public places are embarrassing, and you need to exert almost superhuman willpower not to hit out at him. Just try to remember that the opinion of strangers around you does not matter.

When to consult the doctor
- If you find yourself reacting violently.
- If the child's tantrums irritate you so much that you can no longer enjoy his company.

What the doctor may do
- Listen to you, and help put into perspective what is a passing phase.

Outlook
- The phase should pass by the age of four or five.

TICS

Repeated movements, such as twitching of the mouth, blinking or nodding, of which the child seems to be unaware.

Duration
- Usually a transient stage that rarely persists if treated with understanding.

Causes
- Anxiety.
- An upset or shock.
- Feelings of insecurity.

Treatment in the home
- Do not draw attention to the habit or mock it. This is highly unlikely to bring any improvement.
- Try to discover what lies at the root of the child's insecurity, and give reassurance.

When to consult the doctor
- If the child is caused distress or embarrassment.
- If he seems totally unable to control the tic (there is a rare disease—ST VITUS'S DANCE—which may mimic a tic).

What the doctor may do
- Check on the possibility of St Vitus's Dance.
- Listen to you and the child, and help work out the cause.

Outlook
- Most tics clear up in a month or two, but some last into adult life.

6. NO LONGER A BABY

Rearing the growing child

In the chart on page 163 you will find the earliest age, the average age, and the latest age by which most children are likely to achieve certain tasks. 'Most', not 'all'—and you should not fear the worst if your child does not fit the pattern.

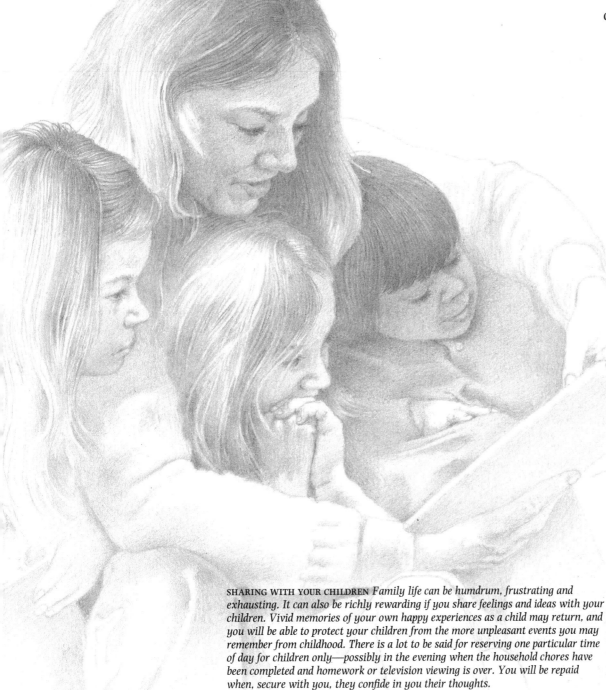

SHARING WITH YOUR CHILDREN *Family life can be humdrum, frustrating and exhausting. It can also be richly rewarding if you share feelings and ideas with your children. Vivid memories of your own happy experiences as a child may return, and you will be able to protect your children from the more unpleasant events you may remember from childhood. There is a lot to be said for reserving one particular time of day for children only—possibly in the evening when the household chores have been completed and homework or television viewing is over. You will be repaid when, secure with you, they confide in you their thoughts.*

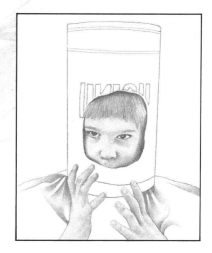

IMPROVISED TOYS *Cardboard boxes, toilet-roll cores, empty yoghurt pots, sticky tape, powder-paints and silver foil are cheaper than manufactured toys and can be just as much fun. You will be surprised at just how inventive your child can be with a few simple props like these.*

LATE TALKERS

There are many late talkers, it is often a family trait, and there is rarely need to worry. The three questions to ask yourself are: Does he seem to understand? Can he hear properly? Is he up to average in other ways? If the answer is 'yes' to all these questions, do not worry. If one or more answers are 'no' or 'not sure', consult your doctor.

REPETITION AND STUTTERING

All pre-school children go through a stage when speech does not flow easily. They repeat syllables or words, they seem to be casting around for the right words, or they trip over words.

It is normal up to the age of six or seven for thoughts to be faster than speech. Correcting the child, making him repeat himself slowly, or making fun of him will make things worse, and could cause a permanent stutter.

If a stutter is persistent, if the child is aware of it, and if he tries, unsuccessfully, to conquer it, you should seek your doctor's advice. *See* SPEECH DISORDERS

LISPING

All small children lisp, particularly over 'r' and 'w' and 's', 'th' and 'f'. In general a lisp disappears by itself, but if a child's lisp is severe enough to make it difficult for others to understand him, ask your doctor for help. If the problem is severe, he may refer you to a paediatrician or directly to a speech therapist. *See* SPEECH DISORDERS

LATE WALKERS

Nine out of ten children walk well by 15 months, although they usually waddle, or turn in their feet, or trip over themselves.

Some children have an unusual, although not abnormal, way of developing. Instead of progressing from rolling over to sitting, then crawling, then walking, some children go from sitting to shuffling along on their bottoms, and absolutely refuse to walk. When held off the ground they 'sit in the air' and will not put their feet down. This is often a family trait; the children may not walk until two and a half years, but they are normal.

Except in the case of a bottom-shuffler, you should see your doctor if a child is not on his feet by 18 months, or walking well by two years.

LATE LEARNERS

Your child may seem to be behind others in learning social tasks—feeding himself, dressing and undressing, learning names of objects, and how to use simple objects such as a brush and comb. But the age chart is only a guide—children whose achievements do not fit the pattern are likely to be perfectly normal. If you are still worried by the child's apparent lack of progress, talk to your doctor.

WHAT YOU CAN DO ABOUT LATE DEVELOPMENT

The best way to encourage a child's development is—quite simply— to talk to him, show him books, point out things in the house or street, play with him and allow him to explore. He should be allowed to do things in his own messy or slow way, rather than have you do them for him neatly or quickly.

WHAT THE DOCTOR MAY DO

He may test the child's development using a kit containing rattles, bricks, pictures and miniature toys. Or he may refer you to a paediatrician or a specialist in child development.

After these tests it may be possible to put your mind at rest—or it may be possible to diagnose a specific problem. On the other hand, the tests may be inconclusive, especially if the infant is tired, angry or shy—and the doctor may arrange to repeat them on a future occasion.

If a specific problem is discovered, arrangements may be made for various experts to see your child. His abilities in movement may be assessed by a physiotherapist, speech by a speech therapist, hearing by an audiologist or teacher for the deaf, and intellect by a psychologist.

TOILET TRAINING

Most mothers think children should be clean by the age of two and dry at night by two and a half. In fact only about half reach these targets, and it is more realistic to add a year to each of these ages.

There is no point in trying to train a child before he is capable of learning—just as there would be no sense in trying to teach him to talk at the age of a few weeks.

If you sit a baby of a few weeks on the pot immediately after a feed, you are likely to succeed. But this is neither training nor learning, merely taking advantage of a reflex in young babies whereby they empty their bowel soon after a feed. This ability will be lost towards the end of the first year as the reflex diminishes.

The best time to introduce a child to the pot is once he is old enough to understand its purpose, but before the onset of his phase of tantrums and other negative behaviour, at

about two years. The best method of teaching is elaborate praise for success, and no comment for failure. If you show any reaction to failure—whether disappointment or anger—your child may be so pleased by the power he thinks he has over you that he will go on failing.

Do not get over-anxious about failure on the pot. Almost the only children who are referred to doctors for failure to learn bowel control are those who have been subjected to excessive training.

If he shows no signs of learning, put the pot away for a month and then try again. Taking him out of nappies may be successful. Mockery, bribery or suggesting he is being a 'baby' are more likely to make things worse than better.

TAKING YOUR CHILD ON OUTINGS

Pre-school children love outings. At first, simple walks, shopping and expeditions to the park are likely to be the limit.

Swimming can start at six months. Playgrounds are unlikely to be suitable for those under a year old, and you should supervise older children carefully, since accidents are common. The children's section of the public library is popular with children as young as two. Museums, concerts and children's theatre come a bit later.

When out shopping, toddlers will naturally take things from super-market shelves. If you did not notice it happening at the time, politely ask the check-out assistant to take charge of the goods. If your child takes sweets placed invitingly at the check-out there is no need for you to pay—simply return them to the assistant.

LANDMARKS IN A CHILD'S GROWTH

MUSCULAR DEVELOPMENT

☐ Copies housework
Earliest 12 months
Average 14 months
Latest 20 months

☐ Uses spoon carefully
Earliest 13 months
Average 14 months
Latest 2 years

☐ Puts on some clothes
Earliest 20 months
Average 23 months
Latest 3 years

☐ Washes and dries hands
Earliest 19 months
Average 23 months
Latest 3 years

☐ Does up buttons
Earliest 2½ years
Average 3 years
Latest 4½ years

☐ Dresses without supervision
Earliest 2½ years
Average 3½ years
Latest 5 years

ACHIEVEMENT
Praise her when she does things for herself.

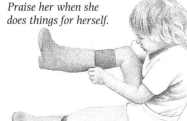

SIGHT AND CO-ORDINATION OF HAND AND EYE

☐ Scribbles
Earliest 12 months
Average 14 months
Latest 2 years

☐ Makes a tower of four bricks
Earliest 15 months
Average 18 months
Latest 2 years

☐ Copies a straight line
Earliest 19 months
Average 22 months
Latest 3 years

☐ Copies O
Earliest 2¼ years
Average 2½ years
Latest 3¼ years

☐ Draws a man (three parts)
Earliest 3¼ years
Average 4 years
Latest 5½ years

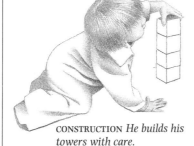

CONSTRUCTION *He builds his towers with care.*

SPEECH AND HEARING

☐ Says three words (not counting 'Mama', 'Dada')
Earliest 11 months
Average 13 months
Latest 21 months

☐ Joins two words
Earliest 14 months
Average 20 months
Latest 2¼ years

☐ Names one picture
Earliest 16 months
Average 20 months
Latest 2½ years

☐ Can give surname as well as first
Earliest 2 years
Average 2½ years
Latest 3½ years

FIRST STAGE *Learning by heart comes first— then reading.*

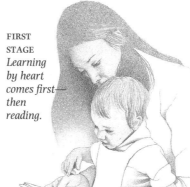

RESPONSE AND PLAY

☐ Walks up steps
Earliest 14 months
Average 17 months
Latest 22 months

☐ Pedals tricycle
Earliest 21 months
Average 2 years
Latest 3 years

☐ Hops on one foot
Earliest 3 years
Average 3½ years
Latest 5 years

☐ Catches bouncing ball (two out of three times)
Earliest 3½ years
Average 4 years
Latest 5½ years

THREE WHEELS *The first tricycle is a great treasure.*

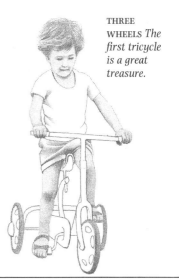

REARING YOUR CHILD

There are no rules which apply to everyone since parents and children are all different; though it is true to say that children are treated less strictly than they were 50 years ago.

You are likely to raise your child as you yourself were raised, so this is a time to think back and decide whether there were aspects of your upbringing that you do not want your own child to experience.

SHOULD I BE STRICT OR LAX?

On each occasion a conflict arises, ask yourself why you want to impose your will on your child. This will help you to decide when to 'put your foot down', and how to do it. Possible reasons are:

1 To stop him getting into danger Once he begins exploring, keep him away from electrical points (for example) by saying 'no' and gently moving him away. Once he is old enough to understand—usually between 15 and 18 months—he will control his exploring impulse.

Sooner or later he will test you by deliberate disobedience: this is normal behaviour and deserves, at most, a firm reproof.

2 To show him what is right and what is wrong What is right and wrong to you may be meaningless to him. For example, to him there is nothing 'wrong' about untidiness or urinating in the street.

He will learn what adults approve and what they disapprove simply by watching and listening. Punishment is unnecessary.

3 Because what he does annoys and angers you If the child goads you to a point at which you cannot restrain your temper, it may do you good to release your anger. It may even do

him a little good to know how far it is permissible to go. But only release your anger in words, and then avoid hurting him emotionally—try not to hit him or otherwise hurt him physically.

4 Because what he does might annoy others A child may have to be restrained in another person's house or presence, so long as you make it clear to the child that it is for the other person's benefit that his freedom is restricted.

5 Because what he is doing is wicked It is wicked if an adult tears apart a child's toy—but it is natural curiosity for a two year old to do so. It is normal behaviour, not wickedness, for a four year old to play with his or her genitals—usually in a fairly casual way. By contrast, adult disapproval can be clearly demonstrated about unkindness, cruelty and bullying. In children old enough to understand, disapproval can be shown towards antisocial behaviour such as lying, deceitfulness, dishonesty and stealing.

In deciding what judgment to make, remember the child's level of development. No one would punish an 18-month-old baby for being unable to walk; but a surprising number of adults will punish a four year old for wetting the bed. Yet the cause of the two events may be exactly the same—the child's body has simply not matured sufficiently.

STRIKING THE BALANCE

Try to imagine that you are the child; put yourself in his shoes, try to decide whether punishment was justified, and whether it is likely to make you a better person.

There are many ways of correcting a child without causing physical or

emotional pain. Children cannot have free rein; there must be certain clear limits for children old enough to understand, allowing parents time to themselves, excluding children from certain rooms, the necessity for orderly mealtimes. If the number of restrictions and prohibitions grows larger or—worse—if they keep changing, the likely result will be resentful children, temporarily obedient but eventually taking out their pent-up anger on somebody. Children learn by example, so one who experiences anger and pain is likely to grow up to inflict them on others.

NEGATIVE BEHAVIOUR

At about the age of two there is often a dramatic change in a child's behaviour. Up to then he has learned to accept the limits you put on him, and seems happy to do so. Now he appears to be deliberately uncooperative and awkward. Tantrums become more frequent and 'No' seems to be his favourite word.

None of this is 'naughtiness' or 'spite'. For the first time he is really aware that he is a separate person from his mother, with a right to express likes and dislikes. The trouble is he has not yet learned to do as adults usually do when they disagree with each other—to compromise. Even if he could, he probably would not do so, because this is his time for working out how to express his will and state his cause.

HOW YOU SHOULD COPE WITH THIS

First, accept it—do not hanker for the easy child he was. Secondly, live through it—once he is satisfied he has made his point, he will relax and

be reasonable. Thirdly, do not clash head-on—use your superior understanding to head off fights, distract him, make him laugh his way out of a confrontation, or gently deceive him into what you want him to do.

If he develops a particular trait—such as refusing food—do not be misled into joining battle. A child usually refuses food because it has been forced on him. He will not starve, and you will only make a fool of yourself by getting agitated. Ignore this behaviour, and he will probably lose interest in it.

THE STRICT FATHER

Fathers generally feel they should be firmer than mothers. If you and your husband cannot agree on discipline it is vital for you to compromise, and your arguments should take place out of earshot of the children.

INDEPENDENCE

Can a child get too much attention? Children learn by doing things themselves, not by having them done for them. If you constantly fuss round a child who has passed the age of total dependence—about two —you will restrict his development. This might mean, for example, letting him make a mess when feeding himself; or letting him open a boiled egg even if he takes a long time and his meal gets cold.

Older children need time to themselves. If you notice your child playing in a world of his own, talking to imaginary people, performing complicated rituals, do not interrupt. But if he is bored, mooning around or goading you, perhaps he needs some organised play with paints, bricks or clay.

WHY PLAY IS MORE THAN JUST A WAY OF FILLING TIME

Play is the method by which your child learns to gain control over his body. A baby reaching for a mobile is learning to co-ordinate the movements of his eyes and hands; a 15 month old playing 'peek-a-boo' is working out that when you cannot see something it has not necessarily vanished.

Later, physical games teach him how to use his new-found skills of balance control.

Play also develops a child's powers of imagination. Watch a three year old with his soft toys in long, earnest conversation—this is not 'dreaming', it is practising speech, working out relationships with other people, determining how the world works.

Finally, play develops the child's reasoning; his curiosity—his need to work things out—is given free rein. A four year old constructing a 'house' or 'machine' out of household junk is learning about how things are put together.

TOYS AND BOOKS

Most children tend to make their own playthings out of household objects, such as cardboard boxes. The best toys are those which the child can use to do many things—a doll, a farm, a garage or bricks. Toys designed for a single task where no imagination is needed are soon discarded.

Almost all children love books— and you cannot introduce them too early. For those who cannot read,

bold, bright pictures are preferable to complex illustrations.

If you can spare the time, almost all children love the evening ritual of reading a story aloud in bed.

Clay, bricks, Plasticine and paint are enjoyed by most children.

TABLE MANNERS

The sole reason for encouraging good table manners in toddlers is to protect them from criticism and you from embarrassment. Be guided by age: a two year old can be forced to wait patiently for each course, but he cannot see the reason for it.

WHEN HE SHOULD DRESS HIMSELF

As soon as he is able to put on clothes, let him do it. The result will be jumpers back-to-front and ludicrously unsuitable combinations of clothes. His pride in the achievement is far more valuable than your pride in his neatness and tidiness. Therefore, congratulate him and, some time later, try to correct his wilder flights of fancy.

WHEN HE SHOULD TIDY HIS OWN ROOM

Children are capable of tidying their rooms from about three onwards, but they need help—otherwise they become discouraged, or distracted by a toy. Turn tidying-up into a game, but allow them a room or a corner where their mess is tidied up only once a day. Constant clearing away of toys clears away their fantasies, their imagination and, consequently, their learning capability.

WATCHING TELEVISION

Television can be entertaining and educational. It can also be frightening and can introduce him to

ideas—particularly about violence— from which he needs protection.

Television can also be used as a substitute for doing other more active things which are not so simple as turning a switch. And it can be used so that a parent does not have

to bother to talk to or play with the child.

You should consider which of these uses of television applies to your household. Certainly there is no need for primary school children to watch anything other than children's

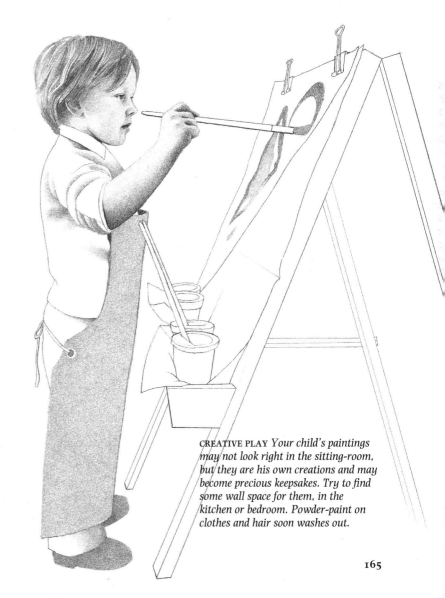

CREATIVE PLAY *Your child's paintings may not look right in the sitting-room, but they are his own creations and may become precious keepsakes. Try to find some wall space for them, in the kitchen or bedroom. Powder-paint on clothes and hair soon washes out.*

programmes; up to teenage years, viewing in the evening should be a privilege restricted to certain programmes so that the child gets sufficient sleep and can complete any homework. The argument that other children will mock him for not seeing certain programmes is tried by most children and can be safely ignored.

PREPARING FOR SCHOOL
You can help to prepare your child for this new stage in his life by talking about school encouragingly; mentioning nice teachers and new friends; showing him books about school; and taking him to visit the school before he begins to attend there.

If you look on his eventual going to school as an extension of your happy home life, then he will regard starting school as a natural transition and will catch your enthusiasm. But if you look on school with fears and worries, your child will be worried also and will suffer unnecessary dread.

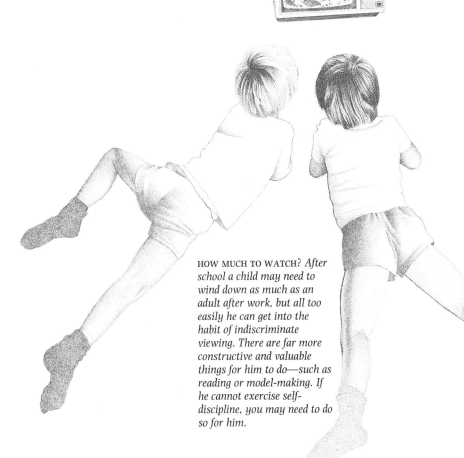

HOW MUCH TO WATCH? *After school a child may need to wind down as much as an adult after work, but all too easily he can get into the habit of indiscriminate viewing. There are far more constructive and valuable things for him to do—such as reading or model-making. If he cannot exercise self-discipline, you may need to do so for him.*

Will separation harm my child?
A pre-school child's best place is with his parents, but in the United Kingdom about 200,000 such children have mothers working full time. Between the ages of about six months and three years, separations can be very distressing for a child. The signs may be obvious—withdrawal or sadness—or less obvious—bed-wetting, stomach pains, headaches, refusal to eat. However, much depends on how consistent the mother-substitute's care is. Recent evidence suggests that provided the child is cared for by a loving, balanced person, he is as well off as he is with his mother, and may grow up to be more independent and stable.

FINDING HELP TO LOOK AFTER YOUR CHILD
Particularly if you work, you will have to face the problem of finding someone suitable to care for your child.

Until eight or nine months, most babies will happily stay with strangers. After that age most babies become more clinging, protest at separation and seem to dislike strangers.

The age varies at which toddlers will once again happily leave their mothers. Some children are clearly ready for playgroup or nursery by three. Others seem scarcely ready for school at five. All children eventually learn how to cope without a parent's constant attendance.

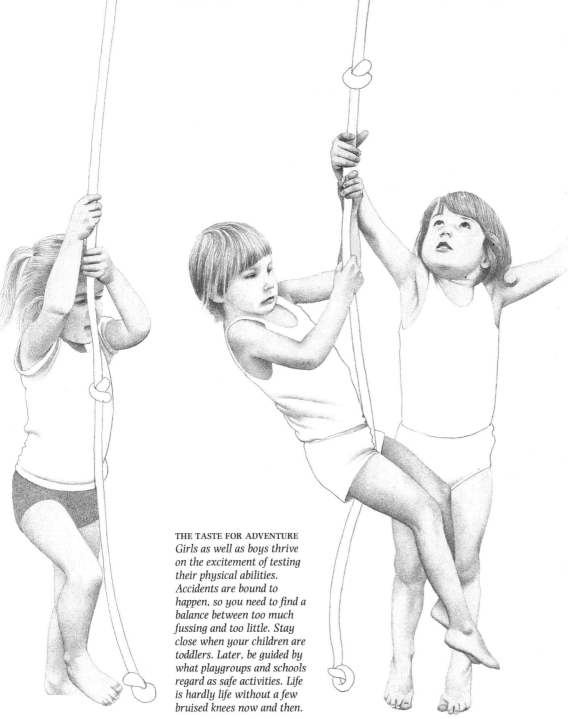

THE TASTE FOR ADVENTURE
*Girls as well as boys thrive
on the excitement of testing
their physical abilities.
Accidents are bound to
happen, so you need to find a
balance between too much
fussing and too little. Stay
close when your children are
toddlers. Later, be guided by
what playgroups and schools
regard as safe activities. Life
is hardly life without a few
bruised knees now and then.*

CHILD-MINDERS

You may hear of someone willing to
take in children, or see an advertise-
ment in a shop window or local
newspaper.

A good minder can be an immense
help. But check carefully before
trusting your child to a stranger.
First ensure that the minder is
registered—the social services
department of your local council will
tell you. Then check the following:
Are the premises large enough?
Are they warm?
Are the lavatories clean and
hygienic?
Are there lots of toys and books?
Is there a garden or a chance to
get outside?
Does the minder seem kind?

Make sure the minder does not
have an unruly animal that might
harm your child.

Avoid minders whose idea of
'minding' is for the children in their
charge to be either eating, in bed or
in front of the television set.

PLAYGROUPS

Most playgroups are excellent and
very cheap, being run by mothers
themselves. It is wise to stay for the
first two or three sessions, perhaps
playing with other children, until
you are happy that your child is
content. Your health visitor, church,
local National Housewives' Register
and Citizens' Advice Bureau are all
helpful sources of information.

STATE NURSERY SCHOOLS

Some local authorities provide
nursery schools for children between
the ages of three and five. There is
no obligation on them to do so,
however, and nursery places are in
short supply. If there is a nursery

school in your area, get your child's name on the waiting list as early as possible.

Some nursery schools are attached to state primary schools, and the children move into the infants' department at the age of five. The hours and holidays in the nurseries are similar to the primary schools, although many nursery schools take children for only half the day. One group attends in the mornings and another in the afternoons. The children are supervised by one qualified teacher and one assistant for every 26 children.

State nursery schools usually give priority to children with special needs, such as children with language difficulties, children living in deprived conditions or children from one-parent families.

If you have difficulty getting your child into a nursery school and you believe that he should have priority, talk to your health visitor, doctor or social worker. They may be able to help.

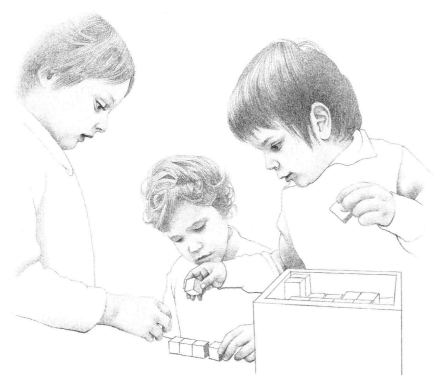

GROUP PLAY *Most playgroups take children from three years; some children are ready before then, others not until four or older. It should be for your child's enjoyment as well as your convenience, so keep an eye open for any distress.*

DAY NURSERIES

Most local authorities also run nurseries catering for children whose parents are in specially difficult circumstances—usually single parents who can find no other help. Most day nurseries care for children between 8 a.m. and 6 p.m., five days a week including school holidays. They are permitted to accept children from six weeks of age, but many will not take children under two.

Children are allocated places by the local authority's social services department, normally on the recommendation of a social worker.

PRIVATE NURSERIES

Privately run nursery schools have to register with the local social services department, which lays down regulations about buildings and teaching. The department can supply you with a list of private nurseries in your area. They may be expensive, however, and if you have the money available you may prefer to employ a mother's help or a nanny. They can be found through the local newspaper, *Nursery World*, or *The Lady*, or in the Yellow Pages of the telephone directory.

HOLIDAYS WITH CHILDREN

Even on holiday, the daily routine for a small child cannot be very much different from that which rules at home. He will need feeding at regular intervals on food he is used to, his nap may be at an awkward time while on holiday, and he still needs to be changed and kept clean. So even if you are going to a hotel where the cooking and domestic work is done for you, do not expect the child to fit in miraculously with your plans. The first holiday with a small child will prove more tiring than you think and you should make due allowance for this.

Self-catering holidays may sound ideal—but they do mean having to shop, cook and clean. Many parents like camping or caravanning, particularly where tents and caravans are already set up. Both offer more freedom than a hotel, friendliness from nearby campers, and lower costs. But if your child is normally unsettled at night, camping may be a nightmare, especially between one year and four years.

Holidays abroad are likely to be very expensive. Babies under two generally travel free or for a nominal sum, but do not expect half-fare for children on airlines. Also, there is no baggage allowance for babies, although they need an enormous amount of baggage.

If you are flying with a small baby, ask in advance for a Skycot—a carry-cot which clips on to the bulkhead. Take plenty of drink and nappies in case of delays at terminals.

If you plan to visit a tropical country, seek the advice of your doctor on inoculations against diseases (*see* TRAVEL AND HOLIDAYS).

CAR TRAVEL

Children should never travel in a front seat. They can distract a driver, and are unprotected in an accident. A baby in a carry-cot or any small child should be strapped in. Take plenty of books, paper and pens and simple toys—not the sort with small pieces that are easily lost. Do not constantly feed a child with sweets—an occasional apple is less likely to cause sickness. (*See also* MOTION SICKNESS.)

The first years—how will they affect you?

Your life changes completely with a toddler in the family. There is much to enjoy, but the sheer physical and mental strain of looking after another human being—if necessary 24 hours a day—can be exhausting and demoralising.

He may wake very early and deprive you of a couple of hours' sleep. You may be unable to have a slow and peaceful start to the day because he has to be changed, dressed and fed first. He may want to be entertained when you want to get on with household or other work.

His daytime sleep and mealtime routines may interfere with your plans. Simple outings become major expeditions because of hunting for clothes, dressing him while he protests, or trying to get somewhere while he explores every gateway and gutter.

If he is a poor sleeper you may have little chance of relaxing in the evening, when you may need to catch up with housework. Your partner may become impatient if he fails to understand why you are tired or preoccupied.

Tiredness—or a child demanding attention—may interfere with your sex life.

If you worked before becoming a mother, you may feel the financial pinch.

How to cope
Do not assume you can go on as before and the baby will just 'fit in'. He has his own ideas, needs and demands.

Learn to build a new routine. For example, you may have to take a nap when he does.

Review your priorities. Keeping a neat and tidy house, having friends over, or going out a lot at night may have been important to you. Decide whether they still are, and if they are not then drop them.

Find other mothers to meet and talk to. You can do this at mother and toddler groups, at the Welfare Clinic, in the park or playground, or while shopping. All mothers have something in common. The National Housewives' Register may help to put you in touch with women in similar situations to your own.

Let your husband know your feelings in a quiet and rational manner—not angrily, or by complaining, or by letting it all come out when you have a row. He may turn out to be your best help and support.

Try to get some time off—using a relative, neighbour or friend as a sitter.

Angry feelings
All mothers have momentarily violent feelings towards their offspring. You may find a toddler's demands almost impossible to cope with, particularly if you are exhausted or ill, or have housing, money or marriage problems. It may help to mention these feelings to someone whom you trust and rely on—a friend, your health visitor or your doctor.

If you find yourself on the point of hurting your child, walk out of the room until you are calmer. Look at your reasons for feeling as you do. Do you get cross because he is still in nappies? Do you think it is a sign of bad behaviour if he wets the bed or is a messy eater? If so, talk to your health visitor or doctor. Different children attain different skills at different ages—they will not develop in the same way, or always in the way you expect.

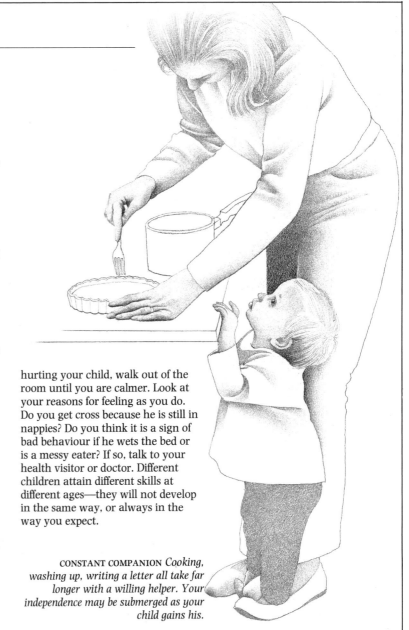

CONSTANT COMPANION *Cooking, washing up, writing a letter all take far longer with a willing helper. Your independence may be submerged as your child gains his.*

CIRRHOSIS OF THE LIVER

A chronic disease often associated with drinking alcohol; knobbly fibrous tissue, like scar tissue, replaces the cells as they become damaged. If the disease can be stopped in time, the undamaged liver can regenerate itself back to a normal state. Cirrhosis is more common in men, with symptoms usually appearing in the thirties and becoming severe in the forties.

Symptoms
- Sometimes there are no obvious symptoms and patients can look and feel well after the disorder has begun.
- A pale, slightly 'dirty' complexion is common.
- Weakness and feeling ill.
- Anaemia.
- Tingling and numbness in feet and fingers.
- Small blood vessels (SPIDER NAEVUSES) show on the skin.
- In men, the breasts may swell as the diseased liver cannot inactivate the female hormones that are present to a small degree in all men.
- Atrophy (shrinking) of the testicles.
- Loss of sex drive.
- Loss of appetite and loss of weight.

Duration
- Cirrhosis caused by alcohol lasts until the patient stops drinking alcohol altogether. If no complications arise within about a year and a half after abstaining, a normal life without drink can be enjoyed.
- If the patient does not stop drinking, liver destruction continues and death will eventually follow.

Causes
- Alcohol is the cause of the majority of cases.
- Alcohol also aggravates cirrhosis from other causes.
- Virus HEPATITIS (type B or C).
- Chemical damage from anaesthetics, cleaning fluids and some drugs.
- Cirrhosis less commonly follows HEART FAILURE, obstruction of bile ducts and poisoning of the liver cells by other substances and infections.

Complications
- PILES.
- Internal haemorrhage from the oesophagus.
- ASCITES, that is, a build up of fluid in the abdomen.
- CANCER of the liver.

Treatment in the home
- None advised. Consult the doctor.

When to consult the doctor
- If drinking is heavy (see ALCOHOLISM), or there is danger

from exposure to industrial solvents.
- If the above symptoms suggest the disease.

What the doctor may do
- Take blood tests to determine the amount of liver damage, and to identify the cause if it is other than alcohol.
- Refer the patient to a specialist physician, psychiatrist or alcoholics support group, depending upon the cause.
- Advise the patient to give up alcohol, and suggest a nourishing vitamin-rich diet, and rest.

Prevention
- Avoid too much alcohol or contact with other potential liver poisons. See ALCOHOLISM.
- Get medical help if you are a heavy drinker.
- Vaccination against hepatitis B for those at risk.

See DIGESTIVE SYSTEM *page 44*

CLAUDICATION, INTERMITTENT

Cramp in the legs while walking.

Symptoms
- Tight, gripping pain in the calves. This pain is clearly related to use and usually comes on after walking a certain distance. It is relieved by rest.

Duration
- The condition is usually steadily progressive and is only partly eased by treatment.

Causes
- ATHEROMA of the main arteries supplying blood to the legs. Usually the arteries are diseased from within the abdomen, downwards to the feet.
- Thrombosis (clotting) of the artery supplying blood to the calf.

Complications
- Limitation of activity and occasionally gangrene of the feet.

Treatment in the home
- Rest the legs. If outdoors, stop walking until the pain is relieved; resume walking at a slower pace.

When to consult the doctor
- As soon as the pain develops.

What the doctor may do
- Determine whether the symptoms are caused by arteries which generally are diseased and narrowed, or by a short block (thrombus) in the artery.

- Arrange X-ray and other hospital tests.
- Arrange, where necessary, to remove part of a blocked artery and have it replaced by an artificial graft.

Prevention
- Stop smoking. This is the most important of all preventive measures.
- Avoid overeating: part of any excess food is deposited as fat in the arteries. A person can be certain of not overeating only if he or she maintains an ideal weight for height and sex. See ATHEROMA.

Outlook
- Treatment modifies but does not cure symptoms.

See CIRCULATORY SYSTEM *page 40*

CLAUSTROPHOBIA
An abnormal fear of enclosed spaces. Claustrophobia is the opposite to agoraphobia, the fear of open spaces. *See* PHOBIA

CLAW FOOT
Excessive arching of the foot, known medically as pes cavus, which is usually congenital. There is a high arch and clawed toes. The symptoms are usually calluses over the prominent bones and pain in the instep. In many cases treatment is not required and mild symptoms can often be relieved by chiropody and pads to distribute the weight more evenly. In severe cases an operation may be necessary.

CLEFT PALATE AND HARE-LIP

A deformity of the lip and palate present at birth. Such deformities are usually obvious, but minor abnormalities can be seen only if the roof of the mouth is inspected while the child is crying. The tendency may run in families.

Symptoms
- Difficulty in sucking from the breast or bottle. (Babies can be spoon-fed from birth if necessary.)
- A characteristic type of speech.

Causes
- In most cases the cause is unknown.
- Medicines in the first three or four weeks of pregnancy

may sometimes cause congenital deformities.

Treatment in the home
• None advised. Consult the doctor.

What the doctor may do
• Arrange for a plastic surgeon to repair the deformity by an operation or series of operations.
• Arrange for the child to have speech therapy.

Outlook
• Operations are extremely successful in most cases.

See RESPIRATORY SYSTEM *page 42*

CLINICAL

Concerning a doctor's examination and diagnosis. For example, clinical signs in a patient are those noted by a doctor, as distinct from, say, radiological signs, which are detected by X-rays.

CLUB-FOOT

An abnormality of the foot joints in which the patient cannot stand with the sole of the foot flat on the ground. In the most common type, which is known medically as talipes equinovarus, the front part of the foot is turned inwards and downwards at the ankle, forcing the patient to walk on the outside of his foot. Some cases are due to the baby lying in an abnormal position in the womb, but in many other cases the cause is not known. Very occasionally the cause is CEREBRAL PALSY.

The condition is usually noted at birth. The doctor will examine the position of the foot to see if it can be corrected by gentle manipulation. If it cannot, he will refer the baby to an orthopaedic surgeon who may apply a splint. In either case, early treatment should eventually result in a complete cure.

CLUSTER HEADACHE

A severe headache which tends to recur nightly for several weeks or months, and then disappear for years. Its name derives from this habit of appearing in 'clusters'. Cluster headaches are four times more common in men than in women.

The headache, which usually begins two or three hours after falling asleep, starts as an intense pain behind one eye which wakens the patient. The pain is continuous rather than throbbing (as in MIGRAINE). The eye fills

with tears, the nose gets blocked on the affected side and then runs. The cheek may swell, too.

The symptoms last one or two hours. Unlike migraine, it is rare for a cluster headache to produce nausea and vomiting.

Bouts of cluster headache may be brought on by stress, or alcohol. They are thought to be caused by a minor temporary disturbance of circulation in the brain.

If the symptoms are reported to your doctor, he is likely to prescribe a painkiller with added ergot, which helps to restore the normal circulation (*see* MEDICINES, 22). Taken nightly before going to bed, this may prevent an attack occurring.

See NERVOUS SYSTEM *page 34*

COARCTATION OF THE AORTA

A congenital narrowing of the aorta within the chest which reduces the circulation to the lower part of the body and also raises the blood pressure. It can be remedied by surgery.

COCCYDYNIA

Pain in the coccyx (the lowest segment of the spine) or surrounding area.

Symptoms
• Pain at the base of the spine, which either occurs when sitting or is made worse by sitting.

Duration
• If injury is the cause, coccydynia may last for several weeks.

Causes
• The condition usually develops after an injury to the coccyx—most commonly after the patient has sat down abruptly on something hard. It tends to occur more often in women, in whom the coccyx is less well protected.

Treatment in the home
• Take a painkiller. *See* MEDICINES, 22.

When to consult the doctor
• If the symptoms are severe or persist and are interfering with activities.
• When pain is not relieved by a painkiller.

What the doctor may do
• Examine the area, perhaps including the rectum, to exclude the possibility of fracture or some other disorder.
• Advise the patient about how to sit.

• Arrange an X-ray, to check that the coccyx has not been fractured. If it has been, occasionally an operation is necessary.

Outlook
• When caused by injury other than a fracture, the condition usually clears up spontaneously.

See SKELETAL SYSTEM *page 54*

CO-COUNSELLING

A type of psychotherapy developed in the United States in the 1950s and 1960s, in which people are taught skills to counsel each other in turn, developing a supportive network that reduces the need for expensive professional psychotherapy. It is claimed to improve an individual's ability to understand and cope with his emotions, and has been used in England in training programmes for doctors.

COELIAC DISEASE

A rare disorder in which the patient is unable to absorb essential food from the intestines. Coeliac disease runs in families, and commonly affects babies, though mild cases might not be diagnosed until adult life.

Symptoms in babies
• Failure to thrive and grow after weaning between the ages six to 18 months.
• The child is often miserable and weak, with wasted, feeble muscles and a distended abdomen.
• Stools are abnormally bulky, soft, pale and exceptionally smelly.

Symptoms in adults
• Unpredictable attacks of diarrhoea.
• Stools are typically pale, bulky, frothy and greasy, and tend to float.
• The patient may suffer badly from wind, and the abdomen is often distended.
• Wasting and weakness of the rest of the body.

Duration
• In children the disease may last into adolescence, when it tends to subside. It may recur later.

Causes
• The disorder is due to an intolerance of gluten (a protein found in wheat, barley, rye and possibly oats), and so symptoms do not appear until flour is added to a baby's diet.

Complications
• If untreated, growth and development may be affected. The child easily contracts infections of all kinds.
• Vitamin and mineral deficiencies may cause anaemia, sore tongue and mouth, thinning of the bones and a tendency to bleed.
When to consult the doctor
• If the symptoms persist for several weeks.
What the doctor may do
• Send the patient for tests to confirm the diagnosis.
• Advise about diet and supply prescriptions for gluten-free dietary products and any necessary vitamins. Rice, corn or soy flour can be substituted for wheat flour.
• Suggest that parents and other children of the family be investigated to see if they are intolerant of gluten.
Outlook
• Once the offending foods are cut out of the diet, the patient will enjoy normal health.

See DIGESTIVE SYSTEM *page 44*

COLD SORES

The virus which causes cold sores, known medically as herpes simplex, is one of mankind's commonest infections. There are two types — HSV$_1$ which carries infections of the mouth, face and eyes, and HSV$_2$ which causes GENITAL HERPES. Over 50 per cent of the adult population have antibodies to HSV$_1$ in their blood, which means that at some time they have been infected; but only a few recall having had the rash. The virus lies dormant in the sensory nerve cells for many years causing no trouble, but it can be activated at any time by stimuli such as fever, menstruation, extreme cold or sunburn. The infection is said to be primary (first attack) or secondary (recurring). Adults who escaped infection during childhood are at risk.

PRIMARY COLD SORES
Children from six months to five years are most liable to this infection.
Symptoms
• Most commonly the child is feverish and unwell for three or four days without any rash. The condition is treated as a cold and only blood tests will reveal cold sores as the cause.
• The less-fortunate child will be ill with blisters, sores and bleeding ulcers of the lips, the lining of the cheeks, the gums and the tongue.

• In a similar way, in girls, the vulva and vagina may be affected.
• In adults, especially nurses, dentists and doctors, the skin round the nail is infected. This is very painful and resembles a whitlow, except that no pus develops.
Duration
• The painful, distressing stage lasts seven to ten days and recovery with healing of the ulcers is complete within three weeks.
Causes
• A virus called *Herpesvirus hominis*.
• In adults primary herpes may be contracted as a venereal disease and spread by sexual intercourse. *See* GENITAL HERPES.
Treatment in the home
• Rinse the mouth frequently with diluted, proprietary mouth washes.
• Sip iced water.
• Use a soothing cream to soften cracked lips.
When to consult the doctor
• If an infected child has atopic ECZEMA, see the doctor at once because the condition can spread rapidly.
• If a child becomes generally more ill and drowsy.
What the doctor may do
• Prescribe antiviral ointment. *See* MEDICINES, 27.
• Prescribe antibiotic ointments as there is usually a secondary infection with bacteria. *See* MEDICINES, 43.
• Blood tests may be needed to confirm the diagnosis.
• In the case of the ill or drowsy child, check for other possible causes of the condition.
Prevention
• Adult sufferers should avoid contact with children.
• Infection of the fingers may be reduced by wearing protective gloves when in contact with possible infected areas in other people.
Outlook
• Complete recovery is usual, although rare complications like MENINGITIS and ENCEPHALITIS do occur.
• The infection may be reactivated again and again as recurrent cold sores.

RECURRENT COLD SORES
The condition usually recurs at the same site, the most common sites being the lips and face, but any part of the skin may be affected.
Symptoms
• The onset is usually sudden. Tingling, burning and itching may be felt for a few hours before the typical blisters appear. These break, crust and become infected by bacteria and cause pain.
Duration
• The crusting develops in three to five days and healing

is usually complete within 14 days.
Causes
• The same virus that causes the primary infection. Previously dormant in the sensory nerve cells of the affected area, it becomes active. Reactivation appears to be produced by stimuli (for example, infection, sunburn, cold, menstruation or an injury).
Complications
• These are rare, but can include herpetic ulcers of the eye and encephalitis, or the virus may spread to others by direct contact, sexual intercourse or during childbirth to the baby.
Treatment in the home
• Application of alcohol, Vaseline and antibiotic creams may all help to soothe or even reduce the size of the cold sore, but there is no cure.
When to consult the doctor
• If the rash is anywhere near the eye, complications must be avoided by seeking early medical advice.
• If the recurrences are frequent, as some underlying medical disorder may be responsible.
What the doctor may do
• Apart from excluding other illness the doctor may prescribe one of the newer antiviral drugs. *See* MEDICINES, 27.
Prevention
• None is known, but the virus is found in the blisters, so avoid direct contact with others if blisters are present or broken.
Outlook
• Each attack will clear, but recurrence is always possible.

See SKIN *page 52*

COLITIS, ULCERATIVE

A chronic inflammation of the large bowel causing ulceration.
Symptoms
• At first, attacks of bloody diarrhoea at intervals. These may be sudden and severe, but more commonly they are mild with cramps low in the abdomen, an urge to defecate, and blood and mucus in the stools.
• If the disease is extensive or severe, diarrhoea may occur ten to 20 times a day. Sometimes the diarrhoea consists of water, blood and pus only.
• Fever, malaise, loss of appetite and weight, and anaemia, may also occur.

Causes
- The cause is unknown, though the disorder may occur in other members of the family.

Complications
- The disease may be localised in the rectum, in which case it is known as PROCTITIS, and be very mild with few complications.
- It may spread to involve the whole colon.
- Haemorrhage is common.
- The ulcers may perforate the bowel causing sudden, severe, abdominal pain from PERITONITIS, which requires instant medical treatment.
- Non-cancerous growths may occur.
- ARTHRITIS, eye inflammation and skin disorders may also occur.
- If colitis begins in childhood, involves the whole colon and lasts more than ten years, the risk of cancer of the bowel developing is high (nearly 200 times the usual rate) and more than half the patients will develop cancer after 30 to 40 years of colitis. These risks may be reduced by proper treatment.

Treatment in the home
- Mild disease can be managed by taking a normal diet apart from cutting out raw fruits and vegetable roughage.
- Avoid stress and anxiety.
- Rest in bed during acute flare-ups.
- Take simple antidiarrhoea preparations in recommended doses to help lessen bowel activity. *See* MEDICINES, 2, 4.

When to consult the doctor
- If there are severe, rapidly progressing symptoms, or if there are recurrent or prolonged bouts of diarrhoea, lasting more than two or three weeks.
- If blood or pus is present in the stools.

What the doctor may do
- Send the patient for a barium enema and internal examination of the bowel with a sigmoidoscope (a device with a light attached) to confirm the diagnosis and assess the extent of the disease.
- Prescribe drugs to help reduce the number of attacks. These may include steroids in the form of tablets, suppositories or enemas. Such enemas may be self-administered and retained in the bowel overnight.
- Advise suitable diet to rest the bowel and reduce diarrhoea.
- In severe or prolonged disease, a blood transfusion may be necessary to combat anaemia and help healing.
- An ileostomy may be necessary. In this operation the colon is totally removed and the small bowel (ileum) brought out on to an opening in the abdomen, where it empties into special disposable plastic bags sealed to the skin. *See* COLOSTOMY and BOWEL OBSTRUCTION.

Outlook
- About 10 per cent of patients completely recover after a single attack.
- Very severe first attacks with haemorrhage, perforation and infection may cause serious complications in another 10 per cent.
- In the remainder of cases the symptoms may grumble on, with bad and good periods.
- It is rare for the disease to appear in people over 60, but when it does it is dangerous and more severe.

See DIGESTIVE SYSTEM *page 44*

COLLAGEN DISEASES

A group of rare disorders marked by a breakdown of collagen. This substance forms connective tissue, which binds together the cells of the skin, tendons, ligaments, cartilage and bones. Collagen diseases vary widely in type and effect. They include lupus erythematosus, scleroderma and dermatomyositis.

COLLAPSE

A loosely used term, meaning different things to different people. Medically it always refers to loss of consciousness. *See* SYMPTOM SORTER—CONSCIOUSNESS, DISTURBANCES OF

COLON, INACTIVE

A condition in which the large bowel is sluggish in its response to overfilling, is slow to pass on its contents, and fills with soft, putty-like faeces. It is also known as sluggish bowel.

Symptoms
- Constipation, but with soft and not hard faeces present.
- Futile efforts to defecate are made. Watery diarrhoea may occur because the bowel produces fluid in response to continual irritation.
- Cramps due to wind may occur in the abdomen and rectum.

Duration
- The condition may be lifelong, and although harmless may be annoying and difficult to cure.
- It may persist in older people.

Causes
- Confining old and infirm patients to bed and letting them get constipated.

- Using bedpans, instead of the lavatory or a commode, may inhibit normal defecation.

Treatment in the home
- Use a mild laxative. *See* MEDICINES, 3.
- Train the bowels to open up at regular times (for example, half an hour after breakfast), and use the lavatory or a commode.
- Eat plenty of roughage—for example, bran, fruit and vegetables.
- Regular exercise may be helpful.
- Abdominal cramps can often be helped by lying face down on a bed, this allows the passage of wind. *See* CONSTIPATION.

When to consult the doctor
- If symptoms do not respond to the simple treatment described above.

What the doctor may do
- Advise you about diet, exercise and the use of suppositories or enemas where necessary.
- Arrange nursing care with enemas or removal of the faeces by the fingers.

Prevention
- Suitable diet and exercise.

Outlook
- The tendency is usually lifelong.

See DIGESTIVE SYSTEM *page 44*

COLOSTOMY

An operation in which part of the colon (the large intestine) is pulled out through a cut in the abdominal wall to make an artificial anus. The pulled-out colon is cut into and joined to the skin of the abdomen. This makes a new exit for the faeces (motions). A colostomy bag, that is a plastic or rubber bag with an adhesive rim, is fixed to the skin surrounding the new opening to collect the faeces. The bags can be removed for disposal and replaced as necessary.

A colostomy may have to be performed if the lower bowel is obstructed, gangrenous, inflamed or has to be removed because of cancer. Although most colostomies are permanent, they can sometimes be closed and the bowel allowed to work normally when the diseased area has been removed or the inflammation has cleared.

It should be stressed that when an ileostomy or colostomy is permanent, proper regulation allows complete personal freedom in almost all activities (including sex), with no offence to others. *The Colostomy Association*, 15 Station Road, Reading, Berkshire RG1 1LG (Tel. 0734-391537), provides advice and help.
See DIGESTIVE SYSTEM *page 44*

COLOUR BLINDNESS

Difficulty in distinguishing between colours, particularly red and green, is an inherited defect. It is much more common in males and affects about 8 per cent of all men, as opposed to about 0.4 per cent of women.

Colour blindness rarely causes problems. As a child the individual learns that grass is green and pillar-boxes are red, and is therefore able to tell them apart. As a car driver he will know that red is at the top and green at the bottom of the column of traffic lights.

Problems will arise only if a person wishes to follow an occupation for which perfect colour vision is essential, such as an aeroplane pilot, naval communications operator, or electrician. For these, and similar occupations, a doctor will test a recruit for colour blindness.

The doctor will probably test the type of colour blindness with a special series of colour plates (known as Ishihara tests). These are cards covered with irregular spots of different colours. On some of these cards, only colour-blind people can detect certain patterns, while on others, different patterns can only be seen by people with normal colour vision. Certain employers (for instance, the Royal Navy and British Rail) may require other tests.

TEST YOUR COLOUR VISION
How the numbers you see add up

The test plates should be viewed in a room lit by natural daylight. Seen under electric light or in direct sunlight the different shades of colour used in the dots may appear to vary, producing discrepancies in the results of any test. The plates should be viewed from a distance of 30 in. (75 cm.) with the line of vision at right-angles to the plate. You have to give the reading for each plate within three seconds. The correct reading for each plate is given below it. Correct readings for plates 1-6 show that you have normal vision. If you read any of the plates incorrectly, you should see your doctor or an ophthalmic optician for a full test of your colour vision. Plates 7 and 8 are used for those who cannot read—young children, for example.

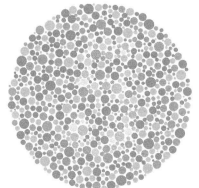

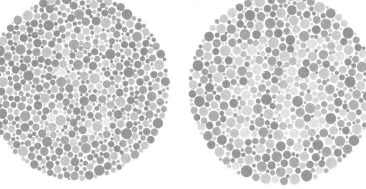

3 The normal see 5. Those with a red-green defect see 2. The totally colour blind cannot see a numeral.

5 The normal see 16. People with all types of colour-vision defects either see no numeral or the wrong one.

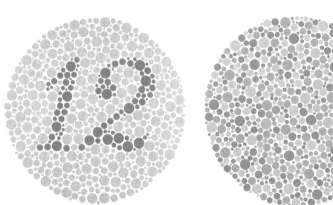

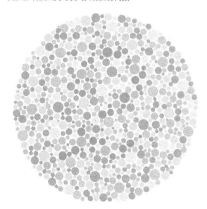

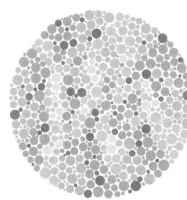

1 People with normal colour vision and those with all types of defects in their colour vision see 12.

2 The normal see 8. Those with a red-green defect see 3. The totally colour blind cannot see a numeral.

4 The normal see 2. People with all types of colour-vision defects either see no numeral or the wrong one.

6 Whether you have normal colour vision or are colour blind you will be unable to see a numeral on this plate.

For most people there are no difficulties in living with colour blindness. It does not prevent a person becoming a lorry driver or bus driver. No link has been shown between defective colour vision and road-traffic accidents. Some colour-blind people even become painters. It is believed by some that the great English artist John Constable was colour blind.

See EYE *page 36*

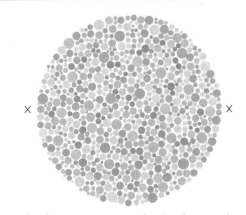

7 The object is to trace a winding line between the two Xs. The normal trace the orange line. The colour blind cannot see it.

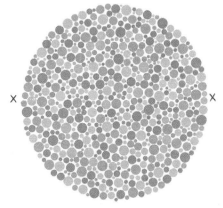

8 The normal connect the purple and orange dots. Those with a red-green defect connect the purple and green dots. The totally colour blind see no line.

COMMON COLD

A highly contagious virus infection, more usual in winter months, though common all the year round. It can be caused by many different viruses, and as these are constantly changing, any immunity developed from one infection may not protect against further infection. However, some immunity is developed over the years and adults are usually less vulnerable than children. The following groups of individuals are at special risk: the frail and elderly; babies and the very young; patients who are obviously ill or who have a persistent fever for more than three days.

Mucus from the nose is loaded with viruses, and the air breathed, coughed or sneezed out by an infected person may infect others in the vicinity. Cold viruses are also transmitted by hand-to-hand contact with adults or other children, entering the body when the recipient then rubs his eyes or nose.

Symptoms
- Sore throat, headache and a stuffy feeling in the front of the head.
- Runny nose—the discharge is clear and runny at first, later becoming thicker and greenish-yellow, tending to block the nose. Sneezing is common.
- A cough which may be dry and tickly.
- Lack of appetite.
- Although the patient may feel hot or cold, the temperature if measured is normal or only slightly raised.
- General feeling of lack of energy.

Duration
- The incubation period is approximately two days.
- Symptoms usually last at least three days and subside over the following three to seven days.
- The nose may run or feel blocked for up to three weeks afterwards.

Causes
- Numerous viruses.
- Colds are not caused by getting wet or physically cold, but infection is more likely if the body's resistance is reduced by factors such as chronic illness, fatigue, stress or depression.

Complications
- Colds may trigger off other secondary infections in the lungs, sinuses or ears.

Treatment in the home
- Keep the patient's temperature down. Although the patient may feel cold his temperature may actually be raised.

- *Do not* wrap up in extra clothes or blankets, and *do not* heat up the room excessively or sit in front of a hot fire. Rather, allow the body to lose some of the excess heat being generated. Babies are particularly vulnerable to overheating. They should be kept in a comfortably warm room and wear as little clothing as possible, to prevent dehydration and convulsions.
- Tepid sponging may cool and soothe children.
- Take extra drinks, especially cool drinks, to replace

Cold cures—true or false?

☐ *True* Medicine or nose drops can make the symptoms of a cold easier to bear.

☐ *True* Over-the-counter cold cures are generally safe to use, but some may be unsafe for people with diabetes, high blood pressure, heart or thyroid disease and stomach ulcers.

☐ *True* If you are already taking drugs for another condition, you should check with your doctor or chemist before taking self-medication for a cold.

☐ *True* A cough that produces phlegm is helpful to a cold.

☐ *True* Breathing moist air or steam relieves symptoms.

☐ *True* Over-the-counter medicines may produce unwanted side-effects. Some, for example, can add to the effect of alcohol and make it dangerous to drive.

☐ *False* Medicines can cure a cold or cut short its duration.

☐ *False* Coughing should always be prevented by taking linctus.

☐ *False* Vitamin C is definitely effective in preventing or treating colds.

fluids being lost and to cool the body. Lack of food is not important, but fluid loss makes the patient feel worse, and in babies can be dangerous. Babies should, if possible, be given additional water or diluted fruit juice between milk feeds in sufficient amounts to produce at least three wet nappies in 24 hours.

- Take painkillers in recommended doses (*see* MEDICINES, 22). This helps to keep the temperature down.
- A linctus or cough mixture may ease irritating cough symptoms. *See* MEDICINES, 16.
- Steam inhalation may help. Be careful not to expose children to the danger of scalding if boiling water is used.
- Do not smoke, and avoid tobacco fumes.
- Do not use nose drops. They may appear to give immediate relief but can cause the nose to become more blocked.
- A walk in the fresh air may ease symptoms.
- Extra sleep or rest in bed assists recovery.

When to consult the doctor
Colds get better on their own—doctors cannot cure them. Antibiotics (such as penicillin) are of no value unless there are complications which respond to them. But the doctor should be consulted if:
- There is chronic lung disease, such as EMPHYSEMA.
- Green or yellow phlegm is being coughed up.
- A raised temperature persists for over three days.
- Earache or a runny ear develops.
- A stiff neck develops that cannot be bent forwards.
For children you should consult the doctor:
- If the temperature cannot be reduced by removing clothes, tepid sponging and extra fluids.
- If crying is inconsolable.
- If the child becomes drowsy and unresponsive.
- If the child vomits more than twice.
- If there is difficulty in breathing or noisy breathing.

What the doctor may do
- Look for complications, particularly chest infection or, in children, ear infection.
- If there are complicating infections he may prescribe antibiotics. *See* MEDICINES, 25.

Prevention
- Regular exercise.
- Stop smoking.
- Because colds are often passed by hand-to-hand contact the spread of viruses can be reduced by frequent hand washing, the use of disposable tissues and the avoidance of physical contact with sufferers.

Outlook
- No long-term problems if secondary complicating infections can be avoided.

See RESPIRATORY SYSTEM *page 42*

COMPLICATION
A disorder that develops as the result of some other, already existing disorder. For example, kidney damage can occur as a complication of DIABETES mellitus.

COMPULSIVE OBSESSIONAL BEHAVIOUR

An uncommon and extreme exaggeration of a trait of normal behaviour, in which actions or thoughts are endlessly repeated for no reason. Although the sufferer may be aware of his behaviour, he is unable to control it.

Symptoms
- Repetition of an activity to a degree that interferes with normal living.
- A thought or idea which perpetually breaks through into other thoughts. It can be voluntarily suppressed but will rapidly recur.

Duration
- The state may last from a few weeks to several years unless treatment is given to modify the behaviour.

Causes
- Frequently the condition is triggered off by stress in a thoughtful individual who is over-careful and meticulous in his or her habits. It is six times as common in women as in men.
- Although minor obsessions are present in all of us, doctors do not know what causes the persistent and extreme forms of obsessional behaviour.

When to consult the doctor
- If normal life is being disturbed. Relatives and friends are often the first to report the abnormal behaviour to the doctor.

What the doctor may do
- Discuss the problem with the patient and begin treatment, possibly with tranquillisers. *See* MEDICINES, 17.
- Refer the patient to a psychiatrist.

Prevention
- None known.

Outlook
- Most minor cases settle on their own. Extreme cases, which are rare, may be resistant to all treatment.

See MENTAL SYSTEM *page 33*

CONCUSSION
A head injury which causes any loss of consciousness is called concussion. The loss of consciousness indicates that the brain requires a period of rest to recover completely.
See POST-CONCUSSIONAL SYNDROME

CONFUSION

A state, usually seen in elderly people, in which the sufferer is unable to make sense of the situation in which he finds himself and therefore feels lost and muddled. Sometimes, but not in all cases, confusion may be associated with loss of memory. It can be caused by physical or mental illness.

Symptoms
- Failing to recognise well-known people or places.
- An inability to complete simple tasks.
- Inappropriate response to questions or requests.
- Frequently there are symptoms of other illness such as a high temperature or general feeling of ill health.
- Confusion may come on rapidly or slowly.

Duration
- If due to physical illness, the onset is usually rapid and of short duration.
- In mental illness the confusion may be prolonged over weeks or months.
- If the confusion is produced by senile DEMENTIA, it is liable to increase in severity, and last the remainder of the patient's life.

Causes
When confusion comes on slowly in the elderly this may be due to dementia. When the confusion comes on rapidly, it may be due to any of the following.
- Head injury.
- High fever.
- Epileptic fit.
- Overdose of drugs (for example barbiturates and LSD).
- Mental diseases such as DEPRESSION and SCHIZO-PHRENIA.

Treatment in the home
- Friends or relatives should remain calm, and contact a doctor when reasonably possible. If the confused person is in a strange place, or with strangers, the confusion will be more marked.
- If there is a high temperature, try to reduce it by removing excess clothing and giving soluble aspirin (un-

less there is a history of stomach trouble).

When to consult the doctor
• When the symptoms described occur—unless the condition is long-standing.
• Immediately, if the symptoms develop suddenly and are possibly due to physical causes, such as head injury, or an overdose of insulin or other drugs.

See MENTAL SYSTEM *page 33*

CONGENITAL DISLOCATION OF THE HIP

The dislocation occurs either before or at birth. It is discovered at the routine examination after birth. In the rare cases when it is not detected early, the child will become disabled—though treatment may remedy this.

Girls are affected by the disorder six times as often as boys. In two-thirds of all cases only one hip is affected.

Symptoms
• Symptoms occur only if the abnormality has not been detected and treated at birth. There are no symptoms until the child reaches walking age: then walking is often delayed, and when it starts the child has a limp or waddling gait.

Causes
• Dislocation of the hip can be inherited.
• It can also be the result of a difficult birth.

When to consult the doctor
• Immediately the condition is suspected.

What the doctor may do
• Manipulate the baby's hip joints and listen for a click, which will almost certainly denote dislocation.
• Refer the child to hospital for an X-ray or a second opinion.
• If the diagnosis is confirmed and the baby is less than six months old, the legs are kept widely separated by a splint for three to six months. This is often the only treatment needed to make the hip develop normally.
• If the baby is older than six months, the dislocation may require a different form of treatment, perhaps an operation.

Outlook
• Excellent if the diagnosis is made at birth or before the baby is six months old.

See SKELETAL SYSTEM *page 54*

CONGENITAL HEART DISEASE

Perhaps as many as one child in every 100 is born with a structural abnormality of the heart. Some are slight and do not affect day-to-day living. Others may be too serious for the child to live a normal life. In between are many different abnormalities, of varying degrees of severity.

Symptoms
• Sometimes there are no symptoms, and the abnormalities may be discovered only at a routine medical examination.
• Shortness of breath on exertion.
• Failure of growth.
• Fatigue.
• Blueness of the skin.

Duration
• Unless treated the symptoms persist indefinitely.

Causes
• In most patients there is no known cause.
• German measles and some drugs taken during pregnancy.
• Some chromosome abnormalities.

Complications
• Small abnormalities may become infected. Larger abnormalities may interfere with efficient pumping of the heart and cause progressive shortness of breath and heart failure.

When to consult the doctor
• If the child becomes blue, when at rest, when crying or on exertion.
• If there is undue shortness of breath on exertion.
• If a baby or child fails to develop properly.

What the doctor may do
• Send the child for X-rays and electrocardiograms.
• Arrange for tests in a special heart unit.
• A heart operation may be necessary to improve the health of some patients; for others it will be vital if they are to stay alive.

Prevention
Mothers can reduce the risks to their children if they:
• Try to be as healthy as possible at the time of conception of a baby.
• Avoid drugs, particularly in early pregnancy.
• Do not smoke if trying to conceive, or during pregnancy.
• Be immunised for GERMAN MEASLES (rubella) before

pregnancy. (It cannot be done during pregnancy.)
• Patients with such abnormalities require antibiotics when having operations or teeth removed.

Outlook
• The outlook depends on the type of abnormality and treatment received.
• In general there will be increased strain on the heart as years go by.
• Some abnormalities are completely cured by operation, others can only be improved.

See CIRCULATORY SYSTEM *page 40*

CONJUNCTIVITIS

Inflammation of the conjunctiva, which covers the white of the eye and the inner surface of the lids. Conjunctivitis is the commonest cause of red and/or sticky eyes and is sometimes contagious.

Symptoms
• The symptoms are usually of gradual onset.
• The eyes feel gritty and irritated.
• They look red and congested.
• They become sticky and crusted, especially when waking up in the morning.

Duration
• Untreated, conjunctivitis may last for two or three weeks. With treatment the condition will clear sooner.

Causes
• The most common cause is bacterial or virus infection.
• Other causes are irritants such as tobacco smoke, cosmetics, and some proprietary eye preparations.
• Sometimes conjunctivitis is a sign of serious underlying eye disease.
• Occasionally conjunctivitis may be a sign of an ALLERGY.
• In infants the cause may be blocked TEAR-DUCTS.

Treatment in the home
• Never cover an irritated red eye with an eye patch, as this can encourage further infection with sometimes disastrous results.
• If the eye is sticky, bathe it with warm water.
• In an infant with a possible blocked tear-duct, massaging the lower eyelid near the nose can help to clear the obstruction.

When to consult the doctor
• If the eyes are sticky and feel gritty, and if redness develops and does not clear within two or three days.
• If you have recently been in a tropical country, consult

the doctor as soon as symptoms develop, as the conjunctivitis could be due to the TRACHOMA virus, the one form of conjunctivitis which can eventually affect the vision.

• If there is severe pain, see the doctor as soon as possible, since a more serious disease may be present.

What the doctor may do

• Examine the eyes to confirm the diagnosis, and make sure that there is no foreign body present to cause irritation. He will then probably prescribe drops and/or ointment to be put in the eyes frequently.

• If the conjunctivitis does not clear up, the doctor may suggest that you stop the treatment and bathe only with warm water for 24 to 48 hours. He may then take a swab from the discharge for laboratory examination and if necessary prescribe different treatment.

• If the doctor suspects serious disease he will refer the patient to an eye hospital for specialist treatment.

Prevention

• If the eyes tend to be sore, avoid irritants such as tobacco smoke and do not apply cosmetics near the eyes.

• *Do not* use proprietary ointments, eye drops or eye-washes, as these may be sources of irritation.

• Eye infections can be passed on by direct contact, so wash your hands after applying drops or ointment. The patient should use only his own towel, and nobody else should use it.

Outlook

• A single attack of conjunctivitis will settle down quite quickly with treatment, and even without treatment will subside in a relatively short time.

• The eyesight is never affected, except in the case of trachoma, which is a tropical disease.

• Conjunctivitis occasionally persists, fails to respond to treatment and so becomes chronic. The cause is usually allergic, rarely serious disease.

See EYE *page 36*

CONSTIPATION

Faeces which have been retained in the rectum for several days tend to become dried out and hardened and thus more difficult to pass. Many people have come to believe that a daily bowel action is essential and that anything less is constipation. But normal bowels may empty three times a day or only once every three days, or at any rate in between. In the case of babies it is quite common and normal for a baby not to have a bowel

action for up to a week. Rarely does it cause trouble. Occasionally a fissure, or tear of the anal skin, may occur and a soothing ointment (such as petroleum jelly) placed with the fingertip into the anal canal will assist healing.

Symptoms

• Difficult or infrequent passing of motions.

• In the case of old people or ill patients, persistent failure to empty the bowel may lead to spurious diarrhoea (a watery discharge, often soiling bedclothes), produced by hard faeces blocking and irritating the rectum.

Duration

• The tendency usually persists throughout life unless appropriate changes to the diet are made.

Causes

• Many painkillers are constipating.

• Ill, feverish people taking little food often become constipated, especially if bed-ridden and trying to use a bed-pan rather than sitting on a commode or a lavatory.

• Lack of roughage and fluids.

• Causes such as strictures, cancers, bowel obstruction are rare; but anal fissures are painful and once caused—usually by passing a hard motion—may make the sufferer reluctant to use the lavatory and lead to constipation.

Treatment in the home

• Take extra fluids and eat plenty of vegetables, fruit and other roughage such as bran (one or two 5 ml. spoonfuls of bran sprinkled over each meal). Wholemeal bread and wholemeal flour also give increased roughage.

• Laxatives may help to retrain bowels, though these should be discontinued when normal habits are restored. *See* MEDICINES. 3.

• Some natural materials absorb water, giving soft bulky faeces which are easy and painless to pass. Proprietary bulking agents are useful supplements to high-roughage diets. *See* MEDICINES, 3.

• In the case of babies, increase the amount of sugar in bottles to loosen the motions. About a teaspoon per bottle may be used to adjust the frequency of dirty nappies. Too much sugar will cause diarrhoea.

• If constipation appears to be causing straining and distress the stools can be softened by a paediatric (baby-sized) glycerin suppository, or a small piece of toilet soap, $\frac{1}{2}$ in. (13 mm.) long, inserted into the rectum.

• In the case of old people, ensure regular visits to the lavatory. Use bulking agents or single doses of a laxative, if necessary regularly until bowel habits are re-established. Administer proprietary or soap suppositories if necessary.

• Seek advice from your district nurse or doctor if the problem persists.

When to consult the doctor

• Any change in bowel habit persisting for longer than two or three weeks should always be reported.

• If the constipation is severe or not responding to home treatment, or if there is abdominal pain.

• If faecal incontinence or impaction (blockage) occurs.

What the doctor may do

• Advise the patient on diet and the use of laxatives or suppositories.

• Enemas may occasionally be necessary, but regular washouts have no value in removing 'poisons'.

Prevention

• A diet with plenty of roughage.

Outlook

• Usually good if dietary changes are made.

See DIGESTIVE SYSTEM *page 44*

CONTRACEPTION

The prevention of pregnancy, or conception, by natural or artificial means.

See FAMILY PLANNING

COPPER THERAPY

According to tradition, wearing copper—usually in the form of a bracelet around the wrist—can ease the pain of RHEUMATISM. Scientific tests suggest that rheumatic disease may be accompanied by a deficiency of copper in the body, but the link has not been positively proved.

CORN

A thickening of the outer skin, most commonly on the toes and soles of the feet. The horny layer of the skin becomes thickened over a bone following repeated friction. The corn consists of a central core surrounded by thick layers of skin. Soft corns may develop between the toes due to friction which occurs between the bony points of the toes.

Symptoms

• Corns are painful when pressed, due to the core resting on the nerve endings.

Duration

• Even if treated, corns will recur until there is no longer pressure and friction on the skin.

Causes

• Most commonly, badly fitting shoes.

Complications

• Soft corns frequently become infected.

Treatment in the home

• By changing shoes, wearing sandals, and using corn pads, pressure is removed from the corn.

• Corn plasters and salicylic acid ointment or paint encourage the hard skin to peel.

• The corn may be gently pared with a sharp sterile blade after softening the skin in a bath. Great care should be taken over this procedure which is always best performed by a chiropodist. Self-treatment should never be attempted by elderly or diabetic patients. The core when revealed is clear and may be scraped away. If the core contains black dots in the centre, these are likely to be the small arteries of a VERRUCA and not a corn.

• It is usually worth while to consult a chiropodist.

When to consult the doctor

• If the corn becomes infected or develops into an ulcer.

• If the bones of the feet are so deformed that no shoes are comfortable.

What the doctor may do

• Treat any infection.

• Check for diabetes and disorders of circulation which will make ulcers more likely.

• Severe deformities of the feet and toes may require surgical correction.

Prevention

• Any comfortable footwear which avoids pressure on the feet will prevent corns.

• Poorly fitting shoes in childhood are especially liable to produce deformities and corns in adult life.

Outlook

• Corns will always disappear if the pressure that causes them is removed.

See SKIN *page 52*

CORNEAL ULCERS

Ulcers on the cornea (the front of the eye) are acutely painful, although not common. Consult a doctor without delay, as untreated or improperly treated corneal ulcers may affect the vision.

Symptoms

• Acute pain, usually in one eye, with watering of the eye and spasms of the eyelid, that prevents proper opening.

• When associated with a speck of grit in the eye, or a scratch or chemical burn, the onset of the pain is sudden.

• The rarer but more serious form of ulcer caused by a virus infection can come on more gradually.

Duration

• With appropriate treatment the ulcer will heal in a matter of three or four days.

Causes

• Corneal ulcers can be caused by a virus infection, or by injury—scratching of the eye's surface with a tiny speck of grit or other sharp object.

• Other causes include burning by chemicals or ultraviolet light—either from a lamp or reflected from snow when skiing, for example.

Treatment in the home

• If a speck of grit has entered the eye, try to remove it (or get a friend to do so) with a wisp of cotton wool or the corner of a clean handkerchief. If unsuccessful, seek medical aid.

• If chemicals (for instance, ammonia) get into the eye, immediate first aid is called for in the form of copious amounts of water—the patient's head should be plunged under a tap or into a bucket of water without delay. It may be necessary to force the eyelid open to allow the water to have full effect. *See* FIRST AID *page 585*.

When to consult the doctor

• If you have acute and persisting pain in the eye, whether the cause is obvious (such as after a scratch or a piece of grit in the eye) or not, consult your doctor immediately or go to the hospital Accident and Emergency Department.

What the doctor may do

• The doctor will ask for any history of injury and then look at the eye with a magnifying glass. If he suspects injury to the cornea (or a foreign body on the cornea) he may stain the injured area yellow with drops to make the ulcer visible.

• Once a corneal ulcer has been diagnosed the doctor will probably prescribe some drops and/or ointment, and may recommend that the eye should be covered with a pad for at least 24 hours to allow healing to take place.

Prevention

• Goggles should be worn whenever there is a risk of eye injury from machinery, chemicals or ultra-violet light. This applies as much to working in the home, especially with power tools, as it does in industry.

Outlook

• Provided treatment is given as early as possible, most ulcers will heal quite rapidly and completely without after-effects.

• Virus ulcers can sometimes recur, but once one has been dealt with the patient will be alert to report early if the symptoms should recur.

See EYE *page 36*

CORONARY THROMBOSIS

In the majority of developed countries coronary thrombosis is the most common cause of heart attacks—and is responsible for more deaths than any other single disease. In an attack an artery supplying blood to the heart is obstructed. Attacks are rare in people under 40, and are more likely to affect men than women. The condition is also called myocardial infarction and may sometimes develop in sufferers from ANGINA PECTORIS.

Symptoms

• Severe constricting pain across the front of the chest, often spreading to one or both arms, the neck and the jaw. The pain comes on suddenly and, although it feels like anginal pain, it is not usually related to exertion and does not pass off with keeping still.

• Preliminary symptoms, experienced some weeks before an attack, are: undue tiredness; shortness of breath; unaccustomed indigestion.

Duration

• If untreated, the pain—which is severe at the outset—may continue for many hours. It gradually vanishes within two days.

• Healing of the damaged heart takes several weeks.

Causes

• Thrombosis (clotting) of the coronary artery is the most common cause of obstruction. The thrombus (clot) occurs at the site of plaque. *See* ATHEROMA.

• Blockage of the coronary artery causes obstruction of the blood supply, destroying the heart muscle.

• The likelihood of developing a coronary thrombosis is increased by smoking, obesity, diabetes, raised blood pressure, lack of exercise, high blood cholesterol and a family history of heart attacks.

Complications

• Failure of the heart and death.

Treatment in the home

• Sit down or sit propped up in bed. This position places least strain on the heart.

When to consult the doctor

• Immediately an attack is suspected.

• When a sudden chest pain, as described above, first occurs.

• If someone suffering from angina has a prolonged or unusually severe attack.

What the doctor may do

• Relieve the pain with drugs such as morphine.

- Give aspirin and arrange hospital admission for treatment with a drug such as streptokinase to break up the blood clot.
- Arrange electrocardiograms and blood tests to confirm the diagnosis.

Prevention

- The best prevention is to stay within the limits of your ideal WEIGHT for your height; to give up SMOKING; to take regular EXERCISE; and to comply fully with treatment if you suffer from DIABETES or HYPERTENSION.
- Adopt a healthy daily regime, with a sensible diet and regular physical activity. This will reduce the risk of coronary thrombosis, or of a further attack.
- Your doctor may recommend a regular daily prescription of aspirin and a beta-blocking drug to reduce the risk of another attack.

See ATHEROMA

Outlook

- **Immediate** More than 80 per cent of those who survive the first few hours after an attack will recover.
- **Short term** Even after serious attacks the outlook is very good, particularly if the patient is under 40.
- Most people are able to resume work, however hard.
- A few people will develop angina if they exert themselves.
- In some cases physical activity will have to be severely curtailed.
- **Long term** To reduce the risk of further attacks, it is essential to follow the doctor's advice about diet, losing weight, stopping smoking and taking the right amount of physical exercise.

See CIRCULATORY SYSTEM *page 40*

Do's and don'ts after a coronary thrombosis

☐ *Do* send for medical care without delay.

☐ *Don't* move until medical care arrives.

☐ *Don't*, if possible, take the sufferer to hospital in the first hours after an attack without expert medical attention. Anxiety and movement of the patient may cause changes in the blood pressure and heartbeat, which could be harmful. Movement of the patient is safest after a doctor has given protective drugs and made an assessment.

LOOKING AT THE HEART
Two new ways of detecting heart disease

Every year more people in Britain are killed by heart disease than by any other cause, including cancer. In many cases heart disease can be controlled or even cured, but for this to happen it must be detected early. Until recently detection of heart disease involved methods of examination requiring minor operations; for example, inserting a narrow tube through a blood vessel into the heart. Newly developed techniques allow organs deep inside the body to be examined without the need for internal probes. Two such methods now widely used are 24 hours ambulatory electrocardiogram (ECG) monitoring, and ultrasound—the echocardiogram.

An ECG records the electrical changes in the heart muscle as it works, and shows up abnormalities in its rhythm—arrhythmias. It is often a matter of luck, however, whether the arrhythmia shows up in the hospital ECG which may last only a few minutes. By recording the patient's heart rhythm on a portable ECG for a whole day or more there is a better chance of picking up any abnormalities.

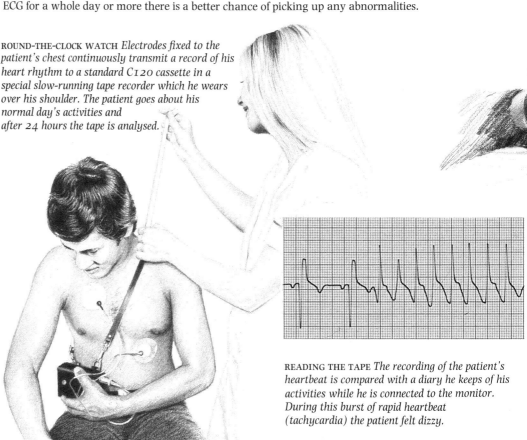

ROUND-THE-CLOCK WATCH *Electrodes fixed to the patient's chest continuously transmit a record of his heart rhythm to a standard C120 cassette in a special slow-running tape recorder which he wears over his shoulder. The patient goes about his normal day's activities and after 24 hours the tape is analysed.*

READING THE TAPE *The recording of the patient's heartbeat is compared with a diary he keeps of his activities while he is connected to the monitor. During this burst of rapid heartbeat (tachycardia) the patient felt dizzy.*

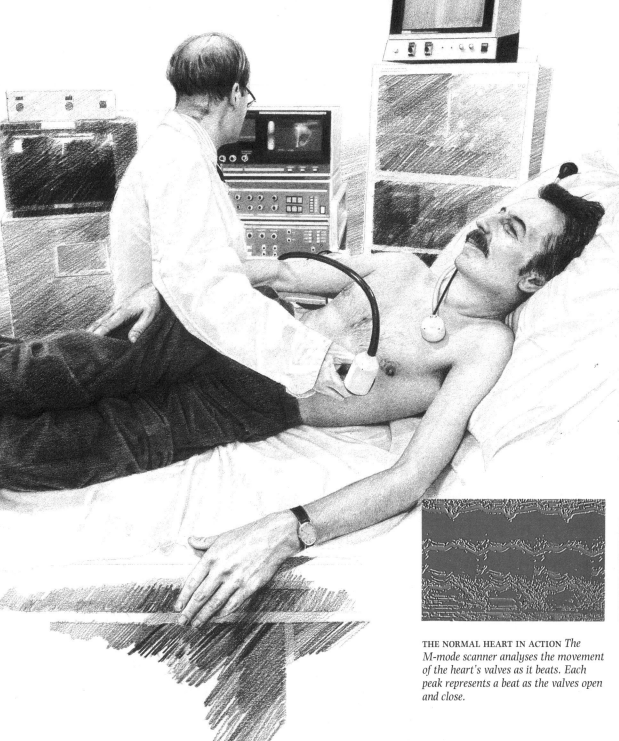

PICTURES FROM SOUND *When a beam of very high-pitched sound— ultrasound—is aimed at the heart, a detailed picture of the heart can be built by analysing the echoes from the boundaries between different tissues. To produce an echocardiogram the doctor sweeps the transducer, or scanning head, over the patient's heart. The transducer gives out pulses of ultrasound, receives the echoes and turns them into electrical signals. These are passed to an analyser and converted into a picture on a screen or a printout. The two main ways of showing the information are Real Time and M-mode. The Real Time scanner gives pictures of the heart moving, very much like a film. These may be colour-coded to show the doctor details of the heart muscle—what it looks like. The M-mode display can show the working of the heart as it beats. By combining the information from the Real Time and M-mode displays the doctor has a full picture of the heart which may pinpoint the cause of the patient's problem.*

THE NORMAL HEART IN ACTION *The M-mode scanner analyses the movement of the heart's valves as it beats. Each peak represents a beat as the valves open and close.*

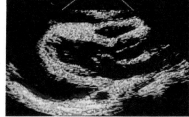

WATER AROUND THE HEART *A Real Time scan of water in the sac around the heart (pericardial effusion) seen, in the elongated black area between the two coloured sections (lower left).*

181

COR PULMONALE

Heart failure which develops when long-standing lung disease has strained the heart and circulation. A poor uptake of oxygen by the lungs causes constriction of the small arteries in the lung, reducing blood flow and increasing the pumping work of the heart.

In people with severe lung disease, heart failure is often brought on by a respiratory infection, exertion, or ascent to altitudes.

Cor pulmonale is sometimes referred to as failure of the right side of the heart, to distinguish it from failure of the left side, which may occur in those with high blood pressure or coronary artery disease (*see* HEART FAILURE). It is more common in men than in women.

Symptoms
- Shortness of breath.
- Blueness of lips and face.
- Swelling of the ankles.

Duration
- With treatment, attacks of cor pulmonale can usually be controlled within seven to ten days, though the risk of recurrence is high since the underlying lung disease is difficult to treat.

Causes
- Chronic bronchitis.
- Asthma.
- Fibrosis of the lung (for example, pneumoconiosis).
- Structural deformities of the chest and spine.

Treatment in the home
- Avoid adding strain to an overloaded heart from overexertion and overweight.

When to consult the doctor
- When shortness of breath develops in those with lung disease, especially if the ankles swell as well.

What the doctor may do
- Treat you with antibiotics and sometimes cortisone and oxygen. *See* MEDICINES, 25, 32.
- Tell you to rest.
- He may also prescribe diuretic tablets to increase the excretion of surplus fluid. *See* MEDICINES, 6.

Prevention
- Stop smoking.
- Reduce weight to ideal. *See* WEIGHT.
- Avoid excessive exertion (if you are still short of breath a minute or two after stopping exertion).
- Always consider respiratory infections to be serious (even common colds).
- Avoid high altitudes.

- Avoid dusty and smoky atmospheres.
- Have an injection in autumn. (This protects against influenza only, not common colds.)

Outlook
- Though cor pulmonale is a late stage in the development of chest disease, it may be treated and controlled for many years.

See CIRCULATORY SYSTEM *page 40*

COSMETIC SURGERY

In recent years there has been an ever-increasing demand for cosmetic surgery in Britain, either performed privately or through the National Health Service. This has emerged from a more liberal social outlook, in which it is no longer considered frivolous or vain to want to correct a blemish, fault or disfigurement in a person's physical appearance.

In seeking to correct such flaws as an unsightly or oversized nose, cosmetic surgery can boost the patient's self-confidence. No longer need he fear, at work or on social occasions, that people are making derogatory remarks about his looks.

The NHS employs more than 80 consultant plastic surgeons, whose work deals primarily with correcting embarrassing disfigurements and deformities. But there are still not enough NHS surgeons to meet the demand. This has led to a profusion of private clinics, some of which are inefficient and which have led the British Medical Association to call for a campaign to educate the public about the dangers of dealing with a clinic without the advice of their own doctor.

Although the General Medical Council forbids doctors to advertise, there is no such restriction on clinics under non-medical management. More and more people are approaching these clinics direct, without consulting their doctor or being referred to a particular surgeon. In so doing they may be exposing themselves to the risk of an expensive and unsuccessful operation—which could result in a series of further operations to correct the one that went wrong.

WHAT COSMETIC SURGERY CAN DO
There are four ways in which cosmetic surgery can help the patient.
1. It can often improve an ugly scar—although it will not remove the scar completely. This is because once the skin

has been cut into deeply, the resultant scar is permanent. But cutting out a scar and sewing the skin neatly may leave the area flat and less defaced.

However, some people—especially those with dark skin—develop thick, raised, itchy red scar tissue called KELOID. This form of abnormal healing is often worse than the original scar. But it is a risk the patient may be prepared to take, and in most cases keloid eventually flattens and fades away. If it persists, then radiotherapy may help it fade.

2. Moles and some birthmarks can be removed with little scarring by surgery or skilled use of an argon laser.
3. Excess skin which may come with advancing years or weight loss can be removed from the face, eyelids, stomach and breasts. The post-operative scars of face-lifting and similar operations will fall into natural crease-lines, be hidden by hair, or be covered by clothing.
4. The nose, chin, breasts and stomach can be reduced in size and made more symmetrical.

WHAT COSMETIC SURGERY CANNOT DO
Despite popular belief to the contrary, cosmetic surgery can rarely be performed without leaving a scar. The few operations in which scars are *not* left are: the sand-papering of pitted facial scars (dermabrasion), which is limited to the top layers of the skin; the use of acid to tighten wrinkled skin, which causes a very mild burn; the reduction of an excessively large nose (rhinoplasty), in which the scars are inside the nose and so are not visible.

1. It cannot make people—men or women—look younger than they are. But it *can* prevent them looking older than they are. It can turn an aged 60 year old into a well preserved 60 year old. Age is not just a matter of years—it is revealed by people's habits, speech, posture and gait, and none of these can be made to seem younger by a surgical operation.
2. By changing a person's face, it cannot necessarily save a marriage, increase job efficiency, or alter personality—although it may make the patient a more contented, happier and therefore nicer person to be with.
3. It cannot cure mental illness or depression caused by brooding about a particular disfigurement—real or imaginary. If the patient is mentally upset by, say, an outsize nose, its reduction will not automatically remove or decrease his obsession. Instead, he may find fault with his 'new' nose or start to worry about some other physical defect which he may or may not have.
4. Cosmetic surgery cannot reproduce an 'ideal' nose from a photograph of an actor or a model in a magazine. And those who expect such perfection are doomed to disappointment.

5. It cannot remove such blemishes as a pink birthmark (haemangioma) or port-wine stain, which if large is better masked by ordinary cosmetics. It is possible to replace a large birthmark—provided it is not on the face—with skin taken from another part of the body and grafted in place. But the graft will not match the colour or texture of the rest of the skin.

WAYS OF USING COSMETIC SURGERY

Cosmetic surgery operations are performed under anaesthetic, either general or local.

Scars and blemishes Scars can be improved and minor skin blemishes such as moles can be removed.

Tattoo marks Tattooing is done by injecting pigment deeply into the skin. A fine needle—and blue, green and red colours—are used to produce a picture. Tattoos can be removed in one of three ways: by cutting out the coloured skin and sewing up the wound to leave a line scar; by cutting out the large tattoo and replacing it with a skin graft; or by using a laser beam to burn out the colour and leave a scar in the shape of the original tattoo. Sandpapering the skin is unsuccessful because the blue dye is always very deep in the skin; it will, however, improve a tattoo by removing the red and green.

Protruding ears Ears that protrude can be set back against the head. The excess skin behind the ears is removed and the cartilage, or gristle, is weakened, allowing the ear to lie flat. The resultant scar is concealed in the crease-line between the ears and the scalp.

Face-lift Excessive facial lines, jowels and a drooping neck can be removed with a face-lift. The incision starts within the hair-line at the temple. It descends in the natural crease-line in front of the ear, curved round the lobe into the crease-line behind the ear, and then follows the hair-line to the nape of the neck. The surgeon gently pulls the facial skin back, making it taut over the cheek-bones. This smooths out the ridges and wrinkles. The excess skin is trimmed off and the edges are stitched together. The wounds are then dressed. The effect of a face-lift can be gauged beforehand by pulling the cheek skin back towards the ears with a finger on each side of the face.

Other techniques use injections and implants to smooth out wrinkles and pad out the face for a more youthful appearance.

Bags around the eyes Excess skin from the upper eyelids can be removed to eliminate bagginess. This leaves the scar in the natural crease-line, about midway between eyebrow and eyelash, when the eye is closed. In the lower eyelid the cut is made immediately below the lower eyelashes, where the resultant scar will not be noticeable. The skin is undercut, pulled upwards and outwards, and the excess is trimmed off, removing the bags under the eyes. The outer part of the scar thus lies in the natural crease-line between eye and temple.

Pockmarks Acne and smallpox scars can be smoothed and removed, provided they are not too deep. The skin is rubbed down with a mechanical abrasive cylinder, or sometimes by using sandpaper. The best results are obtained on the cheeks, forehead and chin; the chest and back are less responsive to treatment.

Where there are many deep scars on the face, a face-lift will make them less noticeable by changing the shape of the pits from round to oval. Acne must always be inactive before an operation takes place—otherwise it will flare up again.

Misshapen chin An over-prominent chin, caused by an over-developed lower jaw, can be rectified. The jaw-bone is divided on both sides and pushed back to a new position. The teeth are then wired together to allow the bone to set and heal. As well as improving the contour, the operation often makes the entire face look rounder and smaller. When only the chin is over-prominent, and the jaw-bone is normally proportioned, the excess bone can be shaved down.

In the case of a receding chin, silicone rubber (or occasionally bone from the hip) is implanted to give the chin thrust and firmness. As the operation is usually performed through the mouth, between the gum and the lower lip, there is no external scarring.

Misshapen nose Noses can be made smaller, shorter, or straight—and these are the most frequently requested operations. All incisions are made inside the nostrils.

With crooked noses, the inner mid-line partition—the septum, which separates the nostrils—is often buckled. This can hamper a person's breathing, and the disability is corrected as part of the straightening operation.

Other noses may be lacking the structural support provided by the mid-line and so have a deformed or 'collapsed' appearance. If the bridge-line is narrow, the deformity is corrected by inserting a silicone or hip-bone strut through a vertical incision made in the mid-line of the columella—the piece of skin between the nostrils. The resultant scar is narrow and hidden by the shadow of the nose.

Small breasts Flat chests in women can be enlarged by means of a silicone rubber implant behind the breasts. An incision is made in the horizontal crease-line beneath the breast. A pocket is then tunnelled behind the breast, but in front of the chest muscles.

The implant fits snugly into the pocket. The scar will lie in the natural crease-line and is hidden by the new breast contour. However, more than half of patients later develop excessive scar tissue around the implant—which makes it hard, round and sometimes uncomfortable.

There is no way of preventing this, nor any way of knowing whom it will effect. However, the scar tissue can be removed by a second operation in which the implant is taken out and then replaced. Even so, there is no guarantee that the trouble will not recur.

Over-large breasts Large and drooping breasts can be reduced and given a firm and shapely contour. The excess skin, fat and tissue are removed, but this causes the nipples to move out of position. They then have to be transferred to their correct sites. This is a more complicated operation than breast enlargement, and the scars are more noticeable. There will be a long scar in the crease-line under the breast. There will also be a cut around the areola—the flat, pigmented part of the nipple. However, as the scar lies at the junction between the pigmented and non-pigmented skin, it will not be too obvious. A vertical scar—partly in shadow—joins the other two. This scar often broadens, but it will fade with time.

In men, the breast may become unnaturally enlarged and so be unsightly. It can be reduced by removing all the breast tissue, by means of an incision through the areola. The resultant scar is unnoticeable.

Big stomachs Excess skin and fat from the front of the abdomen—which cannot be got rid of by dieting—can be removed to give the patient a trimmer figure. The incision goes across the abdomen down almost to the abdominal muscles, and the layer of overlying skin and fat is stripped upwards. The layer is then pulled down, tightening the rest of the skin, and the excess is trimmed off. By then, the navel has become too low and has to be surgically moved back up the abdomen. To relax the wound as it is being stitched, the patient's knees and hips are bent, so he will have to walk bent for the next few days, but he can sit normally. The scar runs from one hip to the other. But while sunbathing, it can be hidden by a pair of shorts or a conventional bathing suit.

Excess fat can also be removed from the thighs, buttocks and hips. However, the resultant scars may stretch and be obvious.

Another method is liposuction, in which fat is sucked out from abdomen, buttocks or hips through a much smaller incision.

Baldness Hair transplants—which are not always successful—are mostly performed on men, who characteristically become bald at the temples and on the crown of the head. Pieces of skin containing hair roots from the sides and back of the scalp are punched out by a sharp, hand-held punch and then planted in punch holes in the bald patches. About 200 transplants are needed and they may be combined with a strip of hair-bearing skin— taken from above the ears—which forms a false hair-line on the forehead. The final result—effective after about a year—is never as thick as a wig or a hair-piece—and the donor sites may look unsightly.

THE HAZARDS OF COSMETIC SURGERY

Before undergoing any form of cosmetic surgery, the patient should be aware of the dangers and drawbacks. They fall into four categories:

Risk As well as the physical risk of infection and excessive bleeding involved in all forms of surgery, cosmetic surgery carries its own hazards. There is a slight risk of wound breakdown and delayed healing, which may spoil the finished result. There is also the risk of a collection of blood under the skin (haematoma). This stretches the skin and spoils the result of, say, a face-lift. It also increases the chance of infection and wound breakdown.

Price Although some cosmetic operations are performed free under the NHS for medical reasons, most cosmetic surgery is done privately. An operation may cost several thousand pounds.

Expectations Some people believe that cosmetic surgery can 'work miracles'. This is not true. It cannot make a person youthful, virile, or professionally successful.

Disappointment Even if the operation is a success patients are often disappointed with the outcome, they feel that their new nose or chin could have been a little 'different' or a little 'better'. The dissatisfaction often stems from a lack of communication between the patient and the surgeon beforehand, when the effects should have been fully discussed.

Ten per cent of all patients suffer from some disappointment; 15 per cent are dissatisfied with their built-up breasts; 20 per cent dislike their reduced breasts, face-lifts and eyelids; and 30 per cent are displeased with their smaller or straighter noses.

Actual failure of the operation in trained hands is only about 2 per cent, but people who embark upon cosmetic surgery with unrealistically high hopes can often have them cruelly dashed.

RULES AND SAFEGUARDS

Do not enter a private clinic for cosmetic surgery without first discussing it with your own doctor. He will advise you whether it is likely to improve your appearance.

If you decide to go ahead your doctor can put you in touch with a reputable clinic and ensure that the consultant surgeon there is fully trained and qualified. You can also look up the surgeon's qualifications in *The Medical Directory* in any public library. You should make sure he is a Fellow of the Royal College of Surgeons, with FRCS after his name; and that he works at a reputable hospital and was trained at a reputable centre.

In addition, the General Medical Council advises surgeons in private clinics to contact the patient's own doctor and ensure that there is no physical reason why cosmetic surgery should not take place.

If you cannot afford private treatment, and your doctor feels that cosmetic surgery would be beneficial, he can put you down for an operation under the NHS. However, there is a long waiting list of a year or even more.

As soon as an operation has been arranged you should discover whether a local or a general anaesthetic will be used, how long you will be in hospital, and what kind of discomfort you will later suffer.

Remember: wounds heal better if they are kept dry; scars are often at their worst in the first three months and—although permanent—they should fade within a year; swelling is common, but disappears in about a month; with nose reductions, it takes almost a year for the skin to shrink fully into place; and bruising fades in about three weeks. Finally, you should realise that the end result of minor cosmetic surgery may not be immediately obvious to relatives, friends and colleagues.

COSTOCHONDRITIS

A painful swelling of the joint between the ribs and the breast plate, also known as 'Tieze's disease'. One or more lumps may develop on the chest wall, and deep breathing or coughing may produce pain. In older people this may be confused with ANGINA PECTORIS. The cause is unknown. Sometimes the lumps go away on their own; more often they persist but become painless. Painkillers or anti-inflammatory drugs may help (*see* MEDICINES, 22).

COT DEATH *See* SUDDEN INFANT DEATH

COUGH

Coughing, although annoying, is a protective response helping to rid the lungs of irritants. Coughing may be a symptom of a wide variety of diseases.
See SYMPTOM SORTER—COUGH

CRAB LICE

Lice that infest the pubic hair and that are usually caught by sexual contact. They are popularly known as 'crabs'.

Crab lice are harmless in themselves, but may indicate the possible presence of another serious sexually transmitted disease.
Symptoms
- Yellowish-brown, round, pinhead-sized lice (about 1 mm. across) can be seen close to the skin, clasping the roots of pubic hairs. They remain still unless they are picked off.
- Crab lice may also infest the hair around the anus, in the armpits and on the abdomen or chest, and occasionally the eyebrows, but they are never found in the hair on the head.
- Itching in the pubic and genital region.
Duration
- The lice will persist until removed by treatment.
Causes
- Crab lice are caught by close, usually sexual, contact with someone who already has them.
Treatment in the home
- A lotion should be applied to the affected area. Ask a chemist, doctor or nurse which is the most effective application.
- Shaving of the pubic hair is not necessary.
When to consult the doctor
- If the problem is suspected.
What the doctor may do
- Prescribe a lotion if one is not already being used.
- Investigate the possibility of the patient having another sexually transmitted disease, and tell him about the risk of infecting others.
Prevention
- The less sexually promiscuous a person is, the less risk he has of catching crab lice.
Outlook
- Treatment clears up the problem.

See MALE GENITAL SYSTEM *page* 50

CRADLE CAP

A scaly, brownish-coloured rash, like dandruff, which often forms on the scalps of babies. The condition is harmless and usually clears up with regular shampooing.
See CHILD CARE

CRAMP

A sudden involuntary contraction of a muscle or muscles, causing acute pain. Writer's cramp is a spasm brought on by constant writing. It is a prescribed industrial disease which may entitle a sufferer to state benefit. Treatment

consists of contracting the opposite muscles to those in spasm. Abdominal pain is sometimes described as stomach cramps.
See FIRST AID *page* 575
SYMPTOM SORTER—ABDOMINAL PAIN

CREUTZFELDT-JAKOB DISEASE

A rare form of pre-senile dementia (see ALZHEIMER'S DISEASE), believed to be due to a virus infection with a long incubation period. It is similar to virus diseases of sheep (scrapie) and cattle (BSE—bovine spongiform encephalopathy), but there is as yet no firm evidence that eating infected meat causes the disease. Human cases may be transmitted when infected tissue is implanted, as in corneal grafting, for instance. And some children have contracted the disease after taking human growth hormone to correct a deficiency and prevent dwarfism.

CROHN'S DISEASE

Another name for regional ileitis, a condition in which the lower part of the small bowel becomes inflamed. Occasionally other parts of the digestive tract are also affected.
See ILEITIS

CROUP

An infectious virus disease of childhood, more common in winter. Viruses can infect any part of the upper respiratory tract. When the infection is mainly in the larynx (voice-box) in a child under the age of five, it is called croup. The word 'croup' (which literally means to croak) describes the characteristic symptoms of noisy breathing and hoarseness, rather than any particular virus. Most cases occur in the first two years of life.

As a child gets older the larynx gets bigger, and infection causes only hoarseness. *See* LARYNGITIS.

Symptoms
- Hoarse, barking cough in children under five.
- A characteristic harsh noise from the voice-box when the child breathes.
- Fever, with a temperature often over 101°F (38°C).
- Irritability and restlessness.
- Exhaustion or confusion.
- Marked indrawing of the chest wall with each breath.
- The child may turn a pale grey-blue colour.

- Dribbling, difficulty in swallowing, painful throat.
- The child insists on sitting up, quite still, with head craned forwards.

Duration
- Croup develops over a period of one or two days.
- Noisy breathing usually lasts only about 12 hours.

Causes
- Several respiratory viruses.

Complications
- PNEUMONIA.
- Most cases are mild and recover quickly. Occasionally, in babies and young children, the small airway can become blocked by severe infection.

Treatment in the home
- Give cool drinks (water, fruit juice, milk—whatever the child will take).
- Steam relieves symptoms. Fill a sink or bath with hot water and close the door to fill the bathroom with steam. Sit the child on your knees so that he is as high as possible. Alternatively, boil water in the kitchen to fill the room with steam. Take great care not to risk scalding.
- Give painkillers in recommended doses to reduce fever and ease discomfort. *See* MEDICINES, 22.

When to consult the doctor
- If the child has a high fever, appears distressed or ill, and breathing is rapid and difficult. Breathing is always noisy in croup, but it should not be difficult.
- If the child is drooling or complains that he cannot swallow, or that his throat hurts.
- If the child insists on sitting up quite still, with his head craned forwards.
- If the child's colour is poor. Children with croup are usually flushed and pink. Call the doctor immediately if the colour becomes pale, grey or bluish.
- If the child is restless and struggling to get air, call the doctor quickly.
- If in any doubt at all about a case of croup, consult the doctor.

What the doctor may do
- Because croup is caused by a virus, the doctor may examine the child and simply recommend continued treatment as above.
- Antibiotics are not normally of value, although they may be prescribed to prevent complications.
- Occasionally it may be necessary to remove a baby or child to hospital for observation.

Prevention
- None known.

Outlook
- Rapid complete recovery is normal.

See RESPIRATORY SYSTEM *page 42*

CUSHING'S SYNDROME

A collection of symptoms produced by an excess of glucocorticoids, one of the hormones secreted by the adrenal glands. These hormones, which are known as steroids, regulate the use of carbohydrates in the body, and too many of them upsets the body's regular pattern of converting food into energy.

Cushing's syndrome is a rare condition which can affect both men and women, but is more common in women over the age of 30. The symptoms include high blood pressure, obese trunk with spindly arms and legs, moon-like face with high colour and acne, and purple streaks on the abdomen. Diabetes may also develop, and in women the periods may stop and hair may grow on the jaw and upper lip.

The overproduction of the hormones can be due to a number of causes—usually tumours in various parts of the body, including the adrenal glands themselves—but the most common cause is a tumour in the pituitary gland (the gland at the base of the brain which produces another hormone that stimulates the adrenal glands). Sometimes a form of Cushing's syndrome is caused by long-term use of hormones in the treatment of RHEUMATOID ARTHRITIS, LEUKAEMIA and serious ALLERGY problems.

Treatment depends upon the cause. A tumour of the pituitary gland may be treated by radiotherapy. Tumours in other parts of the body will be removed surgically. If the adrenal glands need to be removed, the patient will be given steroid tablets or injections to replace those that can no longer be manufactured naturally by the body.

CYANOSIS

Blue fingers or lips due to lack of oxygen in the blood: this is the result either of slowed circulation in cold weather, or of serious heart or lung disease.
See BLUE BABY

CYST

An abnormal cavity, lined with tissue and containing a fluid or semi-fluid substance or air. Cysts occur as lumps in various parts of the body. There are many types and usually they are benign (that is, non-cancerous) and often do not cause discomfort. But some may become malignant (cancerous) or interfere with normal functions by pressing on a neighbouring organ, so it is always wise to seek advice from your doctor as to whether or not they should be removed.

See OVARIAN CYST
SEBACEOUS CYST

CYSTIC FIBROSIS

A hereditary disease that affects about one in every 1,000 newborn babies. It is also known as fibrocystic disease of the pancreas and mucoviscidosis. Symptoms normally appear during the first few weeks of life and very rapidly become severe. In rare cases, the disease appears at puberty. At one time cystic fibrosis caused death in early childhood, but now many children with the disease survive into adolescence.

The condition causes the failure of the glands which produce mucus in the lungs and pancreas, and sweat in the skin. The mucous glands of the lungs produce instead a thick, sticky sputum that clogs and dilates the air passages causing BRONCHIECTASIS. This leads to severe breathing difficulties and respiratory infections. The pancreas degenerates, and the resulting lack of pancreatic digestive juices means that not enough fat is absorbed from the intestines.

Symptoms
• The baby is fretful and fails to thrive and put on weight.
• The baby has a grossly swollen abdomen, but the rest of the body is thin and wasted.
• Steatorrhoea—the baby passes large, clay-coloured stools that are frothy, float on water and have an extremely offensive odour.
• Anaemia—with pallor. Sometimes the baby's cheeks have a blue tinge.
• The baby becomes more and more barrel chested, and has violent fits of coughing with severe breathing difficulties. This may lead to cyanosis, or blueness of the skin.

Duration
• Cystic fibrosis lasts for the life of the sufferer, though the symptoms can usually be relieved by treatment.

Causes
• A defective gene.
• Cystic fibrosis is hereditary, and there is a one in four chance of carriers of the disease having a child who suffers from it.

Complications
• Some babies with cystic fibrosis may have meconium ileus at birth. This is an accumulation of sticky intestinal

debris blocking the small bowel. The meconium is removed in a difficult and hazardous operation.
• Sometimes the large bowel prolapses, or turns inside out through the anus.
• A hard mass of faeces may block the intestines, and this condition may require surgery.
• Respiratory infections—PNEUMONIA, BRONCHIECTASIS, SINUSITIS.
• Heart, liver and gall-bladder disease—CIRRHOSIS.
• Poor food absorption—STEATORRHOEA.
• INFERTILITY.

Treatment in the home
• Parents can be trained to look after a child at home. This will include physiotherapy training on how to massage the chest in order to ease breathing difficulties; and advice on preparing diets and administering drugs and supplementary foods.
• The sufferer must avoid crowds, people with colds, smoking or any other conditions that could be a source of respiratory infection.
• Such children need a great deal of parental support. This has to be emotional as well as physical.

When to consult the doctor
• Immediately the symptoms become apparent, though the condition will often be diagnosed in the maternity hospital.
• Early diagnosis is vital to the child's survival.

What the doctor may do
• Analyse the patient's sweat, which will show an unusually high level of salt if the disease is present.
• Arrange X-rays of the lungs to detect presence of the disease there.
• Examine the patient's stools.
• After diagnosis, treatment in early life is normally in special centres. It will involve a special diet with enzyme, vitamin and mineral supplements, antibiotic therapy, physiotherapy and isolation nursing.

Prevention
• It is not possible to prevent cystic fibrosis occurring. However, if a member of your family has suffered from the disease, it would be sensible to consult a doctor before having children.

Outlook
• There is no known cure for cystic fibrosis, though the symptoms of the disease may be relieved. At present about 75 per cent survive until adolescence. In long-term sufferers, cirrhosis of the liver, diabetes and circulatory problems tend to develop.

Contact: *Cystic Fibrosis Research Trust*, 5 Blyth Road, Bromley, Kent BR1 3RS (Tel. 081-464 7211).

See DIGESTIVE SYSTEM *page 44*

CYSTITIS

Inflammation of the lining of the bladder. It is common in newly married women (when it is called honeymoon cystitis) and in pregnant women. Before puberty it is rare.

There are two types of cystitis: acute, when the inflammation lasts for only a short time; and chronic, when the bladder is permanently inflamed.

ACUTE CYSTITIS
Symptoms
• Pain (often burning) in the genitals on passing urine.
• Pain may also be felt in the lower abdomen, both while passing urine and, often, for a long time afterwards.
• Urine is passed more often than normal, day and night. The urge to urinate is usually sudden, and it may be difficult to hold on before a lavatory can be reached. A child may start wetting pants or bed-wetting.
• Urine may be cloudy, have a fishy smell or contain blood.
• The temperature may be raised.
• In some cases, especially during pregnancy, there are no symptoms, the infection being discovered only after routine examination of the urine.

Duration
• Acute cystitis usually lasts for about four or five days.

Causes
• The usual cause is a germ that lives in the bowel, entering the urethra (the channel through which urine is passed), and reaching the bladder. Because the urethra in the female is closer to the anus and is shorter than in men, cystitis is much more common in women.
• Minor bruising of the female urethra and bladder (which lie close to the vagina) during sexual intercourse. Use of the contraceptive cap may make this more likely.
• An abnormal vaginal discharge.
• Sensitivity to cosmetic or contraceptive products.

Complications
• Chronic cystitis and PYELONEPHRITIS may occasionally develop.

Treatment in the home
• Rest as much as possible.
• Drink plenty of fluids. Adults should drink about 7 pints (4 litres) every 24 hours. Lemon barley-water often provides some relief.
• Take painkillers. *See* MEDICINES, 22.

When to consult the doctor
• If the symptoms described occur. When symptoms are severe, the doctor should be consulted immediately.

- If blood or other changes are noticed in the urine.

What the doctor may do
- Test a mid-stream specimen of urine.
- If the patient is female, he may carry out a vaginal examination.
- With a male patient he may perform a rectal examination.
- In men, boys, and girls who have not reached puberty, the infection is uncommon and he may arrange an X-ray or send the patient to a specialist in order to eliminate more serious disease.
- Encourage increased drinking of fluids.
- Prescribe antibiotics. *See* MEDICINES, 25.

Prevention
- Take plenty of baths; pass water after sex.
- Maintain a good fluid intake.
- Avoid highly perfumed soaps, vaginal sprays or spermicidal jellies.

Outlook
- With treatment acute cystitis usually clears up within five days.
- In women recurrences are common.

CHRONIC CYSTITIS

Symptoms
- As in acute cystitis.

Duration
- For long periods if not treated.

Causes
- The germs that cause acute cystitis can prove resistant to antibiotics; or the full course of antibiotics is not completed.
- Some abnormality in the urinary tract—for example, a STONE, a STRICTURE or a deformity present from birth.

Complications
- If left untreated the infection can spread to the kidneys (PYELONEPHRITIS).

Treatment in the home
- As for acute cystitis.

When to consult the doctor
- As for acute cystitis. Chronic cystitis always needs medical advice, to exclude (and treat) other underlying causes.

What the doctor may do
- In most cases he will send the patient to a specialist to look for pus cells and germs and evidence of damage to the kidneys.
- Arrange a full urine examination.
- Most cases of chronic cystitis are referred to a hospital for investigations to exclude the serious causes mentioned above.
- If there is no evidence of such causes, increased fluids

and antibiotics will be prescribed. *See* MEDICINES, 25.

Prevention
- As for acute cystitis.

Outlook
- With appropriate treatment the outlook for chronic cystitis sufferers is good though recurrences are common.

See URINARY SYSTEM *page 46*

CYTOMEGALOVIRUS INFECTION

A common infection which affects people of all ages without causing symptoms. Up to 80 per cent of adults may show evidence of previous infection in their blood. The disease, which is also known as salivary gland virus disease, is spread by close contact with an infected person, or through the placenta to an unborn child. The disease is diagnosed by blood tests.

Symptoms
- In most cases cytomegalovirus infection is what is known medically as sub-clinical—that is, there are no symptoms.
- Very occasionally, if an unborn baby contracts the disease from its mother during pregnancy, the baby may fail to thrive and may have jaundice, anaemia, pneumonia or eye inflammation. In 10 per cent of such cases the brain will be affected and the baby will be born deaf or mentally retarded.
- If the baby contracts the infection from the mother during birth or in infancy the symptoms will be milder and without the risk of brain damage.
- In older children and adults there may occasionally be an acute feverish illness similar to GLANDULAR FEVER, with headache, pain in the back and abdomen, and sore throat.
- There may be a brief rash, similar to that of GERMAN MEASLES.
- Patients on drugs after transplant surgery may have the illness severely.

Treatment
- When symptoms are present, treatment is the same as for glandular fever, otherwise there is no specific treatment and so far no effective immunisation or preventive measures.

See INFECTIOUS DISEASES *page 32*

D & C
The commonly used abbreviation for dilatation and curettage, an operation in which an instrument called a dilator enlarges the entrance to the uterus (womb) and an instrument called a curette scrapes tissue from the inner wall of the uterus. This is done with the patient under a general anaesthetic. The operation is usually carried out so that the tissue can be analysed for signs of disease, but it is sometimes performed as treatment—for example, to clear out the inside of the uterus after a miscarriage. The operation requires only one or two days' stay in hospital and a week's convalescence.
See FEMALE GENITAL SYSTEM *page 48*

DANDRUFF

Scales of dead skin from the scalp. It is most common in early adulthood, but may occur at other ages.

Symptoms
- Dry scales showering on to clothing and surrounds.
- Less commonly the scales are greasy and stuck to the hair and scalp. These cause severe irritation. If removed by scratching, the skin may bleed.

Duration
- This depends on how the condition is managed.

Causes
- The cause is not known. The tendency is inherited and the greasier the skin the worse the dandruff.

Treatment in the home
- Twice weekly use of detergent shampoo helps; for example, one containing 1 per cent of cetrimide.
- In the more severe forms, proprietary preparations containing salicylic acid, tar or selenium should be tried.

When to consult the doctor
- If the scalp becomes infected after scratching the head.
- If the scales persist or get worse after several weeks of home treatment.
- If the scales appear to be thick.

What the doctor may do
- Check that the scales are not caused by an infection.
- Give further advice on how to treat the dandruff.

Prevention
- No specific steps are available. *See* SEBORRHOEA.

Outlook
- Dandruff can be controlled even if not cured.

See SKIN *page 52*

DEAFNESS

About one in 10,000 of the population suffers from congenital deafness—that is, they are born deaf. Others become deaf as they grow old, a condition known as senile deafness or presbyacusis. Temporary deafness in one or both ears is a symptom of many diseases of the ear.

CONGENITAL DEAFNESS
Congenital deafness may be partial, one-sided or total. In most cases, the auditory nerve is not functioning properly, even though the middle and outer ears may be normal. The main effects of the deafness are on speech development.
Symptoms
• Poor or absent speech development. Normal children vary considerably, but average development is shown in CHILD CARE—FIRST MONTHS *page 141*.
• Retarded general development.
• Lack of response to mother when baby cannot see her.
• Lack of response to sounds and bangs.
Causes
• In most cases the cause is unknown, but deafness can run in families.
• German measles (rubella) in the first 13 weeks of pregnancy.
• Certain drugs (for example, streptomycin) in pregnancy.
• Syphilis in the mother.
• Brain damage at birth.

Do's and don'ts about deafness

☐ *Do* consult your doctor if you think you or your child may be going deaf.

☐ *Do* make sure that you have a proper hearing-aid that suits you. Excellent aids are available from the National Health Service.

☐ *Do* find out about equipment other than hearing-aids. The Royal National Institute for the Deaf offers advice on what is available.

☐ *Do* seek the advice of the *Royal National Institute for the Deaf*, 105 Gower Street, London WC1 (Tel. 071-387 8033), or 9A Clairmont Gardens, Glasgow G3 (Tel. 041-332 0343).

☐ *Don't* be tempted to buy a hearing-aid at an exhibition or from a door-to-door salesman. Seek your doctor's advice first.

☐ *Don't* expect other people to understand your problem automatically. Help them to help you by teaching them to speak to you clearly, slowly and without shouting. Make sure that they are in a good light and do not speak to you while eating or smoking.

☐ *Don't* be shy of approaching your local centre for the deaf—it will have many ways of helping you.

HOW HEARING IS MEASURED
First steps in the fight against deafness

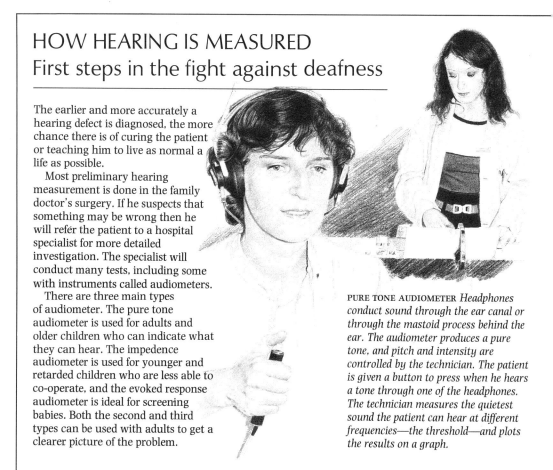

The earlier and more accurately a hearing defect is diagnosed, the more chance there is of curing the patient or teaching him to live as normal a life as possible.

Most preliminary hearing measurement is done in the family doctor's surgery. If he suspects that something may be wrong then he will refer the patient to a hospital specialist for more detailed investigation. The specialist will conduct many tests, including some with instruments called audiometers.

There are three main types of audiometer. The pure tone audiometer is used for adults and older children who can indicate what they can hear. The impedence audiometer is used for younger and retarded children who are less able to co-operate, and the evoked response audiometer is ideal for screening babies. Both the second and third types can be used with adults to get a clearer picture of the problem.

PURE TONE AUDIOMETER *Headphones conduct sound through the ear canal or through the mastoid process behind the ear. The audiometer produces a pure tone, and pitch and intensity are controlled by the technician. The patient is given a button to press when he hears a tone through one of the headphones. The technician measures the quietest sound the patient can hear at different frequencies—the threshold—and plots the results on a graph.*

Treatment in the home

• None. If you suspect that your child may be deaf, consult your doctor or health visitor.

What the doctor may do

• Test the child's hearing. If he suspects deafness, examination by a specialist will be necessary.

• A hearing-aid may be fitted, and special hearing (and speech) training for mother and child may be needed.

• Cochlear implants, tiny devices inserted in the ear by an operation, can improve hearing in some types of deafness.

Prevention

• Take no drugs not prescribed by a doctor.
See PREGNANCY.

Outlook

• Many deaf children attend ordinary school; others require special education. Although learning can be slow and difficult, many congenitally deaf children grow up to become successful in demanding careers.

DEAFNESS OF OLD AGE

Although this condition is known as senile deafness, it can occur any time from the age of 50 onwards.

Symptoms

• Increasing deafness in both ears over the age of 50. The first sign is usually a failure to notice high sounds.

• The deafness is most noticeable when there is background noise, such as television or other conversation in the same room.

• Noises in the ears.

Duration

• Comes on gradually over a period of years, and lasts for life.

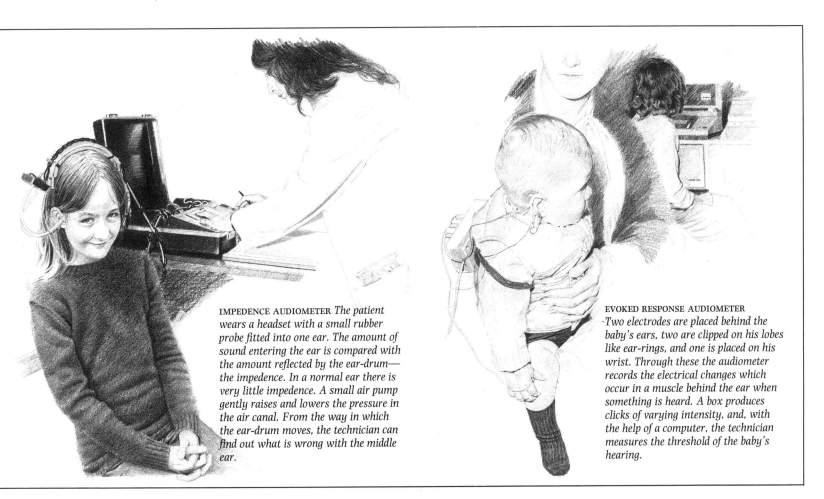

IMPEDENCE AUDIOMETER *The patient wears a headset with a small rubber probe fitted into one ear. The amount of sound entering the ear is compared with the amount reflected by the ear-drum— the impedence. In a normal ear there is very little impedence. A small air pump gently raises and lowers the pressure in the air canal. From the way in which the ear-drum moves, the technician can find out what is wrong with the middle ear.*

EVOKED RESPONSE AUDIOMETER
Two electrodes are placed behind the baby's ears, two are clipped on his lobes like ear-rings, and one is placed on his wrist. Through these the audiometer records the electrical changes which occur in a muscle behind the ear when something is heard. A box produces clicks of varying intensity, and, with the help of a computer, the technician measures the threshold of the baby's hearing.

Causes
- The inner ear ceases to function properly as the person gets older.

Treatment in the home
- Do not try to clean wax out of the ears yourself—you will probably make it worse. *See* EAR WAX.
- Two or three warm, wax-softening ear drops or olive oil in the ears may soften any wax and be helpful.
- Do not buy a hearing-aid without first consulting the doctor.
- In severe cases, various aids such as an amplified telephone earpiece may help.

When to consult the doctor
- If deafness is interfering with normal activities.

What the doctor may do
- Examine your ears and remove any wax.
- Arrange for a hearing-aid to be fitted. This will help only if deafness affects both ears. It will be fitted in the better ear.

Prevention
- None known.

Outlook
- Although there can be no improvement in the deafness, deterioration may be very gradual.

See EAR *page 38*
NERVOUS SYSTEM *page 34*
RESPIRATORY SYSTEM *page 42*

DEATH AND BEREAVEMENT

Many old people accept the prospect of death calmly, without fear. During their final illness, they may gradually lose interest in life and contact with those around them, and death may be welcomed as a release from suffering.

Younger people who learn that they are suffering from a terminal illness generally react differently from the old. They will usually show several reactions: refusal to face the likelihood of their own death, anger, depression, and finally acceptance. Sometimes the reactions occur in that order, sometimes they are mixed.

A person's conscious or unconscious refusal to admit that he is going to die from his illness is an extremely valuable defence mechanism. Shutting out reality protects a terminally ill person from emotional suffering. The patient may become quiet and withdrawn and avoid answering questions, or may behave cheerfully and be overactive, as if to prove that everything is normal. If a person is denying death, he should be allowed to do so and not be forced to face reality.

Patients may ask themselves the angry question, 'Why me?' Their anger, particularly if it is allied to physical discomfort or pain, can make them demanding, irritable, aggressive and often ungrateful for the care they are receiving. To cope with behaviour of this kind may well need considerable understanding.

Depression in dying people may not be due simply to the prospect of their own death but to worry about their dependants, pain, weakness or even the inability to look after themselves.

Patients may reach a stage where they no longer deny their death or are angry or depressed about it but instead accept it. Such patients may be weak, sleep a lot, lose interest in their family and visitors and withdraw into themselves.

CARE OF THE DYING

Unless a person has made it obvious that he wishes to be left in peace, he will need the support and comfort of family and friends. If visitors feel awkward and embarrassed in the presence of a dying person, this may make them act in an offhand or glib manner and cut short their visits—which will increase the dying person's feeling of loneliness.

Any visitor should put the dying patient's feelings first, spend time with him and listen sympathetically. Even if the patient is unconscious, he may still be aware enough to appreciate another's presence, another's comforting touch.

Most terminally ill people, especially the old, know that they are dying without being told; and those who suspect the fact and ask questions about it usually know if they are being told the truth or not. For that reason, close relatives or friends should always answer direct questions honestly.

However, such information need not be volunteered—if the person does not ask direct questions, it may well be that he does not want to know the truth about his situation.

Death may be frightening for the patient and his relatives. Every dying person has his own fears, and you may be able to help allay them if you know what they are. Some worries—about the future of dependent relatives and the family, or of 'being a nuisance' while ill—can be discussed with the patient. But other fears—of pain, for example—may be best discussed first with the doctor or nurse, for false reassurance is worse than none.

People who care for the dying must have endless reserves of patience and tolerance. When terminally ill, even the bravest and normally the most agreeable of people may behave very differently. If frightened, worried about others, or in pain, it may be impossible for them to keep a brave face. Children are sometimes angry with their parents for 'allowing' them to be ill. Remember also that family, friends, nurses and doctors may be struggling with their own emotions—they, too, deserve patience and tolerance.

In some cases a dying person may remain buoyant enough to joke or laugh about things. Do not be inhibited about joining in—rather, be glad that the dying person still has the capacity to experience enjoyment during what remains of life.

CARE OF A DYING CHILD

A dying child under the age of five may be aware of the fact of death but will not really understand it, since he has a limited idea of the future. If a pre-school child asks directly if he is going to die, a reply that he is not going to die that day or that week may be completely reassuring, because a month is too long a period for a child of that age to grasp mentally.

An older child, from about five onwards, has a better understanding of time. If he asks whether he is going to die it is best to give some such answer as: 'Some children do die when they are seriously ill, but many others get better.'

The child's main fears will probably be about separation from his parents and other loved ones. It may be helpful, with the doctor's co-operation, to nurse such children at home. Inevitably this puts great strain on parents, and the pros and cons must be carefully considered.

A dying adolescent, often lonely already because he is making himself independent of the family, may feel extremely isolated. He may take refuge from reality by becoming child-like again; and he may also experience any or all of the adult reactions of denial of death, anger and depression.

In such situations, the efforts and time given by relatives and friends are of supreme importance.

The Compassionate Friends is an organisation of bereaved parents who have been through their own heartbreak, loneliness and social isolation, and who can offer comfort and help to others. The address of the current National Secretary is 53 North Street, Bristol BS3 1EN (Tel. 0272 539639).

A PLACE TO DIE

About two-thirds of deaths occur in hospitals or nursing homes, where experienced medical staff are able to provide the necessary care for people with terminal illnesses. Recently there has been a growth in the number of hospices—small hospitals devoted entirely to the care of the terminally ill. They provide expert nursing care, control of pain and other symptoms, and emotional support for the dying.

Much nursing of the terminally ill is carried out in the patient's home, among their family, where many terminally ill patients find it most comforting to die in familiar surroundings.

THE MOMENT OF DEATH

Someone who has never witnessed a death may find it difficult to imagine what actually happens. When death is sudden—for example, following a heart attack or a road accident—there is no time for the patient to suffer. Consciousness is lost immediately.

When death occurs at the end of an illness, it is not usually dramatic. A very ill patient may breathe intermittently (Cheyne-Stokes respiration). The rate of breathing slows down until it stops altogether, for perhaps half a minute or so, only to restart at an increasing rate; then the breathing slows down and the cycle starts again. Cheyne-Stokes respiration may last for days and does not always mean that death is near. When death actually occurs, the patient becomes limp. Patients often die in their sleep—a painless end.

BEREAVEMENT

The loss of a loved one, particularly a husband, wife, parent or child, is a traumatic experience. However, most people, no matter how heartbroken and desperate they feel, manage to find the strength to cope with their loss—though it may take as long as two years to adjust to it.

Even when death is expected, the first reaction is usually one of shock and numbness. This may last from one or two days to several weeks. Emotions are vivid yet at the same time muddled and unexpected; details may be difficult to take in and remember.

As the finality of loss sinks in, grief becomes intense. The mind becomes preoccupied with thoughts of the dead person, and sometimes there are feelings that he is still present, so that the table may continue to be set for him or conversations started with him. Familiar sights and sounds may keep conjuring up the dead person. Such behaviour—which may last for months—may seem strange to others, but it is in fact quite a normal reaction to loss.

Deep depression often follows. It may show itself in any or all of the following ways: loss of interest in life, lack of energy, poor sleeping and weight loss or increase. Support and understanding from family and friends are the best help for the bereaved person, but if, despite such help,

depression persists, medical treatment with antidepressants may be needed. *See* DEPRESSION.

Physical illness is not unusual in a bereaved person during the year following loss, particularly loss of a husband, wife, parent or child.

In older people loss of a life partner appears to

Coming to terms with bereavement

Coping with the death of a close relative or friend is a very personal matter, but experience has shown that the following can help:

☐ Seeing and touching the body of the dead person and attending the funeral acknowledges the fact of death—which can be a first step to accepting it.

☐ Not taking alcohol, sedatives or antidepressants routinely, but only if they are absolutely necessary and recommended by the doctor.

☐ For those who wish to support and help a bereaved individual the time of greatest need is on anniversaries of the death, birthdays, Christmas and other times when memories become strongest. At this time loneliness is greatest.

☐ A close relative who has to deal with the practical matters after a death—registration of the death, funeral arrangements, insurance claims—may need guidance from the undertaker.

☐ A leaflet, *What to do after a death*, is published by the Department of Health and Social Security, and is available free from DHSS offices, doctors, hospitals and undertakers.

☐ *Cruse: Bereavement Care* offers all the bereaved and their families help and encouragement in emotional and practical matters. Local branch addresses are obtainable from Cruse House, 126 Sheen Road, Richmond, Surrey TW9 IUR (081-940 4818). Help line: 081-332 7227.

increase the likelihood of death from other natural causes—there is some truth in the expression 'dying from a broken heart'.

DECOMPRESSION SICKNESS

A hazard of diving that can occur when surfacing from a dive deeper than 50 ft. Gas bubbles form in the bloodstream, and can cause serious illness ('the bends'). Affected divers may need several days of treatment in a pressure chamber.

See OCCUPATIONAL HAZARDS

DEGENERATIVE DISEASES

A general term describing diseases associated with ageing. The two most common degenerative diseases are OSTEOARTHRITIS and ATHEROMA. There is little that can be done to prevent them—they occur to a greater or lesser extent as a part of the natural process of ageing—though it is known that obesity, which is avoidable, is an aggravating factor in osteoarthritis. The ageing process cannot be reversed, but the problems caused by ageing can sometimes be cured—worn-out hip and knee joints, for example, can be replaced with artificial joints.

DÉJÀ VU

Déjà vu is a French term meaning 'already seen'. It describes the strange feeling which sometimes occurs, that you are seeing or doing something you have seen or done before, though no such episode ever occurred. Almost everybody has had this experience, which has no significance in itself.

See NERVOUS SYSTEM *page 34*

DELIRIUM

An acute mental state in which normal thought and consciousness is disrupted. Delirium may involve terrifying visual hallucinations, impairment of memory, disorientation, lack of comprehension, PARANOIA, INSOMNIA and restlessness. It is associated with slurred speech, rapid eye movements, tremors and a general physical restlessness that may vary from tossing and turning to repetitive actions such as hand-washing.

The condition may have a number of causes. When delirium is the result of alcoholism it is known as DELIRIUM TREMENS, but the symptoms are usually little different from those of delirium caused by other conditions, such as brain damage, serious vitamin deficiency or a shortage of oxygen in the brain due to heart failure.

DELIRIUM TREMENS

People who have drunk excessively and steadily for many years may develop severe symptoms if alcohol is withdrawn. Delirium tremens (DTs) is a particularly severe complication of withdrawal. It can be fatal.

Symptoms
- Confusion and sleeplessness occurring two to four days after stopping drinking.
- Hallucinations—these are usually visual and often frightening.
- The patient trembles and is agitated.
- The patient may be feverish.
- DTs are most likely to occur after a patient has been deprived of alcohol through being admitted to hospital because of injury or infection or taken into police custody.
- In less-severe cases of alcohol withdrawal, when delirium tremens does not develop, there may be a state of tremulousness or nervousness that is relieved by a further intake of alcohol. This condition is known as 'the shakes'.

Duration
- Most episodes of DTs end as abruptly as they begin within about three days. The patient has no memory of the episode.

Causes
- Alcohol withdrawal in a sufferer from chronic alcoholism.

Treatment in the home
- None is advised.

When to consult the doctor
- Immediately the condition is suspected.

What the doctor may do
- Exclude other possible causes.
- Send the patient to hospital for expert care. Treat infection (such as pneumonia), head injury or certain blood disturbances.
- Prescribe sedative drugs to calm the patient and reduce the severity of symptoms brought on by withdrawal of alcohol. *See* MEDICINES, 17.
- Prescribe extra vitamins, because an alcoholic's diet is high in carbohydrate (from alcohol) but relatively low in B vitamins particularly thiamine, which is needed to regulate the intake of essential nutrients.

Outlook
- The condition may recur.

See NERVOUS SYSTEM *page 34*
ALCOHOLISM

DEMENTIA

Because of the death of brain cells through normal ageing, many people develop some loss of memory, confusion and odd behaviour as they get older. When many brain cells die rapidly the result is dementia. Although it can occur in middle age, it is usually a disease of old age. Six per cent of people over the age of 65 and 20 per cent of the over 85s become demented. Caring for a loved one with dementia is a difficult and demanding job that is both physically and psychologically exhausting.

Symptoms
- Confusion, particularly in new surroundings or with new faces. Later on, this occurs in well-known places.
- Lack of initiative and loss of interest in life.
- Loss of sense of time. The patient may wander in the middle of the night, and not know what the day or date is.
- Inability to think clearly or to understand complex ideas.
- Forgetting people's names—even those of close members of the family.
- Loss of memory of recent events (although memory of distant events may be good). For example, events of 50 years ago may be quite clear in the person's mind, but he has no idea what he had for breakfast.
- The limbs may become stiff.
- Deterioration in the patient's ability to cope with the problems of normal life.
- Inability to carry on a conversation.

Duration
- The symptoms get worse over a period of years. Eventually the patient is bed-bound, talks little or not at all, is incontinent of urine and faeces, does not eat unless fed and is at risk of catching pneumonia because of moving about so little.

Causes
- Dementia is usually caused either by multiple small STROKES which damage brain cells, or by Alzheimer's disease in which brain cells become tangled. If caused by strokes, the disease usually progresses in a step-like way, whereas Alzheimer's disease is more gradually progressive.

Treatment in the home
- With domestic support, a sufferer from mild dementia may live a normal life at home.
- Help will be required with shopping and finance.
- Open fires must be guarded. Electric cookers are safer than gas.
- Arrange for regular visits to be made by neighbours, relatives, home helps and later by social services and health visitors.

When to consult the doctor
- If any of the above symptoms are interfering with normal activity or are clearly causing social problems.

What the doctor may do
- As there is no cure yet, personal care, and attending to the patient's everyday needs are all that can be done.
- Prescribe drugs to help ease some of the symptoms.
- Ask social services to assess the sufferer and carers' needs for care at home, or a nursing home if necessary.

Prevention
- None.

Outlook
- Rapid development of the symptoms is rare. Usually progressive degeneration continues until death.

See NERVOUS SYSTEM *page 34*
ALZHEIMER'S DISEASE

DENGUE FEVER

A common virus disease of the tropics and subtropics which causes severe pain in the joints and muscles. It is also known as dandy fever or breakbone fever. The infection, which can be caught even by casual visitors to countries where the disease occurs, is transmitted to man by a bite from an infected mosquito. The incubation period is five to eight days. Symptoms come on suddenly and are severe.

Symptoms
- Headache.
- Raised temperature.
- Pain behind the eyes.
- Backache.
- Muscle and joint pains.
- A widespread skin rash, often intensely irritating, may appear on the third day. This rash distinguishes the disease, which initially resembles influenza.

Duration
- After two or three days the fever drops and symptoms disappear for a few days, and then return with a lower fever and a rash.
- Although recovery can be prolonged, dengue fever is rarely fatal.

Causes
- A virus transmitted by the mosquito.

Treatment

• There is no specific treatment, but the patient should have complete bed-rest and be given plenty of fluids. Aspirin, in recommended doses, can be given to relieve the headache and fever.

See INFECTIOUS DISEASES *page 32*

DENTURES

False teeth. Dentures may be partial, with just one or several teeth, or they may be complete, replacing all the teeth in both upper and lower jaws. Many people wear dentures. In Britain alone, nearly 2 million sets are supplied each year.
See TEETH

DEPERSONALISATION

A state in which a person loses his sense of self. He may feel so detached from his own body and actions that he seems to be observing those of some other person. The condition can be a form of mental illness or may be a feature of EPILEPSY.

DEPRESSION

A state of low spirits felt by most people at some time in their lives, but which becomes an illness if prolonged or severe. Frequently a cause can be recognised, but sometimes the symptoms just develop without obvious cause. About 2 per cent of the population get depressed each year to the point of needing medical help. Recent work suggests that women between the ages of 20 and 45 are particularly vulnerable, especially if they have become isolated from their usual 'confidants' by the presence of a young family or the death of a mother.

Symptoms

• Lack of interest in normal activities.
• A feeling of worthlessness.
• Poor performance at work.
• Frequent crying, often for no reason.
• Loss of appetite, concentration and memory.
• Disturbed sleep, often with a tendency to wake early in the morning and stay awake.
• Mood variations, sometimes with improvement as the day progresses.
• If severe, there is a risk of SUICIDE.

Duration

• Depression may last from a few days to many months. Initially it may seem to get worse, but even without treatment most cases will eventually get better.

Causes

• It is often brought on by some major event in a person's life such as bereavement, divorce or loss of employment. Sometimes job failure follows, rather than precedes, the depression.
• Some people get repeated attacks for no obvious reason, and these often alternate with times of over-activity. *See* HYPOMANIA.
• Many women become depressed before their menstrual periods.

Treatment in the home

• Encourage the sufferer to carry on a normal life.
• Reassure the depressed person that he or she is loved and needed.
• Remember that depression gets better in time. Previous personal experience of getting through a depression will often help the patient's understanding.

When to consult the doctor

• If the illness has lasted more than two weeks without improvement.
• If the general health of the patient or family is suffering.
• If the depressed person cannot cope.
• If SUICIDE is considered a possibility.

What the doctor may do

• Take a careful history and discuss the problems and possible solutions.
• Prescribe small quantities of drugs or psychotherapy. *See* MEDICINES, 19.
• Refer the patient to a psychiatrist if the depression is severe, particularly if there is talk of suicide.

See MENTAL SYSTEM *page 33*
NERVOUS SYSTEM *page 34*

DERMATITIS

Another name for eczema; a form of inflammation of the skin. There are a number of different types, each with its own cause or causes.
See ECZEMA

DERMOGRAPHIA

Weals produced on the skin by gentle pressure. The phenomenon occurs naturally in certain people with hypersensitive skin but in others it may be the first sign of a drug allergy.

DETACHED RETINA

The retina is the inner light-sensitive lining of the eye and is formed from two layers. If a hole or tear develops in the inner layer, fluid enters and separates the two layers and causes the detachment.

Symptoms

• A sudden painless loss or change of vision, sometimes preceded by a sensation of flashing lights.

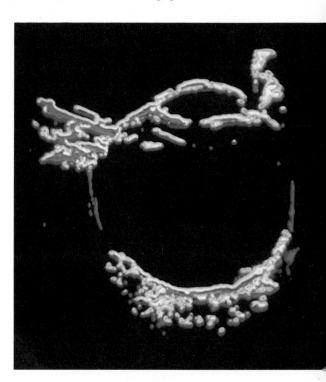

LOOKING INTO THE EYE *In this ultrasound scan of the eye the front is at the top with the upper eyelashes (yellow) to the left. To their right is the black disc of the iris with the eyeball below. The yellow line at the bottom of the eyeball is the inner layer of the retina. The thin red line below this is fluid that has penetrated the two layers of the retina causing them to become detached. The mass of yellow below this is optic fat.*

- The patient may perceive what appears to be a curtain coming across the field of vision.

Duration

- The detachment persists unless treated.

Causes

- Although retinal detachment may follow injury, the immediate cause of the detachment cannot usually be identified. The condition occurs more commonly in short-sighted people and it may follow an operation for the removal of a cataract.

Complications

- Partial or complete loss of vision.

When to consult the doctor

- At once.

What the doctor may do

- The doctor will test the eyesight by means of a chart, test the field of vision and look into the inner eye with an ophthalmoscope. If a detachment is suspected he will refer the patient to a specialist for immediate treatment to heal any detachment and prevent it from spreading.

Outlook

- Provided treatment is undertaken within a few days, successful restoration of the eyesight is usual.

See EYE *page 36*

DEVIATION OF NASAL SEPTUM

A condition in which the nasal septum (the wall between the nostrils) is bent to one side.

Symptoms

- Blocked nose, usually on one side.
- If the cartilage (the front part of the septum) is bent, the nose may appear deformed.

Causes

- Injury to the bone or cartilage, which heals in its deformed position.
- The bones growing unevenly.

When to consult the doctor

- If the symptoms are troublesome, particularly if one nostril is persistently blocked.

What the doctor may do

- Send you to hospital to arrange for an operation under general anaesthetic to correct the condition.

See RESPIRATORY SYSTEM *page 42*

DIABETES

A condition in which the body cannot properly use sugar and starches (carbohydrates) from the diet, because the pancreas is not producing enough of the hormone insulin. As a result, sugar accumulates in the blood and tissues and this causes defects in various parts of the body.

This condition is medically known as diabetes mellitus to distinguish it from an extremely rare disorder, diabetes insipidus.

All types of diabetes can be controlled with diet, tablets or insulin replacement. Provided the diabetic plays his part in helping himself and working with his doctor he can enjoy a normal life.

Symptoms

- Thirst and passing excessive amounts of urine. The large amounts of sugar in the blood cause the kidneys to produce huge amounts of urine. Because of the loss of body fluids in this way, the patient becomes thirsty, but drinking does not reduce the feeling of thirst.
- Loss of weight, because of the loss of fluids and inability of the body to use carbohydrates.
- Itching of the vulva in women.
- Itching of the penis in men.
- Tiredness and irritability.
- A tendency to suffer from boils, skin infections and infections of the vulva and penis.
- Cessation of periods in women.
- Disturbances of vision with difficulties in focusing.
- Ulcers on the feet.
- Pins and needles and numbness of the hands and feet.

Duration

- There is no cure for diabetes. Once present it is there for life; but it can be controlled by proper treatment and self-care.

Causes

- Failure of the pancreas gland to produce insulin, the hormone that organises the proper storage and use of sugars in the body. Diabetes is a different condition in children and young adults from that in older people. In the young diabetic there is very little insulin produced in the body and it has to be replaced by insulin injections. In diabetics aged 50 and over there is partial production of insulin, and treatment can usually be by diet and tablets without insulin.

The exact cause of failure of the pancreas is unknown, but there may be some inherited predisposition to diabetes. If two diabetics marry and start a family, the chances are one in four that one of their children will also be a diabetic.

- Some virus infections may also initiate diabetes.

Complications

- Most diabetics do not develop any complications, but those complications which do appear tend to be related to the duration of the condition, and may take 20-30 years or more before occurring. Parts of the body that may be adversely affected by diabetes include:

Blood vessels Small blood vessels may become blocked because of thickening of their walls; or weakened, forming micro aneurysms (minute bulges that may burst). These defects of the small blood vessels may affect the eyes, legs, nerves, heart and kidneys.

Eyes Cataracts are more likely in diabetics. Retinopathy (haemorrhages in the blood vessels) may occur, and may affect the vision.

Legs Arteries may become blocked, leading to coldness, pain on walking, and ulcers. In rare cases gangrene may develop.

Nerves Numbness and deadness in the feet and hands may result from involvement of the sensory nerves.

Heart Damage to the heart may lead to angina, heart attacks, breathlessness and swelling of the legs.

Kidneys Blockage of the small arteries and other changes may damage the kidneys. Very rarely this may lead to kidney failure.

Complications in pregnancy, stillbirths and malformations are more likely in diabetic women. Close medical attention is needed to keep diabetes under control in pregnancy and ensure the best prospects for mother and baby.

Treatment in the home

- None is possible until diabetes is diagnosed. Once identified as a diabetic, the patient has to take on many responsibilities for self-care:
- Visit the doctor for regular check-ups.
- Keep to the diet advised by the doctor.
- Eat regularly—do not miss out meals.
- Take tablets or insulin.
- Make regular checks on the urine and/or blood to make sure that the sugar levels are being adequately controlled.
- The diabetic's family can play an important part in providing him with support by helping him to keep to his diet, encouraging him to lead a normal life, and by reporting unusual reactions to treatment.

When to consult the doctor

- Immediately if persistent thirst, passing excessive amounts of urine or other symptoms suggestive of diabetes develop. Take a sample of urine to be tested.
- If there are any unusual symptoms or if you may be pregnant, once the diagnosis of diabetes has been made.

What the doctor may do
• Place a special dipstick into some urine. If there is sugar present—a sign of diabetes—there will be a change of colour. Confirmation is by a blood test to measure the level of sugar in the blood.
• Manage the case himself or send the patient to a diabetic clinic at a local hospital.
• All diabetics need proper medical treatment. If neglected the disease can kill, blind and maim. The aims of treatment are to restore levels of sugar in the body to normal and to prevent complications.
There are three main forms of treatment:
Diet to reduce the amount of sugar-containing food in the diet, such as bread, cakes, biscuits, sweets, sugar, potatoes, so that the body can cope better with lessened demands. Those diabetics who are overweight must reduce weight—this may be all that is necessary to control the disorder. *See* OBESITY.
Tablets may help the older 'mature' diabetic. *See* MEDICINES, 30.
Insulin injections may be given to replace the insulin that is missing in a patient who has severe diabetes. It may be possible to control the blood sugar by one injection daily, but often better control is achieved by two injections, one in the morning and one in the evening. Insulin has to be given by injection because it is destroyed in the stomach and so cannot be taken by mouth. Injections are usually self-administered, sometimes using a convenient insulin 'pen', and most diabetics soon learn how to do this, but the family should also know how to cope.
  All diabetics on insulin at times experience symptoms of low blood sugar of hypoglycaemia (due to excess insulin); the symptoms are faintness, sweating, unsteadiness and disturbed behaviour. The patient himself may recognise the warning signs and cut short the attack by taking sugar. If he does not, he may appear to be drunk and there is a risk of coma. It is never safe to assume that the patient is drunk, and immediate medical help should always be sought.
Prevention
• Diabetes cannot itself be prevented or anticipated, except by avoiding overweight, but diabetic complications can be prevented by good control of the condition.
Outlook
• Bad in the untreated, unstable and unco-operative case.
• Good in those whose condition is controlled by co-operation with the doctors, regular checks, and strict adherence to the treatment advised.
• Insulin cell transplants may be available.

See DIGESTIVE SYSTEM *page 44*

Living with diabetes

Most important of all is to learn all you can about your condition—how the body controls blood sugar, the effects of insulin, different foods, exercise, illness and so on. Pamphlets and a list of book titles are available from the *British Diabetic Association*, 10 Queen Anne Street, London WIM OBD (Tel. 071-323 1531).

☐ Do not let your life be ruled by your condition. Provided you stick to the simple rules of management which you have been taught, there are few activities the diabetic cannot do, including vigorous sport.

☐ Make sure friends understand you cannot join them in an eating or drinking free-for-all. Make particularly sure teachers, relatives and close friends of a diabetic child understand what is inadvisable.

☐ A diabetic on insulin should avoid driving or using dangerous machinery unless he has had some food in the previous two hours. For this, and other reasons, regular mealtimes are important.

☐ Particularly if you are prone to hypoglycaemic attacks it is useful to carry a card or wear a bracelet stating your diagnosis and emergency instructions. It is embarrassing and could be dangerous to be mistaken for being drunk when all you need is some sugar.

☐ The older diabetic is very prone to foot troubles because of poor circulation and nerve damage: daily washing, warm clean socks and well-fitting soft shoes are essential. Any sign of a foot problem, such as a corn or ingrowing toe-nail, should be reported to the doctor or chiropodist as soon as possible.

☐ Problems can be encountered on long plane journeys or in coping with foreign menus: the BDA provides an excellent leaflet for diabetics going abroad. The association also runs holidays for diabetic children.

DIAPHRAGM
A flexible, dome-shaped muscle between the chest and the abdomen, attached to the lower ribs at the sides and the breastbone and backbone at its front and back. Openings in the muscle allow large blood vessels, nerves and the oesophagus to pass through into other organs. The purpose of the diaphragm is to work the lungs in the breathing process. As the diaphragm contracts, its shape becomes flatter increasing the volume of the chest cavity. Atmospheric pressure then forces air into the lungs which expand to fill the space. The diaphragm then relaxes and pushes upwards, deflating the lungs and causing the person to breathe out.

DIARRHOEA
An extremely common symptom which is caused by a great variety of conditions.
See SYMPTOM SORTER—DIARRHOEA
CHILD CARE—CHILDHOOD ILLS *page 151*

DIASTOLE
The resting period of the heart after each muscular contraction, or SYSTOLE. Each diastole and systole lasts about two-fifths of a second.

DIATHERMY
The generation of heat in the tissues by electricity passed between two electrodes placed on the skin. The procedure, which is painless, is used to destroy diseased tissue, to relieve muscular disorders or to stop bleeding during surgery.

DIET
The food a person eats. A well-balanced diet contains all the nutrients required by a healthy person.
See NUTRITION

DIPHTHERIA

Until recent times diphtheria was a dreaded killer, claiming one-third of its victims. But immunisation has made the disease, which is highly infectious, much less common in the Western world. In Britain, where an immunisation campaign was launched in 1940, diphtheria now occurs only rarely. It is caused by bacteria called *Corynebacterium diphtheriae*, which produce a toxin (poison) that destroys tissue. The heart and kidneys may be affected, and if antitoxin is not given immediately, permanent damage may result.

The toxin may also affect the nerves, causing double vision, difficulty in swallowing and paralysis of the breathing muscles and the limbs. In extreme cases, the toxin may cause death, particularly in very young and old patients. Although immunised people can catch diphtheria, they are less likely to die from it than non-immunised patients.

The infection, which usually starts in the throat, is spread by germ-laden air breathed out by patients or carriers. Carriers carry the infection but do not have any symptoms. Sometimes the infection can begin in the skin, nose or other parts of the body, and in this case can be spread by direct contact with towels or other belongings used by the patient.

Symptoms
- Sore throat.
- A bluish-white, grey or blackish film at the back of the throat. The film grows bigger and thicker for up to 24 hours, and attempts to wipe it away cause bleeding.
- If the site of infection is the skin, there may be an ulcer with a film across it.
- Fever, malaise and prostration usually follow.
- Toxins may affect the heart muscle or nerves any time after the fourth day, causing heart failure or paralysis of the muscles of breathing, swallowing or eye movement.

Incubation period
- One to seven days.

Duration
- One to three weeks.

Causes
- Bacteria.

When to consult the doctor
- Immediately if diphtheria is suspected.

What the doctor may do
- Take a throat swab to confirm the diagnosis.
- Arrange for admission to hospital.
- Give immediate injections of antitoxin.
- Perform a TRACHEOTOMY if necessary to maintain an airway for breathing.
- Order complete bed-rest.
- Prescribe antibiotics, although these are less important than the antitoxin injections.

Prevention
- The surest prevention is immunisation. The current practice of giving three injections of diphtheria toxoid in the first year of life, with a booster dose upon starting

school, gives good protection. The toxoid is usually given together with tetanus, polio and whooping-cough vaccine in one immunisation known as DPT. A child should not be immunised when it has a feverish illness, otherwise there is no danger in diphtheria immunisation.

Outlook
- Although immunised individuals can catch diphtheria, most recover without complications.
- In non-immunised patients, the outlook is always serious.

See INFECTIOUS DISEASES *page 32*

DISABILITY
With the help of specialist organisations and the aid of modern equipment, disabled people can cope with everyday life better than ever before.
See DISABILITY *page 198*

DISSEMINATED SCLEROSIS
Another name for multiple sclerosis. A chronic disease of the nervous system in which the nerves of parts of the brain and spinal cord are damaged.
See MULTIPLE SCLEROSIS

DIVERTICULAR DISEASE OF THE COLON

Diverticula are pouches in the mucous lining of the large gut wall in which faeces may gather. They tend to be pushed outwards through weak spots in the muscle coat and cause bulges in the wall of the bowel. Since they have no muscle coat of their own, they cannot empty by normal muscular contraction. The contents may harden, block the mouth of the pouch and become infected, causing diverticulitis.

Diverticula generally have short necks and wide mouths, and so drain easily. They vary from $\frac{1}{5}$ to $1\frac{1}{5}$ in. (5 to 30 mm.) or more in diameter and arise most frequently in the lower (sigmoid) colon, where they are more likely to have long narrow necks which are more prone to blockage.

Diverticular pouches are present in four people out of every ten by the age of 50, but only cause symptoms (diverticulitis) in a few of these.

Symptoms
- Diverticula produce no symptoms in the majority of people.
- Where symptoms occur they may begin with wind, discomfort and a feeling of distension. These are hard to distinguish from symptoms of indigestion, hiatus hernia, ulcers or disorders of the gall-bladder, any of which may be present as well.
- Distension of the abdomen is eased by defecation or passing wind.
- Severe symptoms are aching pains in the lower left abdomen.
- Diarrhoea or constipation may occur.
- Blood or pus may be passed.
- Heavy bleeding occasionally occurs.

Duration
- The diverticula persist for life, but symptoms usually settle with rest.

Causes
- The causes of both the diverticula and why they should suddenly become infected are uncertain, but sudden muscular contractions, constipation and the low-roughage Western diet are all thought to be possible contributors to the initial pouch formation.

Complications
- Diverticulitis. This occurs when the pouch becomes inflamed, giving rise to feverish symptoms and attacks of abdominal pain and tenderness. Diverticulitis results from a blockage by hardened faeces or by inflammatory swelling at the neck of the blow-out causing an abscess. When diverticulitis occurs near the bladder it may cause symptoms like those of CYSTITIS.
- The inflamed pouch may burst through the gut walls forming an abscess (like an appendix abscess, but situated in the left of the abdomen.)
- A burst abscess may also lead to local or general PERITONITIS.
- Perforations in the wall, resulting from a burst abscess, may issue into the bladder, vagina or other part of the intestine. Intestinal obstruction may follow.

Treatment in the home
- Mild symptoms can be relieved by bed-rest and by placing a hot-water bottle over the ache.
- Mild painkillers may be taken if the diagnosis has been clearly established.

When to consult the doctor
- If there is severe pain or feverishness, or if blood or pus are passed with the motions.

What the doctor may do
- Prescribe antibiotics, stronger painkillers and anti-spasmodics. *See* MEDICINES, 1, 22, 25.
- Advise for more detailed examination if the diagnosis

is in doubt or if there are severe symptoms or complications.

Prevention

• A high-roughage diet helps to prevent attacks, wind and abscess formation. Rough vegetables, meat, wholemeal bread and bran are recommended.

See DIGESTIVE SYSTEM *page 44*
NUTRITION

DIVERTICULITIS

Inflammation of one of the pouches formed in the intestine by DIVERTICULAR DISEASE OF THE COLON.

DNA

The abbreviation for deoxyribonucleic acid, a substance found in the nucleus of every living cell. It contains the genetic information that causes characteristics to be passed on from parent to child. The single cell of a fertilised egg, which contains DNA from both parents, reproduces itself—and becomes a new living being—by dividing into two cells, which in turn divide into two, and so on. The DNA in each of these cells ensures that they are all of the same kind. *See* CELL and CHROMOSOMES.

DOCTOR

A good relationship between doctor and patient is essential if the best use is to be made of the doctor's skill. For a relationship to be successful the patient must have faith in the doctor, and the doctor must feel that the patient trusts him.

See YOU AND YOUR DOCTOR *page 220*

DO-IN

A form of self-massage developed in the East, and based on the same principles as SHIATSU and ACUPUNCTURE, although needles are not used.

DOUBLE VISION

Permanent double vision is usually caused by a defect in the muscles that co-ordinate eye movements. The condition is known medically as diplopia. Temporary diplopia sometimes occurs in a child recovering from illness and may also be caused by drugs or alcohol.

See NERVOUS SYSTEM *page 34*
EYE *page 36*
SYMPTOM SORTER—EYE PROBLEMS

DOUCHE

A jet of water or chemical solution for washing out the vagina. Douches have little to recommend them. Hygienic douches are not necessary if a woman bathes and washes herself regularly; and contraceptive douches, used after sexual intercourse, are less than 70 per cent effective.

DOWN'S SYNDROME

This condition is caused by an abnormality of a baby's chromosomes; there are 47 instead of the normal 46. These babies (sometimes called mongols) suffer from a variable degree of mental retardation and are usually recognisable at birth by a number of definite physical characteristics. The children are of a happy disposition and have a great sense of humour. The condition arises in one in 660 births but the frequency increases with maternal age, especially after 35. Two tests (amniocentesis and chorionic villus sampling) can detect the condition during the early stages of pregnancy. Older parents and those with previous Down's babies can, if they wish, get such a test. If positive this provides legitimate grounds for a parental request for the pregnancy to be terminated.

Symptoms

• The face is flat with slit eyes and a broad ridge to the nose.

• Flattening of the back of head and neck.

• The baby is unusually floppy when handled.

• The fifth finger is short with only one transverse crease on the palm of the hand.

• Mental retardation and slow physical development.

Duration

• The condition is lifelong.

Causes

• Chromosome abnormalities which affect all cells of the body. Mothers over 35 and those who have had one Down's baby are at highest risk.

Complications

• Many Down's babies may have associated congenital defects in the heart and other organs.

Treatment in the home

• Parental support and the maintenance of Down's children at home is the largest contribution that any individual can give to a Down's baby. Parents who have to face the sadness and problems posed by the birth of a Down's baby should remember:

• The immediate parental grief and feeling of failure is considerable, especially for the mother. If the baby is to stay at home, both its parents should face together, as soon after birth as possible, the implications for the years to come.

• Down's children are affectionate and rewarding to look after. Often, in spite of many problems, they strengthen family ties, not the reverse.

• Many contribute much to family life. Some may even perform simple supervised jobs.

• Down's children develop better mentally in a happy family than in a happy institution.

• Not all Down's babies and not all families are suitable for home care.

• Any family proposing to undertake the responsibility for a Down's baby should first discuss the problem fully with the doctor or paediatrician and then contact the appropriate supporting agencies, through the *Down's Syndrome Association*, 155 Mitcham Road, Tooting, London SW17 9PG (Tel. 081-682 4001). Other parents of Down's children are a helpful source of information.

When to consult the doctor

• The diagnosis is made by doctors at the birth of the child.

What the doctor may do

• Support the parents at all times, but especially in the early days of decision.

• Give advice about development and handling as the baby develops.

• Reassess the problems of home care if they become too much for the family.

Prevention

• None, apart from early diagnosis and termination of pregnancy in appropriate cases.

Outlook

• There is no treatment, and life expectancy is variable. Many Down's babies die within five years of birth because of heart disease. However, if they survive the first five years, life expectancy is now almost the same as that of anyone else in the community.

• There is no record of a male affected by Down's syndrome having fathered a child.

• Girls can menstruate and may be fertile.

See MENTAL SYSTEM *page 33*

DROPSY

An abnormal accumulation of fluid in the tissues of the body, causing swelling. It is known medically as oedema.
See OEDEMA

Disability

HOW DISABLED PEOPLE CAN LEAD ACTIVE AND USEFUL LIVES— THE AIDS AND EQUIPMENT WHICH HELP THEM

A disabled person is someone who, because of physical or mental impairment, cannot function properly in a society designed for fit people. Some people are born disabled; others become disabled by an accident or disease, and for them coming to terms with disability resembles adjusting to life after a bereavement. The afflicted person has to go through a period of shock and grief, often mixed with anger, in order to adjust to his loss. He may need to experience these emotions many times before he gains the strength to accept his limitations and establish a new identity for himself. At this time of major crisis he needs strong emotional and social support.

The person who is born with a disability will have just as difficult a path to self-acceptance. His feelings of loss may be less intense because he has never known full physical freedom, but he will still experience great frustration. Over-protection by parents and segregated schooling may result in the disabled person not becoming fully aware that he is 'different' until he is a teenager. And then his sudden awakening to being set apart may be complicated by the first confused feelings of sexual awareness and arousal.

The parents of someone disabled from birth have a difficult task: they need to give unlimited patience, understanding and support, while at the same time making sure they do not stifle the development of independence and initiative. Indeed, they must encourage as much self-reliance as is possible.

AIDS

Today a wide variety of aids is available to help disabled people. They range from simple devices that assist walking, eating, dressing, and going to the lavatory, to electronic equipment that enables severely disabled people to control a wheelchair, operate a typewriter, switch the television or lights on and off and answer the telephone.

Many disabled people experience unnecessary difficulties in their daily lives because they are unaware of the existence of these aids, which can revolutionise not only the disabled person's life but that of his family as well.

There are various ways in which a disabled person and his family can adapt their home to make it easier for the disabled person to use. If the person walks unsteadily, rails can be fitted in the hallway, on the landing and around the bathroom and lavatory. For wheelchair users, the problem of negotiating steps can be overcome by fixed, folding or portable ramps. Getting up and down stairs, however, presents a bigger problem. It may be decided to avoid the problem altogether by building an extension on to the ground floor to house a bedroom and lavatory. A disabled person can claim an improvement grant from his local authority when his existing home is inadequate to his needs. On the other hand, some wheelchair users have a strong desire to carry on having access to their upstairs rooms. For these people a lift is the ideal answer. The standard type of lift is open-sided, compact and unobtrusive (built into the corner of the downstairs and upstairs rooms it connects). An alternative is a lifting platform mounted on a track on the side of the stairs.

To adapt a kitchen for wheelchair users, shelves can be lowered and knee space provided under the sink and working surfaces. For those with weak hands, special tin openers, tap turners and other equipment are available.

The use of hoists can be of immense help to those caring for disabled people. There are fixed hoists, which travel on tracks and which carry the disabled person from one particular place to another— from bedroom to bathroom, for example. And there are hoists that can be moved from place to place and can be used to transfer the disabled person from his wheelchair to a bed, lavatory, bath or anywhere else.

Some local authorities provide such aids and adaptations, but this varies greatly from area to area according to resources and the amount of money available. In some cases voluntary organisations concerned with specific disabilities may be able to give financial and practical help.

Helpful guidance and advice can also be obtained from local authority workers or occupational therapists. To meet temporary needs, items like wheelchairs and commodes can be borrowed from social service departments and they are sometimes available from local branches of the Red Cross.

Aids can also enable disabled gardeners to continue their hobby. Window-boxes can be easily reached, and in the garden raised flower beds can be built for the wheelchair-bound gardener to tend. Again, many special tools such as one-hand operated shears are available to make up for lack of physical strength or dexterity.

Special equipment makes it possible for disabled people to pursue many other leisure activities, including photography, bowls, fishing, archery, board games, sailing and swimming.

Full information about the aids and equipment is available from the organisations and books listed at the end of this section.

Sometimes the standard aid does not meet a disabled person's needs. In such a case, the Rehabilitation Engineering Movement Advisory Panel (REMAP) may be able to devise an individually designed aid to meet a particular need. No charge is made for labour, but there is sometimes a small charge for materials. Contact can be made direct to REMAP in London, or through a local social worker.

Organisations

Disabled Living Foundation, 380–84 Harrow Road, London w9 2HU (Tel. 071-289 6111). Provides advice, aids, information sheets and books, and will supply a list of provincial aid centres providing similar services. Visits may be made by appointment.
Centre on Environment for the Handicapped, 35 Great Smith Street, London SWIP 3BJ (Tel. 071-222 7980).
Rehabilitation Engineering Movement Advisory Panel, Hazeldene, Ightham, Sevenoaks, Kent TN15 9AD (Tel. 0732 883818).

Exhibition

The Naidex exhibition, organised by the Royal Association for Disability and Rehabilitation, 25 Mortimer Street, London WIN 8AB (Tel. 071-637 5400), is held annually in various parts of Great Britain. The exhibition has an extensive display of specialised equipment, including the most recently developed apparatus.

Aid centres

There are aid centres with a wide range of aids on display in many towns, including: Belfast, Birmingham, Caerphilly, Edinburgh, Glasgow, Liverpool, London, Newcastle upon Tyne, Sheffield, Southampton, Stockport and Wakefield. Details from the Disabled Living Foundation (*see* **Organisations** above).

Publications

Equipment for Disabled People, 13 separate booklets including *Furniture* and *Home Management* available from Mary Marlborough Lodge, Nuffield Orthopaedic Centre, Headington, Oxford OX3 7LD.
Equipment and Games, illustrated catalogue available from the Royal Institute for the Blind, 224 Great Portland Street, London WIN 6AA.
In Touch, printed, Braille and tape versions available from Broadcasting Support Services, PO Box 7, London W3 6XJ.
Aids for the Disabled, Department of Health and Social Security leaflet HB2, available from local DSS offices, libraries and post offices.
Designing for the Disabled, available from RIBA Publications Ltd, 66 Portland Place, London WIN 4AD. Fuller details appear in section two of *Directory for Disabled People*, available from Paramount Publishing International. Campus 480, Maylands Avenue, Hemel Hempstead, Herts HP2 2EZ (Tel. 0442 881900).

MOBILITY

The aids available for people who have difficulty in walking include sticks, tripods, crutches, frames and trolleys. Many people who can walk with such aids are naturally reluctant to take to a wheelchair. However, taking to a wheelchair for distances can enable a disabled person to save limited energy and so live a fuller life. For those who cannot walk at all and are not bedridden, a wheelchair is a necessity.

In the United Kingdom everyone who needs a wheelchair can obtain one of a wide range free from the Department of Social Security (DSS), but this does not include powered outdoor wheelchairs or four-wheeled buggies.

Before selecting a chair, one should ask the following questions: Is the chair for indoor or outdoor use or both? If it is to be used at an office or factory, will it fit under a desk or work bench? If it is to be carried in a car, will it fit into the boot or body of the car? It is often best to acquire two chairs, keeping one permanently at home and the other at the place of work or in the car. The DSS will sometimes provide two chairs in cases of special need.

For many disabled people the use of public transport is impossible, and the only answer is to travel by car—preferably one with automatic transmission. When choosing a car, a disabled person needs again to ask himself various questions such as: Is the door wide enough to get in and out easily? (Two-door cars usually have wider doors than four-door cars.) Does the door open out enough? If not, is it possible to loosen the restraining strap? (A swivel seat or a car-top hoist may help ease any difficulties of entry and exit.) If a wheelchair is to be carried, can it be lifted into the car behind the front seats or fit into the boot? If the boot is big enough, is the sill so deep that considerable strength is needed to lift the wheelchair over it?

Once all these matters have been settled, there remains the question of what kind of controls are needed. Controls are available to suit practically every disability, including sophisticated controls for those who have arm disabilities. Some types of hand controls (that will fit most models of car) are available in kit form, and a local garage may be able to fit them. Costs vary considerably, according to the complexity of the controls required and the work involved in fitting them. Before making a decision, drivers are advised to contact the local branch of one of the disabled drivers' organisations listed below, which will give advice and often demonstrate various types of controls.

Organisations

The Mobility Information Service and Disabled Motorists' Federation,
Unit 2A, Atcham Estate, Upton Magna, Shrewsbury SY4 4UG
(Tel. 0743-761889).
Disabled Drivers' Association,
Ashwellthorpe Hall, Ashwellthorpe, Norwich NR16 1EX
(Tel. 050-841 449).
Disabled Drivers' Motor Club Ltd,
Cottingham Way, Thrapston, Northants NN14 4PL
(Tel. 08327 34724).

Publications

Equipment for Disabled People, 11 booklets including *Hoists and Lifts, Walking Aids,* and *Outdoor Transport* (see **Publications,** *page 199*).
Motoring and Mobility for Disabled People, by Ann Darnbrough and Derek Kinrade, from Royal Association for Disability and Rehabilitation (see **Exhibition,** *page 199*).
Door to Door – A guide to transport for disabled people, available without charge from FREEPOST, Department of Transport, Building 3, Victoria Road, Ruislip, Middlesex HA4 0NZ. The booklet is also available free from DSS offices, Citizens Advice Bureaux and doctors' surgeries.
So you're Paralysed, by Bernadette Fallon, Spinal Injuries Association, 76 St James' Lane, London N10 3D7.

Getting out of the house and about in the world

Just because a disabled person is confined to a wheelchair, this does not mean that he or she must be totally housebound. Disabled people can learn to drive a specially equipped car at local training centres, and this new skill makes it possible for them to lead much fuller, more useful and stimulating lives— to go shopping, drive to work or go to the cinema. The garage and the entrance to the house will need careful planning if wheelchair users are to get the full benefit from a car.

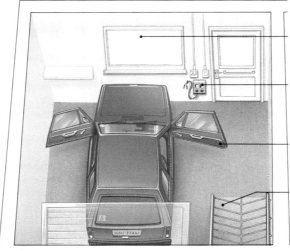

Check-list for entrance and garage

VENTILATION *To ventilate the battery unit a window should always be provided. It can have remote-control gear so that it can be opened by someone in a wheelchair.*

BATTERY-CHARGING EQUIPMENT *Electric wheelchairs need to have their batteries re-charged regularly. The plug-in point for the charging unit should be easy to reach from the wheelchair. Check on safety regulations with the fire brigade.*

WHEELCHAIR ACCESS *There must always be enough space at the sides of the car so that the doors can open fully and allow a wheelchair to enter.*

RAMP PLATFORM *To prevent any petrol from running into the house, the garage floor must legally be at least 6 in. (150 mm.) below the floor level of the house. So a ramp is needed linking the two areas. It should not be steeper than one in 12, with a level platform at the top.*

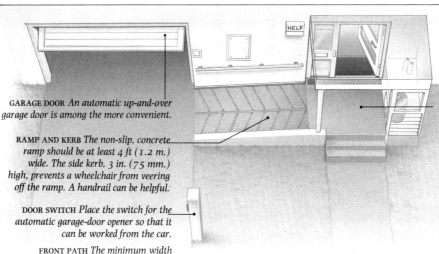

GARAGE DOOR *An automatic up-and-over garage door is among the more convenient.*

RAMP AND KERB *The non-slip, concrete ramp should be at least 4 ft (1.2 m.) wide. The side kerb, 3 in. (75 mm.) high, prevents a wheelchair from veering off the ramp. A handrail can be helpful.*

DOOR SWITCH *Place the switch for the automatic garage-door opener so that it can be worked from the car.*

FRONT PATH *The minimum width should be about 4 ft (1.2 m.). Do not put down rough or loose surfaces.*

FRONT DOOR AND PORCH *There should be no step outside the front door—which should have a minimum width, when open, of 30 in. (75 cm.). Fix a draught seal at the bottom of the door, and a drainage channel and grid to stop water from entering. An illuminated 'Help' sign–operated from within the house and garage—can be placed near the porch.*

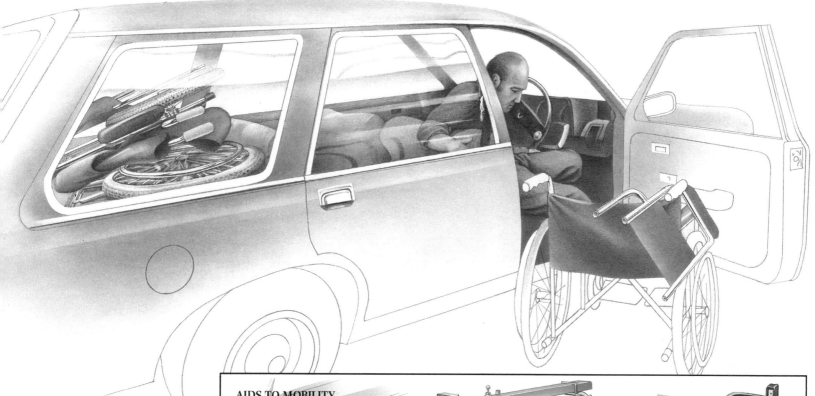

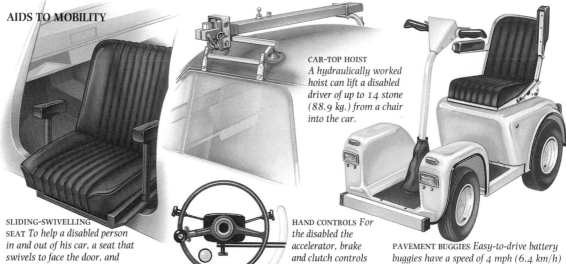

GARAGES AND VEHICLES *Some garages can be extended to accommodate a car and wheelchair. But where this is not possible, a car port is a suitable alternative. In either case, the minimum dimensions should be about 12 ft (3.6 m.) wide and 19 ft (5.7 m.) long. Some people choose to leave their regular wheelchair at home and carry a second chair in the car for use at their destination. The chair is folded and kept in the back of the car, or else placed in the boot by a helper. In either case, a helper is needed at the other end.*

AIDS TO MOBILITY

SLIDING-SWIVELLING SEAT *To help a disabled person in and out of his car, a seat that swivels to face the door, and then slides over the sill, can be fitted.*

CAR-TOP HOIST *A hydraulically worked hoist can lift a disabled driver of up to 14 stone (88.9 kg.) from a chair into the car.*

HAND CONTROLS *For the disabled the accelerator, brake and clutch controls can be attached to the steering-wheel.*

PAVEMENT BUGGIES *Easy-to-drive battery buggies have a speed of 4 mph (6.4 km/h) and a range of up to 18 miles (29 km.). They can climb 5 in. (130 mm.) kerbs.*

Getting around the house—downstairs and up

Since a disabled person may have problems in adapting to the physical limitations of a house, it is the house that must be adapted. Some ideas on how this can be done are described below.

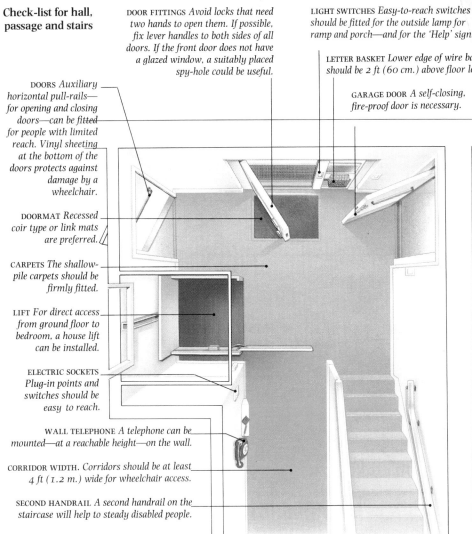

Check-list for hall, passage and stairs

DOOR FITTINGS *Avoid locks that need two hands to open them. If possible, fix lever handles to both sides of all doors. If the front door does not have a glazed window, a suitably placed spy-hole could be useful.*

LIGHT SWITCHES *Easy-to-reach switches should be fitted for the outside lamp for ramp and porch—and for the 'Help' sign.*

LETTER BASKET *Lower edge of wire basket should be 2 ft (60 cm.) above floor level.*

GARAGE DOOR *A self-closing, fire-proof door is necessary.*

DOORS *Auxiliary horizontal pull-rails—for opening and closing doors—can be fitted for people with limited reach. Vinyl sheeting at the bottom of the doors protects against damage by a wheelchair.*

DOORMAT *Recessed coir type or link mats are preferred.*

CARPETS *The shallow-pile carpets should be firmly fitted.*

LIFT *For direct access from ground floor to bedroom, a house lift can be installed.*

ELECTRIC SOCKETS *Plug-in points and switches should be easy to reach.*

WALL TELEPHONE *A telephone can be mounted—at a reachable height—on the wall.*

CORRIDOR WIDTH. *Corridors should be at least 4 ft (1.2 m.) wide for wheelchair access.*

SECOND HANDRAIL *A second handrail on the staircase will help to steady disabled people.*

STAIRLIFT *Electrically powered stairlifts can be installed for the disabled. Some of the lifts can go round corners and others have seats. Before choosing either a stairlift or a personal lift—for houses where the stairs cannot take a stairlift—discuss the matter with your doctor and an occupational therapist. They will advise on such matters as the type of controls to be fitted and so on. With personal lifts, most disabled people find it easier to use touch-light controls than buttons.*

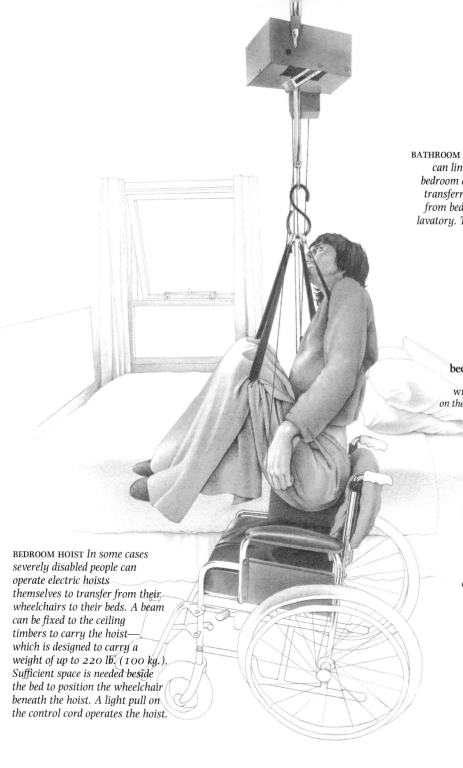

BATHROOM HOIST *A ceiling track can link a hoist between the bedroom and the bathroom for transferring a disabled person from bed to the bath or to the lavatory. The track should pass near to the lavatory.*

BEDROOM HOIST *In some cases severely disabled people can operate electric hoists themselves to transfer from their wheelchairs to their beds. A beam can be fixed to the ceiling timbers to carry the hoist—which is designed to carry a weight of up to 220 lb. (100 kg.). Sufficient space is needed beside the bed to position the wheelchair beneath the hoist. A light pull on the control cord operates the hoist.*

Check-list for bedroom and landing

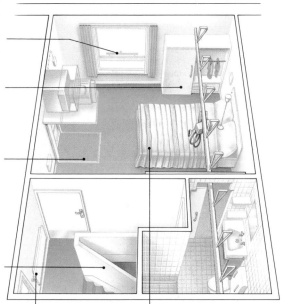

WINDOW BAR *A push-bar on the bottom of the window makes it easy to open.*

STORAGE SPACE *The shelves and hanging rails should be at an accessible height for the user.*

LIFT LEVEL *Lifts should be automatically self-levelling and stop exactly at floor level. There must be enough space in front of the door for the wheelchair to enter the lift.*

HANDRAIL *A rounded handrail is easy to grasp.*

RADIATOR PANEL *Disabled people may have a limited sense of touch and can easily be harmed by a hot radiator. A covering outer panel gives protection.*

BED SPACE *Position beds away from window glare—and allow plenty of space on both sides.*

203

Planning a comfortable, adaptable bathroom—a key area in the home

The essential factor in planning a bathroom for someone in a wheelchair is that there should be enough room for the wheelchair to turn around. Sometimes a shower is better than a bath, as some people find it comparatively easy to transfer from their chairs to a shower area. A bathroom should be kept comfortably warm at around 72°F (22°C). A well-equipped bathroom restores a disabled person's independence and reduces the amount of assistance he needs.

ELECTRIC HOIST *Bathroom hoists have their electricity supply transformed to a lower and safer voltage. The power supply must be placed outside the room. The hoists can be used with or without a helper.*

WASHBASIN AND MIRROR *The washbasin should be securely bracketed to the wall so there is space for the wheelchair foot-rest to fit underneath. The bowl should have lever taps and be positioned so that the user can get close to it. Fit the mirror at a convenient height to look into.*

AUTOMATIC TOILET-AND-BIDET *The disabled person need only lean against the back panel to flush the toilet, and then be washed by the bidet's automatic arm and dried by hot air.*

FOLDING GRAB RAIL *When not in use, the rail can be swung to rest in a vertical position.*

VENTILATION CONTROL *The bathroom window can be opened and closed by a remote-control winder. An extractor fan keeps the air fresh.*

BATH PLATFORM *A waterproof platform at the head of the bath can be used for getting into and out of a wheelchair.*

GRAB RAIL *Most disabled people find it easier to push themselves upright, rather than to pull. So a horizontal grab rail should be fitted above the platform.*

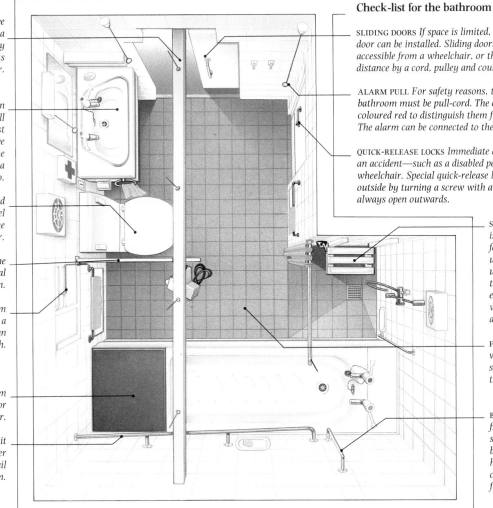

Check-list for the bathroom

SLIDING DOORS *If space is limited, a single leaf, straight sliding door can be installed. Sliding doors can have a pull-handle accessible from a wheelchair, or they can be controlled from a distance by a cord, pulley and counterweight.*

ALARM PULL *For safety reasons, the alarm controls in a bathroom must be pull-cord. The cord and knob should be coloured red to distinguish them from the electric-light controls. The alarm can be connected to the outside 'Help' sign.*

QUICK-RELEASE LOCKS *Immediate access is needed in the event of an accident—such as a disabled person falling out of his wheelchair. Special quick-release locks can be opened from the outside by turning a screw with a coin. The doors should always open outwards.*

SHOWER FITTINGS *The shower is thermostatically controlled for safety. Have the control unit fitted within reach of the user. A hinged bench seat fixed to the approach wall allows easy transfer from a wheelchair. Support rails are advisable.*

FLOOR SURFACE *Non-slip, waterproof tiles or welded sheeting are installed throughout.*

BATH FITTINGS *If necessary, fit extra grab rails on the sides of the bath. Portable bath seats can be used for handicapped people who cannot transfer directly to or from the bottom of the bath.*

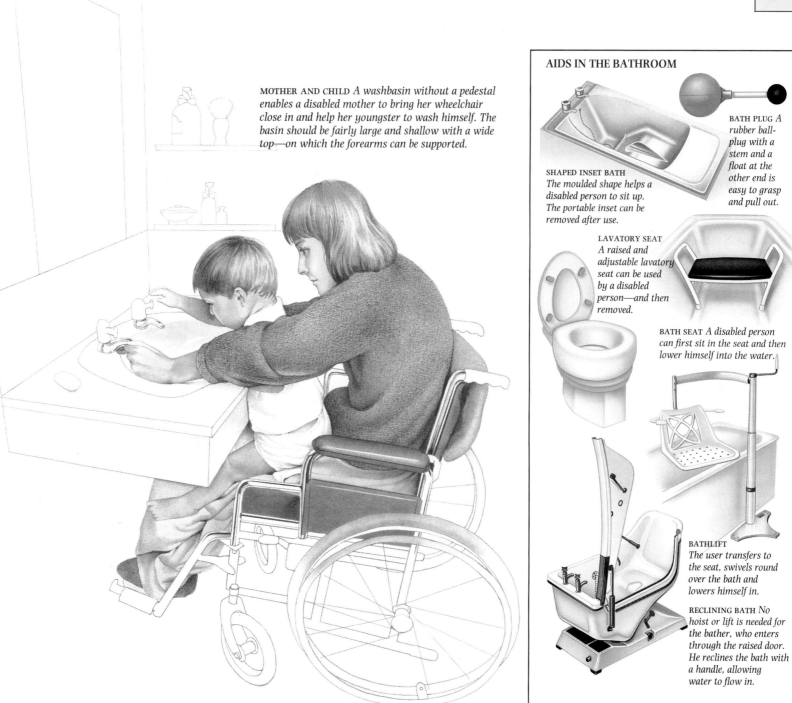

MOTHER AND CHILD *A washbasin without a pedestal enables a disabled mother to bring her wheelchair close in and help her youngster to wash himself. The basin should be fairly large and shallow with a wide top—on which the forearms can be supported.*

AIDS IN THE BATHROOM

SHAPED INSET BATH *The moulded shape helps a disabled person to sit up. The portable inset can be removed after use.*

BATH PLUG *A rubber ball-plug with a stem and a float at the other end is easy to grasp and pull out.*

LAVATORY SEAT *A raised and adjustable lavatory seat can be used by a disabled person—and then removed.*

BATH SEAT *A disabled person can first sit in the seat and then lower himself into the water.*

BATHLIFT *The user transfers to the seat, swivels round over the bath and lowers himself in.*

RECLINING BATH *No hoist or lift is needed for the bather, who enters through the raised door. He reclines the bath with a handle, allowing water to flow in.*

Planning a safe and convenient kitchen with everything to hand

Plan a kitchen layout to keep as much as possible of the work and storage space within easy reach. The best arrangement is: worktop-sink-worktop-cooker-worktop. Worktops, cookers and sinks should be at the same level and at an appropriate height for the user taking safety and efficiency into account. A disabled person with weak hands or arms needs to slide pots and pans along the worktop, from

preparation area to oven or hotplate. Allow ample knee space under the fittings, but install adequate insulation to avoid burning or scalding the knees on the underside of a cooker or sink. The fittings should rest on chromium-plated legs 6 in. (150 mm.) tall, which allow space for the wheelchair foot-rest and so prevent damage. The floor area must be large enough for a wheelchair to turn around and manoeuvre.

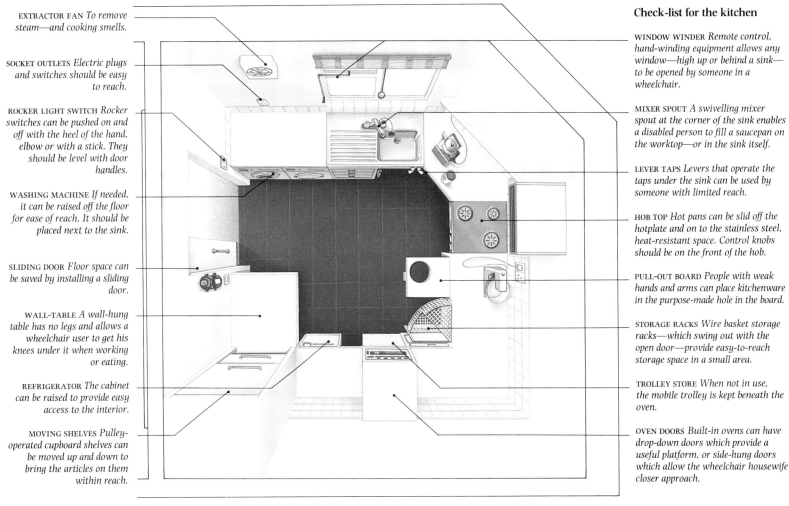

EXTRACTOR FAN *To remove steam—and cooking smells.*

SOCKET OUTLETS *Electric plugs and switches should be easy to reach.*

ROCKER LIGHT SWITCH *Rocker switches can be pushed on and off with the heel of the hand, elbow or with a stick. They should be level with door handles.*

WASHING MACHINE *If needed, it can be raised off the floor for ease of reach. It should be placed next to the sink.*

SLIDING DOOR *Floor space can be saved by installing a sliding door.*

WALL-TABLE *A wall-hung table has no legs and allows a wheelchair user to get his knees under it when working or eating.*

REFRIGERATOR *The cabinet can be raised to provide easy access to the interior.*

MOVING SHELVES *Pulley-operated cupboard shelves can be moved up and down to bring the articles on them within reach.*

Check-list for the kitchen

WINDOW WINDER *Remote control, hand-winding equipment allows any window—high up or behind a sink—to be opened by someone in a wheelchair.*

MIXER SPOUT *A swivelling mixer spout at the corner of the sink enables a disabled person to fill a saucepan on the worktop—or in the sink itself.*

LEVER TAPS *Levers that operate the taps under the sink can be used by someone with limited reach.*

HOB TOP *Hot pans can be slid off the hotplate and on to the stainless steel, heat-resistant space. Control knobs should be on the front of the hob.*

PULL-OUT BOARD *People with weak hands and arms can place kitchenware in the purpose-made hole in the board.*

STORAGE RACKS *Wire basket storage racks—which swing out with the open door—provide easy-to-reach storage space in a small area.*

TROLLEY STORE *When not in use, the mobile trolley is kept beneath the oven.*

OVEN DOORS *Built-in ovens can have drop-down doors which provide a useful platform, or side-hung doors which allow the wheelchair housewife closer approach.*

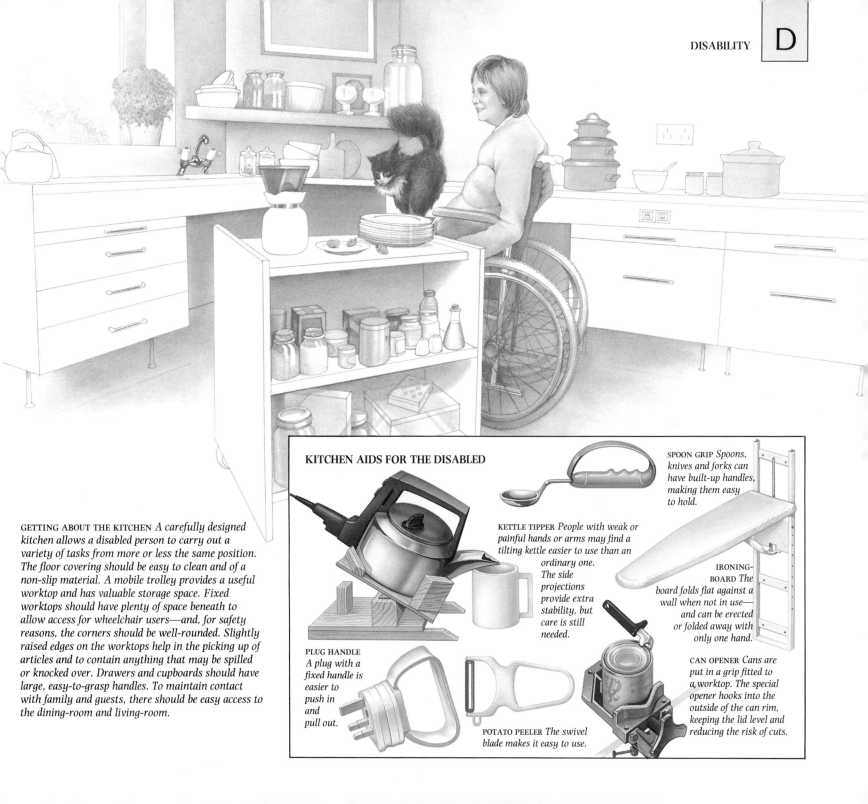

GETTING ABOUT THE KITCHEN *A carefully designed kitchen allows a disabled person to carry out a variety of tasks from more or less the same position. The floor covering should be easy to clean and of a non-slip material. A mobile trolley provides a useful worktop and has valuable storage space. Fixed worktops should have plenty of space beneath to allow access for wheelchair users—and, for safety reasons, the corners should be well-rounded. Slightly raised edges on the worktops help in the picking up of articles and to contain anything that may be spilled or knocked over. Drawers and cupboards should have large, easy-to-grasp handles. To maintain contact with family and guests, there should be easy access to the dining-room and living-room.*

KITCHEN AIDS FOR THE DISABLED

SPOON GRIP *Spoons, knives and forks can have built-up handles, making them easy to hold.*

KETTLE TIPPER *People with weak or painful hands or arms may find a tilting kettle easier to use than an ordinary one. The side projections provide extra stability, but care is still needed.*

IRONING-BOARD *The board folds flat against a wall when not in use— and can be erected or folded away with only one hand.*

PLUG HANDLE *A plug with a fixed handle is easier to push in and pull out.*

CAN OPENER *Cans are put in a grip fitted to a worktop. The special opener hooks into the outside of the can rim, keeping the lid level and reducing the risk of cuts.*

POTATO PEELER *The swivel blade makes it easy to use.*

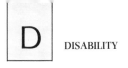

Working in the garden and the greenhouse

A properly designed and equipped garden can provide hours of creative pleasure, and allows a disabled gardener to do a great deal of work without undue effort. Since he cannot get down to his plants to tend them, they must be brought up to his level in raised beds. And since he cannot bend and stretch in order to dig, weed and prune, special lightweight tools have been developed to aid him with these tasks.

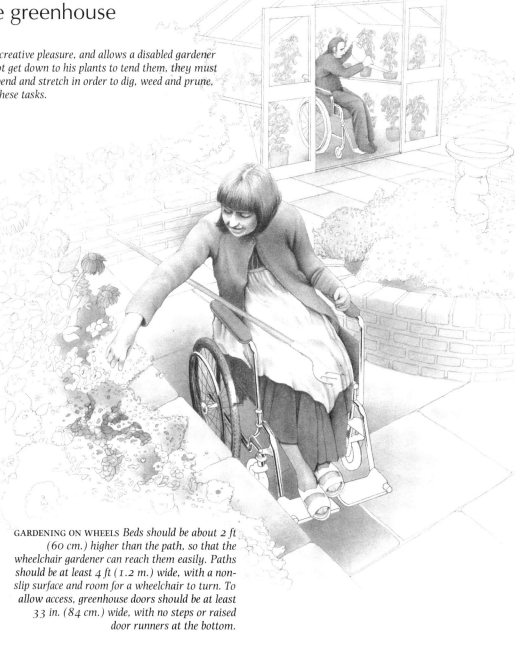

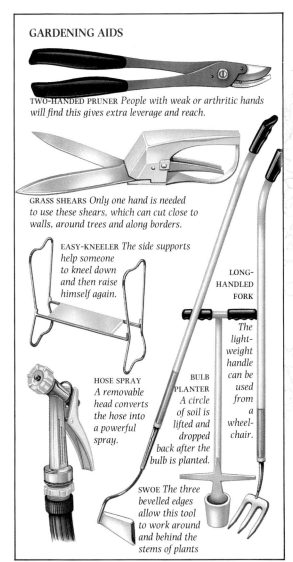

GARDENING AIDS

TWO-HANDED PRUNER *People with weak or arthritic hands will find this gives extra leverage and reach.*

GRASS SHEARS *Only one hand is needed to use these shears, which can cut close to walls, around trees and along borders.*

EASY-KNEELER *The side supports help someone to kneel down and then raise himself again.*

LONG-HANDLED FORK *The lightweight handle can be used from a wheelchair.*

HOSE SPRAY *A removable head converts the hose into a powerful spray.*

BULB PLANTER *A circle of soil is lifted and dropped back after the bulb is planted.*

SWOE *The three bevelled edges allow this tool to work around and behind the stems of plants*

GARDENING ON WHEELS *Beds should be about 2 ft (60 cm.) higher than the path, so that the wheelchair gardener can reach them easily. Paths should be at least 4 ft (1.2 m.) wide, with a non-slip surface and room for a wheelchair to turn. To allow access, greenhouse doors should be at least 33 in. (84 cm.) wide, with no steps or raised door runners at the bottom.*

Check-list for gardens

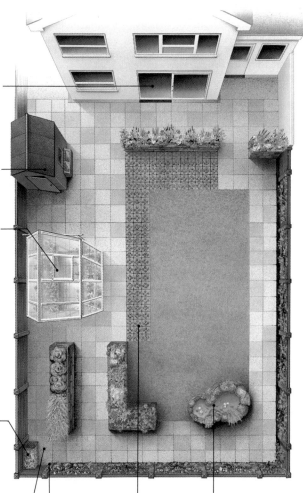

SLIDING DOORS *Glass doors that slide allow easy wheelchair access between house and garden.*

POTTING SHED *It is situated within easy reach of the greenhouse.*

GREENHOUSE *The centre path should be at least 30 in. (75 cm.) wide, and the shelves 2 ft (60 cm.) wide on either side. An approach area of 4 ft 6 in. (137 cm.) square allows a gardener to manoeuvre his wheelchair sideways to open the sliding door.*

COMPOST HEAP *A neat wire mesh in which compost is packed in small layers and kept well watered. This reduces the amount of turning needed.*

CONCRETE PATHS *As well as looking attractive, the surface must provide a good grip for walking and for wheelchair tyres.*

NARROW BEDS *Where beds can only be reached from one side, they should be no more than 2 ft (60 cm.) wide.*

GRASSY PATH *Hollow concrete blocks allow grass to grow between the gaps. The path can be used to avoid making tyre marks on a wet lawn.*

WATER GARDEN *A raised water garden, with waterfall, should be 2 ft (60 cm.) above path level.*

EMPLOYMENT

Disabled people are often denied work through prejudice or because employers do not want the bother of making special arrangements for them. And those who do succeed in getting work are often employed below their true potential. Yet research has shown that, in general, disabled people have less time off than able-bodied workers, have fewer accidents, are just as productive and tend to be more conscientious.

A wide range of specialised aids is available to employers to enable them to take on disabled workers. They include special fitments for tools, purpose-built desks and electric typewriters and accessories that enable the disabled person to use the telephone.

Such aids may be supplied on free permanent loan from the Manpower Services Commission, which can make grants of up to £6,000 to employees towards the cost of adaptations for disabled people such as ramps and special toilet facilities. Applications should be made to the local Disablement Resettlement Officer through any Jobcentre or employment office.

Because opportunities for employment are so limited for disabled people, they need to obtain the best qualifications they can. A newly disabled person may need to consider a change of occupation, which may entail retraining. Some disabled people set up their own business, often working from home.

For the severely disabled who cannot undertake normal employment there exist opportunities to work under special, sheltered conditions, either for certain commercial organisations or in workshops run by local authorities and charities with government help.

Organisation

Disablement Resettlement Service (contact through Jobcentres, listed under Employment Service Division Manpower Services Commission in local telephone directories). Helps disabled people to find suitable training and employment.

Publications

Able to Work, by Bernadette Fallon, published by the Spinal Injuries Association, 76 St James' Lane, London N10 3D7.
Creating your own work, by Micheline Mason, The Gresham Press. Now out of print—consult your local librarian.
Working for yourself, The Daily Telegraph Guide to Self-Employment, by Godfrey Golzen, Kogan Page Ltd, 120 Pentonville Road, London N1 9JN.

INCONTINENCE

Loss or weakening of control of the bladder or bowel is termed incontinence. It may be caused by a stroke, childbirth, infection of the urinary tract or uterus, an enlarged prostate gland, disease or injury of the spinal cord.

Incontinence of the bladder can show itself in various ways: a need to urinate more often than usual; very little warning of the need to urinate; a constant leakage of urine with little or no awareness of the fact; some people find that a slight exertion, such as coughing, sneezing or laughing, causes such a leakage.

Bowel incontinence may take the form of permanent diarrhoea, which should always be treated by a doctor, or diarrhoea following severe constipation, which can be rectified by a diet including plenty of fibre and liquid. *See* NUTRITION. In disabled people incontinence is made worse by the fact that often the lavatory cannot be reached in time.

The disabled person is usually embarrassed by incontinence. It is vital that one is sympathetic towards his problem, since lack of understanding can only make him more anxious—and consequently more incontinent. In all cases, consult a doctor, since a wide variety of aids is available on prescription. Treatment of the underlying condition ensures that in most cases these aids need only be used temporarily.

The unpleasant smell created by wet or soiled clothes or bed linen causes considerable distress to the incontinent person. For this reason he should use one of the special deodorants that can be applied to affected articles to get rid of smell. Whoever is looking after the disabled person should change the articles as soon as possible. *See* HOME NURSING.

Publication

Incontinence and its Management, by Dorothy Mandelstam, Chapman & Hall, from Haigh Hockland Ltd, Booksellers, The Precinct Centre, Oxford Road, Manchester M13 9QA.

SEX
Sexual intercourse presents practical problems for some physically disabled people and is impossible for others. For those who are able to have

intercourse, problems can often be overcome by an imaginative and flexible approach to lovemaking, with a knowledge and acceptance of various positions and sexual techniques—and, if desired, the use of aids. Counsellors with the Sexual and Personal Relationships of Disabled People organisation take a particular interest in the special needs of disabled people.

Those for whom sexual intercourse is impossible can still lead sexually fulfilled lives through alternative ways of giving and receiving sexual satisfaction.

Even in cases where the genitals are part of an area that is paralysed and that has lost all sensation, sexual feelings can still be expressed. Many other parts of the body can be stimulated by caresses.

Disabled people who are able to have children but are concerned about whether their disability can be passed on should consult their doctor, who may refer them to a genetic counsellor.

Organisations

Sexual and Personal Relationships of Disabled People (*SPOD*), 286 Camden Road, London N7 0BJ. It provides advice and help on sexual and personal relationships of disabled people.
The Outsiders Club, Box 4ZB, London W1A 4ZB (Tel. 071-837 3559). A club that encourages personal relationships between disabled men and women.

Publications

Entitled to Love: the sexual and emotional needs of the handicapped, by Dr Wendy Greengross, Malaby Press.
Not Made of Stone, by K. Heslinga,

A. M. C. H. Schellen and A. Verkuyl, Woodhead-Faulkner, Cambridge.
The Sexual Side of Handicap, by W. F. R. Stewart. Woodhead-Faulkner, Cambridge.

BLINDNESS AND PARTIAL SIGHT
The three most common causes of blindness are macular degeneration, cataract and glaucoma.
See BLINDNESS.

As well as those who are totally blind, there are many people whose vision is so impaired that glasses or other optical treatment cannot help them to see effectively.

Local authorities maintain a register of blind people and another register of those who are partially sighted. Both groups are entitled to a wide range of local authority services, though many authorities will give help whether the visually impaired person is registered or not. Social services departments can arrange for aids to help with self care and home management, better home lighting and instruction in Braille.

Most local authorities employ instructors who will train blind people to use the 'long-cane'—a white cane 45–55 in. (114–140 cm.)—which helps blind people to find their way. For those who have some residual sight, a white 'symbol-cane' may be all that is required, but users will need training in how to move about outdoors.

Many blind people find that a guide dog gives them both confidence and companionship, and greatly enhances the range of their mobility and personal safety. In the United Kingdom, guide dogs are provided by the Guide Dogs for the

Blind Association. Only people who are fit enough to be taught to use a guide dog effectively and who can provide adequate care for the dog can be accepted for training.

Sonic travel aids have been developed to guide blind people by sound reflections, and these include devices for fitting to wheelchairs. However, the uses are limited.

Of all the skills a physically active blind person needs to acquire, probably the most important is that of mobility. Good training can prove invaluable. There is much to be learned, not least the degree of assertive independence and courage which will be so necessary if the person is to make successful forays outside his home. Many people who are registered blind in fact have guiding sight but need encouragement to use it.

Much information, instruction and enjoyment is available to the blind and partially sighted through the medium of Braille or Moon. In Braille, combinations of raised dots are used to represent letters which can be 'read' by the fingertips; it can also be 'written' by the visually impaired. The clear, bold symbols of the Moon system are easier to learn and follow, but it is much slower to produce than Braille, so there is far less literature available in Moon. A number of services exist to translate an individual's special requirements—from knitting patterns and instructions for domestic appliances to textbooks and study courses. They can be obtained through the Royal National Institute for the Blind.

Also available are aids to help the blind and partially sighted with such things as dressing, eating and drinking, going to the lavatory, driving and housework.

In seeking employment, blind and partially sighted people can use the Disablement Resettlement Service of the Manpower Services Commission and its Blind Persons' Resettlement Officers. There are also Blind Persons' Training Officers who provide initial training on the job and advise on technical matters and aids for the blind. These include talking calculators, Braille measuring equipment, tape-recorders and Braille computer terminals.

Organisations
Royal National Institute for the Blind, 224 Great Portland Street, London WIN 6AA (Tel. 071-388 1266). It provides training for a number of occupations, including computer programming, physiotherapy, shorthand and typing, audio typing and telephony. It also promotes education, training, rehabilitation, employment and welfare of blind people.
The Royal National College and Academy of Music for the Blind, College Road, Hereford HR1 1EB (Tel. 0432 265725) offers various courses in piano tuning and commercial training, and tuners can also be trained at the *London College of Furniture*.
The Guide Dogs for the Blind Association, Head Office, Hillfields, Burghfield, Reading, Berks RG7 3YG (Tel. 0734 835555).

Publications
Blindness and Partial Sight (a guide for social workers and others concerned with the care and rehabilitation of the visually handicapped), by Astrid Klemz, Woodhead-Faulkner, Cambridge.

Equipment and Games, available from the Royal National Institute for the Blind.
Directory of Agencies for the Blind, published by the RNIB, contains over 1,300 entries covering the national state and voluntary agencies concerned with blind people as well as regional and local associations, schools, ophthalmic hospitals, homes and hostels. It includes information about periodicals in Braille and Moon, and about publishers of large-print books.

DEAFNESS AND HEARING IMPAIRMENT
People are considered deaf if they cannot hear speech even when it is amplified. People who are hard of hearing can make out speech, but often only in fragments. Deafness of any degree may be due to a defect in the conduction of sound to the inner ear; to a defect in the perception of sound by the inner ear; to a defect in the auditory nerve leading to the brain; or to brain damage or mental abnormality. *See* DEAFNESS, *page 188*.

Anyone who suspects his hearing has become impaired or who has a child they suspect may have a hearing problem should see their doctor, in order to be referred to an ear specialist. In addition, anyone with a long-standing hearing impairment who has not seen a specialist for years should see their doctor about arranging a visit, since it is possible they can be helped by one of the latest developments in hearing-aids.

Many people who are hard of hearing, find every attempted conversation ends in misunderstanding and sometimes

ridicule. This makes normal communication impossible and may lead to depression, a withdrawal from life and a feeling of total isolation. Therefore it is essential to seek help.

Surgery or a hearing-aid can improve many people's hearing. For those who cannot be helped in these ways, lip-reading and sign language are skills which can be acquired with patience and training. They are best learned by joining classes which are provided by most local adult education services and some special colleges, usually at modest cost.

It is essential that children who are found to be partially deaf are spoken to much more than children with normal hearing would be. This lessens the child's isolation and makes the fullest use of residual hearing at a stage when they are most open to learning. This is especially important if the child is at the age when he is learning to speak, but is necessary at any age if the child is to acquire a normal speaking vocabulary.

Organisations
Royal National Institute for the Deaf, 105 Gower Street, London WC1E 6AH (Tel. 071-387 8033). It promotes the prevention and relief of deafness and helps the welfare of deaf people.
Breakthrough Trust Deaf/Hearing Integration, Charles W. Gillett Centre, Selly Oak Colleges, Birmingham, B29 6LE (Tel. 021-472 6447).
Hearing Concern (BAHOH), 7–11 Armstrong Road, London W3 7JL (Tel. 081-743 1110).

Publications
Your Hearing Loss and How to Cope with It, by Kenneth Lysons,

David & Charles.
The Hearing Loss Handbook, by Richard Rosenthal, St James Press.

SPEECH IMPAIRMENT
Inability to speak usually occurs in those who have been completely deaf from birth or who have disease of the left side of the brain. Speech handicap can also arise through accident, illness (such as stroke), for psychological reasons or through congenital mental handicap. The person may be capable of thinking normally, but unable to express his thoughts; or he may have difficulty in learning and in assembling accurate and coherent messages.

Speech impairment may be accompanied by a difficulty in writing. For those who can understand speech and use language, communication aids range from a simple letter board to an electronic keyboard that will display words on a television screen. Those whose powers of understanding are limited and who cannot use language can sometimes be helped to communicate by systems in which symbols take the place of words.

Whatever the method of communication, it is bound to be slower than speech, and the 'listener' must be prepared to spend considerable time in ensuring that he understands exactly what the 'speaker' is trying to communicate. When a method is chosen, therefore, it is essential that the 'listener' as well as the 'speaker' is taken into account.

There remain many people for whom existing communication aids are of little or no help. However, even in cases where they are of limited help they should still be used, since they serve to bring the afflicted person into closer contact with others and so lessen his feelings of isolation.

Organisation
International Society for Augmentative and Alternative Communication (ISAAC), 25 Mortimer Street, London WIN 8AB (Tel. 071-637 5400). It promotes international co-operation in the field of communication aids.

THE DISABLED CHILD
Today's disabled child is tomorrow's disabled adult. The aim must be to prepare him as efficiently as possible to face the challenge of the future. In the first place, although he needs special help and understanding, it is vital that he is not over-protected and shielded too much from the harsh realities of life. He should be encouraged to do as many things for himself as possible. He must be allowed to make his own special contribution to family life, to take part as far as possible in its everyday activities, to share in its worries and joys and to take risks and accept disappointments as all children must. Any brothers and sisters should be encouraged to support the disabled child and to share in the joy of his major achievements. At the same time, they too will need their share of attention if resentment is to be prevented.

Play is an essential element in any child's development; for the disabled child, it can provide the best possible form of exercise and therapy. Many aids and imaginatively designed toys are available to encourage a disabled child to amuse himself or to join in

the fun of his companions. Children who cannot move need to be seated comfortably. Special chairs can be obtained to suit specific handicaps. Bean bag chairs are particularly useful; they can be placed in a variety of positions to allow for different activities and also be used by other members of the family. Specially designed go-karts and trolleys enable the disabled child to enjoy a certain degree of mobility.

Other vehicles, designed to look like racing cars, encourage children who have enough co-ordination and power of movement to explore their surroundings. Many types of wheelchairs and pushchairs are made for the disabled child, and special car seats are also available.

Every piece of equipment the child uses should be a positive aid to development and not reinforce any undesirable postures. The child's therapists will advise on this matter.

It is vital that the disabled child's educational needs are assessed by teachers, psychologists, therapists, social workers, doctors and the parents as early as possible; and these needs should be regularly reassessed as the child develops.

Children with disabilities of mind or body need specially trained teachers and educational aids. For many years disabilities have been classified and largely provided for in special schools. But it has recently been felt that such disabilities cannot be neatly categorised. Many children have multiple handicaps, and every disabled child has his own particular problems and needs.

There is also an argument that it is unwise to segregate disabled children, since they then lose valuable contact with able-bodied children and

are cut off from normal life. As a result of these powerful arguments it is likely that there will be an increasing integration of disabled children into ordinary schools supplied with special teaching resources.

The parents of the child must continually seek, and if necessary demand information as to the best available provision for the child's needs at all stages. It is only by such planning—and by accepting their child's limitations— that parents can help him to achieve his potential.

Organisations
Disabled Living Foundation, 380–84 Harrow Road, London W9 2HU (Tel. 071-289 6111). Provides advice and information on services and aids for the disabled.
Council for Disabled Children, 8 Wakley Street, London ECIV 7QE (Tel. 071-278 9441). Provides information on all aspects of childhood disability.
MENCAP—The National Society for Mentally Handicapped Children and Adults, 123 Golden Lane, London ECIY ORT (Tel. 071-454 0454). Provides a wide range of services for mentally handicapped people and their families. Local groups offer personal support.
Advisory Centre for Education Ltd, IB Aberdeen Studios, 22 Highbury Grove, London N5 2EA (Tel. 071-354 8321). Provides information and advice for everyone involved in education, including the education of disabled children.

Publications
The Wheelchair Child, by Philippa Russell (Souvenir Press).
The Warnock Report: Special Educational Needs (HMSO).

The Disabled Schoolchild and Kitchen Sense, by S. Foott, S. Handscombe and M. Lane, Heinemann Health Books. Now out of print, but your local library should either stock a copy or be able to order one for you.

STATUTORY SERVICES IN THE UNITED KINGDOM
Both the National Health Service and Local Authority Social Services provide training and support to help disabled people to cope with daily living. For newly disabled people, the process usually begins in hospital, where an occupational therapist will instruct the patient in techniques for overcoming physical handicaps.

At first, the disabled person needs to readjust to routine tasks such as washing, dressing and shaving. A physiotherapist will help to maintain and improve bodily movements as far as possible.

Community health services provide health visitors and district nurses; health centres and clinics; incontinence and chiropody services; and treatment and therapy in specialist hospital departments.

Social services departments also provide extensive facilities through social workers and help to co-ordinate the various welfare services. They can aid handicapped people on a personal basis especially when difficulties arise through illness, stress or other domestic problems.

In addition, social services offices can advise and assist in such matters as aids and adaptions, financial benefits, home-help, meals-on-wheels, holidays, long and short-term residential care, the issue of orange badges (for parking concessions) and concessionary travel passes.

Statutory benefits—standard and special—available to disabled people

Attendance allowance
For severely mentally or physically disabled people over 65 who need prolonged care.
DS 702 (DSS).

Dental treatment
Free if on income support or family credit. Free or reduced cost if on a low income. Free for pregnant women or those who have had a baby in the previous 12 months.
D 11 (DSS).

Disability Living Allowance
A tax-free benefit for disabled people under 65 who need help with personal care and with getting around. It is not dependent on national insurance contributions.
DS 704 (DSS)

Disability Working Allowance
For people over 16 who work at least 16 hours a week, but have an illness or injury which limits their earning capacity. It is tax free and does not depend on having made national insurance contributions.
DS 704 (DSS)

Family credit
For working people having care of one or more children at home where total family income is low.
FC1 (DSS).

Glasses
NHS lenses and frames free if you are on income support or family credit. Free or at reduced cost if on a low income. G 11 (DSS).

Hospital fares for patients
Full refund if on income support or family credit. Full or partial refund if on a low income. H 11 (DSS).

Income Support
For people whose total income falls below minimum requirements prescribed by the Government. Additions can be made for certain necessities and some other expenses incurred through disability.
IS 1 (DSS).

Industrial injuries disablement benefit
For those who cannot work through industrial injury or prescribed industrial disease.
NI 2: Industrial diseases
NI 3: Pneumoconiosis & byssinosis
NI 6: Disablement benefit
NI 207: Occupational deafness
NI 237: Occupational asthma
(all DSS).

Invalid care allowance
For people of working age who cannot work because they have to care at home for a relative or friend (for at least 35 hours a week) who is so severely disabled as to qualify for attendance allowance.
FB 31 (DSS).

Invalidity benefit
The follow-on to sickness benefit or Statutory Sick Pay for those remaining incapable of work after 28 weeks and who are covered by the National Insurance contributory scheme.
NI 16A (DSS).

Milk and vitamins
Pregnant women and children under school age in families on income support can each get one free pint of milk a day and free vitamins. Those receiving family credit get a cash allowance instead.
AB 11 (DSS).

Prescription charges
Exemption for people on income support, on family credit, on a low income, or over pension age, or who suffer from certain prescribed medical conditions.
P 11 (DSS).

Severe Disablement Allowance (SDA)
For people over the age of 16 who are incapable of work, but whose National Insurance contributions do not qualify them for sickness or invalidity benefit. People over 20 who claim must also be 80 per cent disabled and incapable of work.
NI 252 (DSS).

Sickness benefit
For people covered by the National Insurance contributory scheme who become incapable of work through sickness or disablement, and cannot get statutory sick pay from their employer. Sickness benefit ceases after 28 weeks, but may be followed by invalidity benefit.
NI 16 NI 253 (DSS).

Statutory Sick Pay (SSP)
People who are sick when employed receive from their employers statutory sick pay for up to a total of 28 weeks in a tax year. When SSP runs out, they can claim state sickness benefit or invalidity benefit.
NI 244 (DSS).

Therapeutic earnings concession
Disabled people may in certain circumstances derive limited earnings from work without affecting their right to sickness or invalidity benefit. Contact local DSS office.

War-disablement pensions
For people disabled as a result of military service and civilians disabled in the Second World War.
MPL 152, 153, 154 (DSS).

Further information
Disability Rights Handbook available for £2, including postage, from Disability Alliance, 25 Denmark Street, London WC2 8NJ.

Most DSS leaflets can be obtained from local offices of the Department of Social Security. War Disablement leaflets are also available at war pensions offices.

DRUG ABUSE

In the broad sense, the word drug means any habit-forming substance. Medically, it means any medicine taken to combat an illness. Almost any mood-changing drug can be misused—and most people take such drugs in one way or another. They take aspirins because they feel run down; they drink coffee so they can finish a piece of work without falling asleep, they drink alcohol to relax after a long day. Only in extreme circumstances—alcoholism or heavy smoking—does this amount to serious abuse.

The popular picture of drug abuse encompasses heroin and cocaine addiction, glue-sniffing, taking LSD or amphetamines, and smoking cannabis. This area of abuse is peopled very much by the young. They start taking drugs as an experiment, as the result of group pressures to conform, or as an escape from the problems of becoming adult. For many teenagers this is a brief phase, for a few it leads to a drug habit and sometimes to addiction.

However, it is not only the young who abuse drugs. Older people may not experiment, but they do use drugs as a response to the problems they face. They tend to turn to less-publicised types of drug abuse, such as tranquillisers, sleeping-pills and alcohol.

The many drugs that are commonly abused can be divided roughly into five groups:

Stimulants make people more active mentally and physically, and they prevent sleep. They include cocaine and amphetamines (appetite suppressants).

Sedatives calm anxiety, reduce activity, and induce sleep. In larger doses they produce loss of feeling or coma. They include heroin, morphine, barbiturate sleeping-pills and strong tranquillisers.

Hallucinogens bring about a mental change known as a trip consisting largely of colourful hallucinations. The main types are chemical, like LSD, or from plants such as certain fungi.

Cannabis is mainly sedative but can also induce hallucinations. It is used in the form of dried leaves or resin from the cannabis plant.

Solvents are very unpredictable. Most act as sedatives, but they can also stimulate and induce hallucinations. Glue, dry-cleaning fluid and paint thinners are three examples.

Drugs of different kinds are often taken together. Sometimes this is done deliberately, as when stimulants are taken to enhance an LSD trip or to counteract sedatives. Haphazard combinations of sedatives with alcoholic drinks can be particularly dangerous, leading to rapid intoxication, accidents, coma and even death.

What all drugs of abuse have in common is that they alter the mood or perceptions of the people who take them. They make them feel happier, or more relaxed, or provoke hallucinations. It is this change that people are looking for when they first start taking drugs.

PATTERNS OF DRUG-TAKING

Most young people are naturally curious and may want to try any drug that is fashionable or available, especially if the offer is a friendly one. Group pressure, the risk of being thought 'chicken', and a wish to defy authority and make a protest may be some of the factors that influence the decision to try a drug. The elements of danger are attractive to those who start taking drugs for 'kicks'.

The first experience may, in fact, not live up to expectations or may even be unpleasant. The taker may feel ill or frightened, or may have a bad hangover afterwards. The imagined attractions of taking drugs may be replaced by worries about being involved with pushers and drug takers, and by fear either of prosecution or of the bad effects of the drugs. Most young people who experiment soon decide that drugs are not for them.

For some, however, young and old, drugs appear to fill a gap in their lives. Cannabis and sedatives may ease their anxieties, stimulants overcome their inhibitions and LSD relieve boredom. For many, drug-taking may be just a form of social relaxation or a passing phase, but the few who habitually take drugs lack self-esteem, friends, motivation, and any positive expectations for the future. At first drugs appear to fill these gaps, providing the taker with the social role he lacked before.

The pattern may then develop towards stronger preparations, a greater variety of drugs, bigger doses more often, intravenous injection and physical dependence.

The taker is totally unaware—until he misses a dose—that he has crossed the dividing line between abuse and addiction. Physical dependence develops when the body and brain become so chemically adjusted to the presence of the drug—usually heroin, barbiturates or alcohol—that they cannot function 'normally' without it. Missing one or two doses is then followed by the onset of the withdrawal syndrome, called 'Cold Turkey' by heroin addicts. This is extremely unpleasant and occasionally causes death. From agitation and symptoms like a running head cold, it soon progresses to headache, muscle cramps, abdominal pain and vomiting, sometimes accompanied by orgasm, or even epileptic fits. This can last for as much as three days and nights if the drug is withdrawn from severe heroin addicts.

Once established, addiction is extremely hard for the addict to break, with its mixture of craving, fear of withdrawal and established life-style. The addict's life is concerned solely with obtaining further supplies of the drug. Many addicts are at the mercy of drug pushers, and the high cost of illicit supplies often leads to money-raising crime, prostitution and theft of drugs, and introducing novices to the habit as potential future customers.

Not all drug dependents follow this pattern, however. Those who reach middle age, or become dependent comparatively late, are more like alcoholics of the same age, and less likely to introduce others to their habit or become involved in crime. Older addicts are usually more controlled in their drug-taking, and a few seem to mature out of their addiction altogether.

Very few people become addicted because they are tricked into taking drugs by a pusher. Some dependency can, however, develop insidiously and only be recognised as such when the taker attempts to stop taking the drug.

People with long-term prescriptions for sleeping-pills or tranquillisers may find, when they stop taking them, that they are suffering withdrawal symptoms. Similarly, a person who uses tranquillisers or stimulant drugs as a prop to enable him to get through the day may find himself unable to function normally without them. Even where physical dependence is not present, all drug habits produce psychological dependence.

HOW DRUG-TAKING CAN BE RECOGNISED

It is not easy to recognise drug-taking in the early stages: the signs are slight and the taker will try to hide what is happening. It is always dangerous to jump to conclusions, and what seem to be signs of drug abuse may be misleading, but early diagnosis is vitally important. If any evidence of drug-taking comes to light, at whatever stage, it should be checked and discussed with the person concerned or through an intermediary, who may be a family member, friend or professional (such as general practitioner, probation officer or social worker).

Behaviour The first sign of drug abuse is often a shift in behaviour. Changes in friends, attitudes, dress, mood, interests, punctuality and performance at school or at work are some of the signs that something may be amiss.

Physical clues Tablets, capsules, powder, seeds, greenish-brown 'tobacco' or growing plants that may be cannabis, hypodermic syringes and home-made cigarette stubs all provide evidence. However, drugs of abuse may not be involved even if the owner thinks they are. Illicit supplies sometimes consist of dried plant material masquerading as cannabis, for example, or tablets that simply resemble stimulants or sedatives and can be sold more profitably.

Herbal cannabis produces aromatic smoke, something like a bonfire, that may cling to sweaters and curtains or linger in an unventilated room.

Health and appearance The depressed 'hangover' after stimulants have worn off may be accompanied by a dry cough, slight peeling around the lips and thirst.

Sedative abuse may be accompanied by unsteadiness, trembling, confusion, even coma. Intoxication with sedatives often resembles drunkenness. Heroin and morphine make the pupils of the eye contract to a pin-point, in addition to their sedative effects.

Cannabis smokers become relaxed and drowsy. Sometimes their eyes go red and their appetite increases.

A person who has taken LSD may appear to be disorientated or giggly, living in a world of his own. Since, however, the taker usually retains some control over his actions, an unsuspecting watcher may not realise when someone is hallucinating. Someone experiencing a 'bad trip' will normally appear to be terrified by nightmarish visions.

Late evidence Needle marks on the inside of the elbow are evidence of someone who injects himself. Such marks are a sign that addiction is well established.

In general the habitual drug taker becomes unreliable and lazy. He may neglect his food and himself. He may appear 'other worldly' and secretive.

Criminality is often associated with theft of drugs or money-raising offences to buy them, especially among addicts who steal to obtain a supply.

TREATMENT AND REHABILITATION
The most important aspect of any attempt to treat drug abuse is early diagnosis. In the early stages, experimentation and occasional misuse of drugs may correct itself or respond to everyday measures such as informed discussion and a change of friends, locality or work-place. The longer drug-taking goes on, the more established it becomes and effective treatment becomes more difficult. Treatment is always a matter for specialists.

Sudden withdrawal of a drug from someone who is physically addicted to it will lead to unpleasant and possibly dangerous withdrawal symptoms. No drug should ever be withdrawn from a habitual taker without a doctor's advice. In the few addicts with a genuine will to reform, withdrawal may be carried out gradually and without too much pain.

Whether a drug is physically addictive or not, there is always the difficult problem of psychological dependence. Habitual drug-taking is a warning sign that all was not well with the taker before it began and that he took the drug to fill some need. It is therefore seldom sufficient to withdraw the drug. The addict is likely to feel that he cannot continue without it. Only by helping him to regain self-esteem, and a positive outlook, can the desire for drugs, and the risk of relapse, be eliminated.

How to help the young addict

If you are worried that your teenage son or daughter might be taking drugs, do not rush to the doctor or the police. Except in emergencies like an overdosage, coma or a bad LSD trip, it is seldom necessary to act quickly. Usually there are many factors to consider, including the following.

☐ Try to establish confidence between yourself and the teenager—via a close friend or relative.

☐ The drug-taking may not be particularly serious, and adopting too hard a line may push a teenager into deeper involvement. In considering what, if anything, needs to be done always try to involve the teenager.

☐ There may be a need for medical or psychiatric advice about the effects of the drugs or about an underlying state of depression. If so, a general practitioner should certainly be consulted.

☐ In other cases, there may be no need for medical advice. The drug-taking may have been just a brief experiment that is already over. If drugs are still being taken, they will be associated with a particular teenage group, and a period away from home may be the remedy.

☐ In more difficult cases, when drug-taking is established, there is usually little that can be done to stop an older teenager continuing to take drugs if he wants to. The object must be to spot drug-taking early, and also to discuss the question of drug abuse with young teenagers before they have become involved.

☐ In particular, drug-taking should always be regarded as a warning sign that there may be other things amiss in a teenager's life. Drugs, and the people who go with them, may be filling gaps—in self-esteem, in satisfying relationships with real friends, and in rewarding experiences at home, at school, at work, in sport or hobbies.

WILL TO SUCCEED
To give up a drug habit successfully requires a very strong desire to succeed on the part of the addict. Unfortunately most addicts seek help only when they are unable to find drugs or have become ill, and they accept help only until the immediate crisis has passed.

In addition, there is no known method of medical or psychiatric care that has a high success rate in curing addiction. If addicts are malnourished, anaemic, physically ill, or suffering from mental disorder, they can be treated medically or psychiatrically, provided they play their part. Treatment of addiction itself usually comes down to prescribing habit-forming drugs, in limited amounts, often in the form of less-harmful substitutes.

Most of the heroin addicts who attend clinics—and only a minority do so—receive limited supplies of methadone. This is a synthetic substitute for heroin and is also physically addictive, but it is less harmful to health, can be taken orally, and the period between doses can be 24 hours against heroin's eight hours. This allows some addicts to work and live a more normal life rather than looking for supplies. Unfortunately methadone treatment rarely breaks the addiction altogether, and may even help to perpetuate dependence on drugs.

The best hopes rest with early identification of young drug takers and intervention well before they become addicted. Where medical or psychiatric help is required it can be obtained by seeing the family doctor, who may refer the drug taker to a hospital specialist. Addicted drug takers can apply directly to the special clinics, which will not normally take on other drug takers.

There are a small number of rehabilitation centres which aim to reintegrate the former addict into society and restore his psychological balance.

HOW THE DRUGS ARE TAKEN
The speed of action and effects of drugs depend on how they are taken. There are three usual ways:

Swallowing Most sedatives, stimulants and hallucinogens such as LSD are taken in the form of tablets or capsules. After swallowing, absorption in the stomach may take half an hour or more and may not be complete. The absorbed drug then passes first to the liver, where it may be modified chemically before circulating to the rest of the body. These delays act as a safety mechanism, but there is also the risk that an appreciable amount of the drug may remain in the stomach, to be absorbed later. This poses an additional danger of coma or even death from overdosage. Any suspicion of unabsorbed alcohol or drugs calls for an emergency stomach wash-out.

Sniffing and inhalation Absorption from the nose and lungs is generally more complete than absorption after swallowing, as it allows drugs to reach the bloodstream directly and without having to pass through the liver. Powdered cocaine ('snow') and sometimes amphetamine are sniffed up the nose. Solvents are often both sniffed and inhaled, but smoking—whether of tobacco, cannabis or opium—is the commonest form of inhalation. Drugs taken this way act almost immediately.

Injection There are two ways of injecting drugs: 'skin popping'—under the skin; and 'mainlining'—directly into a vein. Heroin addicts often start by skin popping but most soon start mainlining. Barbiturates, morphine, cocaine and amphetamines may also be injected.

Injection directly into the bloodstream generally produces the most potent effect of all because the entire dose acts at once. Some drugs, like amphetamines, considered moderately harmful when misused by mouth, become at least as addictive and hazardous as heroin when injected.

Dividing drugs into 'hard' and 'soft' therefore makes little sense; too much depends on the dose and how it is taken. In the development of a serious drug habit, progression from swallowing to mainlining is as great a hazard as increasing the strength or taking more potent drugs. Worst of all, addicts desperate for supplies sometimes turn to injection of alternative drugs without thinking of their suitability. Examples include impure heroin, more suitable for smoking or taking by mouth, and injection of the powder from barbiturate sleeping capsules—which only partially dissolves and is caustic and unsterile. Injection of questionable drugs, often with unsterile water and careless technique, can lead to septicaemia, infective HEPATITIS and other infections, while barbiturates burn through the skin from beneath if they fail to enter a vein, causing deep ulcers. The sharing of needles is a major cause of HIV-infection, and hence of AIDS. Some addicts seem to be more hooked on the act of injecting than on some particular drug. They will turn to any alternative, even injecting water or air if they can get no drugs.

THE STIMULANT DRUGS

The chief stimulants to be abused are amphetamines (and other drugs prescribed to slimmers for reducing appetite), ephedrine and adrenaline (and related drugs, used against asthma), and cocaine (formerly used as a local anaesthetic). Very occasionally strychnine, better known as a poison, is also abused; it may be present in LSD, unknown to the taker. Nicotine (in tobacco) and caffeine (in coffee, tea and cola drinks) are also stimulants on which people become dependent. But they are not usually regarded as drugs of abuse, partly because they are so widely accepted.

The slang term 'speed' is used for stimulants in general,

or for particular types, especially amphetamines taken by injection. Amphetamines are usually taken as tablets or capsules. Many of these 'pep pills' or 'uppers' are coloured and have slang names to match, such as 'blues' and 'black bombers'.

How stimulants act The stimulant drugs all mimic the natural effects of adrenaline—one of the body's hormones which keys up the body for instant action. Stimulants increase activity and reduce hunger—because eating is relatively unimportant at moments of crisis. They brighten a person's mood and many takers feel sexually stimulated. There is increased mental alertness and a feeling of physical strength.

All the stimulants are habit-forming. This is primarily because when the effects of the drug wear off they are replaced by a feeling of deep depression and fatigue (the 'rebound'). The user will take the drug again not only to regain the original feeling of elation but also to relieve the depression.

Excessive dosage eventually produces a mental state in which the taker becomes unaware of what is going on around him or the consequences of his actions. This mentally disordered state sometimes lasts for several days. Accidents may be caused and crimes committed under the influence of stimulants, which are sometimes taken by young delinquents to give them 'Dutch courage'.

With repeated doses of amphetamines, whether for slimming or in the case of abuse, the stimulant effect soon declines. 'Tolerance' is said to have developed. Larger and more frequent doses may be taken and a drug habit becomes easily established.

Cocaine, known as 'coke', 'crack', or 'C', is obtained from the leaves of the coca bush that grows in the Andes. People there chew the leaves to obtain the drug, but it is supplied on the black market as a much more potent white powder, 'snow'. Cocaine is usually taken by sniffing, but can also be injected.

In small doses cocaine, like other stimulants, produces a pleasurable state of well-being. In larger doses it acts as an intoxicant and produces excitement, mental confusion and, rarely, convulsions.

Regular use leads to severe personality disturbances, inability to sleep, loss of appetite and consequently weight, increased tendency to violence, and hallucinations—especially tactile ones such as the feeling that bugs are crawling under the skin. Prolonged sniffing of cocaine can eventually damage the nose, by impairing its blood supply. Other organs, including the brain, can also be damaged.

SEDATIVES

When abused, sedatives are the most dangerous of all the

mood-changing drugs. They are physically addictive and may kill if taken in overdose.

Sedatives fall into three main groups: barbiturates and other sleeping drugs, and tranquillisers; the opiates (heroin, morphine, codeine and methadone); and alcohol.

How sedatives act Sometimes referred to as 'downers', sedatives change mood in the opposite direction to 'uppers'—calming and relaxing rather than stimulating. Stimulants and sedatives, however, do not counteract all one another's effects. Their combined intoxicant effects tend to be cumulative. The 'purple hearts' of some years ago seemed to be all the more habit-forming because they contained both a barbiturate sedative and an amphetamine. Many patients complaining of anxiety or difficulty in sleeping are prescribed regular sleeping-pills or tranquillisers and become to some extent mentally dependent on them. Tolerance may also develop, with a need for larger doses, but this hardly amounts to addiction. It may not be ideal to rely on such drugs, but they do help people cope with life's stresses. Very few patients become physically dependent on prescribed barbiturates, morphine or heroin.

All three groups of sedatives have much in common. Moderate doses produce a relaxing effect and relieve stress. Larger doses of barbiturates and tranquillisers tend to be misused for their intoxicant action, often together with alcohol, which intensifies the effect. Accidents under their combined influence, on the road and elsewhere, and accidental overdosage are among the main hazards of drug abuse.

All sedatives are physically addictive, some more so than others. The physical dependence can be overcome relatively quickly by gradual withdrawal of the drug over three weeks or so, though this usually requires constant supervision. But psychological dependence is much more difficult to overcome.

Heroin addiction in girls often leads to their periods stopping, but some nevertheless become pregnant. Babies born to mothers who are addicted to heroin or barbiturates at the time of delivery are themselves physically dependent on the drug, and are likely to die unless they receive gradual withdrawal treatment during the first week or two after birth. Provided that is done, there seem to be few if any further ill effects on the child's development.

Other hazards of heroin abuse are respiratory failure from overdosage, collapsed veins, and infections resulting from the use of unsterile syringes and needles. Sharing needles can spread infective hepatitis and even malaria from one addict to another. Some heroin addicts are badly fed and live in poor conditions. This gives them limited resistance to infection and inclement weather.

An overdosage of any of the sedative drugs leads to unconsciousness or coma, which demands emergency care. The main thing is to ensure a clear airway for the unconscious patient to continue breathing. But if the breathing actually stops after mainlining heroin or a barbiturate, it is vital to perform mouth-to-mouth resuscitation promptly. *See* FIRST AID *page 555*.

How sedatives are taken Barbiturates and other sleeping-pills, and tranquillisers, are nearly all made chemically, and are usually taken as tablets or coloured capsules, but some can be injected.

The opiates include heroin ('H', 'horse'), morphine, codeine, methadone, and other strong analgesics (pain-killers) such as pethidine and pentazocine. Some are still obtained from the opium poppy; others are synthetic drugs with similar effects. *See* MEDICINES, 22.

Heroin and morphine, often in the form of white or off-white powder for dissolving in water, are usually injected by addicts. They may also be sniffed, though this has a less-powerful effect.

Raw opium is traditionally smoked, but can also be eaten. Some opiates are available in cough mixtures or linctuses, or diarrhoea preparations.

Alcohol, which is commonly regarded as a social 'stimulant', is actually a sedative which only appears to stimulate in the early stages of intoxication, when it overcomes inhibitions. *See* ALCOHOLISM.

HALLUCINOGENS

There are two main groups of hallucinogens—those that are chemically produced, and those that come from plants.

LSD (lysergic acid diethylamide, or 'acid'), the best-known hallucinogen, is illicitly produced, although it was originally derived from ergot—a fungus on rye and wheat. Other chemically synthesised hallucinogens include DMT, STP and PCP ('angel's dust').

Chief among the natural hallucinogens are mescaline (usually in the form of dried buttons from the peyote cactus which grows in the south-west USA and Mexico), and psilocybin and psilocin which come from Mexican mushrooms. Many other natural hallucinogens exist, however, some found growing in Britain, such as 'magic mushrooms'.

How hallucinogens act Hallucinogens all produce a wide range of effects, but there is apparently no reaction that is distinctive for a particular drug. They are now usually taken in the form of tablets or capsules. LSD is so powerful that it may be prepared in 'microdots' not much larger than a full stop.

Hallucinogens all produce a 'trip' which usually comes on within 40 minutes of taking a dose by mouth and lasts for several hours. A typical trip consists of a weird mixture of distorted reality, chiefly in the form of highly coloured, rapidly changing images, intermingled with dreams or nightmares. It amounts, in effect, to temporary mental disorder.

'Good' trips are exciting and colourful, and give many takers an illusion of creativity and insight, even of being all-knowing.

'Bad' trips can be extremely frightening, with the 'tripper' terrified by nightmarish experiences, and may call for emergency measures. However, ambulances with

Drugs and the law

The Misuse of Drugs Act 1971 is intended to limit the availability of drugs of abuse and to stop trafficking. Although the law is directed mainly against criminal 'pushers', most of the 15,000 people convicted or cautioned for drug offences each year in Britain are takers rather than suppliers.

☐ The 'controlled' drugs are divided into three classes, depending on how dangerous they are judged to be. The seriousness of any offence depends on the quantity of the drug involved and its class.

☐ Class A drugs are officially considered to be the most dangerous. There are 99 drugs in the group, including heroin, morphine, cocaine, LSD, injectable amphetamines, cannabinol, opium and mescaline. Class A drugs attract maximum penalties of life imprisonment and an unlimited fine for trafficking, and seven years for simple possession. The other classes attract lesser penalties.

☐ Class B contains 13 drugs including amphetamines, herbal cannabis, cannabis resin and codeine.

☐ Class C contains ten drugs including several amphetamines.

☐ Not all drugs of abuse are controlled by the Act. For example, it does not cover barbiturates or most tranquillisers, but the law may be changed.

☐ It is an offence to possess, import, supply, produce, or—in the case of cannabis—grow a controlled drug unless you have the authority to do so. It is not an offence in itself to take drugs, but when a blood or urine test reveals a controlled drug in someone's body this may be counted as possession.

☐ If a person is found with a controlled drug in his possession he will have to prove that he is entitled to have it—by producing a medical prescription, for example—or that he was unaware that he had taken the drug or had it in his possession.

☐ If a policeman has reasonable grounds for suspecting that someone is in possession of a controlled drug he can stop and search him without a warrant.

☐ To search a person's home or any other building, the police need a search warrant. They do not need a warrant to search vehicles, and the Customs and Excise have wide powers of search inland as well as at ports and airports, and on board can search ships or aircraft.

☐ If you are in charge of premises it is an offence knowingly to allow the production of drugs, supplying of drugs, preparing opium for smoking or the smoking of opium, cannabis or cannabis resin. If an offence is committed on your premises without your knowledge you have not committed an offence. A person in charge of premises is not obliged to report evidence of drug practices to the police, but if he does not, he runs the risk of being charged as an accessory.

☐ If you know, or suspect, that someone is taking drugs you are not obliged to report the matter to the police, or to report suspected possession.

☐ If you take a controlled drug away from another person to prevent him from committing or continuing to commit an offence you are not guilty of unauthorised possession, provided that you deliver it to someone legally entitled to take control of the drug—usually the police—or destroy it, as soon as possible.

flashing lights, agitated people and constant movement can make a bad trip more terrifying. It is generally better to get the tripper into a quiet, darkened room and try to 'talk him down' into a calmer state. If medical help is needed, try to get the doctor to visit. If the tripper becomes violent, more than one person may be needed to restrain him. Trips seldom last longer than four or five hours, passing into sleep.

Accidents are a major hazard of taking hallucinogens—particularly accidents in traffic, or when trippers believe they can fly from a high window or walk on water.

Physical tolerance to hallucinogens develops quite rapidly—reducing the intensity of successive trips—and disappears as rapidly after a few days off the drug. There is no real addiction to hallucinogens, and no withdrawal symptoms after long use.

Persistent mental disorder has, however, been reported after trips. People with a previous history of mental instability appear to be particularly vulnerable.

Some psychologists have related the effects of the hallucinogens to schizophrenia. The strychnine sometimes taken to intensify the effect can be a major hazard, and 'flashbacks' (like replays of short sequences) can happen days or weeks after a trip. They also appear to be brought on by smoking cannabis. The effective dose of LSD is very low compared to the lethal dose, and so there is little danger from accidental overdosage.

CANNABIS
Two preparations are produced from the Indian hemp plant: herbal cannabis, known as 'pot', 'grass' or 'marijuana', consists of the dried leaves and flowering heads of the plant; cannabis resin, called 'resin' or 'hash' (from hashish), is the more concentrated dried sap of the plant.

Some cannabis is imported in traditional forms such as 'Thai sticks' (dark in colour and resembling a slender stick) and a small amount as extracts in oil. The drug in cannabis can be dissolved in many oils, such as salad oil or cooking oil, which can be dropped on to a tobacco cigarette. These oil extracts are made to escape detection by customs or police.

How cannabis acts The active ingredient in all types of cannabis is tetrahydrocannabinol (THC). The different types vary widely in strength—from some herbal cannabis that is too weak to have any appreciable intoxicant effect, to the strongest resin that may contain as much as 100 times more THC. The strength differs with the preparation and the climate in which it is grown.

In Britain, with its cool climate, only a very weak form of cannabis can be grown. This is of similar strength to the weakest Indian preparation, bhang, made of cannabis leaves. The most potent form of cannabis is hashish (or

charas), made of pure resin. Ghanja, which is made in India from the flowering tops, stems, leaves and twigs, contains less THC than hashish but is still one of the more potent forms. Cannabis reaches Europe illicitly from many sources in North Africa, the Middle and Far East, and Central and South America.

Cannabis is generally smoked. The dried leaves or crumbled resin are sometimes mixed with tobacco in home-made cigarettes ('joints' or 'reefers'), which are usually large enough to be shared by several smokers and have a filter to cool the hot smoke of herbal forms. The strength of cannabis is very hard for the inexperienced taker to assess. Some herbal forms weak in THC make hot pungent smoke, while strong resin with a more intoxicant effect may smoke cooler and milder when added to tobacco.

THC is rapidly absorbed from smoke, but cannabis is also taken in the form of sweets or cake, and in this form absorption is unreliable and may be delayed for several hours. THC is longer acting than most drugs because, being insoluble in water, the body has difficulty in excreting it or breaking it down. Consequently, the after-effects of a bout of cannabis-smoking slowly decline over several days, and repeated doses have a cumulative effect.

The cannabis smoker typically becomes relaxed and drowsy. Cannabis has a pain-killing effect. There may be alterations in mood—euphoria and increased sociability. Occasionally the taker may experience fear and anxiety. Distortions of space and time occur. Reactions may be slowed and the taker may be clumsy. Commonly there are feelings of depersonalisation, detachment, and a loss of a sense of reality. With some novices, and especially with large doses, hallucinations develop. Hashish, for example, can sometimes produce effects rather similar to those of LSD.

The main immediate risk with cannabis is that of accidents, particularly traffic accidents, as judgment, reactions and manual skills are impaired. It is as dangerous to drive under the influence of cannabis as under the influence of alcohol.

True addiction does not develop, and there are few withdrawal symptoms when the drug is discontinued, but an established cannabis habit can be hard to break, and seriously affects capacity for work or study. Drowsiness seldom progresses to coma, but large doses can provoke an acute mental derangement (with confusion, drowsiness and irrational behaviour which may require restraint). Known as cannabis psychosis, this may last for several days as THC is slowly eliminated.

Regular smoking lowers resistance to infections (by reducing the stomach acid and hindering production of antibodies). It reduces blood levels of the male sex

hormone testosterone. Habitual smokers may show some signs of mental slowing.

SOLVENT SNIFFING
A wide variety of solvents like benzene, trilene and carbon tetrachloride are sniffed or inhaled from many household products, including cleaning fluid, glues, nail-varnish remover, contact adhesives and paint thinners. All these products give off vapours. Most have a sedative effect like alcohol, and some act as anaesthetics, but takers sometimes describe stimulation, and hallucinations may also occur.

There are frequently distressing physical and psychological symptoms interfering with normal living—persistent pains, double vision, buzzing sounds, numbness and frightening mental images.

Many solvents are intoxicants not only in the sense that they make the sniffer 'drunk', but also because of their actual toxicity to body tissue, which may damage organs like the brain, liver and kidneys and also prevent normal production of blood cells. Some of the solvents—including petrol, the propellants in aerosols, or the contents of fire extinguishers—are very dangerous, and the safety margin between the dose that produces an effect and an overdose is hazardously narrow.

Solvent sniffing ranks as one of the most life-threatening forms of drug abuse—especially when a paper or plastic bag containing toxic solvents is held up to the nose and mouth for maximum effect, introducing the danger of asphyxiation.

Some sniffers also develop a habit that can be as hard to break as other forms of addiction.

DRUGS MISUSED BY ATHLETES
Two entirely different types of drugs are misused by some athletes and sportsmen to try to improve their performance: stimulants, such as amphetamines, and anabolic steroids. See MEDICINES, 20, 32, 33.

The stimulants simply stimulate the whole body to extra effort and stave off exhaustion for a few hours after a dose. They are therefore taken shortly before a game, competition or race. In rare cases, overstimulation of this kind has resulted in death while competing.

Anabolic steroids act more slowly to build extra muscle over a training period of weeks or months. They are therefore taken regularly, starting a considerable time before a competition, and often stopping for the last days or weeks to escape detection.

Both stimulants and steroids have been banned by all responsible international and national sporting bodies. Taking these drugs not only amounts to cheating; it can also seriously damage the health of athletes.

DRUG RASH

A rash brought on by an allergic reaction to a drug or combination of drugs. In some cases the drug or drugs may have been taken for years before causing a rash.

Symptoms
The rash, which is often accompanied by itching, may take various forms. The following are some of the more common:
- Generalised rash as in measles.
- Acute URTICARIA with wheals and puffy eyes.
- Unusual sensitivity to sunlight.
- A generalised redness or fine rash as in scarlet fever.
- Large blisters.
- An ECZEMA-like rash with small blisters and scales.

Duration
- The rash will persist until all of the drug has been passed out of the body; this can take many days, occasionally weeks.

Causes
- It is not known why some people are allergic to certain drugs.

Treatment in the home
- An irritating rash may be soothed by sponging it with cool water or applying calamine lotion.

When to consult the doctor
- If any rash persists for longer than two days.

What the doctor may do
- If he suspects the rash is caused by a drug or combination of drugs, he will stop the drug or drugs.
- He may prescribe antihistamine tablets to soothe severe discomfort and itching. In a few cases steroid drugs will be needed. *See* MEDICINES, 14, 32.

Prevention
- Do not take more than one drug at a time without first consulting a pharmacist or doctor.

Outlook
- The allergy and rash normally clear when the drugs are stopped and have no long-term effects.

See SKIN *page 52*

DUMPING SYNDROME
Faintness and nausea that sometimes occur after a meal in a person who has had a stomach operation, particularly partial removal of the stomach. The feelings are caused by the sudden emptying of the stomach contents into the small intestine.

DUODENAL ULCER

Gastric juices are most acidic in the outlet where the stomach joins the duodenum (the first few inches of the small intestine) and in the duodenum itself. Ulceration which occurs here is three or four times more common in men, particularly young men, than in women. Patients with duodenal ulcers, like those with gastric ulcers, tend to have group O blood and to come from families with ulcer histories.

Symptoms
- Burning, gnawing pain below the ribs, which may wake the patient in the early hours of the morning.
- Pain tends to start one or two hours after meals and continues up to the next meal, being relieved by food, milk and antacids.

Duration
- Bouts of indigestion after most or all meals recur for four to six weeks and are followed by pain-free intervals of months or even years. Milk or antacids temporarily relieve the pain but do not prevent it recurring.

Causes
- Stress, anxiety, overwork and smoking.
- Excess acid in the stomach. In addition there is often more pepsin, a digestive enzyme which breaks down protein in the stomach.

Complications
- Bleeding, perforation as in GASTRIC ULCER.
- Penetration backwards into the pancreas may cause PANCREATITIS with pain in the back.
- PYLORIC STENOSIS (the closure of the outlet from the stomach), caused by scarring and inflammation.

Treatment in the home
- Stop smoking and avoid stressful situations.
- Take small, frequent, milky, bland meals and antacids. These will help to neutralise acidity throughout the day.
- Avoid fried foods.

What the doctor may do
- Prescribe tablets to block the release of acid.
- Prescribe an antacid, or an antispasmodic. *See* MEDICINES, 1.
- Send you to hospital for a barium meal and examination with an endoscope, a device passed through the mouth to enable the doctor to see inside the stomach.

Outlook
In most cases the outlook is good. But severe ulcers may need an operation.

See DIGESTIVE SYSTEM *page 44*

DUPUYTREN'S CONTRACTURE

A fixed bending forward of one or more fingers, usually the ring finger and little finger. The condition is the result of thickening and shortening of the fibrous tissue under the skin of the palm. It usually develops from middle age onwards and is more common in men than in women. One or both hands may be affected.

Symptoms
- The first sign is a small lump that develops under the skin in the middle of the palm, usually opposite the base of the ring finger.
- Eventually, hard, fibrous, cord-like bands run under the skin from the palm into the affected fingers.
- Often the skin puckers over the areas of thickening.
- At first it is impossible to open the fingers fully; then over a period of months or years the fingers gradually close over the palm in a fixed position.
- In severe cases the fingers and hand may be unable to function properly.

Duration
- Unless treated, the condition is permanent.

Causes
- A predisposition to the disorder can be inherited, possibly through a slight defect in the body's immune system.
- It is more common in patients suffering from EPILEPSY and alcoholic CIRRHOSIS OF THE LIVER.

Treatment in the home
- None.

When to consult the doctor
- When the deformity starts to affect the function of the hands.
- Earlier treatment, by surgery, may only make the trouble worse.

What the doctor may do
- Refer the patient to a hospital outpatients department.
- The only effective treatment is by an operation that restores the ability to open the hand fully. But surgery may not be indicated in every case. In the elderly the condition may best be untreated.

Prevention
- None is possible.

Outlook
- Treatment usually restores the use of the hand, but complete correction of the deformity may not be possible.

See SKELETAL SYSTEM *page 54*

You & your doctor

SUCCESSFUL HEALTH CARE DEPENDS ON MUTUAL TRUST AND ON FOLLOWING A FEW SIMPLE RULES FOR CONSULTATIONS AND VISITS

Every successful relationship between patient and doctor is based on mutual trust. The patient needs to have confidence in his doctor. The doctor needs to feel that his patients trust him and will try to follow the advice given.

Building up a relationship requires time, understanding, tact, and an appreciation of the difficulties that both doctor and patient face.

In many instances contact with your doctor will be through his reception staff—and a friendly relationship should be established with them.

Do's and don'ts when registering with a new family doctor

□ *Do* register as soon as you can after moving into a new district. Avoid waiting until someone in your family is ill. Except in emergencies it may take two to four months for your medical records to be transferred.

□ *Do* ask your previous doctor to give you a letter with details that you can pass on to your new doctor if any member of your family is receiving treatment before your move. This is vital if you are moving to a new country.

□ *Do* take time and trouble when you first register. You may not see your doctor, but you can develop friendly relations with the reception staff. Remember that all future requests to see the doctor will probably be through them— and they will help you in every reasonable way.

□ *Don't* worry if it takes several contacts with the new doctor and his staff before you begin to feel relaxed and confident with them. This is quite usual.

CHOOSING YOUR DOCTOR

Many patients have definite ideas about the kind of doctor that they want—for example, the doctor must be young, must be a woman or must be 'like my last doctor'. Satisfying all these desires is rarely possible, and sometimes there may not be a choice. Apart from knowing his job, the two most important requirements are that the doctor should give the patient confidence, and that he should be easily available.

If you have moved into a new district find out as much as you can about the local doctors. A list is kept in the local post office, and the chemist will often give very helpful advice. Discover the views of your new neighbours and friends. Find out what sort of person their doctor is, how to get to his surgery, how easy it is to see him, and what arrangements are made when he is away.

When you have decided, visit the surgery and register all the members of your family who wish it. Find out from the reception staff surgery times, how to make appointments and when to put in calls; and also about any other services, such as antenatal clinics, that may be available. Doctors like to see patients when they first register. Practices provide a leaflet or brochure for patients, giving details of telephone numbers, surgery times and how to contact the surgery. If you have any difficulty in registering or obtaining a doctor you should consult your local Family Health Services Committee. You will find the address in the telephone book or at the police station, public library or Citizens Advice Bureau.

ARRANGING TO VISIT THE DOCTOR'S SURGERY

Many patients feel concerned when making a request to see their doctor that they may be bothering him over something that will turn out to be trivial. This is quite natural, and the doctors and staff prefer to deal with patients who are diffident, rather than over-confident, about medical matters.

Requests can be divided into four groups of increasing urgency:
1 Non-urgent requests for an appointment at the surgery when reporting progress or for a repeat prescription.

2 Requests for an early or immediate appointment for medical (or other) urgent reasons when reporting a possibly serious symptom for the first time.

3 Requests for the doctor to visit a patient at home when a child or old person is too ill to report to the surgery.

4 Emergency calls that require the doctor to stop what he is doing and visit immediately. For example, when a patient has suffered any possibly serious accident, is unconscious or bleeding heavily and is unable to be moved.

It is important to both the doctor and his reception staff that the patient makes it clear which of these categories is involved. It may be difficult for the patient to strike a balance between exaggerating the problem and understating it. Individual doctors and practices differ in their way of handling this problem, but the following points may be helpful.

NON-URGENT REQUESTS

For all requests, be prepared to give the following information:

1 Full name and address of the patient. Telephone number if there is one.

2 Full details of the nature of the main problems for which you wish the doctor's help. Such details should include the chief symptoms and how long they have been present. Be prepared to give all details (even personal ones) to the reception staff. Remember that they will have instructions to obtain this information and it will be treated in absolute confidence.

3 Give the age of the patient if under 15 or over 60.

4 Make it clear if you wish to see a particular doctor.

5 Describe any difficulties that you may have, such as transport or timing of the appointment.

Example 'This is Mrs Anne Stuart of 9 Orchard Road. My telephone number is 6688. I was discharged from hospital yesterday after an operation on my womb two weeks ago. I still have a slight discharge and may need a certificate for my work. I'm not sure if I can get to surgery by bus, but I have the chance of a lift on Thursday afternoon. I usually see Dr Able, who arranged the operation.'

URGENT OR SAME-DAY APPOINTMENTS

If you consider an appointment is needed urgently or on the same day, make this clear by stating your reasons and what is worrying you. Doctors and reception staff understand such fears very well.

Example 'This is Mrs Anne Stuart of 9 Orchard Road. My telephone number is 6688. My son, Steven, has a pain in his stomach which has been going on since late yesterday afternoon. This kept him awake last night and made him sick. The pain stopped an hour ago, but I am worried that he might have appendicitis. My husband could bring him down to see any doctor in the next two hours. Steven is eight years old.'

HOME VISITS

Doctors vary about the number of home visits which they consider necessary. In the USA house calls are rare, and expensive. But in Britain most family doctors consider that some home visits are essential. A first-hand knowledge of the patient's background is often an important aspect of

care. There is no legal obligation for the doctor to visit. Patients cannot insist that a doctor must visit, but if the doctor refuses to visit and the patient suffers as a result of his refusal, the doctor might legally be considered negligent and can be reprimanded.

The doctor needs clear, accurate information so that he can decide if a home visit is needed. Be prepared to discuss the details over the telephone with either the doctor or the reception staff.

Get in touch with the doctor yourself whenever possible. Mistakes and dangerous delays may occur if messages are left with neighbours and are then forgotten or misunderstood.

Give the doctor your full name, address and telephone number. Tell him how long the symptoms have been present and why you think a home visit is necessary.

Example 'This is Mrs Diana Smith of 12A Orchard Road. My telephone number is 5521. Could you ask the doctor to call and see my mother, Mrs Elizabeth Robinson, at my home. She is 66 years old. She has been having dizzy attacks for the past five days. She finds walking difficult since she fell two days ago, and she cannot manage to go out. She last saw the doctor with arthritis of her knees four months ago. She usually lives at 6 Station Road.

'We live in the top flat—I'll leave the bottom door open for the doctor.'

EMERGENCY CALLS

It may be difficult for patients to assess the urgency of medical emergencies. Sometimes it is obvious if, for example, the patient is unconscious. At other times it may be necessary to telephone the doctor with details and let him

decide how the emergency is best handled. For this reason it is essential that whoever calls the doctor should have full knowledge of the relevant details:

1 Full name, address and age of patient.

2 Exact nature of emergency.

3 Exact place that emergency has occurred and how to get there.

Example 'This is Mrs Anne Stewart. My mother, Mrs Elizabeth Robinson, has fallen while visiting my sister at 12A Orchard Road. Her telephone number is 5521. My mother cannot move her right leg and is in great pain. She fell at 10.15 a.m. (an hour ago). She was sick at 10.30 a.m. We have had to make her comfortable on the floor, as she is very heavy. Can the doctor come at once?'

Sometimes the doctor may decide to send an ambulance and not to visit himself. Alternatively, he might decide that the patient can safely be brought to the surgery or he might visit immediately.

An ambulance can be called without involving the doctor by dialling 999. This method should only be used in true emergencies where immediate hospital admission is considered likely.

ON SEEING THE DOCTOR

Patients are often uncertain about when to ask a doctor's advice. They may be afraid of bothering him unnecessarily, or afraid he is going to tell them something unpleasant. Doctors are used to such fears.

In most instances the doctor will

need the following information:

1 When the symptoms started.

2 Where and how bad the symptoms are.

3 What, if anything, makes them better or worse.

The doctor may wish to know other details about personal and general health, especially if the patient has ever been in hospital or has had treatment from other doctors. The doctor may also ask about the medical problems of your parents and family. Patients often find it helpful to write down a brief summary of such information before they visit.

Remember that all you tell your doctor is in the strictest confidence.

EXAMINATIONS AND EXPLANATION

Once the required information has been obtained and assessed, the doctor may wish to make an examination. Patients are wise to wear clothes that are easily removed. When the examination is completed, most doctors like to tell the patient what the medical problems are and what should be done. In some cases the doctor may perform further tests, send the patient to a consultant or hospital. In most cases such extra examinations eliminate the possibility of serious disease.

Patients often say that doctors do not explain what is going on. There may be several reasons for this: the doctor may think the patient knows already; the doctor may not be absolutely sure himself and be waiting to see how the situation develops. Only rarely is a patient kept in the dark because the doctor suspects serious disease. If not already told, the patient should make a point of asking what the doctor thinks is the matter when treatment or further action are prescribed.

TAKING MEMBERS OF YOUR FAMILY TO THE DOCTOR

Babies are difficult patients because they are frightened, cannot communicate and do not understand. Reception staff, nurses and health visitors are very helpful. They do not mind being asked to help, because they are usually as anxious as you for a trouble-free visit. Bring another member of your family to help if necessary.

Toddlers may be suspicious or frightened. Threats, bribes and suggestions that the doctor will do something unpleasant make matters worse. Even telling the child that the doctor is not going to hurt adds to suspicion. A brief explanation with a matter-of-fact parental attitude is usually best.

In the case of older children, parents should never worry if the doctor wishes to question a child alone. Later, the doctor will want to hear the parent's story. The same applies when an elderly parent visits the doctor.

WHEN THE DOCTOR SEES A PATIENT AT HOME

Whenever possible the patient should be alone in a quiet, warm room where it is possible to remove clothes for an examination. Turn off the television and radio and remove all cats, dogs and other pets. Curious children and friendly neighbours should be asked to leave.

REQUESTING A DOCTOR'S ADVICE BY TELEPHONE

This can be extremely helpful for both patients and doctors—especially when patients are ill at a weekend or during the night. There can, however, be difficulties because the patient's relatives are left with the main responsibility for care. The caller is wise to make a list beforehand of the questions he wants the doctor to answer. Sometimes it is helpful to ask the doctor if you can ring again if the problem has not settled after an appropriate lapse of time.

CERTIFICATES AND SICK NOTES

There is a special form to fill in to cover the first seven days of illness. The forms are obtainable from doctor's surgeries, DSS offices, hospitals and employers. After seven days' illness a sick note signed by a doctor is necessary.

REPEAT PRESCRIPTIONS

Modern drugs are very powerful, and their use must be carefully monitored. This is why drugs are available only on prescription. If a patient finds a particular drug helpful—a tranquilliser, for example—it does not follow that a repeat course is advisable.

Repeat prescriptions, which are those obtained at the patient's request without seeing the doctor, can save both time and trouble, but their issue must always remain under the doctor's control.

When the main cost of any prescription is borne by an insurance

---

Do's and don'ts when making appointments and putting in calls

□ *Do* make requests, whenever possible, during office hours and as early as you can.

□ *Do* make requests through reception whenever possible.

□ *Do* make a list or write down what you want to say. This will prevent you from omitting an important fact—and is especially helpful if you have to deal with an answer-phone. If you are not used to using an answer-phone, replace the receiver, write down your message, make a second call and dictate your message to the answer-phone.

□ *Do* make separate appointments for each patient who is to be seen. This ensures that the doctor will be prepared and have the correct medical records to hand.

□ *Do* make sure the doctor knows exactly how to get to your house if he is making a home visit. If you live in a flat, state which floor.

□ *Don't* exaggerate or minimise the reasons for calling to justify your action or get quicker service. The doctor has other patients to care for and may have to base important decisions on what you say.

scheme, including the NHS, the pre-scribing doctor is bound to prescribe only for the patient's current condition.

SOME DIFFICULTIES AND PROBLEMS

Despite good intentions on both sides, the relationship between a doctor and his patient can go wrong. But such difficulties can be solved. Here are some typical 'problem' situations.

SECOND OPINIONS
Asking any doctor for a second opinion may sometimes be both sensible and wise, but the decision should never be taken lightly because it implies a lack of confidence in your present doctor's advice. If, after careful consideration, this decision is taken, most patients find it easier and more tactful to bring a close relative or friend who can then ask for a second opinion on the patient's behalf. Ulti-mately, the patient's peace of mind is more important than the feelings of the doctor.

OBTAINING A DOCTOR WHEN AWAY FROM HOME
There are three ways of obtaining medical advice when you are not in your home area.

You can register as a temporary resident with any NHS general practitioner of your choice. You are then treated for a fixed period of weeks as being registered with that doctor. If required, you can also obtain medicines and NHS hospital treatment just as if you were at home. University students regularly use this process; they register with a doctor in the university town and then register as a temporary resident with another doctor if they need medical attention during the holidays.

You can report to the accident and emergency or out-patient department of any NHS hospital anywhere at any time. This department may treat you or may refer you to a local general practitioner, depending on your complaint.

You can see a doctor privately. In this case you will be expected to pay for both doctor and the medicines prescribed. If hospital treatment is needed your private doctor can still, if you ask, arrange this through the NHS.

When you leave home for any length of time it will be helpful to take your NHS card with you.

CHANGING FAMILY DOCTORS IN YOUR AREA
A patient may wish to change his doctor because it is no longer easy to get to see him, because another doctor provides a special service such as antenatal classes, because he does not get on with his doctor or the receptionist; or, more seriously, because he believes the doctor is pro-viding the wrong treatment.

CHANGING TO ANOTHER PARTNER IN THE SAME PRACTICE
Ask the reception staff how to change to another partner. This should not upset the doctor/patient relationship.

CHANGING TO ANOTHER PRACTICE
If you are not currently receiving treatment, it is not difficult to change to another doctor in your area. Make sure the new doctor will accept you as a patient, hand in your medical card (if it is available), and complete certain forms.

If you are receiving treatment, it may be difficult to change your doctor because it usually implies lack of con-fidence. Under certain circumstances a change may be wise, and every patient has this right. Careful con-sideration of the disadvantages is essential. You may be wise to discuss the change with a friend or relative.

First see the new doctor of your choice. Give him details of your present treatment and make sure he will accept your case.

RECEPTION STAFF
Receptionists and all staff who accept messages from patients are in a responsible and difficult position. They must always transmit essential information accurately and quickly to the doctor, while at the same time they should ensure that the doctor is not interrupted by less important or non-urgent messages.

The best way to gain the co-operation of reception staff is to state your problem frankly, openly and as briefly as possible, and let the recep-tionist then tell you what you should do.

Remember that your medical problems (and fears) will always have greatest priority, while the problems of your own convenience, such as the timing of appointments or difficulties of transport, will be balanced against the availability of the doctor.

Do's and don'ts when visiting the doctor

☐ *Do* make a list of all the matters on which you need advice.

☐ *Do* state the main reasons for your visit.

☐ *Do* tell the doctor of any fears or worries, however trivial they may seem to you. They are often important.

☐ *Do* give precise and accurate information. Avoid the often natural tendency either to minimise or to exaggerate information. Let the doctor decide whether something is important or not.

☐ *Do* be ready to undress quickly for an examination. Doctors appreciate patients who are prepared for this.

☐ *Don't* be afraid to ask the doctor to explain in ordinary language anything he may have expressed in medical terminology that you have failed to understand.

☐ *Don't* fail to tell the doctor if you are allergic to certain treatments or drugs—such as penicillin.

DYSENTERY

An infection of the bowel causing severe diarrhoea. There are two forms, one caused by bacteria and the other by an amoeba. Their initial symptoms are the same, so identification of the cause is important in order to determine treatment. The amoebic form is very rare in Britain but is more serious because the parasite is hard to kill, and may cause abscesses in the liver and lungs.

Symptoms
- Frequent bowel movements—as many as 20 a day in the case of children.
- Watery stools, often streaked with blood, pus or mucus.
- Griping pains in the abdomen and urgent desire to defecate.
- Vomiting.
- Wind.
- Tenderness and swelling in the abdomen.
- Children may suffer from high temperature, irritability and loss of appetite.

Duration
- Mild bacillary dysentery may settle, with rest and fluids, in four to eight days. Severe cases, however, may last for weeks before the diarrhoea stops and the stools are free of the bacillus responsible.
- Amoebic dysentery (also known as AMOEBIASIS) needs at least ten days' treatment. Since relapses are possible, the condition may require prolonged treatment.

Causes
- *Shigella bacillus*.
- *Entamoeba histolytica*.
- Both types of dysentery are spread by infected food and poor hygiene. Amoebic dysentery is also spread by water.

Treatment in the home
- Replace food with sips of water.
- If the symptoms are not too severe, try a simple anti-diarrhoeal medicine. *See* MEDICINES, 2.

When to consult the doctor
- If symptoms are severe, persistent or getting rapidly worse.
- If symptoms occur in a country where amoebic dysentery occurs.
- If blood, pus or mucus occur in the stools, especially after travel abroad or contact with other cases.

What the doctor may do
- Have the stools examined to identify the cause.
- Recommend a fluid diet and advise on hygiene.
- Prescribe antimicrobial drugs such as metronidazole in cases of amoebic dysentery and sometimes antibiotics in cases of bacillary dysentery.
- Arrange for specialist treatment.
- Follow-up treatment and tests are essential to ensure that the disease is eradicated. Bacillary dysentery may be considered cured if the stools passed on three successive days contain no *Shigella bacilli*. For amoebic dysentery, however, the doctor may advise six months of follow-up.

Prevention
- Boiling all food and water is advised if contact with dysentery sufferers is likely or if you are eating in a country where amoebic dysentery is known to occur.

Outlook
- In bacillary dysentery, good. For amoebic dysentery complete cure may be more difficult to achieve.
See DIGESTIVE SYSTEM *page 44*

DYSLEXIA
Word blindness.
See LEARNING DIFFICULTIES

DYSPEPSIA
Pain or discomfort in the upper middle part of the abdomen. It usually occurs after eating unwisely and is sometimes accompanied by belching and nausea.
See INDIGESTION

EAR
The ear may be affected by many different conditions including earache, discharge and hearing difficulties. These are symptoms of a wide variety of diseases.
See SYMPTOM SORTER—EAR PROBLEMS

EAR INJURY

Head injuries and loud or sudden noise can cause serious damage to the middle or inner ear or the nerve of hearing. Injury to the ear-flap alone is unlikely to affect hearing.

Symptoms
- Deafness in one ear following injury.
- Earache.
- Bleeding or discharge from the ear.

Causes
- Head injury with fractured skull.
- Loud noise. *See* NOISE INJURY.
- Sudden blast or explosion. *See* PERFORATED EAR-DRUM.
- Poking objects such as matchsticks or hairclips in the ear to try to remove hard lumps of wax or a foreign body.

Treatment in the home
- None advised.

When to consult the doctor
- As soon after the injury as possible, or if any of the above symptoms occur.

What the doctor may do
- Stitch the ear-flap if necessary.
- Look into the ear to check for internal damage.
- Send you to hospital if there is internal damage.
- If the ear-drum has a large hole in it (perforated ear-drum), it may need repair with a graft of tissue. If the bones of the middle ear have become dislocated, an operation may be necessary.

Outlook
- A damaged ear-flap should heal without side-effects. If the damage is severe or recurrent (as it sometimes is with boxing or rugby injuries) the flap may be deformed (cauliflower ear) but hearing will not be lost. It will remain even if the flap is totally removed by injury.
- Damage to the outer ear canal should heal without loss of hearing unless the canal is severely distorted or there is damage elsewhere as well. There may be increased tendency after injury to OTITIS EXTERNA or EAR WAX.
- Damage to the middle ear may result in partial or complete loss of hearing depending upon the severity of the injury.
- Damage to the inner ear will usually cause permanent loss of hearing. There may also be disturbance of balance, dizziness or vertigo.
- Damage to the nerve of hearing and balance will usually result in permanent loss of hearing.
- Skull fractures usually heal without treatment, although hearing may return only over a period of months or years, if at all.
See EAR *page 38*
FOREIGN BODY IN EAR, NOSE OR THROAT

EAR WAX

Small glands in the outer ear canal ('ear hole') continuously produce wax which protects the sensitive ear lining from infection. Tiny hairs (cilia) in the outer ear constantly force out the soft, moist wax. Sometimes the wax becomes hard and immobile, and blocks the outer ear canal. This causes deafness, particularly in the elderly.

Symptoms
• Deafness in the affected ear.
• Sometimes there is a feeling of fullness in the ear.

Duration
• Hard wax may remain indefinitely unless removed by a doctor or nurse.

Causes
• In the elderly, it is a normal part of ageing.
• Some people, particularly those with a narrow or long, external ear canal, are prone to the build-up of wax.

Treatment in the home
• Soften the ear wax by applying two or three drops of wax softener such as olive oil twice a week and keeping it in overnight with a small plug of cotton wool. This may reduce the need for syringing.
• Put oil in the ears for at least three consecutive days before having ears syringed.
• Do not attempt to clean the ears with cotton-wool buds.

When to consult the doctor
• If deaf in one or both ears.

What the doctor may do
• Syringe the ears.
• Remove hard lumps of wax with a small probe.

Outlook
• Although hard wax is easily removed, the blockage may recur after a period of months or, more usually, years.

See EAR *page 38*

ECTOPIC PREGNANCY

A pregnancy in which the fertilised ovum grows outside the uterus—usually in one of the Fallopian tubes. For a few days the tube enlarges with the developing fetus, then as the tube stretches and finally splits an acute abdominal emergency or 'ruptured ectopic' develops.

Symptoms
• Sudden, severe pain in the lower abdomen, or a less-severe pain in the lower abdomen with slight bleeding from the vagina.
• For one to three days before the tube ruptures there may be attacks of increasingly severe abdominal pain simulating that of acute APPENDICITIS. The pain may be on the left or right side of the abdomen.

• A period that is overdue by two or three weeks.
• Sudden collapse due to excessive blood loss into the abdomen.

Duration
• The length of time the pain lasts varies.

Causes
• It is more likely to occur in a tube that has been damaged by infection.
• A contraceptive coil (IUD) in the uterus.

Complications
• If the condition is not treated the tube may rupture, causing sudden collapse and even death.
• Occasionally the embryo dies in the tube, leaving an abnormal swelling known as a mole.

Treatment in the home
• None advised. Seek medical advice.

When to consult the doctor
• Immediately a woman in early pregnancy collapses or suffers pain in the lower abdomen.

What the doctor may do
• Admit the patient to hospital immediately for an operation to remove the embryo or tube.
• Arrange for a blood transfusion.

Prevention
• Avoid IUDs for contraception.
• The dangers of rupture can be reduced if, in pregnancy, any abdominal pain localised to the right or left side of the abdomen is reported to the doctor early.

Outlook
• Since only one tube is affected it is still possible to conceive.

See FEMALE GENITAL SYSTEM *page 48*

ECTROPION AND ENTROPION

These two conditions of the lower eyelids are sometimes experienced in older patients. Entropion is a turning in of the eyelid. Ectropion is a turning out of the eyelid. They are rarely dangerous, but can cause discomfort and inconvenience if not treated.

Symptoms
• In entropion: sore, watering red eyes.
• In ectropion: watering of the eye occurs because of the inability of the tears to drain away normally down the passage into the nose.

Causes
• Both conditions may be caused by inflammation or scarring following injury, but the commonest cause is either spasms or a slackening of the lid muscle, which can occur as the muscles age.

Treatment in the home
• None advised.

When to consult the doctor
• If you have persistent eye discomfort and redness, or persistent watering, especially in one eye, consult the doctor.

What the doctor may do
• He is likely to refer you to an eye surgeon. The treatment in each case is by a minor operation.

Outlook
• If entropion is untreated, the persistent rubbing of the eye by the inturned lashes can cause infection and later scarring, and so interfere with sight. Success with minor surgery in this condition is very high.
• An untreated ectropion, although unsightly, does not usually cause any damage, but it is better to have it operated on to relieve the discomfort of a persistently watering eye.

See EYE *page 36*

ECZEMA

There are five types of eczema (also known as dermatitis). They are all forms of inflammation of the skin, each of which passes through several stages. Initially there is redness due to the skin blood vessels dilating. Fluid accumulates in the skin causing swelling, itching and blisters. These burst quickly if the skin is thin, but much later if the skin is thick, as on the palms and soles.

This weeping stage may become infected but eventually dries with scabs and crusts. As the reaction subsides it may become chronic; the epidermis (outer layer of the skin) thickens with mild inflammation, leaving red patches of skin covered with flakes or scales. One or several combinations of these features may occur in any one person.

The five types of eczema—contact, atopic, seborrhoeic, discoid and varicose—develop at different ages in clearly recognised patterns. The site of the eczema varies according to the type.

Factors common to all eczema:
• Itching is very troublesome, but less so in most

seborrhoeic eczema. Scratching further damages the skin, which becomes infected and painful.

• When eczema affects the palms and soles it may form small blisters like sago beneath the thick skin. This is called cheiropompholyx.

• The dry, scaly, thick skin of chronic eczema exaggerates the normal skin markings. It may become cracked and bleed.

CONTACT ECZEMA

This develops in the exposed skin of persons sensitive to particular irritants. Even a few minutes' contact with the irritant can produce a rash as, for example, happens when people sensitive to surgical tape have it applied to their skin.

Symptoms
• Itching, small blisters, and redness at the site of contact.
• Weeping as the blisters are scratched or burst followed by flaking as the affected skin dries.

Duration
• The condition persists until the cause has been identified and removed.

Causes
Some of the commoner causes at different sites include:
• Head and neck: cosmetics (especially around the eyes), hairsprays, chemical dust, and plants such as chrysanthemums and primulas.
• Armpits: perfumes, antiperspirants and deodorants.
• Trunk: nickel fastenings and elastic on underwear.
• Between the buttocks and around the genitals: douches, powders, contraceptives.
• Hands: washing powders, many industrial chemicals (especially oils), dyes, flour, cement, garden plants, nickel in rings, bracelets and watch straps.
• Ankles and feet: dyes and chemicals in leather, rubber boots and gloves.

Treatment in the home
• Remove the cause when it has been identified and avoid further contact with the irritant substance.
• Report skin sensitivities to your doctor and at your place of work. If the irritant is a chemical or other substance that is used in industry, a worker may be able to claim compensation from his employer if the irritant is legally recognised. See OCCUPATIONAL HAZARDS.

When to consult the doctor
• If your symptoms are severe or interfering with daily living or work.

What the doctor may do
• If uncertain about the cause of the eczema the doctor will arrange for you to have 'patch testing' of the skin using different common irritants.
• Advise about protection and treatment.

Prevention
• Avoid direct contact with the irritant by wearing gloves, protective clothing or goggles.
• Do not use or wear articles known to cause eczema.

Outlook
• Contact eczema will clear, but is likely to recur if there is further exposure to the irritant.

ATOPIC ECZEMA

This type often affects people with a family history of disorders such as asthma or hay fever. Most cases of eczema in children are of this type.

Symptoms
• The skin is usually very dry.
• Itching is often intense.
• In infants, eczema usually develops about the age of two months on the face and head. Occasionally patches appear on the outside of the forearms and lower legs. It seldom involves the nappy area.
• In later childhood eczema is most commonly found in the elbow creases, behind the knees, and in front of the wrists.
• The older the child, the more likely is the eczema to become chronic with thickening of the skin, cracking and scaling.
• Acute eruptions with weeping and crusting develop in some people with chronic eczema.

Duration
• Of young children with eczema, half will have recovered completely by two years of age. In most cases the condition improves and then recurs unpredictably.
• In extreme cases, atopic eczema persists throughout life, but this is unusual.

Causes
• Atopic eczema is an inherited tendency associated with certain antibodies in the blood.
• Cold, wind and sometimes emotional stress often aggravate or precipitate attacks.

Treatment in the home
• The early inflammation, before blisters form, may be treated with calamine lotion to soothe the irritation. See MEDICINES, 43.
• Once blisters form, do not apply lotions which leave an irritant powder when dry. An oily calamine lotion with ichthyol added is soothing.
• The dry, thickened skin of chronic eczema will be helped by zinc and crude coal-tar ointment.
• Do not allow vaccination against smallpox as this can be dangerous to life. Other immunisations carry no additional dangers for people with eczema.
• Do not scratch.
• Regular use of a bath oil will help very dry skin.

When to consult the doctor
• If patches of rough irritant skin persist for more than two or three weeks in a baby or child, especially if there is much irritation or a family history of eczema or asthma.

What the doctor may do
• Prescribe corticosteroid creams to promote healing of the skin. See MEDICINES, 43.
• Prescribe sedatives to reduce irritation and scratching, especially at night when the patient is warm.
• Prescribe other medications, depending upon the progress of the skin.

Prevention
• With present medical knowledge, it is not possible to prevent this type of eczema.
• Avoiding climatic or emotional factors which are known to precipitate attacks may help prevention.

Outlook
• Although atopic eczema may persist for life, all cases will improve with treatment and most will eventually clear.

SEBORRHOEIC ECZEMA

This eczema develops where the sebaceous glands are numerous. When it occurs in the external ear canal it is called OTITIS EXTERNA; on and around the eyelids it is known as BLEPHARITIS.

Symptoms
• On the head 'cradle cap' in infancy is the earliest form. This varies from a few scales to a greasy cap of thick scales covering the scalp.
• Red scaly areas with cracks frequently appear in the creases above, below and behind the ears.
• On the front of the chest below the breastbone and on the back between the shoulder-blades greasy, red scaly patches often develop.
• Irritation is only slight or is absent. Greasy red patches of eczema occur under the breasts, in the armpits, around the navel and in the groin. These areas are normally moist and occasionally become infected.

Duration
• Response to treatment is usually good within a month. Without treatment the condition may persist for months or years into adult life.

Causes
• It is not known what causes seborrhoeic eczema.

Treatment in the home
• Regular washing will help reduce the chance of infection. Try to use coal-tar soap, as some soaps irritate the skin.
• Mothers of babies with cradle cap can be assured that the condition is not a result of poor motherhood. Proprie-

tary scalp preparations for babies are normally adequate, and the condition will often clear in a few months.

When to consult the doctor
- If the condition is not clearing up with simple remedies.
- If you have a discharge of pus, tenderness or boils associated with eczema, you should go to your doctor immediately.

What the doctor may do
- Prescribe the appropriate skin cream or lotion, steroids and antibiotics if necessary.

Prevention
- Seborrhoeic eczema cannot be avoided, but the frequent attacks can be treated early.

Outlook
- The condition responds to treatment but frequently recurs.
- Although annoying, this condition, unlike atopic eczema, rarely causes distress.

DISCOID ECZEMA
Patches of coin-shaped eczema, 2-4 in. (50-100 mm.) across, which usually occur in young adults and in middle life.

Symptoms
- The discs of eczema occur along the outer surface of the arms and legs and less often on the buttocks and lower trunk.
- Blisters, weeping and crusting are common.
- Infection of the patches may give the appearance of impetigo or insect bites.

Duration
- The discs, which do not usually grow in size, last from a few months to two or three years.

Causes
- It is not known what causes this type of eczema.

Treatment in the home
- Avoid scratching and treat as for atopic eczema.

When to consult the doctor
- If you suspect you have discoid eczema.

What the doctor may do
- Prescribe skin cream or lotion.

Outlook
- The condition will eventually clear itself in all but a very few cases.

VARICOSE ECZEMA
This type of eczema frequently develops on the lower third of the leg in later life.

Symptoms
- The eczema is a dark brown colour with much scaling and flaking of the skin, and is often around an ulcer.
- Varicose veins are usual but not always obvious.

- Weeping and crusting are common.
- Intense irritation.
- Secondary patches of eczema may occur elsewhere.

Living with eczema

☐ While nine out of ten cases of eczema begin in early infancy, the vast majority improve and clear before adulthood.

☐ Most eczema sufferers are treated with steroid skin preparations. It is important to know how to use these safely, not to assume that more is better, and to avoid lending them to friends 'to try out'.

☐ Many sufferers will want to try special diets or 'fringe' treatments, when conventional treatments fail to cure. It is wise to seek your doctor's advice first and not to expect too much.

☐ Itching and scratching can distress parents, infuriate teachers, provoke schoolfriends and embarrass the sufferer. Children should not be made to feel guilty: if itching is unbearable they must learn to rub, not scratch, be allowed to leave the class to cool down.

☐ Teachers need to know how to cope—and may need to explain to other children or assure their parents that eczema is not contagious.

☐ Eczema sufferers should avoid wool next to the skin and have a bedroom similar to that described for ASTHMA, otherwise few changes in life-style are necessary. Eczema is made worse by stress, so a calm and happy atmosphere is helpful.

☐ The more outside activities the child with eczema undertakes, the better: explanation in advance to instructors or leaders is important.

☐ The *National Eczema Society* produces leaflets for children, parents and teachers and sponsors numerous local self-help groups. Their address is 4 Tavistock Place, London WC1H 9RA (Tel. 071-388 4097).

Duration
- The condition may last for many years with a tendency to improve, then recur.

Causes
- Poor drainage of blood from the skin, due to stagnation in the varicose veins is thought to be the cause.

Complications
- Varicose ulcers may develop.

Treatment in the home
- Protect the skin from injury, as ulcers may develop in the eczema and these are slow to heal.
- Do not use strong ointments such as lanolin and preparations containing antibiotics.
- Wherever possible rest the foot on a stool to encourage drainage from the veins.
- Gentle washing and bathing will do no harm, but dab, rather than rub, the skin dry.

When to consult the doctor
- If the condition is spreading or very irritating, or changing colour, or if ulcers are forming.

What the doctor may do
- Advise a strict pattern of treatment combining rest, exercise, using elastic bandages to aid circulation, and special dressings. Treatment may fail, usually because the patient has failed to follow instructions.
- If varicose veins are present, the doctor will advise treatment by injection or surgery.

Outlook
- The brown colouring of the skin will be permanent but with patience the eczema will heal.
- Recurrence is probable at some future date.

See SKIN *page 52*

EJACULATION
The discharge of sperm from the penis into the vagina during the sex act. Ejaculation occurs when the climax, or orgasm, is reached.
See SEX PROBLEMS

ELECTROCARDIOGRAM (ECG)
A record of the minute electrical impulses generated by the HEART, used to determine the condition of a patient's heart. Electrodes are placed on the chest and limbs, and the impulses which they detect are amplified by an instrument called an electrocardiograph, to which the electrodes are connected. The electrocardiograph records the impulses as a tracing on graph paper. Deviations from normal in the tracing reveal the presence of any heart disorder. Electrocardiography involves no risk.

ELECTROENCEPHALOGRAM (EEG)
A record of the electrical activity of the brain, used to determine whether or not any brain disorder exists. The brain produces minute electrical waves whose patterns are altered recognisably by disorders such as EPILEPSY. The waves are detected by electrodes attached to the scalp. The electrodes are connected to a machine called an electroencephalograph, which produces a tracing of the wave patterns on graph paper. The procedure is painless and without risk.

EMPHYSEMA
Inflation of the tiny air sacs in the lungs. They become distended, their walls become thin and rupture. Any recurrent or severe infection of the lungs may lead to a loss of general elasticity; the lung then becomes over-distended and ineffective.

The most common cause is chronic bronchitis. In old age, another form may develop when the tissues of the lung wither.

Emphysema is usually part of another condition (bronchitis and old age) and accentuates symptoms already present, such as breathlessness and blueness of the lips. Most cases are diagnosed when a chest X-ray is taken.

Because the blood flow through the lungs is slowed down by the destruction of the lung tissue, an added strain is put upon the heart, and sometimes leads to heart failure. If emphysema becomes established, there is little that can be done to undo the process.

See RESPIRATORY SYSTEM *page 42*

ENCEPHALITIS

Inflammation of the brain, usually caused by a virus infection. It is a very rare complication of many common and otherwise harmless viral infections such as MUMPS, MEASLES and COLD SORES. Usually encephalitis develops during an acute infection. Occasionally, as in RABIES, symptoms take weeks or even months to develop.
Symptoms
- Headache.
- Fever.
- There is neckache or backache. The patient dislikes bending the neck or back forwards. The neck may be held rigid.
- Fits may occur.

- There may also be muscle ache and weakness, odd movements, and lack of co-ordination. These symptoms are variable, depending upon which part of the brain is affected.
Duration
- Usually several weeks rather than days or months.
Causes
- Virus infections such as mumps, measles, rabies and poliomyelitis can all cause encephalitis, as can several other viruses.
- The commonest cause in the United Kingdom is the cold sore virus. However, although cold sores are common, encephalitis caused by them is not.
Treatment in the home
- None advised.
When to consult the doctor
- Immediately for anyone who has severe headache together with a stiff neck and fever.
- A patient with encephalitis will be quite ill, and there will be no doubt that medical attention is necessary.
What the doctor may do
- Send the patient to hospital.
- The hospital will make tests which may include an ELECTROENCEPHALOGRAM, a CAT scan and possibly a lumbar puncture (testing fluid from around the spinal cord and brain) to confirm the diagnosis.
- Treat the symptoms, by providing painkillers for headache and anticonvulsant drugs to prevent convulsions.
- Prescribe antiviral drugs.
Outlook
- Most patients recover completely in a matter of weeks.
- A minority of patients (about 5 per cent) may die of the illness even with treatment, and others may suffer permanent effects such as poor memory or partial muscle weakness.

See NERVOUS SYSTEM *page 34*

ENCOUNTER GROUPS
A form of group psychotherapy in which participants are encouraged both to discuss their feelings and to touch and embrace each other. The object is to improve the individual's mental and, by extension, physical state, and his ability to form well-balanced relationships with others.

Various versions of it have been developed, chiefly in the United States.

One of the most publicised variants is EST, whose name comes from the Latin word for 'is'. Followers of EST say it is not therapy as such, though it may incidentally benefit health.

ENDOCARDITIS

A rare but serious and sometimes fatal infection of the lining of the heart cavity (the endocardium), the heart valves and the bloodstream.
Symptoms
- Unexplained persistent or recurring high temperature.
- Later there may be signs of rash, arthritis, strokes or mental confusion.
Duration
- Some weeks: depends on how soon treatment starts.
Causes
- Organisms enter the bloodstream and infect the inner lining of the heart. A normal heart may become infected, but usually the heart is congenitally deformed, or has been previously damaged by RHEUMATIC FEVER.
- Tooth extraction and other dental treatment is probably the most common cause of infection; but other medical procedures can introduce the infection into the bloodstream.
Complications
- If untreated with antibiotics the infection may spread by the blood to damage many organs.
Treatment in the home
- None advised. Consult a doctor.
When to consult the doctor
- When a high temperature lasts more than two or three days without apparent cause.
What the doctor may do
- Examine specimens of blood in hospital to see if there is any infection. He may then prescribe drugs.
Prevention
- Special care should be taken during dental and surgical treatment with anyone known to have a diseased heart or a congenitally abnormal heart.
Outlook
- Even with antibiotics, recovery is not always sure.

ENDOCRINE SYSTEM

The endocrine glands manufacture hormones—chemical substances that carry out work essential to the body's operation, and to life itself. The glands pass hormones into the bloodstream, by which they are distributed to the organs and tissues.

The 'master' endocrine gland is the pituitary gland, a pea-sized organ at the base of the skull. The release of its hormones is regulated by an adjoining part of the brain, the hypothalamus.

The pituitary not only makes growth hormone, which promotes bone growth, but also produces hormones that 'trigger' other glands into making their own hormones. Some, for instance, stimulate the thyroid gland to make the hormones regulating the body's metabolism—the process of chemical change that allows it to use energy and function. They are essential for both mental and physical development. Other pituitary hormones stimulate the sex glands—the testes and ovaries—to make the hormones that control sexual development and produce sperm and ova. Still more pituitary hormones stimulate the adrenal glands to make corticosteroids—hormones that, among other functions, allow the body to utilise the essential foods, sugar and starch, and permit a normal response to stress.

The adrenal glands also produce one hormone—adrenaline—without stimulation. Adrenaline prepares the body for 'fight, fright or flight' by strengthening heart, lung and muscle action, and slows the onset of fatigue. The parathyroid glands make a hormone that controls the level of calcium and phosphorus in the body—elements essential to bone building, the working of the nerves and muscles, and the conversion of food into energy. The placenta is, in part, an endocrine gland that regulates pregnancy.

When the endocrine glands do not work properly, drugs must be used to correct the condition and repair the deficiencies it has caused. For instance, the pancreas manufactures insulin, a hormone that regulates the use of blood sugar by the body—its source of energy. If the pancreas is not producing enough insulin, diabetes results, and insulin must be administered by injection. If the adrenal glands are not making corticosteroid hormones, preparations containing cortisone—one of the corticosteroid hormones—may be prescribed.

See MEDICINES, 30–34.

ENDOSCOPY

Viewing internal organs, usually through a flexible fibre-optic instrument. For example, an endoscope can be passed through the mouth, anus or penis, or through a cut in the abdominal wall. The doctor can inspect internal organs (for example to diagnose an ULCER), take specimens for diagnosis, and, if necessary, undertake 'keyhole surgery' such as the removal of GALLSTONES, female sterilisation, or treatment of enlarged PROSTATE GLAND in men.

ENDOMETRIOSIS

A condition in which cells from the lining of the womb occur in an abnormal position outside it, usually in the Fallopian tubes, in the ovaries or behind the uterus.
Symptoms
- Pain or aching in the lower abdomen or lower back, which worsens during menstruation.
- Pain during sexual intercourse.

Duration
- Until the condition is treated.

Causes
- Unknown.

Complications
- Infertility often occurs.
- Cysts may form in the pelvis.

Treatment in the home
- Take painkillers in recommended doses. *See* MEDICINES, 22.

When to consult the doctor
- If the symptoms occur for two or three menstrual cycles.

What the doctor may do
- Carry out an INTERNAL PELVIC EXAMINATION.
- If this confirms the diagnosis he may send the patient to a gynaecologist who may prescribe progestogens or oral contraceptives, which help endometriosis, or the drug danazol (*see* MEDICINES, 34).
- Alternatively, the gynaecologist may advise an operation to remove the abnormal tissue.

Prevention
- None.

Outlook
- Each attack of endometriosis settles after a few days.
See FEMALE GENITAL SYSTEM *page 48*

ENTERITIS
Strictly, enteritis refers to any infection or food poisoning causing diarrhoea; while the term GASTROENTERITIS indicates that vomiting as well as diarrhoea is present. Wrongly, the terms are used synonymously.

ENTROPION
An eye condition in which the lower lid and lashes turn inwards. It is not a dangerous condition, but is uncomfortable and causes sore, watering, red eyes.
See ECTROPION AND ENTROPION

EPIGLOTTITIS

A relatively rare but serious illness that strikes suddenly, mostly in children aged one to six years (principally in the second year). It occasionally occurs in older children and adults.

The infection causes inflammation of the pharynx, and swelling of the epiglottis.

Although it is a bacterial infection, other children in contact with an affected child are unlikely to be infected.
Symptoms
- Fever.
- Noisy breathing.
- Excessive mucus in the mouth with drooling.
- Difficulty in breathing, which often makes the child want to sit up.
- Cough, which is often hoarse or 'brassy'
- Rapid heartbeat and pulse.
- The symptoms develop rapidly over a few hours.

Duration
- With treatment, recovery begins within 24 hours.

Causes
- A bacterial infection of the epiglottis.

Treatment in the home
- None. This is an emergency: consult the doctor without delay.

When to consult the doctor
- You should consult the doctor if a child with croup is having difficulty in breathing.
- If the child's colour changes from pink and flushed to grey, pale or blue.
- If the noisy breathing is not relieved by steam inhalation. *See* CROUP.

What the doctor may do
- If epiglottitis is suspected by the doctor, he will send the child to hospital immediately for X-rays and treatment.
- The infection responds to antibiotic medicines, but if breathing is difficult a tube may have to be passed into the trachea. Sometimes a TRACHEOTOMY may need to be performed.
- Fluids are usually given into a vein, through a 'drip', to maintain adequate body fluids.
- Oxygen is often given.

Outlook
- Once the danger of obstruction to breathing is past, recovery is complete.

See RESPIRATORY SYSTEM *page 42*

EPILEPSY

A condition in which the sufferer has recurrent seizures. There are three main types of epilepsy: grand mal, petit mal and temporal lobe epilepsy (also known as psycho-motor epilepsy). A further category is the Jacksonian fit, which may occur by itself or be followed by a grand mal seizure. The symptoms differ for each type.

Epilepsy is not a mental illness and its victims are no more likely to suffer mental illness than anyone else. Although sufferers may not drive cars within three years of a daytime attack, they can usually lead an otherwise normal life. Epilepsy occurs in about four people in 1,000. In children—particularly under the age of three—convulsions indistinguishable from epilepsy may be brought on by a high temperature. *See* CHILD CARE—CHILDHOOD ILLS *page 151*.

Symptoms

GRAND MAL

• Sometimes there may be a few seconds warning of an attack. This warning, which is called an aura, may take the form of ringing in the ears, seeing flashing lights or a sensation of smelling, hearing or taste.

• Sudden loss of consciousness and stiffening of the limbs and neck, followed by rhythmic twitching or shaking of the whole body.

• During an attack, the epileptic will often bite his tongue, froth at the mouth and pass water—his face is either normal-coloured or red, not pale as in a faint.

• Once movements have stopped, the patient remains unconscious for anything up to half an hour.

• After an attack, there may be a period of confusion and drowsiness lasting a few hours.

• A series of fits, without the patient regaining consciousness in between them, is called status epilepticus. It is a serious condition and can be fatal.

• In babies under six months, fits may occasionally be confused with colic.

PETIT MAL

This occurs mainly between age four and adolescence.

• There is a brief loss of consciousness (without falling or loss of position), lasting a few seconds, when the eyes may blink or flicker. The patient regains full consciousness and carries on, unaware that there had been an interruption in consciousness.

TEMPORAL LOBE EPILEPSY

There may be an aura, as in grand mal, but the symptoms that follow are less dramatic to the onlooker. The patient does not lose consciousness or fall to the ground.

• The patient may have a feeling of unreality or DÉJÀ VU.

• Objects and people may seem far away or unreal.

• The patient may not be able to communicate properly during a seizure, although he may run, speak or even drive automatically as though sleepwalking.

• The patient may display temper or act violently.

JACKSONIAN FIT

• Twitching usually starts in one hand or foot or one side of the face.

• The twitching spreads to the rest of the muscles on the same side of the body.

• Unconsciousness and a grand mal seizure may follow.

Duration

• The possibility of having an attack always remains, but some epileptics (particularly children) can stop taking anticonvulsant drugs (*see* **What the doctor may do**, below) after a few years without a fit.

Causes

• An abnormal discharge of electrical activity from part of the brain. The electrical discharge can spread throughout the brain causing a grand mal seizure.

• In many cases the cause of epilepsy is unknown. Causes which can be identified include: birth injury,

---

Living with epilepsy

☐ As with many chronic disorders, the attitude of other people can make a world of difference to the patient. Like diabetics or the deaf, those who have seizures need to reassure others that they need not be frightened of the unfamiliar.

☐ Epilepsy can frequently be controlled well by anticonvulsant drugs, so it is wise to take prescribed drugs without missing doses. If unhappy with the treatment, do not be nervous of asking to see a specialist.

☐ Fits can be provoked in some people by stress, alcohol, fluorescent lights or watching television. Try to discover if any of these are harmful in your own case. Some people with epilepsy find that going without food for long periods or becoming overtired also brings on attacks. If you are one of these, eat regularly and get plenty of sleep.

☐ You must decide for yourself how much to tell others: knowledge is better than secrecy. Certainly a future marriage partner or employer should know, although if you have been free of fits for some years it could be a mistake to endanger your employment prospects by being too frank.

☐ It is not necessary to go to hospital if a fit occurs, and relatives and friends should be informed of this. If fits begin to occur more frequently than usual, consult your doctor.

☐ Young people entering a career should avoid working on heights and near unprotected machinery or fire. If epilepsy is controlled for three years, the only banned careers are the armed forces, flying and driving public transport or heavy goods vehicles.

☐ It is illegal to hold a driving licence after epilepsy while awake has been diagnosed, but it may be restored after two years' freedom from further fits. After a fit while asleep, the period is three years. Minor attacks, causing even very brief loss of consciousness, feelings of unreality or dizziness are as important as grand mal seizures when it comes to driving. Epileptics owe it to themselves and others to be honest about this.

☐ If you have a child who has fits it is vital to make sure his head teacher and class teacher understand how to react and what to do. If you do not feel capable of explaining, get the help of the school doctor or your family doctor.

☐ Epileptics need not avoid sport—although swimming by yourself could be a hazard, in case you have a fit when there is no one available to help you. Other potentially dangerous sports such as climbing or skiing are best avoided.

☐ Learn about your condition by contacting the *British Epilepsy Association*, Anstey House, 40 Hanover Square, Leeds LS3 1BE (Tel. 0532 439393).

infection (MENINGITIS or ENCEPHALITIS), STROKE, ALCO-HOLISM or DRUG ABUSE, BRAIN TUMOUR and degeneration of the brain in old age.

Treatment in the home
- Lay the patient on his side, without a pillow.
- Loosen clothing around the neck.
- Make sure there is enough space around the patient so that he cannot injure himself.
- *Do not* try to prise open his mouth, or try to give fluids, or try to force anything between his teeth.
- *Do not* try to restrict his movements.
- Once the movements have stopped and the patient is asleep, make sure his airway is clear. Grasp him under the jaw and extend the neck. *See* FIRST AID *page 612.*
- Allow the patient to rest if he wishes.

When to consult the doctor
- After a first convulsion.
- If the convulsions last more than five minutes, or are getting more frequent despite treatment.
- If there are two attacks within 24 hours.

What the doctor may do
- Take a careful history and examine the patient.
- Confirm the diagnosis with brain tests such as an ELECTROENCEPHALOGRAM.

- Prescribe anticonvulsant drugs. *See* MEDICINES, 23.
- Stress the need for regular meals and plenty of rest.

Prevention
- Because epilepsy sometimes runs in families intermarriage in two such families increases the risk of epilepsy in the offspring, and genetic counselling may be helpful.

Outlook
- Sometimes, particularly in children, treatment can be stopped after a few years and fits do not recur. But usually treatment for life is advisable.

See NERVOUS SYSTEM *page 34*

A WINDOW INTO THE BRAIN
The Cerebral Function Monitor

By monitoring electrical activity in the brain the Cerebral Function Monitor provides doctors with information about the condition of an unconscious patient which may help to prevent brain damage or even save his life.

The CFM is used in hospital intensive care units to monitor people with epilepsy, and, during operations, to check the depth of anaesthesia or warn when the blood supply to the brain is failing. The CFM is also used to monitor babies during birth, to call attention to any drop in the baby's oxygen supply.

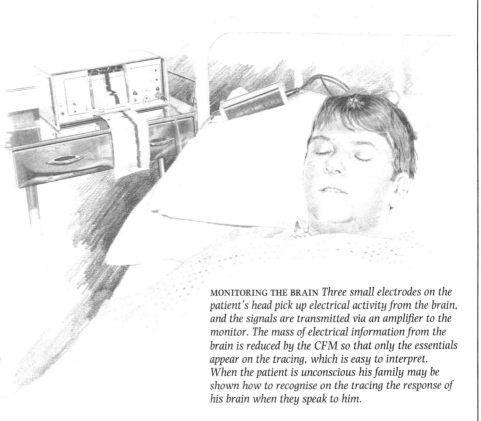

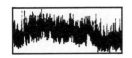

AWAKE AND ASLEEP *Recording of brain activity in a normal person falling asleep. The pattern varies slightly from person to person.*

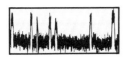

EPILEPSY *Each peak represents the disturbance of the brain during a fit. Between fits the level of activity returns towards normal.*

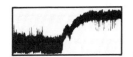

IMPROVEMENT *First signs of recovery in an unconscious patient who has taken a drug overdose. The patient first moved two days later.*

MONITORING THE BRAIN *Three small electrodes on the patient's head pick up electrical activity from the brain, and the signals are transmitted via an amplifier to the monitor. The mass of electrical information from the brain is reduced by the CFM so that only the essentials appear on the tracing, which is easy to interpret. When the patient is unconscious his family may be shown how to recognise on the tracing the response of his brain when they speak to him.*

EPISCLERITIS

A fairly uncommon cause of persistent redness of the eye.

Symptoms
- Episcleritis usually occurs only in one eye. It develops gradually with a dull ache being felt, rather than the irritating grittiness of CONJUNCTIVITIS.
- The eye becomes red and sometimes there is a little raised dull red patch on the white of the eye.

Duration
- With suitable treatment most cases of episcleritis clear up in a few days, although it is a condition which may recur.

Causes
- The cause is not well understood, but episcleritis can sometimes be a symptom of one of the rheumatic conditions which can affect joints and muscles in other parts of the body.

When to consult the doctor
- Any persistent red eye or ache in the eye should be reported to the doctor.

What the doctor may do
- The doctor will probably examine the eye with a light and a magnifying glass. He may then apply yellow drops to make the cornea visible and examine it for damage.
- If he diagnoses episcleritis he will probably prescribe drops and/or ointment.
- He may also carry out further tests (possibly blood tests and X-rays) to check if there is any other form of rheumatism elsewhere.

Outlook
- Episcleritis often persists despite careful treatment, but does not affect the eyesight.

See EYE *page 36*

ERYSIPELAS

A bacterial infection of the skin which rapidly spreads to the deeper tissues and caused many deaths before the advent of penicillin and the knowledge of necessary ordinary hygiene. Now it is serious but very rarely fatal. Erysipelas is spread by direct contact, and is seen in those between 40 and 60 years of age often during spring or autumn. Alcoholics are prone to the disease.

Symptoms
- The patient experiences a general feeling of ill health for about 24 hours.
- A red spot, usually on the face or scalp, enlarges rapidly over three or four days to form a red area of skin with a raised edge and a diameter of several inches that is painful, swollen and hot.
- The patient develops a fever with a high temperature, chills and vomiting.
- The inflamed patch of skin spreads, and the tissues beneath become swollen. The lymph glands in face and neck that drain the affected area enlarge, and become painful to the touch.
- Blisters may form in the centres of the patches.
- Sometimes the rash starts round a wound.

Causes
- A bacterium called *Streptococus pyogenes*.

Complications
- If untreated, the infection may spread to cause blood poisoning and inflammation of lungs, brain and kidneys. These complications may prove fatal.

Treatment in the home
- None possible. If the condition is suspected, consult doctor.

When to consult the doctor
- As soon as the disease is suspected.

What the doctor may do
- Take a sample of the fluid from blisters to confirm the diagnosis.
- Prescribe antibiotics such as penicillin or erythromycin. *See* MEDICINES, 25.
- Send the patient to hospital, if the condition is severe. The patient is kept in bed while the inflammation lasts. Dead skin is removed and blisters drained.

Prevention
- Avoid direct contact with known sufferers from the disease.

Outlook
- If erysipelas is recognised and treated immediately, the inflammation usually clears up within ten days and recovery is complete. Sometimes the disease recurs after a few months or years.
- If the patch appears on the legs, and the patient is elderly, there may be a long period of convalescence while the legs are swollen.

See INFECTIOUS DISEASES *page 32*

ERYTHROBLASTOSIS FETALIS
A rare blood disorder of the newborn, in which the baby's red blood cells are destroyed. It is usually caused by the incompatibility of the mother's and baby's blood. *See* RHESUS (Rh) FACTOR

ERYTHROMELALGIA

Attacks of red, warm and painful blotches on the hands and feet, mainly affecting the middle-aged. Attacks are triggered off by warming not cooling the limb.

Symptoms
- Burning sensation associated with red blotches on the hands and feet.

Duration
- A few minutes to several hours.

Causes
- Unknown.

Treatment in the home
- Cool the hands and feet with a fan and raise them.
- Remove clothes or bedclothes and cool the room temperature with a fan.
- Wear sandals and avoid the tight or thick clothing which triggered off attacks.

When to consult the doctor
- If symptoms arise.

What the doctor may do
- Test your circulatory system to exclude any serious disease.
- Prescribe to ease symptoms. *See* MEDICINES, 8.

Prevention
- Keep hands and feet as cool as possible. Stay out of the sun and do not wear thick gloves and socks.

Outlook
- The condition is harmless but is often difficult to cure.

See CIRCULATORY SYSTEM *page 40*

EUSTACHIAN TUBE, BLOCKAGE OF

The Eustachian tube is a narrow canal that joins the middle ear to the throat. In normal circumstances, air can pass through the tube to maintain equal pressure on both sides of the ear-drum and so allow it to pick up sound most effectively. Air can sometimes be felt passing through the Eustachian tube, for example when ascending or descending a hill, when flying, or when diving or swimming underwater.

If the tube is obstructed, the pressure becomes unequal and causes discomfort or pain. The ear-drum is also unable to function properly, and temporary deafness results. The normal flow of air is up the tube, into the middle ear, usually when swallowing. When the tube is blocked the ear-drum often cannot vibrate normally, and temporary deafness follows.

Symptoms
- Earache or a sensation of fullness in the ear.
- Temporary partial deafness in one or both ears.
- If the blockage is partial, and brought on by activities such as flying or diving, symptoms are more pronounced on descent than on ascent.
- Symptoms may come on quite suddenly when flying, but may take several days to appear if the cause is a common cold.

Causes
- Common cold.
- Chronic rhinitis.
- In children, enlarged adenoids.
- Flying or diving.

Treatment in the home
- Try to breathe out forcefully with the mouth and nose closed.
- Swallowing, moving the jaw and other movements of the head may help.
- Do not use ear drops.
- Steam inhalations may help, but be careful to avoid scalding. See HOME NURSING.

When to consult the doctor
- If earache persists for more than a day.
- If deafness persists for more than seven days.
- If the blockage is on one side only, and persists for more than seven days.

What the doctor may do
- Examine your mouth and ears.
- Test your hearing with a tuning-fork.
- Prescribe decongestant medicines. See MEDICINES, 41.

Prevention
- Avoidance of swimming, diving and flying may be necessary.

Outlook
- Most blockages last only a few hours, but if symptoms persist it may mean that fluid is collecting in the partial vacuum in the middle ear, and this can result in secretory OTITIS MEDIA.

See EAR *page 38*

EXCHANGE TRANSFUSION

A form of blood transfusion in which all the patient's blood is withdrawn and simultaneously replaced with new blood. A single syringe, fitted with a three-way tap, is used for both procedures. Exchange transfusions are given in certain cases of erythroblastosis fetalis, poisoning and liver disorders and RHESUS INCOMPATIBILITY.

EXERCISE

The daily routine for modern men—and women—often lacks the vigorous exercise for which their bodies are adapted. Regular exercise with specially arranged exercises can help make up the deficiency.
See KEEPING FIT *page 234*
POSTNATAL EXERCISES *page 248*

EXTRADURAL HAEMATOMA

A serious complication of head injury. The head injury causes unconsciousness (CONCUSSION) and also fractures one of the bones of the skull. This in turn ruptures one of the internal arteries which runs across the cracked bone. Extensive bleeding inside the skull occurs and a large clot of blood (haematoma) then builds up and exerts pressure on the brain. Death will follow if the pressure is not relieved by an immediate operation.

Symptoms
- The initial head injury causes unconsciousness (concussion). This may last for a few seconds or continue for several minutes or even hours. When the initial unconsciousness lasts for longer than two or three minutes the injury is usually recognised as being serious and the victim is sent to hospital at once.
- A more dangerous situation may arise if the initial unconsciousness is shorter. Then the patient, who may be a child, regains consciousness after the knock and is assumed to be all right. The possibility of a skull fracture and internal bleeding is not considered until the enlarging haematoma and increasing pressure on the brain cause drowsiness then further unconsciousness some two to four hours later.
- One side of the body may be noticeably affected by stiffness or paralysis.
- Pupils may be unequal in size.

- Vomiting may occur.

Duration
- Symptoms may develop over a period of two to six hours, but in severe cases their onset is more rapid. Death may result before any attempt can be made to save the patient.

Causes
- The skull is fractured over the middle meningeal artery. This runs in front of the ear just inside the wall of the skull. A mass or clot of blood builds up between the skull and brain. Continued bleeding brings increasing pressure on the brain, and an even deeper state of unconsciousness.

Complications
- Without treatment, the haematoma results in death.

Treatment in the home
- If anyone falls unconscious after a head injury, emergency first aid treatment is needed. The patient should be laid down and given plenty of room to breathe. Stop people from crowding round; the air must be allowed to circulate freely. If breathing stops, give artificial respiration. See FIRST AID *page 554*.
- Call an ambulance or doctor immediately. Even if the patient recovers consciousness after the initial blow and appears perfectly normal, he or she will need to be examined in hospital and possibly undergo a period of observation.

When to consult the doctor
- Immediately, if a person has been unconscious, even for a short time, after a head injury.

What the doctor may do
- Arrange for the skull to be examined by X-rays or scanning. If a haematoma is present an immediate operation will be necessary to remove it and release the pressure on the brain.

Prevention
- Most head injuries result from road accidents. The risks are reduced by driving carefully and wearing a seat belt.
- Observe speed limits. Whenever a speed limit is imposed on a stretch of road, the number of serious injuries falls.
- Motor-cyclists should wear an approved crash helmet and receive proper driving instruction.

Outlook
- In cases where the haematoma develops slowly and the patient is got quickly to hospital, an operation produces a cure. In severe cases, the pressure on the brain may build up so quickly that death results before treatment is possible.

See NERVOUS SYSTEM *page 34*

Keeping fit

AN ACTION PLAN TO BUILD UP YOUR SUPPLENESS, STRENGTH AND STAMINA

Man's body is adapted for regular, vigorous exercise, but in today's push-button, microchip, automated world it all too often does not get it. Exercise helps to keep bones, joints and muscles young. It can reduce the risk of heart attacks, and increase the chances of survival if you suffer one. It helps slimming by burning up the energy in food, and works off the tensions of everyday living. It can help to keep you in a healthy state of mind and cut down anxiety and depression. Above all, it promotes fitness.

Do's and don'ts about exercises

☐ *Do* consult your doctor before starting an exercise programme if you have a history of heart disease, high blood pressure, dizzy spells, blackouts, diabetes, persistent back trouble, arthritis, are convalescing, or are worried about the effect of exercise on some other aspect of your health.

☐ *Do* start gently and build up your efforts gradually over about six weeks. Stay comfortably within your limits.

☐ *Do* rest immediately if you feel pain or discomfort.

☐ *Don't* make the mistake of thinking that exercise must hurt to do you good.

☐ *Don't* take exercise if you feel physically tired—you are more likely to pull a muscle or sprain a joint.

☐ *Don't* take vigorous exercise within two hours of a heavy meal —you risk indigestion or abdominal cramps.

☐ *Don't* exercise if you have a heavy cold, feel ill, or are at all feverish.

WHAT IS FITNESS?

There is no scientific definition of fitness, but, as those who are fit will vouch, it is more than the mere absence of illness or disease, more than simply feeling well. It is a manifestation of *positive* health, the physical expression of vitality. It is having the capacity to cope with the physical demands most people face each day . . . and having a little extra left in reserve.

The fitness programme outlined here will not turn you into Superman or Superwoman. It will help anyone— from the youngest to the oldest— establish how fit he or she is and build up from there, in gentle stages, to a basic level of fitness which can be further developed, or simply maintained.

TEST YOUR OWN FITNESS

Here is a simple fitness test to try at home. Before tackling it, read the 'Do's and don'ts' panel on this page.

Stand with your feet together in front of a step 8 in. (200 mm.) high. For three minutes, step up and down at the rate of two complete movements every five seconds. A 'complete movement' means one foot up, the other foot up, then one foot

Building up to basic fitness

This exercise plan is suitable for all but the very young and the very old.

Before carrying it out, study the Do's and don'ts panel and the fitness test on the left.

The plan is based on 25 minute sessions—
two minutes for suppleness, three minutes for strength and 20 minutes for stamina. Plan at least two sessions a week.

The suppleness exercises warm up the muscles, reducing the risk of muscle pulls. They involve slow, gentle stretching, keeping within your limits of comfort.

The strength exercises build up power in your arms, trunk and legs.

The stamina exercises form the core of any fitness programme. Any activity that makes you moderately breathless, will have a stamina-building effect.

SUPPLENESS EXERCISE 1

Side bends

Time allowance: 30 seconds

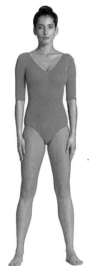

In doing this exercise, push the palms of your hands as far down the outside of your legs as is comfortable.

1 Stand with your feet about 12 in. (300 mm.) apart and your arms by your sides.

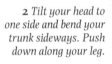

2 Tilt your head to one side and bend your trunk sideways. Push down along your leg.

3 Repeat to the other side. Alternate the movement from one side to the other for 30 seconds.

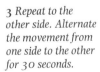

235

down, the other foot down. *Stop if you begin to feel uncomfortable.*

When the three minutes are up, sit and rest for exactly one minute. Then take your pulse-rate (see below). If you are fit, it should be more or less back to normal. Check your fitness level according to the table below.

Your test result will decide at what level you start the basic fitness programme on this and the following pages.

Pulse-rate (beats per minute)		Fitness level
Men	Women	
Under 79	Under 84	Very fit
80–89	85–94	Fit
90–99	95–109	Unfit
100 plus	110 plus	Very unfit

Note: the figures do not apply to children.

THE COMPONENTS OF FITNESS
The three basic components of physical fitness are suppleness, strength and stamina.
Suppleness Suppleness means flexibility or mobility of the neck, trunk and limbs. The more supple you are, the more easily you can move your joints without discomfort. Suppleness exercises stretch and loosen the various muscles that work the joints. The joints themselves are tightened and toned up, while the ligaments that support them are shortened and strengthened.

Suppleness allows you to twist and

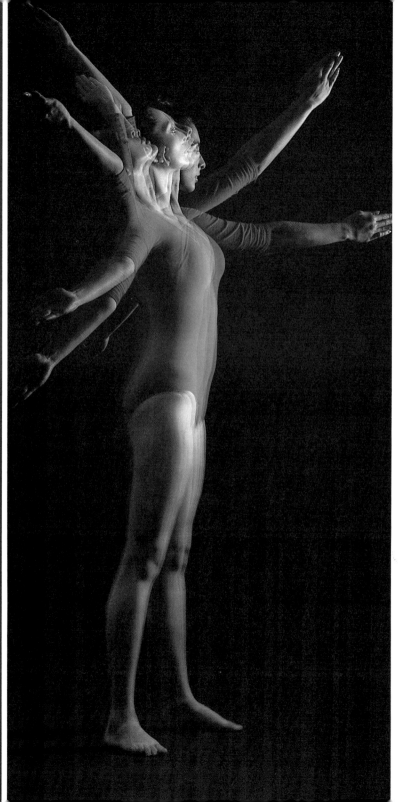

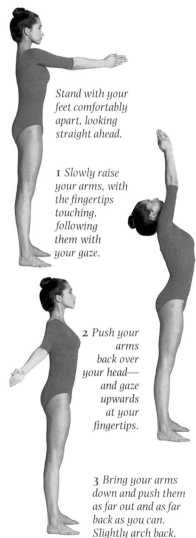

SUPPLENESS EXERCISE 2
Arm circles

Time allowance: 30 seconds

Stand with your feet comfortably apart, looking straight ahead.

1 *Slowly raise your arms, with the fingertips touching, following them with your gaze.*

2 *Push your arms back over your head— and gaze upwards at your fingertips.*

3 *Bring your arms down and push them as far out and as far back as you can. Slightly arch back.*

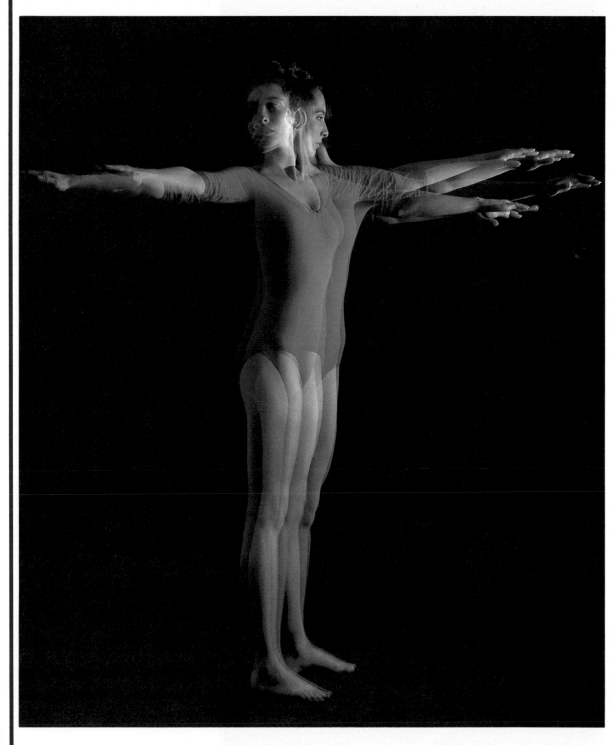

SUPPLENESS EXERCISE 3
Trunk twists

Time allowance: 30 seconds

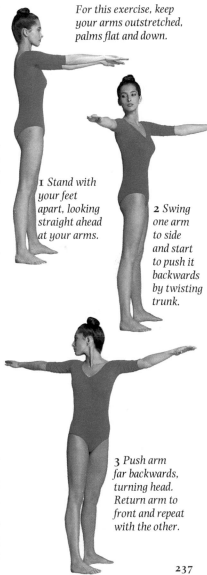

For this exercise, keep your arms outstretched, palms flat and down.

1 *Stand with your feet apart, looking straight ahead at your arms.*

2 *Swing one arm to side and start to push it backwards by twisting trunk.*

3 *Push arm far backwards, turning head. Return arm to front and repeat with the other.*

237

turn and bend and stretch without strain or sprain. It is an important component of fitness, especially for elderly people, whose muscles easily stiffen, making it difficult to cope even with ordinary activities such as getting out of bed, bathing, dressing and doing housework.

Activities that develop suppleness include dancing, YOGA, and gymnastics.

Strength Strength is simply muscle power—the maximum force that a group of muscles can apply to an action. Strength is needed for pulling, pushing, lifting and shifting. Strength of forearm muscles gives a strong hand-grip. Strong shoulder muscles make light work of lifting children or loading shopping into the car. Elderly people need to maintain the strength of their limbs so that they can get in and out of chairs or the bath with ease.

Strength is developed by exercising muscles against resistance—for example, by weightlifting, press-ups or bicycling. Broadly, the more resistance a muscle meets when it contracts, the more its individual fibres are brought into play. Muscles that are regularly exercised against resistance respond by becoming bulkier and stronger.

Stamina Stamina means endurance or 'staying power', and it is the most fundamental component of fitness. It is the capacity to keep going without gasping for breath or going weak at the knees. Any activity involving the rhythmic contraction of large muscles, such as those of the legs, requires stamina.

Running and swimming are examples. They are sometimes known as 'aerobic'—from the Greek words for air and life—because the working

238

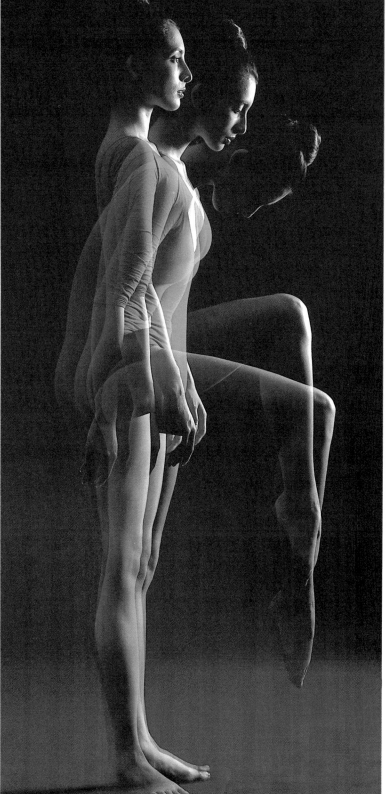

SUPPLENESS EXERCISE 4
Leg flexes

Time allowance: 30 seconds

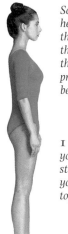

Some people may find it helpful, at first, to use the back of a chair to aid their balance while doing this exercise. But with practice the chair can be dispensed with.

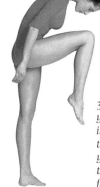

1 *Stand with your back straight and your feet together.*

2 *Slowly raise one knee, keeping your toes slanting down.*

3 *Continue raising your knee as high as is comfortable. At the same time lower your head and try to bring together forehead and knee.*

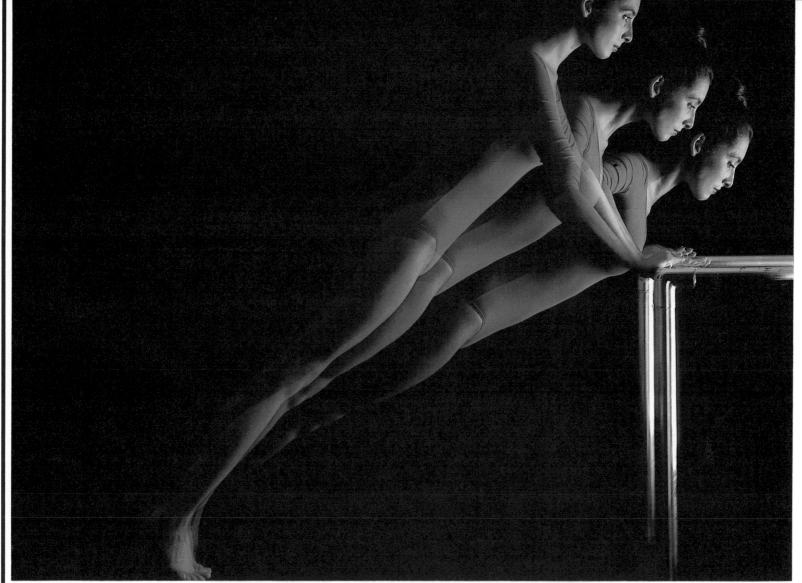

STRENGTH EXERCISE 1

Basic push-ups

Time allowance: 1 minute

To begin with, you should do all the strength exercises at the rate of ten a minute. Gradually speed up over several sessions to 30 a minute.

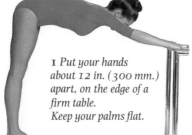

1 Put your hands about 12 in. (300 mm.) apart, on the edge of a firm table. Keep your palms flat.

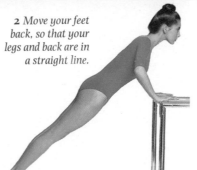

2 Move your feet back, so that your legs and back are in a straight line.

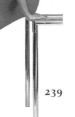

3 Bend your elbows and try to touch the table with your chest. Then straighten up.

239

muscles need a plentiful supply of oxygen. That puts extra demand, not only on the heart, lungs and circulation, but also on the muscles themselves, which must be able to extract oxygen from the bloodstream rapidly and efficiently. All these functions can be improved by exercising energetically and frequently.

WHY BE FIT?
For many people, the words 'fitness' and 'exercise' conjure up visions of agonising physical-training sessions in the school gym or the loneliness of the long-distance runner. In fact, far from being unpleasant, the whole point of exercise and fitness is to increase your enjoyment of life.

There are so many different ways to exercise and keep yourself in good physical shape that it is not difficult to find an activity or mix of activities that you really enjoy. Because keeping fit means taking regular, moderately vigorous exercise, it is important to choose something that gives you an incentive to continue. The table below lists a selection of activities and their exercise value.

Apart from the physical benefits of exercise, research has shown that exercise can help to relieve anxiety and lift depression. Athletes describe the 'natural high' that they get from vigorous exercise, and that is a very apt description of what happens in their brain. Scientists studying this effect have found that exercise seems to stimulate the release of certain natural hormones within the brain which mimic the action of morphine and have a pleasurable and pain-suppressing effect.

Being fit can also help to combat degenerative diseases. Inactivity can

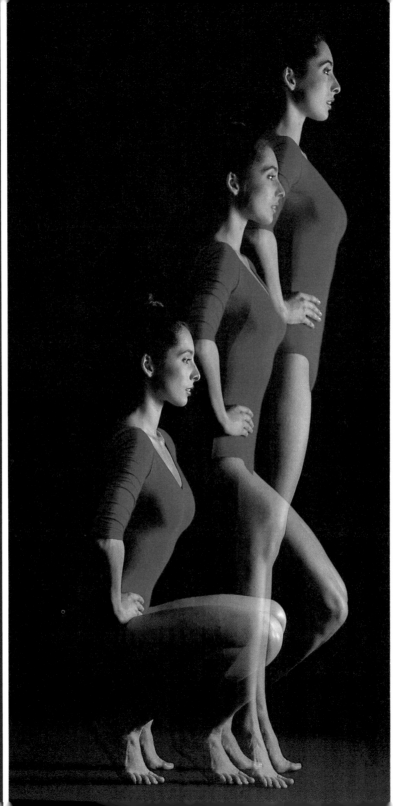

STRENGTH EXERCISE 2
Basic squat-jumps

Time allowance: 1 minute

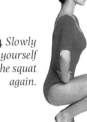

This exercise should be done hands-on-hips. But if this proves too difficult at first, use the back of a firm chair for support.

1 *Squat with hands on hips.*

2 *Slowly rise to a standing position. Hold this pose.*

3 *Keeping the standing position, now move up on to your toes.*

4 *Slowly lower yourself to the squat again.*

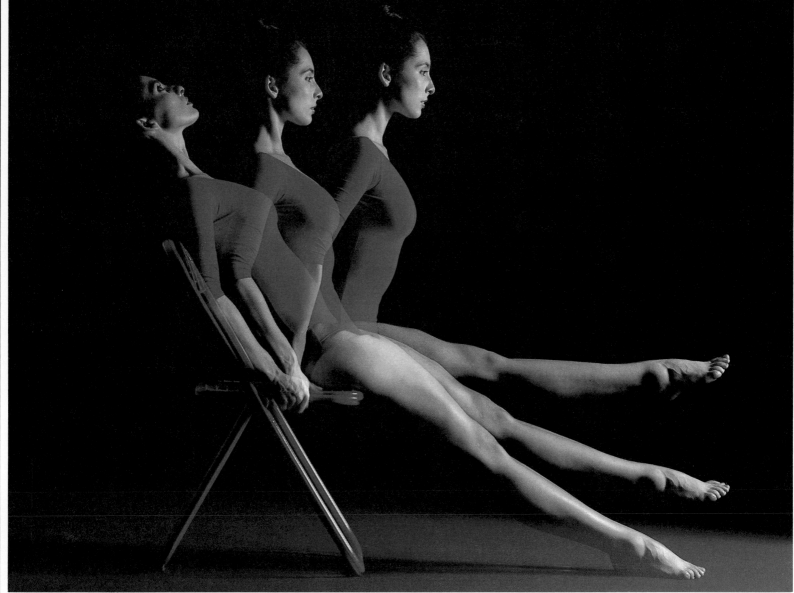

STRENGTH EXERCISE 3

Basic sit-ups

Time allowance: 1 minute

Use a firm chair—one that will not slide or slip about. Support yourself with your hands on the edge of the seat.

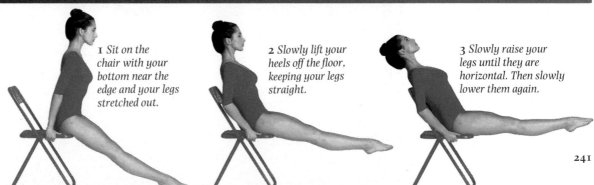

1 Sit on the chair with your bottom near the edge and your legs stretched out.

2 Slowly lift your heels off the floor, keeping your legs straight.

3 Slowly raise your legs until they are horizontal. Then slowly lower them again.

241

lead to problems ranging from muscle and joint stiffness to obesity, or from palpitations to an increased risk of heart attack. Regular, moderately vigorous activity with at least 20 minutes of stamina-building exercises twice a week, and preferably more often, reduces the likelihood of these conditions.

GETTING STARTED

The first and most crucial step to fitness is making the decision to get started. Obviously, it is going to mean extra effort—there is no lazy way to get fit. But that does not mean that you have to launch yourself into a rigorous physical-training programme. The essential thing is to start gently and build up gradually over the weeks.

While deciding which activities to pursue and how much time to devote to them, you can take the first steps to fitness by making a few changes in your lifestyle. Here are some:

Use your legs Walk more each day to work or to the shops. Use the stairs instead of the lift. Get off the bus a stop or two sooner. Take every opportunity to use your legs.

Sustained brisk walks of five or ten minutes are an excellent introduction to fitness. Each day, put a little more effort into your walking. Tackle more stairs and hills. Aim to spend at least five or ten minutes a day performing some activity that makes you moderately breathless—by putting a little more effort into the housework or do-it-yourself jobs, by playing tag or another active game with the children or by towelling briskly after a bath or shower.

Even standing still is better exercise for your heart and circulation than sitting or lying.

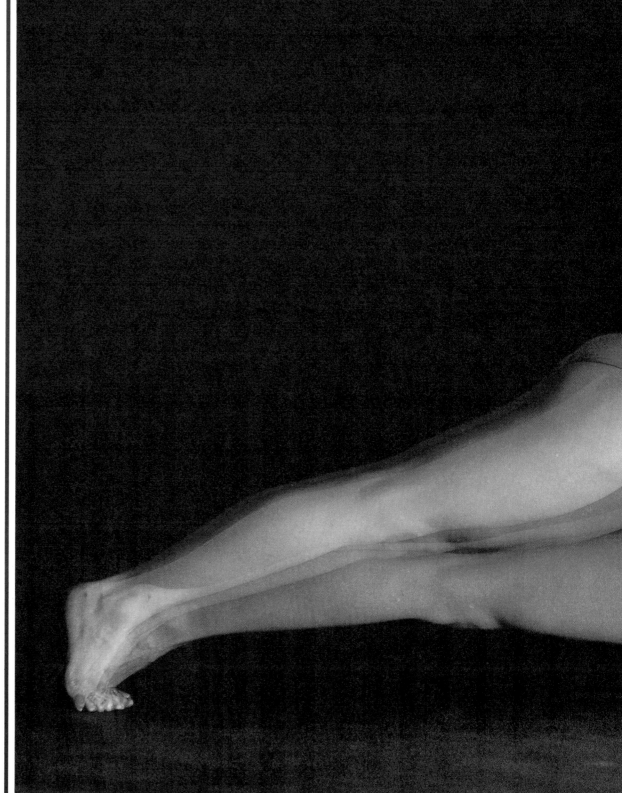

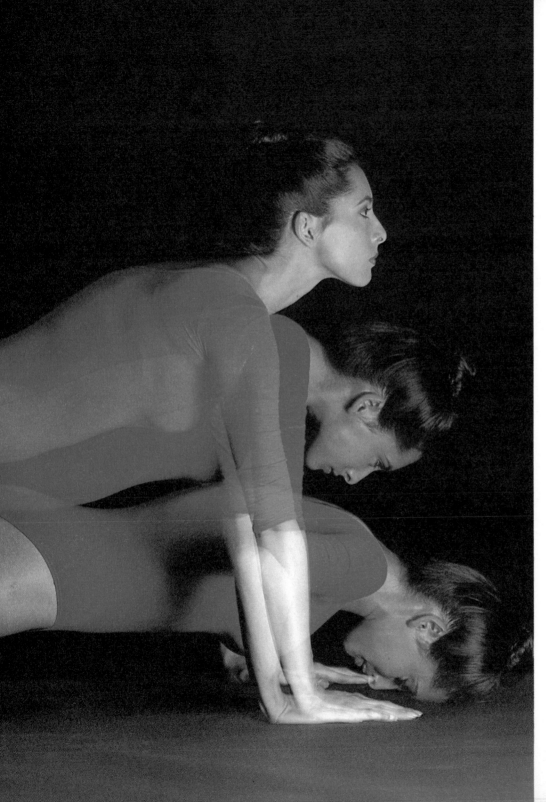

STRENGTH EXERCISE 4

Advanced push-ups

Time allowance: 1 minute

As with all the advanced strength exercises, this more strenuous version should not be attempted until you can cope comfortably with the basic version.

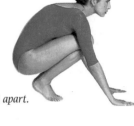

1 Crouch down, legs together, and put your palms on the floor about 12 in. (300 mm.) apart.

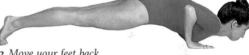

2 Move your feet back until you are flat, with your legs together and body straight.

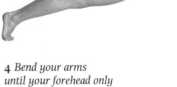

3 Push your body up until your arms are straight.

4 Bend your arms until your forehead only touches the ground.

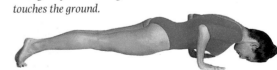

How your hobbies, sports and activities rate as exercise

Four dots means excellent effect; three, very good effect; two, beneficial effect; one, of no real effect, though it may aid relaxation.

Activities	Suppleness	Strength	Stamina
Badminton	•••	••	••
Canoeing	••	•••	•••
Climbing stairs	•	••	•••
Cricket	••	•	•
Cycling (hard)	••	•••	••••
Dancing (ballroom)	•••	•	•
Dancing (disco)	••••	•	•••
Digging (garden)	••	••••	•••
Football	•••	•••	•••
Golf	••	•	•
Gymnastics	••••	•••	•
Hill walking	•	••	•••
Housework (moderate)	••	•	•
Jogging	••	••	••••
Judo	••••	••	••
Mowing lawn by hand	•	•••	••
Rowing	••	••••	••••
Sailing	••	••	•
Squash	•••	••	•••
Swimming (hard)	••••	••••	••••
Tennis	•••	••	••
Walking (briskly)	•	•	••
Weightlifting	•	••••	•
Yoga	••••	•	•

Information from the Health Education Council

Stop smoking Cigarette smoking reduces stamina. A few minutes after

STRENGTH EXERCISE 5
Advanced sit-ups

Time allowance: 1 minute

To perform this exercise properly, it is vital to have your feet tucked to the ankles under a heavy piece of furniture. A low bench or sofa would be suitable.

1 *Lie flat on your back on the floor with your feet in place and your hands clasped behind your head.*

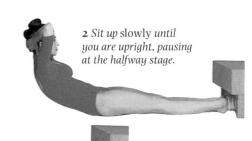

2 *Sit up slowly until you are upright, pausing at the halfway stage.*

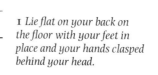

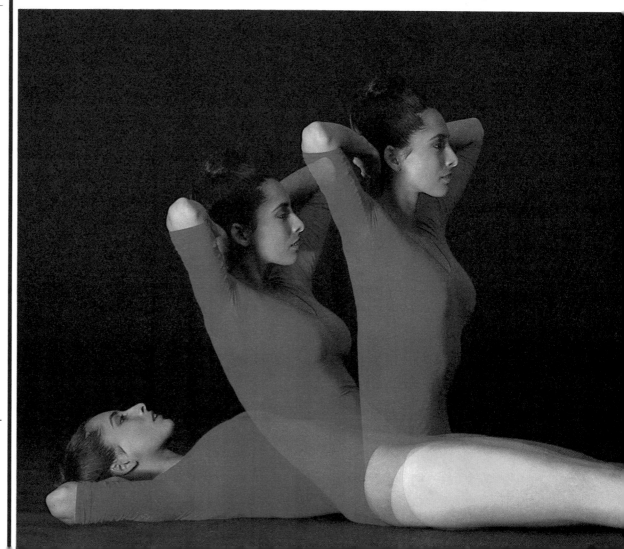

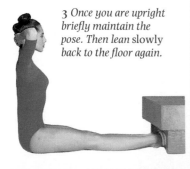

3 *Once you are upright briefly maintain the pose. Then lean slowly back to the floor again.*

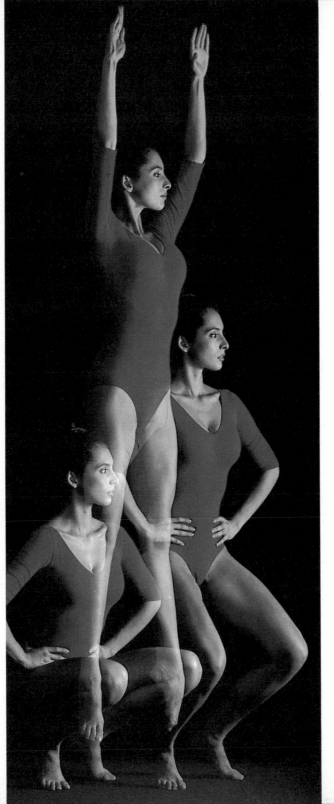

STRENGTH EXERCISE 6

Advanced squat-jumps

Time allowance: 1 minute

In all the strength exercises —advanced and basic— muscular force is built up. You should start by doing each exercise ten times a minute and gradually speed up over several sessions to 30 times a minute.

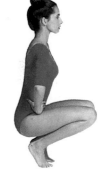

1 *Squat with your hands on your hips. Prepare to straighten rapidly.*

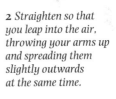

2 *Straighten so that you leap into the air, throwing your arms up and spreading them slightly outwards at the same time.*

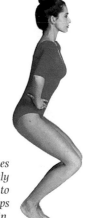

3 *Land on your toes with your knees slightly bent. Then bob down to the hands-on-hips squat again.*

someone smokes a cigarette, the air-tubes (bronchioles) in the lungs shrink, almost doubling the resistance to airflow. While that makes little difference at rest, it leads rapidly to breathlessness during exercise. Smoking raises the heart-rate by about 20 or 30 beats a minute, which reduces stamina. Nicotine in the bloodstream is also associated with the silting up of arteries with fatty deposits, reducing the blood flow to active muscles including the heart, and increasing the risk of thrombosis. The fewer cigarettes you smoke, the more good exercise will do you. Exercise cannot cancel out the effects of smoking. *See* SMOKING.

SHED EXCESS WEIGHT
Exercise helps you to lose weight, but equally, staying slim helps you to benefit more from our fitness programme. The more surplus fat you lose, the more comfortable you will be when exercising, and the less likely you will be to suffer injury. So combine your fitness programme with sensible eating. *See* NUTRITION.

ADVANCED EXERCISE PROGRAMMES
Once you have reached basic fitness, you may want to develop particular muscles to improve your performance in some specific activity—for example, tennis, or judo. One of the most efficient ways of doing that is 'weight training'—exercises using weights, such as barbells or dumb-bells, or even plastic bottles filled with water or sand. The benefit comes from the repetition of exercising your muscles against the resistance of the weights. Different exercises develop different muscles so take advice from a trainer or a training manual.

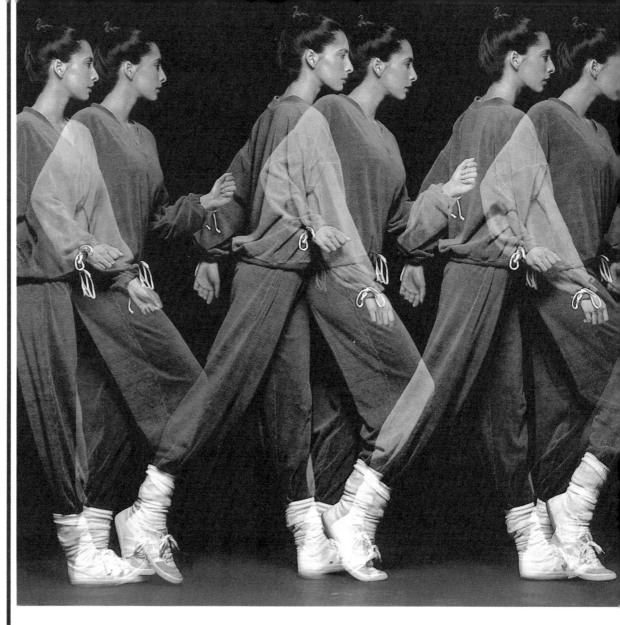

STAMINA EXERCISES
Walking and jogging
Time allowance: 20 minutes

The following stamina-building programme is based on a combination of walking and jogging. The build-up programme has four stages, corresponding to the four levels of fitness in the 'pulse-rate' test on pages 234 and 236. Stage 1 is suitable for those who score 'very unfit' in the test; stage 2 is for the 'unfit'; stage 3 is for the 'fit'; and stage 4 is for the 'very fit'. These categories apply to both sexes and all ages.

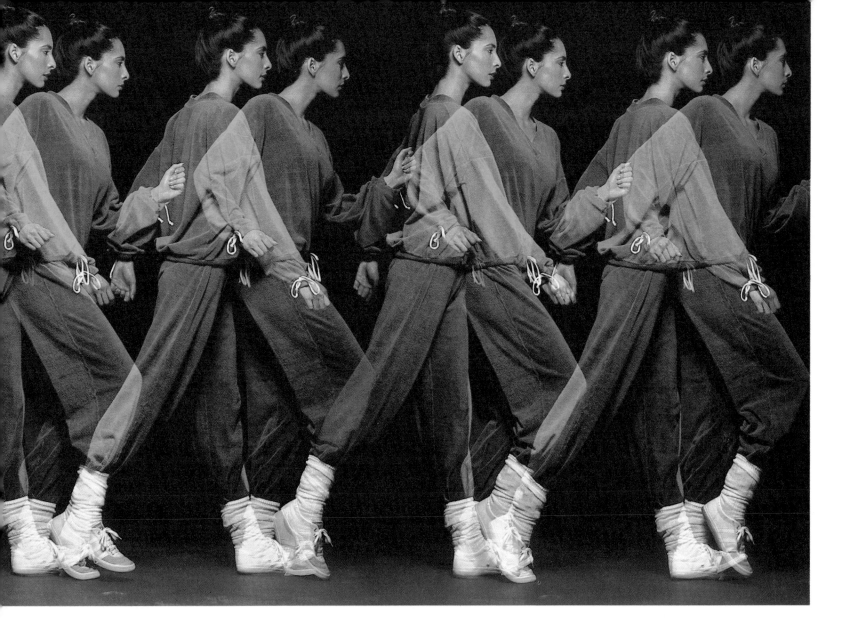

Stage 1 *Walk briskly for four minutes. Then jog and walk alternately for 15 seconds each for a total of four minutes. Then walk another four minutes. Then jog/walk (15 seconds each) for four minutes. Finally, walk four minutes.*

Stage 2 *Walk briskly for two minutes. Then jog two minutes, walk 30 seconds, jog two minutes, walk 30 seconds, jog two minutes. Now walk two minutes before starting new jogging/walking sequence. Finally, walk two minutes.*

Stage 3 *Walk briskly for one minute. Then jog for four minutes, walk for 30 seconds, jog four minutes, walk 30 seconds, jog four minutes, walk 30 seconds, jog four minutes. Finally, walk one minute.*

Stage 4 *Jog the whole 20 minutes at a comfortable speed, taking a breath every six paces. If you need more breaths, slow down; if you need less, speed up. Gradually, you will be able to move faster for a given breath rate.*

CARING FOR YOURSELF AFTER CHILDBIRTH
Four simple exercises to help restore your figure and tone up your abdominal muscles

During pregnancy and childbirth the pelvic floor muscles and the abdominal muscles become very stretched. They stay like that after the baby is born and consequently do not function properly. The longer the muscles are left slack the longer it takes to restore them to normal. So that you will be fit to look after your baby and resume your everyday activities, it is important to begin the exercises in hospital within a few hours of giving birth.

The pelvic floor muscles surround the anus, the vagina and the urethra—the tube through which urine is passed from the bladder. They support the contents of the pelvis, the womb, the bladder and the bowel. When weakened, they can give rise to incontinence and uterine prolapse.

The abdominal muscles are split into three groups; those which run straight up and down the abdomen; those which run horizontally across the abdomen; and those which run obliquely across the abdomen. Altogether, they form a 'corset' which supports the abdominal organs and the spine. After childbirth the stretched and weakened muscles often cause backache.

The following exercises—performed on a firm surface during the first week after childbirth—will tone-up and strengthen the affected muscles. If it is not practical for reasons of space or hygiene to exercise on the floor, do so on a firm bed. Once you have got into the habit, you should continue the exercises for the rest of your child-bearing life. But remember, plenty of rest is just as important as exercise. To achieve the right balance, you should seek advice from the maternity hospital.

AN EXERCISE TO STRENGTHEN THE PELVIC FLOOR MUSCLES

Clench and draw in the muscles in and around your anus and vagina. Continue to clench the muscles while counting slowly up to four. Relax, pause and repeat four times. At first you may not be able to get beyond a count of one. But by the third or fourth day after childbirth you should be able to do the full count without causing strain. The exercise is performed at hourly intervals during the day in the following three positions:

Position one

Lie on your side on the floor or bed, with your head on a pillow. Bend your right leg and rest it on another pillow. Then perform the exercise.

Position two

Turn on your back and lie with your arms outstretched at your sides and your knees raised. Keep your feet flat. Then perform the exercise.

Position three

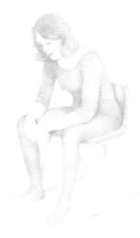

Sit on a chair, or a lavatory seat, and lean slightly forward. Then perform the exercise.

EXERCISES TO STRENGTHEN THE ABDOMINAL MUSCLES

Exercise one

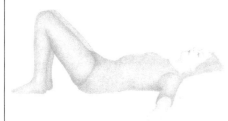

*Lie on your back with your knees bent, your feet flat and your arms outstretched at your sides.
Clench your buttocks and simultaneously draw in your abdominal muscles.
Continue until the small of your back is pressed against the floor or bed and then relax.
Perform the exercise five times running, twice a day, building up to 20 times running, twice a day.*

Exercise two

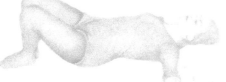

*Lie on your back with your knees bent, your feet flat and your arms outstretched at your sides.
Tilt your pelvis backwards.
Put your heels and ankles close together.
Then swing your knees as far as possible to one side.*

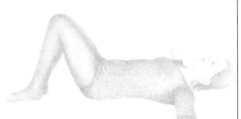

Return to your original position, relax and repeat to the other side. Perform the exercise five times running, twice a day, building up to 20 times running, twice a day.

Exercise three

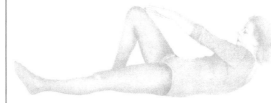

Relax and repeat to the other side. Perform the exercise five times running, twice a day, building up to 20 times running, twice a day.

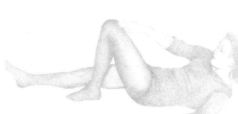

Lie on your back with your right leg straight, your left leg bent and your arms outstretched at your sides. Tilt your pelvis backwards. Then lift your head and touch your left knee with your right hand.

EXTRASYSTOLES

An irregularity in the heart rhythm in which a beat occurs immediately after a normal beat, followed by a longer interval before a regular rhythm resumes. Extrasystoles may be very infrequent, or occur several times a minute, even as often as every other beat. Occasional extrasystoles may occur in otherwise healthy people.

The individual may not be aware of the irregular beat. In other cases it feels as though the heart 'jumps', 'bumps', or 'thumps', or 'misses a beat'. The 'thumps' are also called 'palpitations' by sufferers.

The causes are numerous. In many cases no significant cause is found; sometimes excessive intake of alcohol, tea, coffee or smoking may be suspected; in other cases the symptom indicates the presence of serious disease and for this reason should be reported to a doctor.

See CIRCULATORY SYSTEM *page 40*

EXUDATE
A liquid containing white blood cells that seeps through blood vessels into inflamed tissue. The white blood cells, which are the body's chief defence mechanism, attack any bacteria in the inflamed area.

EYE
The eye and eyelids may be affected by many different conditions ranging from redness of the eye to swellings on the eyelid. These are symptoms of many diseases.
See SYMPTOM SORTER—EYE PROBLEMS

EYE, FOREIGN BODY IN

The commonest emergency eye condition is the minor injury caused by a foreign body. The amount of irritation and discomfort which can be caused by a tiny speck of dust, grit or metal is out of all proportion to its size.
Symptoms
• Pain with watering.
• If the foreign body is not dislodged fairly promptly irritation will be set up and the white will become congested and red as in CONJUNCTIVITIS.

Causes
- Tiny specks of dust, metal or grit blown into the eye by the wind or when using tools.

Treatment in the home
- Pull down the lower eyelid (or get a friend to do so) and gently remove the foreign body with a wisp of cotton wool or with the corner of a clean handkerchief. If the speck comes away easily, no further action is required. The eye may remain uncomfortable, especially if there has been a little scratching of the surface, but this should settle in a couple of hours or so.

When to consult the doctor
- If the foreign body appears to be stuck under the upper lid, or if it is still lying on the cornea (the surface of the eye), a doctor or nurse should be consulted.
- If the injury has been caused by a fragment of metal or glass at high speed (for example, when using a chisel or power drill or by a shattered windscreen) seek medical help urgently, either by going to a doctor or going to a hospital accident and emergency department.

What the doctor may do
- The doctor will look first under the lower lid by pulling it downwards, and then under the upper lid by rolling it backwards (often using a cotton-wool bud or a matchstick to help). This procedure may look unpleasant to anyone watching but it is only slightly uncomfortable. If the foreign body is located the doctor will lift it off with a wisp of cotton wool.
- If the particle cannot be seen under the eyelids the doctor may stain the front of the eye with drops of dye or with a paper strip impregnated with dye, and then examine the surface of the eye with a light and a magnifying glass. If he sees the fragment he will probably put a drop or two of local anaesthetic on the eye and then lift off the foreign body gently with the tip of a needle. He will then put in some drops or ointment to guard against infection, and he may put a pad over the eye for a period of 24 hours or so.
- If he cannot remove the fragment, or if he suspects that the injury has been caused by metal or glass travelling at speed, he will send the patient urgently to a specialist.

Prevention
- If you are travelling on a motor-cycle, welding or working with power tools, wear protective goggles.

Outlook
- The eye will recover rapidly after a speck of grit or dust has been removed.
- If an eyeball injured by a high-speed foreign body is not treated at once, the sight in both eyes might be seriously damaged.

See EYE *page 36*

FACE
Changes in the face are a symptom of many diseases and include pallor, change in expression, change in colour, becoming fatter or thinner, weakness and pain.
See SYMPTOM SORTER—FACIAL PROBLEMS

FACE-LIFT
Surgical removal of wrinkles and sagging skin of the face and chin. The operation is performed by a plastic surgeon.
See COSMETIC SURGERY

FAECAL IMPACTION

A mass of faeces lodged in the rectum. It usually affects invalids confined to a chair or bed, especially the elderly.

Symptoms
- Constipation of four or five days or more.
- Liquid faeces, which have pushed past the impacted mass, leaking uncontrollably from the anus.

Causes
- Inactivity.
- Illness.
- Ignoring the need to open the bowels.
- Allowing severe constipation to persist.

Treatment in the home
- It may be possible to scoop out some of the faeces by slipping a finger into the rectum. Wear a rubber glove and lubricate the finger with cream or soap. Put plenty of paper under the patient and have some ready for cleaning the glove.
- When the faeces are partly removed, insert two glycerin suppositories high up in the rectum to soften the motion more. These will often stimulate the bowel to evacuate in an hour or two. The loaded bowel may continue to work for a day, on and off, causing soiling.
- If suppositories are not available, a 1 in. (25 mm.) long piece of soap, as thick as a pencil, is often effective.

When to consult the doctor
- If there is constipation lasting more than two or three days in an old person or someone immobilised by injury or illness.

What the doctor may do
- Try to remove more of the faeces with a glove-covered finger, using a local anaesthetic jelly if necessary, and inserting laxative suppositories.
- Ask a nurse to give the patient an enema—either of plain water, soap and water, or a laxative.
- Prescribe a bowel stimulant. *See* MEDICINES, 3.

Prevention
- Avoid inactivity in the elderly.
- Do not let constipation persist for long.

See DIGESTIVE SYSTEM *page 44*

FAINTING ATTACK

Temporary loss of consciousness and collapse, known medically as syncope, or a vasovagal attack.

Symptoms
- Often fainting occurs without warning, but may be preceded by a sensation of lightheadedness or dizziness associated with feeling cold or clammy.
- Yawning, sometimes sighing, nausea, perspiration, weakness or rapid heartbeats precede the faint.
- When a patient has fainted, the pulse may be slow.
- Marked pallor of the face.

Duration
- A simple fainting attack lasts only a few minutes, provided the person is laid flat.

Causes
- A hot, stuffy atmosphere.
- Temporary decrease in blood supply to the brain.
- Emotional reaction to shock, sight of blood, or fear. Some people are especially sensitive and may faint even when sitting down, for example, in a dentist's chair.
- Prolonged standing in one position.
- Suddenly standing up, especially soon after getting out of bed when the body is warm, and more likely if followed by straining, such as passing urine, opening the bowels or coughing.
- Obstruction to the arteries of the neck on turning the head or looking upwards, as when hanging out washing, decorating or reaching to a high shelf.
- Poor output of blood from the heart, due to heart attack, disturbance of heart rhythm (arrhythmia) and disease of the heart valves.
- ANAEMIA and other blood disorders.
- FEVER or other debilitating illness.
- PREGNANCY or a heavy period.
- Hunger.
- Prolonged bout of coughing.
- EPILEPSY sometimes occurs with slight twitching.

Treatment in the home
- Lie down flat immediately there is any warning.

Ignoring early symptoms may result in collapse and injury.

• If you see someone faint, lie him down flat and loosen his clothing, at neck, chest and waist. Do not put his head between his legs and do not support him in a sitting or upright position.

• Make sure he has a clear airway. Grasp the jaw beneath the chin, then pull the jaw forwards and upwards.

• If he has a pulse and is breathing but does not regain consciousness in one or two minutes, put him in the unconscious position and call a doctor. If he stops breathing, start artificial respiration at once. If he has no pulse, start external cardiac massage.

• When the patient comes round, give sips of water if he asks for them. Do not give alcohol. *See* FIRST AID *page 611.*

When to consult the doctor

• If there is no obvious explanation for the faint.

• If there are abnormal movements during the faint which may suggest epilepsy.

• If the faint was a symptom of an illness such as anaemia or blood loss.

• If faints recur.

What the doctor may do

• The person will usually have recovered when first seen by the doctor, who will then exclude the possibility of any serious cause.

• Blood tests may be taken to see whether the patient is anaemic.

Prevention

• Avoid sudden changes of posture, prolonged standing, and emotional situations which may cause a faint. Older people are particularly prone to fainting attacks on suddenly standing up or on making sudden movements of the neck.

Outlook

• If no serious disease is present, recovery will be complete.

See CIRCULATORY SYSTEM *page 40*

FAITH HEALING
A belief that illnesses can be cured by harnessing 'spiritual forces' is probably as old as mankind. A form of faith healing was practised by the ancient Egyptians and Greeks, and the idea is familiar to millions in the Christian world through the miracles attributed to Jesus in the New Testament.

Some modern 'healers' have undoubtedly achieved successes. But their failures tend not to be publicised, and

medical experts remain sceptical, because there is no generally accepted scientific explanation of how such healing may work.

One theory is, that as many illnesses are psychosomatic, that is, the physical symptoms have an underlying mental cause, a believer in the powers of a healer may be cured simply because he believes that he will be cured.

However, the opinion fails to explain reported cases of 'absent healing', in which the sufferer was 'cured' by a healer practising many miles away and was apparently unaware that healing was being attempted.

Modern healers have not helped their cause in the eyes of orthodox doctors by retreating into mysticism when questioned about their powers. Most simply say that the abilities they claim to possess are a 'gift' which they prefer not to analyse too closely.

Although the term 'faith healing' is generally used for all types of healing associated with a belief in a spiritual force, it properly applies only to healing linked to Christianity. The major Christian churches, while recognising the healing miracles of Jesus, are unenthusiastic about endorsing those who claim similar powers today.

In the Roman Catholic Church, shrines such as Lourdes in France are visited annually by thousands of people seeking the intercession of the Virgin Mary to cure their ailments.

Christian Scientists—members of the Church of Christ, Scientist—rely heavily on a belief in the healing teaching of the Christian faith.

Outside Christianity, there are 'spiritual healers' who say that the world is controlled by some omnipotent force, whose spirit may be invoked to restore health, provided that the sufferer is willing to believe in the spirit and to receive it.

'Spirit healers' claim to be able to invoke the 'powers' of a dead person to assist in a cure, and often say they have clairvoyant abilities or 'psychic sensitivity' as well. There are no reliable records of their achievements in diagnosis or cure, and in some countries they are officially discouraged from practising.

FALLOT'S TETRALOGY
A heart disorder, present from birth, in which the heart has a combination of four particular defects: a narrowing of the pulmonary valve; a hole in the partition between the two ventricles (the lower chambers); enlargement of the right ventricle; and the aorta over-riding both ventricles instead of only the left one. The baby looks blue and is breathless. Surgery can correct, or at least improve, the condition in many cases.

FALLS

Many old people have falls. Sometimes they are the result of tripping or slipping but often they occur for no apparent reason or are due to sudden, passing deficiencies in cerebral circulation. Once falls begin they are liable to happen with increasing frequency.

Causes

• Failure to notice or react quickly enough to hazards, such as slippery floors.

• General ill health and muscle weakness.

• Minor blackouts due to poor circulation.

Treatment in the home

• An old person who has suffered a fall should not be lifted off the floor unless the helper is experienced at doing this or has another person's help; otherwise both the helper and the fallen person may suffer injury. Roll the fallen person on to his side and bend the lower knee. Place a chair within reach of the fallen person's upper arm; by pressing with the forearm or the upper arm on the chair and with the other forearm on the floor, the person can then pull himself up into a kneeling position—from which he can be helped on to the chair.

• If the fallen person feels cold, give him a hot-water bottle, cover with a blanket and check for HYPOTHERMIA.

When to consult the doctor

• If there is any suspicion that the person has been unconscious or has broken a hip or other bone.

• If there is no apparent reason for the fall.

What the doctor may do

• Arrange treatment in hospital for any injury or broken bone.

• If he suspects a blackout, he will investigate the possible causes.

• Look for evidence of a STROKE or any other serious disease and, if necessary, arrange treatment.

• Check the blood pressure and heart function.

Prevention

• Make sure that floor surfaces and footwear are safe and that the home is well lit. Outside the home, old people should take care in badly lit or icy conditions.

Outlook

• If an old person has recurrent falls and finds difficulty each time in regaining mobility, this may be a sign of general breakdown of health and the doctor's advice should be sought.

See NERVOUS SYSTEM *page 34*
OLD AGE

FAMILY PLANNING

If no contraception at all is used for one year there is an 80-90 per cent chance of becoming pregnant.

The ideal method of contraception does not exist. For most people there is some inconvenience involved. Couples should consider the full range, as different methods are suitable for different phases of a man or woman's fertile life. Certain methods of contraception are suitable only for women after childbirth; others may be harmful to particular individuals.

Sexual intercourse needs to take place only once for pregnancy to result, and full penetration is not necessary. Even sperm left on the woman's skin can find their way to the uterus and, if she is fertile, make her pregnant. Pregnancy cannot be prevented by having intercourse in certain positions; nor by careful washing or douching afterwards.

Breast-feeding a baby does not prevent another pregnancy, as some people believe, although it does reduce the possibility.

NATURAL FAMILY PLANNING
By recognising the 'rhythm' of their menstrual cycles, women can calculate the time when the egg is produced by the ovary and can be fertilised by the man's sperm. During this 'unsafe time' (about ten days in each month), the couple need to abstain from intercourse. Natural contraception is the only method generally approved by the Roman Catholic Church.

There are three ways of estimating the 'safe' period: the calendar, temperature and ovulation techniques. A combination of all three is the most reliable.

Calendar (rhythm) method In a menstrual cycle the first day of menstruation is counted as Day 1. A woman with an absolutely regular 28 day cycle will have her unsafe time between Day 11 and Day 18. During that time she needs to abstain from intercourse.

However, if the menstrual cycle is not regular (as it rarely is) the unsafe time must be worked out more precisely. The woman makes a note of the length of each cycle over a period of 12 months.

The first unsafe day is obtained by deducting 19 from the shortest of the last 12 cycles. So, if the shortest cycle was 25 days, 25−19 = 6, and conception is possible from Day 6.

The last unsafe day is obtained by deducting 11 from the longest of the cycles. If the longest was 31 days, 31−11 = 20. In this example, conception would be possible from Day 6 until Day 20. Intercourse would only be safe from Day 1 to Day 6 (there is no reason why intercourse should not take place during menstruation) and from Day 21 to the end of the cycle.

The calendar method is very risky for women with short cycles, and for those whose cycles are very irregular. To detect the time of ovulation it is wise, therefore, to use other methods as well.

Temperature method A woman's temperature rises a small amount at the time of ovulation—0.5 to 1°F (0.2 to 0.5°C). The temperature must be taken by mouth, and recorded each morning before getting out of bed and before taking food or drink. The thermometer must be left in place for at least three minutes, and the temperature reading recorded on a chart made for the purpose. Of course the temperature may rise for other reasons, such as an infection. If there is no rise, ovulation has not taken place—this happens increasingly with advancing age.

Ovulation thermometers which are clearer and larger than normal thermometers can be obtained from chemists and family planning clinics. The clinics will also provide the charts.

Ovulation (Billings) method Many tell-tale biological changes occur at ovulation. The easiest to detect is in the mucus usually seen at the entrance of the vagina. This is a jelly-like substance, similar to egg white, produced by the cervix (the neck of the womb). Around the time of ovulation it becomes more profuse and watery, the wettest day being the fourth day after ovulation.

Women can learn to watch for these symptoms and, with the temperature chart, can predict ovulation.

The disadvantage of the rhythm method is that it does not actually prevent conception, it just warns a woman when intercourse is risky.

It is then up to her to refrain from intercourse, which may be difficult.

Further advice about natural family planning can be obtained from *The Catholic Marriage Advisory Council*, Clitherow House, 1 Blythe Mews, Blythe Road, London W14 0NW (Tel. 071-371 1341).

Coitus interruptus Male withdrawal—coitus interruptus—is the oldest method of contraception. It is simple, cheap, and without the undesirable side-effects of more sophisticated methods. The couple have intercourse normally until the moment of the man's climax, when he withdraws his penis before ejaculation.

There may be disadvantages to both the man and woman using this method. The man may find it inhibiting to withdraw before ejaculation, and the woman may not reach a climax as a result of his withdrawal. Furthermore, it is not effective as contraception, because sperm may be released before ejaculation.

ARTIFICIAL PLANNING—BARRIER CONTRACEPTION
Barrier contraceptives prevent live sperm from entering the womb either by killing them (spermicides) or by obstructing them (condoms and diaphragms).

Spermicides These are chemical contraceptives intended for insertion high into the vagina just before intercourse. They should be used either with condoms or diaphragms as they are less effective by themselves. They are available in the form of creams and jellies; aerosols (foams); suppositories or pessaries; foaming tablets; and incorporated into soluble plastic C films.

Home-made spermicides of strong soap, soap powder or detergents, mustard oil or strong salt solutions will irritate the vagina and should not be used.

The vaginal sponge This is a sponge impregnated with spermicide which is inserted high into the vagina. It may be left in place for 24 hours with no need to add more spermicide.

Condoms The condom, or sheath, was known in Europe in the 16th century and was made of animal gut or linen. Now condoms are made of rubber or plastic, and may be lubricated (sometimes with spermicide). The condom also affords some protection against sexually transmitted disease. Male and female versions are available.

The teat, or end of the male condom, should be pinched to expel air as the condom is rolled on to the erect penis before penetration, or else it may burst during intercourse. On ejaculation, the semen stays inside the condom; the penis should be withdrawn while still erect, the rim of the condom being held to prevent it slipping off.

A condom should be used only once. If lubrication is needed, KY jelly should be used. Petroleum jelly or oil destroy the rubber. The condom is more effective if the woman also uses spermicide. Short condoms (American tips) covering only the tip of the penis are unreliable, as they easily slip off, and do not protect against disease.

The diaphragm The rubber cap, or diaphragm, inserted in the vagina, blocks the passage of sperm into the womb. It is simple to use, but should be fitted the first time by a doctor or nurse to establish the correct size. As an added safeguard, it is covered with a spermicide before insertion; and it should not be removed for at least six hours after intercourse, to ensure that all the sperm are dead. Once removed the cap should be washed in warm soapy water and carefully dried to prevent it perishing.

ARTIFICIAL PLANNING—INTRA-UTERINE DEVICES
A variety of plastic devices, including coils and loops, can be placed in the womb to prevent the fertilised egg becoming implanted in the wall of the womb where it would grow. These intra-uterine devices (IUD) are inserted in the womb by a nurse or doctor. They should

never be given to a woman who has had an infection of the pelvic region, and preferably not to those who have never been pregnant. They are usually not advisable in the case of women with heavy or painful periods, as these may become worse.

The device is pulled straight for insertion, and reverts to its shape once inside. Insertion is quick and usually painless. The device has a small thread hanging from it through the cervix and into the vagina, so that it can be pulled out. Care must be taken not to pull the thread when removing a tampon. The device should be removed only by a doctor or nurse.

Devices with copper around the plastic stem usually need to be changed every five years, as the copper wears away. Others can be kept in for as long as there are no

Which method of contraception?

If a normal young woman has regular intercourse without using any sort of contraception, there is an 80-90 per cent chance that she will get pregnant within a year. All types of contraception have some limitations or disadvantages. This chart can be used to select the method most appropriate to a person's circumstances.

☐ **Breast-feeding**
Reliability Poor.
Advantages No preparation before intercourse.

☐ **Douche**
Reliability Nil.

☐ **Natural family planning (rhythm method)**
Reliability Fair.
Advantages No artificial aids required. No preparation before intercourse.
Disadvantages Needs careful calculation, probably by more than one method. Limits occasions when intercourse may occur. Requires male co-operation.

☐ **Withdrawal**
Reliability Poor.
Advantages No preparation needed before intercourse.
Disadvantages Satisfaction reduced. Requires male co-operation.

☐ **Spermicide only (suppositories, foaming tablets, etc.)**
Reliability Poor.
Advantages Easily available.
Disadvantages Requires preparation before intercourse. Intended for use with diaphragm or condom.

☐ **Condom (sheath)**
Reliability Fair.
Advantages Easily available for both male and female. Protects against sexually transmitted disease, cervical cancer and AIDS.
Disadvantages May interfere with satisfaction.

☐ **Diaphragm (cap)**
Reliability Fair when used with spermicides.
Advantages No side-effects. Easily available. Male co-operation not required. Protects against cervical cancer.
Disadvantages Needs to be fitted first by a doctor or nurse. Requires preparation before intercourse.

☐ **Vaginal sponge**
Reliability Poor
Advantages Easily available.
Disadvantages Requires preparation before intercourse.

☐ **Intra-uterine device (loop, coil, etc.)**
Reliability Fairly good.
Advantages Once inserted no further preparation needed. Male co-operation not required.
Disadvantages Needs to be fitted by doctor or nurse. Unsuitable for women with heavy periods. Increased risk of infection and ectopic pregnancy.

☐ **Progestogen-only pill**
Reliability Good.
Advantages Can be taken while breast-feeding, and by women over 35. No preparation before intercourse. Male co-operation not required.
Disadvantages Must be taken every day. Periods irregular.

☐ **Progestogen injection**
Reliability Good.
Advantages Lasts up to three months. No preparation before intercourse. Male co-operation not required.
Disadvantages Irreversible for three months. Periods irregular.

☐ **Combined pill**
Reliability Very good.
Advantages Predictable, light periods with few cramps. No preparation before intercourse. Male co-operation not required. Reduces risk of some cancers (ovary, endometrium).
Disadvantages Must be taken regularly. Can have side-effects. Not suitable for women over 35 years if they smoke, are obese, or suffer from raised blood pressure (HYPERTENSION) or DIABETES. May increase risk of some cancers (breast, cervix) and of thrombosis.

☐ **Vasectomy (sterilisation for men)**
Reliability Very good.
Advantages No preparation before intercourse.
Disadvantages Irreversible minor operation. Only for men who want no more children.

☐ **Tubal ligation (sterilisation for women)**
Reliability Very good.
Advantages No preparation before intercourse. Male co-operation not required.
Disadvantages Irreversible operation. Only for women who want no more children.

☐ **Hysterectomy**
Reliability 100 per cent.
Advantages Totally reliable. No preparation before intercourse.
Disadvantages Major operation. There must be other reasons apart from contraception.

side-effects; though all devices should be checked every year to ensure that they have not shifted.

Possible side-effects following insertion of the device include cramps resembling period pains. These should stop after a few hours. Sometimes the device is expelled by the womb soon after insertion and a new one has to be fitted.

Pregnancy can occasionally occur even with the device in place, and if it does, there is a greater risk of abortion between the fourth and sixth months, and an increased chance of the pregnancy being ectopic (at a site outside the womb).

About 2 per cent of women with an intra-uterine device can be expected to develop infection of the pelvic region during the first year of using it, and infection can reduce fertility. Any woman who develops pain in the lower abdomen or a vaginal discharge should see a doctor.

There is no evidence that women with an intra-uterine device run an increased risk of cancer of the cervix or womb.

ARTIFICIAL PLANNING—PILLS AND INJECTIONS
The first pills—oral contraceptives—were sold in 1959. It is estimated that there are now 80 million users of oral contraceptives throughout the world. In Britain the pill can be obtained only with a prescription.

There are two types. The combined pill consists of the hormones oestrogen and progestogen, and the mini pill consists of progestogen only. These pills can be taken only by women.

Combined pill The oestrogen in the combined pill works by stopping the ovaries from shedding their eggs. The effect of the progestogen is to make the mucus of the cervix hostile to sperm, and change the character of the womb lining so that it is unfavourable for implantation of the fertilised egg. It is important to take the pill at the same time every day to maintain constant hormone levels. If the pill is forgotten for more than a few hours, it is no longer reliable.

The pill is taken for 21 or 22 days within a regular 28 day cycle, but each make of pill differs slightly in its instructions. Pills are an unreliable contraceptive during the first two weeks of taking them, and when taking antibiotics or suffering from diarrhoea.

Check your usage of this pill with your doctor or local family planning clinic. *See* MEDICINES, 33. It should not be taken by any woman who has had a blood clot or PHLEBITIS as it may cause clots to occur more readily, or any woman who has liver disease. It can sometimes make MIGRAINE headaches worse. And it is not recommended to women over the age of 35, if they are overweight or if they smoke as it may make them more liable to heart attacks. In fact, no one on the pill should smoke or become overweight.

Taken regularly, the combined pill is one of the most reliable of contraceptives. Menstruation is regular, much lighter, and usually painless. There is less likelihood of ANAEMIA and also less PREMENSTRUAL TENSION.

The combined pill can contain many different combinations of the two hormones. Their side-effects vary with their ingredients, and with the person taking them. When first taking the pill a woman may experience nausea and

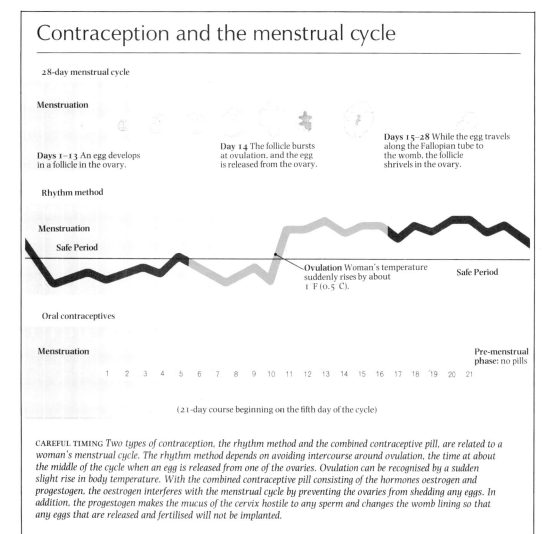

Contraception and the menstrual cycle

28-day menstrual cycle

Menstruation

Days 1–13 An egg develops in a follicle in the ovary.

Day 14 The follicle bursts at ovulation, and the egg is released from the ovary.

Days 15–28 While the egg travels along the Fallopian tube to the womb, the follicle shrivels in the ovary.

Rhythm method

Menstruation

Safe Period

Ovulation Woman's temperature suddenly rises by about 1 F (0.5 C).

Safe Period

Oral contraceptives

Menstruation

Pre-menstrual phase: no pills

1 2 3 4 5 6 7 8 9 10 11 12 13 14 15 16 17 18 19 20 21

(21-day course beginning on the fifth day of the cycle)

CAREFUL TIMING *Two types of contraception, the rhythm method and the combined contraceptive pill, are related to a woman's menstrual cycle. The rhythm method depends on avoiding intercourse around ovulation, the time at about the middle of the cycle when an egg is released from one of the ovaries. Ovulation can be recognised by a sudden slight rise in body temperature. With the combined contraceptive pill consisting of the hormones oestrogen and progestogen, the oestrogen interferes with the menstrual cycle by preventing the ovaries from shedding any eggs. In addition, the progestogen makes the mucus of the cervix hostile to any sperm and changes the womb lining so that any eggs that are released and fertilised will not be implanted.*

headaches, but these usually improve after the first month. There may be breast enlargement, and some women retain fluid, causing weight gain. Different pills may have to be tried before finding the ideal one.

Sometimes there may be irregular menstrual bleeding, in which case a different combination of hormones is called for. There can be an increase in blood pressure, and for this reason doctors check it every six months. Combined pills are not recommended during breast-feeding, as they can lessen the supply of milk.

After stopping the pill, periods may not return for several months. It is therefore wise to stop taking it some months before wanting to conceive.

Progestogen-only pill (mini pill) These pills are taken every day. Their main action is to make the cervical mucus hostile to sperm and to make the lining of the womb unfavourable for implantation of the egg. Though slightly less reliable than the combined pill, they become effective after one week, and can be taken when breast-feeding. Periods can become irregular, and may be no lighter than usual.

Some research has suggested that the contraceptive pill, when taken over many years, may increase the risk of developing BREAST CANCER. All women using oral contraceptives are advised to check with their doctor or local family planning clinic that they are using a pill that is safe, and suitable for their age group.

Progestogen injections A single progestogen injection is an effective contraceptive for a period of one to three months. Injections, are administered by doctors, with whom you should first discuss the advantages and disadvantages fully. The menstrual cycle is frequently disrupted —about one-third of women stop periods altogether after a year of injections. Some women gain weight.

See MEDICINES, 33

Morning-after contraception An intra-uterine device inserted up to seven days after sexual intercourse can prevent implantation of the fertilised egg in the womb. Also, a high-dose morning-after pill can be effective. It should be obtained from a doctor or family planning clinic within 72 hours of intercourse taking place. There may be nausea and vomiting.

Neither method should be employed regularly.

STERILISATION

This is a simple operation for both men and women. The operations are not easily reversible, and should take place only if neither partner has any doubts.

Male sterilisation—vasectomy—takes 15-30 minutes. The tubes which carry sperm from the testes to the penis are tied and cut. There should not be any change in sexual feelings or sex life after the operation, as there will

still be an orgasm; but the fluid will not contain sperm.

In female sterilisation, the Fallopian tubes which carry the egg from the ovary to the womb are tied and cut. This is done with the help of ENDOSCOPY through a very small incision in the abdomen near the navel. There should be no side-effects, though some women have irregular and slightly heavier periods.

Hysterectomy is surgical removal of the womb. Women with heavy periods or FIBROIDS may prefer it to cutting the Fallopian tubes, but it is a major operation.

Contraception should be re-started a month after childbirth. If breast-feeding, the progestogen-only pill is suitable, otherwise the combined pill can be taken. An IUD can be inserted at the post-natal visit.

ADVICE ON FAMILY PLANNING

NHS family planning advice is available from more than 23,000 family doctors and 2,000 family planning clinics. British hospitals also provide facilities for male and female sterilisation. All consultations are confidential.

Further advice can be obtained from *The Family Planning Association*, 27-35 Mortimer Street, London WIN 7RJ (Tel. 071-636 7866), and from the FPA's regional centres and local clinics.

In addition, male and female condoms and spermicides are sold by chemists and mail-order firms. Diaphragms may be bought from chemists once a woman has been fitted by her doctor and knows the size she needs. Intra-uterine devices and contraceptive pills and injections are obtainable only through your doctor or family planning clinic.

THE FUTURE OF CONTRACEPTION

Researchers are working on a cervical cap which may be left in place for several months, and on hormone preparations which can be taken as snuff, or by injection, or as implants under the skin, or as inserts in the vagina.

For men, more acceptable condoms are being developed. In addition, various ways are being explored of preventing sperm production, but so far these have had unacceptable side-effects, so there is no immediate prospect of a 'male pill'.

Different methods of sterilisation for men and women are being investigated—in particular a reversible method, in which a plug or valve can be surgically inserted in the tubes of a man or woman, and removed as required.

FARMER'S LUNG

An occupational lung disease caused by an allergy to the spores of fungus growing in mouldy hay or straw.
See OCCUPATIONAL HAZARDS

FERTILITY

Ability in a woman to conceive a child, or in a man to induce conception. Inability to conceive or to fertilise an ovum may be due to a number of causes.
See INFERTILITY

FEVER

Many lay people associate the word fever with specific illnesses such as scarlet fever or malaria. To a doctor it means raised temperature which may be accompanied by shivering, headache and other symptoms.
See SYMPTOM SORTER—FEVER

FIBROADENOMA OF THE BREAST

A soft, sometimes intermittent lump in the breast that is usually non-cancerous. The lump is also known as a 'breast mouse', since it slips away from the fingers when the breast is being examined.

Symptoms
- A soft, tender lump comes and goes in one breast.
- The lump is likely to be larger and more tender before a period and may disappear at the onset of a period.
- The condition may be accompanied by tenderness and lumpiness in both breasts. *See* MASTITIS, NODULAR.

Duration
- The tendency persists indefinitely; surgical removal is usually needed to ensure it is not a cancer.

Causes
- The condition is due to glandular changes in the breast.
- It is most common in women between 20 and 40, women who have not breast-fed their children and childless women.

Treatment in the home
- Wear a firm bra.

When to consult the doctor
- Immediately any lump in the breast is noticed.

What the doctor may do
- Examine both breasts and also the armpits for any signs of swelling there. He may then suggest another examination after the woman's next period.
- Arrange for an examination by a surgeon.
- It is often necessary to remove the lump by surgery to

make certain that it is not cancerous.

Prevention

• Prevention is not possible, but early detection of all breast lumps can be ensured if a woman examines her breasts regularly.

Outlook

• Good.

See FEMALE GENITAL SYSTEM *page 48*

FIBROIDS, UTERINE

Benign (non-cancerous) tumours of the muscle wall of the uterus. One-third of women over the age of 35 will have one or more fibroids. They do not necessarily cause any symptoms and never become cancerous.

Symptoms

• Heavy periods in women between 30 and 50.

• Painful periods.

• Backache.

• In some cases there is swelling in the lower abdomen.

Duration

• Fibroids persist once they have developed and may slowly grow larger unless removed.

Complications

• Anaemia may develop if the periods are heavy.

• Rarely, degeneration of the muscle wall of the uterus occurs, causing more pain.

• Infertility may be associated with fibroids.

Treatment in the home

• None.

When to consult the doctor

• If periods become heavier than usual or painful.

• If there is swelling in the lower abdomen.

What the doctor may do

• Carry out an INTERNAL PELVIC EXAMINATION.

• Give a blood test for anaemia.

• Arrange for an examination by a gynaecologist.

• If there is infertility or annoying symptoms present the fibroids may be removed under general anaesthetic. If the patient is past child-bearing age and there are many fibroids a HYSTERECTOMY may be performed.

Prevention

• There is no way of preventing fibroids forming.

Outlook

• Excellent with treatment.

See FEMALE GENITAL SYSTEM *page 48*

FIBROMA

A benign, that is non-cancerous, tumour which is sometimes found in fibrous tissue, particularly in tissue surrounding the nerves.

See NEUROFIBROMATOSIS

FIBROSITIS

Inflammation of the fibrous connective tissue of muscles. Fibrositis is a common, painful but harmless complaint about which the medical profession knows very little at the present.

Symptoms

• Pain and tenderness in certain muscles—usually those of the shoulder, the base of the neck and the lower back—when the muscles are used.

• Sometimes nodules, little hard lumps, can be felt in the affected muscles.

Duration

• Home treatment usually clears up the condition within a few weeks.

Causes

• What causes fibrositis is not known. It tends to occur more often in those who are suffering from anxiety and whose pain threshold is therefore lowered.

• Damp weather and damp conditions also seem to bring on the disorder.

Treatment in the home

• The pain can be relieved with heat from a hot-water bottle or some other source.

When to consult the doctor

• If the pain does not go after four to seven days of self-treatment.

What the doctor may do

• Check, by examination, questions and possibly X-rays, that some more serious disorder is not causing the symptoms.

• If fibrositis is diagnosed, arrange heat treatment and deep-massage treatment for the patient to carry out himself or at a hospital out-patient department.

Prevention

• Damp conditions should be avoided if possible.

Outlook

• Attacks are usually over within a few weeks, but they tend to recur.

See SKELETAL SYSTEM *page 54*

FISTULA IN ANO

An abnormal extra channel that is created between the ano-rectal canal and the skin around the surface of the anus.

Symptoms

• There may be pain and slight bleeding from the anus.

• Discharge of pus and sometimes faeces.

Duration

• The fistula persists until treated.

Causes

• Usually faecally contaminated abscesses alongside the lower bowel discharging into the bowel or on to the skin of the anus.

• ILEITIS, REGIONAL.

Treatment in the home

• Frequent baths will help to clear the discharge and lessen the smell.

• Wearing protection, such as nappy pads and plastic pants, will help to absorb the discharge and prevent seepage on to clothing.

When to consult the doctor

• If any discharge from the anus persists for more than seven days.

What the doctor may do

• Send the patient to hospital for surgical treatment.

Prevention

• None.

Outlook

• Good with treatment.

See DIGESTIVE SYSTEM *page 44*

FIT

A disturbance of consciousness which may last for a few seconds or for several minutes, and which may be followed by further fits. Fits, or convulsions, have different causes at different ages.

See SYMPTOM SORTER—DISTURBANCES OF CONSCIOUSNESS

FLAT FEET

Feet that lie flat on the ground due to a lack of arching. All children have flat feet for a year or two after they begin to stand, but by the time the child has reached the age of 16 both feet should have developed a well-marked arch.

Symptoms
- In adults there is foot strain and pain.
- In children there is usually no discomfort. The characteristic sign of the condition is a bulge on the inner side of the foot just below the ankle bone. The child's shoe bulges inwards over the heel, which becomes worn down on the inner side.

Duration
- In the many children who have only slightly flat feet the condition disappears without treatment after a month or two.
- Children who have more marked symptoms need treatment to bring about a complete cure.
- In many adults treatment is less effective, and the condition persists throughout life.

Causes
- In children the cause is often slow development of the muscles used in walking.
- In adults excessive walking, standing and weight bearing may cause the arches of the feet to drop.

Treatment in the home
- In children with slightly flat feet, plenty of walking quickly clears up the condition.
- Children and adults with markedly flat feet should practise exercises that involve repeatedly rising up on their toes.

When to consult the doctor
- If the feet are painful.
- If the symptoms described persist.

What the doctor may do
- Arrange physiotherapy to strengthen the muscles of the feet.
- Prescribe arch supports to be worn in the shoe, or special shoes with a wedge to raise the inner side of the foot.
- Refer severe cases for a second opinion.

Prevention
- Plenty of walking and other exercises during childhood prevent flat feet from developing.
- Properly fitting shoes should always be worn.
- Obesity places a great load on the feet, and adults who can prevent it should do so.
- If possible, adults should also avoid strain on the feet caused by excessive standing.

Outlook
- In children the condition usually clears up. In adults it is often difficult to cure.

See SKELETAL SYSTEM *page 54*

FLOATERS

This is the name given to the sensation of threads or black dots floating in the field of vision.

Symptoms
- There is a gradual awareness that the vision is not completely clear and that a small black dot or filament appears to be floating in front of the eyes.

Causes
- The small threads are caused by tiny leakages of blood into the fluid of the eyeball.
- There is no need to worry about floaters unless they are accompanied by other symptoms (such as partial loss of vision or pain) or are due to obvious injury such as a blow on the eye. Floaters may disappear, but then reappear.

When to consult the doctor
- If you are worried about any aspect of vision, you should consult your doctor. Simple floaters do not require medical treatment, but if the eye is painful, or the vision impaired, the doctor should be consulted.

What the doctor may do
- After taking the history the doctor will look at the inside of the eye through an ophthalmoscope (a magnifying glass with a light). If the presence of floaters is confirmed, or if the doctor sees nothing abnormal (floaters cannot always be seen through an ophthalmoscope) he is likely simply to reassure the patient.

Outlook
- The outlook is excellent. The floaters may disappear in a few weeks, though they may recur.

See EYE *page 36*

FLOODING
1. Extensive bleeding from the uterus (womb). This may be due to PERIOD PROBLEMS, or the sign of a spontaneous ABORTION, or miscarriage.
2. A psychiatric technique for treating a PHOBIA (an irrational fear of a certain object or situation). The sufferer is exposed at length to whatever he fears.

FONTANELLE
Any of the areas of CARTILAGE between the unfused bones on the skull of a young baby. Most babies have two main fontanelles. The larger, about 1 in. (25 mm.) across, is on the top of the head towards the front. The smaller is

towards the back of the head. The smaller is closed by the end of the first year. The bones surrounding the larger fontanelle have fused by the time the baby is aged 18 months.

FOOD POISONING
An acute illness caused by eating contaminated food. There are various forms of food poisoning with varying degrees of severity.
See GASTROENTERITIS

FOOT
Injury, weightbearing, wear and tear, and disorders of the circulation affect the feet and toes in a variety of ways including pain, numbness, swelling and itching.
See SYMPTOM SORTER—FOOT PROBLEMS
FOOT CARE *page 258*

FOOT STRAIN

A disorder in which prolonged walking or standing strains ligaments in one or both of the feet and causes pain.

Symptoms
- Pain is felt mainly in the middle of the foot.
- It may extend along the inside of the foot and into the calf.

Duration
- The condition usually subsides with rest.

Causes
- Unaccustomed or excessive walking or standing.

Treatment in the home
- Rest the feet and avoid ill-fitting shoes.

When to consult the doctor
- If the symptoms do not clear up after resting the feet.

What the doctor may do
- Arrange a course of exercises and electrical stimulation to strengthen the muscles of the foot and leg.
- Suggest that the patient wears arch supports.
- If the strain is severe and due to the person's work, advise a change of occupation.

Prevention
- Excessive, unaccustomed walking or standing should be avoided.

See SKELETAL SYSTEM *page 54*

Foot care

HOW TO TAKE CARE OF YOUR FEET—FROM YOUR CHILDHOOD TO YOUR OLD AGE

In supporting the weight of the body, the feet have to take a considerable strain. To cope with this they have a complex structure of bones, muscles, sinews and nerves. Each foot contains 26 small, very delicate bones—the highest concentration of bone structure in the human body. To keep the bones in their correct position and provide elasticity, there are four times as many ligaments and muscles as there are bones—all of which need looking after if they are to work properly.

A once-a-week home pedicure

For people who are prone to develop foot problems, the following pedicure and exercises may help. The equipment consists of: bowl, nail cream, hoof stick, cotton wool, nail clippers, emery boards, hard-skin remover and hand cream. There are 11 stages.

1 *Remove nail varnish. Wash each foot in turn in a bowl of warm water. Clean the nails with a brush. Rinse in cold water and dry thoroughly, particularly between the toes.*

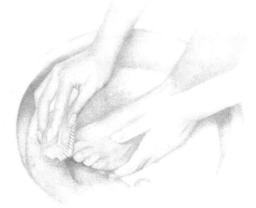

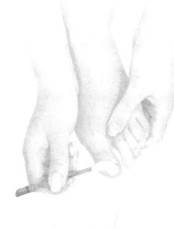

2 *Apply nail cream with the sharp end of the hoof stick wrapped in cotton wool. Ease back skin from the half moons. Massage cream into the sides of the nails.*

3 *Gently massage the cream into the nails. This stops them from becoming dry and flaky. Allow the cream to soak into the nails for at least three minutes.*

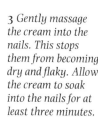

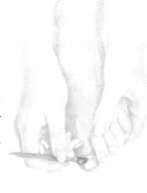

4 *Using the blunt end of the hoof stick, ease the cuticle down— away from the nail. This allows the nail to grow freely.*

5 *Finish cleaning the nails with the sharp end of the hoof stick, wrapped in cotton wool.*

WALKING AND WORKING

The main strength in the foot comes from the big toe, and a person's true centre of balance is the ball of the foot.

As well as bearing the body's weight, the feet have to do a great deal of work. By the time their 'owner' is 70 years old, they will have walked the equivalent of three times around the world. Yet, in spite of all the work they have to do, they are—along with the hands—among the most neglected parts of the human body.

Ninety per cent of foot trouble is caused by wearing the wrong shoes.

If shoes are too tight or too narrow, they cause BUNIONS, CORNS and CALLUSES. If they are worn for a long time they will also cause malformation of the feet.

Shoes that are too big and which do not support the feet correctly will result in blisters and possible flattening of the arches.

Heels more than 2 in. (50 mm.) high, worn constantly, cause an extra load on the transverse arch and the front of the longitudinal arch. *See* FLAT FOOT.

They can also lead to backaches as they disturb your natural posture.

When trying on new shoes, check these essential points:
Do they grip your heels?
Can you wiggle all your toes? If you cannot, the shoes are too tight.
Do the shoes pinch or cut into the feet at any point?
Do they give full support to the arch?

Another way of ensuring healthy

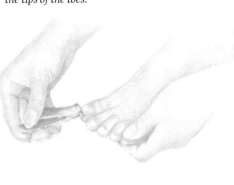

6 *Trim the nails with steel clippers, making sure to cut straight across to discourage ingrowing nails. Leave the nails level with the tips of the toes.*

7 *Rinse off all traces of nail cream with warm water, and pat dry with cotton wool. If left wet, the feet could become chapped.*

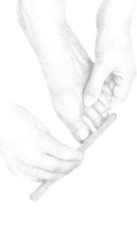

8 *Gently file away the rough edges of the nails with an emery board. Take care to retain the square shape of the nail—as 'shaped' edges encourage ingrowing toe-nails.*

9 *Wrap clean cotton wool round the hoof stick and clean down the sides of the nails. If the nails grow inwardly, do not dig into the skin in case infection sets in.*

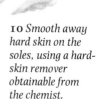

10 *Smooth away hard skin on the soles, using a hard-skin remover obtainable from the chemist.*

11 *Massage hand cream thoroughly into the whole foot. Use gentle circular motions, working from toes to the ankle.*

feet is occasionally to walk barefoot outside—especially on sand, or on grass in good weather. This makes the toes more mobile, reduces bodily tension and helps you to relax. Taking off the shoes at home in the evening and wiggling the toes also has a relaxing effect.

PREPARING FOR LONG WALKS
Many country holidays are spoiled by people—who are not used to walking long distances—developing painful blisters. To avoid blisters, you should start treating your feet a fortnight before the holiday begins. Each night

liberally pat on surgical or methylated spirit and let it dry. If, despite this, blisters do occur, paint them with a weak solution of iodine and cover them with a piece of elastic adhesive strapping. Blisters should never be deliberately broken.

Comfortable, well-fitting boots or shoes should be worn for country walks, and two pairs of socks will greatly reduce friction on the feet. They can be two medium-weight pairs, or a thin cotton pair next to the feet and a thicker pair of woollen oversocks. The oversocks should fit comfortably over the undersocks.

Implements for looking after the feet

NAIL BRUSH *The firm nylon bristles are ideal for cleaning the toes and the toe-nails.*

EMERY BOARD *Files the nails without breaking them.*

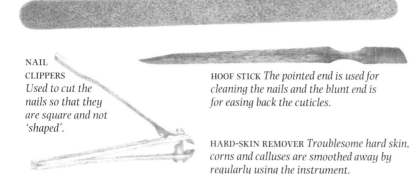

NAIL CLIPPERS *Used to cut the nails so that they are square and not 'shaped'.*

HOOF STICK *The pointed end is used for cleaning the nails and the blunt end is for easing back the cuticles.*

HARD-SKIN REMOVER *Troublesome hard skin, corns and calluses are smoothed away by regularly using the instrument.*

Wash your feet and put on clean socks every day. For washing, use lukewarm water and finish with a cold rinse. The feet should be thoroughly dried and dusted—especially between the toes—with talcum powder. A little talc should also be shaken into a fresh pair of socks before putting them on. *See* BLISTERS, FIRST AID.

DEALING WITH SWEATY FEET
Many people suffer from sweaty feet both in hot and cold weather—especially if they are moving about in stuffy offices or factory buildings. The condition is dealt with by washing the feet morning and evening with soap and comfortably warm water—very hot water stimulates the sweat glands. After the warm bathing, the feet should be dipped into cold water.

They should be thoroughly dried with a rough towel, and an astringent—either a powder or a deodorised spray—should be applied. A liberal application of surgical or methylated spirit is equally effective. After the astringent or spirit has dried, lightly dust the feet with talcum powder or an astringent foot powder.

Socks should be changed at least twice a day, and sufferers should change into sandals or soft shoes when they return home from work.

Although sweat itself is free of odours, some of the bacteria ever-present on the skin produce the unpleasant smell associated with sweaty feet. This is made worse by wearing enclosed footwear that does not allow the feet to breathe, particularly shoes with plastic or rubber uppers. Open sandals can be the solution in summer. Medicated insoles fitted into normal shoes have a deodorising effect, and insoles

containing activated charcoal also absorb odours. Both types of insole are quite cheap, easy to fit and can be bought from a chemist or some supermarkets.

SOME COMMON FOOT AILMENTS
Chilblains Exposure to cold causes itchy, inflamed patches on the toes. They should not be scratched and usually disappear within three weeks. To prevent recurrence, keep the feet warm and dry. *See* CHILBLAINS.
Plantar warts People can contract these very contagious and frequently painful warts—also known as verrucas—at swimming baths. They usually appear on the toes or the soles of the feet. Sometimes they disappear naturally after a few months, but if they persist they can be removed by a doctor. The sufferer should not spread the infection by walking about barefoot. *See* WARTS.
Athlete's foot The main symptoms of this fungus infection are cracked and itchy skin—especially between the toes and on the soles. Athlete's foot is aggravated by perspiration and the feet should be kept as clean and as dry as possible. Socks of natural fibre—cotton or wool—should be worn to allow the feet to breathe. An anti-fungal foot powder, obtainable from the chemist, should be used. *See* ATHLETE'S FOOT.

FOOT CARE FOR THE ELDERLY
Elderly people should take particular care of their feet, as they are especially susceptible to corns, calluses, bunions, and horny and deformed toes and nails. Sloppy, ill-fitting shoes—though they may be old favourites—can pinch the toes and give no help to aged feet, which need more support than young ones. Firm, well-fitting shoes should

be worn and advice on which to choose will be given by a shoe shop.

All foot problems affecting old people can be treated by a National Health Service chiropodist.

FOOT CARE FOR THE YOUNG

Children's feet grow quickly, and it is a false economy to buy very expensive shoes which will soon become too small. It is better to buy cheaper shoes that can economically be replaced as soon as they are outgrown. Young bones are soft and can be forced out of shape by badly fitting footwear, so the shoe size should be regularly checked.

To ensure that you buy the correct size, you can measure the child's feet at home before going to the shoe shop. Stand the child on two strips of paper about $\frac{1}{2}$ in. (13 mm.) wide and cut them to the exact length of the feet when standing. Mark the strips 'Left' and 'Right'. Slip each one into the appropriate shoe until it touches the toe-cap. Make sure there is $\frac{3}{4}$ in. (19 mm.) to spare between the end of the paper and the heel of the shoe.

Never buy shoes without the child being present and do not buy footwear for 'Sunday best' or as 'party' shoes. They will be infrequently used and will be outgrown long before they are outworn.

For the summer and for playing about the house or garden, sandals with open toes and firm straps are the best buy. But whenever possible—in a carpeted room, in the garden or on the beach—children should go barefoot as this allows their feet to develop naturally.

Remember that a baby's feet can be damaged by 'baby grow' garments that are too small, and that a child's feet can be damaged by wearing socks that are too short.

Exercises to benefit the feet

To keep your feet supple and in good condition, the following exercises should be practised two or three times a week. Wear clothing that does not restrict leg movements, such as a leotard or shorts.

THE STEP RAISE
Stand barefoot on the edge of a step at the bottom of a flight of stairs. Hold on to bannister for support.

1 Lower the heels slowly and hold the position.

2 Slowly raise the feet and stand on tiptoe.

THE FOOT REVOLVE
Sit barefoot in an upright chair and cross one leg over the other.

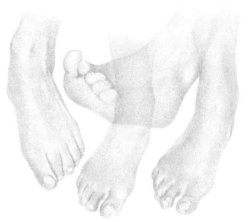

1 Keep the uppermost leg as still as possible and point the toes.

2 Draw large circles in the air with the foot.

THE LEG STRETCH
Sit barefoot on the floor, bracing yourself with the palms of your hands.

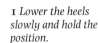

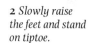

1 Move the knees apart and place the soles of the feet together.

2 Without separating the soles, slide the legs along the floor.

3 Straighten the legs as far as possible.

FORCEPS

A tongs-like instrument for holding an object firmly or pulling it. There are many different types. Obstetrical forceps are used to grasp a baby's head during labour when the baby needs help to emerge from the birth canal. Surgeons use many kinds of forceps, to separate tissue, to hold it in position and to compress blood vessels. Dental forceps—short, powerful instruments—are used to pull out teeth.

FOREIGN BODIES IN THE EAR, NOSE OR THROAT

A foreign body in medical terms means anything found in the body that should not naturally be there, such as a thorn in the skin, a bead in the nose or ear, or a fish-bone in the throat. Children particularly have a habit of pushing objects into their ears and noses, or swallowing things while they are playing.

FOREIGN BODY IN THE EAR

Symptoms
- There may be no symptoms—only the knowledge that the object is in the ear.
- Discharge from the ear.
- Earache.
- Deafness on the affected side.

Treatment in the home
- Go to the doctor—within 24 hours if there are no symptoms, sooner if there are symptoms.
- Do not try to remove the foreign body. You risk causing OTITIS EXTERNA or a PERFORATED EAR-DRUM.

What the doctor may do
- Remove the foreign body by syringing the ear, or retrieve it with forceps.
- If the foreign body is stuck deep inside the ear, it is necessary for it to be removed in hospital under an anaesthetic.

Prevention
- Do not put anything in the ear, and discourage children from doing so.
- Do not attempt to clean the outer ear canal. It will usually clean itself, and wax can be wiped off the outside opening of the ear with a flannel. It is better to have the ears syringed from time to time by a doctor or nurse than to attempt to clean the wax out with cotton-wool buds.

Using buds pushes most wax further in, and there is the risk of losing the cotton wool in the canal.

Outlook
- Excellent after removal.

FOREIGN BODY IN THE NOSE

Symptoms
- The child playing with its nose.
- Obstruction of one nostril with blood, discharge or both.
- Discomfort or pain in the nose.

Treatment in the home
- Go to the doctor—within 24 hours if there are no symptoms, within 12 hours if there are symptoms.
- Do not attempt to remove the object yourself.

What the doctor may do
- Gently remove the foreign body with a pair of forceps.
- If the child is struggling, and removal of the foreign body would risk damaging the nose, it may be necessary to remove the object under anaesthetic in hospital.

Prevention
- Discourage children (and adults) from putting things into the nose.
- If the nose is runny or dirty, clean around the outside only. Do not poke inside.

FOREIGN BODY IN THE THROAT

Symptoms
- Discomfort in the throat. The patient can usually indicate the exact site.
- Difficulty and pain on swallowing.
- Excessive saliva.
- Difficulty in breathing.
- Inability to speak.

Duration
- Because a foreign body may scratch the delicate mucous membrane of the throat, symptoms may continue for up to 72 hours after the foreign body has been removed or swallowed.

Treatment in the home
- If the patient is able to breathe, speak and swallow slap him several times vigorously on the back. The slaps should be firm enough to force air out of the lungs, but not fierce enough to cause pain or leave a mark. If the patient cannot breathe, *see* FIRST AID *page 572.*
- If the slaps do not dislodge the foreign body, apply the abdominal thrust, *see* FIRST AID *page 572.* If the first aid does not work get *immediate* medical aid. Go to the doctor, or straight to the hospital accident and emergency department as soon as possible.
- Do not attempt to remove the foreign body with your fingers. This may push it into a more dangerous position.

- A child can be turned upside-down before slapping the back, as this helps to remove the object.

When to consult the doctor
- As soon as possible.

What the doctor may do
- Check the breathing.
- Examine the throat.
- Try to remove the object with forceps after spraying the throat with local anaesthetic to numb the area.
- If the object is not easily visible through the mouth, removal may require a general anaesthetic.
- Send the patient for an X-ray if the foreign body is metal or bone, such as a coin or fish-bone.

Prevention
- Give small children large, well-made toys that they cannot swallow.
- Take care to remove fish-bones from fish before swallowing.

Outlook
- Once the foreign body is removed or swallowed, the mucous membrane usually heals completely in about three days. After that, there should not be any long-term effects.

See EAR *page 38*
RESPIRATORY SYSTEM *page 42*
EYE, FOREIGN BODY IN

FRACTURE

A break or crack in a bone usually caused by injury. Less often a fracture may be the result of repeated stress to a bone (fatigue) or weakening by disease (a pathological fracture). The more common fractures are described below according to site and illustrated according to type. A fracture is 'simple' or 'closed' if the skin above the break is not broken, and 'compound' or 'open' if the bone is exposed, in which case there is greater risk of infection. The healing process varies greatly according to the site and age of the patient. In children a break may heal in four to six weeks, in adults it may take three or four months.

It is usually clear when a bone has been broken (*see* FIRST AID *page 588*), but occasionally a fracture goes unsuspected because the patient can still use the injured part. Consult the doctor after any injury—especially one caused by a fall or severe blow—which causes pain or a large bruise for more than a day or so.

FRACTURED ANKLE

The three bones that form the ankle (fibula, tibia and talus) are fractured more often than any bone, apart from the radius in the forearm.

Symptoms
- Immediate pain, which is often severe.
- The ankle soon becomes swollen or bruised.
- Pain when moving the ankle.
- It may be impossible to stand on the affected leg.

Duration
- The ankle is usually in plaster for about six weeks.

Causes
- An awkward fall or stumble that makes the foot bend excessively.
- Falling on the foot from a height.

Complications
- OSTEOARTHRITIS may follow several years after if the joint is injured.

Treatment in the home
- Rest the ankle. Do not place weight on it.
- Apply a cold compress to help reduce swelling.

When to consult the doctor
- As soon as a fracture is suspected.

What the doctor may do
- Send the patient to the nearest hospital.
- At the hospital the type and extent of the fracture will be determined by examination and X-rays.
- In the case of a simple fracture, a plaster will be applied to the leg below the knee.
- If the fracture is severe, the ankle may be manipulated with the patient under a general anaesthetic, or an operation may be necessary to pin the fractured bone together. Then a plaster is applied.
- Arrange intensive exercises before and after the plaster is removed to restore the strength of the muscles in the foot and leg.

Outlook
- With a straightforward fracture of the ankle, normal function of the joint nearly always returns with treatment in two or three months.
- If a fracture is severe, there may be permanent stiffness in the ankle after healing.

FRACTURED COLLAR-BONE

A common fracture that usually follows sporting injuries. There is a partial or complete breakage of one of the two bones that extend from the top of the breastbone to the shoulder-blades.

Symptoms
- Pain, often severe, over the collar-bone.
- A tender swelling, usually in the middle of the bone.
- Inability to lift the arm on the affected side.

Duration
- With treatment, the bone usually heals within four weeks.

Causes
- The fracture is almost always caused indirectly by an impact elsewhere: a fall on the hand or on the point of the shoulder.

Treatment in the home
- Putting the arm on the affected side in a sling often relieves the pain in the injured area.

When to consult the doctor
- Immediately a fracture is suspected.

What the doctor may do
- Send the patient to hospital.
- At the hospital the collar-bone will be examined and X-rayed in order to discover the type and the extent of the fracture.
- The shoulders are forced back by bandaging. This

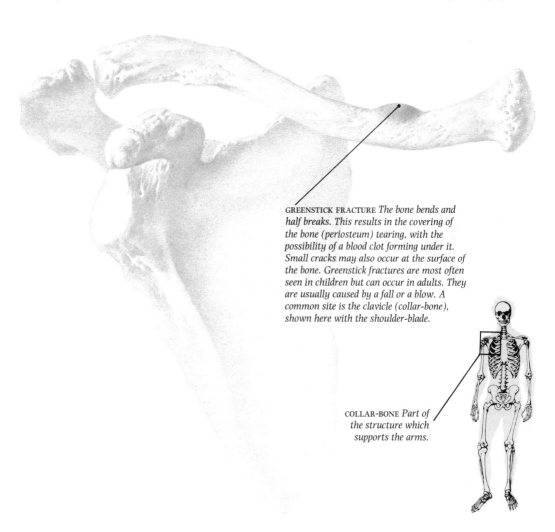

GREENSTICK FRACTURE *The bone bends and half breaks. This results in the covering of the bone (periosteum) tearing, with the possibility of a blood clot forming under it. Small cracks may also occur at the surface of the bone. Greenstick fractures are most often seen in children but can occur in adults. They are usually caused by a fall or a blow. A common site is the clavicle (collar-bone), shown here with the shoulder-blade.*

COLLAR-BONE *Part of the structure which supports the arms.*

brings the fractured parts of the bone into line so that the bone can heal.

- If there is excessive pain, the arm may be put in a sling.
- Elderly patients will be given shoulder exercises to do after the bone has healed. This is to prevent stiffness in the shoulder joint.

Outlook

- The bone usually heals completely with no after-effects, other than a bump in the bone at the site of the fracture.

COLLES' FRACTURE

A partial or complete breakage of the lower end of the radius (one of the two bones of the forearm) just above the wrist. It is the most common fracture and occurs most often in elderly women, in whom the radius is particularly brittle.

Symptoms

- Pain, deformity and swelling at the wrist follow the injury immediately.
- The affected hand cannot be used.

Duration

- Recovery of the full use of wrist and hand usually takes about ten weeks.

Causes

- Falling on an outstretched hand is the most common cause.

Treatment in the home

- A cold compress helps to immobilise the wrist or reduce swelling while waiting to see a doctor.

When to consult the doctor

- Immediately the symptoms occur.

What the doctor may do

- Put the arm in a sling for support and reduction of pain.
- Send the patient to a hospital accident and emergency department.
- At the hospital the wrist will be X-rayed to determine the extent of the fracture. Then the displaced ends of the broken bone will be realigned after the patient has been given a general or local anaesthetic: a doctor manipulates the bone ends into position, feeling through the skin with his fingers. Afterwards a back slab is applied to immobilise the wrist and is kept in position by firm bandaging. The arm is then supported in a sling for two or three days until the swelling has died down. From time to time the sling is removed and the patient does elbow and shoulder exercises. Finger movements are also performed to encourage the return of full use of the hand.
- When the swelling has subsided, the forearm is put in plaster for six weeks.

- Some fractures may still become displaced and require further immobilisation or an operation.

Prevention

- Elderly people should make sure there are no loose-fitting carpets or dangerous stair treads in the house. When walking outside they should take care and use shorter steps in the dark and in icy conditions.

Outlook

- The recovery of wrist movement and use of the hand takes about ten weeks. Complications are rare.

FRACTURED HAND

Five metacarpal bones support the palm of the hand and join the wrist (carpal) bones to the finger bones (phalanges). One or more of these metacarpal bones may be partly or completely fractured by crushing or punching.

Symptoms

- Acute pain and tenderness following injury are felt in the palm and back of the hand at the site of the fractured metacarpal bone. Several bones may be fractured.
- Swelling of the hand.
- The knuckles of affected bones become less prominent than usual.

Duration

- According to the extent of the injury, the hand will be out of action for about ten days to a month.

Causes

- The commonest causes are a fall on the hand or a blow on the knuckles, as may happen, for example, during fist fighting or skiing.

Treatment in the home

- Apply a firm cold compress to support the hand and reduce swelling.

When to consult the doctor

- As soon as a fracture is suspected.

What the doctor may do

- Send the patient to a hospital accident and emergency department.
- At the hospital, the hand will be examined and X-rayed to determine the type and severity of the fracture.
- Most cases are mild, and after a period of rest exercise of the hand will be encouraged.
- If splinting is required, then a light plaster on the back of the arm can be applied for several weeks.
- If the ends of the broken bones are displaced (out of alignment), they will either need to be manipulated into place with the patient under a general anaesthetic, or require an operation to pin them together.

Outlook

- The hand usually returns to full use after most fractures.

FRACTURED BONES IN THE LOWER LEG

Partial or complete breakage of the shafts of the tibia (shin bone) and the fibula, which run from knee to ankle. Often both bones are fractured.

Symptoms

- Immediate severe pain.
- Sometimes a 'crack' is heard on injury.
- Swelling and deformity of the leg.
- An inability to place weight on the leg.
- The ends of the broken bones often pierce the skin (compound fracture).

Duration

- If the bones are not displaced out of alignment, the fracture usually takes at least four to six weeks to heal. If they are displaced, it can take 12-20 weeks for them to mend.

Causes

- A road accident is the most common cause. There is a high incidence of the fracture among motor-cyclists who crash.

Complications

- Road traffic accidents often cause severe fractures, including multiple and open breaks, which give rise to complications. These may include damage to blood vessels and nerves, infection, difficulty in setting the bones and difficulty in immobilising the bones—all of which may mean that the bones fail to knit and recovery is delayed. If this happens, it may be necessary to operate in order to fix the break.

Treatment in the home

- The patient must be handled with great care, otherwise a simple fracture can be turned into a compound one or a compound fracture made worse.
- When there is an obvious fracture of this type, the patient should be made comfortable and warm where he is—in the open or on the roadside—until emergency medical help is available.

When to consult the doctor

- Immediately.

What the doctor may do

- Send the patient to the nearest hospital accident and emergency department.
- At the hospital the leg will be X-rayed. If the bones are not displaced the leg is put in a plaster that immobilises the bones and allows the patient to walk. It is applied above the knee if both bones or the tibia alone is fractured, below the knee if the fibula is fractured. Weight-bearing and walking in a suitable plaster will be encouraged as early as is feasible.
- If displacement of the bones has occurred, the patient is given a general anaesthetic and the doctor manipulates the separated parts of the bone together by feeling

through the skin of the leg. Sometimes the bones need pinning. Then a plaster is applied to immobilise the leg. After two weeks this plaster is replaced by an above-the-knee plaster that allows the patient to walk.

• A compound fracture may become infected and require antibiotics which may delay healing.

Prevention

• During icy or wet conditions on the road motor-cyclists in particular should take great care. The leg guards of motor-cycles should never be removed for the sake of speed. Seat belts should always be worn in cars.

Outlook

• For undisplaced fractures and displaced fractures that are successfully manipulated, the outlook is good.

FRACTURED (NECK OF) THIGH BONE

The neck of the thigh bone (femur) is at the top of the bone, where it joins the pelvis. It is commonly fractured in elderly people, especially women, whose bones have become brittle.

Symptoms

• Pain, which is usually made worse by movement of the leg.

• In cases when the ends of the broken bone are displaced (out of alignment), the person cannot put any weight on the affected leg, and, if the fracture was caused by a fall, cannot stand up unaided.

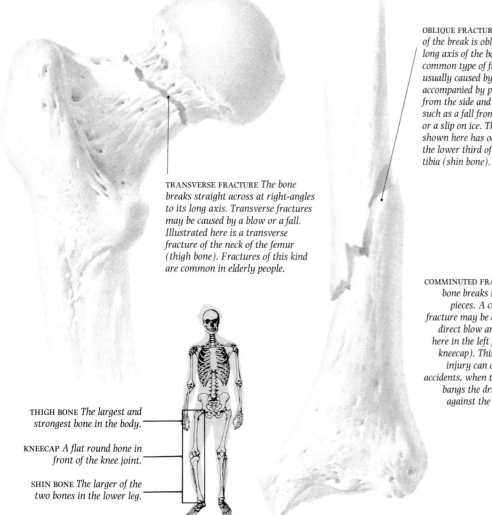

TRANSVERSE FRACTURE *The bone breaks straight across at right-angles to its long axis. Transverse fractures may be caused by a blow or a fall. Illustrated here is a transverse fracture of the neck of the femur (thigh bone). Fractures of this kind are common in elderly people.*

THIGH BONE *The largest and strongest bone in the body.*

KNEECAP *A flat round bone in front of the knee joint.*

SHIN BONE *The larger of the two bones in the lower leg.*

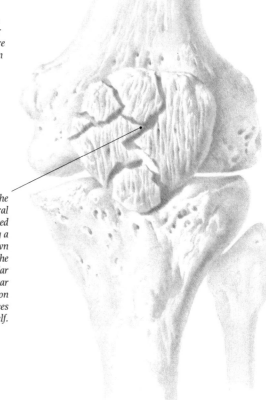

OBLIQUE FRACTURE *The line of the break is oblique to the long axis of the bone. This common type of fracture is usually caused by a fall accompanied by pressure from the side and twisting, such as a fall from a ladder or a slip on ice. The fracture shown here has occurred in the lower third of the left tibia (shin bone).*

COMMINUTED FRACTURE *The bone breaks into several pieces. A comminuted fracture may be caused by a direct blow and is shown here in the left patella (the kneecap). This particular injury can occur in car accidents, when the collision bangs the driver's knees against the glove shelf.*

- When the bones are impacted (wedged together), walking is not affected but there is pain in the knee.
- The affected leg (and foot) is turned outwards when the patient lies on a bed or sits in a chair.

Duration
- The fracture generally takes about three months to heal, but the patient may not be fully mobile until several months after that.

Causes
- The most common cause is a fall, but often a fracture in an elderly person is simply the result of a slight knock.

Complications
- Pneumonia and respiratory complications can occur.

Treatment in the home
- All attempts to move the leg (or patient) should be avoided.

COMPRESSION FRACTURE *The bone is squashed and the resulting deformation causes a fracture. Compression fractures may be caused by the impact force of a vertical drop, such as a jump from a high window to escape fire. In this illustration the force transmitted up the spine as a result of jumping from a height has caused the fourth lumbar vertebra to be compressed and fractured.*

SPINE *The five lumbar vertebrae form the inwards curve in the lower back at waist level.*

When to consult the doctor
- Immediately if a fracture is suspected.

What the doctor may do
- Arrange for the patient to be taken to a hospital accident and emergency department. In the meantime he may tie the patient's ankles and knees together, so that the unaffected leg provides a splint for the injured one; this prevents further movement of a displaced fracture.
- At the hospital, several X-rays will be taken to determine the nature of the fracture.
- An impacted fracture will usually heal of its own accord and will need no treatment. The patient will be allowed to walk on the affected leg with the aid of sticks.
- For a displaced fracture an operation will be needed to pin the broken bones together. After that the patient will not be allowed to put weight on the affected leg for two or three months.

Prevention
- Elderly people should make sure there are no loose-fitting carpets or unsafe stair treads in the home. They should walk carefully with short steps when outside, especially after dark and on icy pavements.
- Hormone replacement therapy slows bone-thinning in women after the MENOPAUSE.

Outlook
- Pinning together displaced bone ends is successful in 70 per cent of cases. In the rest a further operation will be needed.
- ☐ Mobility after treatment is usually excellent.

FRACTURED SPINE
The spine may be fractured in the neck (cervical spine), the back (thoracic spine) or waist (lumbar spine). All are potentially serious fractures because the spinal cord may be injured either by the original injury or by subsequent moving of the patient. The spinal cord carries the nerves which control breathing, the bladder, bowels and movements of the limbs. These and many other bodily functions can be permanently paralysed. Do *not* attempt to move a casualty after an accident if there is pain on moving or twisting the spine (neck, back or waist).

Symptoms
- Pain on moving or twisting any part of the spine.
- Paralysis or numbness of the limbs or trunk.
- Difficulty in breathing or passing water.

Duration
- Three months, if there is no injury to the spinal cord.

Causes
- Falls, accidents in vehicles, at work or in sport.
- Impact injuries such as those from fast-moving traffic

or falling masonry on building sites.
Complications
- Permanent paralysis of one or more limbs.
- INCONTINENCE of urine or faeces.
- Injuries to the cervical spine can cause death.

Treatment in the home
- Make the casualty warm and comfortable where he is.

When to consult the doctor
- Immediately.

What the doctor may do
- Confirm the diagnosis and check on possible injury to the spinal cord.
- Supervise transfer to ambulance and hospital.
- Arrange X-rays and immobilisation of the spine in hospital.
- Arrange rehabilitation.

Prevention
- Car drivers and all passengers should always wear seat belts.

Outlook
- Good, unless the spinal cord is injured, in which case paralysis may result.

FRACTURED NOSE

The bones at the bridge of the nose may be broken or displaced by injury. There is then a danger that the deformity may be permanent as is seen in the case of some boxers.

Symptoms
- Severe pain.
- Irregularity of shape.
- Severe nose-bleed.

Duration
- A fractured nose usually takes about two weeks to heal.

Causes
- Most commonly, a blow with a fist or blunt instrument, or a road traffic accident.

Treatment in the home
- Bleeding can often be stopped by gauze packed into the nostrils.

When to consult the doctor
- If the symptoms described occur.

What the doctor may do
- Inspect the nose carefully. If there is no deformity causing obstruction of the nose or no dislocation of the septum (thick elastic tissue which divides the top of the inner nose into two chambers), treatment is usually unnecessary apart from an X-ray to check that there is no displacement.
- In cases of deformity, obstruction or dislocation, the trouble will be corrected by an operation, with the patient

under a general anaesthetic.

Prevention
- Anyone travelling in a car should wear a seat belt.

Outlook
- A nose knocked out of shape can usually be corrected if operated on at an early stage.

FRACTURED SCAPHOID

Partial or complete breakage of the scaphoid, a bone in the wrist, following injury. This fracture is easily overlooked.

Symptoms
- Painful, swollen wrist. Tenderness is most pronounced below the base of the thumb.

Duration
- With treatment the fracture usually heals after about eight weeks.

Causes
- The most usual cause is falling on an outstretched hand; this is most common in young adults.

Treatment in the home
- Take painkillers in recommended doses to relieve pain. See MEDICINES, 22.

When to consult the doctor
- Immediately a fracture is suspected.

What the doctor may do
- Refer the patient to a hospital accident department.
- At the hospital the wrist will be X-rayed. (In some cases, however, the fracture is not immediately revealed by X-ray and there is a failure to diagnose the injury.) A further X-ray after ten days usually reveals the fracture.
- The wrist is put in a plaster, which leaves the fingers free, for eight weeks, after which time the wrist should have healed. However, healing may be delayed if the fracture has interfered with the blood supply to the scaphoid, or if splinting has been delayed because no fracture showed on early X-rays.

FRACTURED SKULL

Partial or complete breakage of one or more of the bones forming the skull, due to a head injury. A fractured skull is usually serious because there is associated damage to the underlying organs. There may be concussion (bruising of the brain), intracranial haemorrhage, damage to brain tissue, its coverings (meninges) or other structures within the skull. All may be dangerous.

Symptoms
- Bruising of the skull.
- Bleeding from the ear.
- In many cases, the associated concussion at the time of the head injury causes dizziness, unconsciousness, loss of memory, abnormal behaviour or vomiting.

Causes
- The most common causes are a road traffic or riding accident, a fall from a height (in children, often from a swing or roundabout), boxing or an assault.

Treatment in the home
- Place the injured person at rest with the head in a comfortable position.
- Do not give food or drink.
- If the patient is unconscious, ensure a clear airway. See FIRST AID page 611.

When to consult the doctor
- Immediately a head injury has occurred, accompanied by any of the symptoms described.

What the doctor may do
- Send the patient to a hospital accident and emergency department.
- At the hospital the skull will be X-rayed, and if there is any possibility of complications developing the patient may be admitted for 24-48 hours for observation. Complications may need to be treated by surgery.

Prevention
- Wear a seat belt during car journeys.
- Adequate protective headgear (hard hats) should be mandatory for all jobs and sports such as riding, cricket and motor cycling in which head injury is a potential hazard.
- Do not box.

Outlook
- Every head injury is potentially serious. If there is no prolonged concussion or other evidence of damage to underlying structures the outlook of a fractured skull is good.

See SKELETAL SYSTEM page 54

FRECKLES

Brown spots on the skin due to over-production of pigment. Fair-skinned people have a considerable variation in the amount of skin pigment. The pigment-producing cells are stimulated by sunlight so that freckles appear on the face, forearms and wherever pale skin is exposed. The number of freckles depends on the amount of sun received, but those who develop freckles are also easily sunburnt. See SKIN page 52

FRIGIDITY

Lack of sexual desire, or inability to achieve full sexual excitement. Frigidity can affect both sexes, but the term is usually applied to women only. See SEX PROBLEMS

FROZEN SHOULDER

A disorder of the shoulder that develops gradually, usually over several weeks, in the middle-aged and elderly.
Symptoms
• A severe aching pain in the shoulder and upper arm that tends to be worse at night.
• Restriction of shoulder movements.
Duration
• From two months to two years.
Causes
• Not known.
Treatment in the home
• Rest the arm in a sling.
• Take painkillers in recommended doses for relief of pain. *See* MEDICINES, 22.
• Do not force movements to get the joint 'working'
When to consult the doctor
• If the pain interferes with activities or sleep.
What the doctor may do
• After examining the shoulder, he may arrange for a blood test and an X-ray.
• Prescribe tablets for pain relief.
• Arrange physiotherapy or demonstrate simple graded exercises to relieve the condition.
Prevention
• There is no way of preventing the disorder.
Outlook
• Recovery can take as long as two years but always eventually occurs, and is usually complete.

See SKELETAL SYSTEM *page 54*

FUNGUS
A small organism of the plant family. Some types of fungus are valuable sources of food, vitamins and drugs. Others cause disease such as RINGWORM and THRUSH.

GALLSTONES

Solid masses, like pebbles, found in the gall-bladder and in the bile duct leading from the liver. Gallstones (known medically as calculi) form as a result of chronic inflammation of the gall-bladder called cholecystitis. The causes, symptoms, outlook and management of gallstones and cholecystitis are similar. One person in ten has gallstones, and one in five of the over-40s.
Symptoms
• Often none, and the gallstones are discovered only after an X-ray for other purposes. When there are symptoms they often start after a fatty meal.
• Mild, upper abdominal discomfort.
• Wind.
• A bloated feeling.
• Bouts of pain in the upper middle and right abdomen, going through to the shoulder-blade, associated with sickness and vomiting.
• Stones in the bile duct cause attacks of severe intermittent pain with vomiting.
Causes
• Too much fat in the diet.
• Chronic infection of the gall-bladder (cholecystitis) is usually present.
Complications
• JAUNDICE and PANCREATITIS may develop if a stone in the bile duct blocks the outflow of bile.
Treatment in the home
• Take sips of water.
• Take painkillers in recommended doses to relieve bouts of pain. *See* MEDICINES, 22.
• A hot-water bottle over the ache will help to relieve the pain.
When to consult the doctor
• If you have abdominal pain, which does not settle down within four hours.
What the doctor may do
• Send you to hospital to have an X-ray or ultrasound scan.
• Give advice about diet.
• Prescribe drugs to try to dissolve the gallstones.
• Refer the patient to hospital where the stones may be disintegrated by powerful sound waves (lithotripsy) or removed by an operation.

See DIGESTIVE SYSTEM *page 44*

GANGLION

A harmless swelling in the sheath of tissues that contains tendons. It is usually found near a joint, most commonly on the back of the wrist. A ganglion may also occur on the palm, finger, heel or ankle.
Symptoms
• A swelling usually about $\frac{1}{2}$ in. (13 mm.) across. In rare cases it is painful.
Duration
• In many cases the swelling disappears of its own accord within two or three months.
• In other cases it has to be cut out.
Causes
• The cause is unknown.
Treatment in the home
• The swelling can be dispersed by firm finger pressure or by a blow with a large flat object, such as a book. But with either method the ganglion tends to recur, and if it is painless it is best left alone.
When to consult the doctor
• If the ganglion is getting bigger and pressing on nerves, causing pain.
What the doctor may do
• Send the patient to a hospital out-patients department, where the ganglion will be numbed with a local anaesthetic and cut out.
Prevention
• Prevention is not possible.
Outlook
• Ganglions may recur after disappearance or removal.

See SKELETAL SYSTEM *page 54*

GANGRENE

Death and decay of the fingers, toes, limbs or other parts of the body that occurs when their blood supply is cut off.
Symptoms
• The affected tissue or extremity becomes suddenly pale and cold.
• After a few days the part—which may be dry or moist—turns black.
• In moist gangrene, the surrounding tissue may be infected and painful.
• Pain at the edge of the affected area may be intense.
Duration
• The dead part is shed from the body over a period of weeks or sometimes months.
Causes
• Faulty circulation—constriction or blockage of the arteries from any cause.
• DIABETES, atherosclerosis of arteries (*see* ATHEROMA, BUERGER'S DISEASE) and thrombosis may damage and block

arteries and cause gangrene.
- Frost bite. *See* FIRST AID.
- Pressure—such as BEDSORES, or tight bandages.

Complications
- Infection and loss of a limb.

Treatment in the home
- Avoid pressure, friction and extremes of temperature until medical advice is given.

When to consult the doctor
- Immediately if a limb or part of a limb suddenly becomes pale and cold and remains in this state for over two hours, despite rest.
- If there is persistent discoloration, or ulceration, of smaller areas such as the tips of the fingers or toes which does not clear up after one or two days.

What the doctor may do
- Advise careful nursing in mild cases.
- In more severe cases, further investigation in hospital may be necessary.
- Surgery may be considered, either to improve the circulation or to remove dead tissue.

Prevention
- Keep the extremities of the body warm.
- Avoid tight-fitting shoes.
- Treat minor infections of hands and feet, particularly in old people and those with faulty circulation.
- Cut toe-nails carefully.

Outlook
- This depends upon the cause. But with care the condition can usually be controlled.
- With advanced arterial disease, however, it may be necessary to amputate the affected parts.

See CIRCULATORY SYSTEM *page 40*

GAS GANGRENE

Tissue destruction caused by the soil germ *Clostridium welchii* entering a wound, usually on a hand or foot. The disease is so named because the decay of tissue in and around the wound produces gas beneath the skin. In most cases the diseased area is removed surgically.

GASTRECTOMY

Surgical removal of part or all of the stomach. Partial gastrectomy is usually carried out as treatment of severe DUODENAL ULCERS, and the lower, acid-secreting part of the stomach is removed. More common alternatives to partial gastrectomy are vagotomy and GASTROENTEROSTOMY. Total gastrectomy is performed in many cases of STOMACH CANCER.

GASTRIC ULCER

Ulceration of the lining of the stomach, penetrating into the outer muscle coats of the stomach wall. Gastric ulcers are more likely in middle age or later, and men are more susceptible than women.

Symptoms
- Burning, gnawing pain in the upper abdomen or below the left ribs. The pain often comes in bouts and may occur in the early hours of the morning.
- Pain or nausea may follow soon after taking food.

Duration
- Bouts of pain lasting four to eight weeks may recur every few months and continue intermittently for years.
- Treatment usually helps to relieve discomfort in one or two weeks, but healing may take six weeks or more.

Causes
- Ulcers occur where the protective mucous layer of the stomach breaks down, as in chronic GASTRITIS. The unprotected stomach wall may then itself be digested.
- Alcohol, tobacco, irregular meals, anxiety, stress and overwork may all provoke symptoms.
- Some drugs, especially aspirins, steroids, indomethacin and phenylbutazone may precipitate an ulcer in susceptible people. *See* MEDICINES, 22, 32, 37.

Complications
- Erosion of the blood vessels may cause sudden bleeding and vomiting of blood, either bright red or brownish, like coffee grounds. Later, the sufferer may pass black tarry stools.
- PERITONITIS. The deepest ulcers may perforate through the stomach wall and release acid contents into the abdominal cavity with sudden severe pain.
- Chronic gastric ulcers rarely become cancerous, but full investigations are usually necessary to distinguish simple ulcers from STOMACH CANCER if they do not respond rapidly to treatment.

Treatment in the home
- Take small, frequent milky meals and simple antacids.
- Stop drinking alcohol; and stop smoking, as this causes damaging muscular contractions.

When to consult the doctor
- If symptoms are progressive or persist for longer than two or three weeks.
- If there is sudden pain or blood in the stools or vomit.

What the doctor may do
- Prescribe drugs to promote healing, tablets to block the production of acid and antacids to neutralise the acid. *See* MEDICINES, I.

- Send the patient to hospital for a barium meal or ENDOSCOPY through a gastroscope (a device with a light which can be passed into the stomach to see what is happening there). Tissue can be removed for tests to establish the nature of the disease.
- If the ulcer resists other treatment, surgery may be necessary to remove part of the stomach. lifelong check-ups will be needed then to detect vitamin-deficiency anaemias, which might develop slowly.
- Advise about diet and life-style.

Prevention
- Avoid gastric irritants such as alcohol, tobacco and drugs such as aspirin, steroids and certain arthritis drugs.
- Avoid rushed meals and erratic life-style.

Outlook
- Non-cancerous gastric ulcers should heal completely in three months.
- May recur if the old life-style is resumed.

See DIGESTIVE SYSTEM *page 44*

GASTRITIS

Inflammation or irritation of the stomach lining. There are two forms of gastritis: acute, which is triggered by something the victim has eaten or drunk, and chronic, which may persist, especially in old people, without being limited to a specific incident.

ACUTE GASTRITIS

Symptoms
- Pain in the upper abdomen.
- Nausea and vomiting.
- Blood in the vomit which may be fresh red or look like coffee grounds.
- Diarrhoea.

Duration
- An attack usually settles when the cause is removed.

Causes
- Alcohol. A hangover is an attack of acute gastritis.
- Food infected with staphylococci (germs) from handlers with boils and sores. Cream and undercooked or reheated foods are particularly susceptible. An attack caused in this way starts four to six hours after eating.
- Irritants such as aspirin, or poisons such as cleaning fluid, antiseptics or paraffin.

Complications
- None.

Treatment in the home
- Rest. Give sips of water only.

When to consult the doctor
- If abdominal pain does not settle within four hours.
- Any blood in the vomit should be reported to a doctor.
- If vomiting and diarrhoea are severe and the patient's general condition is causing concern.
- If a number of people are affected. *See* GASTROENTERITIS.

What the doctor may do
- Investigate to exclude the possibility of serious disease.
- Give dietary advice.

Prevention
- Avoid dietary and alcoholic excesses.

Outlook
- Acute gastritis usually clears up with simple treatment.

CHRONIC GASTRITIS

Symptoms
- Vague discomfort. Nausea.
- Often none, and the condition will come to light only when a doctor examines a patient for some other reason.

Duration
- The condition tends to persist despite treatment.

Causes
- Breakdown of the stomach lining in old age.

Complications
- Iron and vitamin deficiency. ANAEMIA.

Treatment in the home
- As for acute gastritis.

When to consult the doctor
- If symptoms persist.

What the doctor may do
- As for acute gastritis.

Prevention
- As for acute gastritis.

Outlook
- While treatment eases the symptoms, the condition is likely to persist.

GASTROENTERITIS

Inflammation of the lining of the stomach and intestines.

Symptoms
- Acute vomiting and diarrhoea, usually with abdominal cramps and colicky pains.
- Mild temperature and perspiration.
- Prolonged loss of fluid may lead to dehydration and shock.
- Traces of blood may be seen in the vomit and stools.

Duration
- Most attacks of vomiting and diarrhoea are over after two to four days, though sometimes there are more prolonged bouts. Bacterial (salmonella) infections may persist for months, or even years; the person affected may hardly notice the symptoms but still act as a carrier and transmit the condition to others.

Causes
- Bacterial infections, especially from reheated or half-cooked food, are among the most common causes. Food left at room temperature, especially cream fillings, milk, processed meat and fish, may develop a heavy bacterial contamination. Bacteria of the staphylococcal, shigella and salmonella groups are the common causes. Staphylococcal infections cause acute symptoms within two to eight hours. Salmonella and shigella bacteria infection usually comes from food handlers, flies and unhygienic cooking utensils and develops after 12 to 36 hours.
- Campylobacteria are present, especially in contaminated poultry, meat and fish. They are a common cause of diarrhoea, and may produce severe abdominal pains.
- *Escherichia coli:* these are normally harmless bacteria, but certain types may cause acute gastroenteritis in newborn babies, the infection spreading in nurseries.
- Listeriosis infection comes from contaminated foods. Sometimes it causes an influenza-like illness with fever and sore throat, headaches, swollen glands or skin rash. Pregnant women, children, the elderly and the sick are the most vulnerable to infection.
- Virus infections often cause both gastroenteritis and ENTERITIS. Rotavirus is the most common form of diarrhoea in children. Many types of virus may cause gastroenteritis. Symptoms may develop within two days.
- Poisons occurring naturally in plant life: yew, deadly nightshade, morning glory and horse-chestnuts are all examples. The green parts of potatoes are poisonous.
- Chemical poisons such as arsenic, lead and insecticides. Symptoms develop within hours of intake.
- Certain diseases such as AMOEBIASIS and GIARDIASIS may cause symptoms of gastroenteritis.

Complications
- Gastroenteritis generally has a poisoning effect. In most cases, the poisoning is mild, and the body is quite capable of coping without treatment. However, BOTULISM and certain plant and chemical poisons may prove fatal if early action is not taken.

Treatment in the home
- If acute vomiting and diarrhoea occur, take lots of sips of water. Do not take food or milk drinks. The stomach is trying to get rid of an irritant; do not irritate it more.
- A medicine containing antidiarrhoeal and painkilling elements may be taken by adults. *See* MEDICINES, 2.
- Antidiarrhoeal medicine is suitable for children under five years old (but not babies). This will help to absorb irritants and soothe the aches caused by muscular activity in the stomach.
- When the stomach begins to settle for a few hours, begin nourishment again with dry biscuits, cornflour, jellies, blancmanges, and clear soups. Avoid tea and coffee, or acid drinks such as lemon or orange juice; they may cause irritation and vomiting to recur.
- Most bouts of gastroenteritis settle after one to three days, and a patient can be put back on a fuller non-irritating diet as the symptoms die down.

When to consult the doctor
- In mild cases it may not be necessary to report symptoms to the doctor.
- If there is associated abdominal pain, blood in the motions or other unexpected symptoms.
- If symptoms are severe, or prolonged.
- Consult the doctor immediately if a plant or chemical poison has been taken.
- Consult the doctor immediately if there is any difficulty in focusing the eyes, double vision, fits or paralysis.

What the doctor may do
- Send you to hospital for investigation and treatment if symptoms are severe, or if a plant or chemical poison is known to have been taken.
- The doctor may inject an antiemetic to treat retching which persists after the stomach has been emptied.
- Where diarrhoea persists, the doctor may prescribe antispasmodics or antidiarrhoeal mixtures.
- The doctor may prescribe a sugar and electrolyte solution, such as Dioralyte, to be taken by mouth to replace lost body fluids.
- In young, old or weak patients, he may recommend transfusions of fluid to replace those which have been lost.

Prevention
- Wash your hands carefully before preparing food, before eating meals and after using the toilet.
- Wash salads, and fruit and vegetables that will be eaten raw.
- Keep food for as short a time as possible, follow storage instructions carefully and observe 'best-by' and 'eat by' dates on labels.
- Avoid eating raw eggs or uncooked food made from raw eggs, such as home-made mayonnaise or ice cream.
- Do not use cracked eggs.
- Refrigerate food if you are not going to eat it immediately. Make sure the refrigerator works properly.
- Cook poultry thoroughly.
- Do not allow uncooked poultry to contaminate other foods in the kitchen or refrigerator.

- Kill germs by re-heating food until it is piping hot all through. Avoid inadequately re-warmed food.
- Do not eat food from damaged tins.
- Pregnant women should avoid soft cheeses and pâté.

Outlook
- Gastroenteritis is very common, and hardly ever results in anything worse than a few days of feeling sick. Vomiting and diarrhoea are unpleasant, but they are mechanisms by which the body gets rid of acute infections or poisons.

See DIGESTIVE SYSTEM *page 44*

GENITAL HERPES

A recurring infection of the genitals, transmitted during sexual intercourse. Most primary (first) infections occur in teenagers and young adults.

Symptoms
- Both primary and recurrent infections produce a crop of tiny blisters like a cold sore on the genitals and surrounding areas. In the first attack the blisters usually appear two to 12 days after intercourse with an infected partner. They burst in one to three days and form ulcers with a crust, healing in seven to 20 days.
- While the rash is developing, intercourse is painful and there may also be a burning pain in the infected area.
- There may also be frequent and painful urination and a slight watery discharge.
- In a primary infection there is often a general feeling of ill health, low fever and tender swellings in the groin.

Duration
- Symptoms of an attack usually subside within three weeks, but sometimes the ulcers persist for several weeks longer. Attacks can recur at intervals. The patient is infectious during all attacks.

Causes
- The herpes simplex virus HSV₂, which is only transmittable by direct sexual contact. *See* COLD SORES.

Complications
- These are rare, but include two serious complications, CORNEAL ULCERS and ENCEPHALITIS, both of which may occur in babies born to infected mothers. Such babies are infected in passing through the birth canal of a mother with active infection.

Treatment in the home
- Keep the affected area clean.
- Avoid intercourse.

When to consult the doctor
- As soon as any sore or rash appears on the genitals.
- Recurrent attacks usually require medical advice to confirm the diagnosis and oversee treatment.
- Every attack suffered by a mother during pregnancy should be reported to the doctor.

What the doctor may do
- Make an examination to determine the cause of the symptoms.
- Check for other sexually transmitted infections.
- Prescribe analgesic ointment and tablets (*see* MEDICINES, *43, 22*). In the course of numbing local pain, ointments may also numb the sensations needed to produce an erection.
- Prescribe antiviral drugs such as Acyclovir (*see* MEDICINES, *27*).

Prevention
- Avoid casual sex.
- Use a condom if spread of infection is likely.
- Caesarean section, may be necessary to protect unborn babies of mothers with active infection.

Outlook
- The infection may clear completely after a single attack never to recur, but in most cases it reappears at intervals over many years, and at present there is no effective treatment.

See SKIN *page 52*

GERMAN MEASLES

A common infectious disease, known medically as rubella, which is spread by close contact, that is working with or living alongside infected people. It is not serious in itself, but if it occurs in a woman during the first 16 weeks of pregnancy it may affect the unborn child. A baby with congenital rubella may be stillborn, or born deaf, blind or with heart disease. About 25 per cent of babies whose mothers get German measles during the first 16 weeks of pregnancy are likely to be affected. In very early pregnancy the risk is as high as 60 per cent.

Symptoms
- A characteristic rash of tiny, pink, slightly raised spots, which begin behind the ears or on the face, then spread downwards to the rest of the body.
- Swollen glands, particularly behind the ears.
- Joint pains which may be quite severe, especially in young women.

- The patient may feel unwell for a few days before the rash develops.

Incubation period
- Fourteen to 21 days.

Duration
- The rash lasts from one to five days.
- Joint pains may last up to 14 days.
- The patient is infectious to others from five days before until four days after the rash appears.

Treatment in the home
- Stay indoors for four days from the onset of the rash.
- Keep away from pregnant women.
- If necessary take painkillers to ease discomfort.

When to consult the doctor
- If severe joint pains develop.
- If diagnosis is in doubt and there is a danger of infecting others, especially adults.
- If German measles is suspected in early pregnancy in a woman not known to be immune. (Routine blood tests in pregnancy will show up immunity.)
- If the patient develops a high temperature, severe persistent headache or becomes drowsy.

What the doctor may do
- Take blood tests to confirm the diagnosis, since several other viruses cause symptoms similar to those of German measles.
- If German measles is confirmed in early pregnancy, he may ask the patient if she wishes to terminate, rather than risk bearing a child with congenital deformities.

Prevention
- Since German measles is very serious in pregnant women, it is better for children, especially girls, to obtain immunity from catching the disease.
- Women of child-bearing age who have not had German measles, and who may wish to become pregnant at a later stage, should be immunised. After immunisation a rash and joint pains, like those of German measles, may occur. Pregnancy should be avoided for at least three months after the injection, since immunisation can affect an unborn child during this period.
- Immunisation is now routinely offered to all children in the MMR vaccine given in the second year of life.
- Before their first pregnancy, all women should have a blood test to confirm that they are immune.
- Immunisation after childbirth is offered to women who have no immunity.

Outlook
- One attack of German measles usually ensures immunity for life. Apart from its effects on the unborn child, the outlook is good and complications are rare.

See INFECTIOUS DISEASES *page 32*

GERSON THERAPY

A dietary approach to the prevention and treatment of cancer. Exponents of the theory believe that all denatured or artificially processed foods are potentially harmful to the body.

See NUTRITION

GIARDIASIS

Infection of the digestive system by a microscopic parasite called *Giardia lamblia*. The disease affects people who have returned from Mediterranean countries or other parts of the world, although it does occur in Britain. Symptoms usually develop a few weeks after infection.

Symptoms
- Diarrhoea with bulky, foul-smelling stools.
- Discomfort and distension of the stomach.
- Nausea.
- Inability to absorb food.

Duration
- The condition may last for several weeks or more.

Causes
- The parasite *Giardia lamblia*.

Treatment in the home
- Kaolin or other simple antidiarrhoeal mixtures may be used to settle symptoms. *See* MEDICINES, 2.

When to consult the doctor
- If you have diarrhoea after travelling abroad.

What the doctor may do
- Examine your stools to confirm the diagnosis.
- If you have the disease he will prescribe tablets to kill the parasite.

Prevention
- Other members of the family should be tested and treated.

Outlook
- With treatment, cure is usually complete.

See DIGESTIVE SYSTEM *page 44*

GINGIVITIS

Inflammation of the gums. The disease, which can start at about the age of seven, is treatable until about the age of 18. After that, damage is irreversible and the teeth may eventually be lost.

See TEETH

GLANDULAR FEVER

A disease of children and young adults, more prevalent in the 15-25 age group, particularly among students.

Although also called infectious mononucleosis it is not particularly infectious, and in many cases there has been no obvious contact with other patients. The incubation period (time from catching the infection to first symptoms) is uncertain, but may be one to six weeks.

Glandular fever is probably diagnosed less often than it occurs. In many cases, particularly in children, it may be indistinguishable from other upper-respiratory infections.

Symptoms
- The symptoms may come on suddenly, or gradually develop over four or five days.
- Sore throat or tonsillitis, often severe and persistent, and sometimes with yellow spots on the tonsils and little red spots at the back of the throat.
- Feeling of lethargy, poor appetite and of being unwell.
- Fever, headache and swelling around the eyes.
- Swollen glands in the neck, armpits and groins.
- The spleen may be enlarged enough to be felt by the doctor, and jaundice may occur.
- In about 15 per cent of cases there is a fine red rash similar to GERMAN MEASLES.
- Ampicillin causes a severe rash if given to patients with glandular fever. This does not mean that the patient is allergic to this drug at other times. *See* MEDICINES, 25.

Duration
- Symptoms often persist for two or three weeks, followed by six to eight weeks before the patient feels completely well again.
- Younger children recover more quickly.

Causes
- A virus known as the Epstein Barr virus. This is found in the saliva of an affected person, and may lead to infection of others by kissing or other close contact.

Treatment in the home
- Rest in bed during the acute phase.
- Take painkillers in doses recommended on the container. *See* MEDICINES, 22.
- Stay in cool surroundings.
- Take extra drinks, but do not drink alcohol until fully recovered, as the liver is usually involved in the infection.
- Avoid blows to the abdomen to prevent damage to the enlarged spleen.

When to consult the doctor
- If a severe sore throat in the 15-25 age group persists for more than five days.
- If there is a severe headache and stiff neck.
- If swallowing is painful and not relieved by painkillers.
- If the patient is unable to drink adequately.

What the doctor may do
- Take blood tests to confirm the diagnosis.
- In severe cases prescribe a course of steroid tablets, otherwise there is no specific treatment other than the above.

Prevention
- None is known.

Outlook
- In children recovery is complete in two to four weeks. Older patients may take six to eight weeks. During this time the patient should avoid sports and other violent activities that could lead to abdominal injury and rupture of the spleen.
- It is extremely rare to develop the clinical symptoms of glandular fever more than once.

See RESPIRATORY SYSTEM *page 42*

GLAUCOMA

A disease of the eye, usually affecting elderly people. The condition can be acute or chronic. Both types are serious because unless treated early, duration is indefinite and irreversible—blindness may develop.

ACUTE GLAUCOMA
This is a rare but serious eye emergency. It occurs most often in elderly patients, especially elderly women.

Symptoms
- Acute pain in and around the eye, sometimes severe enough to cause vomiting.
- Blurring of the vision.
- The attack often comes on in the evening and may be caused by excitement.
- Often there is visual disturbance with earlier blurring of the vision and discomfort in the eye. The disturbance is better after sleep.
- Sometimes rainbow-like 'haloes' are seen around lights at night-time. These may start with short-lived attacks which gradually become longer.

Causes
- A blockage of the channel which runs around the edge of the inside of the iris, and drains off fluid from the front of the eye between the lens and the cornea. Pressure rises inside the globe of the eye causing the pain and ultimately

pressing on the nerve fibres at the back of the eye and thus threatening the eyesight. This blockage is made worse by the pupil dilating as it does in response to darkness and to excitement.

Treatment in the home
• None.

When to consult the doctor
• Acute eye pain and blurring of the vision is an emergency and the doctor should be consulted at once.
• If there is any delay in getting medical help, keep the patient calm and reassured and in a well-lit environment.
• If there is discomfort in the eye (especially in the evenings) and 'haloes' around lights.

What the doctor may do
• If the history suggests possible glaucoma, the doctor will probably examine the eye with a torch (to see if the chamber between the lens and the cornea is narrow) and look in the eye with an ophthalmoscope (to see if there is increased pressure). He is likely to send the patient for specialist treatment and observation.
• If the doctor diagnoses acute glaucoma he is likely to put drops in the eye to make the pupil smaller, and so reduce the pressure on the drainage channel.
• He may also give a painkilling injection.
• Send the patient to hospital, where treatment will continue with drops and drugs to reduce the pressure inside the eye. An operation on the eye may be needed.

Outlook
• With modern treatment and surgery the damaging effects on the vision can be lessened.

CHRONIC GLAUCOMA
This is a serious condition affecting the vision of both eyes and which can eventually cause blindness. It usually affects elderly people, and there is often a family history of the condition.

Symptoms
• There are no obvious warning symptoms in chronic glaucoma and this is its great danger. Gradually, over a period of months or years, vision is lost at the edges of the visual fields. The disease often progresses slowly, perhaps for several years, and loss of vision is not noticed until a good deal of incurable damage has occurred.

Causes
• The cause is a build up of excess pressure inside the eye. The pressure increases because the part of the circulation which drains the fluid from the front of the eye begins to fail. Why it fails is not usually clear—it may simply be part of the diminished efficiency of the circulation generally in some people as they grow older, although it does tend to be commoner in relatives of other sufferers from chronic glaucoma.

When to consult the doctor
• If you have any difficulty in seeing, especially at the edge of the visual field, or if the optician suggests that a consultation is desirable.

What the doctor may do
• The doctor will probably test your fields of vision by asking you to look with each eye in turn at a fixed point and telling you to say when you can see his hands moving in from different points on the edge of the area of vision.
• He will then probably look into your eyes with an ophthalmoscope to try to detect any deepening of the optic disc (the bundle of nerve fibres at the back of the eye which carry the light messages to the brain).
• The doctor may also test for hardness of the eyeball by lightly pressing his fingers over the upper eyelid.
• If he suspects chronic glaucoma he will probably send you to a specialist.
• The specialist will usually measure the visual fields, and also the pressure in the eyeballs.
• If chronic glaucoma is confirmed, the specialist will probably prescribe treatment with eye drops to try to reduce the pressure in the eye and keep the pupil small to help the drainage at the front of the eye.
• Sometimes a special drainage operation is needed.

Prevention
• There is no way of preventing either acute or chronic glaucoma from developing, but there are important steps to take to prevent it from developing to a stage where sight is seriously threatened.
• Have regular eye check-ups every two years after the age of about 40. If there is a history of glaucoma in your family, you may be eligible for free eye tests.
• Consult a doctor if the vision appears to be deteriorating on the edge of the visual field, especially if there is any family history of glaucoma.
• Co-operate closely in any treatment that is prescribed and any follow-up examinations that are arranged. Many people fail to understand the importance of regular check-ups.

Outlook
• With present-day treatment the outlook is good, but failure to persist with treatment can lead to blindness.

See EYE *page 36*

GLUE EAR
The common name for chronic-secretory otitis media. The condition mainly affects children, especially between the ages of five and seven.
See OTITIS MEDIA

GONORRHOEA

A sexually transmitted disease that is transmitted by the gonococcus bacterium during intercourse. It can affect both the male and female genitals, and it may damage the eyes of babies born of infected mothers, leaving a scar at the front of the eyeball.

In rare cases arthritis may develop as a complication. In women, gonorrhoea often affects the Fallopian (egg-carrying) tubes and may, as a result, cause severe pelvic inflammation or PERITONITIS.

In both men and women gonorrhoea can cause INFERTILITY.

Contrary to much popular supposition, the disease cannot be caught from lavatory seats.

GONORRHOEA IN THE MALE
Symptoms
• An intense burning in the penis, three to ten days after sexual intercourse, followed by a profuse yellowish discharge of pus.
• Untreated, the symptoms gradually subside, and the person may be misled into believing the problem has cleared up.
• In some cases there are no symptoms.

Duration
• If the disease is not treated, symptoms tend to disappear within six months. But symptom-free people are still infectious if untreated: they act as carriers of the disease and are responsible for most new cases of infection.

Causes
• Transmission of the gonococcus bacterium by sexual intercourse.

Treatment in the home
• None is possible.

When to consult the doctor
• See the doctor as soon as possible if symptoms develop or if contact with an infected person is suspected. Alternatively, if anonymity is desired, go to a special clinic for sexually transmitted diseases.

What the doctor may do
• Take samples of the discharge and of blood. These will help to determine whether SYPHILIS has been contracted at the same time as gonorrhoea.
• Prescribe antibiotics. The patient must continue taking these until all the follow-up tests show that he is completely free of infection.

Prevention
• The less promiscuous sexual activity is, the less risk

there is of contracting gonorrhoea.
- Condoms (sheaths) should be used as a safeguard, but will not always prevent infection.

Outlook
- Prospects are very good if treatment is early and the patient follows the doctor's instructions exactly.
- Untreated or inadequately treated men will be prone to INFERTILITY, arthritis and constriction of the urethra, the tube through which urine is passed.

GONORRHOEA IN THE FEMALE
Symptoms
In women gonorrhoea often presents no symptoms, with the result that a woman may have the disease without knowing it and may unknowingly infect her sexual partner(s).

If symptoms occur, they include:
- Pain on passing urine.
- Urinating more often than usual.
- A discharge from the urethra, the channel through which urine is passed.
- These symptoms usually start three to ten days after the infection was contracted.

Duration
- As for gonorrhoea in the male.

Causes
- As for gonorrhoea in the male.

When to consult the doctor
- If any possibility of infection in the least is suspected.

What the doctor may do
- Examine the patient to determine whether gonorrhoea is present or not. If it is, he will prescribe antibiotics. These must be taken until tests show the patient is completely free of infection.
- Carry out tests to see if any other sexually transmitted disease is present.

Prevention
- The less sexually promiscuous a woman is, the less risk she runs of catching gonorrhoea.

Outlook
- As for gonorrhoea in the male.
- In addition, untreated women are prone to SALPINGITIS with INFERTILITY.

Warning: In both men and women, cases occur with slight or absent symptoms. These people remain infectious unless treated. For this reason, even the slightest suspicion or fear of infection should always be reported to a doctor.

See FEMALE GENITAL SYSTEM *page 48*
MALE GENITAL SYSTEM *page 50*

GOUT

A disorder in which the chemical processes of the body are upset, resulting in an excess of uric-acid salts collecting in various organs. Men between the ages of 20 and 60 are the most susceptible to gout. The condition rarely affects women.

Contrary to popular belief, gout is not caused by high living and over-indulgence. Nor is it solely a rheumatic disorder, although joint pains are the most dramatic symptom. The kidneys may be affected and stones may form causing severe pain. Deposits of urates collect, causing inflammation and pain in the ears, tendons, knees, elbows, hands and feet.

Symptoms
- Very sudden onset of severe pain, swelling, redness and tenderness of affected joint. For some reason the big toe joints are the most likely to be affected—but knees, ankles, wrists and elbows may also be affected.
- In cases of chronic gout, deposits of urates or tophi may form as hard lumps on the ears, hands and feet. If untreated, the pain may last for a week or more and then pass. As well as suffering pain, the victim feels very ill.

Duration
- Once the condition has started, the sufferer is liable to attacks for the rest of his life.
- Acute attacks may be few and far between or they may be frequent.

Causes
- The precise causes are uncertain, but sufferers have an inherited inability to eliminate the urates from the body.
- Some attacks of gout may be side-effects of diuretics used in the treatment of high blood pressure and heart failure. *See* MEDICINES, 6.
- The condition itself is not caused by over-indulgence of food and alcohol—although these may trigger off some attacks.

Complications
- Repeated attacks may lead to joint damage and cause arthritis.
- Deposits of urates in the kidneys may lead to the formation of kidney stones, causing severe pain and kidney damage.
- If untreated, minute urate crystals may destroy the kidney tissues, causing HYPERTENSION and HEART FAILURE.

Treatment in the home
- There is no effective home treatment until the diag-

nosis is confirmed by a doctor.

When to consult the doctor
- As soon as the condition is suspected.

What the doctor may do
- Take a blood test to show the levels of uric acid in the blood, and possibly arrange for X-rays.
- Prescribe anti-inflammatory medicines to control acute pain and inflammation in the joints. The patient should take them at the start of each attack. Relief should occur within 24-36 hours. *See* MEDICINES, 37.
- Those who suffer from repeated attacks and high levels of uric acid in the blood may need long-term treatment with drugs to keep uric acid at more normal levels.
- Give general advice on how to avoid aggravating the condition—keeping fit, not being overweight, and avoiding certain foods, drinks and activities which may trigger off attacks.

Prevention
- Avoid those foods, drinks or activities that have been found to start attacks.
- Have 'anti-attack' drugs ready and take them as soon as an attack starts.
- If prescribed, take long-term drugs to keep levels of uric acid down.

Outlook
- Attacks tend to get less severe and less frequent as the sufferer gets older.
- Acute attacks can be effectively controlled by treatment.
- Serious complications can be prevented by long-term medication and treatment.

See SKELETAL SYSTEM *page 54*

GUILLAIN-BARRÉ SYNDROME

A rare inflammation of nerves which complicates an earlier, usually milder, infection. It has also developed following immunisation against certain strains of influenza, and can occur as a reaction to some malignant diseases, including Hodgkin's disease.

Symptoms
- The condition usually begins one to three weeks after an infectious illness such as PHARYNGITIS or GASTROENTERITIS.
- Muscle weakness develops usually in a limb over a

period of days. In severe cases, the patient rapidly becomes paralysed.
- Discomfort, tingling and numbness of the skin in the limbs.

Duration
- Weeks to months, sometimes longer.

Causes
- The cause is unknown. Patients seem to develop antibodies against their own nerves.
- About half the cases follow a minor infection or surgical operation.

Treatment in the home
- None possible.

When to consult the doctor
- If weakness in the limbs develops.

What the doctor may do
- Send the patient to hospital for expert nursing care.
- Steroids may be prescribed, but their value is unproven.

Prevention
- None known.

Outlook
- More than 75 per cent of patients make a complete recovery within 18 months. Of the remainder, most have only mild muscle weakness, despite the severity of the illness. Only about 5 per cent of cases are fatal.

See NERVOUS SYSTEM *page 34*

HAEMOPHILIA
A hereditary disorder of blood clotting, almost exclusively affecting males. In the past, sufferers often died in childhood from bleeding after minor trauma, but modern treatment supplements clotting factors and offers a much improved outlook. Before the supplements (Factor VIII) could be prepared synthetically, haemophiliacs were at risk of transfusion-associated diseases, particularly HEPATITIS B and C. Some patients contracted the AIDS virus before its links with blood transfusion were recognised and safeguards taken.

HAEMORRHAGE
Heavy internal or external bleeding. Any visible haemorrhage is an emergency.
See SYMPTOM SORTER—BLEEDING ENTRIES

HAEMORRHAGIC DISEASE OF THE NEWBORN
A rare condition which may occur within the first few days after birth. It is caused by a failure of the digestive system to produce vitamin K, which is essential for blood clotting. As a result, there is bleeding in the bowel, the skin and the brain. The disease is treated with vitamin K.

HAEMORRHOIDS
Varicose veins outside or inside the anus, which often cause bleeding. Haemorrhoids are usually caused by straining to pass stools.
See PILES

HAIR
There is more to looking after hair than brushing, combing or occasional washing.
See HAIR CARE *page 276*

HAIRY PIGMENTED NAEVUS

An area of skin, hairy and pigmented to dark brown, usually 1 in. (25 mm.) or more in diameter, and sometimes covering large areas.

Duration
- The naevus is present at birth. It grows with the growth of the body, but does not spread.

Causes
- None known.

Treatment in the home
- No home treatment should be attempted.

When to consult the doctor
- As soon after the birth as possible.
- If there is any change in the naevus during childhood or adult life, as skin cancer is a possibility. Such changes are: any increase in size, any alteration in colour or bleeding from the naevus.

What the doctor may do
- Send the patient to a plastic surgeon, who may remove the naevus and carry out skin grafting.
- Send the patient for an X-ray. A hairy naevus in the lower back is sometimes associated with bone abnormalities found in mild spina bifida.

Outlook
- The naevus will not spread.
- The chances of skin cancer starting in the naevus are higher than for normal skin, but early treatment will usually prevent such serious complications.

See SKIN *page 52*

HALLUCINATION
False perception by an individual of events that have never occurred. Vision, hearing and other senses may be involved. Hallucinations usually suggest serious mental or brain disorders and should always be reported to the doctor.
See SYMPTOM SORTER—BEHAVIOUR, ABNORMAL, IN ADULTS

HAND
Injury, excessive use and certain chronic diseases of the joints and circulation may affect the hands and fingers in many ways.
See SYMPTOM SORTER—HAND PROBLEMS
HAND CARE *page 282*

HAND, FOOT AND MOUTH DISEASE
A minor virus infection which usually affects young children. Blisters appear on the hands, feet and buttocks, and the inside of the mouth.
See MOUTH ULCERS

HARE-LIP
A deformity of the upper lip present at birth. It occurs when the two sides of the face fail to unite completely in a baby before it is born. The condition is often associated with a cleft palate.
See CLEFT PALATE

HAY FEVER
An allergic condition affecting the eyes and nose, usually brought on by grass pollen.
See RHINITIS

HEADACHE
A very common symptom, usually of trivial origin. Headaches vary greatly in intensity and location and have many different causes.
See SYMPTOM SORTER—HEADACHE

HEAD BANGING
Sometimes children rock their cots backwards and forwards, banging their heads on the bars to the rhythm. Often the only reason for this is that it is a pleasurable sensation, but there may be an underlying cause.
See CHILD CARE

Hair care

HOW TO ACHIEVE AND MAINTAIN A HEALTHY HEAD OF HANDSOME HAIR

Three main things are needed for a good-looking head of hair—good health, the right attention to cleanliness, and caution when using cosmetic treatments.

Severe illnesses, particularly if they involve a high temperature, can cause the patient's hair to become lifeless and very thin. A major surgical operation, or even severe emotional stress, can have the same effect. The lifelessness and loss of hair occurs several weeks after the incident that provokes it. The hair usually takes several months to recover, but nearly always does so.

ADEQUATE DIET

Hair growth depends on an adequate diet. People in famine areas of the world who suffer from severe protein deficiency lose large amounts of their hair. This is unlikely in the Western world, but slimmers in the United States who have received too little protein on drastic reducing diets of 800 calories a day have suffered loss of hair a few months later. *See* NUTRITION.

A more widespread diet problem which causes loss of hair is iron-deficiency ANAEMIA. It is quite common in Britain, particularly among women. The cause is too little iron in the blood, brought on by a diet containing too little meat, eggs, cereals or peas and beans. Fresh fruit and vegetables are also needed to provide vitamin C, which enables the body to absorb iron. If you suspect anaemia, see your doctor.

WASHING THE HAIR

The scalp produces scales and grease like the rest of the skin and these need to be washed off. How often you should wash your hair depends upon how greasy your scalp is and the kind of work you do. If you work on the coal-face or in a steel works you will get much more dirt in your hair than if you work in an office, and you may need to wash it daily. For most people a weekly wash is sufficient.

Hair can be washed with soap, although this is difficult to rinse out completely. It is better to use a shampoo, which usually consists of detergent, soap, water and oils. As well as being easy to rinse off, it will make a better lather. Shampoos are sold containing numerous additives, such as tar extracts, egg, beer, herbs, cucumber and every sort of perfume and colouring. As the visible hair

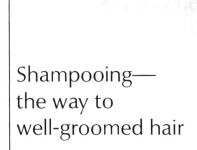

Shampooing— the way to well-groomed hair

The main purpose of shampooing the hair is to remove grease and dirt and provide a clean, well-groomed appearance. Shampoos can be given weekly, although very greasy or dirty hair can be shampooed daily.

1 The hair should be thoroughly brushed or combed to loosen the dirt and scales—or dead cells—on the scalp. For this you may use a brush with natural bristle, or a comb with widely spaced, smooth teeth. Do not brush or comb too vigorously, as this can thin the hair. For hygienic reasons the brush and comb should be thoroughly cleaned after use.

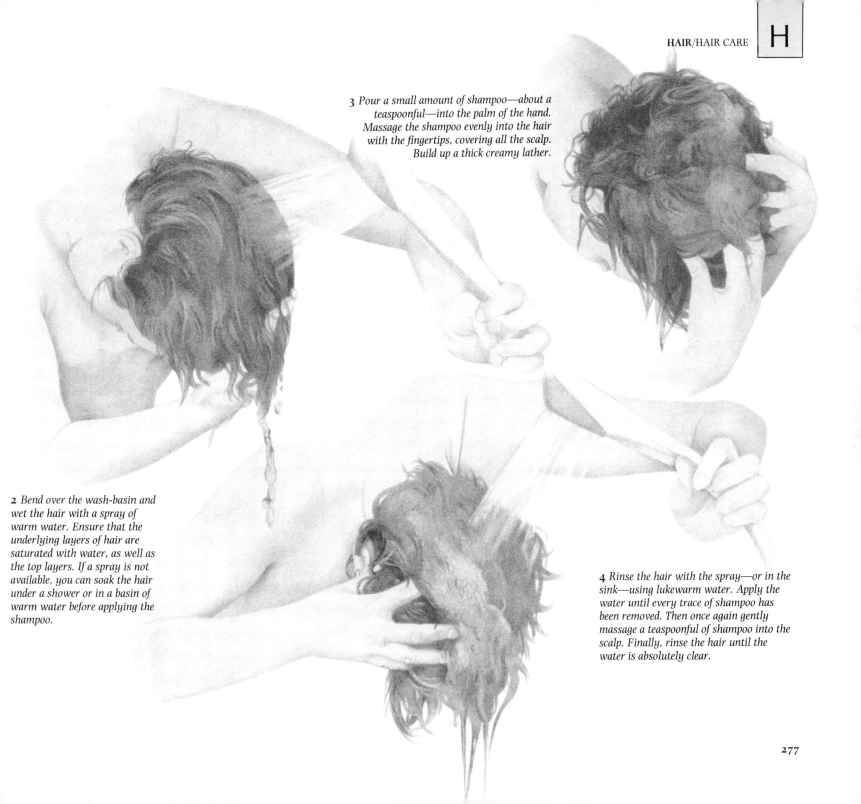

3 *Pour a small amount of shampoo—about a teaspoonful—into the palm of the hand. Massage the shampoo evenly into the hair with the fingertips, covering all the scalp. Build up a thick creamy lather.*

2 *Bend over the wash-basin and wet the hair with a spray of warm water. Ensure that the underlying layers of hair are saturated with water, as well as the top layers. If a spray is not available, you can soak the hair under a shower or in a basin of warm water before applying the shampoo.*

4 *Rinse the hair with the spray—or in the sink—using lukewarm water. Apply the water until every trace of shampoo has been removed. Then once again gently massage a teaspoonful of shampoo into the scalp. Finally, rinse the hair until the water is absolutely clear.*

shafts are dead fibres, they are not influenced by the 'extras'. Expensive and 'different' shampoos are not necessarily better than cheap and simple ones. Any other effects caused by shampoos—such as making the hair shine—are only temporary.

When washing your hair, use moderately warm water. After washing, rinse the hair until it squeaks as it is pulled gently through the fingers. Do not rub it roughly with a towel to dry it, but pat it to remove some of the moisture and then comb in place. Use gentle heat to dry it, or, in the summer, dry it in the sun.

Conditioners—which usually consist of a mixture of oil, emulsifier and waxes—are often applied by hairdressers. The conditioners may be helpful if the outer layer of hair, the cuticle, is damaged. The cuticle is made up of minute, overlapping scales, which protect the inner layers of the hair. The scales can be roughened by frequent washing, permanent waving, or bleaching. By coating each strand with a fine film, the conditioner makes the hair easier to comb after washing and gives it an appearance of smoothness and thickness—which is washed away by the next shampoo.

CUTTING THE HAIR

Although cutting the hair is not essential to its well-being, it is easier to keep the scalp clean if the hair is kept reasonably short. Regular cutting does not make the hair grow strong or faster. And shaving a beard does not stimulate its growth; it merely makes it feel more bristly as it grows again.

HOW HAIR CAN BE DAMAGED

Although scalp hair is hardy, and can withstand a lot of abuse, it can be damaged by too much—or inexpertly applied—perming, dyeing, bleaching and massage. The amount of 'beautifying' the hair can take varies from person to person.

In permanent waving, the hair is first softened by breaking some of the links in the protein bonds which form the hair shafts. This is done either with heat and chemical applications or with cold chemicals alone. The softened hair is then suitably re-shaped and the protein bonds are linked together again by means of an oxidising agent.

There are many ways of perming the hair, which retains its new shape through several shampoos. None of the techniques is harmful if carried out by an experienced hairdresser—or if the instructions for a home perm are carefully followed.

Today, synthetic hair dyes have largely replaced the harmless but messy vegetable dyes used in the past. Temporary dyes, or rinses, which simply coat the hair and are removed by shampooing, are not destructive. However, permanent dyes (usually composed of aromatic benzines) can be harmful to the scalp. These dyes penetrate the hair shafts and form chemical compounds within them. They produce natural-looking colours and are proof against shampooing—although the hair slowly grows out, revealing the undyed 'roots'. Occasionally, the scalp is allergic to the dye and becomes inflamed and swollen.

To prevent this occurring, the dye should be tested by applying it to a small area on the arm (if there is an allergy the skin on any part of the

Equipment used in grooming the hair

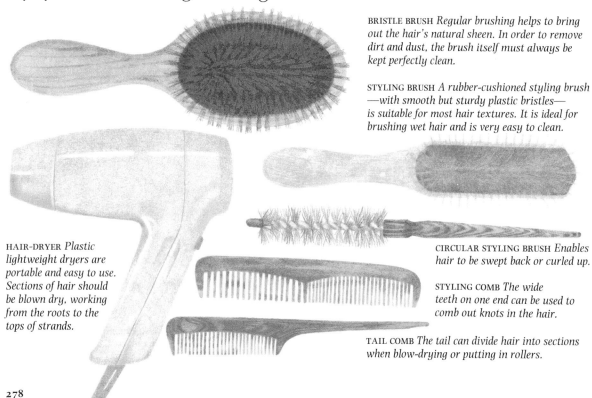

BRISTLE BRUSH *Regular brushing helps to bring out the hair's natural sheen. In order to remove dirt and dust, the brush itself must always be kept perfectly clean.*

STYLING BRUSH *A rubber-cushioned styling brush —with smooth but sturdy plastic bristles— is suitable for most hair textures. It is ideal for brushing wet hair and is very easy to clean.*

HAIR-DRYER *Plastic lightweight dryers are portable and easy to use. Sections of hair should be blown dry, working from the roots to the tops of strands.*

CIRCULAR STYLING BRUSH *Enables hair to be swept back or curled up.*

STYLING COMB *The wide teeth on one end can be used to comb out knots in the hair.*

TAIL COMB *The tail can divide hair into sections when blow-drying or putting in rollers.*

body will show a reaction). The area should be examined after 48 hours—and if a patch of inflammation has developed, the dye must not be used on the hair.

Most people who bleach their hair do so with hydrogen peroxide. If the peroxide is repeatedly applied, it may make the hair brittle—and so less able to tolerate the effects of permanent waving and tinting. If this happens the hair may turn rough, develop split ends, or become thinned or shortened.

GREY HAIR

The hair's colour is determined by the proportion of two pigments—one brown-black, the other red-yellow—which are deposited in the hair shafts. Greying hair is part of the natural ageing process, in which less and less pigment is laid down in the shafts. Grey hairs usually first appear on the temples and then spread over the scalp. Beard and body hair may become grey later on. The age at which greyness begins and its extent depends upon heredity.

AILMENTS THAT CAN AFFECT YOUR HAIR

The hair can be affected by a number of ailments—some of which may require professional treatment.
Hair loss Women may lose hair several weeks after childbirth, or after giving up the contraceptive pill. Hair loss can also occur in patients taking certain anticancer drugs. In all these cases the hair will gradually grow back again as the body returns to normal health.

Many women going through the menopause find that their hair becomes much thinner—and stays that way.

Very tight hair-styles such as a pony-tail—if worn repeatedly or for long periods—can also cause hair loss. And rollers applied too tightly or too frequently can make the hair thin. Repeated massage of the scalp (often done to try to reverse natural baldness) can actually cause hair to fall out. Vigorous and repeated brushing can also make the hair thinner instead of thicker. Nervous children sometimes twist and pluck at an area of their hair, causing thin patches. However, in all these cases, the hair grows back to normal once the tight hair-style or other cause has been abandoned.

Hair grows most luxuriantly in early adulthood. But the rate of growth slows and the hair becomes thinner as men and women get older. This applies to the entire body, on which the hair grows at varying rates on different parts. It grows fastest on a man's beard, slowest on a woman's thigh, and for both sexes the scalp growth averages something in between—about $\frac{1}{64}$ in. (0.3 mm.) a day.

The average scalp contains about 100,000 hair follicles—five out of six of which are growing hairs, while the sixth is at rest. The cycle slowly changes and the previously active follicles enter a resting state and shed their hairs before becoming active again. In this way, just under 100 hairs are shed each day from a normal scalp.

Male baldness Loss of hair from a man's temples and crown is determined by heredity. But it does not necessarily follow that because a man did not go bald his son will not either. Baldness can be inherited from the female side of the family, or from male grandparents or great-

Making the hair manageable

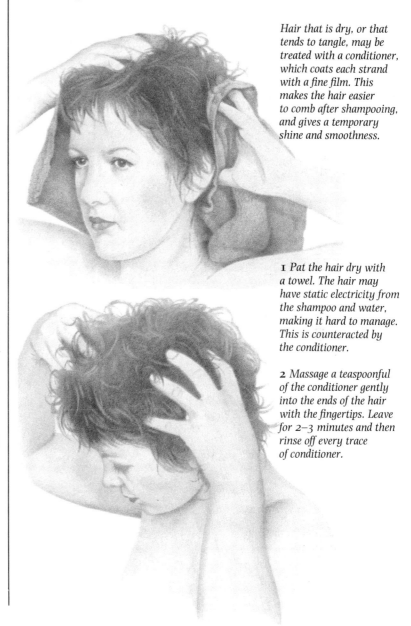

Hair that is dry, or that tends to tangle, may be treated with a conditioner, which coats each strand with a fine film. This makes the hair easier to comb after shampooing, and gives a temporary shine and smoothness.

1 *Pat the hair dry with a towel. The hair may have static electricity from the shampoo and water, making it hard to manage. This is counteracted by the conditioner.*

2 *Massage a teaspoonful of the conditioner gently into the ends of the hair with the fingertips. Leave for 2–3 minutes and then rinse off every trace of conditioner.*

grandparents. *See* BALDNESS.

Dandruff The scalp, like the skin in general, continually produces dead scales. If the scaling is rapid, it may gather on the scalp, or fall on to the shoulders. *See* DANDRUFF.

Split hair Unruly, fuzzy hair which is split at the tips is often the result of damage by too much perming or too strong a bleach. The only answer to split ends is to have them cut away by a hairdresser.

Avoid using sharp combs and brushes that can tear the hair—and dry the hair gently after washing as it is most vulnerable when wet.

Lice and nits The head louse is a tiny, parasitic insect that lives on the human scalp. It lays greyish-white eggs—or nits—which are attached to the hair. Head lice are particularly prevalent in 'closed' communities such as schools.

In common with other insects, lice are becoming resistant to insecticides such as DDT. However, the lice and their eggs can be killed with lotions containing malathion. *See* LICE.

Blow-drying—to give the hair bounce

When blow-drying your hair, hold the dryer about 6 in. (150 mm.) away from your head. If held any closer it can dehydrate and possibly singe the hair. By using a styling brush with the dryer you can give your hair added 'lift' and bounce.

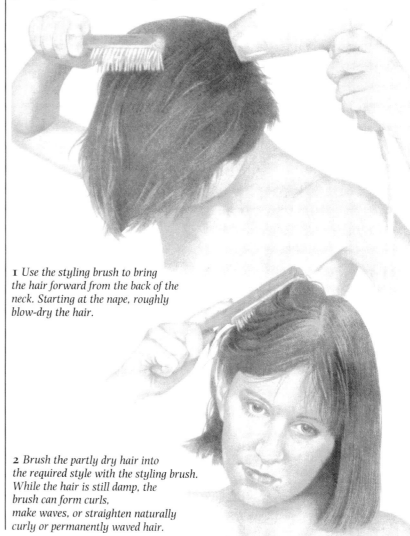

1 Use the styling brush to bring the hair forward from the back of the neck. Starting at the nape, roughly blow-dry the hair.

2 Brush the partly dry hair into the required style with the styling brush. While the hair is still damp, the brush can form curls, make waves, or straighten naturally curly or permanently waved hair.

Beliefs about hair—True or false

☐ **Beer is good for the hair**—*True*
Pale ale makes an excellent setting lotion. Apply it to the hair before putting in rollers or blow-drying.

☐ **Brushing hair 100 times a night makes it shine**—*True*
Thorough brushing stimulates the oil glands in the scalp and makes the hair shinier than normal. However, too much brushing can split and thin the hair.

☐ **Baldness is a sign of virility**—*False*
Baldness may be partly caused by the male sex hormone testosterone circulating in the body. It can therefore be regarded as a sign of virility by those who wish to do so. But men with full heads of hair can be just as virile as those who are bald.

☐ **Hair can turn white overnight**—*False*
Because of the slow growth of hair—about $\frac{1}{2}$ in. (13 mm.) a month—it is impossible for anyone to go white overnight from shock or grief.

☐ **Singeing the hair makes it grow**—*False*
Visible hair is made up of dead cells and singeing only causes split ends. Live hair is under the skin and is unaffected by singeing.

☐ **Hair continues to grow after death**—*False*
The shrinkage of skin surrounding the hair follicles might reveal a further $\frac{1}{16}$ in. (1.5 mm.) or so of hair after death, but hair growth—like nail growth—ends once the body stops functioning.

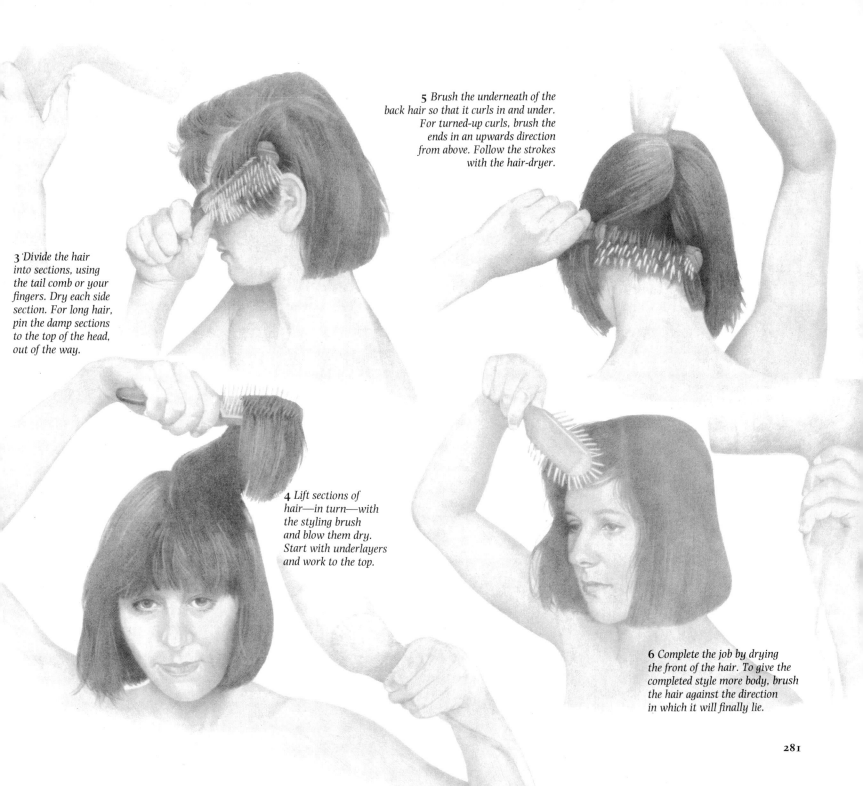

5 Brush the underneath of the back hair so that it curls in and under. For turned-up curls, brush the ends in an upwards direction from above. Follow the strokes with the hair-dryer.

3 Divide the hair into sections, using the tail comb or your fingers. Dry each side section. For long hair, pin the damp sections to the top of the head, out of the way.

4 Lift sections of hair—in turn—with the styling brush and blow them dry. Start with underlayers and work to the top.

6 Complete the job by drying the front of the hair. To give the completed style more body, brush the hair against the direction in which it will finally lie.

Hand care

HOW TO TAKE CARE OF YOUR HANDS—IN DOMESTIC, WORKING AND EVERYDAY SITUATIONS

For many people, especially housewives and manual workers, the hands are the most overworked and ill-used part of the body. They are exposed to all kinds of wear and tear; to the effects of temperature and climate; to frequent wetting; to the onslaughts of harsh chemicals; and to the risk of minor injury and subsequent infection. Yet the care of the hands is often completely overlooked until, say, the skin becomes rough and cracked or a nail is broken.

How to perform a home manicure

Nails should be kept clean by daily brushing with a nail brush. You can perform a home manicure once a week. A basic manicure kit consists of cotton wool, emery boards, a hoof stick shaped at one end for cleaning and with a rubber tip at the other end for easing back cuticles, nail or cuticle cream, a nail buffer, and an oily nail-varnish remover.

2 Wash hands thoroughly in warm soapy water. Do not soak the hands as this will soften the nails too much.

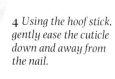

4 Using the hoof stick, gently ease the cuticle down and away from the nail.

1 Remove all trace of nail varnish with an oily nail-varnish remover.

3 Massage nail or cuticle cream all over the nail and cuticle. Wait for three minutes.

CHAPPED HANDS

For everyday hygienic reasons hands should be clean and germ-free. However, the repeated use of soap and water (and even more so of detergents in washing-up water) damages the horny top layer of the skin, and can cause excessive scaling, or chapping. Some skins are more susceptible to chapping than others, and in some cases the skin may develop painful cracks. The problem is aggravated by cold weather and inadequate drying.

When washing hands, lukewarm water and the simplest soap should be used. The soap should be employed sparingly and the hands thoroughly rinsed. They should be completely and gently dried with a dry towel—including between the fingers. Before washing, any rings should be removed as soap can be trapped beneath them, causing irritation.

Exposing unprotected hands to bleaches and other kitchen chemicals, and also to shampoos, can aggravate chapping. These products should not be used any stronger than recommended by the makers.

Bare hands should not be exposed to solvents such as white spirit, turpentine, petrol and dry-cleaning fluid.

To protect hands, wear plastic gloves (some people are allergic to rubber gloves, especially if they have eczema). If you wear gloves while washing clothes or dishes, do not keep them on for more than 10-15 minutes—as they become wet from

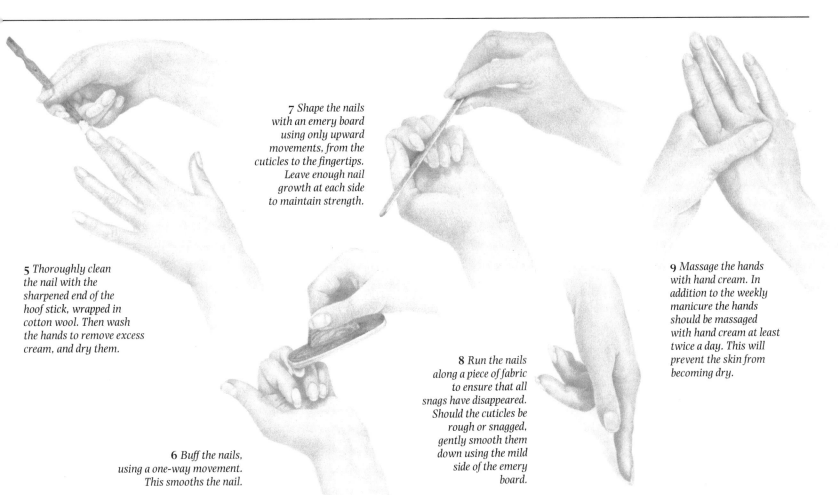

7 *Shape the nails with an emery board using only upward movements, from the cuticles to the fingertips. Leave enough nail growth at each side to maintain strength.*

5 *Thoroughly clean the nail with the sharpened end of the hoof stick, wrapped in cotton wool. Then wash the hands to remove excess cream, and dry them.*

9 *Massage the hands with hand cream. In addition to the weekly manicure the hands should be massaged with hand cream at least twice a day. This will prevent the skin from becoming dry.*

8 *Run the nails along a piece of fabric to ensure that all snags have disappeared. Should the cuticles be rough or snagged, gently smooth them down using the mild side of the emery board.*

6 *Buff the nails, using a one-way movement. This smooths the nail.*

the sweat of the hands, brought on by the heat of the water.

If water, soap or detergent get inside a glove it should immediately be taken off, and not used again until it has been dried by sprinkling the inside with talcum powder.

Although it is helpful to wear protective gloves while doing dirty work, many jobs—such as a car mechanic's—cannot be done with them on. In these cases a barrier cream should be applied to the hands before starting work.

Cold weather can also cause chapping of the hands. The skin becomes sore and red and may begin to crack. To ease the soreness caused by chapping, massage with cold cream. Until the condition has cleared up, avoid using a perfumed hand cream—as the perfume could set up an additional irritation.

ECZEMA
In some extreme instances, chapping can lead to eczema, or inflammation of the skin. Eczema can also affect people who are allergic to certain materials. A reaction can arise from anything that has been handled.

As the hands are almost always in contact with some material, the condition can persist. Eczema should be treated by a doctor or skin specialist, and the patient can help himself by rigorously following the advice given for chapped hands.

WHITLOWS
People who often have their hands in water may get whitlows, or small abscesses, at the sides of the nails. The folds of skin around the nails become soft and open to infection. In acute cases, treatment is by cutting the inflammation and letting out the pus. Antibiotics are also used and the hands should be kept as dry as possible.

People with whitlows should not handle food, or dress wounds.

Equipment used in caring for the hands

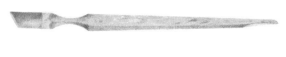

HOOF STICK *The rubber end is used for easing back cuticles—and the other end for cleaning.*

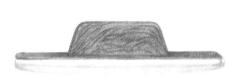

EMERY BOARD *Nails can be filed and shaped by using firm upward movements.*

NAIL BUFFER *To smooth and polish the nails use a brisk, one-way movement.*

CALLUSES
Thickened skin develops as a form of protection where the hands are subjected to constant pressure or friction. Many occupations produce different patterns of calluses on the palms and fingers.

Calluses usually do not need to be removed or treated. Sometimes, however, the thickened skin splits and becomes sore. The calluses should be rubbed twice a day with a pumice stone and cracked skin softened with cold cream.

WARTS
Children in particular are affected by warts, which develop on the hands or fingers and are contagious. Most warts disappear spontaneously, as immunity develops, though they often persist for a year or more. There is no way of preventing them and if they persist and cause concern they should be seen by a doctor, who can destroy them with corrosive or freezing fluids. *See also* WART.

LIVER SPOTS
Large brown spots on the back of the hands are caused by the ageing effects of climate. They particularly affect fair-skinned people who have spent much of their lives in the sun. As well as spots, wart-like growths, called keratoses sometimes appear. *See* KERATOSIS.

If the spots or warty areas appear on the hands before old age, you should not try to remove them with bleaches or creams. They should be examined by a doctor, as in rare instances they could be malignant.

NAILS AND THEIR PROBLEMS
The main function of finger-nails is to protect the sensitive tips of the fingers and concentrate the sense of touch. The exposed part of the nail is inert and consists of a protein called keratin—which is also the chief component of hair and the outer layer of skin.

Nails grow continually throughout a person's life. But the rate of growth differs greatly between individuals according to their age and state of health. On average, a nail grows from its base to its top edge in about six months.

If nails are not cut, they will become split and broken. They can be kept at a suitable length by cutting with scissors or clippers, or by filing.

Flaking nails The top layers of nails can separate and start to flake off if they are exposed to too much soap and water or detergent. If flaking occurs, wear plastic gloves when washing dishes or clothes, and massage nail cream into the nail base each day.

Brittle nails When nails easily crack or break they can be a permanent worry. Weak nails are caused by general ill health or a protein deficiency in the diet. You can increase your nutritional intake by eating more lean meat, fish, fresh fruit and vegetables.

Brittle nails could also be suffering from extreme dryness and, if this is the case, rub in a nail cream every morning and night and keep the nails fairly short until the condition improves.

Loose nails The excessive use of nail hardeners containing formaldehyde can cause the nail plate to separate from the nail bed. The space beneath the nail may then become infected, causing discoloration.

The trouble is slow to heal, although it may be restricted by trimming the affected nail very short.

The condition occurs mostly in women, who—as well as using nail hardeners with formaldehyde—generally keep their nails longer than men. This makes them more likely to be broken or torn. Loose nails can also accompany skin diseases such as eczema and PSORIASIS.

Hang nails If the hands are frequently immersed in water the outer skin layer may split away from the cuticle. The splits, or hang nails, are painful and can become infected. They can be snipped off with sharp nail scissors. To prevent them occurring the skin should be kept flexible by nightly applications of cold cream.

Pitted nails A few isolated pits or dimples in the nails are common and do not indicate any physical disorder. Home treatment consists of keeping the affected nails clean, using nightly applications of an anti-irritant made up of glycerine and boracic (boric) acid. These can be bought separately from a chemist and mixed at home according to his instructions. Do not use nail varnish or nail-varnish remover until the condition clears up.

Nail furrows A minor external injury, or a CYST near the cuticle, can make vertical furrows or grooves appear on the nail. The furrows may split open causing pain, and an infection could occur if dirt enters the split. In the case of swelling and inflammation—or the presence of a cyst—consult your doctor. Home treatment consists of keeping the split nail clean and trimming off any loose nail.

On women's hands, less severe ridges between the furrows can be smoothed by regularly using a nail-buffer, or by using a ridge-filling base coat from the chemist. This is applied under nail varnish and helps to create a smooth finish for the varnish. New growth gets rid of the problem.

Black nails A heavy blow on the nail—or jamming it in a door—can cause bleeding under the nail which eventually turns black. If the bleeding is extensive the nail may eventually fall off. New growth will cure the condition.

If the injury is very painful the nail may have to be removed surgically.

Yellow nails Some nail varnishes—especially if used without a base coat—can produce yellow stains on the nails. The stains are harmless and will disappear with new growth.

White spots The little white flecks that occur in the nail are sometimes the result of a minor injury, such as a damaged cuticle. On some people, however, they appear spontaneously. They are harmless and will grow out.

NAIL-BITING

In both adults and children, nail-biting is a common habit, sometimes stemming from insecurity, boredom, anxiety or excitement. Excessive nail-biting results in very weak nails and, in extreme cases, damaged fingers caused by chewing the nail down to the quick—the sensitive skin beneath the nail.

There is no guaranteed cure for nail-biting. One possible solution is to find something that occupies your hands when they are idle—a creative hobby such as building model aeroplanes, painting, knitting or sewing.

But the best remedy is often to appeal to the individual's vanity. With a girl who bites her nails it can be a good idea to give her a manicure set to make her 'nail conscious'. Failing this, the person concerned must use willpower to conquer the habit.

Hand exercises

People suffering from ARTHRITIS *or* RHEUMATISM *can benefit from the following exercises. The first increases the strength of the hands and wrists and makes them more flexible. The second increases the flexibility of the hands and fingers and improves the circulation.*

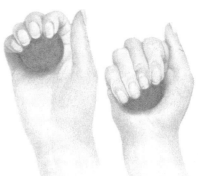

THE SQUEEZE *Place a squash ball in the palm of the hand and firmly squeeze it with your fingers. Repeat until you feel the strain. Then rest and repeat with the other hand.*

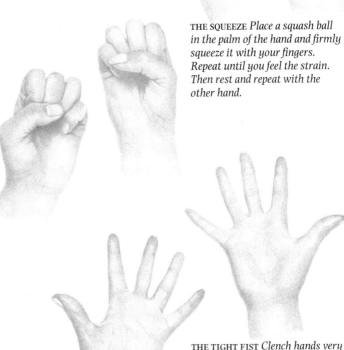

THE TIGHT FIST *Clench hands very tightly then fling the fingers wide and hold for two seconds. Repeat six times.*

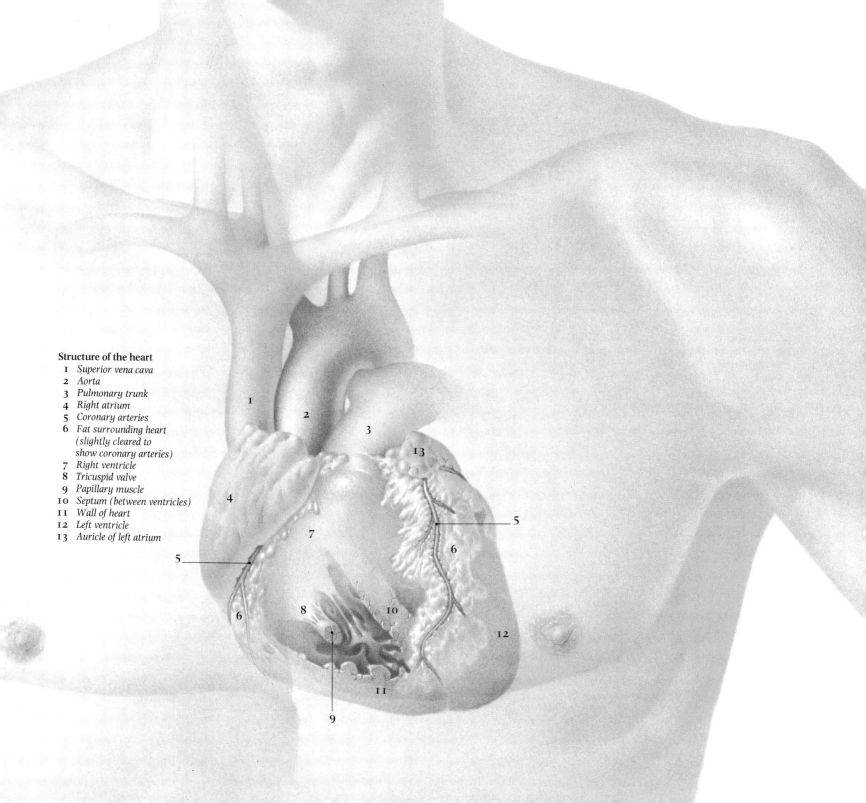

Structure of the heart

1 *Superior vena cava*
2 *Aorta*
3 *Pulmonary trunk*
4 *Right atrium*
5 *Coronary arteries*
6 *Fat surrounding heart
   (slightly cleared to
   show coronary arteries)*
7 *Right ventricle*
8 *Tricuspid valve*
9 *Papillary muscle*
10 *Septum (between ventricles)*
11 *Wall of heart*
12 *Left ventricle*
13 *Auricle of left atrium*

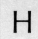

THE HEART

The heart is the strongest muscle in the body. Its job is to pump blood through the hundreds of miles of linked arteries, veins and smaller vessels which reach out to every part of the human body. The blood, in turn, carries oxygen and nutrients to the body's tissues and removes waste products. Every minute of every day the blood is in constant motion, driven by the heart.

The heart starts to beat in the womb within a month of conception and ceases only with death. In the resting adult it pumps 8-9 pints (4.5-5.1 litres) of blood in the body on a complete circuit every minute. This amounts to something like 8 tons of blood every day—or a staggering lifetime total of more than 200,000 tons.

This remarkable organ is a pear-shaped muscle, about the size of a man's fist and weighing 12-14 oz. (340-396 g.) It is behind the breastbone and extends over to the left side of the chest, where the heartbeat is felt.

HOW THE PULSE VARIES
The heartbeat is measured by the pulse, best located on the radial artery on the inner side of the wrist at the base of the thumb, or at the carotid artery on the side of the neck below the chin. The rate at which the heart beats varies throughout life. In a baby's first weeks it may beat 140 times per minute, but by the age of ten the rate will have dropped to an average of 90 per minute. In the adult male, awake but at rest, it beats an average of 70-72 times per minute. The woman's rate is slightly higher—78-82 per minute. For the sleeping adult of either sex the rate is 60-65 per minute. These are average figures, but the heart has a big reserve of capacity. It is capable of rising to 140 beats a minute to cope with extremes of physical activity or anger. Thanks to its reserve capacity a heart that is healthy cannot be over-loaded.

AVOIDING HEART TROUBLE
Heart trouble can start in the womb—some congenital defects are known to be related to harmful influences, such as German measles, during pregnancy. The effect of smoking by the expectant mother is now widely known—it has a toxic effect on her circulatory system and results in a smaller, potentially less-strong baby. Less well known is the risk of damage to the unborn baby's heart by drugs such as aspirin, which are freely available and widely used for the relief of everyday aches.

For those born with healthy hearts the object must be to avoid the process of degeneration which has turned heart disease into the major cause of death in the Western world. Such degeneration is not inevitable—it is the result of a number of harmful environmental factors operating over many years—possibly since birth. Diet is known to be important—but the precise harm caused by individual items of food is not fully understood. Smoking is known to have a damaging effect on the arteries—both within the heart itself and in the general circulation.

In trying to avoid degeneration, no single measure is enough. What is needed is a package of preventive measures which must include: sensible diet, controlling the quality as well as the quantity of what is eaten (see ATHEROMA, NUTRITION); maintaining an ideal WEIGHT; not SMOKING; regular, moderate EXERCISE.

THE HEART AND GREAT VESSELS *The inside of the heart is divided down the centre by a partition called the septum. Each side is subdivided into an inner chamber called an atrium and a lower chamber called a ventricle. Each atrium is linked to its ventricle by a one-way valve. The right atrium and ventricle deal with deoxygenated or 'used' blood and those on the left with oxygenated blood. The septum prevents the two types of blood from mixing.*

The heart wall is made of cardiac muscle (myocardium) which is partly covered on its outside by fat and on its inside by a smooth lining (endocardium). The illustration shows the general form of the heart and the inside of the right ventricle.

Deoxygenated blood is brought to the right atrium by the two largest veins in the body, the superior vena cava and inferior vena cava. From the right atrium the blood passes to the right ventricle between the three cusps of the tricuspid valve. Little muscles, called papillary muscles, attach part of the cusps to the ventricular wall. When the valve closes, the blood in the right ventricle is pumped out through another one-way valve, into the pulmonary trunk which takes it to the lungs to be oxygenated.

Oxygenated or 'fresh' blood returns along two pulmonary veins which feed it into the left atrium, part of which, a pouch called the auricle, is shown. From there it passes through the mitral valve into the left ventricle which pumps it via a fourth valve (the aortic) into the aorta. The major arteries to the head, neck and arms are shown branching off from the aorta. Also issuing from the aorta are the coronary arteries, which supply the heart itself with blood. The aorta arches over the back of the heart to carry blood down to the abdomen and legs.

Heart disease

The principal diseases of the heart are listed below. Each has its own entry where its symptoms are described and you are told what to do about it.

ANGINA PECTORIS
AORTIC INCOMPETENCE
AORTIC VALVE STENOSIS
ATRIAL FIBRILLATION
ATRIAL FLUTTER
CARDIOMYOPATHY
CONGENITAL HEART DISEASE
CORONARY THROMBOSIS
COR PULMONALE
ENDOCARDITIS
EXTRA SYSTOLES
HEART BLOCK
HEART FAILURE
ISCHAEMIC HEART DISEASE
MITRAL INCOMPETENCE
MITRAL STENOSIS
MYOCARDITIS
PERICARDITIS
RHEUMATIC FEVER
TACHYCARDIA
VENTRICULAR FIBRILLATION

See CIRCULATORY SYSTEM *page 40*

HEART ATTACK

A loose term, that doctors try to avoid, meaning many different things. A lay speaker usually intends CORONARY THROMBOSIS, but heart attack also covers other acute heart emergencies.
See CIRCULATORY SYSTEM *page 40*

HEART BLOCK

A block, or partial block, at one of the places in the heart muscle where the electrical impulses occur that keep the pumping system of the heart working at a regular speed. The block makes the different pumping chambers of the heart act independently of each other. The two main pumping chambers (ventricles) and pulse then beat at a much slower rate than usual.

Symptoms
• Partial blocks may not affect the heart's pumping rate and therefore cause few symptoms. The condition is then discovered only after an ELECTROCARDIOGRAM.
• When occasional beats (ventricular contractions) are missed out (dropped), the patient may be aware of the irregularity.
• With more severe blocks, the circulation to the brain is reduced. This can cause dizziness, disturbance of behaviour, and sometimes fainting and a small fit.
• All types of block reduce the usual performance of the heart and may result in chest pain (ANGINA PECTORIS), breathlessness and ankle swelling (HEART FAILURE).

Duration
• This depends on the underlying cause. Both partial and complete blocks may last only seconds or minutes. After attacks of CORONARY THROMBOSIS and in MYOCARDITIS (inflammation of the heart muscle) the blocks are often permanent.

Causes
• Coronary thrombosis.
• Myocarditis.
• Congenital heart disease.
• Degeneration of the nerves which stimulate the heart muscle to contract.
• Some drugs. *See* MEDICINES, 5.

When to consult the doctor
• If the patient is aware of an irregularity in the heartbeat.

What the doctor may do
• He may arrange for an electrocardiogram to reveal the size and seriousness of any block present.
• If symptoms are slight and there is no evidence of heart failure, the doctor may do nothing else.
• With more severe blocks, the doctor will consider whether fitting an artificial PACEMAKER would help temporarily or permanently.

Prevention
• This must be related to the underlying cause of the condition.

Outlook
• This is always dependent on the basic cause, which is frequently due to old age or degenerative conditions. In such cases symptoms can be completely relieved and the full pumping action of the heart restored by fitting an artificial pacemaker.

See CIRCULATORY SYSTEM *page 40*

HEARTBURN

A hot sensation behind the breastbone coming on after meals. It occurs in most forms of INDIGESTION.
See ACID REGURGITATION

HEART FAILURE

Failure of the heart to cope with the pumping demands placed on it: the heart may become weak and unable to pump blood around the body; or an obstruction in the heart may reduce the amount of blood returning to it; or both conditions may occur.

The onset of heart failure is usually slow, and the heart compensates for the failure by beating more forcefully and strengthening its muscle. In some cases, however, the heart is weakened suddenly—as, for example, by a severe CORONARY THROMBOSIS—and then shock and collapse may follow.

Heart failure interferes with the functioning of other organs. The kidneys in particular are affected, with the result that excessive amounts of fluid are retained in the blood; these overload the circulatory system and so increase the strain on the heart.

Symptoms
• If heart failure is mild the following symptoms occur only on exertion, but if failure is severe they are present all the time.
• Progressive breathlessness. This is sometimes accompanied by wheezing, which can be severe, as happens when a patient suffers an attack of asthma.
• Unexplained or persistent coughing. In severe cases there may be attacks of bronchitis.
• A preference for sleeping propped up by pillows.
• Swelling of the feet and ankles which is worse in the evening or after activity.

Duration
• Depending on the severity and cause of the heart failure, it may take the form of attacks lasting only a few hours or, at the other extreme, be a permanent condition.

Causes
• HYPERTENSION (high blood pressure).
• Severe ANAEMIA.
• Disorder affecting the regularity and rate of the heart's pumping action (ATRIAL FIBRILLATION and HEART BLOCK).
• Advanced lung disease, chronic BRONCHITIS, ASTHMA.
• Diseases of the AORTIC and MITRAL heart valves (stenosis and incompetence).
• Disease of the heart muscle (CARDIOMYOPATHY).
• CONGENITAL HEART DISEASE.
• Inflammation of the heart (MYOCARDITIS, PERICARDITIS).
• CORONARY THROMBOSIS.
• ISCHAEMIC HEART DISEASE, in which the supply of blood to the heart is restricted.
• Overactive thyroid gland (THYROTOXICOSIS).
• SMOKING, being overweight, and many serious illnesses can overload the heart and precipitate failure.

Treatment in the home
• If an attack starts, sit down and rest.

When to consult the doctor
• If there is undue breathlessness.
• If there is unexplained or persistent coughing.
• If the feet or ankles swell.

What the doctor may do
• He will give drugs to make the patient pass more fluid, to bring down high blood pressure and to control irregular or rapid heart beat. *See* MEDICINES, 5, 6, 7.
• If heart failure has been sudden and severe he may give the patient an injection of morphia to relieve breathlessness and diminish activity and anxiety.
• After these immediate measures, the doctor will try to discover the cause of the heart failure. To do this he may have to send the patient to hospital for tests.

Prevention
• Give up smoking. This is the best way of preventing or at least delaying the onset of heart failure and many of its causes.
Those who have already had an attack of heart failure or who have been told they are liable to have one should act on the following advice:
• Keep weight down to normal.

- Avoid excessive or unnecessary physical activity. If such activity is essential, take it more slowly.
- Be cautious about climbing stairs, walking uphill or walking against the wind.
- Do not drink large amounts of fluid.
- Keep strictly to the treatment prescribed for any underlying disorder.

Outlook

- Prospects depend on the cause of the heart failure. They are favourable when the underlying disorder is one that can be treated—for example, thyroid disease, valvular disease, congenital heart disease or hypertension. The outlook is less good for those underlying conditions in which the heart has already compensated for the increasing strain as much as possible. These conditions include severe lung disease, ischaemic heart disease and other similar disorders.

HEMIPLEGIA

A paralysis that affects one side of the body only. The cause is usually a STROKE.

HEPATITIS

Inflammation of the liver which can be caused by at least five different viruses.

Hepatitis A, or infectious hepatitis, has an incubation period of 14-42 days, and is most common in children and young adults. The virus is found in the patient's faeces and is transmitted by contaminated food or water.

Hepatitis B, or serum hepatitis, has an incubation period of six to 26 weeks and can occur at any age. The virus has a number of different particles (antigens) which cause the formation of antibodies in the blood. These antigens and antibodies can be detected by special tests, and help doctors to monitor the course of the disease.

The virus may stay in the blood for months, possibly for life, and for this reason people with B virus cannot give blood for transfusions and are a risk to dentists, doctors and nurses, as well as laboratory staff who may handle blood samples.

Hepatitis B is spread by contact with blood or body fluids. Male homosexuals, drug addicts, babies born to infected mothers and patients given transfusions and injections with incompletely sterilised needles and syringes are at risk. With modern tests and disposable syringes

and needles, the risks to most people in developed countries are now low.

Hepatitis C This virus causes most cases of hepatitis spread by blood transfusion. It also occurs in drug addicts, and after sexual or household contact with an infected person. Its incubation period is five or six weeks, and it may occur at any age.

In addition, **hepatitis D (Delta)** virus may infect patients who already have hepatitis B, usually making the disease worse, and **hepatitis E** virus is transmitted by contaminated water or food.

Symptoms

- Flu-like symptoms of raised temperature, headache and joint pains. In some patients these may be mild, in others they may be severe and may be accompanied by jaundice.
- Early symptoms are headache, loss of appetite with a general feeling of illness, nausea and vomiting. There may be a rash and a distaste for smoking.
- After three to ten days jaundice develops, with dark urine and light-coloured stools. The patient may then feel better.

Duration

- Jaundice may increase over about three weeks, then fade over two to four weeks.

Complications

- In 5 to 10 per cent of cases hepatitis B infections may progress very rapidly and seriously to cause drowsiness, confusion and even unconsciousness, with bleeding from various sites and acute atrophy (shrinkage) of the liver, sometimes progressing to liver failure and death.
- Relapses, slow recovery and progressive liver damage can occur in hepatitis B or C.

Treatment in the home

- Not advised until the doctor has been consulted.
- Complete isolation is unnecessary for hepatitis.

When to consult the doctor

- If any hepatitis symptoms develop.

What the doctor may do

- Take blood tests to confirm the diagnosis.
- Recommend bed-rest until any fever has settled.
- Suggest a high-calorie, low-protein and low-fat diet for the patient.
- Send the patient to hospital for specialist treatment.

Prevention

- Urine and faeces, saliva and blood should be considered infective. Wash the hands carefully after handling bedpans, the patient or his clothes.
- If you are travelling to a tropical or subtropical country where hepatitis A is common, get immunisation.
- Avoid homosexuality, promiscuity and drug abuse, especially in foreign countries.

- A vaccine is available to protect those at the greatest risk of hepatitis B infection, such as health workers.

Outlook

- Most patients recover completely from hepatitis A, but a minority of patients with hepatitis B or C may have long-term liver damage.

See INFECTIOUS DISEASES *page 32*

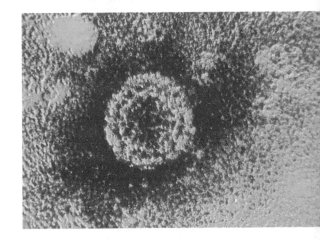

HEPATITIS B VIRUS *Magnified 240,000 times by a transmission electron microscope, the active part of the hepatitis B virus has a double-walled outer coating and inner core.*

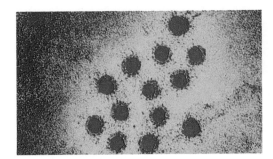

HEPATITIS A VIRUS *Magnified 120,000 times, the virus cells are clearly differentiated from those of hepatitis B by their uniform outer coating and dense core.*

HERBALISM

The use of plants, or substances extracted from them, to try to cure illness is probably the oldest form of treatment known to man. Herbal medicine was practised in prehistoric times, and herbal treatments formed the basis of medical care in most ancient cultures, as they do among many primitive peoples today.

In Western civilisations, the decline of herbalism began with the rise of alchemy, which advocated the use of inorganic substances, in the 16th century. Nevertheless, it continued to flourish widely for another 200 years, and in rural and remote areas it never really died out. In addition, many drugs used by doctors today are derived from plants—for example digitalis from the foxglove and opium from the poppy—and related products.

Modern scientific interest in herbalism stems from a growing awareness that man-made drugs may have unpleasant, and sometimes serious, side-effects. Extensive research is being carried out into the plant-based folk medicines of the native peoples of South America, Africa, China, Siberia and elsewhere.

Although some plant-based treatments for minor ailments—particularly herb 'teas', or infusions—are widely available and are generally regarded as harmless, many other plant derivatives are potentially dangerous and some could prove fatal. Therefore, anyone seeking a remedy from a herbalist should obtain the endorsement of a doctor as well, and herbal treatments should not be self-administered without the advice of a qualified person.

HEREDITY

The passing on of physical and mental characteristics from parents to their children. The process is brought about by CHROMOSOMES, the structures in each human cell that carry hereditary information. At conception the 23 chromosomes in the male sperm cell are united with their 23 counterparts in the female egg cell. This provides the fertilised egg with characteristics from both parents, in the form of the 46 chromosomes that all human cells except sex cells contain.

HERNIA

A protrusion of abdominal organs through a gap in the abdominal wall, commonly called a rupture. Hernias are usually described according to the site in and around the abdomen at which they occur.

Inguinal hernia is the most usual type and most common in males. The bulge, which can be very large—up to 6 in. (152 mm.)—occurs above the groin crease and tends to go into the scrotum.

Femoral hernia is most common in women. The bulge, which may be only the size of a cherry, occurs just below the middle of the groin crease.

Umbilical hernia is most common in babies. It is noticed as a round swelling near the navel. As the baby grows the swelling usually disappears without treatment in one to four years. Pads and strapping are of no value. Large umbilical hernias or those developing in adults may need surgical treatment.

Midline hernia occurs in women who have had several pregnancies, stretching may cause the muscles to diverge in the midline and produce a bulge which becomes evident when sitting up from a lying position.

Hiatus hernia is a bulging of the stomach through the diaphragm at the weakest point where the oesophagus (food pipe) passes through. The hernia is not visible and often symptomless. Symptoms when present are those of indigestion. See OESOPHAGITIS.

Incisional hernia is a bulge beneath an abdominal scar, where the muscles or deep tissues have failed to knit together. It is commonest after an abdominal wound has been infected.

Symptoms
- Bulging, particularly when pressure within the abdominal cavity is raised, as in standing, coughing, crying or straining over a bowel motion.
- Discomfort at the site.

Duration
- Hernias last until treated.

Causes
- Internal pressure acting on a weak point in the abdominal muscles, especially at the edges of muscles. Weak points occur naturally at points where organs are linked, or they can appear on the sites of operation scars. The tendency remains until surgically repaired.

Complications
- If the hole through which the hernia pushes is small the blood supply to the contents of the sac may become blocked and the hernia will eventually die and become gangrenous. This is called strangulation.
- An immediate operation is needed to prevent gangrene.

Treatment in the home
- Some hernias can be reduced (pushed back into the abdomen) by lying back, relaxing the abdominal muscles, and using the fingertips gently to knead the bulge back into place. The patient can safely do this.
- If you wear a truss, you should push the hernia back before fixing the truss into place.
- If the opening through which the hernia bulges is wide, strangulation is unlikely to occur, and trusses are less likely to work.
- Strangulated hernias are painful, tense and tender and cannot be pushed back. There is no increase in bulging on coughing.

When to consult the doctor
- If there is tenderness and pain in a hernia that cannot be easily pushed back, the doctor should be contacted at once. This is treated as an emergency, because strangulation may cut off the blood supply to the bowel and cause gangrene.
- Any hernia, even if not causing pain, should be seen by the doctor to advise about treatment and eliminate the risk of complications.

What the doctor may do
- Send you to a surgeon for an opinion and possibly an operation.
- In some cases (for example, hernias with wide necks, and in elderly or infirm patients and those who refuse an operation), the doctor may prescribe a truss, usually consisting of an appropriately shaped leather-covered pad held in the correct place by straps. Trusses are used mainly for inguinal hernias.

Outlook
- Trusses when advised should control the hernia. In many cases surgery is indicated, but even after operation the hernia may recur.

See DIGESTIVE SYSTEM *page 44*

HERPES

A term used loosely to describe several localised infections of different parts of the body, such as face, lips, eyes and genitals. These infections are caused by two types of the herpes simplex virus. Herpes zoster is the medical term for SHINGLES, which is caused by the closely related chicken pox virus.

See COLD SORES, GENITAL HERPES

HICCUPS

Repeated and involuntary spasms of the diaphragm.
Duration
- An attack is usually over in ten to 20 minutes, though prolonged bouts may occur. Persistent hiccups suggests there are underlying abnormalities.

Causes
- Irritation of the diaphragm by overfilling the stomach after swallowing an excess of food or drink—especially hot fluids.
- Some bouts seem to have no cause.
- Rarely, kidney, liver, lung and abdominal disorders.

Treatment in the home
- Carbon dioxide inhibits hiccups, and simply holding the breath several times will allow carbon dioxide to build up in the body.
- Breathing in and out of a paper bag works the same way. *Do not* use a plastic bag as this may fatally obstruct respiration. Most other successful home remedies act by making the patient hold his breath.
- Sucking ice, drinking water slowly, inducing vomiting, and pulling on the tongue are ways of trying to stop hiccups.

When to consult the doctor
- If you have persistent or recurrent bouts of hiccups that last more than a day.

What the doctor may do
- Prescribe a sedative by mouth or injection. *See* MEDICINES, 17.
- Arrange a supply of 5 per cent carbon dioxide for you to inhale.

See DIGESTIVE SYSTEM *page 44*

HIP *See* SYMPTOM SORTER—LIMP

HIRSUTISM

Hirsutism, the excessive growth of hair, in men is considered a sign of virility and does not cause problems. In women, extra growth of hair on the face or limbs can cause unhappiness and embarrassment. It is usually an inherited condition.

Symptoms
- The extra growth of facial hair in women may start at about 30 and usually before the menopause. It can start with pregnancy and then continue.
- The hair grows in the same places as on a hairy man— on the face, chest and limbs.
- In elderly women, strong coarse hairs often grow on the face. These are quite different from the hairs on younger women.

Duration
- Lifelong.

Causes
- Often there is no obvious cause.
- Hirsutism may be due to hormone imbalance or to over-reaction of the hair follicles to male hormones.
- Some rare glandular disorders.
- Certain drugs such as phenytoin and some steroids provoke hair growth. *See* MEDICINES, 23, 32.

Treatment in the home
- The woman who is unusually hairy needs to be reassured of her femininity and to understand that she is unlikely to have any disorder of the glands.
- The simplest approach is shaving, which does not increase the growth of hair or make the hairs stronger, or bleaching or waxing.
- If there are only a few hairs they may be pulled out with tweezers at the roots, but will regrow in six weeks.
- The hairs can be permanently destroyed with electrolysis. This must be done with skill to avoid scars. As each hair is treated separately it is an exhausting and expensive process.
- Proprietary cosmetics are available which destroy the hairs. All the chemicals, while effective for a time, may cause skin reactions with prolonged use.

When to consult the doctor
- If there are any symptoms of glandular disorder such as lack of menstrual periods.
- If an increase in the growth of body hair coincides with a course of medication.

What the doctor may do
- Take blood and urine tests to exclude any gland disorders.
- Sometimes he will arrange more complicated investigations in hospital.
- Prescribe a special hormone preparation (Dianette), which also acts as an oral contraceptive.

Prevention
- None is possible.

Outlook
- Suitable advice enables most women to find the treatment that suits them and minimises embarrassment.

See SKIN *page 52*

HISTOPLASMOSIS
The fungus that causes this infection grows in surface soil in many parts of the world. The spores thrive in bird droppings particularly and humans contract the disease by breathing in the spores. Symptoms are ill-defined or absent. Diagnosis is by blood tests, or by growing the fungus from sputum specimens. Most cases do not require treatment, but antifungal drugs are effective.

HIV *See* AIDS

HIVES
A condition in which fluid accumulates in the skin and its underlying tissues, causing swelling.
See URTICARIA

HODGKIN'S DISEASE

A tumour of the lymph glands or organs rich in lymphatic tissue such as the spleen. The disease mainly affects young people.

Symptoms
- Swelling in the neck, usually on one side.
- Enlarged glands in the armpits and groin.
- Fever, night sweats and excessive tiredness.
- Loss of appetite.
- Abdominal pain.
- Anaemia, loss of weight.

Duration
- Sufferers may survive for years without treatment, but only treatment can effect a cure.

Causes
- Unknown, although recent research indicates that a virus may be responsible.

Complications
- Infections.

When to consult the doctor
- As soon as the condition is suspected.

What the doctor may do
- Send the patient to hospital. There, samples from enlarged lymph glands and bone marrow will be examined to check diagnosis.
- If the diagnosis is confirmed early enough, arrange radiotherapy—treatment with X-rays.
- For more advanced cases, a complex course of drug treatment lasting six to nine months will be necessary.

Prevention
- Not possible.

Outlook
- If the disease is caught early, most patients are cured. Those with advanced disease benefit rapidly from drug treatment, and about half are cured.

Home nursing

A PRACTICAL GUIDE TO CARING FOR A SICK PERSON AT HOME— SO THAT HE IS MADE COMFORTABLE IN BODY AND MIND

Most people who are ill would rather stay at home to recover than go into a hospital. Doctors recognise that a sick person feels happier in an environment he knows, where he can see relatives and friends when he chooses. However, nursing a sick person at home puts mental and physical strains on all the other members of the household. The stresses cannot be eliminated entirely, but the problems can be kept to a minimum by following a few rules.

Do's and don'ts of home nursing

There are six basic principles to follow in home nursing.

☐ *Do* encourage the sick person to be as independent as possible, and to perform those tasks of which he is capable—such as washing. Too much fussy care can destroy the patient's sense of initiative, and delay or even prevent a return to normal life.

☐ *Do* help to preserve the patient's dignity and self-esteem, for example, by ensuring that he is well-groomed and that his clothes and bedclothes are changed as soon as they become soiled.

☐ *Do* watch the patient's progress. Record pulse, temperature and respiration rates, and the times at which they were taken. Call the doctor immediately if the condition worsens or recovery seems to be delayed.

☐ *Do* make sure that the treatment prescribed by the doctor is carried out.

☐ *Do* take time to show love and affection for the patient.

☐ *Do not* do anything to make the patient more anxious or nervous than he is already.

CHOOSING THE SICKROOM
Anyone suffering from more than a minor ailment needs a special room in which to recover. It should be large enough to contain a bed which is accessible from both sides, warm, about 60°F (15.5°C) is ideal, 65°F (18.3°C) for babies and old people (or those with chest complaints), well-ventilated, well-lit and quiet.

Usually, the patient's own bedroom is the best place if the illness is likely to be brief, or if he is able to move around easily on his own when he is not in bed.

But if the illness is prolonged or permanent, or if the patient has difficulty in walking, the usual bedroom may not be suitable, particularly in houses or apartments with more than one storey. Staircases and long passageways are both a physical and a psychological barrier. A patient confined to a remote room may feel cut off from the rest of the household, and the person doing the nursing may become overtired from frequent trips to and from the sickroom, even if she is young and fit.

In such cases, particularly if the patient has a disability affecting the legs or heart, or a severe breathing

2

Furnishing the sickroom
1 *Bed, accessible from both sides.*
2 *Armchair for patient to sit on.*
3 *Two high-backed chairs for visitors or placing blankets on.*
4 *Chest of drawers for linen.*
5 *Surface for toiletries.*
6 *Bedside table for books, radio, water carafe, lamp and alarm intercom.*
7 *Cantilevered bedside table for meals.*
8 *Pictures, flowers and plants.*
9 *Wardrobe.*
10 *Carpet, for a warm floor.*
11 *Windows low enough for the patient to see out of, but not draughty.*

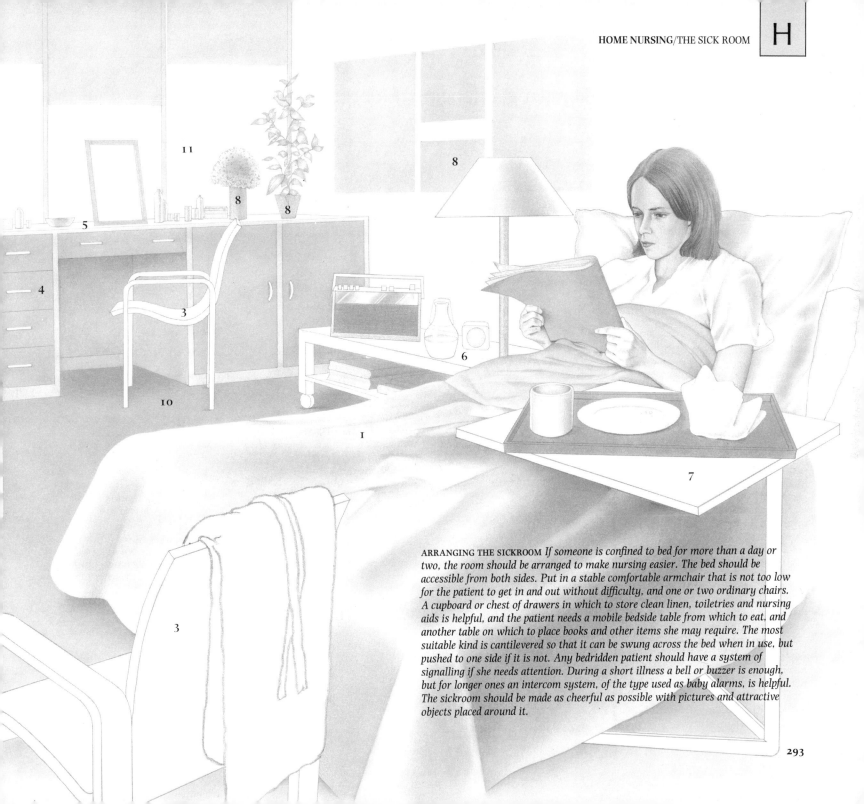

11

8

8

8

5

4

3

10

6

1

7

3

ARRANGING THE SICKROOM *If someone is confined to bed for more than a day or two, the room should be arranged to make nursing easier. The bed should be accessible from both sides. Put in a stable comfortable armchair that is not too low for the patient to get in and out without difficulty, and one or two ordinary chairs. A cupboard or chest of drawers in which to store clean linen, toiletries and nursing aids is helpful, and the patient needs a mobile bedside table from which to eat, and another table on which to place books and other items she may require. The most suitable kind is cantilevered so that it can be swung across the bed when in use, but pushed to one side if it is not. Any bedridden patient should have a system of signalling if she needs attention. During a short illness a bell or buzzer is enough, but for longer ones an intercom system, of the type used as baby alarms, is helpful. The sickroom should be made as cheerful as possible with pictures and attractive objects placed around it.*

293

disorder, it is better to use a room closer to the centre of family activity—for example, by adapting the dining-room in homes that have a separate one. Ideally, the room chosen should be within easy reach of a lavatory, but if that is not possible, and the patient is at least partly mobile, it may be necessary to install a commode.

If the patient needs frequent attention during the night, as well as in the daytime, the person doing the nursing may need to sleep near by.

BUZZERS AND ALARMS
Any bedridden patient should have a system for signalling if he needs attention. During short illnesses a bell or buzzer is enough, but for longer ones an intercom system of the type used as baby alarms is helpful.

In some types of illness—for example, relatively mild infections—the patient can sleep in his own bedroom at night, but have a day-bed on which to rest at other times, nearer the rooms the family uses. The day-bed can be made-up on a comfortable sofa, or on a sun-lounger, provided it is stable. This arrangement is particularly helpful for mothers looking after small children who need frequent attention to stop them from getting bored.

EQUIPPING THE SICKROOM
In general, the sickroom should be functional without being too clinical. Pictures and other attractive objects create a pleasant environment.

Many people tend to keep medicines in the sickroom, either on the bedside table or the dressing-table. But this should *not* be done. Patients—particularly the elderly

Bedmaking: changing the bottom sheet

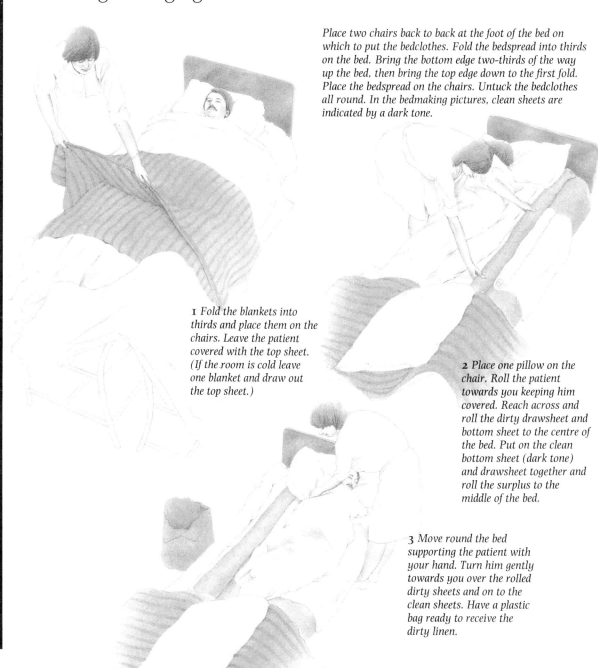

Place two chairs back to back at the foot of the bed on which to put the bedclothes. Fold the bedspread into thirds on the bed. Bring the bottom edge two-thirds of the way up the bed, then bring the top edge down to the first fold. Place the bedspread on the chairs. Untuck the bedclothes all round. In the bedmaking pictures, clean sheets are indicated by a dark tone.

1 *Fold the blankets into thirds and place them on the chairs. Leave the patient covered with the top sheet. (If the room is cold leave one blanket and draw out the top sheet.)*

2 *Place one pillow on the chair. Roll the patient towards you keeping him covered. Reach across and roll the dirty drawsheet and bottom sheet to the centre of the bed. Put on the clean bottom sheet (dark tone) and drawsheet together and roll the surplus to the middle of the bed.*

3 *Move round the bed supporting the patient with your hand. Turn him gently towards you over the rolled dirty sheets and on to the clean sheets. Have a plastic bag ready to receive the dirty linen.*

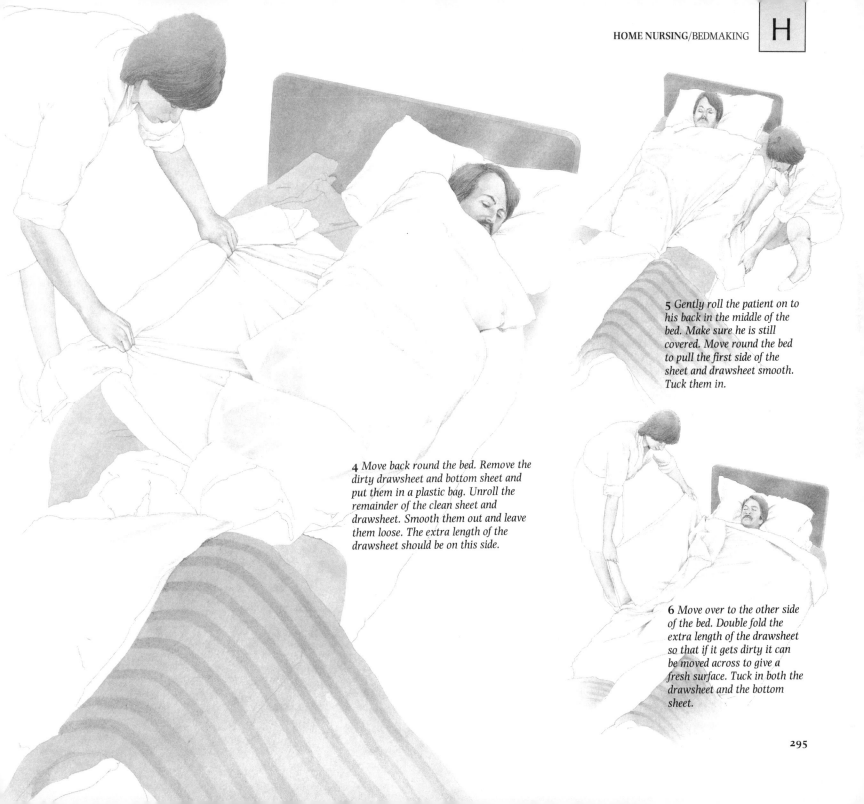

5 *Gently roll the patient on to his back in the middle of the bed. Make sure he is still covered. Move round the bed to pull the first side of the sheet and drawsheet smooth. Tuck them in.*

4 *Move back round the bed. Remove the dirty drawsheet and bottom sheet and put them in a plastic bag. Unroll the remainder of the clean sheet and drawsheet. Smooth them out and leave them loose. The extra length of the drawsheet should be on this side.*

6 *Move over to the other side of the bed. Double fold the extra length of the drawsheet so that if it gets dirty it can be moved across to give a fresh surface. Tuck in both the drawsheet and the bottom sheet.*

295

and confused—can easily take an overdose by mistake, possibly with serious results. All medicines, therefore, should be kept in the family medicine chest, and should only be taken out when it is time to administer the dose.

FLOWERS AND PLANTS

If the patient is likely to be bedridden for a long time, or permanently, put in cheerful curtains and other furnishings. It is also a good idea to supply him with notepaper and envelopes and materials for handicrafts, particularly if he is convalescing. Flowers and plants can be used to brighten the sickroom of many patients during the day, but they should be taken out at night. Never put them in the room of someone with a respiratory ailment.

CHOOSING THE BED AND BEDDING

Ideally, a sick-bed should be about 28 in. (71 cm.) high, with a firm mattress. If it is much higher or lower, the patient will have difficulty in getting in or out, and if it is lower it is also awkward to make. In some illnesses—for example, a SLIPPED DISC—the bed should be made extra firm by putting boards along its full length underneath the mattress.

The bedding should be comfortable and easy to look after. Polyester/ cotton sheets and pillowcases wash and dry well. If possible, use lightweight blankets. They do not press down uncomfortably on the patient, and remove some of the exertion from bedmaking. Alternatively, use a duvet with a polyester/cotton cover.

If the patient is incontinent, protect the mattress and under-blanket or ticking with a

Bedmaking: changing the top sheet

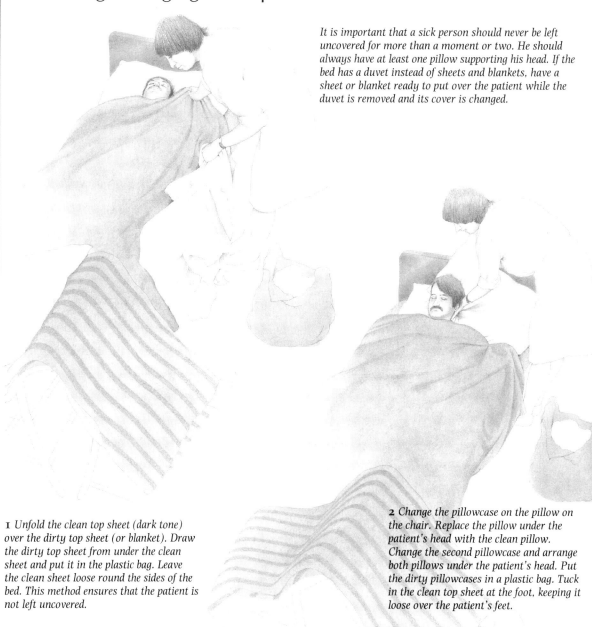

It is important that a sick person should never be left uncovered for more than a moment or two. He should always have at least one pillow supporting his head. If the bed has a duvet instead of sheets and blankets, have a sheet or blanket ready to put over the patient while the duvet is removed and its cover is changed.

1 *Unfold the clean top sheet (dark tone) over the dirty top sheet (or blanket). Draw the dirty top sheet from under the clean sheet and put it in the plastic bag. Leave the clean sheet loose round the sides of the bed. This method ensures that the patient is not left uncovered.*

2 *Change the pillowcase on the pillow on the chair. Replace the pillow under the patient's head with the clean pillow. Change the second pillowcase and arrange both pillows under the patient's head. Put the dirty pillowcases in a plastic bag. Tuck in the clean top sheet at the foot, keeping it loose over the patient's feet.*

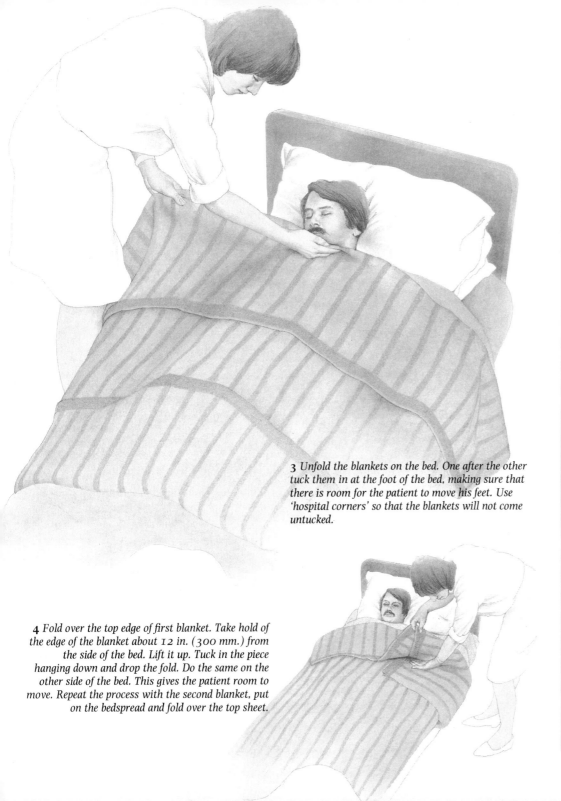

3 *Unfold the blankets on the bed. One after the other tuck them in at the foot of the bed, making sure that there is room for the patient to move his feet. Use 'hospital corners' so that the blankets will not come untucked.*

4 *Fold over the top edge of first blanket. Take hold of the edge of the blanket about 12 in. (300 mm.) from the side of the bed. Lift it up. Tuck in the piece hanging down and drop the fold. Do the same on the other side of the bed. This gives the patient room to move. Repeat the process with the second blanket, put on the bedspread and fold over the top sheet.*

Making 'hospital corners'

Make hospital corners in each sheet or blanket as you put it on so that they do not come untucked.

1 *Tuck the blanket under the mattress along the foot of the bed.*

2 *Pick up the edge of the blanket about 18 in. (450 mm.) from the foot of the bed. Tuck in the piece hanging between the foot of the bed and your hand.*

3 *Tuck in the side of the blanket to make an 'envelope corner'.*

purpose-made waterproof cover or with a sheet of polythene large enough to cover the whole mattress. Put a normal sheet on top of that. Next, you will need a smaller waterproof sheet of rubber or plastic, about 3 ft (90 cm.) wide, to lay across the bed under the patient's buttocks. It should be long enough to tuck in at the sides of the bed. Finally, cover the upper waterproof sheet with a drawsheet, also about 3 ft (90 cm.) wide and placed across the bed. It should be as long as possible, with the surplus tucked in at one side. As the drawsheet becomes damp it can be moved across the bed, and the spare portion used as needed to provide a clean, dry section for the patient to lie on.

The drawsheet can be made either by folding an ordinary sheet to the right width, or by cutting a sheet in half. If you use a folded sheet, make sure that it is not so thick that it causes the patient discomfort or irritation that might lead to bedsores.

CLOTHING

Pyjamas and nightdresses should be light, warm and large enough to make it easy to put them on or take them off. They should not have thick seams or patches against which the patient's body may press, causing discomfort or sores.

A neat, fresh appearance helps the patient's sense of self-esteem, so keep a good supply of clean pyjamas or nightdresses. They can then be changed frequently if they become soiled or damp with perspiration.

If the patient is out of bed only for short intervals, he should wear a dressing-gown, slippers and, if necessary, a rug over the knees. But if he is up for longer, it is both more

Lifting a patient up the bed when he is lying flat

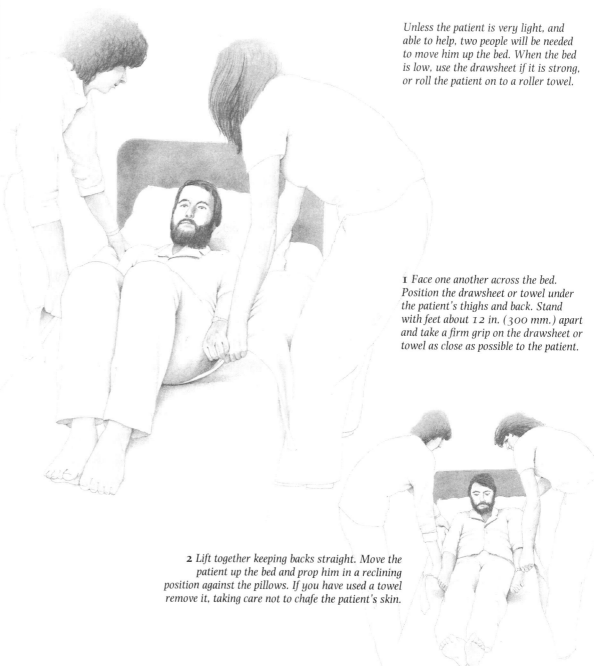

Unless the patient is very light, and able to help, two people will be needed to move him up the bed. When the bed is low, use the drawsheet if it is strong, or roll the patient on to a roller towel.

1 *Face one another across the bed. Position the drawsheet or towel under the patient's thighs and back. Stand with feet about 12 in. (300 mm.) apart and take a firm grip on the drawsheet or towel as close as possible to the patient.*

2 *Lift together keeping backs straight. Move the patient up the bed and prop him in a reclining position against the pillows. If you have used a towel remove it, taking care not to chafe the patient's skin.*

Lifting a patient when he is sitting up

If the patient is sitting up, an alternative method of lifting can be used which has the advantage of leaving each helper with one hand free to steady herself if necessary. This method should not be used for chest or heart patients. Two helpers stand one on each side of the bed facing the head of the bed with feet about 12 in. (300 mm.) apart and knees bent.

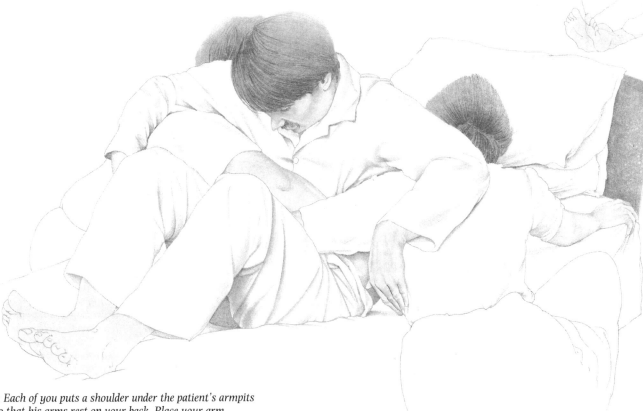

2 *Keeping the back straight and taking the strain with the legs, lift and straighten the patient to raise him. Make sure that the patient's buttocks are lifted well clear of the mattress and bottom sheet to prevent chafing. Move the patient up the bed and prop him against the pillows.*

1 *Each of you puts a shoulder under the patient's armpits so that his arms rest on your back. Place your arm round the patient's body. If the patient is very heavy, place your free hand on the mattress to provide leverage.*

practical and better psychologically for him to wear day clothes.

HOW TO PREVENT BEDSORES

Someone who is confined to bed or to a chair for more than a few days runs the risk of developing bedsores—painful places where the skin breaks down and weeps. The main causes are:

• Pressure and friction from a resistant surface—for example, the bed itself—which restricts the blood supply to the skin. The most vulnerable points of the body are those where the bones lie near the skin—the buttocks and lower spine, hips, knees, ankles, heels, elbows, shoulders, the top of the spine and the back of the head.

• Skin damage caused by rubbing or scratching.

• The chafing of skin surfaces together—as between the ankles.

The less a patient moves around, the more likely he is to develop bedsores, particularly if his skin is already in poor condition because of age or inadequate diet. The problem may also be made worse by incontinence, heavy perspiration, poor circulation and external irritants, such as crumbs in the bed or patches or raised seams on the patient's clothes or on the sheets.

To reduce the likelihood of bedsores:

• Make sure the patient changes position frequently. If he cannot do that for himself, turn him at least once every two hours.

• Massage the vulnerable parts of the body with lanolin or soap when the patient is given an all-over wash or bed bath.

• Keep his skin clean and dry.

• Take care that you do not damage

Turning a helpless patient in bed

If the patient cannot move himself he will have to be turned in bed at least once every two hours to give him a change of position and prevent bedsores. He will also have to be moved when the bed is being made.

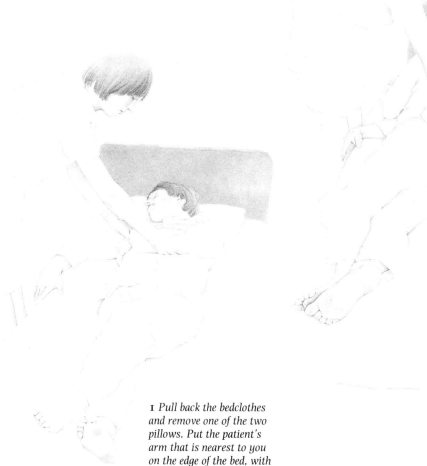

1 *Pull back the bedclothes and remove one of the two pillows. Put the patient's arm that is nearest to you on the edge of the bed, with the elbow slightly bent. Bring his other arm across his body. Turn his head towards you and cross his farther leg over the nearer one.*

2 *Place one hand under the shoulder that is farther away from you and one under the farther buttock. Gently roll the patient over towards you so that he is lying comfortably on his side. If necessary prop him in position with pillows to stop him rolling on to his back.*

Moving a patient from bed to chair

A bedridden patient who is not seriously ill should spend at least part of the day sitting in a chair. Place a chair at 45 degrees to the edge of the bed in line with the top of the blankets. Put your arms under the patient's armpits and gently raise him to a sitting position.

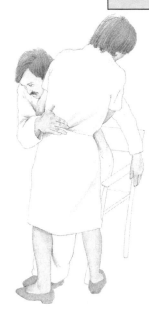

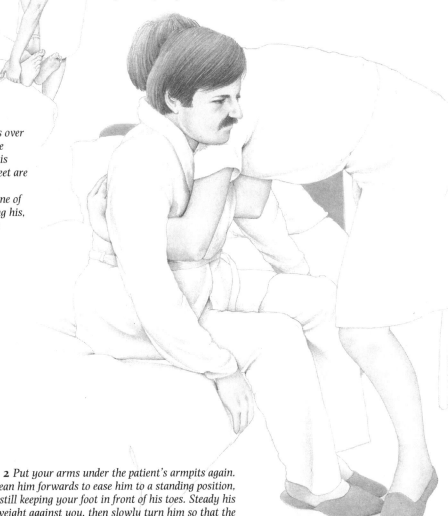

1 *Turn the patient and lift his legs over the edge of the bed so that they are pointing towards the floor and he is sitting on the bed edge. Once his feet are on the floor, put on the patient's dressing-gown and slippers. Put one of your feet in front and just touching his, at right-angles, to stop them from slipping.*

3 *Gently lower the patient into the chair. Put a pillow behind his head and a blanket over his knees. To move the patient back from chair to bed, follow the same process in reverse. Lift him with your arms under his armpits and your foot in place to stop him slipping. Turn him on to the bed and lift up his legs.*

2 *Put your arms under the patient's armpits again. Lean him forwards to ease him to a standing position, still keeping your foot in front of his toes. Steady his weight against you, then slowly turn him so that the chair is directly behind him, ready for him to sit in.*

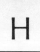
his skin with your fingernails or by careless handling of the bedpan if one is used. Do not wear rings when moving the patient.

• Make sure that the patient has a suitable diet, with plenty of fluids. *See* NUTRITION.

• Encourage frequent visits to the lavatory or commode, or use the bedpan to lessen the chances of the bedsheets becoming wet and chafing the skin.

• Look out for discoloured patches or cracks in the skin, the first sign that a bedsore is developing.

There are various aids that can be used to prevent bedsores.

VULNERABLE AREAS

Sheepskins are widely available, and provide a soft, resilient surface on which the patient can lie or sit. Full-size sheepskins cover the whole bed, but you can also buy smaller pads for particularly vulnerable areas, such as elbows and heels. If they are not already fitted with a fastening arrangement, they can be kept comfortably in place by a 'bandage' of elasticated tubular stockinet.

A ripple bed may be borrowed from some local community nursing services or from the Red Cross medical loan service. It consists of a mattress of air-filled cells, and is placed on top of the normal mattress. A small electric motor alternates the air pressure in the cells, which has the same effect as gently shifting the patient's position.

Heavy bedclothes can restrict the patient's movements considerably, particularly if they are tucked in too firmly. A bed cradle takes the weight of sheets and blankets off the body. You can buy a cradle, or improvise one with a stool or fireguard.

Giving a bed bath

To give a bed bath you will need soap and an ample supply of hot water; three flannels, one each for the face, body and genital region; three towels for the same regions; two large bath towels; and talcum powder to dust each part of the body as you dry it. Put one bath towel under the patient, remove the upper bedclothes and her clothing, and cover her with a second large towel.

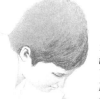

1 Squeeze excess water out of the flannel to prevent drips. Wash the face, neck and ears. Dry gently and thoroughly with a hand towel.

2 Wash, rinse and dry each arm from the fingers to the armpits, keeping the rest of the patient covered. The patient will feel refreshed if she puts her hands in the water bowl.

3 Take the patient's nightclothes off. Wash the chest, abdomen and sides of the body. Make sure that all the skin creases are carefully dried. Keep the rest of the body covered.

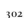

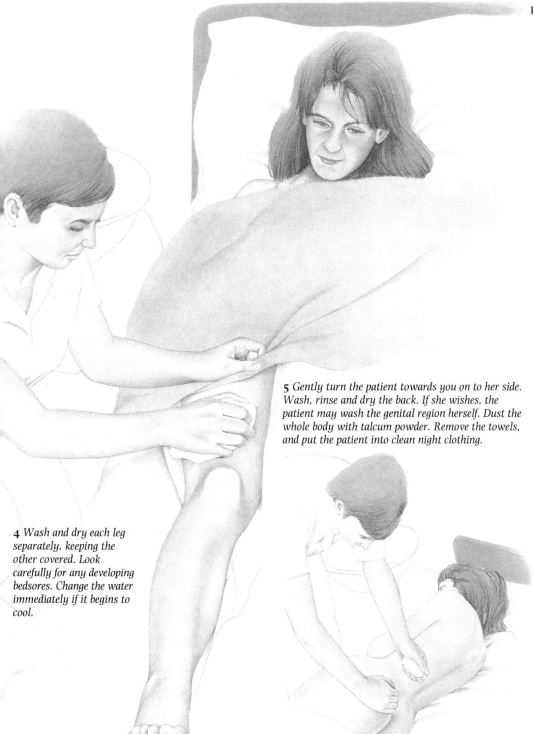

4 *Wash and dry each leg separately, keeping the other covered. Look carefully for any developing bedsores. Change the water immediately if it begins to cool.*

5 *Gently turn the patient towards you on to her side. Wash, rinse and dry the back. If she wishes, the patient may wash the genital region herself. Dust the whole body with talcum powder. Remove the towels, and put the patient into clean night clothing.*

Cleaning teeth and gums

The patient should clean her teeth at least twice daily. If she cannot go to the bathroom to do it, give her a bowl of water, a toothbrush, toothpaste, a towel and a glass of water to rinse her mouth. If necessary, clean her teeth for her.

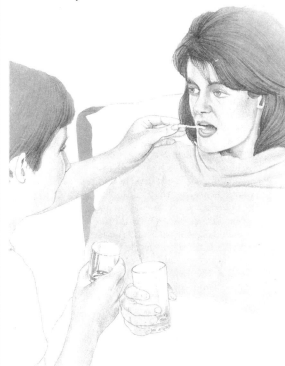

In some illnesses the mouth may become unpleasantly dry or crusted. In such cases clean the inside of the patient's mouth with cotton buds dipped in glycerin thymol solution. The patient should rinse her mouth afterwards with plain water and spit it out into a bowl.

MAKING THE BED

If the patient cannot get out of his bed while it is being made, follow the step-by-step bedmaking procedure used in hospitals.

The steps listed on pages 294–7 incorporate all the basic principles of hospital bedmaking, but the order may vary slightly according to the way in which the bedding is arranged, and according to whether the patient is capable of sitting up and moving by himself.

FOLDING THE BLANKETS

If the patient is incontinent, the rubber sheet and drawsheet should be replaced, or the drawsheet moved across to give a fresh surface, when the bottom sheet is changed or straightened.

Bedmaking is easier if sheets and blankets are correctly folded after they have been washed, dried and ironed. Bring one side two-thirds of the way across to the other, and bring the other side across to the edge of the first fold. Then fold the sheet or blanket into thirds again, from top to bottom.

HOW TO MOVE THE PATIENT FROM BED TO CHAIR

A bedridden patient who is not acutely ill should spend at least part of the day sitting in a chair. He should be encouraged to move his muscles and joints. That benefits the circulation, helps to lessen the chance of bedsores developing and reduces the risk of chest infections.

If the patient cannot move from the sickroom, and is unable to reach the chair unaided, put it near the bed, so that the seat is at an angle of 45 degrees to the bed. Put your arms under the patient's armpits, and

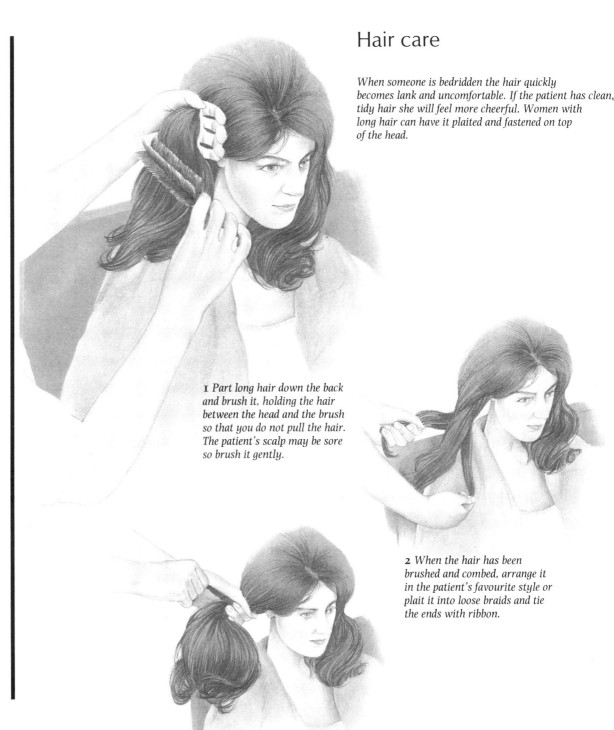

Hair care

When someone is bedridden the hair quickly becomes lank and uncomfortable. If the patient has clean, tidy hair she will feel more cheerful. Women with long hair can have it plaited and fastened on top of the head.

1 *Part long hair down the back and brush it, holding the hair between the head and the brush so that you do not pull the hair. The patient's scalp may be sore so brush it gently.*

2 *When the hair has been brushed and combed, arrange it in the patient's favourite style or plait it into loose braids and tie the ends with ribbon.*

Washing hair in bed

The patient's hair should be washed at least once a week. Place a sheet of waterproof plastic covered with towels under the patient. Wrap towels round the patient so that she does not get wet or cold. She should lie on her back with her hair over the side of the bed.

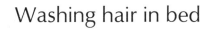

2 *Shampoo the hair and rinse it carefully and thoroughly. Shampoo left behind can irritate the scalp.*

3 *Dry the hair with a warm towel immediately you have rinsed it. Do not let the patient's head get cold.*

4 *Complete drying the patient's hair with a hand dryer and comb it into the patient's favourite style.*

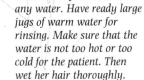

1 *Place a bowl on the floor beneath the patient to catch any water. Have ready large jugs of warm water for rinsing. Make sure that the water is not too hot or too cold for the patient. Then wet her hair thoroughly.*

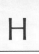
gently raise him. Turn him and lift his legs over the edge of the bed so that they are pointing towards the floor, and he is sitting on the bed edge. Once his feet are on the floor, put one of yours in front and just touching them, at right-angles, to stop them from slipping.

With your arms still under the patient's armpits, lean him forwards to ease him into a standing position, and then turn him through 90 degrees so that the chair is behind him and you can lower him to sit.

To move the patient from chair to bed, follow the same technique, lifting him with your arms under his armpits and putting one foot in front of his to prevent them from sliding. Turn him to sit him on the bed.

COMMODES AND BEDPANS

Encourage the patient to use the lavatory, unless he is completely physically incapable of making the journey. It is more comfortable for him than either a commode or a bedpan, helps to preserve his sense of dignity and is easier for those who are nursing him. The walking involved is also a stimulus to recovery.

If the patient is only partly mobile, but can get out of bed with assistance, use a commode. If you do not want to buy one, ask your local social services department or community nursing services where you can borrow one. Several types are available, but whichever you choose, make sure that it is stable, with a wide base, and preferably has a back and arm rests. It should also be easy to keep clean and fresh. For long-term invalids, a lavatory designed for use in a caravan or

Giving medicines

Keep all medicines out of reach of a patient who is seriously ill, very young or old. Medicines should be administered by the person doing the nursing, giving the right dose at the right time. If you forget on one occasion do not try to compensate by giving a double dose later. Always read the instructions on the bottle first.

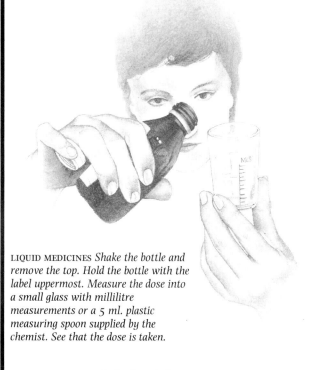

LIQUID MEDICINES *Shake the bottle and remove the top. Hold the bottle with the label uppermost. Measure the dose into a small glass with millilitre measurements or a 5 ml. plastic measuring spoon supplied by the chemist. See that the dose is taken.*

PILLS AND TABLETS *Shake the pills from the container into a spoon or small glass. Give the spoon or glass to the patient with the pills in it and a glass of water. Make sure that he swallows them.*

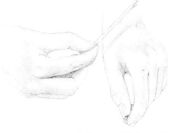

Taking temperature and pulse

In some illnesses temperature, pulse and breathing rate may give the doctor information about the patient's condition. Record them twice a day—about an hour after breakfast and again at 4 p.m.

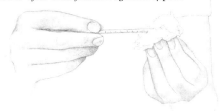

1 *Take the thermometer from the holder in which it is kept. Rinse it under cold water and dry it with a tissue.*

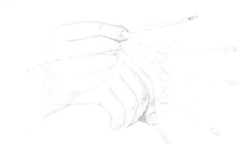

2 *Hold the thermometer at the unshaped end and shake it down sharply two or three times to return the mercury to the bulb.*

3 *Check that the mercury is below 95°F (35°C). To see the line of the mercury, hold the thermometer over the back of your hand.*

Taking temperature under the arm

If the patient is severely ill, has difficulty breathing or is very young it may be safer to take the temperature under the arm. There is less risk of the thermometer breaking.

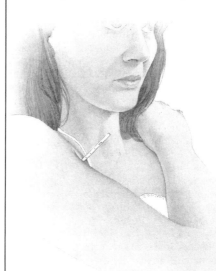

Rinse, dry and check the thermometer. Place the bulb in the patient's armpit and gently fold the arm across the patient's chest so that the bulb is in contact with the skin all around. Wait five minutes and then record the temperature.

4 *Place the bulb under the patient's tongue and tell her to close her lips but not her teeth. Wait for two minutes. Remove the thermometer and record the reading. While waiting for the temperature to register take the patient's pulse and breathing rate. Position the patient's wrist and hand across her chest. Place the tips of your first three fingers on the line of the patient's artery in the wrist, and your thumb behind the wrist. Take a watch with a second hand, hold it in your free hand and count the pulse for 30 seconds, and the breathing rate for 30 seconds. Double and record both figures.*

trailer, with a built-in flushing mechanism, is most suitable. Empty it regularly.

When the commode is needed, put it next to the bed and assist the patient on to it, raising him in the same way as you would move him to a chair.

If the patient is unable to get out of bed, you will need to provide a bedpan. Disposable pans are available from chemists.

When putting the patient on to a bedpan, take care. It is a hard surface which causes pressure that may lead to bedsores, and it may be left in place longer than it is needed. Before use, make sure the pan is slightly warm, though not hot, by running some hot water into it. Then dry it thoroughly.

Help the patient to raise his buttocks. Put the bedpan in place and roll him back on to it.

Male patients need a urinal. Those made from polypropylene are best for home use, as they are light, easy to clean, warm to the skin and relatively cheap.

Female urinals are also available. They are smaller and lighter than a full-size bedpan, and easier for the patient to get on and off.

If the patient is incontinent, make up the bed with waterproof protection for the mattress and rubber cross-sheet covered with a drawsheet.

Alternatively, use incontinence pads, which are available in Britain from local community nursing services.

BATHING THE PATIENT

Encourage and help the patient to use the bath at least two or three times a week—more often if he is able. Non-slip mats in the bottom of the bath and firm handrails along the sides or on the adjoining wall make bathing safer. For severely disabled people, there are several patent forms of sling to transfer them from chair or wheelchair to the bath. *See* DISABILITY.

When the patient is unable to take an ordinary bath, give him a bed bath every two or three days, or daily if he is perspiring heavily or asks for one. Before starting, make sure that the room is warm and that all the necessary equipment is to hand.

See that the sick person's finger and toe-nails are clipped as necessary and that his teeth are cleaned and his hair kept tidy. Male patients will need a shave. Most men prefer to do this themselves, but if they are too ill, do it for them carefully with an electric razor.

Face and hands should be washed frequently. Use soap, a flannel, a towel and a plastic bowl of warm water, and encourage the sick person to wash himself if he can.

LOOKING AFTER THE MOUTH AND TEETH

False teeth should be soaked overnight in water or denture cleaner. *See* TEETH.

FEEDING THE PATIENT

Your doctor will tell you if the patient needs a special diet. Otherwise, make sure that meals are well-balanced, with plenty of bulk—bran, cereals, fruit and vegetables—to prevent constipation. Make the food look as appetising as possible, and vary it regularly. If no special instructions have been given about fluids, these can be taken according to the patient's wishes. *See* NUTRITION.

Giving nose and ear drops

Only administer those nose and ear drops prescribed by your doctor. Do not exceed the given dosage and do not put any other medicines in the ear, as they may be dangerous. Sodium chloride nose drops are sometimes given to try to relieve nasal congestion, as they help to liquefy the secretions of mucus. Ear drops are sometimes given for skin disorders or local infections. But they are usually not applied if the ear-drum is defective.

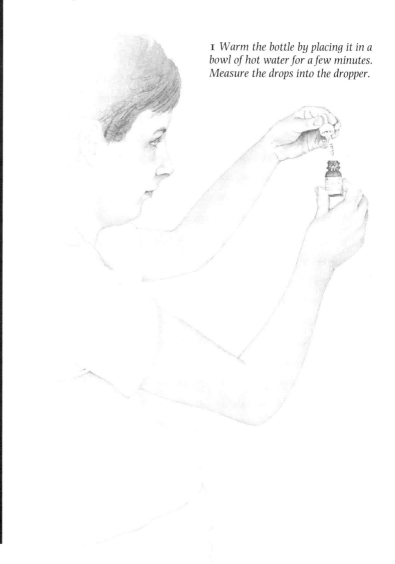

1 *Warm the bottle by placing it in a bowl of hot water for a few minutes. Measure the drops into the dropper.*

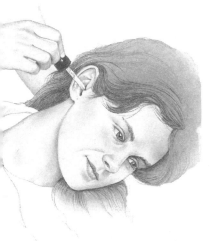

2 For nose drops: the patient should lie face down with head projecting over the edge of the bed, or kneel with the head well forward, and sniff the drops well up into the nose before sitting up.

3 For ear drops: tip the patient's head well to one side so that the ear is almost horizontal. Put a towel over the patient's shoulder. Put the drops into the patient's ear. Wipe away any dribbles.

Caring for a sick child

Most of the general principles of home nursing apply to young children as well as to other age groups. But parents are often given well-meant advice that is totally wrong. Some of the most common fallacies are:

□ A feverish child needs to be wrapped up
On the contrary, if the child has a high temperature, he should be kept cool. One covering sheet is enough and regular sponging with tepid water helps to keep the fever down. Some children who are feverish and become overheated may be liable to fits. These are frightening, but rarely harm the child. There is no reason to believe that fever fits will lead to EPILEPSY. If a fit occurs, put the child on his side, remove from his reach anything on which he might injure himself, and *do not give him anything by mouth* or attempt to restrain him. Call the doctor if the fit lasts longer than five to ten minutes, or if fits are repeated or occur frequently. *See* CHILD CARE—CHILDHOOD ILLS.

□ A child must eat to get better
If a sick child does not feel like eating, do not force him. It does not matter if he goes for a day or two without solids, so long as he has plenty to drink such as fresh fruit juice.

□ A sick child must be kept in bed
Young children are happier nearer their parents than confined to a bedroom. Make up a day-bed on a sofa in the living-room, or on a stable sun-lounger, or simply allow the child to sit in a comfortable chair. Very young children may lose newly acquired skills—for example, bladder control or the ability to drink from a normal cup—while they are ill. Be patient with them. They will re-learn quickly once they are better.

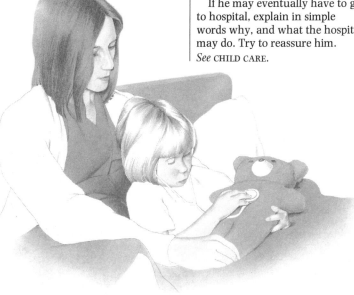

PLAYING AT PATIENT AND DOCTOR
To get your child used to the idea of the doctor's visits, let her play with a toy stethoscope, or pretend to take her own temperature.

□ The child should be sheltered from the facts of his illness
Never try to deceive a child. Many medicines do taste unpleasant, and you risk destroying the child's faith in you if you pretend otherwise.

Explain, so that he can understand, the nature of his illness. If you can, as in the case of most childhood illnesses, give him some idea of how long it will be before he is better—that is, give him something to look forward to. Young children often do not know why they are ill, and can feel that it is a punishment for some real or imagined naughtiness. Reassure the child, and do not become upset if he shows unusual aggression towards you.

If he may eventually have to go to hospital, explain in simple words why, and what the hospital may do. Try to reassure him. *See* CHILD CARE.

HOMEOPATHY

A philosophy that 'like may cure like', also written 'homoeopathy', first suggested by Hippocrates, the father of ancient Greek medicine. It diverges from orthodox medicine, which in general treats diseases with drugs that have the opposite effect to the patient's symptoms, and many doctors dismiss homeopathy as unscientific.

Nevertheless, it cannot be written off as simply another form of 'fringe' medicine. It is widely practised in Europe, India and South Africa, often by physicians holding orthodox medical qualifications. Homeopathy is available under the National Health Service, and the Queen, in addition to two orthodox physicians, has a specialist in homeopathy on her medical establishment.

Homeopaths emphasise that they treat people rather than diseases, and that a human being is more than simply the sum of his physical parts. They say that the medicines they use stimulate the natural forces of recovery within the body. Homeopathic medicine, according to its advocates, is suitable for both acute and chronic conditions, and may, if properly applied, avoid the need for surgery, although it is not a substitute for surgery or a treatment of such injuries as fractures.

One of the features which most orthodox doctors find hard to accept is the belief that the potency of a medicine is actually increased by diluting it. Sometimes remedies are diluted to such an extent that the substances put into them cannot be detected by ordinary analytical means.

Because of the dilution, and because most homeopathic medicines are derived from plants and natural minerals, the risk of side-effects is greatly reduced. Contrast the side-effects of man-made pharmaceutical products, which now cause a high proportion of hospital admissions. On the other hand, money, effort and time are wasted if homeopathic treatment has no effect.

HOOKWORM

Known medically as ancylostomiasis, hookworm is widespread throughout the tropics and subtropics. It is associated with poverty and bad sanitation and particularly affects children and agricultural workers. The worms, which are about $\frac{1}{8}$ in. (3 mm.) long, have four prominent hook-like teeth with which they attach themselves to the small intestine, where they suck blood and produce an enormous number of eggs. The eggs, which are excreted in the faeces, develop in the soil. The larvae then find their way back into the human body, usually through the skin of bare feet, and travel via the bloodstream and the lungs to the small intestine where the cycle begins again. Symptoms are those of chronic

ANAEMIA, but may include a skin rash at the site of entry of the larvae, bronchitis, abdominal pain and diarrhoea. Drug treatment is effective and wearing shoes helps to prevent the disease.
See INFECTIOUS DISEASES *page 32*

HORMONES

Chemical substances in the blood that control the functioning of the body's organs. Most hormones are produced by the endocrine glands. Among the most vital hormones are: sex hormones, pituitary hormones, thyroid hormones, insulin, cortisone and adrenaline.
See STEROIDS *page 487*

HORMONE REPLACEMENT THERAPY *See* MENOPAUSE

HOUSEMAID'S KNEE

An inflammatory condition of the knee caused by excessive kneeling. The bursa, or fluid sac, in front of the kneecap becomes inflamed and excess fluid forms and interferes with the normal lubrication of the joint.
See BURSITIS

HUNTINGTON'S CHOREA

An uncommon inherited disease which produces gradual mental deterioration and eventually results in death.

Its visible symptoms are involuntary facial grimaces, with uncontrollable movements of the arms and legs.

Huntington's chorea is particularly distressing since the symptoms only begin to appear in middle age. This means that a person inheriting the disease is unlikely to be aware of the fact until his or her children have been born. Each child of an affected person has a 50-50 chance of developing the disease.

There is no cure for Huntington's chorea, though certain sedatives and tranquillisers may reduce the intensity of the involuntary movements, as may brain surgery.

If there is any family history of Huntington's chorea, it is wise to consult a doctor before having children.
See NERVOUS SYSTEM *page 34*

OESTROGEN *One of the group of hormones that control female sexual development. Hormones are normally invisible even when viewed with conventional microscopes, but by using polarised light, rotating the sample under the microscope and studying the range of colour and shape of the crystals seen, particular hormones can be identified. Differentiating hormones in this way is important in detecting hormone imbalance problems.*

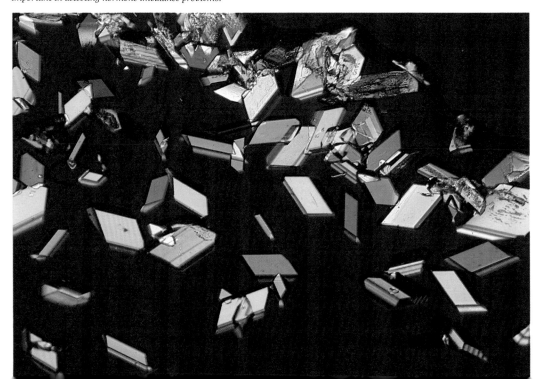

HYDATID CYST

A rare infectious disease, known medically as echinococ-ciasis, and found in communities where sheep and cattle-raising is carried out with the help of dogs. Eggs of a small tapeworm carried by the dogs are excreted in their faeces. The eggs then fall on the ground, and if they are swallowed by man or another animal in contaminated food or water they enter the bloodstream and form cysts, usually in the lung or liver. The cysts are easily over-looked and difficult to diagnose.
Symptoms
• Often there are no symptoms and the disease is usually discovered when chronic ill health or vague abdominal pains are being investigated.
Causes
• A tapeworm called *Taenia echinococcus*, which is a parasite of dogs.
Treatment
• Surgery may be necessary to remove the cysts from the body tissue.
Prevention
• Avoid close contact with dogs which may have tape or other worm infections.
• Never allow dogs to lick plates or other utensils used by the family.

See INFECTIOUS DISEASES *page 32*

HYDROCELE

A collection of fluid in the layers of tissue surrounding the testicle. It is harmless.
Symptoms
• A swelling in the scrotum. This is painless but may cause some discomfort.
Duration
• The swelling persists indefinitely unless treated.
Causes
• The cause of a hydrocele is usually not known.
Treatment in the home
• Once a hydrocele has been diagnosed, support the scrotum with Y-front pants or a jock strap.
When to consult the doctor
• As soon as any swelling in the scrotum is noticed.

What the doctor may do
• Examine the scrotum, possibly by shining light through it in a darkened room.
• If a hydrocele is diagnosed, the fluid will need to be drawn off with a needle and syringe (a fairly painless procedure). The doctor may refer the patient to a hospital.
Prevention
• There is no way of preventing a hydrocele from developing.
Outlook
• Treatment will clear up the problem, but in some cases repeated drainage of the fluid is needed and in others an operation is required to remove the swelling.

See MALE GENITAL SYSTEM *page 50*

HYDROCEPHALUS

A rare condition also known as water on the brain. It results from an excessive build up of cerebrospinal fluid, a watery substance which surrounds the brain and spinal cord. The surplus fluid collects in cavities in the brain, generally resulting in an abnormally enlarged head. The condition usually develops after birth, but is also known to affect the unborn child.
Symptoms
• In babies and young children the head grows larger than normal. The forehead expands and may overhang the face (which is not itself affected). The soft spots on a baby's skull (fontanelles) are tense and swollen. The veins running over the scalp stand out.
• When hydrocephalus develops in later childhood or adult life there may be no enlargement of the head, be-cause the skull is more firmly formed. Instead, the excess fluid raises the pressure inside the skull, causing headache and vomiting.
Causes
• Hydrocephalus results when the circulation of cere-brospinal fluid gets blocked. When the condition is present at birth, it may be associated with SPINA BIFIDA.
• Occasionally the condition occurs in later life, it may follow MENINGITIS, or results from a BRAIN TUMOUR.
Complications
• Brain damage, blindness, mental handicap and spas-ticity may result if the condition is not treated, or fails to clear up of its own accord.
Treatment in the home
• None is advised.

When to consult the doctor
• Hydrocephalus present at birth will normally be noted by the doctor or midwife.
• If any abnormal swelling of the head occurs.
• If poor vision, persistent headaches or vomiting occur.
What the doctor may do
• Recommend an operation to drain the fluid into the bloodstream. This is done by inserting one end of a tube in the skull behind the ear, with the other end draining into the abdomen or a vein in the neck. The small plastic tube is placed beneath the skin.
Prevention
• None.
Outlook
• Mild cases of hydrocephalus often clear up of their own accord: some 40 per cent of cases in infants require no treatment. If an operation is necessary, it will succeed as long as it is performed before permanent damage is done by the pressure of fluid on the brain.

See NERVOUS SYSTEM *page 34*

HYDROTHERAPY
Strictly, hydrotherapy refers only to the external use of water in various types of bath and shower or through the application of high-pressure jets, but in many spas, where water contains natural salts reputed to have health-giving properties, it is drunk as well. Hydrotherapy has also come to include underwater massage and the application of mud poultices or seaweed compresses.

Scientific research has not yet yielded any convincing explanation for the apparent successes of 'water cures', but there is no doubt that they produce a psychological benefit; or that exercise in water aids recovery from a variety of physical illnesses. Hot baths and mud poultices also seem to help to combat rheumatism and arthritis.

HYPERACTIVITY
Hyperactive children are fidgety, impulsive, easily dis-tracted, clumsy, and unable to remain still for any length of time. They have a short attention span and have diffi-culty completing tasks. Hyperactive behaviour may reflect high energy in a well-adjusted child, or may be a symptom of agitation and anxiety in a child with an emotional disorder or brain damage. Living with a hyperactive child is stressful for the rest of the family; and stress and dis-agreement at home tend to make hyperactivity worse.

Treatment includes creating a structured routine for the child, with firm limits to acceptable behaviour. Psycho-logical, or sometimes drug therapy may be necessary, with treatment often involving the whole family.

HYPERTENSION

This term describes a state of higher blood pressure than is normal. It occurs in about 10 per cent of middle-aged people.

Symptoms
• The condition rarely causes symptoms and is usually discovered when the patient is examined for other reasons.

Duration
• This can persist indefinitely.

Causes
• There are genetic and environmental causes. People living in underdeveloped countries, or with a low salt intake, are less likely to develop hypertension. Related causes include obesity, and heavy drinking, taking the contraceptive pill, and smoking. Rarely, it is caused by kidney disease.

Complications
• The complications of hypertension are many. ATHEROMA, STROKE, ANGINA. CORONARY THROMBOSIS and HEART FAILURE are the most important.

Treatment in the home
• Cut down on drinking and stop smoking, lose weight, and stop using the contraceptive pill. Take regular physical exercise, and reduce salt intake.

When to consult the doctor
• Because hypertension rarely causes symptoms, make sure that your blood pressure is checked every few years. especially if you are over 35.

What the doctor may do
• A doctor will take several tests of your blood pressure to find out if it is abnormally high over a period of time.
• If the patient has hypertension, the doctor will find out if it has damaged the heart, lungs, eyes and kidneys by taking blood tests, X-rays and ELECTROCARDIOGRAMS.
• If he suspects kidney disease he will arrange for the patient to visit hospital for tests and X-rays.
• Advise on diet (see ATHEROMA), including cutting out excessive salt, alcohol and smoking.
• Prescribe antihypertensive drugs. See MEDICINES, 7.

Prevention
• Follow the advice given under **Treatment in the home**.
• There is evidence that regular moderate exercise such as jogging or swimming is an effective added method of preventing hypertension.

Outlook
• Hypertension encourages hardening of the arteries (atheroma). It can lead to heart failure, coronary artery disease and strokes. If the hypertension is controlled, these risks are lessened.
See CIRCULATORY SYSTEM *page 40*

HYPERTHERMIA OR HYPERPYREXIA
A dangerously high temperature—one above 106°F (41°C). Babies with fever are vulnerable to overheating. Parents should resist the desire to pile on clothes and warm up the room in which a feverish baby is being nursed. *See* CHILD CARE—CHILDHOOD ILLS *page 151*.

HYPERTHYROIDISM *See* THYROTOXICOSIS

HYPOTHYROIDISM *See* MYXOEDEMA

HYPNOSIS
An artificially created state of altered consciousness that is neither wakefulness nor sleep, in which the subject is susceptible to suggestion. Hypnosis is increasingly, although not generally, accepted as an aid to orthodox medicine, and many doctors are qualified hypnotists.

Some psychiatrists use hypnosis to try to relieve mental conditions—for example, a PHOBIA—or physical ailments such as ASTHMA, which may have an underlying mental cause. It has also been successfully employed to combat mild addictions. *See* SMOKING.

But it works less well with stronger addictions, such as ALCOHOLISM or dependence upon narcotics. It is also helpful during labour and dentistry.

The essence of hypnotic technique lies in persuading the patient to relax and to focus on an object or the hypnotist's instructions.

It is generally believed that a patient under hypnosis will not do anything against his conscience. Most people are susceptible to hypnosis, but it is difficult, if not impossible, to hypnotise a subject against his will, and very few people—about 5 per cent—are susceptible enough to go into a deep trance in which, for example, major surgery would be possible. During hypnosis there are measurable changes in a patient's brainwaves.

HYPOMANIA
A mild form of mania with extreme restlessness and elation occurring in someone who may also suffer from DEPRESSION. Unusually excessive energy and restlessness causes INSOMNIA. Behaviour may be bizarre, with the sufferer dressing flamboyantly, being excessively generous or grossly overspending. In severe cases, the patient may become confused and behaviour become so antisocial that admission to hospital is required.

If untreated, hypomania may last weeks or months before settling spontaneously or reverting to a depressive state. The period between attacks varies from some months to many years. The cause is unknown, but the condition may be brought on by drugs. Management, prevention and outlook are the same as for MANIC DEPRESSION.
See MENTAL SYSTEM *page 33*

HYPOSPADIAS
An abnormality of the male urethra, the passage through which urine is passed, in which its opening lies on the base of the penis. The condition usually occurs together with chordee, curvature of the penis. Surgery is usually performed after the age of 12 months to straighten the penis and reconstruct the urethra. Normal urination and, later, sexual activity are then possible.

HYPOTHERMIA
An abnormally low temperature—below 95–97°F (35–36°C). Newborn babies and old people are most usually affected. In babies the cause is often a cold room at night. Premature babies and those suffering from illness are most susceptible. Signs are a bright red appearance, lethargy and refusing food. In old people, hypothermia is generally the result of inadequate food, clothing and heating in cold weather. MYXOEDEMA, or immobility due to illness or an accident, can be a contributory cause. Tiredness, muscle stiffness and a confused mental state are the first signs of the condition. In both young and old, unless hypothermia is recognised and action taken, unconsciousness will eventually occur, followed by brain damage, then death.

Hypothermia can also occur accidentally, for example in climbers and fell walkers, or those who have been submerged in water. Treatment of all cases is by slowly rewarming the casualty, administration of oxygen where available, and avoiding alcohol.
See EXPOSURE *page 584*

HYSTERECTOMY
An operation to remove a woman's uterus (womb), cervix (neck of the womb), Fallopian tubes (egg-carrying ducts) and sometimes ovaries (egg-producing organs). If the ovaries are removed, part of an ovary is usually left

in the body to continue producing female hormones. The operation is performed to treat cancer of the uterus or cervix, or certain non-cancerous tumours—for example, FIBROIDS; and is also sometimes performed if excessive menstrual bleeding is causing ANAEMIA.

The operation, which requires a general anaesthetic, is performed through the lower abdominal wall, or through the vagina. In certain cases, after hysteroscopy (a type of ENDOSCOPY), TCRE (trans-cervical resection of the endo-metrium) can be performed under local anaesthetic, avoiding the need for hysterectomy.

See FEMALE GENITAL SYSTEM *page 48*

HYSTERIA

A condition in which the sufferer displays unusual behaviour in order to attract attention or to avoid an unpleasant situation. It is brought on by stress in an immature person who is extremely vulnerable to sugges-tion. It is more common in women than men, and may recur. The term is also used to describe a situation in which members of a group exhibit a similar symptom for which no cause can be found. The symptoms are pro-duced unconsciously and the motives, although obvious to others, are not faced by the patient.

Symptoms
- Almost any symptom can be caused by hysteria, ranging from pain to loss of sensation, and loss of use of any part of the body.
- The response of the sufferer can range from great concern to sublime indifference to the symptom.
- Acute reactions can result in total loss of control over the emotions and loss of memory.

Causes
- Not known. The sufferer, unlike the deliberate malin-gerer, is unaware that his symptoms are not due to physical illness.

Treatment in the home
- Resolve the conflict or cause of the anxiety.
- Use firm reassurance with minimal fuss.
- Symptoms may be aggravated by both too much or too little sympathy.

When to consult the doctor
- On the appearance of any symptom that cannot be explained, as the doctor may discover a physical basis for the trouble.

See MENTAL SYSTEM *page 33*

IATROGENIC DISEASE

Any disorder caused by medical treatment. For example, in some people parts of the body swell in reaction to penicillin given to treat an infection; in others regular aspirin prescribed for arthritis causes stomach bleeding.

ICHTHYOSIS

An inherited skin disorder which may run in families, in which the skin is rough and looks like fish scales. It may be obvious at birth or become apparent a few weeks later. In mild cases it involves just a very dry skin; in severe cases the skin is a mass of loose scales which fall off when dressing and can be shaken off clothing.

Symptoms
- Rough skin that looks like fish scales.
- The person with ichthyosis is extra sensitive to chem-icals and infections which affect the skin.
- In cold weather, the skin cracks and becomes painful.
- The skin may look dirty, although it is not, and the patient is often self-conscious about undressing or bathing in public.

Duration
- The condition is lifelong.

Treatment in the home
- The skin can be temporarily softened by using a bath oil and rubbing in an oily cream after a warm bath.
- Cover as much of the skin as possible with appropriate clothes, such as long-sleeved blouses or shirts. Removing scales from clothing will help reduce social embarrass-ment.
- Warm climates are more agreeable to people suffering from ichthyosis, as skin cracks are less likely in such conditions.

When to consult the doctor
- As soon as any abnormality of the skin has been noticed.

What the doctor may do
- Recently some cases appear to be helped by urea cream (10 per cent) applied daily after a bath. This is not a permanent cure, but sufferers should ask their doctor for a trial.

Outlook
- The condition is incurable, though the scaliness may improve with treatment or age.

See SKIN *page 52*

ID

A psychiatric term meaning the unconscious, instinctive part of the human mind, as opposed to the ego, the conscious, rational part, and the super-ego, the moral conscience. This concept of the mind was formulated by Sigmund Freud (1856-1939), the Viennese founder of psychoanalysis.

ILEITIS, REGIONAL

An inflammation that usually affects the ileum (the lower part of the small bowel) and occasionally other parts of the digestive tract. The condition is also known as Crohn's disease. Parts of the intestine wall grow thick, fluid accumulates, ulcers and infection develop in the lining of the walls. The ulcers may penetrate the wall and lead to peritonitis. Scarring may lead to ring-like constrictions. Most cases occur in the 20s. The disease, which may run in families, particularly Jewish families, affects both sexes equally.

Symptoms
- Chronic diarrhoea, associated with loss of appetite, fever and weight loss, which all may occur in attacks, or continuously, for weeks or months.
- Abdominal pain may be intermittent or continuous and varies in severity.
- The disease may mimic acute APPENDICITIS.

Duration
- Complete recovery may follow a single isolated attack.
- Chronic regional ileitis may be lifelong.

Causes
- The exact cause is not known.

Complications
- Ulcers may cause narrowing and bowel obstruction. Perforation of an ulcer may lead to PERITONITIS, abscess or fistula, that is, an opening into another organ or on to the skin through operation scars.
- The lower bowel may become inflamed. *See* PROCTITIS.
- Mouth ulcers, skin rashes, eye disorders and joint pains may occur.
- Kidney stones and gallstones may result from poor food absorption by the bowel.

Treatment in the home
- Rest during feverish flare-ups.
- Avoid mental or physical overstrain leading to exhaus-tion.
- Simple antidiarrhoeal medicines may help to limit

attacks of diarrhoea and cramps. *See* MEDICINES, 2.
• Water-absorbing bulking agents, which you can buy from the chemist, help to prevent irritation of the bowel and make stools firmer. *See* MEDICINES, 3.
When to consult the doctor
• If there are persistent or recurrent bouts of diarrhoea, fever or abdominal pain.
What the doctor may do
• Send the patient to hospital for tests to confirm the diagnosis.
• Prescribe long-term stronger antidiarrhoeal drugs to reduce inflammatory flare-ups.
• Prescribe short courses of steroids in severe acute stages. *See* MEDICINES, 32.
• If there are complications, such as obstruction or an abscess or fistula, the doctor may suggest an operation to remove the affected gut section.
Prevention
• None known.
Outlook
• Even after surgical removal the condition may recur and require further treatment.

See DIGESTIVE SYSTEM *page 44*

ILEOSTOMY
An operation in which a loop of the ileum, the major part of the small intestine, is brought through an incision in the abdominal wall and opened to create an artificial anus. The operation is performed when acute ulcerative colitis necessitates the removal of the large intestine.

People who have had an ileostomy are able to live a completely normal life. Any advice or information they want can be obtained from the *Ileostomy Association*, Amblehurst House, Black Scotch Lane, Mansfield, Notts NG18 4PS (Tel. 0623 28099).

IMPETIGO

A highly contagious skin infection common in children. It usually affects the face, hands or knees.
Symptoms
• First a red spot appears. This becomes a blister, which quickly breaks down and discharges, causing yellow crusts to develop.
• The crusts spread and other spots then develop near to the earlier infection.

Duration
• With antibiotics, cure is rapid; without antibiotics the sores can fester for many weeks.
Causes
• Bacteria, usually the streptococcus or staphylococcus.
• Dirty hands rubbing the face is a common source of infection.
Treatment in the home
• Bathe the crusts with an antiseptic diluted in warm water.
• Painting the sores with antibacterial paint, such as gentian violet, is very effective and cheap, but also embarrassing. *See* MEDICINES, 43.
When to consult the doctor
• As soon as possible, to avoid spreading infection.
What the doctor may do
• Prescribe antibiotic ointment to treat the spots.
• Give antibiotic tablets or injections if the lymph glands are very tender and the person is ill.

Do's and don'ts about indigestion

☐ *Do* work out what foods make the pain worse and avoid them. Alcohol provokes indigestion and should never be taken in excess.

☐ *Do* tell your doctor if symptoms worsen or change in nature.

☐ *Do* try to avoid stress.

☐ *Do* raise the head of your bed with a couple of telephone directories.

☐ *Don't* have irregular meals or miss a meal.

☐ *Don't* smoke.

☐ *Don't* stoop and bend if the cause of your trouble is hiatus HERNIA or peptic OESOPHAGITIS.

☐ *Don't* take aspirin or any drug containing it unless instructed to do so by your doctor, because aspirin irritates the stomach.

Prevention
• Cleanliness and good food give the best protection, but even a well cared for child may develop impetigo.
Outlook
• With proper treatment rapid recovery can always be expected.

See SKIN *page 52*

IMPOTENCE
Inability in a man to have sexual intercourse. Impotence may be due to failure to achieve an erection or failure to ejaculate.
See SEX PROBLEMS

INCONTINENCE
Inability to control the discharge of faeces from the anus or urine from the bladder.
See SYMPTOM SORTER—INCONTINENCE

INDIGESTION
Discomfort in the upper middle part of the abdomen, sometimes spreading up behind the breastbone. It is often associated with belching wind, which may bring acid up to the mouth, and nausea. There are many causes.
See SYMPTOM SORTER—INDIGESTION

INDUSTRIAL DISEASE
One of a group of diseases to which workers in certain industries are at risk, such as skin diseases caused through handling chemicals, or lung diseases which affect miners.
See OCCUPATIONAL HAZARDS

INFANTILE PARALYSIS
Another name for poliomyelitis, now commonly known as polio. It is a virus infection caused by one of three different viruses.
See POLIOMYELITIS

INFECTIOUS MONONUCLEOSIS
The medical name for glandular fever. A common virus disease of children and young adults that affects the glands of the neck, armpits and groin. Despite its name it is not particularly infectious.
See GLANDULAR FEVER

INFERTILITY

One of the most basic human urges is to reproduce; to have a family is usually regarded as a blessing, and to be denied one, a misfortune. But if 100 young, apparently normal couples have regular sexual intercourse for a whole year, without any sort of contraception, on average only 85 of the women will be pregnant at the end of that time. Seven or eight of them will never become pregnant, however hard they try.

At each intercourse many millions of sperm are deposited in the upper part of the woman's vagina, but they move randomly, in all directions. Few find their way through the narrow neck of the cervix and into the womb, along the fluid lining the womb and up the Fallopian tubes, where the woman's egg may be awaiting fertilisation (*see* PREGNANCY). The vast majority of sperm fail to complete the journey. They die and are discharged. This is to be expected and accounts for the normal delays in becoming pregnant. It is not a sign of infertility.

Most doctors agree that the question of infertility arises only if a normal young couple have had intercourse for more than a year without contraception, and without producing a pregnancy. Infertility may be due to problems in any of four areas—poor sperm production, poor egg production, blockage of the passages between sperm and egg, and a hostile response to sperm by the woman's body.

POOR SPERM PRODUCTION

Sperm are manufactured in the testes from puberty until a man is in his 60s or later. While still immature, they pass up narrow tubes to the seminal vesicles—storage sacs behind the prostate gland. There the sperm mature. During intercourse, just before ejaculation, fluid is pro- duced in the prostate gland and passes down the urethra (the tube to the penis). As this fluid passes the mouths of the seminal vesicles, a jet of sperm-rich liquid is injected into it. The mixture now passing along the urethra is called semen.

Poor sperm production may be due to damage to the cells making sperm. This may then lead to too few sperm in the semen; or the sperm may lack the mobility they need to help them on their journey to the eggs; or they may be deformed or dead. Owing to infection, the tubes between the testes and the seminal vesicles may be blocked; or the sperm may become infected once they are in the vesicles.

The fluid from the prostate may be insufficient or may be unable to sustain live sperm.

Lastly, the man may have problems in obtaining a complete erection, so that he cannot deposit the semen at the upper end of the vagina, from where it has the best chance of sending sperm to meet the eggs.

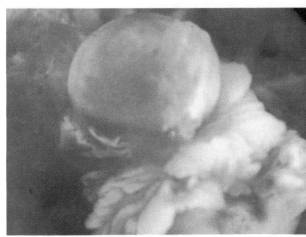

ACTIVE SPERM READY FOR FERTILISATION *About 500 million sperm are introduced into the vagina at intercourse, but only one can penetrate and fertilise the waiting egg. This seemingly simple process involves a vast network of chemical controls, and if even one of these becomes disturbed the chances of fertilisation are reduced.*

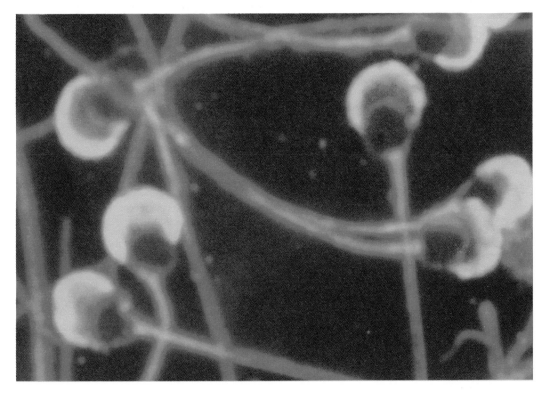

THE BEGINNING OF LIFE *Inside the ovary, a tiny pink follicle nurtures the immature egg for two weeks until it is the size of a pea and mature enough to be released.*

POOR EGG PRODUCTION

The egg cells that a woman needs for the manufacture of eggs are present in her ovaries. The eggs mature from the cells in response to the stimulation of gonadotrophins—hormones released from the pituitary gland beneath the brain. This causes usually one—or occasionally two—eggs to be made in the middle of each menstrual cycle. The mature egg emerges from the surface of the ovary. Finger-like fimbria at the end of the Fallopian tube close round the ovary and catch the emerging egg, which passes into the first inch of the tube and there awaits the sperm that may be coming to meet it.

The pituitary gland may fail to stimulate eggs to develop regularly during each menstrual cycle. Even if a woman has a regular release of normal pituitary hormones, the egg may be resistant to stimulation; or there may not be enough egg cells in the ovaries, so no eggs are made. Even if eggs are made, the fimbria may be unable to close round the ovary and so receive the egg

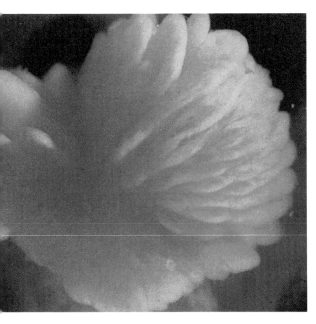

RECEIVING THE MATURE EGG *As the time of maturity draws near, the Fallopian tube becomes erect and its splayed end closes round the ovary to catch the mature egg as it emerges from its follicle.*

into the Fallopian tube to await the sperm.

BLOCKAGE BETWEEN THE SPERM AND THE EGG

Even if some sperm succeed in finding their way from the vagina into the cervix, they may still encounter an obstruction which prevents them from reaching the egg.

The mucus made by the glands of the cervix and the womb may be so thick and tenacious that it will not allow sperm to pass through it. Sperm may penetrate beyond the cervix to the womb, but adhesions in the womb—fibrous tissues resulting from old operations or damage—may prevent them passing through it. Adhesions may also form on the outside of the Fallopian tubes, kinking them and so closing them off.

More likely, the sperm that reach the Fallopian tubes may be stopped by a blockage of the tube itself, due to a past inflammation or infection. Less commonly, the sperm may pass up the tube to the egg, but the lining of the tube will have been damaged, preventing it from propelling the fertilised egg to the womb. In an undamaged tube, thread-like cells wave to set up a current, and muscles in the tube lining contract, so that the lining ripples and moves the egg on its way. Without this assistance, the egg stays in the tube, and the result is an ECTOPIC PREGNANCY, in which the fertilised egg begins to grow in the tube but generally dies after about two months.

HOSTILE RESPONSE TO SPERM

Having received and absorbed a few sperm from a man, a woman may produce antibodies to them in her blood. This is the immune process—part of the body's defences against 'foreign' invaders, such as disease bacteria. The antibodies react against sperm arriving during subsequent love-making, sticking them together. This makes them less active, and less able to travel to the egg.

Or the man himself may produce antibodies to his own sperm. His body becomes unable to distinguish between invaders and its own products. Normally his sperm are isolated from the rest of his body in the tubes of his reproductive system. But if there is a break in the walls of these tubes, the sperm may enter the man's blood which produces antibodies against them. As a result, sperm maturing subsequently will be inactive.

FINDING THE CAUSE

Before action is taken to cure infertility, checks are made and tests are conducted to identify the cause. The hospital fertility clinic and the couple themselves participate in the investigation. The hospital doctor checks the medical history of both partners. He asks for the approximate dates of the woman's periods over the previous year, to

be sure that she is menstruating regularly—this implies regular egg production. The doctor will also ask whether intercourse has been reasonably frequent; and he will examine the woman for any abnormalities of her reproductive organs.

Having made these preliminary checks, the doctor will arrange tests designed to narrow down the problem areas to one or more.

Is the problem poor sperm production? The man is usually asked to produce one or more sperm specimens. The laboratory will check these for the number of sperm in each specimen and their degree of activity. The more active they are, the more likely they are to reach their destination and achieve their purpose. The semen may also be checked for antibodies, and for acidity.

Is the problem poor egg production? When an egg is shed from the ovary, it creates a yellow tissue called the corpus luteum—Latin for 'yellow body'—at the spot where it was attached. This tissue produces the hormone progesterone, which is distributed through the bloodstream and has the effect of raising body temperature. Therefore, if a woman takes her temperature every morning throughout the menstrual cycle and finds it rising consistently in the second half of the cycle, it is probable that an egg has been made. At the same time in the cycle, the doctor can also carry out tests to measure her progesterone level.

Alternatively, by means of dilatation and curettage (D & C), a small strip of the lining of the womb can be removed. Under the microscope the cells in the sample show whether the hormones are being produced and circulating normally, and whether eggs are being made.

Is there a blockage between sperm and egg? Doctors can check for a blockage by means of LAPAROSCOPY. A laparoscope is a fine, illuminated viewing tube which is inserted through the abdominal wall under a general anaesthetic. A blue dye is injected through the cervix, and the doctor can tell if the way is clear by watching its progress through the laparoscope. With the same instrument, he can check that the Fallopian tubes can catch the eggs that are released by the ovary, and that no adhesions on the outside of the tube are kinking it.

Alternatively, a solution that shows up under X-rays can be injected into the womb. Its progress through the womb and Fallopian tubes can be seen on an X-ray screen, or on a series of X-ray photographs.

Is the problem a hostile response to sperm? Antibodies to sperm can be detected in the male or the female partner. The doctor tests samples of the woman's cervical mucus, the man's sperm, or the blood of either partner.

FINDING A REMEDY

Having identified the problem causing infertility, the

doctor can recommend treatment to rectify it.

Poor sperm production A man's testes can be stimulated to manufacture sperm if he is given injections of testosterone, a male sex hormone.

A blockage of the narrower tubes in the male reproductive organs cannot be cleared, but one in the wider pipe carrying semen to the penis may be removed by surgery.

Production of sperm can be improved by lowering the temperature of the testes, if it is too high. As the testes hang outside the body in the scrotum, their temperature is slightly lower than internal body temperature. If the lower temperature is not maintained, sperm production is reduced.

To give the sperm the maximum chance of fertilising an egg, couples should have intercourse within 24 hours of ovulation (*see* FAMILY PLANNING—Rhythm Method).

Poor erection can often be helped by psychological counselling. *See* SEX PROBLEMS.

Poor egg production Under-active ovaries can sometimes be stimulated to produce eggs, either by pills that stimulate the pituitary gland and ovaries, or by injections of gonadotrophins given at the right stage of the menstrual cycle. Both treatments require close medical supervision, and increase the chances of multiple pregnancies.

Blockage between sperm and egg An obstruction between the sperm and the egg in the woman may be cleared with surgery. This has a 25-30 per cent chance of success; but a couple wanting a child are likely to regard a small chance as better than none.

Hostile response to sperm With the use of immuno-suppressive drugs, the body can be helped to reduce the antibodies to sperm—the immune process can be suppressed. But these drugs have potent side-effects, such as lowering the body's resistance to all invaders—including the organisms carrying disease. The doctor will prescribe such drugs only if the benefits are greater than the disadvantages.

The outlook for a couple with infertility problems is now greatly improved compared with 20 years ago. About 60 per cent of couples attending fertility clinics are found to have problems that can be diagnosed, and about 30 per cent of these produce a baby after treatment. Medical research is far from the end of its investigations into treatment of infertility, and there are still great advances to be made.

OTHER REMEDIES

Artificial insemination When an egg is fertilised inside the woman's body by semen which has not been introduced into the vagina at intercourse the process is known as artificial insemination. Instead the semen is introduced with a syringe into the region of the neck of the womb in the hope that the sperm will then travel up to fertilise the egg. There are two types of artificial insemination—by the husband (AIH) and by a donor (AID).

Artificial insemination by the husband can be used if

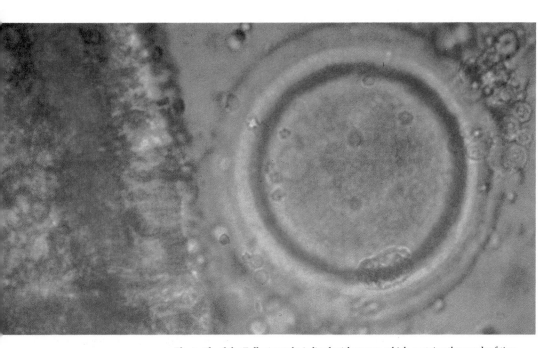

THE EGG ENTERS THE FALLOPIAN TUBE *The inside of the Fallopian tube is lined with mucus which contains thousands of tiny vibrating hairs. When the mature egg is caught, the tube contracts and the hairs vibrate to suck the egg into the mucus, wher it is protected while it awaits fertilisation by one of the millions of male sperm which will come to meet it.*

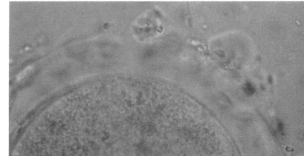

A HUMAN LIFE IS CREATED *The mature egg waits in the outer part of the Fallopian tube (above). Six hours after fertilisation there is an explosion of life, and the now-human egg (below) begins its four-day journey to the uterus.*

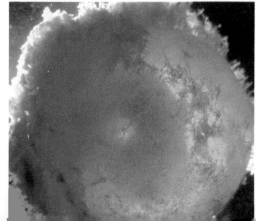

the husband cannot maintain an erection and so cannot deposit semen at the upper end of his wife's vagina. This also happens with premature ejaculation and other neurological states. He produces semen by masturbation, which is collected in a syringe and introduced straight away into his wife. AIH has a high success rate when done at the exact time of the menstrual cycle when the egg is being made. This will require some preliminary investigations of the woman by her doctor. Sometimes, doctors encourage couples to do it themselves, giving them a plastic syringe and showing them how to use it. From a psychological point of view, this is better than going into hospital and having to produce specimens under cold clinical conditions.

AIH may also be used if the woman is producing mucus from the neck of the womb (cervix) which is hostile to the semen. In some cases, fertilisation can be achieved by introducing the semen above the hostile secretions.

Artificial insemination by donor's semen is a bigger step for a couple to take. It is used when a man produces semen but there is no sperm in it and so cannot fertilise his wife. The couple, in consultation with their doctor and a specialist in the field, may feel that they would prefer to have a baby who is at least half theirs (that is the mother's part) than not have a baby at all. The procedure is similar to that for AIH, but is always done at a hospital or clinic. AID has a high rate of success.

Donors are anonymous and not known to the parents, but there must be some match between the physical characteristics of the donor and those of the husband so that the child will have some resemblance to the father in the family. It is probably wise not to use a donor for more than ten to 15 successful donations, otherwise there may be too many of his offspring in his community who could grow up to marry each other and thus unknowingly risk multiplying any defective genes they may have.

Couples should think deeply about AID, both before they go for professional advice and afterwards. Counselling is essential and full agreement must be voluntary on both sides. AID can put a strain on a marriage and may be used as a lever later in domestic battles.

Most people concerned with AID consider it wise to tell the child about the background as soon as he or she is of mature age.

In vitro fertilisation When an egg is removed from a woman and fertilised by the father's sperm outside her body, the process is known medically as in vitro fertilisation. This Latin term, literally 'in glass', describes a biological process made to occur in an artificial environment, outside the living organism. The popular term 'test-tube baby' for the resulting child is a misnomer, since test-tubes are not used in the procedure. The first baby to be produced by in vitro fertilisation was born in 1978. There have been many such births since.

Couples who can benefit most from in vitro fertilisation are those where the woman is making eggs normally, the man is making normal sperm, but the passage between the two is blocked, most commonly by damage or removal of the Fallopian tubes. In such cases, a laparoscope can be introduced into the woman's abdominal cavity under anaesthesia to see if an egg is developing in the ovary. If an egg is present, a long hollow needle is passed into the abdominal cavity to suck it out into a specially prepared chamber. It is then transferred to a flat open dish under sterile conditions and a dilute solution of the father's semen is added to the dish. One of the sperm soon fertilises the egg. Development proceeds by the fertilised egg dividing into two cells. Then the two become four and the four become eight. When the eight-cell stage has been reached, after about 40 hours, the egg is usually returned to the mother's body by a fine plastic tube being inserted through the neck of her womb. If the timing has been correct, the lining of the woman's womb is ready to receive the fertilised egg so that it will implant and develop in the same way as a naturally fertilised egg.

Techniques like this require special research and scientific back-up for the surgeon performing the operation, and at present can be done only in a few centres of the world. Usually the egg can be fertilised and made to grow to the eight-cell stage, but the difficult part is reintroduction and getting the egg to implant in the uterus. This is done blindly and is probably the reason why only 25 per cent of women who accept in vitro fertilisation actually have a child. There are still the risks of spontaneous abortion which may occur in the first 12 weeks of gestation, but once that hurdle is passed, the baby seems to develop like any other. The proportion of twins is slightly higher than for natural births, since many surgeons like to reinsert two fertilised eggs into the uterus in the hope that one will survive; occasionally both do.

In vitro fertilisation is a new development, but as techniques improve it may in the future be made available at regional centres throughout the country.

Embryo freezing It is also now possible to take an embryo, fertilised in vitro, and freeze it in a tank of liquid nitrogen at about −200°C in a state of 'suspended animation'. The frozen embryo can be thawed out later and introduced into the mother's womb, where the postponed pregnancy can continue.

Surrogate motherhood Sperms collected from the husband of an infertile woman can be introduced, by AID, into the womb of another, normal woman. If this 'surrogate mother' becomes pregnant, she carries the baby in her womb until it is born. The baby is then handed over to the infertile woman and her husband. The baby has genes from the husband but not the wife.

Surrogate motherhood is fraught with potential difficulties, particularly if the baby turns out to be abnormal, or if the surrogate mother decides that she does not want to part with the child.

Womb leasing When a woman can produce eggs but is unable to carry a baby throughout pregnancy, an embryo produced from her egg and her husband's sperm can be introduced into another, healthy woman's womb. Unlike surrogate motherhood, the baby in womb leasing is genetically the child of both the husband and wife, and has no genes from the woman who carried it during pregnancy. In womb leasing fertilisation is in vitro, whereas in surrogate motherhood it is usually by AID.

Embryo donation If a woman is incapable of producing eggs, an egg can be taken from the woman of a donor woman and fertilised in vitro with the sperm of the husband. The fertilised embryo is then introduced into the infertile wife's womb, and she proceeds with the pregnancy as if it were her own baby. The child has genes from her husband, but not from her.

Although surrogate motherhood, womb leasing, and embryo donation are now technically possible, there are difficult moral issues involved. The fact that a procedure is possible does not necessarily mean that it is advisable.

Coping with infertility

☐ Remember that infertility is a shared problem. It is often not possible, even after full investigation, to say with certainty that one partner alone is responsible.

☐ Open discussion between partners is the best way of dealing with the disappointments, fears and worries that both may have.

☐ Do not be afraid of discussing your difficulties with a doctor or someone else whom you trust.

☐ Remember that one-third of all couples attending fertility clinics eventually have a baby. Many others achieve a baby after treatment by their family doctor alone.

INFLAMMATION

The reaction of body tissues to infection or injury. The blood supply to the affected area is increased, so that extra white blood cells are available to promote healing. The area becomes red, swollen, hot and tender. Any disorder that is an inflammation is denoted by the ending 'itis'—for example, laryngitis, inflammation of the larynx (voice-box).

INFLUENZA

A virus infection occurring in epidemic form, mostly during the winter months. Many people refer to a COMMON COLD as flu, but this is incorrect. True influenza is caused by three groups of viruses, identified as A, B and C, that can be typed by blood tests. Group A viruses produce Asian flu and Hong Kong flu. Most major epidemics or pandemics (epidemics occurring in many different countries at the same time) are caused by the A viruses. The virus changes from time to time, so immunity does not last indefinitely. But each year a vaccine is produced against the viruses that are expected to be prevalent the following winter. High-risk groups, that is people with heart disease or chronic lung disease, diabetics, and people over the age of 65, should be immunised in September or October.

Epidemics start abruptly, reach a peak in two or three weeks, then rapidly subside. Infection is passed from one person to another by the germ-laden air breathed, coughed or sneezed out by patients.

Symptoms
- Headache.
- Aching muscles and back.
- High temperature with sensation of feeling cold.
- Sweating.
- General weakness.
- Cough, sometimes producing sputum.
- Pain behind the breastbone, which is made worse by coughing.
- Nasal catarrh and sneezing.

Incubation period
- Eighteen hours to three days.

Duration
- The worst of the illness is over within two or three days.
- Aching muscles, headache and fever may persist for a week.
- General weakness may persist for a few weeks.

Causes
- Influenza viruses.

Complications
- Pneumonia is common. In some epidemics it can be severe and lead to death, especially in the elderly and in those with chronic heart or lung disease.

Treatment in the home
- During an epidemic it will not be possible for every case to be seen by a doctor.
- Go to bed.
- Drink extra fluids to replace losses caused by fever.
- Take paracetamol in recommended doses. Children with influenza should not take aspirin.
- Hot lemon and honey drinks or a proprietary cough mixture may help to ease coughing and chest pains. See MEDICINES, 16, 22.
- Do not struggle to work. You will spread the disease and increase the risk of complications.

When to consult the doctor
- If the patient is in a high-risk group—that is, has heart disease, chronic lung disease or diabetes, or is over the age of 65.

What the doctor may do
- Prescribe antibiotics to prevent complications.
- Prescribe antiviral drugs. See MEDICINES, 25, 27.

Prevention
- Annual vaccination against influenza is recommended for people at high risk such as those with diabetes or chronic heart, kidney or lung disease.

Outlook
- In most cases, recovery from influenza is complete, although the patient may suffer a period of depression for a short while afterwards.

See INFECTIOUS DISEASES *page 32*

INGROWING TOE-NAIL

A toe-nail (usually that of the big toe) whose front corners grow inwards, cutting into the surrounding skin.

Symptoms
- Pain at the corners of the nail.
- Inflammation where the corner of the nail digs into the skin.

Duration
- The condition will persist unless treated.

Causes
- Shoes that are too tight.
- Cutting off the corners of the nail instead of cutting the nail straight across.
- Digging down the sides of the nail in order to remove dead skin.
- There may be bacterial infection.

Treatment in the home
- Tuck pieces of gauze soaked in surgical spirit beneath the corners of the nail twice a day.
- Make a V-shaped cut in the middle of the top edge of the nail; this lessens the pressure of the ingrowing sides of the nail.

When to consult the doctor
- If the condition does not respond to home treatment, and the pain becomes worse.
- If there is any discharge or bleeding from the affected area.

What the doctor may do
- Prescribe an antiseptic ointment to be applied to the affected areas.
- If the toe is infected, the doctor may also prescribe an antibiotic. See MEDICINES, 25.
- He may also make arrangements for the toe to be dressed daily.
- If the problem persists, a minor operation will be performed.

Prevention
- Avoid tight-fitting shoes.
- Cut toe-nails straight across.
- Do not dig down the sides of toe-nails to remove dead skin.

Outlook
- Treatment usually clears up the problem.
- As the nail grows, the edges project beyond the skin fold at the corner and stop cutting into the skin.

See SKELETAL SYSTEM *page 54*

INHIBITION

1. The prevention of, or interference with, the functioning of a part of the body by some disorder of a nerve. For example, an injured nerve can inhibit movement of a limb.
2. In psychiatry, excessive restraint by a person of a normal, spontaneous reaction.

INSANITY

A state of serious mental illness in which a person is incapable of distinguishing right from wrong or managing his legal affairs. The term is now much more used in law than in medicine.

INSECT BITES AND STINGS

Insect bites and stings are minor hazards of everyday life, especially common in the summer months. There is no insect native to Britain whose bite or sting contains dangerous poison. However, serious problems may result from a local infection, or an allergic reaction.

Symptoms

• Discomfort or pain following the bite or sting. With a bee or wasp sting, pain is immediate and sometimes intense. In contrast, a midge or mosquito bite may pass unnoticed at first, irritation following later.

• Swelling and inflammation. The swelling may be hard, red and shiny, or capped by a blister.

• The swelling may itch, either mildly or intensely.

• If a bite or sting becomes infected, the symptoms spread and intensify.

• If a person is allergic to a particular insect bite or sting, severe swelling may occur rapidly, and be followed by swellings occurring elsewhere on the body. There may occasionally be additional symptoms such as difficulty in breathing.

Duration

• A normal bite or sting is rarely painful for more than three to six hours. Itching, however, may persist for two or three days afterwards.

• If the bite or sting becomes infected, inflammation and pain spread, rather than clear up, after two or three days.

Causes

• Poison is injected into the skin, either from the sting or the bite. Itching and swelling occur as antibodies present in the blood are stimulated to counteract the poison.

Complications

• An infected bite or sting may result in more widespread evidence of infection such as fever or joint pain.

• In rare cases, anaphylaxis may occur. This is an acute allergic reaction to a poison. The patient may find it hard to breathe, or collapse. In extremely rare instances, an attack may prove fatal before help can be sought. See ALLERGY.

Treatment in the home

• When a young child is bitten or stung, pain and fright can cause real distress. Calm reassurance is the first form of treatment.

• Inspect the affected area. If the sting of a bee or wasp is visible, remove it, preferably with a fingernail.

• Clean the site with antiseptic to prevent infection, and bathe it in cold water to give relief.

• Avoid scratching, as infection may result. Irritation can usually be relieved by applying a calamine lotion.

• If there is any difficulty in breathing, the patient should be carefully watched and kept still in the position of maximum comfort until the doctor or ambulance arrives. Immediate first aid may be necessary.

When to consult the doctor

• If itching becomes unbearable.

• If the local swelling begins to spread elsewhere.

• If the joints, tongue or lips become swollen.

• Call the doctor or an ambulance *immediately* if breathing becomes difficult, if a sting occurs inside the mouth or throat, or if there are symptoms of acute allergic reaction.

What the doctor may do

• Prescribe antihistamine tablets.

• Prescribe steroids, to relieve itching.

• Prescribe antibiotics if the bite or sting has become infected.

• In cases of acute allergic reaction the doctor may inject an antihistamine and arrange for immediate admission to hospital. See MEDICINES, 14, 25, 32.

Prevention

• A few obvious precautions may be taken to avoid the likelihood of being bitten or stung. For example, avoid picnics on sites where mosquitoes and gnats will be found. Parents should be vigilant about wasps, which can be swallowed while feeding on sweet food or drinks.

• Insect repellents are available from chemists and may reduce the attacks.

• If any severe allergic reaction has occurred, particular care should be taken to avoid being bitten or stung. It is wise to consult the doctor about emergency medication to be kept ready in the event of an attack.

Outlook

• In almost every case, a bite or sting will be harmless, and symptoms will clear up within a few days. In the rare cases of allergic reaction, complications may be serious and require immediate treatment.

See SKIN *page 52*
FIRST AID *page 563*

INSOMNIA

No one knows why we sleep, but it is certain that we need to. People who are prevented from sleeping begin to suffer obvious effects after a few days—they think less clearly, and they fall asleep at the slightest opportunity. Some have hallucinations. The fact that all mammals sleep also suggests that sleep has a definite purpose.

There are no rules about how much sleep is necessary. On average, adults sleep about seven and a half hours each night, but 8 per cent are happy with five hours or less, and 4 per cent want ten hours or more.

Children sleep more than adults—perhaps 14-18 hours soon after birth, going down to adult levels by early teens. Sleep patterns also tend to be different in the elderly, who may sleep less at night than they did when young. They may find sleep getting more broken, and make a daytime nap part of their normal routine.

Missing out on more than a couple of hours sleep a night may affect your concentration and efficiency—and make you feel sleepy, nervy and irritable the next day—but it does not seem to cause any physical harm.

The body makes up for the loss without needing to catch up on all the hours of sleep missed. People who have been kept awake for several nights usually feel well recovered after a single sleep of about 12 hours.

Altering the time of going to bed may make sleeping more difficult. This is because your body keeps to a regular 24-hour cycle—the circadian rhythm—during which body temperature rises and falls at fixed times. Normally, it is lowest in the middle of the night and highest in the afternoon. When body temperature is low, most people are asleep—but if you are awake at this time your physical and mental performance are relatively poor. When body temperature is highest you are at your peak of alertness and efficiency for the day. This is why sleeping during the day may be difficult.

The circadian rhythm can adjust itself in time so that its low point coincides with your normal sleeping hours. This may take a week or more. This is what needs to happen, for example, after a long air journey, when the move from one time zone to another means that your circadian rhythm does not coincide with the normal night and day times in the place you have travelled to.

Research has shown that normal sleep is made up of two quite distinct alternating phases—orthodox sleep, which occurs mostly in the early part of the night, and paradoxical or rapid eye movement (REM) sleep, which is associated with dreaming. Both phases appear necessary for normal well-being. Some sleeping tablets (such as barbiturates) appear to suppress the REM phase. This does not matter for a few nights but probably explains why such drugs when taken for longer periods lose their effect and may become harmful.

SLEEP PROBLEMS

People with sleep problems find that they cannot get to sleep, or they wake up frequently in the night, or they wake up too early in the morning. Sometimes they may have more than one of these problems.

Poor sleeping can have a number of causes. By far the most common is worry—preventing you from going to sleep, or from getting back to sleep after waking during the night. Depression often disturbs sleep, especially through early waking.

You may be disturbed by your environment—most commonly by noise, but also by someone else in the room, by light, heat or cold, or by the unfamiliarity of new surroundings (especially when travelling).

Irregular hours can set off sleep problems—shift-work, travelling, or feeding a baby at night. Some illnesses may make sleep difficult, usually because of pain.

Most people probably accept the occasional bad night. But if poor sleep goes on for weeks you may start to worry about whether it is affecting your health and to search for ways of getting more sleep. The Do's and don'ts for poor sleepers box lists some techniques to try.

But before starting on any of these, see if you can accept the number of hours you do sleep as normal for you. You may need only five or six hours' sleep each night—in which case it is fruitless to search for ways of getting eight hours. Think yourself lucky that you have an extra two hours in each day. And remember that sleep tends to become more broken over the age of 55.

HOW YOUR DOCTOR MAY BE ABLE TO HELP

Doctors have no certain cures for sleep problems. But they may be able to offer help by prescribing sleeping-pills, or treating an illness which is keeping you awake, or helping you to work out what is causing the sleep problem—or whether there is a problem at all.

A common difficulty with people who have persistent sleep problems is that they overestimate their sleeplessness. Laboratory tests have shown that people who believe they have chronic insomnia may be sleeping for only 40 minutes or so less than 'normal sleepers'. They may also blame daytime symptoms—including tiredness and headaches—on their lack of sleep when it is uncertain which started first. You may be able to sort out your sleep problem by talking it over with a friend or relative instead of your doctor.

THE BENEFITS AND HAZARDS OF SLEEPING-PILLS

About 5 per cent of British people over 30 regularly take drugs to help them sleep, and as many again take tranquillisers to calm them during the day.

Sleeping-pills work by slowing down the body's central nervous system. In the right dose, they will send you to sleep. But the sleep they produce is different from natural sleep, because abnormal ratios of the two phases (ortho-dox and REM) are produced. Also the effect of the drug can last for several hours after you have woken up. In addition, your body may gradually get used to the drug, so that you have to take more to have the same effect. You may also find it difficult to stop taking these drugs because without them it can take days or even weeks for normal sleep patterns to return. And it is quite likely that you will sleep badly and perhaps get nightmares during that time. Sleeping-pills may make you drowsy the next morning—which can be dangerous if you operate machinery or drive a car. They can react badly if taken with some drugs. And they must not be mixed with alcohol: this combination can even kill you.

The most common sleeping-pills and tranquillisers are barbiturates and benzodiazepines. See MEDICINES, 17.

Barbiturates and the non-barbiturates Doriden and Mandrax are the most likely to suppress REM sleep and become addictive. They also have more side-effects and are much more dangerous if an overdose is taken than benzodiazepines and other non-barbiturates. Because of these problems, many doctors have now stopped prescribing barbiturates. But the benzodiazepines and other non-barbiturates also interfere with the normal phases of sleep and can still cause some of the same problems.

Sleeping-pills may be useful in some situations, perhaps to see someone through a bad period of stress. But insomnia almost always has a cause, and sleeping-pills do not do anything to deal with it permanently. So avoid sleeping-pills if you possibly can.

To sum up: If you have difficulty sleeping—and you are not just overestimating the amount of sleep you need—the first step is to find and remove the problems which keep you awake. If you cannot do this, try to develop a relaxation technique. Sleeping-pills cannot deal with the causes of insomnia. The best advice is to avoid them if you possibly can.

Do's and don'ts for poor sleepers

☐ *Do* ask your doctor for treatment to relieve pain or depression.

☐ *Do* try to go to bed at the same time as your partner if you share a double bed.

☐ *Do* wear ear-plugs or install double glazing to deal with noise. Wear an eyeshade or hang thick curtains to keep out light.

☐ *Do* take steps to be comfortable in bed. This may mean buying a new bed as old ones eventually sag.

☐ *Do* develop a night-time routine. For example, taking the dog for a walk, locking up the house, cleaning your teeth, reading in bed.

☐ *Do* try a relaxation technique after turning the light out. For example, counting sheep, making up stories, reciting poetry.

☐ *Do* try relaxation exercises such as YOGA, deep breathing and tensing and relaxing different groups of muscles around the body.

☐ *Do* try taking exercise in the afternoon.

☐ *Do* take a hot bath.

☐ *Do* read in bed if this helps you to relax.

☐ *Do* try a malted-milk drink (or just warm milk) when you go to bed.

☐ *Do* give up shift-work and frequent travel (if possible) and hectic socialising—you may be trying to sleep when your body feels it is the wrong time of the day.

☐ *Don't* eat anything that you find indigestible before going to bed.

☐ *Don't* take stimulants—coffee, tea, cigarettes—in the evening.

☐ *Don't* get into an excited state—by watching a horror film, for example, or by tackling work problems—just before going to bed.

☐ *Don't* expect to sleep if you are too hot or too cold. Use bedding that is appropriate to the room temperature.

☐ *Don't* take naps during the day.

INTERNAL PELVIC EXAMINATION

This is sometimes described as a vaginal examination, an internal, or a bimanual examination. You will be asked to lie down on the couch, and the doctor will examine you internally, at the same time keeping one hand on the abdomen. In this way all the pelvic organs can be examined. The examination is usually painless provided the patient is relaxed. As part of the examination the doctor may insert a metal speculum, a viewing device, in order to look at the cervix, and may also take a CERVICAL SMEAR.

See FEMALE GENITAL SYSTEM *page 48*

INTERTRIGO

Inflammation of large skin surfaces that are in close contact. A common site is the groin, especially in babies, the elderly and the obese. The condition is common in hot climates.

Symptoms
• An inflamed, unpleasant smelling area of skin.

Causes
• The skin becomes excessively moist due to sweating or incontinence (involuntary passing of urine).
• Friction between the damp surfaces leads to infection.

Treatment in the home
• Bath often, dry yourself carefully, and afterwards apply talc.

When to consult the doctor
• If the simple hygienic measures described do not clear up the problem.

What the doctor may do
• Prescribe an ointment to heal the infected area.
• In rare cases, intertrigo in certain sites is caused by diabetes. If you have intertrigo in one of these areas, the doctor may ask you to provide urine for analysis.

Prevention
• In general, bath often and dry yourself carefully.
• If you are obese, try to reduce your weight.
• If you suffer from incontinence, have this treated.
• For preventing intertrigo in babies, *see* CHILD CARE—CHILDHOOD ILLS *page 151*.

Outlook
• Treatment usually clears up the problem, but good hygiene is required to prevent recurrence.

See SKIN *page 52*

INTRAVENOUS DRIP

The slow introduction of a fluid into a patient's bloodstream by means of a tube inserted into a vein, usually in the arm. The liquid passes into the tube from a bottle on a stand and its rate of flow is controlled by a screw clip on the tube. An intravenous drip may be used to feed a patient who is too ill to eat, or to replace lost body fluids.

INTURNED EYELASHES

This condition is found only with the eyelashes on the lower lid, and causes discomfort. If it is not treated it may scar the front of the eye, which in turn can lead to infection and interfere with the sight.

Symptoms
• The eye becomes irritated, sore and red, and waters persistently. If the predominant symptom is watering, it may be that the lashes are not really turned in, but that one has become loose and is blocking the tear-duct.

Duration
• The condition will persist unless treated.

When to consult the doctor
• If any of the above symptoms occur.

What the doctor may do
• The doctor will examine the eyes and eyelids, possibly with a magnifying glass. If he finds a lash blocking the entry to the tear-duct he will remove it with forceps. If he finds the eyelid turned in, he will probably refer the patient to an eye specialist who may suggest a small operation to correct the eyelid.

Outlook
• Surgery is almost always successful.

See EYE *page 36*

INTUSSUSCEPTION

A twisted gut, a condition in which part of the gut pushes inside the gut beyond it, like a glove finger turning inside itself. It is commonest in babies under a year old and affects boys more than girls, causing severe pain, vomiting and passing of blood and mucus from the rectum. It is less common in adults and then occurs where there is a polyp or cancer within the bowel. A barium enema, given to confirm the diagnosis, may cure the condition but usually surgery is needed.

IRITIS

An uncommon condition, also called uveitis or iridocyclitis, which can cause pain and redness of the eye. It occurs in younger adults more often than elderly people and generally affects only one eye.

Symptoms
• Pain, gradually developing deep in the eye.
• The eye looks red, waters excessively and is tender to the touch. Bright light is irritating and the pupil contracts.
• The vision becomes less acute, though not completely blurred.

Causes
• Although iritis may be associated with some forms of rheumatism, in most cases no specific cause can be found.

Treatment in the home
• None.

When to consult the doctor
• Any persistent pain in the eye or disturbance of vision should be reported to the doctor.

What the doctor may do
• He will probably examine the eye with a torch and possibly look into the interior of the eye with an ophthalmoscope.
• If he diagnoses iritis the doctor may prescribe drops to dilate the contracted pupil.
• He may also prescribe drops to counteract the inflammation.
• He will probably want you to be seen by a specialist at an early stage to supervise treatment.

Prevention
• Since the cause of iritis is not understood, it is not possible to prevent it happening.

Outlook
• With treatment, iritis usually clears in a matter of a week or two, although it may recur. Without treatment there is a danger that the much more serious condition of GLAUCOMA may be brought about by the scarring which can occur as the inflammation settles.

See EYE *page 36*

ISCHAEMIC HEART DISEASE

A general term for any heart condition that is caused by an inadequate supply of blood to the heart. Symptoms include pain in the chest on exertion, breathlessness and

swollen ankles. The reduction of the flow of blood is due to narrowing of the coronary artery walls by deposits building up on them. *See* ATHEROMA. The condition may come on gradually, causing ANGINA or HEART FAILURE, or suddenly, causing CORONARY THROMBOSIS. Cutting out smoking and heavy drinking, keeping the weight down, and taking regular moderate exercise such as jogging or swimming all help to avoid heart disease.
See CIRCULATORY SYSTEM *page 40*

ITCHING

Itching, or pruritis, is a symptom of many skin disorders, particularly ECZEMA, SCABIES and RINGWORM infections. Four types of itching commonly occur in the absence of any other obvious disorders: general itching, itching round the anus (which is more common in men), itching in the region of the female genitals, and chronic irritation (neurodermatitis) of a small, accessible area of skin such as on the neck or legs.

GENERAL ITCHING
Symptoms
• Itching all over the body. Warmth makes the condition worse, and as a result sleep is often disturbed.
Duration
• Unless a cause is found, the problem can continue indefinitely.
Causes
• Drugs, especially barbiturates, cause itching in some people.
• General itching is sometimes an early symptom of DIABETES, obstructive JAUNDICE and other disorders.
• Some pregnancies, which are otherwise normal, bring on general itching, which stops after delivery.
• Ageing of the skin may bring on the problem in the elderly.
• PRICKLY HEAT, ECZEMA and other skin diseases.
Treatment in the home
• If possible, avoid heat and anxiety, which will make the itching worse.
• Try not to scratch the skin hard; otherwise sores may develop.
• Taking antihistamine tablets and applying calamine lotion with added 'coal tar' to the skin may provide relief (the elderly should use an oily calamine lotion). The tablets and lotions are available without prescription from any chemist's. *See* MEDICINES, 43.

When to consult the doctor
• As soon as possible, if a general itching persists for more than two or three days as it may be the sign of some underlying disorder.
What the doctor may do
• Arrange for tests to be carried out, to discover whether the itching is a symptom of any disease.
• Prescribe tablets and/or a lotion to relieve the itching.
Prevention
• None is possible.
Outlook
• Treatment of any underlying disorder will stop the itching. If no cause is found, the complaint may persist for years.
• In the elderly the problem tends to come and go.

ITCHING IN THE REGION OF THE ANUS
Symptoms
• A persistent embarrassing itching around the anus that is worse in warm conditions and when the mind is not occupied. It often keeps the sufferer awake at night.
• Soreness and bleeding, if the anus is constantly scratched.
Duration
• If no physical disorder is discovered, the trouble may persist for years.
Causes
• Any one of a number of disorders may be responsible.
• In many people the problem may be psychological and is often made worse by worry, sweating and hot weather.
Treatment in the home
• Wash the anus at least twice a day.
• Use only soft lavatory paper or, if the anus is very sore, wet cotton wool.
• Change underwear frequently and avoid pants which are too tight.
When to consult the doctor
• If the above measures do not stop the itching.
• If there is any bleeding.
What the doctor may do
• Examine the anus and possibly arrange for tests to discover if there is any underlying cause.
• Prescribe a local application—a lotion cream or an ointment—to relieve the itching. *See* MEDICINES, 43.
Prevention
• Do not become overweight. Obesity increases sweating and depth of skin creases.
• If you are obese, lose weight.
Outlook
• Treatment of any underlying cause will clear up the trouble quickly. If no cause can be discovered, the problem may continue despite treatment for many years.

ITCHING IN THE REGION OF THE VULVA
Symptoms
• Persistent itching which may also affect the opening of the vagina, the anus and the upper thighs.
Duration
• If no cause is discovered, the trouble may persist for years.
Causes
• As for itching in the region of the anus.
• In addition to the disorders listed in the SYMPTOM SORTER any of the following may be responsible:
• Dryness and irritation of the area following the menopause.
• Worry (which may be the result of SEX PROBLEMS).
• An allergic reaction to a particular type of tampon or contraceptive.
Treatment in the home
• If a tampon is known to cause the problem, change to a different type.
• Wash the vulva at least twice a day.
When to consult the doctor
• If the itching persists. It is particularly important to seek treatment if there is discharge or abnormal bleeding from the vagina.
• If a contraceptive is responsible for the trouble.
What the doctor may do
• Examine the affected area, ask for a urine sample and take a swab of any vaginal discharge, to determine whether there is an underlying disorder.
• If a contraceptive is causing the problem, the doctor will recommend the most suitable alternative.
• Prescribe local applications to relieve the symptoms.
Prevention
• None possible.
Outlook
• Treatment of any underlying cause will clear up the problem. When no cause can be found, the complaint may persist on and off for years.

NEURODERMATITIS
A harmless but annoying localised skin condition in which chronic irritation leads to chronic scratching, which in turn makes the skin roughened and ridged by deep, often unsightly skin-folds. The cause is not known, but if the vicious circle of irritation and scratching can be broken the skin returns to normal. The area of skin is always accessible to the hands and rarely large. The back of the neck or legs are usual sites. Women are affected more than men.

See SKIN *page 52*
SYMPTOM SORTER—SKIN ABNORMALITIES

JAUNDICE

Jaundice in adults always indicates serious disease. A yellow discoloration of all the body tissues gradually becomes visible in the skin and whites of the eyes due to deposits of bilirubin. Bilirubin is a yellow pigment which is produced when old or damaged red blood cells are broken down in the spleen. The pigment is then normally removed by the liver and discharged as bile into the intestines to help digestion. Here it contributes to the brown colour of the stools.

A number of diseases may cause an abnormal excess of this yellow pigment to be produced. The excess is then deposited in the body tissues and some passes into the urine, giving it a dark brown colour.

Jaundice may be difficult to recognise in its early stages and may take anything from a few days to several weeks to develop. Often darkened urine and cream-coloured stools are noticed first. The changed colour of the skin may be especially difficult to see in artificial light and in red-haired or dark-skinned individuals. The presence of pigment in the skin often leads to a troublesome itch.

Jaundice may be caused by many different disorders. Excess of yellow bilirubin is produced in three different ways.

JAUNDICE CAUSED BY LIVER DAMAGE
Infections are usually responsible for this type of jaundice, known medically as HEPATITIS. Viral or infective hepatitis is common and occurs in epidemics; a more serious form may occasionally follow blood transfusions and injections. Other infections which may be the cause are GLANDULAR FEVER, LEPTOSPIROSIS, MALARIA and AMOEBIASIS. Jaundice from liver damage may also occasionally follow ALCOHOL-ISM (*see* CIRRHOSIS OF THE LIVER), chemical poisons (*see* OCCUPATIONAL HAZARDS) and pregnancy.

JAUNDICE CAUSED BY EXCESSIVE DESTRUCTION OF RED BLOOD CELLS
This type, known medically as haemolysis, occurs in most normal babies three to five days after birth. Once a newborn baby uses its lungs, less blood is needed and a transient slight jaundice develops as the baby's spleen removes the excess blood. Urine and stools retain their normal colour in all jaundice of haemolytic origin. Apart from the normal jaundice of babies, some less-common disorders may cause haemolytic jaundice. These are sickle-cell ANAEMIA, RHESUS INCOMPATIBILITY and THALASSAEMIA MAJOR.

OBSTRUCTIVE JAUNDICE
Here, jaundice follows disorders in which bile is prevented from being discharged through the bile ducts into the intestines. They include GALLSTONES and CANCER of the pancreas and bowel.

When to consult the doctor
• As soon as jaundice is suspected. Even jaundice of a new baby, which is probably quite normal, should be discussed with the doctor or midwife.

Treatment in the home
• None. Consult your doctor if you suspect jaundice.
• If necessary, take sedatives in recommended doses to relieve irritation. *See* MEDICINES, 17.

What the doctor will do
• Investigate and treat the possible causes. This often requires hospital investigation or treatment.

JOINT

Disease or injury can cause pain, inflammation, limited movement or swelling in the joints.
See SYMPTOM SORTER—JOINT PROBLEMS

KELOID

A harmless tumour-like mass of excess tissue forming in the scar of an injury. Keloids are commoner in black people. The tendency is lifelong.

Symptoms
• Shiny, rubbery-like lumps appear, which later become pigmented and hard.
• Keloids are usually painless unless occurring in tight skin, such as on the face, ears and upper chest.
• The size and shape vary, but they can be large and disfiguring.

Duration
• Shrinkage may occur naturally after months or years, but complete disappearance is unlikely.

Causes
• The underlying cause is unknown, but there is often a family history of keloid formation.
• Dirt or infection in wounds and ornamental colouring, for example, tattoos.
• Stretching of a wound during healing.
• Keloids may develop in any cuts, operation scars or even in severe acne.

Treatment in the home
• Do not try home remedies. There is no simple way to remove keloids, and further injury may make the scars even bigger.

When to consult the doctor
• If the scar is unsightly.

What the doctor may do
• Explain to the patient that recurrences of keloids are common and that any do-it-yourself attempt he may make to shrink an existing growth may result in an even larger one appearing.
• Try to shrink the keloids and alleviate pain by X-ray treatment and repeated injection of steroids.
• Surgical removal and skin grafting are sometimes advised in severe cases.

Prevention
• Do not irritate a wound. The less irritation it receives, the less likely are keloids to form.
• If there is a known keloid tendency, operations should be avoided where possible; if performed then avoid tension on the wound.

Outlook
• Local treatment is not very successful in fair-skinned people, but much better in black people.

See SKIN *page 52*

KERATOSIS, ACTINIC

A hard, dry and scaly, flat brown growth which develops painlessly and suddenly on the skin of individuals in the 30 to 60 age group. The exposed surfaces, such as the face and backs of the hands, are common sites.

Duration
• Actinic keratosis slowly spreads over a period of months or years.

Causes
• Keratoses occur most frequently in males over 40 who have been exposed to prolonged sunshine for much of their working life, for example sailors and farmers.
• Fair-skinned people working in the tropics may develop keratoses at an earlier age.

Complications
• A small percentage of cases will, if left untreated, develop cancer of the skin. Occasionally a little 'horn' of hard skin develops in the centre of such a growth.

Treatment in the home
• None. Do not attempt to treat a newly developed growth on the skin in an adult.

When to consult the doctor
• A person who develops a growth of the skin is always wise to consult a doctor, but this is especially important

if the surface affected has had prolonged exposure to sunlight and the patient is fair-skinned.

What the doctor may do
- Remove the growth for analysis or send the patient to hospital for this. If there are many or large keratoses, plastic surgery with skin grafting may be advised.

Prevention
- Wear clothing that will protect you from the sun.

Outlook
- Early treatment prevents cancer of the skin developing.
- Further keratoses may develop after one has been removed, but treatment can be repeated.
- If skin cancer does develop, complete cure can be expected after surgery.

See SKIN *page 52*
SEBORRHOEIC WARTS

KIDNEY FAILURE
A complication of several kidney disorders, all of which are uncommon. Treatment is by dialysis or a kidney transplant.
See URINARY SYSTEM *page 46*
NEPHRITIS

KNEE
Disease or injury can cause pain, inflammation, limited movement or swelling in the knee.
See SYMPTOM SORTER—KNEE PROBLEMS

KNOCK-KNEE
Known medically as genu valgum, the condition is fairly common in young children and in most cases corrects spontaneously.
See CHILD CARE

KORSAKOFF'S SYNDROME
A brain disorder chiefly marked by the sufferer's inability to remember recent events. He fills in the memory blanks with plausible fantasies that he sincerely believes to be true. Other symptoms are vagueness as to present time and place, a somewhat mindless cheerfulness and an inability to learn simple new tasks. The disorder is most commonly caused by ALCOHOLISM, when it is often accompanied by a nervous disease, Wernicke's encephalopathy, which produces confusion, paralysis of the eye muscles and an unsteady gait. It can also result from a head injury, BRAIN TUMOUR or brain HAEMORRHAGE. Treat-

ment of cases due to alcoholism consists of large doses of B vitamins, particularly B1 (thiamine). But the outlook in these cases and those resulting from a brain tumour is poor. When other causes are responsible the disorder often clears up of its own accord.

KWASHIORKOR
A disease of babies and young children in developing countries where food is scarce. It is caused by a deficiency of proteins and often of vitamins. Symptoms include retarded growth, swellings caused by accumulated fluids in the tissues, swollen abdomen, irritability, loss of skin and hair colouring, anaemia and diarrhoea. The disease strikes when the nutritional value of a child's diet decreases after he has been weaned from the breast. The child may well contract a further debilitating disease, such as HOOKWORM or GASTROENTERITIS.

Treatment consists of an adequate supply of milk, usually in powder form to which proteins and vitamins have been added. Even with treatment, however, many children die, and in those who do not, physical and mental growth are often permanently retarded.
See DIGESTIVE SYSTEM *page 44*

KYPHOSIS
Excessive backward curvature of the spine producing a hump back or a round back. This is an uncommon condition which may be caused by a number of diseases, for example, OSTEOCHONDRITIS or OSTEOPOROSIS. Kyphosis is treated by attacking the underlying condition.

LABYRINTHITIS

Inflammation of the labyrinth, the part of the inner ear responsible for maintaining balance of the body. The labyrinth is sensitive both to the position of the head and to any movement that occurs. Inflammation results in vertigo (unpleasant sensations of movement even when the head is still). The symptoms are similar to motion sickness, which also affects the labyrinth.

Symptoms
- Vertigo—a sensation of turning, falling or spinning.
- Nausea and vomiting.
- Flickering of the eyes when looking from side to side (nystagmus).
- Hearing should not be affected.

Duration
- Symptoms usually clear within ten days.

Causes
- Virus infection—sometimes in an epidemic.
- Spread of bacterial infection from the middle ear, *see* OTITIS MEDIA. This is less common but more serious.

Treatment in the home
- Stay in bed and keep the head still.

When to consult the doctor
- If there is discharge from the ear, or if there is headache or fever, consult the doctor without delay.

What the doctor may do
- Examine the ears and eyes.
- If it is suspected that bacterial infection has spread from the middle ear the doctor will send the patient to hospital for intensive treatment with antibiotics.
- Prescribe medicines to ease the vertigo and vomiting until the inflammation has subsided.
- Tell the patient to stay in bed.

Prevention
- None known.

Outlook
- Viral labyrinthitis resolves in about ten days, the only after-effects being occasional slight deafness.
- Bacterial labyrinthitis, resulting from chronic otitis media, is much more serious. Surgery may be necessary and the inner ear may be permanently damaged, with some permanent deafness.

See EAR *page 38*

LAPAROSCOPY
A technique that enables surgeons to examine the inside of the abdominal cavity without major surgery. A viewing instrument called a laparoscope is inserted through a small cut in the abdominal wall. Laparoscopy may be used to look at the ovaries, Fallopian tubes or abdominal organs, and sometimes surgery can be carried out through the same or another small opening without the need to make a major incision in the skin.

LARYNGECTOMY
Surgical removal of all or part of the larynx (voice-box). The operation is usually carried out when CANCER develops in the organ. The first symptoms of the disease are hoarseness, coughing and difficulty in swallowing. Men over 40 are most commonly affected, particularly heavy smokers or drinkers. After a laryngectomy, a person can learn to speak again by means of breathing in and out of the oesophagus (gullet) and vibrating it.

LARYNGITIS

Inflammation of the larynx (voice-box), producing hoarseness or sometimes loss of voice. There are two types of laryngitis: acute, which is infectious, can strike suddenly and is short-lived; and chronic, which lasts longer or recurs, and is a disease of adults.

ACUTE LARYNGITIS

Symptoms
- Hoarse, squeaky or lost voice and hoarse cough.
- Sore throat with pain on speaking.
- Raised temperature—common in children, occurs in 30 per cent of adults who report to the doctor.
- Because small children have a small larynx their breathing becomes noisy. *See* CROUP.

Duration
- Less than a week.

Causes
- Various respiratory viruses.
- Occasionally bacteria.

Complications
- The infection may spread to the lungs.

Treatment in the home
- Rest the voice—talk as little as possible, do not shout and do not smoke.
- Drink extra fluids. Take painkillers in recommended doses to ease pain and lower your temperature.
- Cough syrup may ease symptoms. *See* MEDICINES, 16, 22.
- Bed-rest will help if you feel ill.

When to consult the doctor
- If the high temperature persists for more than three or four days.
- If you have a hoarse voice for more than three weeks.
- If you cough up blood or green or yellow phlegm.

What the doctor may do
- Prescribe antibiotics if the infection has spread to the lungs. *See* MEDICINES, 25.
- If hoarseness persists, arrange for examination of the larynx using a laryngoscope (a special mirror).
- Send you for a chest X-ray.

Prevention
- Do not smoke.

Outlook
- Recovery is complete, but some people may develop laryngitis when they have upper respiratory infections.

CHRONIC LARYNGITIS

Symptoms
- Loss of voice or hoarse voice.
- There is no difficulty swallowing or breathing and no pain in the throat or ear.

Duration
- May last for days or weeks and recur at intervals.

Causes
- The most common cause is emotional stress or strain.
- Excessive use of the voice, for example, shouting or singing. This can produce 'singer's nodules' or polyps on the vocal cords. These are not cancerous.
- Smoking.
- Exposure to dust or irritants.
- Chronic bronchitis (chronic coughing), or sinusitis.
- Mouth breathing.

Treatment in the home
- Stop smoking.
- Avoid exposure to dust or irritants.
- Rest the voice from shouting or singing.

When to consult the doctor
- If hoarse voice persists for more than 21 days.
- If pain in the throat or ear develops.

Speaking and breathing—the larynx at work

Sound is produced when air vibrates the vocal cords. This happens only when the cords are close but not touching. Fully open or fully closed, the cords cannot vibrate. Nine pictures, taken in the space of one second, show the progression from silence, through speech to silence again.

1-3 *Speech stops as the cords start to open and cease to vibrate.*
4-6 *Silence continues as the cords open fully on breathing in.*
7-9 *Speech resumes on the outward breath as the cords begin to close.*

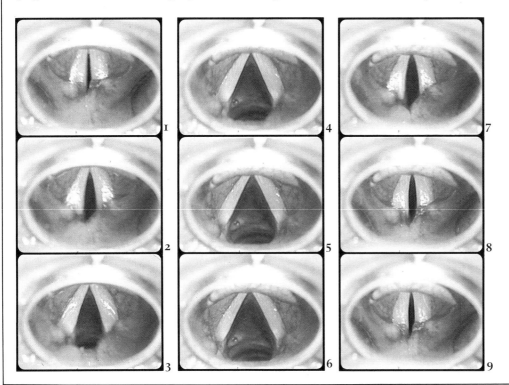

What the doctor may do
- Examine the nose and throat.
- Send you to an ear, nose and throat specialist, who will examine the larynx with a laryngoscope. If a polyp or nodule is seen on the vocal cords, it can then be surgically removed.

Prevention
- Stop smoking.
- Do not abuse the voice.

Outlook
- Chronic laryngitis is not dangerous, but it may recur at times of stress.

See RESPIRATORY SYSTEM *page 42*

LARYNX, GROWTH IN

Growths in the larynx or pharynx need early medical attention. They can occur in men or women, and are more common in smokers, especially if they are male and drink. They rarely occur before the age of 30.

Symptoms
- Hoarse voice that persists for more than three weeks.
- Difficulty in swallowing solid food.
- Weight loss, coughing blood, noisy or difficult breathing, and pain in the ear or throat may arise later.
- A gland or glands swelling in the neck.

Causes
- In most cases the cause is unknown.

When to consult the doctor
- If a hoarse voice persists for more than three weeks.
- If there is difficulty swallowing solid food not associated with throat infection.
- If there is unexplained weight loss, coughing blood, persistent pain in the ear or throat.
- If a gland or glands swell in the neck.

What the doctor may do
- Send the patient for examination by an ear, nose and throat specialist.
- Surgery and/or radiotherapy may be necessary. An operation may involve the removal of the larynx (voice-box). After the operation the patient will be given speech therapy to learn how to speak by breathing in and out of the oesophagus and making it vibrate. Alternatively, he can learn to use a mechanical vibrator held to the throat.

See RESPIRATORY SYSTEM *page 42*

LASSA FEVER

A rare virus disease occurring in West Africa, and involving severe fever with muscular pain and a sore throat. Many of its victims die. A few cases have been seen in Britain among people returning from Africa.

LAXATIVE

A medicine taken to relieve constipation, or to encourage softer or bulkier stools. Laxatives should never be taken regularly without advice from a doctor.
See MEDICINES, 3.

LEAD POISONING

A rare but serious form of poisoning caused by swallowing or inhaling lead, or by absorbing it through the skin. In large quantities, lead is swift-acting, particularly if it is breathed in as fumes. More usually—for example, if drinking water is contaminated—the effects develop slowly. Because the body can get rid of lead only with difficulty, the metal gradually builds up in the bones and tissues of someone who is regularly exposed to it.

A person suffering from slow lead poisoning becomes obviously unwell, but a doctor may not recognise the cause unless he is told or suspects that lead may be involved, because some of the symptoms are like those of other, more common illnesses.

Symptoms
- Repeated attacks of sharp, unexplained pain in the abdomen.
- Increasingly pale appearance or ANAEMIA.
- Weakness of wrist or ankle muscles, making the hands or feet droop.
- A black line along the edge of the gums.
- In children—unexplained drowsiness, unsteadiness and repeated vomiting.
- The temperature generally remains normal.

Causes
The most common sources of lead poisoning are:
- Paints with a relatively high lead content.
- Lead water pipes, particularly in areas where the water is soft or acid.
- Solder.
- Open bonfires on which batteries or accumulators are regularly burned.
- Lead and lead compounds used in factories and industrial processes—for example, glazing pottery—or as fuel additives. Petrol contains a minute quantity of lead, and there is some evidence that it may affect people regularly exposed to the fumes, such as those living on bus routes, main roads, or workmen who clean petrol storage tanks.

Complications
- Severe lead poisoning attacks the nervous system. The victim may suffer from sudden convulsions or lapse into a coma. There may be brain damage.

When to consult the doctor
- Immediately, if lead poisoning is suspected.

What the doctor may do
- Send the patient to hospital for tests and treatment.
- If a large amount of lead has been swallowed recently, the hospital will probably pump the stomach out.
- If the source of possible poisoning is in the patient's home, the doctor will also examine everyone else who lives there.
- If the poisoning could have affected other people—neighbours or colleagues at work—he will warn the local health inspector.

Prevention
- Replace old, peeling paint that may contain high levels of lead, particularly if small children might pick off and swallow the flakes. Since the early 1960s, household paints have contained only a minute quantity of lead, and are considered to be safe. When sanding down old paintwork, wear a protective face-mask to avoid breathing in the dust, and open the windows. Clear up carefully, so that no old paint flakes are left.
- Do not allow young children to play with toys that may contain lead, or be coloured with lead paint.
- Use lead products—for example, solder—according to the maker's instructions in a well-ventilated place, and do not breathe in the dust or fumes. Keep them out of the reach of children.
- Never burn products—for example, car batteries—that contain lead.
- In most areas of Britain, the local water authorities ensure that the chemical content of drinking water stops it from releasing lead from pipes. But that balance can be disturbed if animal or vegetable matter gets into the water system. The decaying body of a dead bird in a cold tank could start a chemical reaction that lets lead into the water, so make sure all tanks are covered.

Outlook
- Mild lead poisoning can be cured if it is treated quickly. More serious cases may leave permanent damage to muscles and nerves, and to the brain. Severe, sudden poisoning can be fatal.

See OCCUPATIONAL HAZARDS

LEARNING DIFFICULTIES

We spend all our lives learning, but the most concentrated period is childhood—early childhood in particular. For most children school presents a few problems, but for some with learning difficulties it may become a place of fear.

A number of factors are important if a child is to learn normally. His mental development must be adequate: major failures of mental and nervous development usually show up in the first few months of life (*see* CHILD CARE), but slight subnormality or specific areas of difficulty such as word blindness (dyslexia) or number blindness (dyscalculia) may not show until he first goes to school.

A child needs a stable environment at home and at school; a broken, or constantly changing home, or many changes of school may cause emotional problems and hold him back.

A child's physical abilities must be adequate, he must have normal sight and hearing—many children have difficulty in learning because they cannot see the blackboard or cannot hear what the teacher is saying. He must also have normal co-ordination of the senses.

Finally, a child needs adequate opportunity to learn at play, school and home. Overcrowding, no place to do his homework, no scope for experimentation and unimaginative teaching will all contribute to learning difficulties. Because a child has difficulty in learning, it does not necessarily mean that he is mentally deficient. Intelligent children have difficulties as well. Obvious symptoms of learning difficulties are poor progress in school—at reading, writing, spelling and sums. Less obvious signs are behaviour problems such as stealing, lying, truancy, ganging, tummy aches and bedwetting.

If you do suspect learning difficulties, go and see your child's teacher, head teacher or family doctor and discuss the problem with them. An educational psychologist may be called in to help. There are a number of tests given to assess verbal and physical performance, reading, writing, arithmetic and other skills, and sight, hearing and muscular co-ordination. Such tests are available in both the educational and national health services.

Physical problems such as deafness or poor sight are easily dealt with, though a child may need special teaching to help him catch up. Special teaching or training may be necessary for other areas of difficulty. If the problem appears to be environmental then counselling may be advised.

If your child is dyslexic contact the *British Dyslexia Association*, 98 London Road, Reading, Berks RG1 5AU (Tel. 0734 668271). They will be able to put you in touch with organisations that may help.

LEG
Pain, swelling, weakness and discoloration are among symptoms affecting the leg—many of which are clearly present in the foot, ankle, knee or hip.
See SYMPTOM SORTER—LEG PROBLEMS

LEGIONNAIRE'S DISEASE

A newly recognised infectious disease, causing pneumonia. It was first identified in 1976 when 29 people died after suddenly becoming ill at an American Legion Convention in Philadelphia. Legionnaire's disease is caused by bacteria, now called *Legionella pneumophilia*, which thrive in warm stagnant water in rain tanks or air-conditioning systems. It may also colonise shower heads. It grows best in temperatures of 68-112°F (20-50°C), and for this reason hotels and large institutions should keep main water tanks and air-conditioning plants above or below these temperatures. Although the disease may occasionally prove fatal, the high death rate at first reported has not been repeated in other outbreaks. Many attacks are probably overlooked because the organism is investigated only if there is an obvious local outbreak of deaths.
Symptoms
- Early symptoms are slight headache, muscle aches and feeling unwell.
- Fever, shaking, chills and cough soon follow.
- Chest pain may accompany cough.
- Nausea, vomiting, diarrhoea or abdominal pain occur in 25 per cent of cases.
Incubation period
- Two to ten days.
Duration
- The illness usually becomes worse over the first four to six days, then after a week begins to improve.
- Fever lasts about 13 days.
Causes
- Bacteria.
Complications
- Severe respiratory failure.
- Kidney failure.

When to consult the doctor
- Immediately, if you suspect you may be suffering from Legionnaire's disease, especially if you have been staying in a hotel, or similar place where other cases are known to have occurred.
What the doctor may do
- Send the patient for a chest X-ray, which will reveal any patches of pneumonia.
- Take blood and sputum tests to confirm the diagnosis.
- Prescribe an antibiotic. *See* MEDICINES, 25.
Prevention
- As yet there is no effective immunisation against Legionnaire's disease.
Outlook
- If contracted, Legionnaire's disease can be fatal, particularly if respiratory failure develops.

See INFECTIOUS DISEASES *page 32*

LEG ULCERS
Ulcers that develop in the lower part of the leg and ankle are very difficult to heal. They usually develop as a result of injuries, or blood clots which block either the arteries or veins of the lower leg. They are most common in people with varicose veins and are fully described in varicose ulcer.
See VARICOSE ULCER

LEISHMANIASIS

An infectious disease which can affect dogs, jackals and foxes, as well as humans. It occurs in parts of China, Russia, India, the Middle East, Africa, South and Central America, and some Mediterranean countries including Greece, Crete and Malta. It has an incubation period of about three months. Leishmaniasis is caused by a parasite and the infection is spread by the bite from sandflies. There are two main types of the disease: visceral leishmaniasis, known as kala-azar or dum dum fever, which affects the internal organs; and cutaneous leishmaniasis, which affects the skin. Symptoms usually develop gradually over a long period. Treatment is essential, as without it the disease can cause death.
Symptoms
- Fever.
- Loss of weight.
- Anaemia.

- Enlarged spleen or liver.
- Pale skin may become darker.
- In cutaneous leishmaniasis, there may be serious skin ulcers which look like LEPROSY. The ulcers may heal on their own or may need treatment. They do not spread to other organs and are rarely fatal.

Causes
- A minute parasite called Leishmania.

Treatment
- Injections of antimony. *See* MEDICINES, 28.

Prevention
- There is no effective immunisation against leishmaniasis, but eliminating diseased dogs and spraying against sandflies with pesticides helps to prevent spread of the disease.

Outlook
- With treatment, the disease is usually curable, although relapses may occur and should be watched for.

See INFECTIOUS DISEASES *page 32*

LENTIGO

These are tiny, flat dark spots, like freckles. They occur in varying numbers anywhere on the body in both children and adults, but especially in old people.

Duration
- The spots are usually permanent.

Causes
- An increase in the number of pigment-containing cells in the skin.
- A few rare disorders may increase the number of spots.

Treatment in the home
- No treatment is necessary.

When to consult the doctor
- If there is any change in the spots or doubt about their origin.

What the doctor may do
- If there is any doubt about the diagnosis, the doctor will send the patient to a specialist to have a spot surgically removed for examination under a microscope.

Prevention
- This is not possible. Unlike freckles, sunlight has no effect on lentigo, so protective clothing does not help.

Outlook
- No complications arise from lentigo.

See SKIN *page 52*

LEPROSY

A chronic inflammation which initially affects the nerves and skin. Contrary to earlier belief, leprosy is one of the least contagious of all infectious diseases. The infection takes several years to show and requires close and prolonged contact with someone who has the disease. Symptoms develop slowly over a period of months or years. It can occur in any country; tropical countries have the highest incidence. It is rare in Great Britain.

Two types occur: a benign type, probably not infectious, with fewer less-distinctive lesions; and a malignant, more destructive type with symmetrical lesions which is probably responsible for the infection of others.

Symptoms
- Colourless blotches develop anywhere on the skin. Their size may vary from about 2 in. (50 mm.) across to the size of the palm of a hand. The centre of the blotch may be numb to heat, cold and light touch.
- The nerves in various parts of the body are often involved, causing gradual loss of sensation, paralysis and deformity. The extremities and parts liable to get cold being affected.

Duration
- The condition is slowly progressive over many years unless treated.

Causes
- Bacteria found in the nerves and skin.
- Infection occurs from direct skin contact with an infected person, but even with prolonged contact is not easily acquired.

When to consult the doctor
- If there is an unusual skin patch that has persisted for several weeks, especially if there is numbness, thickening, discoloration or a history of possible close or prolonged contact.

What the doctor may do
- If leprosy is suspected, send the patient for examination at a centre with experience in the condition.
- Diagnosis is confirmed by biopsies—that is, taking small sections from the nerves or skin for examination under a microscope.
- Prescribe drugs, usually to be taken by mouth.
- Very few patients need to be in hospital during treatment.
- In underdeveloped countries, with shortages of funds and treatment services, severe deformities or destructive lesions may develop. Specialised surgery may then be needed.

Prevention
- With good nutrition, housing and sanitation, leprosy becomes uncommon.
- No special steps need to be taken if an adult comes into casual contact with someone who has the disease.
- If young children are in regular contact with leprosy they should be immunised.

Outlook
- Leprosy can be cured. The drugs need to be taken for three years or more.
- In poor communities this may be extremely difficult to achieve.

See SKIN *page 52*

LEPTOSPIROSIS
An infectious disease, known medically as Weil's disease, caused by one of a group of bacteria called Leptospira. The infection is spread to humans through water contaminated by infected animals, particularly rats. It can occur after swimming or partial immersion in such water. Children and young adults, especially males, are mostly affected.

The incubation period is usually ten days. The symptoms are headache, fever and muscle pains, which may be followed by JAUNDICE, blood in the urine, MENINGITIS or kidney failure. With bed-rest, antibiotics and treatment for complications, the outlook is good and most patients recover.

See INFECTIOUS DISEASES *page 32*

LEUKAEMIA

An uncommon condition in which there is an abnormality in the blood cells. Three main types affect children, the commonest of which is acute lymphoblastic leukaemia—the form where major advances in treatment have occurred. The other childhood forms are acute myeloid leukaemia, which accounts for one in six cases, and chronic myeloid leukaemia, which is responsible for one case in 20. The usual age of onset is between three and six years.

In adults, the acute forms are acute myeloid, and the less common lymphoblastic. The chronic forms are lymphatic, which affects elderly men, and myeloid, which is commoner in the young and middle-aged of both sexes.

Symptoms in children
- Loss of energy, pallor, irritability, fever.
- Persistent or recurrent infections. Nose bleeds.
- Pain in the bones or joints. Bruising.
- The child may develop a limp or refuse to stand.

Symptoms in adults
- Gradual or rapid weakness. Fever and night sweats.
- Loss of appetite and weight loss. Pallor and, in women, excessive periods.
- Pain in the upper abdomen, usually on the left side.
- Bruising of arms and legs.
- Bleeding from the gums. Enlarged lymph glands.

Duration
- With treatment, more than 50 per cent of children can be completely cured.
- With adults, duration can vary according to the type of leukaemia.

Causes
- There is no known cause, but there is a higher incidence after exposure to radiation and benzene.

Complications
- Lowered defences make ordinary infections life-threatening. In children, for example, measles and chickenpox become serious illnesses.
- In adults, excessive bleeding.

When to consult the doctor
- Immediately if the condition is suspected.

What the doctor may do
- Take a blood test and if leukaemia is suspected, send the patient to hospital immediately.
- The hospital will take X-rays and blood and bone-marrow tests to determine the type of leukaemia.
- Treatment will be with blood transfusions, anti-leukaemia drugs, radiotherapy and, possibly, bone-marrow transplants. Antibiotics may also be used to combat infection.

Prevention
- Avoid excess irradiation or exposure to chemicals.

Outlook
- In children, modern treatment can provide a complete cure for more than half those affected.
- With adults, progress has been slower, but many victims can lead a normal life for five years or more.

LICE

Lice are insect parasites which feed by sucking blood. The skin irritation which results is called pediculosis. There are three species of lice which infest human beings: body lice, head lice and pubic or CRAB LICE.

Body lice are pin-head sized and lay their eggs in clothing. Head and pubic lice are smaller. They lay eggs (commonly known as nits) which attach to hair.

Symptoms
- Intense itching at the site of the infestation. Scratching, which is usual, produces a secondary infection similar to IMPETIGO. There may be blisters and yellowish, crusty sores or scratch lines.
- If the head is infested, nits are present. These are grey-coloured eggs attached to the hairs near the scalp. They are clearly visible with a magnifying glass.
- If the pubic region is infested, irritation is particularly intense. The lice, which look like minute scabs, may be seen partially buried in the hair follicles (the indentations out of which hairs grow). The follicles become inflamed, and pus-filled pimples may develop.

Duration
- Infestation persists until treated.
- The eggs take nine days to hatch, and it takes a further nine days for the larvae to become mature.

Causes
- Lice spread by close physical contact. Poor hygiene and overcrowding are conditions in which they thrive.
- Pubic lice are transmitted during sexual intercourse.

Complications
- The irritation may cause secondary skin infections.
- Under conditions of extreme deprivation, TYPHUS FEVER can be spread by the body louse.

Treatment in the home
- Hair combing dislodges nits.
- Change clothes daily—body lice live in them, and die away from the body.
- Effective preparations against lice can be obtained from chemists with directions for use.
- Bedding and clothes should be treated with a fumigant, and then laundered normally. If this is not effective, they should be destroyed. Furnishings may be sprayed with a suitable insecticide.

When to consult the doctor
- If any badly inflamed sores occur.
- If headaches, high temperature, bleeding, rashes or mental disturbances occur.
- If home treatment fails.

What the doctor may do
- In most cases, advise home treatment as above.
- If a secondary skin infection is present the doctor will prescribe antiparasitic and antibiotic applications.

Prevention
- Practise careful personal hygiene, particularly if living conditions are crowded.

Outlook
- Treating lice presents little problem. However, an individual may experience further infestations if living conditions are overcrowded or unhygienic.

See SKIN *page 52*

LICHEN PLANUS

An uncommon condition usually occurring on the front of the wrists and forearms and sometimes the trunk and lower legs. It is very itchy, but not contagious.

Symptoms
- Shiny, purplish, flat-topped, raised spots, usually $\frac{1}{25}$ – $\frac{1}{12}$ in. (1-2 mm.) across at first. Later they get bigger (or several spots may form together), becoming brown with white lines or scales across their surface.
- Itching is intense.
- White streaks may appear on the inside lining of the mouth, with blotches on the tongue.
- Finger-nails may break and be destroyed.
- If a scratch is made, spots may form along the line of the scratch.

Duration
- Usually three to six months—particularly if the onset is sudden and severe. Occasionally years.

Causes
- Unknown.

Complications
- The scalp may be affected with a patchy loss of hair which is occasionally permanent.

Treatment in the home
- None.
- Try not to scratch as this will cause the spots to spread and the skin to break and become infected.

When to consult the doctor
- If there is a persistent, itchy rash.

What the doctor may do
- Prescribe a steroid cream or other preparation.

Prevention
- None is known.

Outlook
- The itching usually stops before the spots disappear.
- Brown staining of the skin may persist for some months but eventually clears. Finger-nails will re-grow.
- Relapses occur in about 20 per cent of patients.

See SKIN *page 52*

LIGAMENT
A band of tough, fibrous, flexible tissue which helps to hold the bone ends together at a joint and to limit the joint's range of movement. Most joints are bound by several ligaments. The overstretching of a ligament can cause a sprain, usually of the ankle or wrist as the result of a fall. Sudden twisting of a ligament can tear it. Torn ligaments most commonly occur in the knee, as sports injuries. They cause severe pain and allow abnormal movement of the joint. The ligament is healed by resting or immobilising the joint.
See TORN LIGAMENT

LIMP
In children the cause is usually trivial, but serious bone disease may be responsible.
See SYMPTOM SORTER—LIMP
CHILD CARE—CHILDHOOD ILLS *page 151*

LIPOMA
A benign (non-cancerous) tumour composed of fat cells. It can be felt beneath the skin as a soft lump that is occasionally painful. Lipomas are more common in women than men. Their cause is unknown. They can be removed by a small operation if they are annoying.

LIVER, CANCER OF
Hepatoma, a primary tumour of the liver cells, is rare. If only a single tumour is present, it may be treated by surgery. Most cancers of the liver, however, are secondaries (metastases) which have spread from other sites. If symptoms such as JAUNDICE then develop, it usually means that there are several tumours of varying sizes and that treatment may no longer help.
See DIGESTIVE SYSTEM *page 44*

LOCHIA
A series of discharges from the vagina following childbirth. The first consists mainly of blood and lasts for about four days. On about the fifth day it gives way to a brown mixture of blood and mucus, and on the seventh day this is replaced by a whitish mixture containing fragments of tissues.

LOCKJAW
The common name for tetanus, a disease causing acute muscle contractions, particularly of the jaw and neck.
See TETANUS

LONG-SIGHTEDNESS
Difficulty in focusing on near objects, while being able to see distant objects quite clearly. The condition is known medically as hypermetropia. The form of long-sightedness that comes with middle age is known as presbyopia.
See REFRACTIVE ERRORS

LORDOSIS
Excessive forward curvature of the spine seen only in the region of the lower back where a slight curve is normal. Lordosis, also known as 'hollow back', is usually a sign of faulty posture caused by a heavy abdomen or weak abdominal muscles, and goes when this is corrected.

LUMBAGO
Severe pain in the lower back (lumbar region) usually felt when lifting or stooping. The pain is often so severe that the patient is stuck in the stooping position. The pain gradually disappears with rest but in some cases it is followed by SCIATICA, in which case there has probably been some pressure on the sciatic nerve. This condition may be an early sign of a slipped disc.

LUNG CANCER

A malignant growth, or tumour, affecting one or both lungs. The growth usually starts on the bronchial tubes which carry air to and from the trachea (windpipe). In such cases its medical name is bronchogenic carcinoma. Other terms sometimes used are pulmonary neoplasm (lung tumour) and respiratory cancer.

Lung cancer kills 32,000 people every year in Britain alone. It is not as common as heart disease, but is more likely to be fatal. The condition is responsible for 6 per cent of all deaths in Britain, making it the fourth most common killer disease after heart disorders, cerebrovascular disease (for example, stroke) and pneumonia. Lung cancer is one of the most common types of cancer among men, and, in the last few years since more women are smoking, it is becoming almost as frequent a killer among women. The disease usually appears in middle to old age, and is 15 times more common among cigarette smokers than among those who do not smoke.

Symptoms
• A dry irritant cough which at first resembles that of a heavy smoker. Later, the sufferer may cough up yellow phlegm.
• Spitting blood (haemoptysis). Pure blood may be coughed up, but more commonly streaks of fresh (red) or altered (brown) blood are mixed with phlegm.
• Shortness of breath, loss of weight, and a dull continuous pain in the chest or shoulders.
• Sometimes the first sign of the disease is a sudden feverish illness which is often mistaken for pneumonia.
Duration
• Lung cancer can become irreversibly established before it is detected, because it can take weeks or even months for the symptoms to reveal themselves. Even regular chest X-rays and sputum tests often fail to detect lung cancer at its earliest symptom-free treatable stage.
• If the cancer is not treated, it progresses steadily.
Causes
• Smoking, particularly of cigarettes. Stopping smoking at any time before the disease has started greatly reduces the otherwise high risks.
• Air pollution. Although the precise connection is not fully understood, lung cancer occurs more frequently in towns than in the country. Prolonged exposure to some industrial dusts (for example, asbestos) increases the risk of lung cancer, particularly in smokers.
Complications
• The cancer may spread to other parts of the body.
When to consult the doctor
• If any of the symptoms appear.
• If the patient's general state of health causes him or his friends or relatives to think of lung cancer.
• Anybody over 35 who has a cough which persists for more than a month should seek medical advice or have a chest X-ray. This applies particularly to smokers or someone who has recently had pneumonia.
What the doctor may do
• After examining the patient, the doctor will probably order a chest X-ray. He may then order further tests in hospital. These may include sputum tests and possibly a biopsy, in which a tiny piece of lung tissue is removed under anaesthetic and examined for cancer cells.
Prevention
• Do not smoke, particularly cigarettes. Pipes and cigars are less likely to cause lung cancer, provided the smoke is not inhaled.
• Smokers and other high risk groups should have regular chest X-rays.
• Observe industrial safety regulations strictly in working areas where there are harmful dusts such as asbestos.

Outlook

• If the disease is detected in its earliest stages it may sometimes be cured by surgery.

• The outlook, despite treatment by surgery or chemotherapy, is not usually good. That is why it is vital to stop smoking in order to reduce the risk of lung cancer.

See RESPIRATORY SYSTEM *page 42*
SMOKING

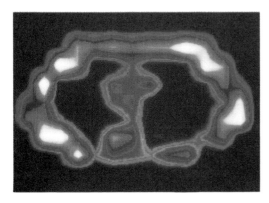

NORMAL LUNGS *The central black areas are the insides of the lungs and the blue outer ones the lung walls. This computer-coded picture was built up from varying signals radiated by body cells of varying density.*

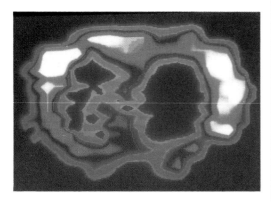

DISEASED LUNG *The greatly thickened blue wall of the left lung represents excess tissue which indicates the possible presence of cancer.*

TEN-SECOND LIFESAVER
Computerised X-ray pinpoints disease

By linking X-ray technology to computer technology the computed tomograph (CT scan) produces a detailed, accurate picture of organs deep inside a patient's body. The tomograph is produced by taking thousands of different readings at a succession of exit points of a narrow X-ray beam as it scans through the patient. Each scan takes a few seconds and produces a picture, like those shown left, of a slice about $\frac{3}{8}$ in. (10 mm.) thick through the patient's body.

The picture is built up by the computer from the X-ray readings and displayed as a pattern of very tiny squares on the cathode-ray tube. Objects of very similar densities can be distinguished one from the other in a way not possible in conventional X-ray pictures, and a cross-section of the body can be seen. More detailed information can be obtained by injecting harmless solutions into the bloodstream which intensify the X-ray pictures. Blood clots, cysts, tumours and a whole range of other disorders and abnormalities can all be detected with no more risk to the patient than any other form of X-ray.

Another scanning technology is magnetic resonance imaging (MRI). Radio waves are intermittently beamed at the body within a strong magnetic field. Because the molecular composition of different types of tissue varies, they give off different vibratory energies in the field, and these signals are built up to form a computer picture of the tissue being studied. MRI has the advantage of not using X-rays, and may allow diagnosis of conditions as varied as heart disease, multiple sclerosis and birth defects.

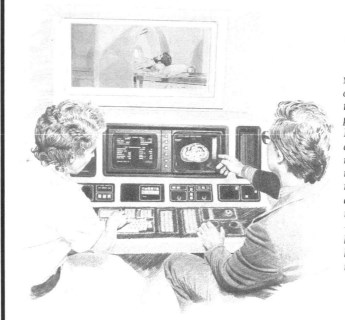

MAKING THE SCAN *The scanning beam of the X-ray operates across the mouth of the tunnel and pictures the part of the patient's body that lies within the circle. His movement into the tunnel and all the operations of the scanner are under the remote control of the doctor and radiographer at the console. Instructions to the scanner are given on the keyboard and recorded on the left-hand screen. The right-hand screen shows the image of a $\frac{3}{8}$ in. (10 mm.) slice through the patient's body. Normally the picture is displayed in black, white and shades of grey, but if necessary it can be shown in colour.*

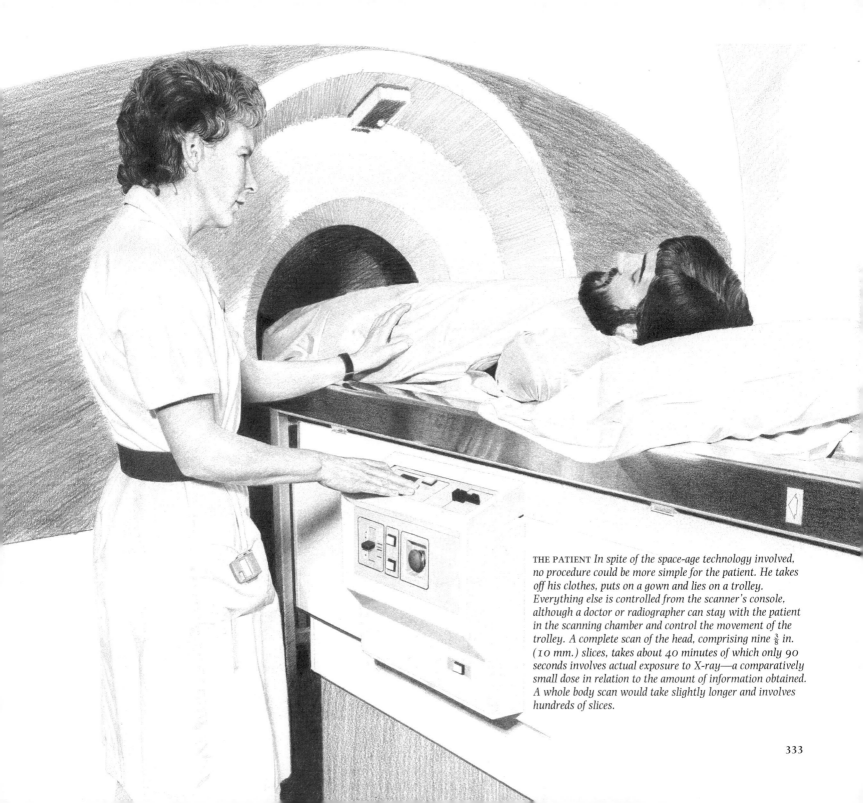

THE PATIENT *In spite of the space-age technology involved, no procedure could be more simple for the patient. He takes off his clothes, puts on a gown and lies on a trolley. Everything else is controlled from the scanner's console, although a doctor or radiographer can stay with the patient in the scanning chamber and control the movement of the trolley. A complete scan of the head, comprising nine ⅜ in. (10 mm.) slices, takes about 40 minutes of which only 90 seconds involves actual exposure to X-ray—a comparatively small dose in relation to the amount of information obtained. A whole body scan would take slightly longer and involves hundreds of slices.*

333

HOW THE BODY FIGHTS INFECTION
A vast army of cells is on constant alert to counter any attack by agents of disease

Most of the germs that invade the body are bacteria and viruses intent on releasing harmful toxins that will cause disease. But wherever the invaders appear, they are immediately attacked by the body's defenders—a task force of tiny, white cells, shown magnified thousands of times.

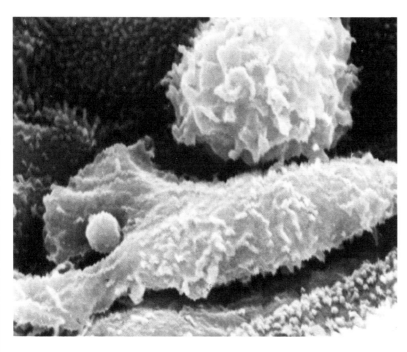

MACROPHAGES DEFENDING THE LUNGS *When a foreign particle enters the lungs it is challenged by one of the mobile macrophage cells. The small, round particle in the lower left of the picture is under attack by an elongated macrophage—while a circular macrophage patrols the upper area. The scavenger macrophages consume bacteria, pollen, dust and parts of tobacco smoke.*

LYMPHOCYTES COMBATING CANCER *The large, round lymphocyte cells home in on an invading cancer cell and try to destroy it. But although they can damage the surface of the cancer cell, they will probably not kill it. Blisters which form on the surface become detached and stick to the lymphocytes, forming a protective barrier for the cancer cell.*

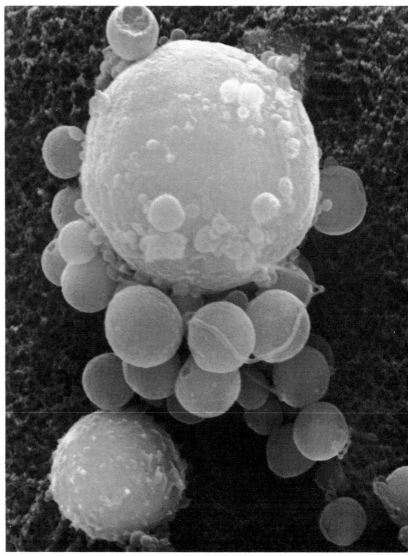

KILLING THE INTESTINAL WORM *The parasitic flatworm seen in the intestine causes schistosomiasis, a tropical disease marked by anaemia and inflammation. The groups of attacking eosinophil cells make a chemical that eats into the worm and kills it.*

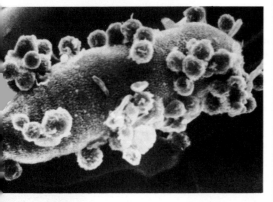

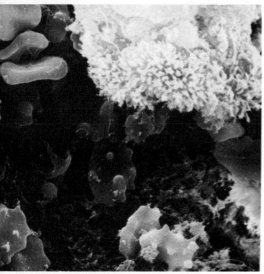

DEFENDING THE INTESTINE *The white amoeboid cells (top right) move in to consume bacteria (bottom right) which cause dysentery in the intestine. The cells also clear up debris. Red cells, which have no protective role, are seen top left.*

LYMPH

Like blood, lymph is a fluid that circulates through the body in a network of vessels. It has two main tasks—to transport certain substances such as fats and other chemicals throughout the body, and to carry the body's mechanisms for defence against disease.

Lymph is a clear or pale straw-coloured fluid which derives from the blood. The vessels through which it flows are much smaller and less obvious than veins and arteries, but they tend to follow their course. Along the course of the lymphatic channels are lymphatic glands. These are about the size of almonds. They consist of tissue cells (lymph cells) that have special abilities to deal with infective organisms and other noxious substances that have been collected from the skin, the breathing apparatus and the gut. Bacteria and viruses are destroyed and dusts and similar substances are broken down in the lymph glands.

In addition to lymph glands, the spleen, liver, tonsils and adenoids are among other organs that contain large amounts of lymphatic tissues and are involved in the body's general defensive mechanisms.

Lymph glands, and this includes tonsils and adenoids, normally tend to become more prominent and enlarged during childhood—between three and eight years of age, and during adolescence. Such enlargement is normal and is probably related to the body's build up of immunity and resistance to common germs. After the age of eight, in most children, the glands that can be felt in the neck and the apparently large tonsils, shrink and decrease in size naturally. Usually, enlarged neck glands and tonsils in children do not in themselves require treatment.

GLANDULAR FEVER is a condition affecting young adults and teenagers, believed to be caused by the EB (Epstein Barr) virus. In it there is enlargement and soreness of most lymph glands in the body with sore throat, fever and general malaise. Recovery takes place without any special treatment, during two to four weeks.

The lymph glands responsible for a particular area may be some distance away in the body. The septic skin infections of the finger, such as a WHITLOW, will produce enlarged painful lymph glands in the armpit; infection of the foot will lead to painful lymph glands in the groin; and throat infections to tender large lymph glands in the neck. Lymph glands responsible for an area of the skin or body will enlarge because they will be dealing with the infecting organisms. Septic skin infections will usually be treated with an antibiotic (*see* MEDICINES, 25).

Diseases of the glands themselves may occur, such as HODGKIN'S DISEASE, lymphoma or certain forms of LEUKAEMIA.

Tumour-affected lymph glands can be diagnosed by biopsy (surgical removal of a small piece of tissue and examination under a microscope) then treated by drugs or surgery.

LYMPHANGITIS
Inflammation of the lymph vessels, usually caused by an infection. When the onset of the disorder is sudden, the inflammation can be seen as patchy areas of redness under the skin. When the disease is gradual in onset and persistent, the inflammation appears as a cord-like swelling beneath the skin. Either type of lymphangitis is nearly always followed by swelling of the lymph glands. Antibiotics are given to treat the disorder (*see* MEDICINES, 25). The chronic form sometimes leads to LYMPHOEDEMA, swelling of all the lymphatic areas of the body.

LYMPHOCYTE
One of the three main types of leucocytes (white blood cells). They are manufactured in lymph glands, bone marrow, spleen, tonsils and other tissue, and their main function is to produce antibodies to fight infection.
See BLOOD

LYMPHOEDEMA

Swelling of arms or legs due to any disease which blocks the circulation of lymph to the lymph glands, which help the body to resist disease.
Symptoms
• Swelling of one or more limbs, which may be considerable.
Duration
• The condition persists whatever the cause and is only partly relieved by treatment.
Causes
• Underdevelopment of the lymphatic channels which drain the limbs. Although present from birth, the condition may not appear until much later.
• Blockage of the lymphatic circulation, caused by surgery, malignant disease, infection or radiation.
Complications
• None.

Treatment in the home
• None is effective.
When to consult the doctor
• If the cause of any swelling of limbs is uncertain.
What the doctor may do
• Arrange for X-rays of the lymphatic circulation.
• Prescribe diuretics to increase the volume of urine produced and reduce the excess fluid in the limbs. *See* MEDICINES, 6.
• Arrange for elastic supports for the limbs.
• Suggest plastic surgery to improve the circulation.
Prevention
• Depends on the cause, but is not usually possible.
Outlook
• Although resistant to treatment, lymphoedema can improve—depending upon the cause.

See CIRCULATORY SYSTEM *page 40*

LYMPHOGRANULOMA VENEREUM

A venereal disease that occurs mainly in tropical regions. It is a viral infection that has an incubation period of one to four weeks. The first symptom is a small short-lived sore that may pass unnoticed. In women it may form in the vagina or on the neck of the womb, in men on the genitals.

The sore is followed by painful swelling of the lymph glands in the groin and then by weeping sores in that region and, in some women, in the rectum. The skin of the genital area may also thicken. Early treatment with antibiotics prevents the formation of abscesses and fistulas that may require surgery. *See* MEDICINES, 25.

MACROBIOTIC DIETS

A way of eating, based on the precepts of Zen Buddhism and Taoism. One aim is to make eating so much a matter of second nature that the eater's mind is left free to concentrate on obtaining spiritual enlightenment. Another is to balance, in the food, the positive and negative 'life forces', yin and yang, in which Taoists believe.

The food itself is largely based on whole grains, cereals, pulses and soya-bean sauces, with little or no meat and no artificially processed constituents. To most Western palates, it seems dull and tasteless.

During the 1970s, the American Medical Association denounced such diets as bad for health and potentially lethal. In their strictest form, they lack vital vitamins—in particular vitamins B12 and C.
See NUTRITION

THE HEALING LIGHT
How lasers can help to save sight

A laser produces an intense beam of light that travels in a straight line. Such a beam can be used to burn a hole in steel or for very delicate operations on the eye.

Certain conditions, such as senile macular degeneration and diabetic retinopathy, result in the little blood vessels in the retina leaking or increasing in number. This may lead to severe deterioration of sight or, in the case of diabetic retinopathy, blindness. To stop the process the doctor will 'photocoagulate', or burn, the abnormal blood vessels with a pinpoint laser.

Laser photocoagulation is performed with a carefully controlled laser connected to a microscope or 'slit lamp'. Green (argon) laser light is usually used in photocoagulation because it specifically affects red pigment in the blood coagulating the blood vessels, leaving the other tissues unharmed. The patient feels no pain, he just sees a flashing light.

Treatment of this kind, given in time, may preserve sight. Lasers are also used in other areas of medicine, particularly in the treatment of cancer and skin disorders.

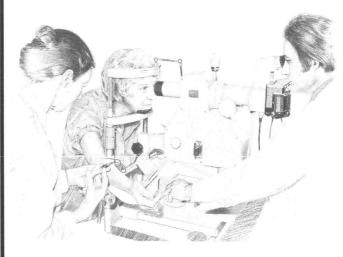

PHOTOGRAPHING THE EYE *Patients with suspected disease at the back of the eye may undergo a fluorescein angiogram. Orange dye is injected into the patient's arm and travels in the bloodstream to the blood vessels at the back of the retina. When the eye is illuminated with blue light, the dye fluoresces green and the abnormal blood vessels show up clearly and can be photographed.*

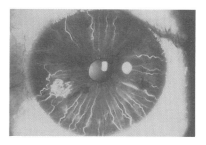

DYE DETECTOR *The irregular patch (left) is an area of disease on the iris, shown up by the dye of a fluorescein angiogram.*

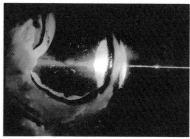

TREATMENT WITH A LASER BEAM *A green laser beam flashes through the eye and painlessly destroys the diseased area of the retina.*

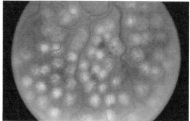

THE EYE AFTER TREATMENT *The yellow spots show the areas that were burned by the laser. Other tissues were unharmed.*

MACULAR DEGENERATION, SENILE

Scarring or swelling of the retina—the light-sensitive membrane at the back of the eye. The macula is the focusing point at the centre of the retina. In disciform macular degeneration, minute blood vessels grow under the retina. They cause swelling, bleeding and scarring, which prevents clear vision. The condition is commonest in people over the age of 55, but it can very occasionally affect young people who suffer from other eye disorders such as severe shortsightedness.

Symptoms
• Blurred and often distorted vision, which makes reading and recognising faces difficult. The onset is quite rapid. Outwardly, the eye appears normal.

Causes
• Although the precise causes are not fully understood, the condition is associated with changes in the tissues behind the retina. The changes are usually related to age, blood pressure or DIABETES.

Complications
• Loss of clear central vision and the ability to do fine work and read.

When to consult the doctor
• If the symptoms described occur.
• If one eye has already been affected; it may be possible to protect the unaffected eye.

What the doctor may do
• Refer the patient to an eye specialist.
• Treat any underlying general causes.
• Enlarge the pupil by administering eye drops, and then examine the eye with an ophthalmoscope. If the blood vessels do not underlie the centre of the macula, the specialist may perform a fluorescein angiogram—a photographic test in which fluorescein (an orange dye) is injected into a vein in the arm to outline the abnormal blood vessels in the macula. These are then photographed and, if possible, destroyed a few days later with a laser. The specialist will observe the patient closely for the next few weeks to make sure that all the abnormal blood vessels have been eradicated.
• If, however, the blood vessels do underlie the centre of the macula, treatment is not possible because the lasers would also damage the vital sensitive part of the macula. In this case, the doctor will advise the patient how best to cope with his sight impairment—how to use a magnifying glass (or some other form of aid) and how to use reading

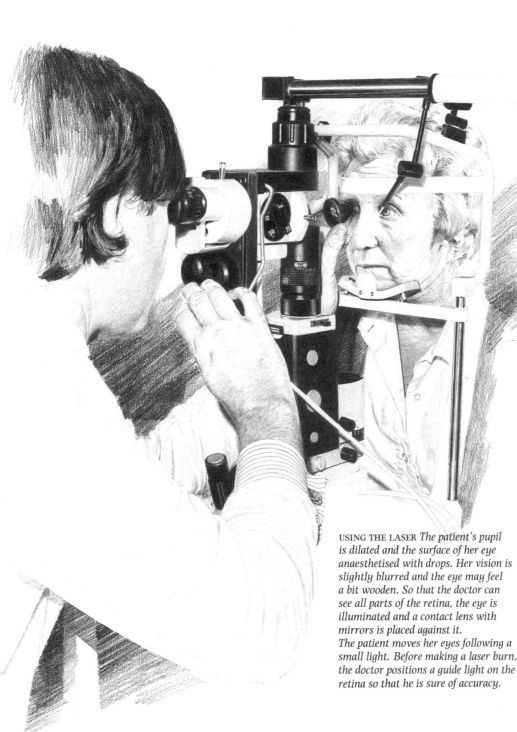

USING THE LASER *The patient's pupil is dilated and the surface of her eye anaesthetised with drops. Her vision is slightly blurred and the eye may feel a bit wooden. So that the doctor can see all parts of the retina, the eye is illuminated and a contact lens with mirrors is placed against it.*
The patient moves her eyes following a small light. Before making a laser burn, the doctor positions a guide light on the retina so that he is sure of accuracy.

lights to their best advantage.

Prevention

• There is none possible. If the condition has already occurred in one eye, the risk to the other eye is increased, and the patient should visit the doctor immediately symptoms develop.

Outlook

• Provided the condition is treated early, the outlook is good. Disciform macular degeneration affects only the macula region and, although it may damage sight, it never causes blindness.

See EYE *page 36*

MALARIA

One of the most widespread and serious infectious diseases in the world. Since 1956, the World Health Organisation has been sponsoring a programme to eradicate it, but malaria remains difficult to control, and the number of cases coming into Britain each year is increasing. There are three major types of malaria—malignant tertian, benign tertian and quartan. They are caused by different species of malarial parasites which are carried by mosquitoes. Infection is transmitted to man by a bite from the female mosquito.

Symptoms

The symptoms are common to all three types:

• Fever that peaks every third or fourth day.

• Headache.

• Muscle pains.

• Bouts of fever with shivering attacks. (Shivering attacks do not usually occur in malignant tertian.)

Incubation period

Time between mosquito bite and onset of symptoms:

• Malignant and benign tertian: ten to 14 days.

• Quartan: 18 days to six weeks.

Duration

• Malignant tertian: with prompt treatment recovery occurs in a few days, although convalescence will probably be necessary. Without adequate treatment infection persists and serious complications can arise.

• Benign tertian: after about a week the fever and shivering attacks begin to occur regularly every other day. Without treatment the infection persists, but it is rarely fatal.

• Quartan: fever and shivering attacks occur every third day and tend to be regular. Although quartan malaria is

more disabling than benign tertian malaria, it responds well to treatment.

Causes

• The malarial parasite.

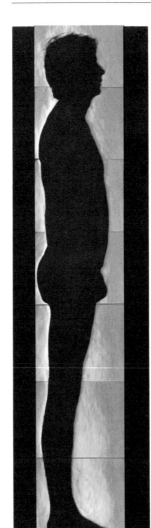

Signal for the mosquito

The air surrounding the human body is constantly moving, sending up a turbulent plume of warm, moist air currents 4 ft (1.2 m.) above the head. The mosquito, first attracted by a rise in the level of carbon dioxide in the area, zooms in on the moist air currents and attacks its victim.

SEEING AIR *This picture, taken by a special photographic method called the Schlieren system, shows the air moving round the body.*

Complications

• The only type likely to cause complications is malignant tertian malaria. Without prompt treatment, ANAEMIA and shock can affect the brain or the lungs and kidneys (*see* BLACKWATER FEVER), and death may follow.

Treatment in the home

• Keep the patient warm, with rest and plenty of drinks.

When to consult the doctor

• Immediately if malaria is suspected, even if it is months after visiting a country that has the disease.

What the doctor may do

• Prescribe chloroquine or another antimalarial drug. *See* MEDICINES, 28.

Prevention

• Travellers to 'at risk' areas should protect themselves by taking chloroquine or other antimalarial drugs from one week before arriving in the area until 28 days after leaving it.

• In certain areas of the world, malignant tertian malaria is not prevented by chloroquine. Seek advice from your doctor, travel agent or employer about appropriate drugs.

Outlook

• With modern drugs the outlook is good, and chronic relapsing malaria should not occur.

See INFECTIOUS DISEASES *page 32*

MALLET FINGER

A finger whose tip cannot be straightened because the tendon controlling it has been snapped by injury.

Symptoms

• The tip of the finger cannot be fully straightened. This may not be noticed until long after the injury.

Duration

• If treated, the tendon heals after about three weeks.

Causes

• The injury is usually caused by stubbing the finger hard or by receiving a forceful blow from a ball when failing to catch it.

Treatment in the home

• Do not use the finger.

When to consult the doctor

• Immediately the symptom is noticed.

What the doctor may do

• Send the patient to hospital for an X-ray to exclude the possibility of a fracture.

- The finger will be straightened and put in splints for three weeks to enable the tendon to heal properly.

Outlook
- The ruptured tendon always heals, even without treatment. However, often it lengthens in the healing, and inability to straighten the joint persists. The patient can accept this or have the tendon repaired by an operation.

See SKELETAL SYSTEM *page 54*

MANIC DEPRESSION

A form of mental illness in which the sufferer's mood swings from profound depression to extreme elation. The manic stage of the illness is described under HYPO-MANIA. The depressive phase of the illness is indistinguishable from ordinary DEPRESSION.

The timing of the swings of mood varies from patient to patient, and many sufferers from the condition may be in good mental health for years between attacks, making the pattern of the illness difficult to recognise.

Manic depression is a rare condition which occurs in one in 2,000 of the population.

MASTITIS, NODULAR

Tender lumps in a woman's breasts. The condition is harmless and is experienced by many women at some time in their life.

Symptoms
- There is a lumpiness of the breasts.
- The breasts feel full.
- Usually one breast is more affected than the other.
- Tiredness, irritability and other feelings associated with PREMENSTRUAL TENSION may be experienced.
- The symptoms of nodular mastitis are usually relieved by the start of a period.

Duration
- The condition usually comes and goes.

Causes
- Nodular mastitis is caused by normal changes in the balance of female hormones.

Treatment in the home
- Wear a brassière that provides a good support for the breasts. This will relieve discomfort considerably.

When to consult the doctor
- Immediately any lump in the breast is noticed.

What the doctor may do
- Examine both breasts, and do so again a few days later, in order to determine whether the lumps are harmless or not.
- Prescribe diuretic tablets, which increase the amount of urine passed (fluid retention seems to make the condition worse). *See* MEDICINES, 6.
- Advise the woman always to wear a well-supporting brassière.
- In some cases the lumps need to be removed to ensure they are harmless.

Prevention
- There is no means of preventing the condition.

Outlook
- Nodular mastitis presents no risk to health and disappears after the menopause.

See FEMALE GENITAL SYSTEM *page 48*

MASTOIDITIS

Inflammation of the mastoid bone. The bone is directly behind the ear-lobe and can be felt through the skin. It is not solid, but contains cells of air which connect to the middle ear.

Since antibiotics have been available for the treatment of ear infections, mastoiditis has become rare in developed countries.

Symptoms
- Mastoiditis is often preceded by earache and OTITIS MEDIA.
- Pain behind the ear. Mastoiditis is usually associated with a PERFORATED EAR-DRUM, and pus drains from the middle ear through the perforation.
- Fever and rapid pulse.
- Increasing deafness in the affected ear.

Duration
- Untreated infection may persist for weeks and spread to surrounding bone and the brain.

Causes
- Mastoiditis, a rare complication of OTITIS MEDIA, is caused by bacterial infection spreading from the middle ear to the mastoid bone.

Complications
- The infection may spread to the nearby bone, blood vessels or brain.

Treatment in the home
- None. Consult the doctor.

When to consult the doctor
- If you have pain in the ear, especially if it is associated with fever, tenderness in the bone behind the ear-lobe, or offensive discharge from the ear.

What the doctor may do
- Examine the ear.
- Arrange an X-ray and admission to hospital.
- Treatment is with antibiotics and often an operation to clear the infection. *See* MEDICINES, 25.

Outlook
- All patients should recover, but there may be permanent partial or total loss of hearing in the affected ear.

See EAR *page 38*

MASTURBATION

Manipulating the genital organs in order to obtain sexual pleasure, or as a means of relieving tension. Despite many theories to the contrary, masturbation does not harm the body in any way.
See SEX PROBLEMS

M.E. *See* MYALGIC ENCEPHALOMYELITIS

MEASLES

A highly contagious disease occurring mostly in childhood. The infection is spread by direct contact, or by germ-laden air breathed out by patients. Measles is one of the commonest diseases in the world, although immunisation programmes have greatly reduced the number of cases and complications. Most victims recover completely, but dangers remain. So attempts are being made, particularly in developed countries, to eradicate it by immunisation. Babies in the first year of life usually have a natural immunity through their mothers.

Symptoms
- A rash of brownish-pink, slightly raised spots starts behind the ears and spreads in blotches over the whole body on about the fourth day of the illness.
- A dry, irritating cough starts one to four days before the rash.
- Temperature rises one or two days before the rash.
- Eyes may be sore and red, or 'heavy', for a few days before the rash.
- Koplik's spots (small white spots inside the cheeks),

occurring about a day before the skin rash appears, are a characteristic sign.

• A child may be quite poorly for two days before the rash appears and while it is developing.

Incubation period

• Usually 12 days, but can range between eight and 15 days.

Duration

• Five to seven days after the first appearance of the rash.

Causes

• A virus.

Complications

• OTITIS MEDIA.

• PNEUMONIA.

• ENCEPHALITIS. This is a rare complication occurring in about only one patient in 1,000. Most patients recover from encephalitis, but there may be some permanent brain damage.

Treatment in the home

• Put the child to bed and give plenty of cool drinks to bring the temperature down. It does not matter if the child does not want to eat, as long as plenty of fluids are taken.

• Keep the child quiet and at rest while there is fever and illness.

• If necessary, give fever-reducing tablets in recommended doses. See MEDICINES, 22.

When to consult the doctor

• As soon as you think the child has measles.

What the doctor may do

• Check to see whether there are complications in the ears, otitis media, or of the lungs, pneumonia. If there are, a course of antibiotics will probably be prescribed. Otherwise antibiotics are of no value in the treatment of measles. See MEDICINES, 25.

Prevention

• Immunisation is the best protection and is effective in about 95 per cent of cases. Although immunisation, like measles itself, can occasionally cause serious complications, immunisation programmes have reduced the incidence of all complications, including encephalitis.

• Most doctors advise routine MMR immunisation of children soon after their first birthday. See CHILD CARE pages 144–5.

• On about the eighth day after the injection there may be a slight fever, rash, sore throat or sore eyes. This is a common reaction to immunisation and is not usually very troublesome.

• If there is a history or close family history of ALLERGY or convulsions consult your doctor before having a child immunised.

• Children with serious blood diseases, such as LEUKAE-MIA OR HODGKIN'S DISEASE, or with feverish illness or allergy to hens' eggs or the antibiotic neomycin, or who are on steroid or similar drugs, should not be immunised without the knowledge of the doctor in charge.

Outlook

• Recovery from measles is usually complete.

See INFECTIOUS DISEASES *page 32*

MECONIUM

The first bowel discharge passed by a new-born baby. It is a soft green mass consisting of mucus, bile and waste products that has collected in the intestine during the baby's last weeks in the womb.

MEDICINES

Which medicine does what? A guide to the thousands of medicines and drugs available today—whether 'over the counter' or on a doctor's prescription—tells you what each preparation is designed to do, together with warnings about side-effects and other problems.

See MEDICINES AND DRUGS *page 342*

MEGALOMANIA

A delusion of grandeur that is common in several psychoses (severe mental illnesses). The sufferer may believe that he has great power, attainments or wealth, or may even claim to be God. A common misuse of the term is to apply it to any politician or businessman who enjoys wielding actual power.

MEGAVITAMIN THERAPY

A method of treatment that advocates massive doses of vitamins as a potential cure for disease. In the late 1960s medical research attempted to prove that large quantities of vitamin C, found naturally in fruit and vegetables, gave protection against the common cold and other virus infections. The research to date has been inconclusive, and is regarded sceptically by many doctors. However, there is no evidence that large doses of vitamin C are actually harmful to health.

That is not true of vitamin A, sometimes used to try to treat arthritis and psychiatric disorders, or vitamin D, occasionally employed for bone ailments. Both can be poisonous in large amounts, although medically qualified megavitamin therapists would not prescribe harmful dosages.

Vitamins B3, B6 and C have, it is claimed, been used successfully in the treatment of ALCOHOLISM and SCHIZOPHRENIA; but research carried out in Canada failed to reach any firm conclusions on their benefits. Similarly, claims made for the use of vitamin E in treating skin disorders and muscle cramps have not been substantiated by independent, properly controlled studies. The belief that vitamin E can improve sexual performance and satisfaction is generally discounted by doctors.

The Journal of the American Medical Association has attacked the commercial sale of multivitamin preparations containing many thousand times the recommended daily intake levels of vitamins. For most people, a well-balanced diet provides all the vitamins they need.

See NUTRITION

MEDICINES, 36.

MEIBOMIAN CYST

These cysts, sometimes called tarsal cysts or chalazions, are little nodules which can form at any age in the supporting gristle layer of the eyelid.

Symptoms

• The patient becomes gradually aware of a small painless nodule or swelling in one of the eyelids.

Causes

• It is thought that such cysts are caused by a minor blockage of the glands in the eyelid.

When to consult the doctor

• If the cyst is very small, not inflamed and not causing any trouble, nothing needs to be done about it. If the cyst grows and becomes embarrassing to look at or irritating, or if it gets inflamed and sore, consult a doctor.

What the doctor may do

• After examining the eyelid, the doctor may recommend that nothing should be done, or he may send the patient to a specialist to have the cyst removed. This will involve a minor operation which can be carried out under a local anaesthetic.

• If the cyst is inflamed and infected the doctor will probably recommend hot bathing to encourage it to come to a head and discharge.

• He may also prescribe antibiotic ointment. See MEDICINES, 38.

Outlook

• Meibomian cysts are harmless and will not affect the eyesight or the general health.

See EYE *page 36*

MELANOMA

A pigmented mole. There are two types of melanoma: the harmless juvenile melanoma, which is common and usually appears in children, and the more rare malignant melanoma. See SKIN CANCER.

JUVENILE MELANOMA
A brownish-red, dome-shaped mole that often develops in children before or at puberty. It is slow-growing and most commonly appears on the face, though it may appear elsewhere and at a later age. Several may appear at one time.

Symptoms
- A small dark brown spot appears and grows for a few months.
- There is no pain or irritation.

Duration
- After initial growth the melanoma remains unchanged for years and may then disappear without trace.

Causes
- Active growth of pigment-containing cells. What stimulates this growth is not known.

Treatment in the home
- Leave the spot alone. Irritating it could possibly cause a cancerous change.
- It is not dangerous to cover the spot with cosmetics.

When to consult the doctor
As soon as possible if the spot:
- Changes shape, size or colour.
- Bleeds.
- Itches.
- Is more than 7 mm ($\frac{1}{4}$ in) in diameter.
- Becomes inflamed or crusted.
- If you are anxious about any growing spot.

What the doctor may do
- Reassure the patient that juvenile melanomas are common and harmless and require no treatment.
- If diagnosis is uncertain the doctor will send the patient to a specialist to have the mole cut out for examination under a microscope.

Prevention
- None is known.

Outlook
- Juvenile melanomas are extremely common and harmless, and often disappear completely. Very rarely a malignant melanoma develops from one of them.

See SKIN page 52

MÉNIÈRE'S DISEASE

A condition in which the body's balance mechanism in the inner ear becomes swollen. It usually affects only one ear, although in 15 per cent of cases both ears are affected. The symptoms come on suddenly and for a few hours are very severe. The patient is helpless and has to go to bed. Ménière's disease does not occur in children.

Symptoms
- Sudden vertigo (giddiness) with a sensation of the room spinning round.
- Vomiting.
- Deafness and noises in the affected ear, which usually persist, and get worse with each attack. Deafness in the affected ear often precedes the attacks.
- Flickering of the eyes (nystagmus) may be noticed.

Duration
- Although the first hours are the worst, symptoms rarely last for longer than 24 hours.
- Attacks may recur, with intervals between attacks getting shorter as time goes on.

Causes
- Not known.

Treatment in the home
- Go to bed and keep still.

When to consult the doctor
- If symptoms are severe when lying quietly in bed.

What the doctor may do
- Examine the ears and eyes and test the hearing.
- Give an injection to relieve symptoms.
- Prescribe tablets or suppositories to use at the onset of any future attack. See MEDICINES, 21.

Prevention
- None known.

Outlook
- Attacks may become more frequent but may suddenly and unpredictably cease altogether.
- The degree of deafness in the affected ear gets worse with each attack, and is permanent.
- Treatment can reduce, but does not always cure, the attacks of dizziness.

See EAR page 38

The inner ear—intricate centre of balance and hearing

Tiny hinged bones transmit sound vibrations from the eardrum to a fluid-filled membrane inside the inner ear. Minute hairs in the fluid convert the vibrations into electrical impulses for onward transmission to the brain.

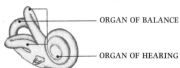

ORGAN OF BALANCE

ORGAN OF HEARING

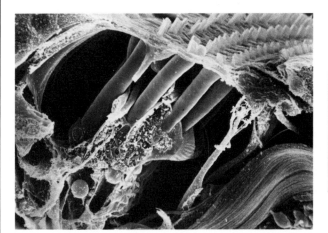

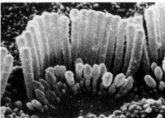

HOW WE HEAR *This cross-section of the membrane shows how the top and bottom surfaces are joined by pressure-sensitive hairs which react to sound waves.*

CONVERTER *Vibration of the fluid moves the hairs which convert the waves into electrical impulses.*

Medicines & drugs

A GUIDE TO THE CAREFUL USE OF OVER-THE-COUNTER REMEDIES AND THE DRUGS YOUR DOCTOR PRESCRIBES

Any medicine, tablet, injection or suppository, whether it be an antibiotic, painkiller or any other, is referred to loosely by both doctors and chemists as a drug. The term drug used in this way has nothing to do with addictive drugs such as heroin or opium.

In the last 100 years a great many chemical compounds have been developed to combat disease by helping the normal bodily functions. Such drugs often have powerful effects and although they may help one function, they may interfere with another. Therefore a careful balance usually has to be reached and *exactly the right dose taken* to ensure that helpful effects outweigh possible harmful side-effects. Instructions must be carefully followed and a medicine prescribed for one person should never be given to another without first asking the doctor.

The drugs described here are listed according to the systems of the body on which they act. The breakdown by numbers allows for easy cross reference from the individual disease entries given elsewhere in the book. For example, MEDICINES 2 refers to drugs used in the treatment of diarrhoea; MEDICINES 20 refers to drugs used to stimulate the nervous system and suppress appetite.

By using this section you will be able to evaluate the drugs which your doctor may prescribe, or which a chemist may recommend.

THE DIGESTIVE SYSTEM

In the digestive system, drugs may be used to treat four main types of disorder: peptic ulcer (peptic is the name given to any ulcer which is produced by normal digestive juices and includes duodenal, gastric and oesophageal ulcers); diarrhoea; constipation; and conditions affecting the large bowel, rectum and anus.

1 DRUGS USED TO TREAT DUODENAL, GASTRIC AND OESOPHAGEAL ULCERS

Antacids
These aim to neutralise the hydrochloric acid produced by the stomach in normal digestion. This helps the ulcer to heal. A great variety of antacids are available. All are effective but each sufferer discovers his own special preference.
Common examples
Aluminium hydroxide; magnesium trisilicate; bismuth compounds; sodium bicarbonate.

Precautions and side-effects
Sodium bicarbonate should not be used repeatedly or for long periods as it may affect the kidneys. Bismuth may stain the motions black.
Obtainable
Without prescription, from chemists.

Antispasmodics (intestinal)
Any peptic ulcer causes a painful muscle spasm which closes the outlet of the stomach. This aggravates the ulceration. Intestinal antispasmodics help by relaxing this spasm.
Common examples
Belladonna; atropine; hyoscine and related compounds. Many antispasmodics are made more effective by combining them with an antacid.
Precautions and side-effects
Belladonna, atropine and many of the related compounds used are poisonous if the prescribed dose is exceeded. Overdosage may cause dryness of the mouth, palpitations, constipation and visual disturbances.
Obtainable
Without prescription, from chemists.

Ulcer healing drugs
Peptic ulcers are greatly helped by these drugs. Symptoms are lessened, healing rates improved and recurrences reduced,
Common examples
Cimetidine; ranitidine; omeprazole.
Precautions and side-effects
These drugs should not be taken intermittently for indigestion, because this could conceal the symptoms of stomach cancer. They should be used with caution by the elderly, those with kidney diseases, and those taking other medicines, particularly anticoagulants and anti-epileptic drugs. They should not be taken within 30 minutes of antacids.

Obtainable
On doctor's prescription only.

2 DRUGS USED TO TREAT DIARRHOEA

Replacement of the fluids and electrolytes lost through the bowel is more important than taking medicines. This is particularly true in infants and in the frail and elderly. If the patient avoids food and milk for 24 hours or until his appetite returns, and takes frequent sips of liquid, the diarrhoea will usually stop fairly soon. Infants and the elderly may benefit from a glucose and sodium chloride powder obtainable from a doctor or chemist, made up with boiled water drunk on its own until symptoms improve. Mild cases in otherwise healthy people may be helped by medicines that either absorb fluid in the bowel or slow down bowel movement.
Common examples
For rehydration: Sodium chloride and glucose oral powder, Dioralyte. To control diarrhoea: kaolin mixture, chalk powder, methylcellulose, codeine phosphate, diphenoxylate, loperamide.
Precautions and side-effects
Diarrhoea accompanied by continuous abdominal pain or bleeding from the rectum, or lasting longer than two weeks, requires medical advice.
Obtainable
Without prescription, from chemists.

3 DRUGS USED TO TREAT CONSTIPATION

Most laxatives act in one of three ways: by increasing 'bulk', by stimulating (or irritating) the bowel, and by softening the motions.

Bulk forming
These act in a passive way and, if effective, are the most satisfactory laxative to use. They are useful for people suffering from chronic constipation and diverticulitis; those who have had colostomies performed; and in many other situations where long-term treatment for the patient is required.
Common examples
Bran, methylcellulose, ispaghula husk; sterculia and similar preparations.
Precautions and side-effects
Side-effects are rare.
Obtainable
At any chemist, without prescription.

Stimulant
These are more varied in their actions and are unsuitable for long-term use.
Common examples
Bisacodyl; castor oil; cascara; fig; senna; Epsom salts; dioctyl.
Precautions and side-effects
Many of these compounds, because of their strength, produce an immediate bowel movement which is then followed by a rebound constipation. They are therefore not helpful in the treatment of long-term constipation. If, however, other laxatives are not effective, they may have to be used, and in this case the milder ones are best—bisacodyl, danthron and senna. They should never be given if there is any abdominal pain.
Obtainable
Available from any chemist, without prescription.

Faecal softeners
These act passively and rarely cause problems even if used for long periods of time.

Common examples
Liquid paraffin; glycerine suppositories.
Precautions and side-effects
Leakage from the anus with irritation and staining of underwear. Occasionally, they may prevent absorption of vitamins and other nutriments.
Obtainable
At any chemist, without prescription.

4 DRUGS USED TO TREAT DISORDERS OF THE LARGE BOWEL (COLON), RECTUM AND ANUS

These include enemas, suppositories and creams which contain soothing agents, steroid substances and antibiotics. They are used mainly in the treatment of ulcerative colitis, piles and pruritus.
Common examples
Soothing compounds include Anusol; Bismodyne; Anodesyn; *Proctosedyl; *hydrocortisone; *prednisolone (Predsol enema).
Precautions and side-effects
Should be used only under medical supervision.
Obtainable
Those marked * need a prescription.

Drugs are used to influence the circulatory system in six different ways: to make the pumping action of the heart more efficient by influencing its rate and rhythm; to reduce the work-load of the heart by getting rid of body fluids; to reduce blood pressure; to dilate the arteries and increase blood supply to heart and other organs; to stimulate the heart; to prevent blood from clotting.

5 DRUGS WHICH AFFECT HEART RATE AND HEART RHYTHM

Drugs which slow the heart rate
These are mainly used in congestive heart failure and atrial fibrillation (irregular heartbeat).
Common example
Digoxin.
Precautions and side-effects
Nausea and vomiting are common. These drugs may slow the heart rhythm too much. They require medical supervision and close co-operation of the patient.
Obtainable
On doctor's prescription only.

Drugs to control rhythm
These are used mainly to control and prevent the occurrence of sudden disturbances of heart rhythm, some of which can be dangerous, and after a coronary thrombosis.
Common examples
Quinidine; verapamil; disopyramide; lignocaine; procainamide; amiodarone; flecainide.
Precautions and side-effects
These drugs require close medical supervision and co-operation between patient and doctor.
Obtainable
On doctor's prescription only.

Beta-blockers
These drugs, besides slowing heart rate and reducing the likelihood of harmful irregularities (arrhythmia), are also used to reduce blood pressure

and pulse-rate in angina and thyrotoxicosis. They have also been used to reduce anxiety and control stage fright.
Common examples
Propranolol; oxprenolol; pindolol; metoprolol; atendol; timolol; acebutalol.
Precautions and side-effects
These drugs should never be stopped suddenly and require close medical supervision and full co-operation between patient and doctor.
Obtainable
On doctor's prescription only.

6 DRUGS USED TO GET RID OF BODY FLUIDS (DIURETICS)

These cause the kidneys to discharge extra water in the urine. This loss of body fluid is especially helpful in congestive heart failure and hypertension, and in treating other conditions in which the amount of body fluid is too great.
Common examples
Bendrofluazide; chlorothiazide; frusemide; bumetamide; spironolactone; ethacrynic acid.
Precautions and side-effects
Many have to be taken with a supplementary tablet of potassium. They should not be taken without medical supervision.
Obtainable
On doctor's prescription only.

7 DRUGS USED TO REDUCE BLOOD PRESSURE (ANTIHYPERTENSIVES)

These act on the heart and arteries at many different points. Most have powerful side-effects which must be

carefully balanced by doctors against the risks of raised blood pressure—which are heart attacks, stroke, and kidney disease.
Common examples
Diuretics: bendrofluazide chlorothiazide (see previous section).
Beta-blockers: propranolol, atenolol.
Vasodilators: hydralazine, diazoxide, verapamil, nifedipine, ACE inhibitors: enalapril, captopril.
Centrally acting drugs: methyldopa, clonidine, reserpine.
Precautions and side-effects
Antihypertensives can cause palpitations, dizziness (or even a faint) after changes of position, mental depression and excessive passage of urine, particularly in elderly patients. Patients may experience other side-effects with some of the drugs. They include: flushing of the skin, cold hands and feet, impotence, gout, or cramps caused by loss of potassium from the body. Careful medical supervision is always necessary. All side-effects should be discussed with the doctor as soon as they occur, before the drugs are stopped.
Obtainable
On doctor's prescription only.

8 DRUGS WHICH DILATE THE ARTERIES AND INCREASE BLOOD SUPPLY (VASODILATORS)

These are used to dilate the coronary arteries of the heart in angina pectoris. They act quickly, the pain is removed and the patient is able to continue normal activity. Vasodilators are also used in the treatment of heart failure, and to improve the peripheral circulation of arms, legs and brain, in the elderly, when arteries are

narrowed by atheroma and the blood supply is therefore restricted.
Common examples
Coronary vasodilators: glyceryl trinitrate; isosorbide mononitrate; trinitrin; verapamil; nifedipine; nicardipine.
Peripheral vasodilators: nicotinic acid; cinnarizine; thymoxamine.
Cerebral vasodilators: co-dergocrine; cyclandelate; naftidrofuryl.
Precautions and side-effects
Any of these drugs may produce flushing, throbbing headache, dizziness or fainting. They should be used only under the guidance of a doctor.
Obtainable
On doctor's prescription only.

9 DRUGS WHICH STIMULATE THE HEART

These are used occasionally in emergencies to stimulate a failing heart during an operation or after a cardiac arrest.
Common examples
Adrenaline-like drugs: adrenaline, isoprenaline, dobutamine.
Precautions and side-effects
These drugs are always given under close medical supervision.
Obtainable
On doctor's prescription only.

10 DRUGS WHICH PREVENT BLOOD FROM CLOTTING (ANTICOAGULANTS)

These are used to prevent blood clots from forming in an artery, or to prevent them from spreading further and cutting off the blood supply to a wider area.

Common examples
Heparin; warfarin; nicoumalone; streptokinase, urokinase; phenindione; aspirin dipyridamole.
Precautions and side-effects
These drugs are always given under close medical supervision. After any anticoagulant has been given, any unexpected bleeding, bruising or sudden pains in joints or elsewhere should be reported immediately to the doctor.
Obtainable
On doctor's prescription only.

THE RESPIRATORY SYSTEM

Apart from the anti-infective drugs (antibiotics—section 25 below), six main types of drug are used to influence the respiratory system and to treat disease: those which dilate the bronchial tubes; drugs which reduce swelling and inflammation of the air passages; those which prevent asthma; drugs used against allergies; those which stimulate the respiratory system; and those which suppress and soothe coughs.

11 *DRUGS WHICH DILATE THE BRONCHIAL TUBES OF THE LUNGS*

In asthma the lungs become overfilled because the bronchial tubes are narrowed by asthmatic spasm (bronchospasm). Bronchodilators widen the bronchial tubes and so allow the lungs to empty properly, giving rapid relief. Such drugs may be given by mouth, by aerosol, by inhalation or by means of an injection.
Common examples
Adrenaline and ephedrine were originally used, but a number of more effective adrenaline-like (sympatho-mimetic) drugs are salbutamol, rimiterol; terbutaline; fenoterol, orciprenaline; aminophylline; theophylline.
Precautions and side-effects
Palpitations, anxiety and dizziness may arise. Bronchodilators should be used with caution if there is any diabetes, thyroid, or heart disease. The chief danger of such drugs is when inhalers are over-used incorrectly in asthma. A single inhalation should produce rapid relief: *if it does not do so, wait for 30 minutes*. Do not take more than eight inhalations in 24 hours. If a larger number of inhalations is necessary to give relief, see your doctor.
Obtainable
On doctor's prescription only.

12 *DRUGS WHICH HELP IN THE TREATMENT OF ASTHMA*

Corticosteroids
These drugs help to reduce the swelling and inflammation in the bronchial tubes of the lungs. They may be given by tablet, or alternatively by injection or aerosol (or rotacap) inhalation.
Common examples
Beclomethasone (Becotide); Budesonide.
Precautions and side-effects
Hoarseness and thrush of the mouth may develop. Medical supervision is essential.
Obtainable
On doctor's prescription only.

13 *DRUGS WHICH PREVENT ASTHMA*

Drugs have recently been developed which decrease the sensitivity of cells lining the lung passages. These drugs greatly reduce the frequency of asthma attacks but are of no value in treating asthma attacks once started. In children especially they are valuable in prevention, but have to be taken over long periods. They may be inhaled or taken as tablets, and are expensive.
Common examples
Sodium cromoglycate, taken by inhalation only; ketotifen; nedocromil.
Precautions and side-effects
There are few side-effects.
Obtainable
On doctor's prescription only.

14 *DRUGS USED AGAINST ALLERGIES (ANTIHISTAMINES)*

These act by neutralising histamine, a substance produced by all allergic reactions, and the cause of the annoying symptoms.
Common examples
Usually obtainable as tablets or syrup: *astemizole, terfenadine, brompheniramine, chlorpheniramine, azatadine, pheniramine, promethazine, *trimeprazine.
Many travel-sickness remedies contain antihistamine drugs.
Precautions and side-effects
Drowsiness is common; the effects of alcohol and sleeping-pills may be aggravated. Antihistamines should not be taken when driving a car or operating machinery. Many remedies for coughs, colds and motion sickness contain antihistamine drugs which may make the taker drowsy.
Obtainable
Only those marked * need a prescription.

15 *DRUGS WHICH STIMULATE BREATHING*

These are a group of life-saving drugs, given only by doctors and paramedics in certain emergency situations where the patient's breathing requires stimulation. These situations include anaesthetic overdose; drug overdose (suicide); cases of asphyxia and in newly born babies who are slow to breathe. Oxygen may be given at the same time.
Examples
Nikethamide, naloxone, doxapram.
Obtainable
On doctor's prescription only.

16 *DRUGS WHICH SUPPRESS AND SOOTHE COUGHS*

Doctors are sometimes reluctant to prescribe cough suppressants since coughing is a protective reflex which prevents infected spit and foreign substances from being inhaled and sucked by the respiratory process deep into the lungs. However, there is a large trade in cough medicine which can be bought over the counter. The benefit they give is doubtful.
Common examples
Codeine phosphate, pholcodine, many soothing linctuses containing syrup or glycerol. There are a great many commercial preparations, many with antihistamine and bronchodilators.

Precautions and side-effects
Drowsiness and constipation may follow excessive use. They should not be given to babies.
Obtainable
A chemist will advise on the cough suppressant to use, and provide it without prescription.

THE NERVOUS SYSTEM

Many drugs have been developed which act on the nervous system. Some of these are of great value, but with others the helpful effects must be carefully balanced against their negative side-effects.

Drugs are used to influence the nervous system in eight different ways: to treat insomnia and anxiety; to treat schizophrenia and similar serious mental disorders; to treat mental depression; to stimulate the nervous system and suppress appetite; to counter nausea and dizziness; to kill pain; to prevent fits; to counter muscle stiffness and tremor.

Sleeping-pills, sedatives and tranquillisers all increase the effects of alcohol, which should be avoided when taking these drugs.·

17 *DRUGS USED TO TREAT INSOMNIA AND ANXIETY*

Hypnotics (sleeping-pills)
These are used for people who have difficulty with sleeping. The same drugs, given in smaller doses, reduce anxiety, but all are addictive.

Common examples
Benzodiazepines (nitrazepam, temazepam) and chloral derivatives (chloral hydrate, triclofos) are the hypnotics now mainly prescribed. Antihistamines (promethazine, trimeprazine) are used for children. All sleeping-pills, including barbiturates such as amylobarbitone and a number of related drugs are now avoided where possible because of the dangers to patients of overdosage and dependence.
Precautions and side-effects
Wherever possible, hypnotics should not be taken for long periods of time. Whenever sleeping-pills are stopped, rebound insomnia—that is, several nights of broken sleep and an increase in dreaming—should be anticipated, even after short periods (three to seven days) of use. After taking any sleeping-pill, drowsiness and impaired judgment may affect driving and work the next day. The elderly and sufferers with severe heart, liver or kidney disease should avoid these drugs: their effects are unpredictable and may be cumulative.
Obtainable
Available on doctor's prescription only.

Sedatives, anxiolytics and tranquillisers
These are used for reducing anxiety and tension. Many drugs have been developed and most of them are similar to sleeping-pills but are given in lower doses. They carry the same risks of dependence as sleeping-pills and there is increasing evidence that their benefits may be outweighed by the long-term disadvantages of making sufferers permanently dependent on them.

Common examples
Benzodiazepines (diazepam, chlordiazepoxide, lorazepam, ketazolam, oxazepam); meprobamate, buspirone.
Precautions and side-effects
As for hypnotics (see preceding section).
Obtainable
Available on doctor's prescription only.

Beta-blockers
These block the effects of adrenaline on the body. Adrenaline is produced in large quantities in anxiety.
Common examples
Propranolol, atenolol.
Obtainable
On doctor's prescription only.

18 *DRUGS USED TO TREAT SERIOUS MENTAL DISORDERS (ANTIPSYCHOTICS)*

These drugs have enabled many thousands of individuals to live safely in the community instead of being confined in mental institutions. How the drugs act is still not certain. Many have a sedative effect, but combined with this they appear to block certain electrical impulses in the brain. This helps to reduce abnormal behaviour and prevent the delusions which are a marked feature of severe mental disease, such as schizophrenia. Long-term, continuous treatment is essential for their effect to be maintained. The danger of side-effects from these drugs is small compared with the benefits.
Common examples
Phenothiazines and related drugs: chlorpromazine (Largactil), benperidol, clozapine, droperidol, haloperidol, pimozide, promazine, thioridazine, trifluoperazine, flupenthixol, fluphenazine; lithium salts.
Precautions and side-effects
These drugs may cause unexpected facial or body movements and dryness of the mouth. Sudden falls in blood pressure with dizziness or even a faint may occur especially in the elderly. Medical supervision is essential. The patient's mental state may prevent the patient from taking the drugs correctly, and they may have to be injected.
Obtainable
Available on doctor's prescription only.

19 *DRUGS USED TO TREAT MENTAL DEPRESSION*

Most antidepressants act by modifying the frequency and extent of mood swings, but how they do this is not certain.

There are three major groups of drugs: tricyclics, monoamine-oxidase inhibitors (MAOI), which are less used because they may have dangerous interactions with foods such as cheese or chocolate, and serotonin uptake inhibitors.

Lithium salts (Camcolit, Liskonum, Phasal) are also used to damp down mood swings in manic-depressive illness.
Common examples
Tricyclics and related drugs: amitriptyline, imipramine (Tofranil); nortriptyline, mianserin. MAO inhibitors: phenelzine, isocarboxazid. Serotonin utake inhibitors: fluroxamine, paroxetine.

Precautions and side-effects
All these drugs may take two to three weeks before they are effective. They should be taken only under close medical supervision. They may affect the heart and cause disturbances of rhythm and falls in blood pressure. Dizziness, blurred vision, drowsiness, dry mouth, constipation and difficulty with passing urine may arise, but pass off if the drug is started gradually. In addition, the MAO inhibitors require special dietary instructions from the doctor.
Obtainable
Available on doctor's prescription only.

20 DRUGS USED TO STIMULATE THE NERVOUS SYSTEM AND SUPPRESS APPETITE

Mild stimulants, such as caffeine, are used to counter drowsiness or fatigue. Amphetamines and related drugs are usually no longer given to suppress the appetite of individuals who wish to lose weight, because of their dangerous side-effects, including dependence and in some instances suicidal depression. Wherever possible the treatment of obesity using appetite suppressants should be avoided. Amphetamines are helpful in narcolepsy.
Common examples
Modern appetite suppressants are either bulk-forming agents such as methylcellulose or sterculia (freely available) or centrally acting drugs such as *fenfluramine (on prescription only).
Precautions and side-effects
Mild stimulants have few side-effects, but equally, because they are mild,

they are of little benefit against drowsiness or fatigue.

21 DRUGS USED TO COUNTER NAUSEA AND DIZZINESS

These are effective in preventing needless disturbance of the balance mechanism as may occur in motion sickness, Ménière's disease and labyrinthitis.
Common examples
Antihistamines: cyclizine; cinnarizine, dimenhydrinate; *metoclopramide, promethazine.
Phenothiazines: *chlorpromazine; *prochlorperazine.
Precautions and side-effects
The dose required to control nausea is small and side-effects are few. Larger doses may cause drowsiness—a fact to be remembered if driving. Vomiting in pregnancy peaks in the first three months. This is the time when certain drugs can affect the baby, so avoid taking drugs to control vomiting in pregnancy if at all possible.
Obtainable
Those marked * need a prescription.

22 DRUGS USED AGAINST PAIN

Analgesics
These are usually divided into two main groups: non-addictive (non-narcotic) and addictive (narcotic).
The non-addictive group are less strong with relatively few dangers. They can be obtained by anyone and can be used with commonsense by any individual in pain. Most such preparations contain aspirin, para-cetamol or related compounds,

which also act to reduce fever.
The addictive group have more powerful painkilling capacity, but are more dangerous to use. They cannot be obtained without a doctor's prescription and must always be used with caution and never taken for long periods of time. This group includes all the opium, morphia, heroin and cocaine narcotics but also many other addictive but less dangerous pain-killers.
A third specialised group has also been developed for special use in migraine and neuralgia.
Common examples
Non-addictive: Aspirin and sodium salicylate compounds; paracetamol compounds; anti-inflammatory drugs such as ibuprofen.
Precautions and side-effects
All the aspirin compounds irritate the stomach and can cause bleeding from the stomach. Neutral aspirin should always be asked for and taken after food or with a glass of milk. Aspirin is not recommended for children under the age of 12. In heavy doses, ringing in the ears and nausea may develop.
Obtainable
At any chemist. Chemists will advise about what is suitable.
Common examples
Addictive: Codeine derivatives are only moderately addictive but must not be taken with alcohol.
Morphine derivatives—morphine, diamorphine (heroin), methadone, buprenorphine, dihydrocodeine, dextropropoxyphene, nalbuphine.
These drugs are all extremely addictive.
Precautions and side-effects
The painkilling capacity, the side-effects and the dangers of addiction all increase together. Drowsiness, nausea,

vomiting, constipation and deficient respiratory activity are all side-effects, the likelihood of which increases with the strength.
Note: The so-called codeine tablets which are sold without a doctor's pre-scription contain only a small, harm-less amount of codeine. Their main effect is from the added aspirin or paracetamol.
Obtainable
Available on doctor's prescription only, except for some mild codeine preparations.

Antimigraine and antineuralgia
A number of drugs have been developed which help to reduce and alleviate attacks of neuralgia and migraine but have little effect on other pain. They are used if ordinary (non-addictive) painkillers are ineffective. Some drugs are intended to prevent migraine or neuralgia, and are taken regularly. Others are taken as soon as there is any symptom of a migraine attack.
Common examples
Antimigraine: Ergot-containing drugs such as ergotamine; also: methysergide; propranolol, pizotifen.
Antineuralgic: Carbamazepine.
Precautions and side-effects
Drugs that contain ergot should not be used if the patient suffers from coronary or vascular disease, has high blood pressure, or is pregnant.
Obtainable
On doctor's prescription only.

23 DRUGS USED TO PREVENT FITS (ANTICONVULSANTS)

These drugs do not cure epilepsy, but they act by preventing fits. For this

reason prolonged treatment is usually required and dosages need careful adjustment to get maximum benefit and minimum side-effects.
Common examples
Phenobarbitone; methylphenobarbitone; phenytoin; carbamazepine; primidone; ethosuximide; clonazepam; sodium valproate; diazepam; vigabatrin.
Precautions and side-effects
Close medical supervision combined with full patient co-operation is essential. Dosage is often increased to the point just before side-effects appear. These may include drowsiness, balance and visual upsets, confusion, skin rashes, dizziness, headaches, nausea, and symptoms of anaemia. *Never attempt to give tablets during or after a fit.*
Obtainable
Available on doctor's prescription only.

24 *DRUGS USED TO COUNTER MUSCLE STIFFNESS AND TREMOR*

Antiparkinsonism drugs
These drugs act on the brain at the site of the disease not on the muscles. They do not cure the disease, but help to make a sufferer's life more bearable.
Common examples
Levodopa with carbidopa; amantadine; benzhexol; orphenadrine; bromocriptine; selegiline; lysuride.
Precautions and side-effects
Maximal effect must be balanced against possible side-effects. Close medical supervision is essential. The drugs should be avoided in many situations including pregnancy, chronic renal conditions and certain

eye diseases. Side-effects include nausea, dizziness and gastro-intestinal upsets.
Obtainable
Available on doctor's prescription only.

INFECTIONS BY MICRO-ORGANISMS

There are many different kinds and sizes of micro-organisms which infect the human body and cause disease, but not all are treatable with anti-infective drugs. There are two kinds of anti-infective agents: viricidal or bacteriocidal, which actually kill the organism, and viristatic or bacteriostatic, which prevent the organism from multiplying, but which require the body itself to kill the organism. In old people and those on immuno-suppressive drugs the body may be unable to kill the organism, so bacteriostatic or viristatic drugs may be ineffective. Anti-infective agents are divided up into five groups for use against five different infections: bacterial; fungal; virus; microscopic parasites; worms and visible parasites. The term antibiotic may be used for all such agents, but it is generally used only for antibacterials such as penicillin.

25 *DRUGS USED AGAINST BACTERIAL INFECTIONS*

Antibacterials
A large number of these have been developed in the last 40 years, and they have greatly reduced the harmful

effects of many previously serious bacterial infections, such as meningitis, pneumonia, gonorrhoea, syphilis and tuberculosis. Different drugs are effective against different bacteria.

The penicillins
The largest group have few side-effects and are effective against many different bacteria.
Common examples
Benzyl-, procaine- and phenoxymethyl-penicillin; amoxycillin; flucloxacillin; ampicillin; methicillin.
Precautions and side-effects
Diarrhoea. The most serious side-effect is penicillin allergy which, in mild cases, causes skin rashes but which, in severe cases, can be fatal. A person allergic to one of the penicillin group of medicines should not be given any other in the same group.
Obtainable
Available on doctor's prescription only.

Tetracyclines
These are effective against a wider range of bacteria than many penicillins.
Common examples
Tetracycline, chlortetracycline, doxycycline, oxytetracycline, minocycline.
Precautions and side-effects
Thrush and diarrhoea (sometimes serious) are common. The drugs stain children's teeth permanently. They should not be taken by children under 12 or by pregnant women.
Obtainable
On doctor's prescription only.

Antituberculous
A special group of antibiotics which, to be effective, must be taken in

maximum strength for many months.
Common examples
Streptomycin; rifampicin; isoniazid, ethambutol.
Precautions and side-effects
Side-effects are common and include skin rashes, upsets of vision and hearing, nausea and diarrhoea. Close co-operation with a doctor is required.
Obtainable
Available on doctor's prescription only.

Other specially developed antibacterials
These antibiotics are used in special situations, such as infections of the kidney and bladder—or if a previous antibiotic has caused sensitivity or become ineffective.
Common examples
Erythromycin; sulphonamides with trimethoprim; gentamicin, neomycin, cephalosporins, aminoglycosides, and metronidazole, which acts against bacteria and protozoa.
Precautions and side-effects
Skin rashes, nausea, diarrhoea are possible side-effects.
Obtainable
On doctor's prescription only.

26 *DRUGS USED AGAINST FUNGAL INFECTIONS (ANTIFUNGALS)*

These are used against several common fungus infections such as ringworm or thrush. Some may be given by mouth; others are applied locally.
Common examples
Amphotericin; terbinafine; fluconazole; itraconazole;

miconazole; clotrimazole; griseofulvin; nystatin.
Precautions and side-effects
When taken by mouth, they should not be used in pregnancy or if there is liver or kidney disease.
Obtainable
On doctor's prescription only.

27 *DRUGS USED AGAINST VIRUS INFECTIONS (ANTIVIRALS)*

Drug treatment of established virus infections is unsatisfactory. Interferon may be helpful in some infections, particularly HEPATITIS B, but it is not yet widely available except for research. At present the best protection against virus disease is by immunisation using a specific vaccine against the virus concerned. An injection of Gamma globulin may give a short period of protection.

Some antiviral drugs appear to depress virus activity in some cases. Idoxuridine if applied locally may help in shingles. Vidarabine may help in chickenpox and shingles. Amantadine may help in influenza and shingles. Acyclovir has been developed against cold sores, shingles, herpes eye infections, AIDS, and genital herpes. AZT also slows the progress of AIDS.

These drugs are only obtainable on a doctor's prescription and require close medical supervision.

28 *DRUGS USED AGAINST PARASITES VISIBLE ONLY BY MICROSCOPE*

Four important infections are caused by these microscopic parasites: malaria, amoebiasis, leishmaniasis and sleeping sickness. All four are essentially tropical diseases. Treatment is specialised and differs according to the place of occurrence as well as the nature and extent of the infection. Treatment for large populations is both expensive and tedious, and is therefore often unobtainable for poor developing countries. For each of these four infections a series of highly effective drugs, of which the following products are examples, has been developed.

Antimalarials
These include chloroquine, primaquine, proguanil, *pyrimethamine, *quinine.

Antiamoebics
These include *metronidazole (Flagyl).

Antileishmaniasis
These include *sodium stibogluconate.

Antitrypanosomiasis (sleeping sickness)
These drugs vary according to the type of organism responsible for the infection.

Apart from the above infections there are two harmless diseases which are caused by microscopic parasites and are not uncommon in all communities. These are giardiasis and vaginitis trichomonas. The same drug, *metronidazole, is used for both. Extent of treatment depends on laboratory tests. The drug is given by mouth, and requires medical supervision. Side-effects include rashes and nausea.
Obtainable
Those marked * need a prescription.

29 *DRUGS USED AGAINST WORMS AND VISIBLE PARASITES*

Many effective drugs have been developed but they usually require laboratory control, prolonged treatment and close patient co-operation. All these factors are expensive and often make it difficult or impossible for communities most in need to eliminate these diseases from their populations. Threadworms are an exception because they are common in all communities, their harmful effects are not great, and they can be easily treated by taking the advice of a chemist.
Common examples
For threadworms and roundworms:
Piperazine; mebendazole.
Precautions and side-effects
Side-effects are rare.
Obtainable
From any chemist.
Common examples
For other parasitic worms
(tapeworms, hookworms, schistosomiasis): piperazine; bephenium, niclosamide; mebendazole; pyrantel.
Precautions and side-effects
Special care must be taken if the sufferer from these parasitic worms is pregnant or chronically ill.
Obtainable
On doctor's prescription only.

THE ENDOCRINE SYSTEM

The secretions of the endocrine or ductless glands, once passed into the blood, function all over the body as hormones or chemical messengers. The bodily functions which they control include the use of energy, the pulse-rate, and many sexual and reproductive activities. Numerous drugs have been developed which act on the whole body either increasing or decreasing the quantity of a particular circulating hormone, and these have been divided into five groups: those which control diabetes; those which either stimulate or suppress thyroid activity; those which simulate the activity of the cortex of the adrenal glands; those which influence the sex glands; and finally the drugs which act on the pituitary gland.

30 *DRUGS USED TO CONTROL DIABETES*

Diabetes develops because the pancreatic hormone, insulin, which controls the body's use of glucose, is either lacking in the body or ineffective.

Insulin
In diabetes, giving insulin by injection is a crude way of achieving normal insulin levels. This is why diabetics have to be so careful about how much insulin they inject, and why doctors have developed many insulins which act at different speeds. Insulin is destroyed if taken by mouth and sufferers from diabetes have to take it by injection.
Common examples
Short-acting: neutral insulin (Human Actrapid).
Intermediate-acting: isophane protamine insulin (Humulin I).

Long-acting: insulin zinc suspension (Human Monotard).
Precautions and side-effects
Close medical supervision and full co-operation between patient and doctor are always essential. Most serious side-effects arise from inadvertent overdosage resulting in lowering of blood sugar to levels which cause sweating followed by abnormal 'drunken' behaviour and coma. These symptoms may develop within an hour or even minutes of an injection that has been incorrectly assessed. Diabetic sufferers who require insulin (and their relatives) should be fully aware of these dangers. If there are doubts, these should be discussed at once with the doctor or diabetic clinic. Such difficulties are especially likely if insulin injections are given at the wrong time of day, on an empty stomach or after a bout of exercise. Fever may upset the dosage of insulin required and should always be reported to a doctor.
Obtainable
Available on doctor's prescription only.

Other antidiabetic drugs
These act by increasing the effect of insulin, and are useful for diabetics who have developed diabetes in adult life or as a result of obesity.
Common examples
Sulphonylureas; tolbutamide; chlorpropamide; gliclazide; glibenclamide; glipizide; tolazamide; Biguanides: metformin.
Precautions and side-effects
Severe side-effects from sudden lowering of blood sugar levels are less likely with these drugs than with insulin, but their possibility means that close co-operation between patient and doctor is essential

for the patient's welfare.
Obtainable
Available on doctor's prescription only.

31 DRUGS WHICH STIMULATE OR SUPPRESS THYROID ACTIVITY

The thyroid hormone controls the rate and energy consumption of the heart and body tissues as a whole. It is essential for both mental and physical development.

Thyroid hormones
These drugs may be prepared from the thyroid of animals, or chemically synthesised. They are used in the treatment of myxoedema and cretinism.
Common examples
Thyroxine; liothyronine.
Precautions and side-effects
These may cause flushing, sweating, palpitations and anginal pain, and should be avoided by people with heart diseases.
Obtainable
Available on doctor's prescription only.

Antithyroids
These act by depressing the activities of the thyroid gland and are used in hyperthyroid states.
Common examples
Iodine; carbimazole; thiouracil compounds.

32 DRUGS WHICH SIMULATE THE ADRENAL HORMONES

These hormones help the body to utilise essential foods, deal with

infection and allow a normal response to stress.

Corticosteroids
These synthetic hormones are used to treat Addison's disease, certain chronic inflammatory diseases such as rheumatoid arthritis, polymyalgia and asthma, and many diseases of the skin.
Common examples
Betamethasone; cortisone acetate; methyl prednisolone; dexamethasone; hydrocortisones; prednisone; triamcinolone.
Precautions and side-effects
When given by mouth or injection, these drugs have many powerful effects. They may have to be increased if there is any acute infection and should never be stopped without consulting a doctor. When used as skin applications, only small amounts are absorbed through the skin, and such precautions are then unnecessary. The risks of taking the drugs must always be balanced against their advantages. Raised blood pressure, diabetes, 'moon face', softening of the bones, and depression are a few of the more serious possible side-effects. Close co-operation between patient and doctor is vital. In children and the elderly such drugs are used only if essential.
Obtainable
Available on doctor's prescription only.

33 DRUGS WHICH INFLUENCE THE ACTIVITIES OF THE SEX GLANDS

The sex hormones control the manufacture of ova and sperms. They also influence the periods and

affect premenstrual tension. *See page 436.*

The contraceptive pill
Female sex hormones consist of oestrogens, which prepare the womb each month for a possible pregnancy, and progestogens, which modify the effects of the oestrogens and assist the progress of pregnancy if conception takes place. Acting together these hormones control the process of ovulation and conception in the female. They are used either in combination or separately as the contraceptive pill, and also to treat menopausal symptoms, dysmenorrhoea, vaginitis, osteo-porosis, endometriosis and abnor-malities of menstruation. Occasionally they are effective in suppressing certain types of prostate and breast cancer.
Precautions and side-effects
Research in the United States and Britain has suggested that certain types of oral contraceptive may, if taken over prolonged periods of time, play a part in causing BREAST CANCER. The harmful effects of the pill are more likely to arise if the woman is over 35, smokes, is obese or suffers from diabetes or hypertension (raised blood pressure). Many other drugs used by doctors may interact with the contraceptive pill, so always tell your doctor that you are taking it, if he prescribes other drugs for you.
Obtainable
On doctor's prescription only.

Hormone replacement therapy (HRT)
Oestrogen, sometimes with progestogen, is taken by mouth or via skin patches to relieve symptoms such as hot flushes and vaginal dryness, and to reduce the risk of OSTEOPOROSIS,

HEART ATTACK and STROKE. HRT usually causes regular vaginal bleeding to continue beyond the menopause, and may slightly increase the risk of BREAST CANCER.
Common examples
Prempak-C, Estraderm, Premarin.
Obtainable
On doctor's prescription only.

Male sex hormones
These all have masculinising effects. They may occasionally make muscles stronger, deepen the voice, increase sweating and stimulate hair growth. Their use in medicine is limited; they do not help males who are impotent or have diminished sperm activity. They are dangerous for both sexes if taken to increase sporting prowess.
Common examples
Testosterones; anabolic steroids.
Precautions and side-effects
Breast enlargement, unwanted weight gain and facial changes may occur.
Obtainable
Available on doctor's prescription only.

34 *DRUGS WHICH INCREASE THE EFFECTS OF THE PITUITARY GLAND*

These are hormone preparations obtained from animals and are used to stimulate growth (pituitary) and other endocrine glands in the human body. They may be used to treat infertility and, occasionally, special cases of asthma, short stature, and in labour.
Common examples
Gonadotrophin; corticotrophin; growth hormone; lypressin;

vasopressin; clomiphene.
Precautions and side-effects
When used to treat infertility in women, twins and triplets are a possible effect of the drugs.
Obtainable
On doctor's prescription only.

BODY CELLS

A number of highly specialised drugs have been developed to suppress the growth of cancer cells (cytotoxic drugs) and to suppress the development of cellular immunity (immuno-suppressive drugs).

35 *DRUGS USED TO SUPPRESS CELLULAR ACTIVITY AND GROWTH*

Cytotoxic drugs
These act by slowing up the division and growth of all cells. They have to be taken over long periods, have many dangers, and require very close co-operation between patient and doctor. Because many cancer cells divide and grow much more than healthy cells, these drugs can be used to suppress some cancers. Cytotoxic drugs also affect healthy cells, so there are many unpleasant side-effects as well as considerable danger of destroying healthy as well as cancer cells. In Hodgkin's disease and a few other cancers a complete cure is becoming increasingly common, particularly in the young.

Immunosuppressive drugs
These are used to suppress the immune process of cellular rejection by which the human body destroys foreign cells. Their uses include the prevention of rejection in transplant surgery. But while these drugs may prevent a kidney or other transplanted organ from being rejected by the body, at the same time they also suppress the body's power to destroy harmful foreign cells such as bacteria or viruses. The benefits of such drugs must, therefore, be very carefully weighed against their dangers. This is a highly skilled medical decision. Like cytotoxic drugs, immunosuppressives have to be taken over long periods, have many dangers, and require very close co-operation between patient and doctor.

DIET

Minerals and vitamins that are essential to the body may be absent from a diet which is otherwise adequate. Deficiency of iron is a common cause of anaemia, but diseases due to a deficiency of any of the vitamins are rare in developed countries. Vitamin A deficiency causes a rare night blindness; vitamin B deficiency causes beri-beri and pellagra, both rare diseases; vitamin B_{12} deficiency causes pernicious anaemia; vitamin C deficiency causes scurvy; vitamin D deficiency causes rickets and poor bone structure. Vitamin E has not been shown to cure deficiency diseases or any other conditions in humans.

36 *DRUGS REQUIRED TO SUPPLEMENT DEFICIENT DIETS*

Iron supplements
These are given by mouth or injection, usually for iron deficiency caused by excessive blood loss.

Common examples
Ferrous sulphate, ferrous gluconate, ferrous fumarate.

Precautions and side-effects
Nausea, diarrhoea and constipation are all common side-effects. Colicky abdominal pain may be noticed but is rarely severe. Motions are always coloured grey or black. Adult doses of iron are harmful to children, and tablets should be kept well out of their reach. Taken before conception and in early pregnancy, Pregnavite Forte F may reduce the risk to the child of spina bifida.

Obtainable
Some on any chemist's advice, without prescription.

Vitamins
Unless taken in excess, these have few side-effects and are frequently included in commercial preparations and sold as tonics. Unless there is clear evidence or likelihood of possible deficiency, as in pregnancy, they are unlikely to do much good because the diet of the taker in most developed countries will be adequate.

Common examples
Vitamin A (cod liver oil and similar preparations).
Vitamin B. Vitamin B_{12} deficiency causes PERNICIOUS ANAEMIA.

Vitamin C (ascorbic acid).
Vitamin D and calcium (cod liver oil; calciferol).
Vitamin E (tocopherol).
Special dietary supplements may also be needed in certain diseases which limit food absorption. These include steatorrhea and coeliac disease.
Precautions and side-effects
Taken in excess, most vitamins can be poisonous.
Obtainable
From any chemist, without a prescription.

MUSCLES AND JOINTS

A great many drugs have been developed for the treatment of diseased muscles and joints. They do not cure the disease and how they act is not fully understood, but their value in reducing pain and damage in the affected joint is undoubted.

37 DRUGS USED TO TREAT DISEASED MUSCLES AND JOINTS BY REDUCING INFLAMMATION

Antirheumatic or anti-inflammatory
These are not antibiotics, but act by reducing inflammation in diseases such as rheumatoid arthritis, osteo-arthritis and gout. Their anti-inflammatory effect appears to be separate from their painkilling effect.
Common examples
Aspirin and other salicylates (benorylate).
Other anti-inflammatory drugs:

ibuprofen, diclofenac, diflunisal, fenoprofen, flurbiprofen, naproxen, indomethacin, mefenamic acid, tenoxicam, piroxicam. Many corticosteroids (*see* MEDICINES, 32). Chloroquine.
Anti-inflammatory drugs prescribed for gout: colchicine, allopurinol, probenecid, sulphinpyrazone.
Precautions and side-effects
Most of these drugs irritate the stomach and may cause bleeding from the stomach and indigestion. They should be used with caution in the elderly, and if there is asthma, duodenal or gastric ulcer, liver disease or anaemia. The dose prescribed should never be exceeded and prolonged use avoided whenever possible. The well-tried aspirin-related drugs may be more effective, cheaper and safer than those introduced more recently.
Obtainable
On doctor's prescription only, except in the case of Ibuprofen and the aspirin and salicylate group, obtainable from any chemist.

THE EYE

Many preparations have been developed in the form of eye drops for the treatment of various eye conditions. A useful method of giving eye drops is to lay the patient flat on his back and to place one or two drops in the inner corner of the affected eye while it is closed. Wait a few seconds, and then pull down the lower lid to distribute the drug over the eyeball.

38 DRUGS USED TO TREAT BACTERIAL AND VIRUS INFECTIONS

Watering of the eye may dilute these drugs when used as drops, and eye ointments are sometimes used.
Common examples
Chloramphenicol; fusidic acid tetracycline; framycetin; gentamicin; neomycin; sulphacetamide; antiviral eye drops used in cold sores include idoxuridine, vidarabine and acyclovir (Zovirax).
Precautions and side-effects
Many eye drops contain corticosteroids which may aggravate an underlying corneal ulcer or glaucoma, therefore *never* use eye drops which have been prescribed for another person or for a previous eye condition.
Obtainable
Available on doctor's prescription only.

39 DRUGS USED TO TREAT CHRONIC EYE INFLAMMATION, REDUCE INTERNAL EYE PRESSURE AND DILATE OR CONTRACT THE PUPIL

All these drugs can be helpful if they are used correctly, but can be harmful to the eye if used incorrectly, therefore extra care must be taken in using them.
Common examples
Betamethasone, atropine; homatropine; pilocarpine; neostigmine.
Precautions and side-effects
Never use eye drops which have been prescribed for another individual or

for a previous eye condition.
Obtainable
Available on doctor's prescription only.

THE EAR, NOSE, MOUTH AND THROAT

40 DRUGS ACTING LOCALLY ON THE EAR TO TREAT INFECTION AND SOFTEN WAX

These are of three types: those for localised eczema of the ear hole (otitis externa); local applications for any chronic infected discharge from the middle ear (otitis media); applications for removing wax.
For eczema or chronic ear infection the following drugs are used. Most of them are corticosteroids, antibiotics or mixtures of these.
Common examples
Aluminium acetate; betamethasone; chloramphenicol; gentamicin; tetracycline and compound preparations. For removal of wax from the ear: olive oil, almond oil, bicarbonate ear drops.
Precautions and side-effects
Some preparations for dissolving wax may cause irritation and are rarely effective—none of these is mentioned above. Any ear drops which cause pain, irritation or aggravate symptoms should be stopped and further medical advice sought. All drops initially may cause temporary deafness.
Obtainable
Many of the above preparations are obtainable only on doctor's prescription.

41 DRUGS ACTING LOCALLY ON THE NOSE

These usually act by reducing congestion and allergic reactions—rhinitis, nasal polyp, hay fever. Many such drops contain an added antibiotic or antihistamine.
Common examples
Corticosteroids: betamethasone, budesonide, beclomethasone, sodium cromoglycate.
Decongestants: ephedrine, oxymetazoline.
Antibacterials.
Precautions and side-effects
Most decongestants should not be used for more than seven days at a time, because they can damage the nostril lining and cause the nose to become more congested and blocked. Corticosteroids, however, should be used regularly for more than seven days.
Obtainable
Only a few of these preparations are obtainable without a doctor's prescription.

42 DRUGS ACTING LOCALLY ON THE MOUTH AND THROAT

These usually act by protecting, soothing or numbing and helping to heal sore spots in the mouth, thus enabling the sufferer to eat. Some preparations contain corticosteroids or antibiotics, others aim to combine all these effects.
Common examples
Benzocaine; salicylates; phenols; thymols; Bioral, Adcortyl, Corlan, Bonjela, Teejel, Peralvex, Orabase, Orahesive, Fungilin, Dequadin, Labosept, Daktarin, Nystan, Anaflex,

Bradosol, Faringets, Hibitane, Strepsils, Tonsillin, Merocets, Tyrosolven, Tyrozets, Betadine, Bocasan.
Precautions and side-effects
Few, but benefits are extremely variable and often a question of personal choice.
Obtainable
Many of these preparations are obtainable without a doctor's prescription.

THE SKIN

Some drugs used in skin conditions act by reducing inflammation, irritation and infection. Others act locally on psoriasis, warts and acne. In all instances two side-effects must be borne in mind; the active ingredient may be absorbed through the skin and have a more widespread effect; the body may develop a general sensitivity to the application and a widespread skin rash and bodily reaction may develop. If any application appears to make a skin condition worse, stop using it at once and consult a doctor. As a general rule, skin creams are more acceptable, but ointments are better for dry skin.

43 DRUGS ACTING LOCALLY ON THE SKIN

Anti-inflammatory applications
These also reduce itching and are extensively used to treat eczema. They are often combined with an

antibiotic to reduce bacterial infection.
Common examples
Corticosteroids (Alphaderm, Calmurid HC, Cobadex, Cortacream, Dioderm, Dome-Cort, Efcortelan, Hydro-Cortisyl, Propaderm, Betnovate, Dermovate, Eumovate, Tridesilon, Nerisone, Temetex, Topilar, Synalar, Synandone, Metosyn, Ultradil, Vioform HC, Ultralanum, Locoid, Adcortyl, Ledercort). Other preparations include: aluminium potassium; permanganate; silver nitrate; zinc oxide; lassar's paste; Viscopaste.
Precautions and side-effects
Stop using the drugs and report to the doctor if application aggravates the condition.
Obtainable
Many of the above are obtainable only on a doctor's prescription.

Antipruritics
These are used to reduce the irritation of itching.
Common examples
Calomine. Local anaesthetic: Xylocaine. Given by mouth (trimoprazine, chlorpheniramine, torfenadine).
Precautions and side-effects
There are few side-effects.
Obtainable
From chemist, without prescription.

Preparations for psoriasis and eczema
Many of the anti-inflammatory preparations above are highly effective against both psoriasis and eczema. Sometimes a plastic cover is also used to increase their effect.
Other common examples
Coal tar preparations (Carbo-Dome, Coltapaste, Alphosyl, Polytar, Psoriderm, Tarband); dithranols

(Dithrolan, Psoradrate, Exolan)—these may stain the skin. Ichthammols (Ichthopaste, Icthaband). Creams containing salicylic acid and urea.
Precautions and side-effects
Stop using and report to the doctor if the application aggravates the condition.
Obtainable
Many on doctor's prescription only.

Preparations for warts and corns
These act by dissolving the skin and therefore may leave a small ulcer after application. The ulcer should then heal to leave normal skin.
Common examples
Podophyllum resin (Posalfilin); salicylic acid (Callusolve, Veracur, Glutarol).
Precautions and side-effects
Apply under dressing to affected area of skin only. Do not apply to normal skin.
Obtainable
From chemist, without prescription.

Preparations for acne
Acne is often best treated generally with antibiotics by mouth, and with sunlight and diet. Local applications are less effective but may help.
Common examples
Preparations containing resorcinal sulphur, benzoyl, aluminium oxide (Acetoxyl, Acnegel, Benoxyl, Panoxyl, Brasivol, Ionax, Retin-A, Eskamel), and many other mixed preparations containing antibiotics and Corticosteroids or the vitamin A derivative tretinoin (Retin-A).
Precautions and side-effects
Stop using and report to the doctor if application aggravates the condition.
Obtainable
Many can be obtained direct from a

chemist, others require a doctor's prescription.

Protective applications

These include sunscreens and barrier creams. The most effective sunscreens are those which act as a barrier to ultra-violet light (Uvistat and Spectraban). These may also prevent a tan from developing. Silicone creams (dimethicone) by repelling water help to protect against chemical skin irritants. For cosmetic purposes also there are many creams which simply cover or camouflage some facial disfigurements.

Precautions and side-effects
There are few side-effects.
Obtainable
On any chemist's advice, without prescription.

Antiseptic cleansing preparations and shampoos

Common examples
Cetrimide and similar preparations (Cetavlon, Cetavlex, Brulidine, Hibitane, Roccal, Rotersept, Dettol, Ster-Zac, Betadine, Merthiolate). Surgical spirit and spirit soaps are effective for dandruff (Lenium, Selsun).
Precautions and side-effects
There are few side-effects.
Obtainable
From any chemist, without prescription.

Anti-infectives

These are antibiotic preparations. They are divided into four groups: antibacterials, used for impetigo and many other skin conditions in which there is evidence of added bacterial infection; antifungals, used for ringworm; antivirals, used for cold sores; and antiparasitics, used for lice and scabies.

Common examples
Antibacterial paints and creams: brilliant green and crystal violet, Castellani's paint, Chloromycetin, Aureomycin, Framygen, Sofra-Tulle, Fucidin, Cidomycin, Genticin, Neomycin, Myciguent, Sulfamylon, Furacin, Anaflex, Ponoxylan.
Antifungals: Benzoic acid, Whitfield's ointment, Fungilin, Mycil, Canesten, Ecostatin, Pevaryl, Daktarin, Dermonistat, Pimafucin, Nystan, Multilind, Tinaderm, Tineafax.
Antivirals: Idoxuridine (Herpid), acyclovir.
Antiparasitics: Benzyl benzoate (Ascabiol, Derbac, Lorexane, Quellada, Prioderm, Tetmosol).
Precautions and side-effects
Few apart from the occasional skin sensitivity.
Obtainable
Antibacterials require a doctor's prescription.

THE FAMILY MEDICINE KIT
Treatment at home for cuts and grazes

A home medical kit is mainly intended for minor injuries and illnesses that you can treat yourself. But it should also be equipped to deal with emergencies and more serious injuries until the victim is seen by a doctor or taken to hospital. *See* FIRST AID.

Because of the possibility of such an emergency it is advisable to have the telephone number of your doctor—and the address of the accident and emergency department of your nearest hospital—written on a piece of paper and fixed to the inside of the kit.

It is also useful to include a brief medical record of each member of your family, giving their allergies, listing any drugs they are already taking and stating their previous illnesses.

Where to keep the kit

Many people keep their medical kit in the bathroom cabinet, but bathrooms can be damp and subject to pronounced changes in temperature. This may affect the strength and durability of some medications.

It is preferable to store the kit in a well-sealed plastic or metal box, which is kept on the highest shelf in the hall cupboard, or in the main bedroom. By keeping the kit in a portable box, it can be taken on family outings or holidays.

Medical kits should always be kept out of reach of children. If you do decide on the traditional wall cabinet, make sure it has either a childproof catch or a lock and key, and that the adults in the family know where the key is kept.

'Short life' of medicines

Even if you store medicines and dressings in a cool, dry and ventilated place, they will not remain in prime condition indefinitely. Certain medicines, including travel-sickness pills and antiseptic cream, have an effective life of less than three years. In Britain and some other countries the expiry date is printed on the labels of some pharmaceutical products.

If the drug's shelf-life is longer than three years—as in the case of foil-wrapped, soluble aspirin—no expiry date is given. Unless other painkillers, such as non-soluble aspirin and paracetamol, are kept in a dry atmosphere in tightly closed containers they can deteriorate after a year, giving a sour, 'vinegary' smell. Cough linctus must also be kept tightly capped. As a general guideline, most family medicines should have an effective life of around a year.

If bottles of patent medicines, such as calamine lotion for sunburn and kaolin-and-morphine mixture for diarrhoea, settle out and do not respond to a rapid shaking, settlement has gone too far and they are no longer effective. Even such standard dressings as adhesive plasters may deteriorate after about two years.

The rule is: when in doubt, throw it out. This particularly applies to any drug and medicines left over from a prescribed course of treatment. These should be flushed down the lavatory, or returned to the chemist. You should *never* pass on to other people medicines that have been prescribed for you.

What to keep in the kit
The most common family ailments are cuts and grazes, splinters, headaches, coughs, indigestion, sunburn, insect bites and stomach upsets. All these can be treated from the basic medical kit which follows. By adding a few extras, you can also deal with toothache, temporary constipation, diarrhoea, strained muscles and travel sickness.

BASIC CONTENTS

□ **Adhesive plaster strips**
Rolls of various widths, for securing or applying dressings.

□ **Antiseptic cream**
Use on cuts and grazes and cover with a dressing. Do not apply cream to burns or scalds.

□ **Antiseptic lotion, or foil-wrapped antiseptic wraps**
For cleaning wounds.

□ **Bandages**
Also used to protect lint dressings. Two rolls 1 in. (25 mm.) wide will meet most needs. A roll of crêpe bandage is useful for awkward shapes such as hands and feet.

□ **Calamine lotion**
For insect bites, bee and wasp stings, nettlerash and sunburn.

□ **Elastic plasters (waterproof)**
A pack of assorted sizes, for small cuts and grazes.

□ **Pain-relieving tablets**
Aspirin or paracetamol. Aspirin should not be given to children under 12.

□ **Safety-pins**
Assorted sizes, for securing bandages.

□ **Scissors**
Blunt-ended, for cutting bandages and dressings.

□ **Sodium bicarbonate**
For relieving indigestion. This should not be taken regularly as—after its beneficial effect has worn off—it can produce stomach acid.

□ **Sterilised lint dressings**
Various sizes; two large and four medium should meet most needs.

□ **Thermometer**
To protect against possible breakage this is best kept in a metal or plastic tube. Normal body temperature is 98.4° Fahrenheit. Thermometers are now marked in centigrade, and the equivalent normal body temperature is 37.0°.

□ **Tweezers**
Square-ended, for removing splinters or thorns.

□ **Eye-bath**
Use with warm water to wash dirt or dust from the eye.

USEFUL EXTRAS

□ **Cotton wool**
Can be used for cleaning wounds, or as a dressing for a sprained ankle, when held in place by a bandage.

□ **Kaolin-and-morphine mixture**
For relieving diarrhoea.

□ **Methyl salicylate ointment**
For easing pain and spasms in strained or bruised muscles.

□ **Milk of Magnesia or Dulcolax**
For relieving constipation and heartburn.

□ **Oil of cloves**
Paint on an aching tooth to give temporary relief.

□ **Sterilised eye-pad**
For covering an infected eye.

□ **Sterilised finger dressing**
Can be applied as a finger-stall with its own bandage.

□ **Sterilised white absorbent gauze**
Use dry to cover a small wound and use wet for cleansing.

□ **Travel-sickness tablets**
Take about 30 minutes before starting a journey, or as directed.

MENINGITIS

An infection of the meninges (the fine membranes that surround the brain and spinal cord). The symptoms are similar in all types, but the severity of symptoms and seriousness of complications depend on the nature of the infecting organism. Viral infections occur in little epidemics, but do not usually cause complications or brain damage. Bacterial infections are rarer, and are more likely to affect children. The commonest type is meningococcal meningitis, also known as cerebrospinal fever. Infections of the bacteria of TUBERCULOSIS cause a disease with less acute symptoms, but it may be fatal unless treated. All the bacterial infections respond to antibiotics and early diagnosis is therefore vital.

Symptoms
The symptoms are similar for all types, and may include:
• Headache, often very severe.
• Painful stiff neck or back.
• Inability to put the head between the knees.
• A rash of tiny, red-purple spots or bruises.
• Vomiting, which may be very severe.
• High temperature.
• Intolerance to bright lights.
• Drowsiness or confusion.
• Small children may have only fever and appear ill. Newborn babies may not even have a fever, and diagnosis can be difficult. The soft spots (fontanelles) on a baby's skull may be swollen and tense.

Incubation period
• The disease is picked up from close contact with a person who is carrying the organism without necessarily having the disease. The incubation period may be from two days to three weeks.

Causes
• Bacteria.
• Many viruses, including those responsible for MUMPS and COLD SORES.

Complications
• Brain damage or EPILEPSY can occasionally occur, particularly if the meningitis is caused by bacteria.

Treatment in the home
• None. Call the doctor immediately if you suspect meningitis.

What the doctor may do
• Send the patient to hospital for treatment.
• Prescribe antibiotics or other drugs if the patient has a bacterial form of meningitis. *See* MEDICINES, 25.
• If the meningitis is caused by a virus no specific

ROUND-THE-CLOCK WATCH ON LIFE
How an intensive therapy unit operates

Severe injury, major surgery or serious illness may all leave the patient in need of round-the-clock medical attention. It is the role of the intensive therapy unit, sometimes called intensive care unit or I.C.U., to provide this attention. Each patient in the unit is connected to a battery of electronic equipment which is used to measure the body's vital functions and to support them if necessary. A nurse is in constant attendance to monitor the equipment, observe the patient and intervene when necessary.

The machines employed in the unit vary from hospital to hospital and according to the patient's condition, but two are found in most—the electrocardiograph and the artificial ventilator. The electrocardiograph gives continuous information on the patient's heart rate and rhythms. If a dangerous abnormality occurs in these the nurse can use an emergency alarm to call the doctor to give appropriate treatment. Sometimes the doctor may use a defibrillator—a machine which gives a carefully measured electric shock to the heart muscle in order to restore it to a regular beat. An artificial ventilator helps the patient to breathe, by intermittently blowing a mixture of air and oxygen into the lungs.

In addition, most units have machines to monitor the pressure in the patient's arteries or veins. They are linked to small tubes inserted into the blood vessels—usually at the wrist for an artery and in the neck or chest for a vein. Drip-feeds are used to replace lost blood or body fluids, or to feed the patient intravenously. Gastric juices may be drained from the stomach through a special tube which is usually inserted via the nose, and secretions from the lungs are removed through a suction tube which is introduced into the windpipe from time to time.

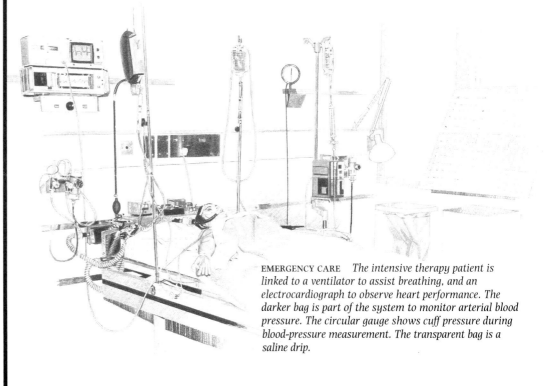

EMERGENCY CARE *The intensive therapy patient is linked to a ventilator to assist breathing, and an electrocardiograph to observe heart performance. The darker bag is part of the system to monitor arterial blood pressure. The circular gauge shows cuff pressure during blood-pressure measurement. The transparent bag is a saline drip.*

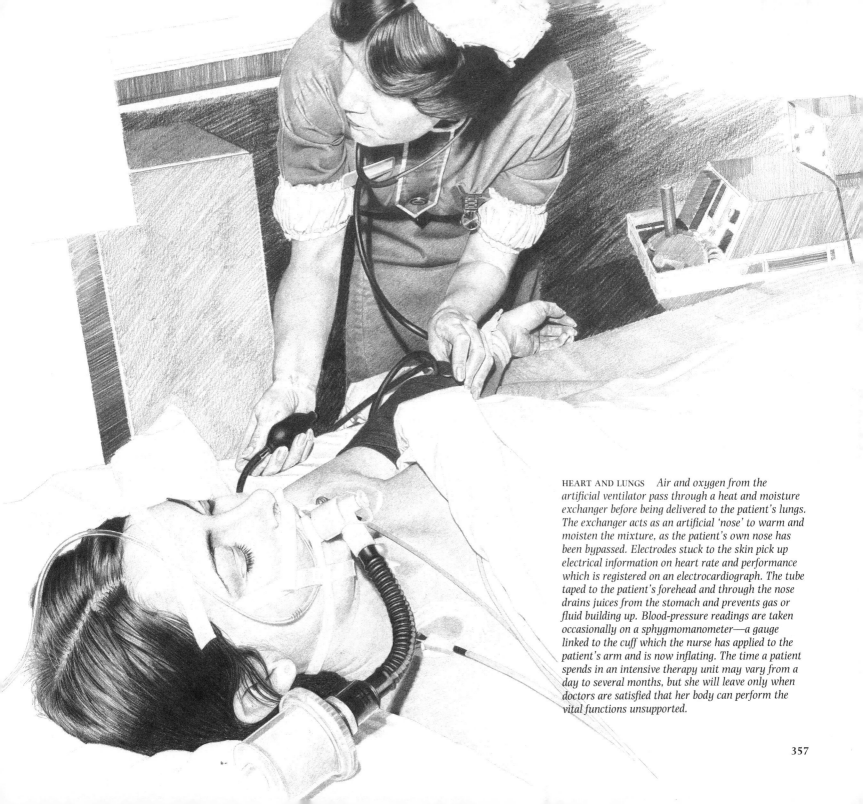

HEART AND LUNGS *Air and oxygen from the artificial ventilator pass through a heat and moisture exchanger before being delivered to the patient's lungs. The exchanger acts as an artificial 'nose' to warm and moisten the mixture, as the patient's own nose has been bypassed. Electrodes stuck to the skin pick up electrical information on heart rate and performance which is registered on an electrocardiograph. The tube taped to the patient's forehead and through the nose drains juices from the stomach and prevents gas or fluid building up. Blood-pressure readings are taken occasionally on a sphygmomanometer—a gauge linked to the cuff which the nurse has applied to the patient's arm and is now inflating. The time a patient spends in an intensive therapy unit may vary from a day to several months, but she will leave only when doctors are satisfied that her body can perform the vital functions unsupported.*

treatment is usually necessary. *See* MEDICINES, 22.
Prevention
• Babies are usually immunised against HiB meningitis in their first year of life.
• Immunisation against meningitis is now possible for certain other people, such as travellers. Consult your doctor. Family contacts of patients with meningococcal meningitis may be given antibiotics in case they are carriers.
Outlook
• Most cases recover provided bacterial infections are diagnosed early and treated promptly.

See INFECTIOUS DISEASES *page 32*

MENINGOCELE
A protrusion of the meninges, the membranes surrounding the spinal cord, through a gap in the bones of the spine, leaving them covered only with thin skin. This is one of the main forms of SPINA BIFIDA. Children born with it need immediate surgery to protect the meninges.

Do's and don'ts about the change

☐ *Do* regard the change as a normal, healthy phase of your life.

☐ *Do* share any worries you may have about it with your husband, or with an understanding friend or relative.

☐ *Do* regard it as an appropriate time to increase outside interests.

☐ *Do* report early any irregular or abnormal vaginal loss of blood, or discharge, to your doctor.

☐ *Do* ask your doctor if you are not sure whether your change is complete.

☐ *Don't* let it interfere with your life and sexual activities.

☐ *Don't* be afraid to ask your doctor about any worries you may have.

MENOPAUSE

The time in a woman's life when the ovaries become less responsive to the pituitary gland, the egg-producing cells begin to disappear, and oestrogen production falls. The menopause, often called the change of life, or the climacteric, is a normal and inevitable event for every woman. The change is rarely for the worse, and for many women it is for the better, because once complete, fears of pregnancy are removed.

The change may begin at any time between the late 30s and late 50s, but for most women the transition occurs during the 40s. The changes are not abrupt and often the gradual lessening of menstrual and ovarian activity lasts for several years.

Less than a quarter of all women going through the menopause have symptoms that are upsetting enough to need medical help. The main symptom for which help is sought is the hot flush, which accounts for 70 per cent of visits to the doctor. This is followed by depression (40 per cent), sweating (30 per cent), abnormal periods (25 per cent), insomnia (25 per cent), fatigue (20 per cent), hair and skin changes (15 per cent), and headache (10 per cent). There are, for most women, some psychological adjustments to be made and these need to be understood.

The implications of the change may be disturbing to a woman's self confidence and are often associated with other symptoms of ANXIETY, which are natural, but unfounded. For instance, there is no evidence that women age more quickly or become less attractive after the change. Surveys suggest that in at least 80 per cent of women, sexual responsiveness is either increased or remains unchanged. Sexual relations should not be restricted and contraceptive precautions should be continued until the change is complete. If you are uncertain about whether your change is complete, you should ask your doctor.

The menopause alters a woman's susceptibility to some diseases. Pre-menopausal women have lower rates of heart disease than men, but this protection is lost after the menopause, so it becomes more important to avoid the risk of CORONARY THROMBOSIS and STROKE. One of the most serious effects of the menopause is loss of bone strength (OSTEOPOROSIS), which can cause hip fractures in later life. To prevent this, some doctors give hormone replacement therapy (HRT) to menopausal women.

HRT is also useful for women who suffer hot flushes (*see* MEDICINES, 33), and sometimes anxiety, DEPRESSION or physical symptoms may be helped. Sometimes, too,

there is dryness of the vagina which may respond to local treatment with oestrogen cream. If there is irregular or abnormal bleeding at this time it must always be reported early to a doctor.

The flushes and sweats associated with the change may persist for a year or so after the periods have stopped. They can usually be helped with treatment and are therefore less upsetting than the less easily treated depression.

Management of the menopause should involve full recognition and understanding by the woman herself, and this recognition should extend to the woman's family, especially her husband, and doctor, whose understanding support can often be of great help.

See FEMALE GENITAL SYSTEM *page 48*

MENTAL AGE
A person's mental age is measured by comparing his mental ability with the age of an average person of the same mental ability. For example, an eight year old who has the same mental ability as an average ten year old has a mental age of ten. Measurement is done by specially devised intelligence tests.

The IQ (intelligence quotient) of a child is measured by multiplying his mental age by 100, then dividing it by his calendar age. For example, a ten year old who has the mental age of a twelve year old has an IQ of 120.

It should be stressed that there are many vital aspects of 'intelligence' which it is impossible to measure. Many individuals with a low IQ have great common sense, for example.

See MENTAL SYSTEM *page 33*

MENTAL SUBNORMALITY
A general name for all conditions in which the brain fails to develop normally, and this results in limited intelligence. Severely subnormal children usually need full-time care in a special home or hospital from an early age. Less severely handicapped children can live at home but will require special schooling.

Adults with mild mental subnormality (an IQ of between 60-70 compared to the normal IQ of 100) can live in the community, if given some extra help and support.

There is no recognised cause for the condition, but it may be due to an injury at birth, or some genetic abnormality. Very occasionally the trouble is due to mental illness, but sufferers from mental subnormality do not suffer especially from other mental illness.

The condition is lifelong and not reversible by medical treatment. In some cases the sufferer may slowly learn

skills and be able to do simple things for himself.
See MENTAL SYSTEM *page 33*
CHILD CARE—FIRST MONTHS *page 141*

MESENTERIC ADENITIS

Inflammation of glands in the abdominal cavity causing stomach pain, sometimes severe enough to mimic APPENDICITIS. The condition chiefly affects children and is sometimes associated with acute TONSILLITIS.
Symptoms
• Abdominal pain and tenderness, usually centred over the navel.
• Often a raised temperature and sometimes vomiting, a cold or sore throat.
Duration
• Three to ten days.
Causes
• Probably a viral infection.
Treatment in the home
• Rest, though not necessarily in bed.
• Drink plenty of fluids. Do not give painkillers.
When to consult the doctor
• If abdominal pain persists for more than four hours.
• If, as well as feeling pain, the child seems unduly ill or vomits a great deal.
What the doctor may do
• Examine the child to rule out appendicitis.
• Possibly take a urine sample to test for infection.
• Advise taking rest and fluids.
Prevention
• None.
Outlook
• Excellent. The condition clears up completely and leaves no after-effects. However, similar further attacks would suggest the presence of appendicitis.

See DIGESTIVE SYSTEM *page 44*

METATARSALGIA

Pain across the ball of the foot. The condition usually affects both feet. Metatarsalgia is common in middle-aged, overweight women.

Symptoms
• The front of the foot is abnormally flattened, with the toes slightly spread out.
• The pain is more pronounced during walking.
• The muscles of the foot become weak.
• A tender callus may form on the sole of the foot, just behind the middle toes.
• Symptoms develop suddenly or over several months.
Duration
• The pain is slow to respond to treatment and can last for many months at a time.
Causes
• Tight-fitting shoes.
• Inadequate exercise which weakens the foot muscles.
• Obesity, which increases the weight on the foot.
Complications
• The condition sometimes leads to fractures of the bones at the front of the foot.
Treatment in the home
• Resting the foot relieves the pain.
When to consult the doctor
• If symptoms occur.
What the doctor may do
• Arrange physiotherapy to strengthen foot muscles.
• Advise the patient to wear well-fitting shoes, and to take regular exercise. If obesity is a cause, the doctor will advise the patient to go on a diet to lose weight.
Prevention
• Always wear properly fitting shoes, take adequate exercise and keep your weight down.
Outlook
• Physiotheraphy and following the doctor's advice about shoes and exercise usually bring about a marked improvement in the condition.

See SKELETAL SYSTEM *page 54*

MICROCEPHALY
The term describes a condition in which a person has an abnormally small head. The forehead is narrow and rather pointed in shape. The brain, too, is unusually small, so that the sufferer is often mentally retarded.

The condition is usually present from birth, sometimes resulting from two parents carrying the same abnormal gene. Microcephaly may also result from severe brain damage occurring in the unborn child, or in infancy. TOXOPLASMOSIS and ENCEPHALITIS are two causes.

Special education and care are often needed for the child with microcephaly, and in severe cases, long-term hospital care may be required.
See MENTAL SYSTEM *page 33*

MIGRAINE

Migraine is a type of recurrent headache, and one of the most common diseases of the nervous system. As many as 5 per cent of the population suffer from it. Women are more prone to migraine than men, and there is a tendency for it to run in families. Attacks usually begin in adolescence or early adult life.

Symptoms vary considerably from one person to another, but there are two broad categories.

In classic migraine there is a severe headache with many or all of the symptoms given below. In common migraine the headache only is present.
Symptoms
• A premonition that an attack is going to occur. This often happens soon after waking. The premonition may be a disturbance of vision such as bright spots or zigzag lines. These are seen with both eyes.
• Minutes after the premonition, numbness, tingling or weakness may be felt in the face, a hand or a leg. It is accompanied by a feeling of confusion and dizziness. There may be a slight difficulty in speaking. The symptoms may spread from one part of the body to another over a period of minutes.
• The early symptoms gradually disappear, to be followed by a severe throbbing headache. This may be felt on the opposite side of the head to the initial numbness or tingling. Often there is dislike of light.
• Nausea and vomiting may occur with the migraine. Children may vomit and suffer pain in the abdomen with or without the headache, a condition known as abdominal migraine.
Duration
• A migraine headache may last anything from a few hours to several days.
• Attacks may come two or three times a week or much less often. Women often get attacks at period times.
Causes
• The initial symptoms are caused by a sudden narrowing of the arteries leading to one side of the head. The headache follows when the same blood vessels widen again, allowing greater blood flow. Exactly why the blood vessels should contract and expand in this way is a subject of much research.
• Migraine is more common in energetic, hard-working people and can be triggered off by overwork or emotional stress. However, it tends to occur after the period of stress is over—at weekends and on holidays, for example.
• The contraceptive pill may cause migraine, while

pregnancy tends to reduce the frequency of attacks.
• Attacks may be brought on by a blow on the head, by bright or flashing lights, or by taking alcohol and certain foods, such as cheese and chocolate which contain phenylethylamine, to which blood vessels are sensitive.

Complications
• Migraine produces no complications apart from the obvious distress caused by an attack. Between bouts, migraine sufferers are perfectly normal.

Treatment in the home
• If a severe attack occurs, lie down in a darkened room and rest.
• Mild painkillers in recommended doses will ease the headache. *See* MEDICINES, 22.
• During a prolonged attack, eat only light, bland meals. These will reduce the risk of vomiting.

When to consult the doctor
• Any severe, recurrent headache should be reported to your doctor. If migraine is diagnosed, it will not normally be necessary to seek further advice.

What the doctor may do
• Ask you to describe the symptoms to find out whether

migraine is the cause. Check to find out whether the headache results from high blood pressure.
• In severe cases which do not conform to the broad pattern of migraine attacks, the doctor may recommend blood tests or X-rays.
• If migraine is diagnosed, and attacks are severe or frequent, the doctor may prescribe special drugs. Some are taken regularly to prevent attacks occurring. Others are taken the moment an attack begins. Do not exceed the prescribed dose. Some, such as those derived from ergot, are effective only if taken minutes after an attack begins, and can themselves cause headaches if taken in excess. Tablets containing ergotamine should not be taken during pregnancy.

Prevention
• In cases where attacks are brought on by overwork or emotional stress, some minor alterations to a sufferer's life-style may prevent bouts occurring.
• It may be possible to identify a specific food or drink which tends to bring on an attack. Once identified, the food can be avoided to prevent migraine occurring.

• In cases where attacks are associated with use of the contraceptive pill, an alternative form of contraception should be considered. *See* FAMILY PLANNING.

Outlook
• In some cases, the methods of prevention described above bring about a complete cure. Attacks tend to become fewer and less severe as a sufferer gets older.
• In women, migraine often ceases completely with the MENOPAUSE.

See NERVOUS SYSTEM *page 34*

MILIA

Small, harmless, pinhead skin cysts which may appear on the face of young adults. The cheeks and eyelids are the most common sites. They are painless and do not itch but sometimes appear after blistering or superficial damage to the skin.

Symptoms
• Small white or yellowish-white nodules.
• Many such pinhead-size white lesions are often noticed on the faces of young babies. These are harmless, require no treatment and will disappear.

Duration
• They persist for many months but eventually disappear without treatment.

Causes
• The cysts develop in damaged sweat ducts, but they also erupt on the face without previous injury or known cause.

Treatment in the home
• There are no simple remedies, and trying different proprietary skin preparations is more likely to produce skin sensitisation than to be of help.

When to consult the doctor
• If the spots are causing anxiety.

What the doctor may do
• Treatment is rarely attempted, but if desired each cyst can be individually incised with a needle and emptied by pressure.

Prevention
• Not possible, apart from the avoidance of injury.

Outlook
• Milia usually disappear completely within two years without the need for treatment.

See SKIN *page 52*

Living with migraine

☐ Keep a diary—not just of events on the day of an attack, but daily over a period of months. Note such details as getting up and bed times, meal times, what you eat and drink, the weather, any emotional stress or extra physical exertion. This may help you to discover some of the things which provoke your migraine.

☐ Avoid chocolate, cheese, citrus fruits and alcohol, unless you are sure they do not affect you.

☐ Low blood sugar—as a result of missing meals—can trigger an attack, so try to maintain regular eating habits.

☐ The contraceptive pill can cause migraine. If you are on the pill and get attacks, seek your doctor's advice.

☐ If you are prescribed a drug for migraine, be sure to read any information supplied with it. Take it exactly as prescribed, remembering that the earlier it is taken

in the attack the better. Ask your doctor if the drug he prescribes could cause drowsiness. If so, avoid driving when taking it. In any case, stop driving if an attack occurs—your vision is likely to be disturbed.

☐ Stress can worsen migraine. You may not be able to change your way of life, but learning how to relax and leading a regular organised life can help.

☐ Migraine is unpleasant but not dangerous. If you are worried that your headaches may have a more serious cause, tell your doctor. He will not think you foolish and will help to put your mind at rest.

☐ Regular exercise, such as swimming or yoga, may help to prevent migraine by relaxing your body. Some people find that meditation also helps.

☐ For further help contact *The Migraine Trust*, 45 Great Ormond Street, London WC1N 3HZ (Tel. 071-278 2676).

MISCARRIAGE

A spontaneous, or natural, abortion. Nature's own way of terminating a pregnancy which may perhaps have been unsatisfactory in some way.

See ABORTION

MITRAL INCOMPETENCE

Failure of the mitral valve to stop blood leaking back out of the main pumping chamber of the heart (left ventricle) into the left atrium with each heartbeat. Consequently, the heart is a far less effective pump. Mitral incompetence is less common than the narrowing of the valve (MITRAL STENOSIS), though the two conditions may be found together.

Symptoms
• Unexplained breathlessness.

Duration
• Permanent.

Causes
• The most common cause is RHEUMATIC FEVER, usually in childhood (*see* MITRAL STENOSIS). Mitral incompetence may follow rheumatic fever immediately.
• More rarely, congenital abnormalities, weakness or rupture of the cords of the valve.

Treatment in the home
• None possible.

When to consult the doctor
• If there is unexplained shortness of breath.

What the doctor may do
If the symptoms are mild:
• Physically examine the heart and lungs.
• Arrange for an ELECTROCARDIOGRAM (ECG), a chest X-ray and an echocardiogram (ultrasound).
If the symptoms are more severe:
• Arrange for special investigations to decide whether surgery is necessary. Artificial valves are available to replace the diseased valve.

Prevention
• The only preventive measures that can be taken are those given under rheumatic fever.

Outlook
• If the condition is causing severe breathlessness, the outlook is poor without surgery. If an artificial valve is fitted the patient is able to live a normal life.

See CIRCULATORY SYSTEM *page 40*

MITRAL STENOSIS

Narrowing of the mitral valve of the heart. Over a period of years the diseased cusps of the valve gradually thicken and fuse. The blood cannot flow forward from the left atrium into the left ventricle, the lungs become congested, and blood vessels within the lungs may bleed.

Symptoms
• Abnormal breathlessness.
• Frequent attacks of BRONCHITIS.
• Spitting of blood often occurs.
• Chest pain on exertion (*see* ANGINA).

Duration
• Permanent and progressive unless treated.

Causes
• Most often RHEUMATIC FEVER where the heart and valves are inflamed. Rheumatic fever usually affects children and attacks may not always be recognised at the time. A proportion of those afflicted suffer permanent heart damage, most commonly at the mitral valve. There may be a latent period of ten to 20 years before symptoms appear. Stenosis (narrowing) is more often found, but a faulty leaking valve (*see* MITRAL INCOMPETENCE) may also have developed. Both conditions may be present.

Treatment in the home
• None possible.

When to consult the doctor
• If there is unexplained breathlessness or spitting of blood.

What the doctor may do
If the symptoms are mild:
• Examine the heart and lungs.
• Arrange for an ELECTROCARDIOGRAM (ECG), a chest X-ray and an echocardiogram (ultrasound).
When the symptoms are more severe:
• Refer the patient to a hospital for further investigations to determine whether surgery will be of benefit.
• If surgery is necessary the surgeon will remove the obstruction, usually by dilating or splitting the valve.

Prevention
• *See* RHEUMATIC FEVER (**Prevention**).

Outlook
• Mild cases may continue to live to an old age with little disability.
• Severe cases require surgery. The benefits of surgery are considerable and the risk very low. If surgery is recommended but declined, the outlook is very poor.

See CIRCULATORY SYSTEM *page 40*

MOLE

A general term used to describe a coloured spot—usually brown—on the body, whether present at birth or developing later in life.

See SYMPTOM SORTER—SKIN ABNORMALITIES
SKIN *page 52*
MELANOMA

MOLLUSCUM CONTAGIOSUM

An uncommon skin infection causing crops of small, painless growths or warts, most commonly on the trunk and buttocks, but any skin may be involved. They usually occur in children, but older persons can also be infected.

Symptoms
• Smooth, shiny growths, about $\frac{1}{8}$-$\frac{1}{3}$ in. (3-8 mm.) across, with small central depressions. They are normal skin colour.

Duration
• The growths may spread to surrounding skin but will usually disappear naturally after some months.

Causes
• A virus growing in the cells of the outer layer of skin.

Treatment in the home
• None.
• The infection can be spread to others by direct skin contact. When the infection is found in schools or camps, the infected person should be isolated from changing-rooms, wash-rooms and gymnasiums until treatment has been completed.
• Simple wart paints are ineffective.

When to consult the doctor
• As soon as possible, as treatment should be carried out only under medical or nursing supervision.

What the doctor may do
• Scratch the top of the growth and apply pure phenol from a stick directly on to its centre.
• Freeze the growth (cryotherapy).

Prevention
• Avoid direct contact with infected people.

Outlook
• The phenol treatment provides a complete cure, otherwise the condition will disappear naturally in time.

See SKIN *page 52*

MONGOLIAN SPOTS

Large blue-grey blotches, often 2 or 3 in. (50 or 75 mm.) in diameter and with unclear edges. They are present at birth and are found chiefly around the buttocks area of babies of Mongolian race, some Negroes, and occasionally Caucasian children.

Duration
- The spots disappear during the first year of life.

Causes
- Collection of pigment-containing cells deep in the under layer of skin.

Treatment in the home
- No action is needed and there is no need to worry about the spots.

When to consult the doctor
- If it is not certain that the blotches are Mongolian spots (sometimes the discolorations may look like bruising).

What the doctor may do
- Confirm the diagnosis.

Prevention
- None.

Outlook
- Once the spots have disappeared they will not recur.

See SKIN *page 52*

MONGOLISM
Another name for Down's syndrome, a form of mental subnormality caused by a chromosome defect. One of the main physical features of the disorder is a slight slant to the eyes, as is seen in the Mongolian races.
See DOWN'S SYNDROME

MONOCYTE
One of three types of leucocyte (white blood cell). It absorbs bacteria, particles of dead tissue and other foreign material from the rest of the blood.

MORNING SICKNESS
Nausea and vomiting in pregnant women, often one of the first signs of pregnancy. Although commonly called morning sickness, the condition often occurs at other times as well.
See PREGNANCY

MOTION SICKNESS

Nausea and vomiting experienced by many people when travelling by road, rail, sea or air. The movement of the vehicle upsets the relation between what the eyes see and what the balance mechanism of the inner ear feels. The eyes adjust to the movement, whereas the inner ear does not, and the resulting 'signals' from eye and ear do not tally. If the eyes can see dry land or the horizon, symptoms are usually less severe.

Symptoms
- Nausea and vomiting.
- Loss of appetite.
- Sweating and feeling faint.
- The face appears pale or sometimes greenish.

Do's and don'ts about motion sickness

☐ *Do* take a travel-sickness tablet (*see* MEDICINES, 21) about ½-1 hour before starting out on a journey. If you are driving, do not take tablets containing antihistamine which can cause the onset of drowsiness.

☐ *Do* take games, toys, puzzles, audio tapes or anything else that might be a distraction for a child sufferer.

☐ *Do* take some waterproof bags in case all else fails.

☐ *Don't* talk about the possibility of being sick in front of someone at risk, as this may cause him to be sick.

☐ *Don't* have a large meal or alcohol before setting out.

☐ *Don't* allow smoking in a car if the passengers include a potential sufferer—it could trigger an attack.

- Abdominal discomfort and diarrhoea.

Duration
- Symptoms may last up to 72 hours on a prolonged journey, but they cease rapidly at the end of a journey or when the motion becomes easier.
- Some people adapt to travel, and the sickness becomes less severe on each subsequent journey.

Causes
- A temporary disturbance of the inner ear caused by unusual motion.

Treatment in the home
- There are several antisickness medicines that help. Some contain atropine, or a related substance, that may cause dry mouth and constipation. Others contain an antihistamine that may cause drowsiness in some people. The first dose should be taken ½-1 hour before departure. *See* MEDICINES, 21.
- Take small amounts of fluid regularly to avoid dehydration, and try to eat small amounts of food regularly, even if you are vomiting. Symptoms are often less severe after vomiting.
- Fresh air helps. If you are travelling by car, make regular stops (every hour with children). If you are at sea, go on deck. Any distraction may help.
- If symptoms are severe, lie down with eyes closed.

When to consult the doctor
- If there is severe pain in the abdomen together with sickness.

What the doctor may do
- Check that the nausea and vomiting are caused by travel sickness and not by any other disease.
- In severe cases, give an injection to stop vomiting.

Prevention
- Prevention is mainly by reducing the expectation of sickness. Be calm and sensible. Do not stimulate the imagination of a possible sufferer.
- Allow time for a stop every hour on a car journey with children or susceptible adults.
- Position children where they can see out of the window.
- Keep warm, with plenty of warm clothing.
- Keep a car window slightly open.
- If you are a passenger in a car, do not attempt to read on the journey.

Outlook
- Most children grow out of car sickness.
- Some adults are always vulnerable to travel sickness, and in the most severe of circumstances (if you are in a small boat that goes straight out of harbour into a gale, for instance) even the hardiest may succumb.

See EAR *page 38*

MOTOR NEURONE DISEASE

The motor nerves are those which carry messages from the central nervous system to the muscles. Motor neurone disease is a condition affecting the units (neurones) of these nerves, causing progressive weakness in the muscles. The disease begins in adult life.

Symptoms
• Increasing muscular weakness. It often begins in the legs or hands. The muscles tend to waste away, sometimes becoming stiff and spastic.
• Some muscles, particularly those around the shoulders, begin to twitch intermittently under the skin. The

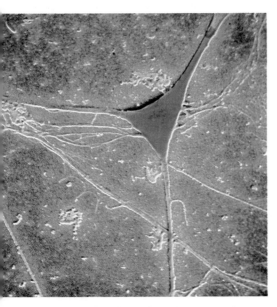

MUSCLE CONTROL *The red triangle with long extensions is a motor neurone, which functions inside the cerebral cortex of the brain. Motor neurones control the workings of the body muscles. They receive messages from sensory nerves via the slender connections on the lower side. Outgoing messages—telling the body what to do—are despatched on a single channel—the thick connection, top right.*

process is known as fasciculation. It begins as a slight, persistent twitching which becomes more obvious as the disease progresses. Skin sensation is not dulled, as it is in many other diseases of the nervous system.
• In severe cases, the disease affects the throat muscles so that sufferers find it increasingly difficult to speak and swallow. There is excessive salivation, and an increasing risk of choking. Food and drink tend to 'go down the wrong way', entering the lungs.

Duration
• The onset of the symptoms is gradual and in some cases they stop getting any worse after a period of months or years. In the most severe cases, however, the patient's condition rapidly deteriorates and 40 per cent of patients die within five years.

Causes
• The cause is not known for certain, but the disease has been linked with virus infection. In rare cases there may be a hereditary tendency.

Complications
• The inability to swallow properly may, in severe cases, cause the lungs to become clogged with saliva and PNEUMONIA may result.

Treatment in the home
• None.

When to consult the doctor
• If symptoms appear.

What the doctor may do
There is no known cure for motor neurone disease, but there are many treatments which may ease distressing symptoms, and facilities to help the sufferer to maintain a full and active life. The doctor may prescribe drugs to reduce problems of muscle stiffness, salivation and shortness of breath. He can also put you in touch with:
• A physiotherapist to help with problems of mobility, breathing and posture.
• An occupational therapist to advise on aids to independence within the home and workplace, and on leisure activities.
• A dietician to advise on suitable food.
• A speech therapist to help with communication difficulties.
• A nurse to give help and advice on general care of the patient. It is often possible to arrange for regular nursing help at home.
• A social worker who can provide emotional support and practical advice on the many facilities available, including financial benefits.

Prevention
• None known.

Outlook
• The symptoms may vary in severity and duration.

Average life-expectancy is two to five years, during which many patients continue to live an active life despite permanent disability.
• In severe cases the disease may be rapidly fatal. In others deterioration slows down or stops. Some patients have lived with motor neurone disease for over 20 years.
• Research is continuing to try to find the cause of the disease and may in future lead to a cure.

The Motor Neurone Disease Association, PO Box 246, Northampton NN1 2PR, provides literature and advice. Freephone helpline 0800-626262.

See NERVOUS SYSTEM *page 34*

MOUTH ULCERS

Mouth ulcers are extremely common. They may be very painful, but they are usually not serious and clear up on their own or with mild home treatments. Occasionally they are persistent or recurring, and may signal some continuing source of irritation, or some other disease or illness.

APHTHOUS ULCERS are the most common, particularly in young people. They are small ($\frac{1}{8}$ in. (3 mm.) across), shallow, round or oval ulcers, often with a white or pale grey base and a slightly raised yellowish edge, surrounded by a thin, red, inflamed border. The most common site is the edge of the tongue, but they may also occur anywhere on the tongue, inside the cheek, on the gums, in the grooves between gum and cheek, and on the roof of the mouth.

STOMATITIS means erosion and ulceration of the mouth or gums. It occurs most commonly at the angles of the mouth (angular stomatitis), and is often accompanied by aphthous ulceration inside the cheeks.

LUMPS in the mouth, with a variety of causes, may get in the way of eating and may form ulcers around the surface.

Symptoms
• An obvious blister or crater, or peeling away of the fine lining of the inside of the mouth.
• Pain on the surface of the ulcer and around it.
• Soreness and sensitivity to hot, acid or spicy foods.
• Discomfort on chewing or swallowing.

- Some ulcers are painless.
- Ulcers may be accompanied by blisters elsewhere on the body, by skin diseases or by symptoms of other illnesses.
- Rarely, ulcers may bleed or become infected and discharge pus.

Duration
- Most ulcers last for a few days only.
- Stomatitis usually clears within four or five days.
- Recurring or persistent ulceration suggests an underlying cause which needs to be identified.

Causes
- There may be some hereditary component—a tendency to ulcers runs in families.
- Ulcers often appear during times of stress, and are made worse by emotional tension.
- Hormones play some part—ulcers often appear first at puberty, may tend to occur with menstrual periods, and usually disappear in pregnancy.
- Diet plays little part in causing ulcers except for strongly irritant foods, but occasionally ulcers or stomatitis may occur in people lacking in B and C vitamins.
- Heat, usually after burning the mouth on hot foods or drinks.
- Trauma from chemicals, including spices, tobacco and alcohol. Prolonged intake of very acidic foods or drinks, or contact with acid stomach contents after persistent vomiting, may also cause ulceration.
- Infections, particularly by minor virus illnesses in toddlers, and in THRUSH, MEASLES and GLANDULAR FEVER. Ulcers may accompany COLD SORES in herpes viral infections. Very rarely mouth ulcers accompany TUBERCULOSIS or SYPHILIS.
- Occasionally mechanical sores develop, most commonly from accidentally biting the cheek or gum or from jagged teeth or ill-fitting dentures. In babies a hard or over-long bottle teat may be responsible.
- Drugs and medicines.
- Cysts, abscesses and growths on tooth roots, gums, tongue or lips.
- Mouth ulcers may accompany skin diseases such as REITER'S SYNDROME, blood diseases such as ANAEMIA, and gastrointestinal diseases such as COELIAC DISEASE.
- Very rarely mouth ulcers occur with cancers of the lips, tongue, mouth or palate. These occur mainly in smokers or people who use chewing tobacco, and in heavy drinkers.

Treatment in the home
- Avoid hot or irritating foods and drink, alcohol and tobacco.
- Remove irritating dentures, or see your dentist about sharp teeth or dental abscesses.
- Use soothing mouthwashes and pastilles, such as glycerin and thymol, to help to relieve pain. *See* MEDICINES, 42.
- Apply glycerin ointments with the fingertip to help to ease soreness.

When to consult the doctor
- With any persistent or recurring ulceration which lasts for more than two weeks.
- With any ulcers accompanied by skin disease or other symptoms elsewhere in the body.
- If ulcers occur in the grooves alongside the gums.
- If there are white patches in the mouth or throat. See THRUSH.
- If ulcers appear while the person is taking any drugs or medicines.
- If ulcers bleed or become infected.
- If there are lumps or growths in the mouth.

What the doctor may do
- Prescribe stronger mouthwashes, pastilles or ointments.
- Advise on diet, perhaps prescribing vitamins.
- Change the tablets or medicine that the patient is taking if the ulcers began during a course of treatment.
- Take a swab from the mouth to test for bacterial infections or THRUSH.
- Examine the skin for rashes elsewhere.
- Test for other diseases, as by blood tests.
- Prescribe antiviral treatment for herpes or other viral ulcers.
- Advise a minor operation to remove cysts or swellings in the mouth.

See DIGESTIVE SYSTEM *page 44*

MUCOUS MEMBRANE
The smooth moist tissue that lines the respiratory and digestive tracts, the urinary tract, reproductive tract and most of the other cavities and passages in the body. It produces a thick fluid called mucus, which lubricates and protects it.

MUCUS COLLECTION IN THE PHARYNX

The natural secretions from the back of the nose and from the salivary glands of the mouth, which are being produced all the time, are normally swallowed. But if they are excessive, as when a person has a cold, or if the swallowing mechanism is not fully developed, as in a small baby, mucus may collect in the pharynx (throat) and cause a cough. The cough is generally desirable, as it helps to prevent the mucus from going down into the lungs.

Symptoms
- A loose cough, especially when lying down.
- The cough is worse at night, and in children can be frightening. Parents may fear that a baby or older child may choke, but this will not happen.
- Sometimes babies sound 'bubbly' as the air they breathe passes through the mucus in the pharynx.

Duration
- Babies can usually swallow adequately by the age of six months and thereafter only cough persistently during a common cold, or if producing extra saliva when cutting new teeth.
- Children and adults may cough for up to ten days after a cold.
- Some children, especially in cold houses, cough at night for months or years without coming to any harm.

Causes
- Irritation by mild infections, dust or allergy may contribute to this condition.

Treatment in the home
- Tilt the head of a baby's cot very slightly upwards by putting blocks under the cot legs.
- Older children and adults may get relief by sleeping with an extra pillow.
- Cough medicines may relieve symptoms; but do not attempt to suppress the cough completely because it is protecting the lungs from infection.
- Do not smoke, and keep children away from tobacco fumes.
- Sleep with a window slightly open.

When to consult the doctor
- If there is chronic disease, such as EMPHYSEMA, BRONCHITIS, SINUSITIS, and the cough is getting worse.
- If green or yellow phlegm is being coughed up and there is a raised temperature.
- If earache or a runny ear develops.
- If breathing is difficult or noisy.
- If a child is ill, feverish, crying inconsolably, off his food, drowsy and unresponsive or vomiting.
- If a baby is restless, pale or unresponsive.

What the doctor may do
- Examine the lungs to make sure that they are clear of infection.
- Prescribe a cough linctus or a decongestant to reduce the amount of secretion. See MEDICINES, 16.

Outlook
- Mucus collection in the pharynx is not really an

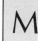

illness, and the symptoms disappear spontaneously in time.

• Once the condition is understood it is often easier to cope with it.

See RESPIRATORY SYSTEM *page 42*

MULTIPLE SCLEROSIS

The condition is also known as disseminated sclerosis, and results from damage to the sheaths surrounding individual nerve cells. The nerves are unable to function properly, causing problems of vision, sensation and muscular control. About one person in 2,000 develops multiple sclerosis. The average age of the onset of symptoms is 30, and women are affected more often than men. The symptoms vary greatly from one patient to another.

Symptoms

• Some 40 per cent of cases begin with some sort of visual disturbance. Sight may be blurred or dimmed in one or both eyes. There may be pain or discomfort behind the eyes, and double vision may develop.

• With or without visual disturbance, the sufferer may feel weakness or loss of control in one or more limbs. Simple tasks can be performed only clumsily. This symptom is known as ATAXIA.

• The sufferer may lose control over bowel movement and urination.

• Physical symptoms are often accompanied by a change of mood. Sufferers often become light-hearted, though some may become depressed.

Duration

• The symptoms usually develop over a period of hours or days, then gradually disappear over the next two to eight weeks. However, they may recur after a period of weeks, months or years, and continue to do so in forms which are increasingly disabling. Eventually multiple sclerosis may prove fatal, but many patients live for 30 or 40 years after the symptoms first appear. In severe cases they may die within two years. The average is more than 20 years.

Causes

• The cause is not known for sure, and is the subject of much research. It may result from a reaction to a virus infection, such as measles, contracted early in life.

• There is a tendency for multiple sclerosis to run in families, but no definite likelihood of its being passed on genetically. The twin of a sufferer is, for example, not specially likely to develop the disease.

Complications

• Infections of kidneys, bladder and lungs may occur.

Treatment in the home

• None possible.

When to consult the doctor

• If any loss of vision, muscular weakness or persistent numbness in the limbs develops.

What the doctor may do

• Perform a physical examination to find out whether multiple sclerosis is present. This will often involve arranging a lumbar puncture. A hypodermic needle is used to draw off some of the fluid surrounding the spinal cord for tests.

• If multiple sclerosis is confirmed, the doctor may prescribe injections of ACTH, a substance which stimulates the adrenal glands and is thought to lessen the damage while the disease is active.

• For long-term treatment, the doctor will recommend rest when the symptoms are present. During periods when they lapse, he will recommend exercises to strengthen the muscles and keep them mobile.

• The doctor will be able to recommend a physiotherapist or occupational therapist to help cope with disabilities arising from the disease. A society exists for sufferers: *The Multiple Sclerosis Society of Great Britain and Northern Ireland,* 25 Effie Road, Fulham, London SW6 1EE (Tel. 071-736 6267).

• Much can be done to minimise the disabling effects of the disease.

Prevention

• None known.

Outlook

• There is no cure for multiple sclerosis at present. Symptoms cause distress and frustration. However, with determination and professional guidance, a sufferer can still live a long and active life.

See NERVOUS SYSTEM *page 34*

MUMPS

Swelling of the salivary glands. This common infectious disease mostly affects children over the age of two, and occurs in epidemics every three or four years.

Symptoms

• The commonest feature is swelling of one saliva-producing gland in front of the ear and over the angle of the jaw. A day or two later the opposite gland may also swell.

• The other saliva-producing glands (under the jaw and under the tongue) may also swell.

• Earache or pain when eating.

• Other glands may also become swollen and painful. Inflammation in the scrotum in males after puberty indicates ORCHITIS. In girls, inflammation of the ovaries or the pancreas may cause pain in the abdomen.

Incubation period

• Fifteen to 21 days. Saliva contains the virus (and the patient is therefore infectious) from approximately six days before the glands swell until about two weeks afterwards.

• Sufferers are infectious before symptoms appear, and it is impossible to prevent spread of infection during this time, therefore isolation is rarely practised.

Duration

• The illness is usually over within a week.

Causes

• Mumps virus, spread by contact with an affected person.

Complications

• Virus ENCEPHALITIS may occur with severe headache.

• OTITIS MEDIA can develop in children.

• ORCHITIS

Treatment in the home

• Rest in bed for a few days.

• If chewing is painful, offer soups and drinks.

• If a testicle is swollen or sore, support the scrotum with a pillow or bandage. Alternatively a towel beneath the testicles with the ends draped over the thighs may help. Leave pyjama trousers off, and give a mild painkiller in recommended doses. *See* MEDICINES, 22.

When to consult the doctor

• If testicles are swollen and sore or there is severe or persistent earache or abdominal pain.

• If headache is severe, with a stiff neck, or if the patient finds light uncomfortable.

What the doctor may do

• Simply advise bed-rest for uncomplicated mumps.

• Prescribe painkillers if necessary.

• Treat complications if suspected.

Prevention

• Vaccination, usually given with measles and rubella vaccine before age 2.

Outlook

• For children excellent. There is a slightly greater risk of complications in adults.

See INFECTIOUS DISEASES *page 32*

MUSCULAR DYSTROPHY

A gradual wasting disease affecting various groups of muscles. Several related types occur. The different types affect different groups of muscles and arise at different ages. In all types the wasting is steadily progressive, no cause has yet been isolated and no treatment appears either to cure or halt the disease. The three main types, which are all genetically inherited and therefore run in families, are: the Duchenne childhood form occurring in boys only, which usually affects the lower limbs and starts in boys between four and ten years old; the facio scapulo humeral form, which affects muscles of the face and upper limbs and starts in the teens or in young adults of both sexes; and limb girdle muscular dystrophy, which affects the muscles of the shoulders or hips, and usually starts in adults of 20-35 of both sexes and runs a slower, less-severe course.

Symptoms
• Weakness of muscles becomes apparent because the child or adult experiences difficulty in walking or using a limb.
• A child may start to waddle, cannot climb stairs properly or can rise to his feet only by using his hands to 'climb up his legs'.
• Adults complain that certain actions have become difficult. There is no pain or tenderness of muscles.
• The muscles affected, though weak, often look enlarged.
• Blood tests reveal raised levels of certain muscle 'enzymes'.

Duration
• The condition is lifelong, with symptoms progressing steadily over the years.

Causes
• The cause is unknown. Most cases are genetically determined and run in families. Some forms arise only in males, but are transmitted through the female line. Others arise only if both parents carry the abnormal gene.
• Any sufferer contemplating marriage should obtain expert advice from a genetic counsellor, to assess the risks of passing the disease to any children.

Complications
• Serious infections, for example PNEUMONIA, are common.

Treatment in the home
None advised. A doctor should be consulted immediately if the condition is suspected.

• Once the condition has been diagnosed, family support and home care provide the essential basis of all treatment. Expert guidance and help is needed.

When to consult the doctor
• If symptoms suggesting muscle weakness are noted in a child or young adult, especially if there is a family history of muscular dystrophy.

What the doctor may do
• Send the patient to hospital for a muscle biopsy—a small operation to remove a piece of affected muscle for examination under a microscope.
• If diagnosis is confirmed, give advice and help about supportive care in the home.
• Arrange for infections to be treated with antibiotics. *See* MEDICINES, 25.
• Advise contact with the *Muscular Dystrophy Group of Great Britain*, 7-11 Prescott Place, London SW4 6BS. (Tel. 071-720 8055).
• Advise genetic counselling.

Prevention
• If the diagnosis is certain, parents (and sufferers) should have the benefit of an expert genetic counsellor.

Outlook
• In some cases, particularly Duchenne type, this is not good. Disability is considerable and walking or use of the affected muscles eventually becomes impossible.
• With modern support and care, most sufferers of limb girdle type can usually be helped to live a happy, modified life for 20-40 years, sometimes longer.
• The best outlook is for those who develop the disease in their teens or later.

MUSIC THERAPY
The soothing or stimulating effects of music have been recognised for centuries. Some therapists have taken the principle a stage further, asserting that listening to or making music can be a helpful additional aid in the treatment of diseases, particularly mental disorders—a technique that is sometimes also called musicotherapy. One practical application of the idea is the broadcasting of soothing music in aeroplanes before take-off and landing, when passengers are expected to be at their most nervous. Doctors and dentists have been known to use music in the surgery to soothe patients. There have also been many documented cases in which the playing of the patient's favourite music has apparently assisted in recovery from coma.

MYALGIC ENCEPHALOMYELITIS
Myalgic encephalomyelitis (ME) is a disorder predominantly

affecting children and young adults, with symptoms that may include muscle weakness and pains, fatigue, exhaustion after only mild exertion, slow recovery after exercise, depression, memory loss, and impaired concentration. Symptoms may last for many months. The muscle fatigue resembles that which follows many viral infections. But as yet no virus has been identified, and the cause remains uncertain. No treatment has proved consistently effective; but other causes of muscle weakness can be excluded by medical examination, and sometimes antidepressant medicines help recovery.

MYASTHENIA GRAVIS

A rare condition in which the muscles all over the body feel weak and tire easily after use. It can occur at any age, in either sex, though women are affected twice as often as men.

Symptoms
• An eyelid may droop, or double vision occur, getting worse as the day progresses.
• There is difficulty in chewing and swallowing, and it becomes worse during the course of a meal as the jaw and throat muscles tire.
• The face becomes smooth and the lips retract, producing an involuntary smile.
• Over a period of months or years, the muscles of the limbs and body become weaker. Finally, the muscles controlling breathing may be paralysed.

Duration
• The condition is chronic, tending to persist over months or years. The symptoms may be mild after sleep or rest, but worsen after any muscular activity.
• In some cases, the disease clears up with treatment, or of its own accord. In others it progresses rapidly, despite treatment.

Causes
• Myasthenia gravis results when an excess of certain antibodies is present in the bloodstream. The antibodies interfere with the normal control of the muscles by the nerves.
• The disease may be caused by a small tumour or other disorder in the thymus gland of the neck. The tumour is not necessarily malignant.

Complications
• In severe cases, paralysis of the breathing muscles may result in death.

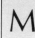

Treatment in the home
- None advised. Seek medical attention.

When to consult the doctor
- If symptoms occur.

What the doctor may do
- Take blood tests to find out whether the disease is present.
- Prescribe drugs which improve the passing of signals between nerve endings and muscles. If the muscles become stronger as a result, a diagnosis of myasthenia gravis is confirmed.
- Prescribe steroids or immunosuppressive drugs. These limit the production of antibodies at the point where the nerve endings and muscles meet. See MEDICINES, 32.
- Recommend an operation to remove the thymus gland.

Prevention
- None.

Outlook
- The condition may clear up of its own accord.
- In more severe cases, treatment will often keep the disease under control, allowing the patient to lead a full and active life.
- In acute cases, prolonged hospital treatment may be needed, and a respirator required to aid breathing.

MYOCARDIAL INFARCTION
A condition in which a segment of heart muscle dies when its blood supply has been cut off by a blocked artery. Myocardial infarction follows a coronary thrombosis and the names are often used interchangeably to describe either condition.
See CORONARY THROMBOSIS

MYOCARDITIS

Acute inflammation of the heart muscle which occurs during the course of other infections or diseases. The heart valves, internal lining and pericardium (the membrane surrounding the heart) may also be affected. Severity will depend on the cause and extent of cardiac muscles affected.

Symptoms
- Shortness of breath.
- Palpitations or pain over the front of the chest.
- Some patients may be ill but not have symptoms specially related to the heart.

Duration
- The acute infection usually lasts for several weeks and then clears up completely. Occasionally the heart muscle is permanently damaged.

Causes
- RHEUMATIC FEVER.
- Bacterial and virus infections (for example, DIPHTHERIA, GLANDULAR FEVER, MUMPS).
- Other causes include TOXOPLASMOSIS and RHEUMATOID ARTHRITIS.

When to consult the doctor
- If you are unusually distressed during the course of a mild illness (for example, a common cold, or flu).

What the doctor may do
- Keep the patient in bed.
- Treat underlying disease.
- Prescribe drugs to relieve the strain on the heart.

Prevention
- As myocarditis may have few or no symptoms, it is wise after any infection to resume full physical activity gradually and not to engage in competitive sport for several weeks.

Outlook
- Most cases of myocarditis recover completely, but because of the risk of heart failure and the danger from disturbances of heart rhythm, including cardiac arrest, the outlook can be serious.

See CIRCULATORY SYSTEM page 40

MYOPATHY
Wasting of the muscles. Myopathy may be hereditary, as in MUSCULAR DYSTROPHY; it may be a complication of another disease—for example, DIABETES mellitus; it may occur during CANCER; or it may be caused by poisoning from drugs used to treat another disorder.

MYOPIA
The medical name for short-sightedness, a focusing problem which makes it difficult to see objects at a distance.
See REFRACTIVE ERRORS

MYOSITIS
Any of a group of muscle diseases which cause inflammation of the muscle. Severe prolonged inflammation may cause scar tissue to replace muscle fibres, resulting in permanent weakness and stiffness. Myositis may occur in some COLLAGEN DISEASES.

MYXOEDEMA

A slowly developing disease caused by deficiency of thyroid hormones leading to lack of energy and thickening of the skin and the tissues beneath the skin with a sticky, jelly-like substance. 'Myx' refers to that substance and 'oedema' means swelling.

Thyroid hormones are essential for normal functioning of the body. Too little thyroid hormone may arise from disease of the thyroid gland itself or from disturbances of areas of the brain (pituitary and hypothalamus) that control the working of the thyroid gland. There are other types of thyroid deficiency—in children it may show itself as cretinism (a condition in which there is mental and physical retardation).

Myxoedema is most common in middle-aged women.

All symptoms come on gradually and may not be noticed for many months.

Symptoms
- Intolerance to cold weather. The sufferer feels cold even in the summer and needs to wear layers of clothing.
- Thickened skin, and changes in the appearance of the face because of thickening of the eyelids and cheeks.
- Dry skin. Thinning and loss of hair.
- Hoarse voice and slow speech.
- Apathy and fatigue.
- Aching muscles and pins and needles in the hands.
- Constipation.
- Periods may become heavier, or may disappear.

Duration
- Myxoedema lasts for life, and the treatment has to be lifelong too. But once treatment is started the symptoms usually disappear in seven to 28 days.

Causes
- An autoimmune disorder—that is, one in which the body reacts against some of its own tissues, in this case the thyroid, destroying essential parts. This is the most common cause.
- Treatment of an overactive thyroid (THYROTOXICOSIS). If too much of the gland has been removed by surgery or destroyed by radioactive therapy, thyroid deficiency may result.
- Disorder of the pituitary gland, which controls the activity of the thyroid gland.

Complications
- Hypothermia (excessive low body heat) in the aged.
- Heart disease.
- If untreated, myxoedema may lead to mental disturbance, self-neglect, coma and death.

Treatment in the home
- None is possible until myxoedema has been diagnosed. After that the sufferer must take the thyroid hormone for the rest of his life and report regularly to the doctor for checks.

When to consult the doctor
- If the symptoms described occur. The early symptoms are vague and difficult to understand by the sufferer—and sometimes even by the doctor—but they should always be reported. Often friends and relatives are the first to realise that the sufferer is ill.

What the doctor may do
- Take blood tests to check whether the thyroid is working properly.
- Prescribe thyroxin tablets. These are synthetic preparations that replace the body's deficiency. *See* MEDICINES, 31.
- Make occasional blood checks to make sure that the correct dose of thyroxin is being taken.

Prevention
- The individual can do nothing to prevent myxoedema, but the doctor may recommend thyroxin tablets after treatment for thyroid overactivity to prevent the condition developing.

Outlook
- Excellent if the treatment is followed. The patient will be able to live a normal life although he will need to have treatment for the rest of his life.

NAPPY RASH
Chafing of the surface layer of a baby's skin. It is caused by contact with ammonia, a chemical produced from urine by bacteria which normally live on moist skin.
See CHILD CARE—CHILDHOOD ILLS *page 151*

NARCOLEPSY

An irresistible tendency to fall asleep. It may occur at any time during the day, but especially in the afternoon. Men are more affected than women, and the condition usually begins in adolescence or early adult life. Seventy per cent of patients also suffer from CATAPLEXY.

Symptoms
- A sudden and irresistible urge to sleep. It may interrupt any normal activity; the sufferer has no choice but to lie down on the spot.
- The sufferer can be temporarily roused. In this respect,

narcolepsy is quite different from fainting or concussion.

Duration
- A bout may last anything from a few minutes to several hours.

Causes
- The condition is caused by a disorder in the part of the brain controlling sleep. This is situated in the hypothalamus, an area near the front of the brain.
- Bouts are not brought on by any of the normal causes of sleepiness, such as overwork, eating, OBESITY, drugs or alcohol.

Complications
- None.

Treatment in the home
- Allow the patient to sleep, taking appropriate precautions to make sure that he is safe from accident while sleeping. Driving may have to be avoided.

When to consult the doctor
- If symptoms recur without any of the normal causes of sleepiness listed above.

What the doctor may do
- Prescribe stimulants to keep the patient awake. *See* MEDICINES, 20.
- Recommend that the patient's daily routine is organised so that he can sleep if the stimulants fail to work.

Prevention
- None.

Outlook
- Narcolepsy is a minor nervous disorder, inconvenient but harmless.

See NERVOUS SYSTEM *page 34*

NASAL POLYP

Shiny polyps, resembling small skinned grapes, can obstruct the flow of air through the nasal passages. They are extensions of the normal mucous membrane lining the nose and contain fluid. They are not cancerous.

Symptoms
- Obstruction to the flow of air through the affected nostril. The polyps are usually found in both nostrils and there are often several in each side. The obstruction is not relieved by blowing the nose.
- They may block the sense of smell (also reducing the taste of food).
- If the polyps extend into the sinuses or obstruct the openings from the sinuses, they may cause SINUSITIS and

headache or pain in the cheeks.
- There is usually a persistent runny nose.
- There may be symptoms of ALLERGY (itchy nose, sneezing, RHINITIS).

Duration
- Polyps persist for years if untreated.

Causes
- Usually an allergy. The cause of the allergic reaction may or may not be obvious.

Treatment in the home
- None. Consult the doctor.

When to consult the doctor
- If the nose is blocked for more than four weeks, and cannot be relieved by blowing.
- If the sense of smell is disappearing and the patient does not have a COMMON COLD.
- If there is increasing headache, worse on stooping, and the discharge from the nose is green or yellow as sinusitis may be developing.
- If the obstruction is in one nostril only and persists for more than two weeks and is not associated with a common cold.

What the doctor may do
- Examine the nose by looking into the nostril and up from the back of the mouth with a mirror.
- Suggest that the polyps be removed under local or general anaesthetic.

Prevention
- Avoid the substances to which the patient is allergic.

Outlook
- Some small polyps disappear without treatment, but most do not disappear spontaneously.
- Polyps tend to recur after removal unless the underlying allergy is treated.

See RESPIRATORY SYSTEM *page 42*

NATUROPATHY
An all-embracing term covering systems of treatment that assume that the body is capable of healing itself through natural processes. Naturopaths, who in general do not hold orthodox medical qualifications, emphasise the importance of diet and exercise to well-being. *See* NUTRITION. They have also borrowed from HERBALISM, HOMEOPATHY, OSTEOPATHY and other forms of unorthodox treatment.

NAUSEA
Feeling sick. Nausea is a very common symptom: causes include MOTION SICKNESS, early pregnancy, and eating

or drinking too much. It is usually temporarily relieved by vomiting.
See SYMPTOM SORTER—NAUSEA

NECK

Stiff or painful neck is a common symptom in both adults and children. It usually clears up in one or two days, but occasionally may be a symptom of infectious disease.
See SYMPTOM SORTER—NECK PROBLEMS

NEGATIVE ION THERAPY

In most atmospheric conditions, unpolluted air contains ions—particles of air molecules with either a positive or a negative electrical charge. But in some circumstances, the proportion of negative ions may drop dramatically, apparently producing headaches, anxiety, depression and similar conditions.

The loss of negative ions occurs naturally in many parts of the world when a rise in temperature and a fall in humidity are accompanied by a high wind—for example, the Santa Ana in California and the Föhn in Switzerland.

In industrial regions, atmospheric pollution destroys the ions, and they are filtered out by the air-conditioning systems of many buildings.

Negative ion therapy uses machines called ionisers or ion generators to increase the proportion of negative ions in the air.

Scientists are experimenting with the technique in the United States, the Soviet Union, Great Britain and Germany to treat not only persistent headaches and the cafard—the name given by French soldiers to the feelings of depression and listlessness brought on by hot dry weather—but also to promote the healing of burns and to cure eczema.

Tests carried out at the University of Frankfurt in West Germany suggest that negative ion therapy can slow down the growth of cancers in mice.

Since the 1950s, commercial companies have sold ionisers for use in the home, office or car. Their sale was banned in the United States in 1961, because the machines that were then available produced ozone as a by-product—in quantities judged to be harmful to health. However, later models do not give off the gas.

Ionisers have been widely used in the US space programme. According to the North American Space Agency, an increase in the negative ions in the atmosphere of a spacecraft improves the metabolism, performance and reaction time of astronauts.

However, most doctors remain sceptical about the alleged benefits of ionisers.

NEPHRITIS

An acute or chronic inflammation of the glomeruli, or filters, in the kidney. As a result, blood escapes through leaks in the damaged filter bed. This rare condition of the urinary system is not usually caused by germs but by a process called autoimmune disease, where the body develops antibodies which attack its own tissue.

ACUTE NEPHRITIS
Symptoms
- Smoky-coloured or red urine.
- Small volume of urine passed.
- Puffy face.
- Severe headache and backache.
- The condition comes on suddenly in children; more slowly in adults.
- It occasionally follows about ten days after an acute throat infection.

Duration
- The condition lasts for about two or three weeks if there are no complications.

Causes
- Autoimmune reaction.
- Some forms of nephritis are triggered by streptococcal infections of the throat.

Complications
- After some years a few cases develop into chronic nephritis, causing eventual kidney failure.

Treatment in the home
- Go to bed and rest immediately.

When to consult the doctor
- Immediately the symptoms described occur.

What the doctor may do
- Test urine.
- Check blood pressure.
- Send the patient to hospital.
- Treat repeated attacks of TONSILLITIS.

Prevention
- Fewer cases now occur—a result of less virulent tonsillitis which follows better living conditions.

Outlook
- In most cases, recovery is complete.

CHRONIC NEPHRITIS
A general disruption of the glomerulus, or filter bed, which eventually leads to uraemia or kidney failure. The condition may follow an attack of acute nephritis, but it can also develop slowly and unnoticed over many years.

Symptoms
- Thirst.
- A lot of pale urine passed.
- Lethargy.
- Swelling of the face and limbs.

Duration
- If untreated, the condition worsens over a few months or years.

Causes
- As for acute nephritis.

Complications
- Progessive failure of the kidneys, which may extend

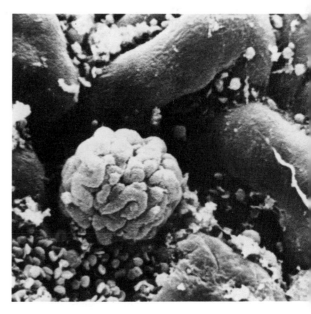

HOW THE KIDNEYS FILTER WASTE PRODUCTS *Inside each kidney thousands of tiny filtration plants are at work to dispose of the body's waste products. The filters (glomeruli) consist of a coil of porous blood vessels which, after straining off the unwanted liquids, reabsorb the useful constituents, such as salts and water, back into the system. The waste liquid, a strong solution of urea, is then passed to the bladder where it is stored before being excreted from the body in the urine, so disposing of unnecessary nitrogen. The picture shows the cauliflower-like coil of a glomerulus set among clumps of folded tissue and stray blood cells.*

over many years and cause HYPERTENSION.

When to consult the doctor
- Immediately the symptoms described develop.

What the doctor may do
- Test urine.
- Check blood pressure.
- Advise on a low-protein diet.
- Send the patient to hospital for further tests to exclude the possibility of a more rare kidney disease.

Prevention
- Routine testing of urine and blood pressure may result in an early diagnosis. Treatment can then begin before the symptoms appear.

Outlook
- The condition may lead to kidney failure. Dialysis or a kidney transplant are life-saving procedures.

See URINARY SYSTEM *page 46*

NEPHROSIS
Also known as nephrotic syndrome, this is a chronic disease of the kidneys in which they fail to process the urine, leading to a chronic loss of protein through the urine. Symptoms include a puffy face, ANAEMIA, and the swelling of all body tissues (dropsy). Nephrosis does not usually respond to medication, and treatment is usually by a high-protein, low salt diet.

LIFE FOR THOUSANDS
Filling the gap when the kidneys fail

Kidneys are responsible for clearing the blood of the poisonous waste products of day-to-day living, such as urea, together with excess salts, minerals and water. Dialysis is used to clear the blood of these wastes when the kidneys fail.

Dialysis works by passing the patient's blood over one side of a semi-porous membrane, while the other side is washed with a solution of similar composition to normal body fluid called dialysate. The small pores in the membrane allow the waste products to pass through into the dialysate while holding back the blood cells and proteins. The waste products are washed away with the dialysate.

There are two systems of dialysis; peritoneal dialysis and haemodialysis. Which is used depends on the doctor's assessment of the patient's condition.

Peritoneal dialysis makes use of the peritoneal membrane which lines the abdomen. On one side of the membrane is the abdominal cavity, and on the other the blood vessels supplying the abdominal wall and the organs in the cavity such as the liver and the stomach. Dialysate is introduced into the cavity via a tube through the abdominal wall. Waste products from the blood filter across the membrane into the dialysate. When the dialysate is saturated with waste, it is drained out and replaced with fresh solution.

In haemodialysis, the blood is cleaned using an artificial membrane made of cellulose. The patient's blood is passed over one side of the membrane, dialysate over the other, and waste products are drained away.

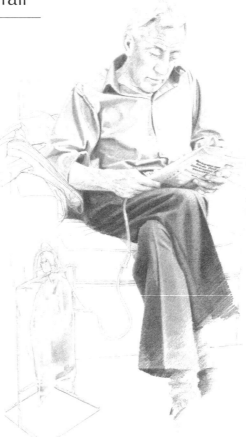

INCREASED FREEDOM *Though peritoneal dialysis is usually carried out in hospital, a new development for suitable patients is Continuous Ambulatory Peritoneal Dialysis (CAPD). This allows the patient to dialyse himself and lead an almost normal life. A catheter is fitted permanently through the patient's abdominal wall into the abdominal cavity. Three-and-a-half pints (2 litres) of dialysate fluid is run by gravity from a plastic bag through the catheter into the cavity. It remains there for four to six hours. At the end of the period the patient drains the fluid back into the bag which is thrown away. Emptying and then filling again takes about half an hour and is done four times a day. While filling or emptying is going on the patient can read, watch television, or listen to the radio. During the rest of the day he follows his normal routine including sleep. The empty bag can be kept in a pocket or strapped to his leg.*

NEPHROSTOMY

Drainage of urine from the kidney by means of a CATHETER which is passed into the kidney through an opening in the skin surface.

NERVOUS BREAKDOWN

A vague, non-medical term for a sudden attack of mental illness. It is loosely applied to a wide range of problems and its use should be avoided.

See MENTAL SYSTEM *page 33*

NETTLERASH

An allergic skin reaction that produces intensely irritating blisters and weals, resembling a sting from a nettle.

See URTICARIA

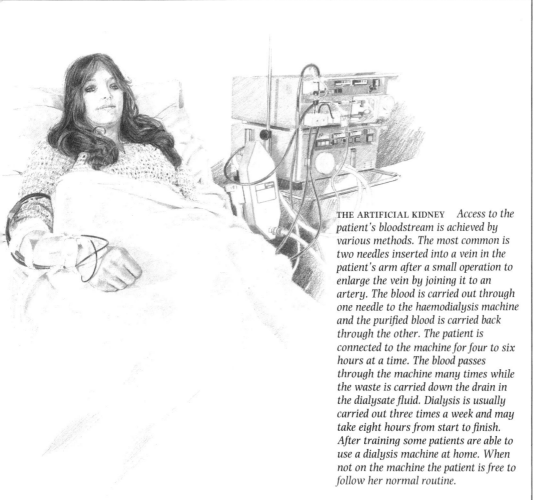

THE ARTIFICIAL KIDNEY   *Access to the patient's bloodstream is achieved by various methods. The most common is two needles inserted into a vein in the patient's arm after a small operation to enlarge the vein by joining it to an artery. The blood is carried out through one needle to the haemodialysis machine and the purified blood is carried back through the other. The patient is connected to the machine for four to six hours at a time. The blood passes through the machine many times while the waste is carried down the drain in the dialysate fluid. Dialysis is usually carried out three times a week and may take eight hours from start to finish. After training some patients are able to use a dialysis machine at home. When not on the machine the patient is free to follow her normal routine.*

NEURALGIA

Pain which results from a nerve being irritated or compressed. This pain is often felt along the full course of the nerve, not only at the point of irritation or pressure.

Symptoms

● The pain may be felt anywhere, depending on which nerve is affected and which area of the body it supplies.

● The pain may be persistent and severe, or felt as a recurrent, excruciating attack.

Duration

● The pain may either persist until its cause is treated or clear up of its own accord.

Causes

● Any inflammation or infection may irritate a nerve, causing neuralgia. SHINGLES is a common cause, producing post herpetic neuralgia. In this condition, pain is felt in the same area as the shingles rash, but may persist after the other symptoms have disappeared.

● A fractured bone or slipped disc may press on a nerve, causing neuralgia.

● Irritation in a sensory nerve to one side of the face produces a condition called TRIGEMINAL NEURALGIA.

Complications

● Neuralgia is a symptom rather than a disease, with no complications of its own.

Treatment in the home

● Mild painkillers may be taken. *See* MEDICINES, 22.

When to consult the doctor

● If any severe, persistent or recurrent pain occurs, especially if associated with other symptoms.

What the doctor may do

● Examine you to find the cause of the pain. If a bone fracture is suspected he may recommend X-rays.

● The doctor may prescribe strong painkillers to ease symptoms.

● For long-term treatment, the doctor will try to cure the cause of the neuralgia. In severe cases he may recommend that the nerve be killed by injection or removed by surgery.

Prevention

● Neuralgia may be prevented by avoiding certain forms of activity which are found to irritate a particular nerve. Going out in cold wind, for example, may trigger off neuralgia in some part of the face.

Outlook

● Depends on the cause.

See NERVOUS SYSTEM *page 34*

NEURASTHENIA

An ill-defined term used to describe a state of low spirits and an inability to cope, which often follows a mild physical illness. The term is also used to describe mild DEPRESSION or a state of ANXIETY.

See MENTAL SYSTEM *page* 33

NEURITIS

A disease of the nervous system which produces muscle weakness and loss of sensation in the skin.

See POLYNEUROPATHY

NEUROFIBROMA

A benign (non-cancerous) tumour of a nerve. It may be symptomless but if it presses on the nerve it can cause pain. Neurofibromas occur most commonly just beneath the skin.

See ACOUSTIC NEUROMA

NEUROFIBROMATOSIS

The condition is also known as von Recklinghausen's disease. Neurofibromas are lumps under the skin, produced by the excessive growth of nerve fibres. A single neurofibroma may arise in anyone. Neurofibromatosis is an inherited disease resulting in multiple lumps affecting nerves all over the body.

Symptoms
• Lumps can be felt under the skin. They are usually smooth, soft, round and mobile. They vary in size from that of a pea to that of a plum.
• Coffee-coloured patches appear on the skin, varying in diameter from a fraction of an inch to an inch or more (a few millimetres to several centimetres).
• Pain may be felt if a neurofibroma presses on a nerve. *See* NEURALGIA.

Duration
• Neurofibromatosis lasts indefinitely, but in most cases there are few or no symptoms. If there are symptoms they will persist unless treated.

Causes
• An inherited genetic abnormality.

Complications
• A neurofibroma pressing on the brain may result in deafness, TINNITUS, blindness or mental retardation.

Treatment in the home
• None possible.

When to consult the doctor
• If any abnormal lump or swelling is found on the body.

What the doctor may do
• Investigate the possible causes.
• Recommend that the lumps be removed by surgery and prescribe painkillers if necessary. *See* MEDICINES, 22.

Prevention
• None.

Outlook
• Neurofibromas are non-malignant and generally painless. (Neurofibromatosis is often found accidentally during the routine examination of a patient.) A few cases may require surgery if they are pressing on vital nerves or structures.

See NERVOUS SYSTEM *page* 34

NEUROSIS

There is much misunderstanding in the minds of both the public and doctors about this over-used term.

Any undue exaggeration of a normal feeling or behaviour may be called a neurosis. Normal individuals can usually recognise neurotic behaviour in themselves. Thus most people will blush when embarrassed, develop undue ANXIETY before taking a driving test or look twice to see that the gas is turned off. If such 'normal' anxiety or obsessional behaviour is extreme enough it can be called neurosis. The term is rightly falling into disuse because it wrongly suggests that such extremes of behaviour are a mental disease.

Neurotic fears are not imaginary and are very real to the sufferer. The term should not be used loosely in a derogatory sense.

NIGHT BLINDNESS

No one can see in total darkness, but provided that there is some light present most people can see a certain amount at night. This is because the eye produces a substance called rhodopsin or 'visual purple' (which in dim light breaks down into chemicals that transfer messages to the brain). Night blindness, a rare condition, occurs when the eye fails to produce visual purple.

Symptoms
• Failing vision in poor light.

Causes
• Severe malnutrition involving vitamin A deficiency. Vitamin A is necessary to replace visual purple.
• A rare inherited disease called retinitis pigmentosa. This may be present from early childhood and will progress, though the rate varies and may be very slow. After many years (10–50) it ends in blindness.

When to consult the doctor
• If difficulty in seeing in poor light persists.

What the doctor may do
• The doctor will probably examine the eye with an ophthalmoscope. If he sees unusual deposits of pigment on the retina (especially if there is any history in the family of retinitis pigmentosa) he will almost certainly refer the patient to an eye specialist. The specialist cannot treat retinitis pigmentosa, but he will follow the rate of progress of the condition, and arrange help for the patient whose sight is deteriorating.

Prevention
• Retinitis pigmentosa cannot be prevented. Genetic counselling may be advised.
• Vitamin A deficiency can be prevented by taking an adequate diet including milk, fish and vegetables. (In fact, vitamin A deficiency is only present in very severe states of malnutrition as found in conditions of severe poverty in underdeveloped countries.)

Outlook
• If the condition is caused by vitamin A deficiency, correction of the deficiency will cure the night blindness.
• Much research is being done into retinitis pigmentosa at present, and in future a cure may be found.

See EYE *page* 36

NIPPLE, CRACKED

Small, barely visible cracks in the nipples that commonly appear in the early days of breast-feeding.

Symptoms
• The nipples feel painful during breast-feeding, especially as the baby starts to suck.

Duration
• The cracks usually last for three or four days.

Causes
• The condition is usually caused by the baby sucking just the nipple instead of the areola as well.

Treatment in the home
• Resting the breast from feeding for 24 hours often

clears up the problem. The milk that fills the breast during this period will need to be expressed; the midwife will show you how to do this.

• Apply a lubricant. such as olive oil, to the nipple after each feed.

• Wear a well-supporting brassière to make the breasts feel more comfortable.

• Do not use nipple shields or breast pumps, they may make the cracks worse.

When to consult the doctor

• If any area of redness or any pain develops in the breast during breast-feeding.

What the doctor may do

• Give advice on how to treat the cracked nipples.

• Prescribe antibiotics if he considers there is a danger of a BREAST ABSCESS developing (through an infection entering the cracks in the nipple). *See* MEDICINES, 25.

Prevention

• Make sure from the start of breast-feeding that the baby is sucking on the areola (the brown or pink ring surrounding the nipple), as well as on the nipple itself.

• For several weeks before the baby is born, keep the nipples soft and supple by regular massage and lubrication.

Outlook

• Cracked nipples usually clear up completely within 14 days, and it is only in a few cases that a breast abscess develops.

See FEMALE GENITAL SYSTEM *page 48*

NOCTURIA

Passing urine at night. It is usually a sign of some disorder since, provided a large quantity of liquid has not been drunk before sleep, a healthy adult has no need to empty his bladder during the night. Among the disorders that can cause nocturia are various forms of kidney disease; bladder infections, such as CYSTITIS; and disorders, especially enlargement, of the PROSTATE GLAND. *See* URINARY SYSTEM *page 46*

NOCTURNAL MYOCLONUS

A sudden jerk of the muscles which occurs when a person is drifting off to sleep. It is usually felt as a single, brief spasm in the arms or legs.

Nocturnal myoclonus is caused by a sudden reactivation of the parts of the brain controlling sleep. Almost everybody has had the experience at some time in their lives. It has no significance in itself, though fright may cause the pulse to race and result in momentary panic.

There is rarely any need to consult the doctor, unless attacks occur night after night, and interfere with sleep. *See* NERVOUS SYSTEM *page 34*

NOISE INJURY

Ear damage caused by noise. Exposure to loud noise for prolonged periods of time, or a sudden blast of extremely loud noise, destroys the delicate cells of the cochlea, the organ of hearing in the inner ear.

Symptoms

• In the early stages there is often a sensation of cotton wool in the ears.

• Ringing in the ears (TINNITUS).

• To begin with, certain high-frequency sounds cannot be heard properly. Later, the deafness extends to all high frequencies and the hearing of speech is affected.

Duration

• Sudden loud noise may produce temporary loss of hearing. More often the damage is permanent.

Causes

• Industrial noise, especially in machine-shops and foundries.

• Prolonged exposure to loud, amplified music.

• Bellringing.

• Gunfire and explosives.

When to consult the doctor

• If deafness is experienced.

What the doctor may do

• Examine the ears and test the hearing.

• Advise on protective measures such as ear-plugs.

• In cases of severe damage, recommend a hearing-aid.

Prevention

• Wear special ear protectors when there is a risk of noise injury. These are often provided by employers and are more effective and more comfortable than ear-plugs.

Outlook

• Although there is no cure, hearing-aids can be a considerable help.

See EAR *page 38*

NOSE

Blocked or runny nose is very common. Other symptoms affecting the nose include bleeding, swelling or deformity, and colour change.

See SYMPTOM SORTER—NOSE PROBLEMS

FOREIGN BODY IN EAR, NOSE OR THROAT

NOSE-BLEED

A common complaint, affecting mainly the young or middle-aged.

Symptoms

• Bleeding from one or both nostrils.

Duration

• Most nose-bleeds stop within an hour.

Causes

• Often none, but common colds, picking, vigorous blowing or sneezing, nose or head injury, pressure changes, HYPERTENSION and SINUSITIS can all cause bleeding. Occasionally BLOOD disorders may be responsible.

Complications

• None likely.

Treatment in the home

• Sit upright in a chair with the head slightly forward and firmly pinch the soft part of the nose for 10 minutes. Swallow or spit out any blood going down the back of the nose. Breathe through the mouth. After 10 minutes release the nostrils and sit quietly. If bleeding restarts, squeeze the nostrils for a further 10 minutes.

• When bleeding stops, sit quietly or lie down for a while. Do not blow the nose for at least three hours.

When to consult the doctor

• If a nose-bleed cannot be stopped by the above measures (particularly in an elderly person), or if so much blood is lost that the patient becomes pale or dizzy.

• If nose-bleeds recur.

What the doctor may do

• Numb the nose with a local anaesthetic and then pack it with gauze or an inflatable balloon.

• Severe cases will be sent to hospital.

• Check the blood pressure for hypertension and provide treatment if necessary.

• CAUTERISE blood vessels that are prone to bleed.

Prevention

• Do not pick the nose or insert foreign objects into it.

Outlook

• *See* FIRST AID *page 597*.

See RESPIRATORY SYSTEM *page 42*

NUTRITION

Good health depends on a balanced diet—that is one that includes a mixture of the five basic nutrients that the human body needs to maintain itself.

See HEALTHY EATING *page 374*

Healthy eating

HOW TO CHOOSE THE BEST FOODS TO BUILD A BALANCED DIET AND A BETTER LIFE FOR YOU AND YOUR FAMILY

Our bodies need food for three main reasons. First, as fuel to keep us warm and supply the energy we need to stay alive and to move about and work. Second, food supplies the necessary materials for growth and to repair worn tissues. And third, we need the vitamins, minerals and other substances that are necessary for the chemical processes that take place inside our bodies.

The energy supplied by food is measured in calories. Two-thirds of this energy is used to maintain our normal body temperature, the normal tone of our muscles and to keep our heart and other organs functioning healthily. So if we did nothing but rest in bed all day, we would still need about two-thirds of our normal food intake to maintain what is known medically as our basal metabolic rate.

To provide this basic energy, an adult weighing 10 stones (about 64 kg.) will require about 1,600 calories each day. The rest of the day's normal activities—dressing, eating, walking, working and playing—require only about 800 calories.

The harder we work and the more we move about, the more calories we use up. For instance, a manual worker standing at his bench and lifting material will expend about 3,000 calories a day, and a very active worker, such as a coal miner or dock labourer, will expend about 4,000 calories. On the other hand, a modern housewife uses only about 2,200 calories. Whatever calories we use up in our daily lives need to be supplied by food, but if we consume more calories than we use we will put on weight. The aim of healthy eating is to get the balance right.

THE FIVE BASIC GROUPS OF NUTRIENTS

No single food is essential to our diet. All the types of nourishment that the body needs are available from many different sources. For example, vitamin C is supplied in varying amounts by cabbages, green peas, potatoes, oranges, lemons and blackcurrants. What is important for good health is that we should eat a variety of foods.

There are five basic groups of nutrients: carbohydrates, proteins, fats, vitamins and minerals. The one food that provides all the nutrients in the correct proportions for good health is mother's milk—but that is only suitable for babies. Everyone else needs to eat a mixture. The more varied the diet, the more likely it is to contain all the nutrients.

PROTEINS FOR BUILDING UP THE BODY

Throughout life, there is a continual breakdown and loss of body tissues. This loss must be made good from proteins in the diet. For this a mature adult needs an average of about $1\frac{1}{2}$ oz.

(40 g.) of protein a day. Meat contains about 60 per cent water, 20 per cent fat and 20 per cent protein, so for a person to obtain his daily minimum requirement of protein from meat alone he would need to eat 7 oz. (200 g.) of meat. Bread contains about 10 per cent protein, so he would need to eat about 14 oz. (400 g.) of bread.

If a person does not get enough protein in his diet to make up for the natural breakdown of body tissues, some of the less vital protein tissues in the body, such as the muscles, are broken down to maintain such vital organs as the heart and kidneys. In the Western world there is no problem about meeting protein needs—so many foods contain protein that people actually consume at least twice as much as they need. Bread and other cereals (such as rice, oats and barley), and peas and beans, are sufficient, without milk, meat, fish, eggs and cheese, to provide plenty of protein.

However, illness causes a considerable loss of protein from the body. Infections, burns, broken bones and the stress of surgery all lead to protein loss. A week in bed with an infection like influenza will lead to a noticeable loss of protein from the muscles of the legs. If the patient has a good appetite when he recovers, he will make up the 1 or 2 lb. (450 or 900 g.) loss of protein in 12–24 days. But as the appetite will probably not be back to normal during convalescence, the process is likely to take longer.

CARBOHYDRATES—TO PROVIDE ENERGY

About 50–60 per cent of food eaten consists of carbohydrate, which supplies much of the energy needed by the body. Carbohydrate is a collective term for sugars, starches and cellulose.

The main sugar in a person's diet is sucrose, obtained from sugar cane or sugar beet. Most sucrose is eaten in the form of sweets, jams, biscuits, cakes and sugar added to drinks; a small amount comes from fruit.

Starch is found in, for example, potatoes, wheat and rice. When we eat these foods the starch in them is broken down and absorbed into the blood as glucose, a form of sugar.

Cellulose is not digested by human beings. It is therefore not a source of energy. However, it is needed in the diet because it is a major form of fibre, or roughage—that is, it remains undigested in the intestines to give bulk to the faeces and so promote regular bowel movements.

FATS—FOR ENERGY AND FLAVOUR

The fats that people eat can come from the food itself or may be added in the cooking process. Fat is contained in milk and cream, cheese, meat (both the obvious fat around the meat and the hidden fat between the fibres of the meat), fatty fish such as herring and mackerel, and eggs. Cooking fats consist of the hard fats, such as dripping and lard, and liquid oils from soya beans, olives and corn.

Fats have several roles in the diet—directly, because of their nutritional value, and indirectly, in improving the palatability of foods and making them easier to chew and swallow. Certain of the vitamins—A, D, E and K—are found in the fatty parts of food and so diets very low in fats are also low in these vitamins. Moreover, they need the fats in order to be absorbed into the bloodstream.

Fats are also important because they are concentrated sources of energy, providing more than twice as much as the same weight of carbohydrate or protein. The addition of a thin layer of butter or margarine to a slice of bread can double the amount of energy (or calories) that the bread alone would have supplied. If a diet is extremely low in its fat content then a greater amount of food must be eaten to provide enough energy.

Fats play an important role in flavour. The taste of many foods depends either on the fats themselves or on other components that are dissolved in the fats.

Finally, fatty foods remain in the stomach longer than low-fat foods, so that they provide a greater feeling of fullness.

VITAMINS—SMALL BUT ESSENTIAL INGREDIENTS

Vitamins are required by the body in only small amounts, ranging from about 30 mg. of vitamin C to as little as 1 microgram (one millionth part of a gram) of vitamin B12. Vitamins play no part in providing the body with tissue or energy, but they are essential to its efficient functioning, in the same way that lubricating oil is to the running of a car.

The discovery of the existence of vitamins began only about 100 years ago, and the first was identified only at the beginning of this century. It is now known that the body requires 13. However, the effects of vitamins have been known for many centuries. Some 3,000 years ago the Greek physician Hippocrates recommended eating the liver of the black cock as a cure for night blindness. It is now known that night blindness is one of the early signs of vitamin A deficiency, and that liver is an especially rich source of vitamin A.

Rickets (a childhood disease of the bones) is due to a deficiency of vitamin D. Cod-liver oil, a rich source

---

True or false?

□ **An apple a day keeps the doctor away**—*False*
A medium-sized apple supplies only 10 mg. of vitamin C compared with about 50 mg. in an orange. Apart from 12 g. of sugar (45 calories), apples have little else other than about 2 g. of dietary fibre.

□ **Large doses of vitamin C prevent colds**—*Probably false*
A few experiments have shown that 1 or 2 g. a day (compared with 30–50 mg. needed for general purposes) seem to reduce colds. But most experiments have failed to show any effect.

□ **Brown bread is more nutritious than white**—*True*
Wholemeal bread made from the whole wheat grain contains a lot more iron, vitamin B1, niacin and other vitamins, and dietary fibre, than white bread. Brown breads are in between.

□ **Fish is good for the brain**—*False*
Unfortunately no food is particularly good for the brain.

of vitamin D, was used to treat the disease at least 100 years before vitamins were discovered.

Scurvy is due to a lack of vitamin C. In 1753, 150 years before the

True or false?

□ **Dark green vegetables are better than light-coloured**—*True*
Dark green cabbage, kale and watercress, for example, contain more carotene (which forms vitamin A in the body), more iron and more folic acid (one of the B vitamins). The green outer leaves of cabbages and lettuces also contain more than the whiter, inner leaves.

□ **Carrots make you see better in the dark**—*Partly true*
If you are short of vitamin A, you cannot see in dim light—an ailment called night blindness. In that case carrots will cure you as they are rich in carotene.

□ **Margarine is not as nutritious as butter**—*False*
Margarine has as much vitamin A added as there is in summer butter (and so is richer than winter butter), and it has more vitamin D than butter. In addition, special margarines are made from polyunsaturated fats and so may be better than butter at keeping down cholesterol levels.

discovery of vitamin C, the disease was cured in sailors by giving them lemon and orange juice.

Some people mistakenly believe that the more vitamins they take, the better their health will be. But that is not true. Once enough of a vitamin has been taken to meet the body's requirements, any extra has no effect. It is true that surplus amounts of vitamins A and D are stored in the body for further use, though taking too much of either can harm the health—but extra amounts of vitamins C, B1 and B2 are simply passed out of the body in the urine.

It is often claimed that large doses of vitamin C will prevent or cure a cold. Despite the wide publicity the claim has received, clinical trials have failed to show any benefit.

The only time that it is useful to take supplementary vitamins is after an illness, in the form of multi-vitamin tablets.

Synthetic vitamins are just as beneficial as natural ones. Chemically, the two are identical.

MINERALS—FOR BONE AND BLOOD

The body needs at least 20 different minerals to function properly. Some of them are required in large amounts—for example, calcium from milk, which makes the hard part of teeth and bones, and iron from meat, which produces haemoglobin, a component of blood that carries oxygen around the body.

Other minerals are needed in small amounts. They include magnesium, manganese, selenium, iodine, sodium, potassium, copper, zinc and chromium. They all help in the production of enzymes (substances that speed up chemical reactions in

the body) and hormones (substances that control the functioning of different organs).

People in developed countries, with access to a wide variety of foods, are unlikely to suffer from deficiency of any essential minerals, unless they limit their foods to a very small selection.

However, a deficiency of iron leads to anaemia. Too few red cells in the blood mean that insufficient oxygen is being carried from the lungs to the organs and tissues of the body. Women of fertile years lose much more iron than men, through menstruation, and consequently they need more iron in their diet than men in order to replace it.

Iron deficiency, producing mild anaemia, is widespread in this country, either because of inadequate iron in the diet, or poor absorption.

Iron from meat is much better absorbed than that from plant foods, so anyone suffering from slight anaemia should eat more meat, especially liver.

Vitamin C helps iron absorption and a glass of orange juice with a meal will help the iron from other foods to be absorbed.

If anaemia is more than mild, it is a medical problem. *See* ANAEMIA.

Iodine is needed to help form thyroid hormone, which controls the body's rate of metabolism. A person who is producing too little thyroid hormone will suffer from hypothyroidism, signified by a goitre—a swelling in the neck. Fish should be included two or three times a week and table salt containing added iodine may be used. But generally there is no problem as other foods, including vegetables contain small amounts of iodine.

In Western society, relatively few people are short of food or lack essential nutrients. Nevertheless, there are some groups of people in this country who are potentially at risk of nutritional deficiency because they have special dietary requirements. They include pregnant and nursing women, infants, growing children, adolescents and elderly people. They are known as the vulnerable groups.

PREGNANT AND NURSING WOMEN
People often say that a woman who is pregnant is eating for two, implying that she should eat more, but this is not true. During pregnancy the mother's body uses food more efficiently, and the extra needs of the growing fetus are therefore taken care of without the mother needing to increase her food intake. However, she must make sure that her diet is of sufficiently high quality to provide herself and her baby with enough proteins, vitamins and minerals. Otherwise the growing baby will satisfy its own requirements at the expense of the mother's tissues—and her health.

INFANTS
Breast milk contains all the nutrients essential for babies, together with substances that protect the baby from infection. *See* CHILD CARE.

The risk to the baby comes when it is weaned. At about three to four months, or when it weighs about 14 lb. (6.3 kg.), it needs more than just mother's milk, so weaning foods are added to its diet, gradually replacing milk. At about nine months of age the baby is eating ordinary foods in ground-up form. If the baby is weaned too late, or weaned on food deficient in protein, vitamins or minerals, its growth or general health can suffer.

CHILDREN
Because children are growing, they require a greater proportion of protein in their food than adults do. Ensure that a child's diet contains plenty of nourishing foods, rather than sweets and sweet drinks that satisfy energy demands without providing any nutrients. Milk, cheese and yoghurt are rich in calcium for building bones and teeth. Meat, especially liver, is a good source of iron for the blood. Fruit and vegetables provide vitamins and minerals. The main source of vitamin D, which is especially necessary for bone formation in growing children, is sunshine.

If a parent cannot be entirely sure that a child is eating the right foods, the child should be given a multi-vitamin and iron tablet two or three times a week.

ADOLESCENTS
In their teens, children undergo a spurt in growth, which slightly increases their need for nutrients. However, at this age they are most likely to feed on snacks. There is nothing wrong with hamburgers, fish fingers, sausages and crisps, provided the teenager eats a variety of foods. But snacking regularly on just one type of convenience food could lead to nutritional deficiency.

ELDERLY PEOPLE
Apathy following bereavement or disability can cut down food intake by old people to a dangerously low level.

Some disabled people lack vitamin D because they are housebound or rarely expose themselves to sunshine (sitting on a park bench on a sunny day will provide the body with vitamin D). There are only a few foods that contain vitamin D in significant amounts: eggs, butter, margarine, and fatty fish such as sardines, herrings, mackerel, pilchards and salmon.

HOW VALUABLE ARE 'HEALTH FOODS'?

The term health food includes organically grown fruit and vegetables, whole foods, various pills and herbs, and foods that are claimed to have mystical properties such as seaweeds, 'live' yoghurt and honey. The term can also include vegetarianism and diets based on oriental philosophy.

Some of these categories, such as whole foods, are nutritionally good; some, such as seaweed and honey, are harmless; and some, such as herbs and ginseng, are quite unproven. Many products sold in health food shops carry claims for non-existent benefits. Even the term health food itself is misleading since it implies that other kinds of food are unhealthy.

VEGETARIANISM
There is nothing nutritionally wrong with being a vegetarian; in fact, the healthy diet recommended by nutritionists is the kind of diet vegetarians already eat—containing less fat, more fruit and vegetables, and more dietary fibre.

Many vegetarians eat eggs and

drink milk. Those who avoid all animal foods are vegans, and so far as is known they are just as healthy as people who eat a mixed diet.

The Zen macrobiotic diet is supposed to offer spiritual enlightenment but has no connection with Zen Buddhism. As you proceed from stage to stage you eat fewer foods until, at stage seven, you live only on brown rice—claimed as a cure-all. Unfortunately some people have died on this diet.

WHOLE FOODS
Whole foods are certainly better than refined foods. This really means wholemeal bread and flour rather than white bread and flour. The amount of rice, maize and other grains that we eat is so small that it makes little difference whether we eat them whole or refined. And brown sugar is very little different from white sugar.

ORGANICALLY GROWN FOODS
Most farmers and gardeners fertilise their soil with sulphate of ammonia, potash and phosphate. They also add as much manure and compost as they can find. Advocates of organic farming claim that the use of chemicals is artificial and that foods that are grown in organically fertilised soil are nutritionally superior. In fact, there is no difference between them. Organic farmers usually avoid all chemicals, including pesticides and weedkillers.

The few controlled tasting trials that have been carried out have shown that people cannot distinguish between organically grown and inorganically fertilised foods.

The same is true for eggs from free-range and battery chickens. Nutritionally they are exactly the

same, and trials have failed to detect any difference in taste.

SEA SALT
Most table salt (sodium chloride) comes from underground mines and is highly purified. It usually has some magnesium carbonate (a harmless mineral salt) added to make it flow freely. Sea salt is made by evaporating sea water and so contains many impurities. Health food advocates claim that these other substances are beneficial to health, but the amounts present in the salt are so small that they have no effect. And sea salt usually costs about twice as much as 'land' salt.

HONEY
Because of the long history of honey as a food, and perhaps because of its pleasant taste, many claims are made for its health benefits. In fact, honey is simply sugar and water with very small traces of several vitamins.

The food value of a teaspoon of honey is exactly the same as that of three-quarters of a teaspoon of ordinary table sugar. You would have to eat pounds a day to obtain a reasonable amount of vitamins.

CIDER VINEGAR, KELP, 'LIVE' YOGHURT, GINSENG
Cider vinegar is vinegar made by refermenting cider—in a similar way to wine vinegar. Nutritionally it is simply acetic acid and water, and so provides a few calories and nothing else.

Kelp is a seaweed. It is a source of iodine—an essential nutrient—and a few mineral salts of lesser importance. It has no special food value.

Live yoghurt contains the bacteria which turned the milk into yoghurt, whereas ordinary yoghurt has usually had the bacteria killed by pasteurisation. The bacteria do not survive inside the human intestines, and do not provide any benefit. If live yoghurt is made from full-cream milk instead of skim milk powder, it is nutritionally better and tastes better, but that is because of the milk not because the bacteria are still alive.

Ginseng is the root of a bush that grows in China and Korea. A vast range of magical properties is attributed to it, but there is no evidence that it has any effect.

'BALANCED VITAMINS'
Most health food shops sell tablets of balanced vitamins that have been extracted from wheat, yeast or liver instead of being synthesised in a factory. They were balanced so far as the wheat plant or the yeast or the animal's liver were concerned but they are not balanced for human needs. Wheat contains very little vitamin B2; the vitamin B1 in yeast extract steadily falls while it sits on the shelf; and the B vitamins in the liver extract will depend on how the animal was fed.

HERBS AND FLOWER PETALS
Herbs have a mystical appeal since they are widely used by primitive people and were used as medicines in this country for centuries. Most of them have no effect; some are poisonous (comfrey, for example, contains alkaloids which damage the liver); and some contain small amounts of drugs (fennel is used in gripe water). Some modern medicines are extracted from herbs—quinine was originally extracted from the bark of a tree—but that is no reason why healthy people should eat small amounts of drugs every day.

Pleasant drinks can be made from some herbs, leaves and petals, but they have no beneficial effects.

True or false?

□ **Meat is essential for strength**— *False*
There are large numbers of healthy (and strong) vegetarians—and even vegans, who eat no animal foods at all.

□ **Honey is especially good for you** —*False*
Honey is only fructose (fruit sugar), glucose (grape sugar) and water, with vitamins present in such small amounts that they make no worthwhile contribution to the diet.

□ **Brown sugar is better than white sugar**—*False*
White sugar is 99.9 per cent pure sucrose; brown sugar is 98 per cent pure sucrose and 1 per cent water, leaving room for only minute traces of mineral salts and protein—too little to do any good.

□ **Jam made in copper pans is better than jam made in stainless steel** —*False*
Copper completely destroys all the vitamin C in the fruit while jam made in stainless steel retains a little vitamin C.

THE DANGERS OF THE WESTERN DIET

Over the last 50 years or so, a number of diseases have become far more common in industrialised countries, and because they are rare in the poorer developing countries they have been called the diseases of affluence. They include coronary heart disorders, diabetes, tooth decay, certain forms of cancer and conditions of the bowel.

Diet seems to play a part in all those diseases because so many changes in Western eating patterns have taken place in parallel with an increase in the diseases.

There is evidence, though not yet proof, that we eat too much fat, sugar and salt and not enough fibre.

IS FAT A CAUSE OF HEART DISEASE?
When people die of heart disease, they are usually found to have fatty deposits on the walls of their arteries. The deposits make the arteries narrower than usual, which can restrict the amount of blood passing along the artery. If a blood clot occurs in the coronary arteries of the heart it will prevent oxygen getting to the heart muscle and the result is a heart attack.

The fatty deposits on the artery walls include ordinary fats (triglycerides), calcium, and a special type of fat called cholesterol. A high fat diet of the type commonly eaten in Western countries will raise the level of blood cholesterol, and this seems to help to cause the fatty deposits. It used to be thought that cholesterol in our food (eggs and meat contain cholesterol) was the major culprit in raising levels of cholesterol in the blood, but this is not so. Dietary cholesterol has relatively little effect, because when more is eaten the body simply makes less cholesterol. So dietary cholesterol is not as important as dietary fat, especially saturated fats.

Fats are referred to as either saturated or unsaturated. Saturated fats come mostly from animals—meat, cream, eggs, cheese, and some margarines. Coconut oil, which is used to make ice cream, is also a saturated fat. Unsaturated fats usually come from vegetables—particularly sunflower and corn oil—and fish.

There is evidence that if the diet includes a lot of saturated (animal) fats there will be higher levels of cholesterol in the blood. It is also suggested that if more vegetable oils are eaten, less cholesterol is produced in the blood. However, the case is far from proven and research work continues.

Until the full facts are known it can do no harm to use vegetable oils for cooking and to cut down on fats in the diet. This means eating less fatty meat, butter, cream, margarine and the foods that contain added fat, such as cakes and biscuits.

It might also be beneficial to use margarine made from sunflower or corn oil to increase the intake of unsaturated fats, but this is still a highly controversial subject.

DIETARY FIBRE: PREVENTION OF BOWEL DISEASE?
During the 20th century, diets in Western countries have become steadily lower in fibre, the indigestible cellulose that gives bulk to the faeces. People have been eating less bread, and a greater amount of the bread they do eat has been white. White

bread is made with flour from which bran, a rich source of fibre, has been discarded. People today also eat less fruit and vegetables, which contain fibre, and more fatty, sugary foods, such as cakes and biscuits, which do not.

As the fibre has decreased, constipation, haemorrhoids, varicose veins and bowel diseases have increased. These disorders are rare among people who have a fibre-rich diet. A high-fibre diet is also thought to make cancer of the intestinal tract less likely.

Many people who have suffered from constipation for years are cured by eating wholemeal bread or bran-enriched breakfast cereals, or by adding bran to breakfast cereals or stewed fruit. To a lesser extent, ordinary brown bread, vegetables and fruit also improve bowel movements.

IS SALT A FACTOR IN HIGH BLOOD PRESSURE?
Small amounts of the mineral sodium are essential to health, but sodium is added to food in large amounts in the form of common salt (sodium chloride) and monosodium glutamate, which is widely used in canned meat and many soups to bring out flavour.

There is evidence that high blood pressure, coronary heart disease and strokes may be associated with too high an intake of sodium, sometimes with a deficiency of potassium. The case against salt is not yet proven, but most people eat far more salt than they need, and it can do no harm to take less—and to increase the intake of potassium by eating more fruit and vegetables.

Excessive sodium intake is more serious for babies than adults, because an adult can excrete the excess in the urine, whereas the baby's kidneys are insufficiently developed for them to be able to do so. For that reason, little or no salt is added to manufactured baby foods.

True or false?

☐ **Fat children become fat adults** —*Possibly true*
Less than 10 per cent of school-children are overweight compared with about 30 per cent of adults, so a fat child might become a fat adult.

Many people are fat because they have a low metabolic rate and so need fewer calories. They get fat on the average diet. A child who is fat for this reason will probably become a fat adult. But a child who is fat because he eats excessively will not be fat when he grows up unless he continues eating excessively.

☐ **Brown eggs are more nutritious than white**—*False*
The colour of the shell is a characteristic of the breed of chicken and nothing to do with nutritive value.

☐ **Margarine is less fattening than butter**—*False*
By law margarine must contain no more than 16 per cent water, the same as butter, and so all margarines contain 84 per cent fat—the same as butter.

SUGAR: DESTROYER OF TEETH
Dental decay is caused by bacteria growing and multiplying on the teeth and producing acids which dissolve the outer surface (the enamel).

To grow on the teeth the bacteria need food. All carbohydrates provide it to some extent, but the bacteria prefer sucrose—ordinary table sugar.

Sweets do most damage as they adhere to the teeth. Sucking sweets means that sugar is kept in constant contact with the teeth for many hours every day.

The best advice is not to have sugar in contact with the teeth except at meal times. But most people, especially children, are unlikely to give up eating sweets entirely, so they should limit the time in which there is sugar in the mouth. Sweets immediately after a meal, or a bout of sweet-eating once a week, are preferable to continuous between-meal snacks of sweet things.

Since the bacteria live as a sticky film on the teeth, called plaque, an obvious remedy is to remove it by regular cleaning. *See* TEETH.

Another safeguard is to remove the carbohydrate from the mouth straight after eating. Saliva helps to dispose of carbohydrate, and a hard food, such as an apple or carrot, after the meal stimulates the flow of saliva. Simply rinsing away the carbohydrate with water also helps.

Small children are at great risk from tooth decay. Bottles of milk containing sugar are often given to babies before going to bed. Even worse, toddlers are 'kept quiet' with a bottle of sweetened fruit drink which they suck at for hours at a time. This leads to rampant decay, and some children have teeth which are half dissolved away.

OBESITY: THE GREATEST ENEMY
The most serious disease of affluence is obesity. Between a quarter and a half of the people in developed countries are overweight, and fat people have an above-average chance of suffering high blood pressure, heart disease, diabetes, gallstones and gout. The extra weight that bones and joints have to bear can also cause osteoarthritis of the knees, hips and the lower back, as well as flat feet. Excess fat around the chest and under the diaphragm may interfere with breathing and create a tendency to bronchitis.

Overweight people also have a lower than average life expectancy. A man aged 45 who is 25 lb. (11.3 kg.) overweight has his life expectancy reduced from 80 to 60. If he reduces his weight to the correct level for his height, he also reduces the risk of premature death.

People become fat by eating more food than they use up in exercise. And people in the rich countries of the Western world have more opportunity than others to eat attractive, sugary foods, such as cakes, biscuits, ice cream and sweets.

A normal amount of fat—10 per cent of body weight for a man and 20 per cent for a woman—provides a reserve store of energy, makes a protective cushion around the vital organs of the body, and acts as a heat insulator (thin people feel the cold much more than fat people).

But if we eat more food than we need the surplus is usually stored as fat. In a grossly obese person, fat can account for 50 per cent of the body weight. But not everyone stores excess food in this way. For a reason that has not yet been explained, some people burn off surplus food as heat.

What are you getting from
your daily food?

The figures in this chart are
rounded off, and are based on
$3\frac{1}{2}$ oz. (100 g.) portions. This is
an average helping, but in some
cases, such as butter or bran, no
one is likely to eat $3\frac{1}{2}$ oz. at a
sitting.
The amount of nutrients varies
according to the amount of water
in the food. For example, the
nutrients in $3\frac{1}{2}$ oz. of chocolate
biscuits are far more concentrated
than in the same weight of cooked
porridge.

A food has been listed as a good
source of vitamins if a normal
portion provides a reasonable
amount of daily needs. 'Nia'
stands for niacin, one of the
B vitamins. 'Tr' indicates a trace
of the nutrient—too small to be
of value.
F stands for folic acid, important
for women planning to have a
baby and in early pregnancy (see
page 423). Bovril and yeast
extract are also high in folic acid.

*Liver contains too much Vitamin
A for pregnant women.

Food	Energy (calories)	Protein (g.)	Fat (g.)	Carbohydrate (g.)	Water (g.)	Fibre (g.)	Vitamin (good sources of)			
Dairy products										
Milk	65	3.3	4	5	88	—	A		B2	Nia
Butter	740	—	82	—	15	—	A			
Cream, single	210	2	21	3	72	—	A			
Cheese, cheddar type	300	23	23	—	37	—	A		B2	Nia
Cheese, Danish blue	350	23	29	—	40	—	A		B2	Nia
Cheese, Stilton	460	26	40	—	28	—	A		B2	Nia
Cheese, cottage	100	14	4	1	80	—				Nia
Cheese, processed	310	22	25	—	44	—	A		B2	
Ice cream, dairy	170	4	7	25	64	—		B1	B2	Nia
Yoghurt, natural	50	5	1	6	86	—		B1	B2	Nia
Yoghurt, flavoured	80	5	1	14	79	—		B1	B2	Nia
Margarine	730	—	81	—	16	—	A			
Low fat spread	370	—	40	—	57	—	A			
Meat and fish										
Bacon, gammon—boiled	270	25	19	—	54	—		B1		Nia
Bacon, streaky—fried	500	23	45	—	28	—		B1		Nia
Eggs	150	12	11	tr	75	—	A	B1	B2	Nia F
Beef, brisket—boiled	330	28	24	—	48	—			B2	Nia
Beef, minced—stewed	230	23	15	—	59	—			B2	Nia
Beef, rump steak—fried	250	29	15	—	56	—		B1	B2	Nia
Corned beef	220	27	12	—	58	—			B2	Nia
Lamb cutlets—grilled	370	23	31	—	45	—		B1	B2	Nia
Pork chop—grilled	330	29	24	—	36	—		B1	B2	Nia
Veal cutlet—fried	215	31	8	—	55	—				
Chicken—roast	150	25	5	—	68	—		B1	B2	Nia
Calf's liver—fried	250	27	13	—	53	—	A	B1	B2	Nia F*
Sausages, beef—fried	270	13	18	15	48	—				Nia
Sausages, pork—fried	320	14	25	11	45	—			B2	Nia
Ham	120	18	5	—	73	—		B1	B2	Nia
White fish, e.g. cod										F
White fish—fried in batter	200	20	10	8	60	—		B1		Nia F
White fish—steamed	80	19	1	—	79	—		B1		Nia F
Fatty fish, e.g. herring										
Fatty fish—fried	230	23	15	1.5	58	—			B2	Nia
Sardines—in oil	220	24	14	—	58	—			B2	Nia F
Sardines—in tomato sauce	180	18	12	—	65	—			B2	Nia
Vegetables and fruit										
Beans, French—boiled	20	2	—	3	90	3	A			F
Beans, baked—canned	60	5	—	10	73	7		B1		
Brussels sprouts	20	3	—	2	88	4	A	B1	B2	C F
Cabbage—boiled	10	1	—	1	96	2.5	A			C F

Food	Energy (calories)	Protein (g.)	Fat (g.)	Carbohydrate (g.)	Water (g.)	Fibre (g.)	Vitamin (good sources of)
Carrots—boiled	20	0.6	—	4	91	3	A F
Cauliflower	10	1.5	—	1	93	2	C F
Cucumber—raw	10	0.6	—	2	96	0.4	C F
Peas—boiled	50	5	—	8	80	12	A B1 B2 Nia C F
Potatoes—boiled	80	1	—	20	77	1	B1 F
Potatoes—roast	160	3	5	27	64	1	B1 F
Potatoes—chipped	250	4	11	37	47	1	B1 F
Tomatoes	15	1	—	3	93	1.5	A C F
Apples	45	0.3	—	12	84	2	
Bananas	80	1	tr	20	70	3	C F
Cherries	50	0.6	—	12	81	2	
Grapes	60	0.6	—	15	80	1	
Oranges	35	1	—	9	86	2	C F
Pears	40	tr	—	11	83	2	
Plums	40	0.6	—	10	84	2	A
Almonds	570	17	54	4	5	14	B1 B2 Nia F
Chestnuts	620	2	3	37	52	7	B1 B2
Peanuts—roasted	570	24	49	9	4	8	B1 B2 Nia F
Peanut butter	620	23	54	13	1	8	B1 B2 Nia F
Drinks							
Beer	30	0.3	—	2	—		
Strong ale	70	0.7	—	6	—		B2 Nia
Wine	70	tr	—	tr			
Spirits	220	—	—	—			
Tea—black	—	—	—	—			
Coffee—black	—	—	—	—			Nia
Sugar—teaspoon	24	—	—	—			
Soup—chicken noodle	20	1	0.3	4		tr	
Soup—cream of tomato	55	1	3	6		tr	
Food from cereals							
Bread, wholemeal	215	9	3	42	40	8.5	B1 Nia F
Bread, white	230	8	2	50	39	2.7	B1 Nia
Rice, white—boiled	120	2	—	30	70	0.8	F
Spaghetti—without sauce	120	4	—	26	72	unknown	
Cornflakes—with milk	205	6.5	4	34.7		1.2	A B1 B2 Nia D F
Chocolate biscuits	520	6	28	67	2	3.1	B2 Nia
Water biscuits	440	11	13	76	5	3.0	B1 Nia
Fruit cake	350	5	13	58	20	3.5	
Sponge cake—with fat	460	6	27	53	15	1.0	Nia
Porridge—cooked	45	1.5	1	8	90	0.8	
Bran—wheat	200	14	6	23	8	44	B1 B2 Nia F

HOW TO LOSE WEIGHT AND STAY HEALTHY

Exercise is not an effective way of losing weight. You would need to walk about 50 miles (80 km.) to use up a single pound of body fat. By far the better way of taking off weight is to eat fewer calories.

That means cutting down on sugar and foods that contain sugar, as they are extremely high in calorific value. Instead, eat more fruit, vegetables and wholemeal bread, which are more filling and contain fewer calories. They will also improve your nutrient intake.

Sugar provides nothing at all apart from calories—and it has been suggested as a possible cause of heart disease and diabetes.

An overweight person who normally eats 2,500 calories a day should reduce his intake by 1,000 calories.

Since 3,500 calories equals one pound of body fat, it will take three and a half days to lose a pound—two pounds in a week.

In the first week the loss may be as much as 5 lb. (2.3 kg.), as the body's first response to the diet will be to lose a great deal of water. But the weight loss will soon settle down to a steady 2 lb. (900 g.).

To lose 1 stone (6.3 kg.) will take about seven weeks.

Losing weight is a long-term process; it takes months. There is no miraculous crash diet to take off large amounts of weight in a few days. Even if a person ate nothing at all for a week—which would be highly dangerous—he could lose only 5 lb. (2.3 kg.) of body fat.

Drugs are not a great help. If you take drugs to reduce the appetite you are likely to go back to the old eating habits when you give them up—and no drugs should be taken for more than a short time.

Other drugs that increase the rate at which the body uses up energy all have serious side-effects, and are dangerous.

If you simply halve your food intake you will also halve your intake of essential nutrients—proteins, vitamins and minerals—and that may pose a serious health risk.

The best way to lose weight is to cut down on foods that supply few nutrients but are high in calories—sugar, fats and alcohol—and to keep consumption of nutrient-rich foods—fish, meat, cheese, fruit and vegetables—at a normal level. But avoid avocados, which are rich in fat, and bananas, dates and figs, which contain a lot of sugar.

Some people find a low carbohydrate diet successful. By reducing their intake of starchy and sugary foods to a low level, but eating plenty of proteins and fats, they usually eat less.

Fats stay a long time in the stomach and provide a feeling of fullness.

Another approach is the low-fat diet which requires the dieter to eliminate most of the fat from his meals.

This makes a substantial reduction in calories without greatly reducing the quantity of food, as a small amount of fat contains a large number of calories.

However hard it is for people to lose weight, it is even harder to exercise the life-long control and restraint needed to keep the weight down to a desirable level.

Many people find it helpful to join a slimming group where fat people—and former fat people—help each other to stick to their diets.

RIGHTS AND WRONGS OF COOKING AND PROCESSING

Certain foods need to be cooked to make them safe to eat. For example, raw minced beef and raw chicken often contain bacteria, which if they were not killed by cooking would cause serious stomach upsets. Certain types of bean are poisonous if eaten raw but completely harmless after they have been cooked.

There are, however, drawbacks to cooking. In all methods there is some loss of nutrients, although in many cases it is too slight to be significant. Some vitamins are destroyed by overcooking. The longer a food is cooked, the lower is its content of vitamin C and, to a lesser extent, of B1 and certain other vitamins. Heat also damages some proteins, so that the nutritional value of the food decreases: the browned exterior of a roast joint and the crust of a loaf are tasty but less nutritious than the rest of the meat or bread.

The biggest loss of nutrients in cooking occurs when the nutrients are washed out into the cooking water. Vitamin C—and to a lesser extent the B vitamins and some minerals—are lost from fruit and vegetables in this way.

The more finely the food is cut up, the greater the amount of water that is used and the longer the food is cooked, the more nutrients will be washed out.

When fruit is stewed, the loss of nutrients into the cooking water is not important, because the juice is normally kept and served with the fruit.

But when vegetables are cooked, the water in which they are cooked is often thrown away, rather than being used to make soups or gravy.

Frying and pressure cooking lead to a much smaller loss of nutrients than boiling. Dropping food into hot fat seals its surface, and in pressure cooking a smaller volume of water is used than in boiling, and the process is more rapid.

A lot of vitamin B1 is lost from potatoes if they are bought ready-peeled or ready-chipped, because they are kept white with sulphite, and this destroys part of the vitamin.

Dietary fibre is not affected by cooking.

It is popular to decry mass-manufactured foods, which are prepared and cooked in factories. But in fact they may well be nutritionally superior to those cooked at home or in canteens. Factory-processed food is partly or wholly cooked under controlled conditions before the public buys it, so that it needs less cooking at home than raw food does. There should therefore be a smaller loss of nutrients, provided the instructions about cooking times are followed exactly.

HOW A BAD COOK CAN RUIN VEGETABLES

A bad cook can destroy every trace of vitamin C in fresh vegetables, such as cabbages.

The process starts when she buys them from the greengrocer. A cabbage fresh from the ground can have about 100 mg. of vitamin C in 100 g. of leaf. When leafy vegetables wilt, enzymes they contain start to destroy the vitamin C.

So a wilted cabbage is already on the way to ruin. If the cabbage is stored in a warm kitchen the process of deterioration will accelerate.

Badly stored cabbage can lose a third of its vitamin C in a day, just from wilting. Before it is prepared for cooking its vitamin C content may

already be down to 40 mg. per 100 g., compared with the 100 mg. it started with.

The cook may cut up the cabbage long before she intends to cook it, allowing the destructive enzymes to attack the vitamin C in each piece. And the value of vitamin C might now fall to 30 mg.

Vegetables should be put into boiling water immediately they are cut, to inactivate the enzymes. But the cook may put the cabbage into cold water and bring it slowly to the boil.

She will cook it until it is soggy—and the longer a vegetable is cooked the more vitamins are lost into the water.

Depending on the time spent on cooking and the amount of water used for the cooking, the vitamin value can be down to 5–10 mg.

She may add a pinch of bicarbonate of soda to the water to retain the vegetable's colour. This increases the destruction of vitamin C—and if the cooking time is short it is not even necessary.

Finally, any vitamin C that has survived can be lost if the food is left standing before it is eaten. The vegetable that is finally served will have little value except as a source of dietary fibre.

Some samples of cooked cabbage that have been kept hot have no vitamin C at all.

All leafy vegetables will behave in the same way; brussels sprouts, cauliflowers and garden peas do not lose as much because they have less surface area.

When vegetables are cooked, part of this loss is inevitable, but we tend to eat more vegetables if they are cooked rather than raw, and that makes up for the loss.

True or false?

☐ **You must not mix protein, fat and carbohydrates because they are digested by different enzymes—** *False*
They are digested by different kinds of enzymes, but the stomach and small intestine produce them at the same time. There are hardly any foods which are not mixtures of protein, fat and carbohydrates.

☐ **Extra vitamins will lengthen your life** —*False*
Once you have enough to maintain health, there is no benefit in having more.

☐ **Vitamin E increases your sex drive** —*False*
A shortage of vitamin E causes different disorders in different animals. Only in rats and mice does a shortage lead to sterility—not in human beings. It has no connection at all with sex drive.

☐ **Red wine gives you a headache—** *True for some people*
Red wine—more so than white wine—has naturally occurring chemicals which do cause headache in some people.

☐ **All refined and processed foods are junk—** *False*
Refined foods certainly have had some of the nutrients removed. The term mostly applies to white flour.

Processed foods, however, are any foods which have been treated

after harvesting, such as frozen vegetables or canned meat. Even butter, bread and pasteurised milk are processed. A well-controlled food factory will produce foods with better nutritional value than a poor home cook.

Convenience foods are foods ready or almost ready to eat. Instant coffee, instant puddings, and fish fingers are all modern convenience foods, but bread and all canned foods are also convenience foods. They can be high in nutritional value.

☐ **Lemon juice or vinegar is good for slimming—** *False*
There is an old tale that they shrink the stomach, but it is untrue.

☐ **Free-range eggs are better than those from battery hens—** *False*
There is no difference.

☐ **Organically grown food is better than food grown with inorganic fertilisers** —*False*
The varieties that grow best under one type of cultivation are different from those that grow best under the other kind, so there is no real comparison.

OBESITY

Probably one in three adults in Britain is overweight. The condition becomes more common with age. Recent surveys show that about 20 per cent of men and women aged 20-30 are obese, a figure which increases to more than 50 per cent of those in their 50s and 60s. Using a chart which relates height to optimum weight, you can work out whether you are one of them (*see* WEIGHT). If you are, you should try hard but not obsessively to achieve your optimum weight.

Symptoms
- Unflattering appearance.
- Finding that your clothes are too tight.
- Discomfort in the abdomen.
- Shortness of breath.
- Aching legs and swollen ankles.

Duration
- Unless steps are taken to lose weight, the condition will persist and probably worsen.

Causes
- There are no easy explanations why some people are fat while others are thin—although they may eat the same amounts.
- Some people are overweight because they eat more than they need to maintain their normal level of activity—this does not mean that they eat a great deal more than other people, but that their food requirements are much less than they think.
- Some people put on weight as they grow older because they continue with the eating habits of earlier, more active, years when their energy output was higher.
- Some people respond to emotional problems, such as DEPRESSION, ANXIETY, boredom or stress, by excessive eating.
- An inherited tendency to obesity.
- Occasionally the condition is caused by disorders of the thyroid, pituitary or adrenal glands.
- Fluid retention due to HEART FAILURE, toxaemia of pregnancy (*see* PREGNANCY, DISEASES OF), and CIRRHOSIS OF THE LIVER.

Complications
- By making people more susceptible to certain disorders, such as DIABETES, HYPERTENSION, and ARTHRITIS of the legs, obesity shortens life expectancy.
- Obesity may also make complications after surgical operations more likely.
- Difficulties with pregnancy, such as VARICOSE VEINS, and low back pain.

- Obesity also worsens the symptoms of many other diseases, for example, ANGINA, heart failure, ANAEMIA and arthritis.

Treatment in the home
- Try to lose weight by dieting and exercise. Diets succeed only if the amount of calories consumed is less than the amount of calories used up by exercise and daily routine.
- Keep a record of everything that you eat and drink each day. This will help to pinpoint any over-eating.
- Eat slowly—it will help you to eat less.

When to consult the doctor
- If you need advice and support in your efforts to lose weight.
- If obesity is making you short of breath, causing any of the above symptoms or interfering with normal activities in any way.

What the doctor may do
- Check your exact weight and physical state. Discuss any emotional problems that may be causing excessive eating.
- Advise on weight-reduction programmes that may help. These are based on:

    Strong motivation to lose weight. The doctor can tell you what to do. Only you can do it.

    Keeping to a strict diet, with no cheating.

    Joining mutual support groups, such as slimmers' clubs, which encourage and advise.

    Cutting down on carbohydrates, such as bread, cakes, biscuits, sweets and sugar; fats, oils and fried foods; and alcohol.

    Increasing proteins, with bulk such as bran, fruit and vegetables.

    Eating small amounts of food often.

    Taking more exercise; but not overdoing it.
- Call you in for a check-up after a couple of weeks or so to see if you are following his advice.
- Occasionally he may prescribe a short course of drugs to help reduce the appetite and remove excess fluid from the body, but this is unwise for many people.

Prevention
- The only prevention is not to eat too much and to watch your waistline and seek your doctor's advice on diet if it starts to grow.

Outlook
- With good motivation and help from friends and relations, weight reduction can be achieved and maintained.

See DIGESTIVE SYSTEM *page 44*
EXERCISE
NUTRITION

OCCUPATIONAL AND ENVIRONMENTAL HAZARDS

For centuries it has been known that people working or living in certain conditions are liable to contract particular ailments as a result. For instance, an inflammation of the skin—ECZEMA—has long been recognised as an occupational hazard among people regularly handling chemicals. The eczema could be seen to worsen when the chemical was handled, and to improve when it was not. But the full extent of occupational lung disease was not recognised until the introduction of X-rays late in the 19th century enabled the damage to the lung to be seen. More recently still, CANCER research has linked a number of occupations directly with the development of cancers of various parts of the body.

Today, medical researchers are discovering more diseases related to contamination of the environment by chemicals and metals, by dust particles, by gases, and by the least tangible of assailants—noise. And it is not only workers amid the pollutants who suffer. Everyone who comes in contact with the pollutants is at risk—the housewife, the young people at a discothèque, the farm worker, the city commuter.

DISEASES OF THE SKIN
Industry uses many chemicals that cause inflammation of the skin, both to the factory workers and to the users of the product. Some act by irritating and damaging the skin. Others make the skin sensitive to contact with metals or light. A third category can cause SKIN CANCER.

Skin damage Some chemicals, including strong acids and alkalis, and the salts of chromium, arsenic and mercury—damage the skin in much the same way as do burns or scalds.

If the upper layers of the skin remain unbroken, blistering develops within a few hours, but more severe damage results in loss of the skin and exposure of the underlying tissue.

The harmful chemicals are encountered by workers producing acids such as sulphuric acid and alkalis such as caustic soda and lime.

Contact eczema After a period of handling, varying between months and years, a small proportion of people engaged in manufacturing paints, chemicals and pharmaceutical products become sensitive to metals. The symptom of this sensitivity is an inflammation called contact eczema—so named because its eczema-like rash is brought on by contact with the metal (for example, nickel). Only the skin beneath the nickel object is affected. Similar problems can arise in the domestic situation. For example, a rash of the ear lobes is produced by ear-rings containing nickel, and small patches of rash on the thighs result from contact with the nickel used to make suspender-belt fastenings.

Handling virtually any of the industrial chemicals causing occupational ASTHMA (including those used in plastics and detergent manufacture) may also cause contact eczema.

Some chemicals, too—such as those in antimalarial drugs (see MEDICINES, 28)—render the skin more susceptible to the ultra-violet radiation in sunlight, so that those taking such drugs or in contact with such chemicals develop sunburn more easily. This condition is known as photosensitivity.

Skin cancer Any chemical which causes prolonged irritation of the skin may eventually cause skin cancer—a condition in which body cells multiply abnormally to invade and destroy healthy tissue. For example, after chimney sweeps have been exposed to soot for many years, they are liable to develop cancer of the scrotum. Some chemicals, called carcinogens, are known to cause skin cancers more quickly than others. Among them are tar, pitch and bitumen—to which building and road construction workers are exposed—and the salts of chromium used in the electroplating industry.

LEUKAEMIA AND OTHER CANCERS
Cancer as an occupational disease can attack other parts of the body.

Some derivatives of petroleum, especially benzene, are suspected as a cause of LEUKAEMIA (cancer of the blood). Benzene is liable to be absorbed by workers in the petroleum refining industry.

The metal cadmium is used in the process of brazing, welding and zinc smelting, among others; and those exposed to it may incur cancer of the prostate gland.

Workers involved in the manufacture and use of organic dyes—especially those derived from the chemical base aniline—are particularly liable to cancer of the bladder.

Asbestos dust is a potent cause of a form of LUNG CANCER known as pleural mesothelioma, as well as of other lung diseases.

People regularly exposed to nuclear radiation, such as hospital workers using X-rays and laboratory workers handling radioactive samples, are more likely than others to suffer cancer of the blood and lymphatic system.

HEAVY-METAL POISONING
The heavier metals—lead and mercury—are present in many industrial processes and products. They are often in a finely divided form, suspended in air or vapour, that is easily absorbed into the body and disperses over a wide area. Rather than being flushed out by the body's waste-disposal system, they accumulate over a period of time, eventually to reach poisonous levels. Consequently they are dangerous not only to people who work with them and are exposed to heavy doses, but also to the public.

Lead-poisoning Lead absorbed into the body causes damage to the nervous system. In children below the age of two years, the outcome is mental subnormality due to inflammation of the nerve tissue in the brain. In adults, only the nerves running into the muscles are affected, resulting in weakness of one or more limbs.

LEAD-POISONING is an occupational hazard of lead smelting, ship-breaking and tin-plating, where the metal is absorbed into the blood after the vapour has been inhaled.

In the past the major cause of lead-poisoning was swallowing lead paints. Children were usually poisoned by chewing painted furniture or playthings. Polyurethane paints are now used in the home.

The environment has been contaminated with lead as a result of the use in petrol of tetraethyl lead, which slightly improves fuel economy. There is now good evidence that children born and raised in urban areas highly polluted by exhaust fumes do less well at school than those who come from rural areas with cleaner air.

Mercury poisoning Like lead, mercury accumulates in the body. Most poisoning results from the inhaling of vapour by people involved in refining mercury, and in the manufacture of scientific instruments containing mercury—such as thermometers and barometers.

Mercury poisoning causes damage to the kidneys and to the nervous system, with symptoms of tremor of the limbs and loss of mental faculties.

At one time powdered toothpaste contained mercury. It caused a disease in children known as 'pink' because of the redness that developed in the skin of the cheeks and the buttocks. In the 19th century, mercury nitrate was used to paint the felt of top-hats. Hatters repeatedly licked their fingers and ran them over the felt before ironing it, swallowing the mercury. The resulting mental damage gave rise to the phrase 'mad as a hatter'.

In 1958 many Japanese people were poisoned with mercury as a result of eating tuna fish, a local delicacy. The source of the trouble was traced to industrial pollution of rivers by factories refining mercury. Micro-organisms in the water absorbed mercury and were swallowed by small fish, that were eaten in turn by the tuna.

REPETITIVE STRAIN INJURY
See TENOSYNOVITIS

HEARING DAMAGE FROM NOISE
The loudness of sound is measured in units known as decibels—dB for short. The background noise of a quiet night in the country is about 20 dB; the sound level beneath a jet aircraft taking off reaches 120 dB.

Permanent hearing damage results from prolonged exposure to sound levels above 88 dB. In a discothèque the level can reach 120 dB, so the hearing of performers and of their audiences is particularly likely to suffer. Their ability to hear high-pitched notes is the first to be lost—eventually they can become deaf to the top quarter or more of the higher notes normally perceptible.

Industrial workers in noisy occupations, such as those using compressed air drills (110 dB or more), are encouraged by their employers to wear ear muffs; but few of them bother. In the cockpit of a military aircraft the noise level can rise well over 100 dB, which can cause both deafness to high notes and fatigue. *See* NOISE INJURY.

OCCUPATIONAL LUNG DISEASE
The largest group of occupational diseases comprises those that affect the lungs. The reason is that the lungs—as part of their normal function—filter impurities from the air they draw in. These foreign bodies are left in the lungs, where many of them cause trouble.

Occupational lung diseases fall into two groups. In pneumoconiosis, the damage is done directly by the dust of the materials inhaled, such as metals, stone, coal or asbestos. In allergic diseases, the materials inhaled do harm indirectly by triggering ALLERGIES that result in damage to the lung.

DUST DAMAGE TO THE LUNGS
Harmful dust particles breathed in by miners and some other workers create little circles of inflammation in the lungs, and each of these eventually forms a solid lump which shows up when the lung is X-rayed. This gives the X-ray picture a spotty appearance, indicating the disease called pneumoconiosis. The lung tissues become thickened and inflexible—a condition known as fibrosis. As a result, the sufferer becomes progressively more and more breathless; and develops a persistent cough.

Once the disease has been allowed to take hold, destruction of lung tissue continues even after exposure to dust has ceased. Eventually the sufferer may become so handicapped that he cannot even leave his home.

In Britain, a certificate from a medical panel to the effect that a patient is suffering from pneumoconiosis entitles him or his widow to a state pension, and to compensation.

The type of dust inhaled can be identified in an X-ray picture because the size and shape of the particle and its distribution around the lung vary according to the dust involved. The different pneumoconioses are named after the type of dust which causes them. The most usual are silicosis, resulting from the dust of rock such as quartz or silica; asbestosis from asbestos, and coal-miner's pneumoconiosis from coal.

Silicosis This disease is found in workers who blast hard rock, for example in mining, quarrying and shaft driving. Others, too, can become exposed to rock dust—stonemasons, men who sand-blast dirty buildings, and people who process certain kinds of clay in the pottery industry. Silicosis sufferers are much more vulnerable than others to infection by TUBERCULOSIS of the lung.

Asbestosis Asbestos is used widely in industry as a heat-resistant material and an electrical insulator. Its dust particles—made up of needle-like crystals—work their way across the lung tissue, and may pierce the lung to scrape against the chest wall. This causes inflammation of the outer lung lining, as well as of the inside of the lung. In many cases the sufferer cannot remember being exposed to asbestos—asbestosis may date back many years, to an incident as trivial as stripping old pipe lagging; and symptoms may not have arisen in the interval.

Exposure to asbestos dust greatly increases the chances of developing cancer of the lung or of its lining. Lung cancer is even more likely if the asbestosis sufferer is a smoker.

Coal-miner's pneumoconiosis Inhaling large quantities of coal dust over a period of ten to 15 years can bring on this disease. It is seen only among coal-miners, but is the commonest kind of pneumoconiosis in Britain—about 500 new cases are diagnosed every year. As with silicosis, there is a greatly increased danger of tuberculosis.

Diagnosis and treatment of dust damage If doctors can diagnose pneumoconiosis early enough—before it has taken hold—it can be checked. Diagnosis is based almost exclusively on chest X-rays, which should be taken once every year. The X-ray tells the doctor which kind of dust is the culprit, and the patient's symptoms tell him how severe the lung disease is.

Treatment consists of stopping the work that exposes the patient to dust before the disease takes a firm hold. Breathing is helped if the sufferer can be persuaded to give up SMOKING. The possible complications of pneumoconiosis— tuberculosis and lung cancer—can be treated with drugs and other therapy under the supervision of experts in chest diseases.

Nowadays the dousing of cutting tools with water and other dust-control measures have greatly reduced the risk of pneumoconiosis in mining. Masks are available to sand blasters, preventing all but the smallest dust particles being inhaled.

ALLERGIC LUNG DISEASES

Sufferers from allergic lung diseases develop antibodies against dusts, irritant gases, and animal or vegetable matter. These antibodies—proteins in the blood that are part of the body's defence system against foreign bodies—attack the invading substances, but at the same time produce the symptoms of allergic disease.

Occupational asthma During an attack, victims of asthma have difficulty in breathing in and out—they are breathless, they cough, and they wheeze. Occupational asthma is an allergic disease, brought on by inhaling chemical, animal or vegetable substances at work. Sufferers might be exposed harmlessly to the material for months or years before asthma develops. But once asthma is established, only the tiniest quantity of the offending material is needed to start an attack—in other words the sufferer becomes sensitised to the substance, so that he reacts to it immediately.

There are seven substances which are the main causes of occupational asthma:

Isocyanate chemicals which are used in the manufacture of polyurethane plastics. Domestic polyurethane paints contain isocyanates, as do some printers' inks, and a wide range of foams used in making furniture, cavity-wall insulation and motor-car upholstery. Asthma usually develops after two or three years of trouble-free exposure.

Attacks begin much sooner if exposure has been very heavy—for example following an accidental spillage of the chemical, or a fire in which plastic foam has been burned. In such cases the firemen called in to deal with the emergency may contract the disease as well. At least 20,000 people in Britain are exposed in their work to isocyanates, and occupational asthma may strike up to 25 per cent of them.

Epoxy resin hardeners—used to harden epoxy resin adhesives—are much more potent causes of asthma than the isocyanates. Symptoms develop within weeks or even days of exposure. One-third or more of people regularly exposed to these hardeners may become asthmatic.

Platinum salts—produced in the process of refining platinum from its ore — cause asthma among workers in the industry. Platinum refiners already suffering from other allergies are two to three times more likely to develop asthma than those with none. In one factory in Britain, between one-fifth and one-quarter of the work-force had to change their jobs each year because of allergy to platinum salts.

Biological detergents contain enzymes—proteins which are capable of digesting other proteins. Among employees of the British enzyme detergent industry exposed to enzymes, nearly one in 20 has developed an allergy to them.

Rosin is a constituent of the sap produced naturally by pine trees. When the sap has been distilled, the liquid forms turpentine, and the solid residue is rosin. It is used most widely in soft solder to assist melting, but it is also put into glue, and is used by wrestlers, dancers, weight-lifters and violinists to give them purchase on the floor, weights or violin strings. When cold, the rosin causes contact eczema and when heated (as in solder) it forms a vapour which can be inhaled and cause asthma. It is most troublesome in the electronics industry, where soft solder is widely used to assemble components. There, occupational asthma can afflict more than one-fifth of the work-force.

Laboratory animals such as rats, mice, guinea-pigs, gerbils, rabbits and domestic pigs can cause asthma when they are handled by workers. Doctors have found that the most potent cause of the asthma is a protein in the urine of the animals. Their fur may also cause trouble, probably because it is contaminated with urine. The people exposed are two or three times more likely to develop occupational asthma if they already have other allergic complaints, such as HAY FEVER or ECZEMA. Between 10-15 per cent of the laboratory workers concerned in handling such animals may develop occupational asthma.

Dust created by harvesting and milling grains—including barley, oats, wheat and rye—can cause allergic asthma, particularly among farm workers. The cause of the trouble may be the dust itself, or contamination by the spores of a fungus which grows on the grain or the faeces of the storage mite, an insect that lives in stored grain.

Diagnosis and treatment of occupational asthma It is difficult to be sure that asthma is the result of exposure to a substance at work, and is not due to allergy to materials in the home. Doctors usually discover the truth by carefully noting the history of the illness. Does it tend to improve when the sufferer is at home, at weekends and during holidays? If so, the harmful material is probably to be found at work. The way to be certain of the diagnosis is to measure what happens to the sufferer's breathing under working conditions. This is usually done in hospital, where work conditions are mimicked as closely as possible—for example, by asking the sufferer to use a paint spray, or by raising dust deliberately. This technique is known as bronchial provocation testing.

Treatment is by antiallergy drugs (*see* MEDICINES, 14), by courses of desensitisation injections, or—if possible—by avoiding the cause of the asthma. If the sufferer is no longer exposed to the substance that brings on an attack, the allergy may disappear.

Occupational asthma has been defined in British law as an industrial injury, and sufferers can claim compensation from the state.

FARMER'S AND BIRD-FANCIER'S LUNG

Diseases that combine allergic asthma with fibrosis of the lungs are grouped under the name of alveolitis. The commonest form is farmer's lung, which is an allergy to the spores of fungus growing in mouldy hay or straw. The

---

Are you entitled to industrial injury benefit?

Anyone who is incapacitated by a disease contracted at work or an accident at work may be entitled to compensation under the industrial injuries scheme.

INDUSTRIAL DISEASES
The following list summarises most of the 51 diseases legally covered by the scheme.

☐ Accidental injuries. Unless an accident is clearly the result of an employee's negligence, most injuries sustained at work are covered by legislation. They may involve cuts, bruises, burns, sprains, broken bones and all head injuries.

☐ Injuries to eyes from accidents, welding flashes, extremes of heat, heat cataract, explosions and miner's nystagmus.

☐ Injuries to ears from explosions, extremes of pressure, excessive noise.

☐ Poisoning by the following substances or related compounds: lead, manganese, phosphorus, arsenic, mercury, carbon bisulphide, carbon monoxide, benzene, nitro, amino or chloro derivatives of benzene, dinitrophenol, tetrachloroethane, tri-cresyl phosphate, tri-phenyl phosphate, dioxan, methyl bromide, chlorinated naphthalene, nickel carbonyl, nitrous fumes, African boxwood, cadmium, acrylamide monomer, beryllium.

☐ Infections caused by organisms that can be traced to the nature of the work: brucellosis, tuberculosis, anthrax, glanders and viral hepatitis.

☐ Some cases of chronic pain or disability that follow repetitive movements over long periods of time: writer's cramp, beat hand, beat knee, beat elbow, and chronic synovitis, affecting some tendons and joints. Only certain occupations are legally considered capable of producing these disabilities.

HAVE YOU A CASE?
In most cases of accidents it is quite clear if an injury has occurred during working hours. If injury or disease becomes apparent only gradually it may be much more difficult to prove that the work is responsible. The following points may help.

☐ Workmates often know if there is a specific hazard related to an occupation. Hearsay is not always reliable but it can be helpful in alerting workers who might be unaware of risks.

☐ The sufferer may note that a particular symptom such as cough or a skin rash only starts after commencing a particular job. Often symptoms will arise only during working hours and will ease during weekends and holidays.

☐ Skin rashes, asthma, difficult breathing, pain in a particular joint that is used at work, allergic symptoms such as sneezing or hives may all suggest—but do not prove—that the sufferer's occupation could be responsible.

☐ Sometimes it is only after a full medical investigation of symptoms that it is possible even to suspect the occupational origin of the disease. This is especially true of infections, growths (either in skin or lungs) and slow general effects of certain metal poisons.

WHAT TO DO
If you suspect that you are suffering from a prescribed industrial disease, you should take the following action:

☐ Report your suspicions to your own doctor. He may be able to say whether work is responsible. Ask his advice about continuing work or for any preventive action you should take. Remember that if work is responsible you will need his opinion later.

☐ If there is a works medical officer report your fears to him.

☐ Consult your union representative or your local social security office if you are in doubt. See DSS pamphlets NI2 (industrial diseases), NI3 (pneumoconiosis and byssinosis), NI6 (disablement benefit), NI207 (deafness), NI16 (sickness benefit), NI16A (invalidity benefit) and NI244 (Statutory Sick Pay).

☐ Always record the time, place and nature of any accident at work. There should be a special book for this purpose at every work place. If there is not, see your employer or your local union representative. As well as recording the injury, record how it happened and the names of any witnesses.

fungus prefers very hot places, and stored hay provides an ideal home. When farmers began to bale hay in large instead of small bales, farmer's lung became more widespread as a result, because the higher temperatures at the centre of the larger bales favour the growth of the fungus. A trend among farmers to store grass (silage) rather than hay is making farmer's lung less common.

The typical symptoms are a cough, shortness of breath and an influenza-like illness developing within four to eight hours of exposure to rotting hay. With each subsequent exposure the breathlessness becomes progressively worse, and ultimately the sufferer is completely incapacitated. Sufferers from farmer's lung may be compensated by the state in the same way as pneumoconiosis sufferers.

Another, less-common form of alveolitis is bird-fancier's lung. This disease is caused by an allergy to the droppings of pet birds. The symptoms are very similar to those of farmer's lung. The harmful substance is a protein of the birds' blood in their droppings. When these dry up, they form a dust which is inhaled, particularly when the bird-fancier cleans out the cage. The treatment for all kinds of alveolitis is to stop exposure to the cause.

MONDAY FEVER
A small proportion of the people exposed in their jobs to the dust of cotton, flax, hemp or sisal develop byssinosis—a condition also known as Monday fever because the influenza-like symptoms typically develop on a Monday, when returning to work from a weekend away from the dust. The symptoms of byssinosis are very like those of chronic BRONCHITIS (persistent coughing and bringing up sputum). They are seen to improve if the sufferer is removed from contact with the harmful dust. Byssinosis is classed as an industrial injury, so compensation may be awarded to the victim.

BRONCHITIS
Prolonged exposure to dust and fumes of any origin causes bronchitis. For instance, the cigarette dust inhaled by smokers is a prime cause of chronic bronchitis. Heavy smokers among coal-miners, who are also exposed to coal dust, are much more likely to suffer from chronic bronchitis than people in less-dusty occupations who smoke similar quantities of tobacco. It is difficult to prove that bronchitis results from exposure to a dust at work rather than to other causes, such as tobacco dust, so no compensation for industrial injury is given to chronic bronchitis sufferers. Bronchitis, like alveolitis, is treated by removing the cause—for instance, by the sufferer giving up smoking or changing his job to some employment that is less dusty.

DECOMPRESSION SICKNESS
The expansion of under-sea oil exploration has increased the number of people exposed to the hazards of deep diving. In the North Sea the working depth ranges from about 500 to 1,000 ft (150 to 300 m). Pressure increases by one atmosphere—the pressure of the earth's atmosphere on the surface—with every 33 ft (10 m.) of depth. The oxygen and other breathing gases (nitrogen and helium) drawn into the diver's lungs dissolve more easily the greater their pressure, so diffuse more readily into the body tissues. If the pressure is removed suddenly—by the diver surfacing quickly—gas bubbles appear in his tissues or blood, as they do in champagne when pressure is relieved by pulling the cork. These bubbles cause decompression sickness, the commonest symptoms of which are pain in the joints (known to divers as 'the bends'), itching of the skin ('the creeps'), and a persistent cough ('the chokes').

To avoid decompression sickness, the diver enters a submersible decompression chamber and surfaces at a fixed, slow rate—perhaps around 90-95 ft (28-29 m.) a day. The rate depends on the length of time the diver has been under water as well as the depth. A diver who has been working at 1,000 ft (300 m.) for more than seven hours must spend at least 10 days decompressing.

The bends, the creeps and the chokes usually develop within four hours of surfacing, but may come on as much as 24 hours later. The same applies in the much more serious symptoms that arise if gas bubbles form in the arteries supplying the brain and spinal cord. These bubbles interfere with the blood supply to the brain, and result in blurring of vision, partial loss of consciousness, confusion, and numbness and tingling or paralysis of the limbs. This is known as a cerebral or spinal bend.

If a diver has been working under high pressure his lung may rupture as he comes to the surface. As a result, large quantities of air suddenly enter the arteries. In this condition—pulmonary barotrauma—the same symptoms develop as in cerebral or spinal bend, but much more quickly.

Decompression sickness may be only one of the consequences of repeated compression and decompression. Evidence is accumulating to suggest that it has long-term effects, in the form of brain damage and bone damage, even among divers who have no history of decompression sickness.

Treatment of decompression sickness The bends, the creeps and the chokes get better slowly if left untreated. But the victim of cerebral or spinal bend must be urgently re-compressed—restored to a pressure close to that of his working depth—in a decompression chamber. The gas bubbles will dissolve back into his blood, and his circula-tion will be restored. He can then be cautiously decompressed again.

All divers, including those diving for sport and recreation, risk decompression sickness when they descend to depths of more than 50 ft.
See DECOMPRESSION SICKNESS *page 191*

OEDEMA
A swelling caused by fluid which has leaked from the circulatory system and accumulated in the body's tissues. It is most commonly seen round the ankles—where it arrives by gravity—but also occurs in other parts of the body. Oedema, which is also known as dropsy, may be the result of injury, but it also occurs in diseases of the circulatory, respiratory and urinary systems.
See SYMPTOM SORTER—ANKLE PROBLEMS

OESOPHAGEAL VARICES
A condition in which the network of veins at the lower end of the oesophagus, or gullet, becomes varicose, or swollen and twisted. It is caused by a rise in blood pressure in these veins due to disorders such as CIRRHOSIS OF THE LIVER. Since the veins have only thin walls, they may bleed dangerously.
See DIGESTIVE SYSTEM *page 44*

OESOPHAGITIS

Inflammation of the oesophagus (the food pipe).
Symptoms
• A burning soreness behind the lower end of the sternum (breastbone), or high in the stomach. The soreness may reach up to the throat and is worse on swallowing, particularly hot, spicy or acid foods.
• Bending forward, especially after meals, and lying flat may worsen the discomfort.
Duration
• The discomfort after swallowing may come and go, or it may last for months or years.
Causes
• A faulty valve at the lower end of the food pipe (often the result of a hiatus HERNIA), which allows acid from the stomach to flow back into the oesophagus.
Complications
• Bleeding, which can result in ANAEMIA or haematemesis (vomiting blood).

Treatment in the home
- *Do not* wear tight clothes or corsets, and avoid bending.
- Eat small, frequent meals and sit upright while eating.
- Avoid being overweight.
- Take milky drinks and an antacid after meals. *See* MEDICINES, I.

When to consult the doctor
- If your symptoms are troublesome, or persist despite home treatment.
- If there is bleeding.

What the doctor may do
- Send you for a barium X-ray.
- He may also request an ENDOSCOPY (examination by an instrument like a telescope being passed down the oesophagus).

Outlook
- Is good with treatment. Occasionally an operation to cure a hiatus hernia is needed.

See DIGESTIVE SYSTEM *page 44*

OESOPHAGUS, CANCER OF

Malignant growths in the food pipe. The disease occurs most commonly in the lowest section of the oesophagus. It is commoner in men than in women and is most likely to occur after middle age.

Symptoms
- Progressive difficulty in swallowing. Meat tends to stick first, then other solids and softer foods.
- The patient can indicate with some accuracy where he feels food is sticking.
- Weight loss may be rapid.

Causes
- Contributory factors may be heavy drinking and SMOKING.
- Untreated COELIAC DISEASE in adults.
- ACHALASIA OF THE CARDIA.

When to consult the doctor
- If difficulty in swallowing lasts for more than two weeks, and particularly if it worsens and feels as if food is sticking.

What the doctor may do
- Send you for a barium-swallow X-ray and an oesophagoscopy (*see* OESOPHAGITIS) to confirm the diagnosis.
- If the tumour is low down in the oesophagus it can be

removed surgically, or a tube may be inserted to prevent the oesophagus from closing.
- Radiotherapy is also used to ease the symptoms.

Prevention
- Avoid smoking or drinking.

Outlook
- The disease usually progresses rapidly to obstruction of the oesophagus, with loss of weight and lack of nourishment. A few cases undoubtedly benefit from therapy or operation, although these are difficult to predict beforehand.

See DIGESTIVE SYSTEM *page 44*

OESOPHAGUS, STRICTURE OF

A stricture is a narrowing in one of the natural passages of the body. In the case of the oesophagus, it is usually due to scarring caused by old injury or disease.

Symptoms
- Vomiting undigested solids, especially bread and meat, soon after swallowing.
- Eventually all food and fluid may be vomited.

Duration
- The condition lasts until treated.

Causes
- Usually ACID REGURGITATION or OESOPHAGITIS (inflammation of the gullet) over months or years.
- Previous ulceration after inadvertently swallowing caustic liquids.
- A growth in the oesophagus.

Complications
- Starvation if not treated.

Treatment in the home
- Not advised. Consult the doctor.

When to consult the doctor
- If solid food tends to stick on swallowing, or is vomited back.

What the doctor may do
- Advise on diet. He may suggest liquidising solid food to help swallowing, or giving tinned baby food or powdered food such as Complan, and milk drinks or soup.
- Send the patient for a barium-swallow X-ray or ENDOSCOPY.
- Send the patient to a surgeon for further investigation and treatment.

- The surgeon may suggest an operation or regular passage of dilators to stretch the oesophagus or remove any obstruction such as a growth.

Prevention
- None possible.

Outlook
- Good with treatment unless cancer is the cause.

See DIGESTIVE SYSTEM *page 44*

OLD AGE

The family is of vital importance in caring for elderly people—and relatives can usually cope with most of the problems of old age. Although the modern family is often criticised for neglecting aged grandparents there is no historical evidence that old people were better cared for by their families in the past. In fact, the care of elderly people by families is now probably better than ever before. One piece of evidence to support this is that the proportion of people over 65 who live in institutions is only about half what it was in 1911.

The diseases that occur in old age are much the same as those that affect younger people, but the attitude of elderly people towards them is different. Often, they believe that failing health is a natural consequence of their age and therefore do not bother to seek help. They accept deteriorating hearing, vision, incontinence, immobility and many other conditions as inevitable, even though they might be cured or improved.

Some people believe that disease is inevitable because it is God's will, and that as God sent the disease, so He will eventually send the cure.

If old people do consult a doctor, they may be reluctant to persevere with the treatment he prescribes because they consider it a waste of time.

It should always be emphasised to elderly people that the problems they may have are not necessarily inevitable —and may be curable if they get medical attention.

WHAT CAUSES AGEING?
Ageing is a normal biological process, but doctors and scientists do not fully understand what causes it. Some believe that it is the result of a gradual accumulation of abnormal body cells. The millions of cells that make up the body are constantly dividing to replace cells that die. The theory is that some of the new cells do not function in the same way as those they replace. When the

abnormal cells in turn divide they produce more abnormal cells. Some of the abnormalities resulting from the process do not affect physical health—for example, the change in the cells making hair protein, which turns the hair white. The increase in abnormal cells in more vital tissues may have more serious consequences. For example, the development of abnormal cells in the liver can result in old people becoming more susceptible to the effects of many drugs.

There are many other theories about ageing, but the experts agree that, whatever the cause, there is no way of stopping it or slowing it down. However, many of the changes that occur in old age are due to disease and physical distress, and to the social and economic consequences of growing old. All these can be prevented, so many of the problems of old age can be prevented and cured too.

Very few people die of old age itself. In fact most of the diseases from which old people die are not related to the ageing process. Heart failure, for instance, which is very common in old age, is not due to ageing of the heart muscle. It may be due to the chronic effects of an attack of RHEUMATIC FEVER that occurred 40 or 50 years earlier or to ATHEROMA, a disease that is aggravated by certain diets. Similarly lung failure in BRONCHITIS or EMPHYSEMA is not due to ageing of lung tissues, but commonly to the effects of atmospheric pollution and cigarette SMOKING.

THE FEARS OF OLD PEOPLE
Old people are usually less afraid of death than young people, but they have many other fears. One of their chief fears is that they will be put in a home, and this may make an old person reluctant to admit that there is something wrong with him. Fear of falling and being unable to get up again often makes an old person reluctant to leave his chair. Blindness is a very common fear, especially among those whose eyesight is failing. Fear of mental deterioration can also cause anxiety and depression.

Fear of loneliness and isolation often reduce an old person's motivation to get better and become independent. While he is disabled and dependent upon others he has visitors, such as the district nurse or home help, and he fears he will lose them if he can cope for himself.

It is essential to find out if any of these fears exist, and if they do, to reassure the old person where possible. Relatives can help considerably by regular visiting, whether or not the old person is in need of help. If visits are made only when help is needed, then calls for help may well increase.

The best way of dealing with a fear is with reassurance

from someone whose opinion the old person respects. No matter how trivial the fear may appear, the elderly person needs to be able to discuss it with someone such as his doctor.

Old people are more pessimistic than young people. This is partly because they assume that their problems are due to old age and so are irreversible. But it is often due to the fact that they are aware of their failings and have lost confidence in themselves and their ability to do new things.

Some may also have experienced broken promises about help and do not believe any new promises that are made to them. It is necessary for anyone trying to help a disabled old person to express optimism openly and frequently, but honestly. Old people easily detect deception and feel patronised by it.

Very often an old person who is obviously in difficulty says that he is all right and refuses to accept offers of help, or even to admit that he has a problem. This attitude is often his way of coping with depression, fear, anxiety or feelings of hopelessness. But while he is denying the existence of the problem to himself, relatives and friends are suffering because of their inability to be of assistance when they know he needs help. This attitude is difficult to influence, and help from a doctor or clergyman is usually needed.

Depression is common in old age. Often an old person will not complain of depression, but observant relatives will begin to see signs. He may begin to neglect himself or his home. He may be losing weight or not bothering to take the medication prescribed for him. Relatives should first try to solve his problems, and give as much love and support as possible.

The help of a clergyman can often be effective. If the depression continues, seek the doctor's help.

Many old people are not afraid of death. Some even say that they look forward to it and hope that they will not wake up when they go to bed at night.

If the old person says that he is thinking of committing suicide, help should be sought immediately from a doctor or social worker.

CONFUSION AND DEMENTIA
The term 'CONFUSION' is used to describe the condition in which an old person's memory is failing, and in addition he is unable to think logically. Some degree of memory failure is normal in old age, and while it can cause a lot of distress to elderly people, it does not necessarily cause practical problems. Failing memory is marked when the old person tries to remember recent events. He may be unable to remember what day it is or who has recently called to see him, but be able to remember his schooldays

clearly. All forms of mental activity—playing bridge, doing crossword puzzles, attending education classes— help to check mental decline.

But the more severe memory failure brought on by disease can cause major problems for the old person and for others. It can cause him to behave in ways that upset other people—for example by getting lost, or by asking the neighbours for sugar at three o'clock in the morning. He may even forget to light the gas after he has turned it on.

If the confusion develops quickly—within a month, or even within 24 hours—it is almost always due to a correctable disease such as a chest infection or a minor STROKE. The victim's doctor should be consulted as quickly as possible.

If the confusion develops over many months or years, it is usually the result of DEMENTIA. This is the name given to a group of diseases in which the brain tissue is destroyed. Only a small proportion of elderly people suffer from it.

Slowly developing confusion, however, is not always the result of dementia. It can be brought on by isolation, family tensions, the failure of sight, hearing or speech, or by some diseases including thyroid disease or severe ANAEMIA. Confusion can also be caused by mistakes in taking medicine and by the damaging effect of excessive alcohol.

DELUSIONS AND HALLUCINATIONS
Confusion can lead to delusions and hallucinations, particularly if the confusion is the result of an infection. But these conditions can also occur in people who are not confused.

A delusion is a mistaken belief. The old person may believe that a dead friend is still alive or that neighbours are conspiring against him. An hallucination is a mistaken perception. The old person sees, hears and talks to the dead friend, or hears the neighbours talking about him when no one is there. Often delusions and hallucinations occur together.

In people who are not confused, delusions and hallucinations can be caused by their feelings of rejection and alienation brought about by isolation, deafness or a recent bereavement. Relatives should prevent isolation by frequent visits, ensure that deafness is properly treated, and offer support after bereavement. If delusions or hallucinations do develop, seek advice from the old person's doctor.

EASING THE STRAIN OF CARING FOR OLD PEOPLE
Encourage old people to be as independent as possible— for example by ensuring that an incontinent person seeks

a cure from his doctor. But even when the old person is as fit as he or she can be, the task and responsibility of caring for him can still be exhausting. Where possible this burden should be shared among his relatives.

Relatives who care for elderly people can be helped in a number of ways. Perhaps the most important is to give them the chance to talk about the tiredness, resentment, frustration and occasional flashes of hatred felt when their lives are dominated by caring for the relative.

THE AVAILABLE HELP

1 Home helps, meals on wheels, nurses, bath assistants—as well as friendly neighbours—may all provide the vital daily support that keeps old people in their own homes.
2 A day centre or a day hospital may provide care of the old person for one or more days each week.
3 A hospital or old people's home may admit him for a few days each month or when his relatives are on holiday.
4 Many councils provide a limited number of holidays each year for old people who are mobile. Infirm elderly people may be considered for a holiday for the disabled. Apply early in the year to the social services department.
5 An elderly couple, or a single person, may be moved into 'sheltered housing' to help them to retain their independence.
6 A relative providing care may be entitled to financial allowances.

The facilities available for the care of old people vary from one district to another. Your doctor, Citizens' Advice Bureau, or the social services department of the local council can provide detailed information.

OLD PEOPLE'S HOMES

Before an elderly person moves to an old people's home, it is very important to be sure that nothing more can be done to keep him going in his own home. First, discuss the idea with a doctor, health visitor or social worker—preferably more than one—to find out what more can be done at home. If it is decided that a move to an old people's home is unavoidable, the local social security department will provide a list of local authority, private and voluntary homes.

THE IMPORTANCE OF FITNESS FOR OLD PEOPLE

Lack of physical fitness is a common cause of disability in old age.

As people grow older they become unfit more easily and find it more difficult to regain their fitness than they did when they were younger. Consequently older people should try to get regular exercise every day. As well as the physical benefits, most elderly people discover a

marked improvement in their mood and morale after starting regular exercise.

For a programme of exercises that can be done by a mobile person at home, see EXERCISE.

All exercise is good for health, including housework and gardening. An old person should get a little breathless every day, and he can achieve this by doing some energetic household job such as polishing a window vigorously or raking the lawn. Relatives should also encourage an old person to do as much as possible around the house to keep him active.

Most local authorities provide a range of classes in keeping fit, music and movement, and YOGA, which provide a good range of exercises and may also broaden an elderly person's social life.

Elderly people with chronic disease or a disability are in special need of group activities and fitness training as their disability may make them immobile. They should obtain advice from their doctor, nurse or physiotherapist for activities appropriate to their condition.

See DISABILITY
HOME NURSING

OLIGURIA

The passing of smaller than normal amounts of urine, which is often darker than usual. Oliguria is often a feature of certain kidney, liver or heart diseases, but it can also occur naturally in people who have not drunk enough to replace water lost by heavy sweating.

OPTIC ATROPHY

Degeneration of the optic nerve, the nerve that connects the rear of the eye to the brain. Atrophy impairs vision irreversibly, in severe cases causing blindness. Causes include certain eye diseases, among them AMBLYOPIA and OPTIC NEURITIS, and some disorders of the nervous system.

OPTIC NEURITIS

Two names are given to the same condition, depending on the parts of the nerve which may be affected. These names are optic neuritis and retrobulbar neuritis. It is a condition which tends to occur in younger adults (unlike circulatory problems causing sudden partial loss of vision,

which occur in older patients).
Symptoms
• The main symptom of optic neuritis is sudden loss of part of the vision in one eye.
• The attack may be preceded by pain behind the eyeball. Movement of the eye is also painful and the eyeball may be tender to pressure.
Duration
• The symptom slowly subsides in a few days, and within a period of one or two months the vision returns, usually completely or very nearly so.
Causes
• The cause of optic neuritis is not known, although in some cases it may be associated with MULTIPLE SCLEROSIS.
• Other possible causes include excess alcohol, methylated spirit, quinine, tobacco or a virus infection.
When to consult the doctor
• If there is persistent pain or difficulty in seeing with one eye.
What the doctor may do
• The doctor will examine the response of the pupils to a light shone in the eye, and look at the interior of the eye with an ophthalmoscope.
• If he suspects optic neuritis he may send the patient to an eye specialist.
• Painkilling tablets may be prescribed, and in some cases a course of steroids to reduce the inflammation, although this is a condition which often settles with time and without active treatment. *See* MEDICINES, 22, 32.
Outlook
• It is unusual for there to be any serious remaining damage once the condition has cleared up.

See EYE *page 36*

ORCHITIS

Inflammation of the testicles. The disorder can occur at any age.
Symptoms
• One or both testicles swell painfully.
• In some cases there is also fever, pain when urine is passed, and, when MUMPS is the cause, swelling of the face.
Duration
• The condition usually lasts for a week or two.
Causes
• The mumps virus is the most common cause.

- In some cases the spread of germs from a urinary infection is responsible.

Treatment in the home

- Rest in bed, support the testicles with a sling or jock-strap and take painkillers in recommended doses. *See* MEDICINES, 22.

When to consult the doctor

- If one or both testicles swell painfully.

What the doctor may do

- Advise rest in bed and prescribe painkillers.

Prevention

- This is difficult, since it is impossible to make sure of avoiding people with mumps, the main cause of the disorder, as mumps has a symptomless incubation period of three weeks.

Outlook

- The condition usually clears up with no after-effects. Rarely, it causes INFERTILITY.

See MALE GENITAL SYSTEM *page 50*

ORF

A skin disease affecting sheep and goats, which is sometimes transmitted to man, usually during lambing time. It is not a serious disease, and although most farmers have their own traditional remedies for curing it, orf gets better on its own without treatment.

Symptoms

- A small lump in the skin on the hand or arm.
- Within one or two weeks the lump forms a blister and later a crust.

Duration

- About four weeks.

Causes

- A virus.

Treatment in the home

- Keep the area clean and dry, and avoid infection.
- Paint the affected skin with gentian-violet solution daily.

When to consult the doctor

- If you are worried about the condition.

What the doctor may do

- Prescribe local creams. *See* MEDICINES, 43.

Outlook

- Recovery is complete and without complication.

See SKIN *page 52*

OSTEOARTHRITIS

Also called osteoarthrosis, osteoarthritis is a degenerative joint disease in which the protective, shock-absorbing cartilage space between the bones of the joint wears away. Osteoarthritis affects mainly the hip, knee, spine and fingers. It is a disorder of late middle age. Women are more likely to be affected than men.

Symptoms

- A slow onset of pain, swelling and deformity in one or more joints. After an initial period of pain, almost half of the sufferers experience no further pain for many years.
- If the fingers are affected, the joints become lumpy.
- In the worst cases, the sufferer finds it increasingly difficult to get around, and there is wasting of the muscles surrounding the affected joints.

Duration

- Osteoarthritis is progressive and irreversible.

Causes

- The ageing process.
- Injury to a joint or an operation on it. In this case osteoarthritis may only develop decades after the injury or operation.
- Abnormal weight placed on a joint. Obesity may cause the disease to develop in the knees or hips.

Treatment in the home

- Avoid over-use of the affected joint.
- Take painkillers in recommended doses for pain relief. *See* MEDICINES, 22.
- Go on a diet if overweight.

When to consult the doctor

- If symptoms are interfering with normal activities.

What the doctor may do

- Arrange for a blood test and X-rays to check that no other disorder is responsible for the symptoms.
- Prescribe pain-relieving tablets. *See* MEDICINES, 37.
- Advise on reducing abnormal weight on any joint.
- He may arrange physiotherapy to strengthen weak muscles.
- In cases of severe disability he will send the patient to hospital. There an operation may be carried out to re-fashion the joint or insert an artificial one.

Prevention

- Keep the weight down and avoid excessive use of any joint.

Outlook

- Favourable, as most patients respond to the treatment given and the condition takes many years to develop fully.
- In severe cases requiring an operation, surgery removes pain and usually restores the mobility of the joint.

See SKELETAL SYSTEM *page 54*

ARTHRITIC JOINT *Pitted and crusted by osteoarthritis, this joint at the head of the thigh is so deformed that it can no longer move smoothly in the hip socket. The white curved line to the left marks the original outline of the bone. The dark spots represent pitting and the yellow patches are areas of abnormal growth of bone. An artificial replacement would give years of trouble-free mobility.*

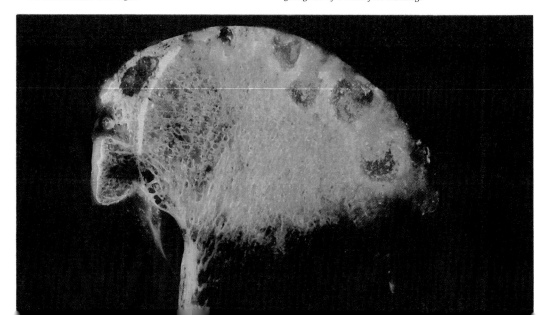

NEW JOINTS FOR OLD WITH MODERN TECHNOLOGY
Relief from pain and restored mobility

People who were once confined to wheelchairs or even bed by the crippling effects of osteoarthritis have been given new mobility thanks to modern techniques of joint replacement. The artificial joints are made from special alloys of steel and specially formulated plastics which do not react to the body's tissues or provoke rejection by the body's immune system.

Many major joints can now be replaced, including shoulders, elbows, hips and knees. In addition, a whole new field of surgery has developed in recent years specialising in the replacement of the small joints of the hand to such good effect that people who once could not open their hands can now thread needles. The artificial joints will give years of mobility.

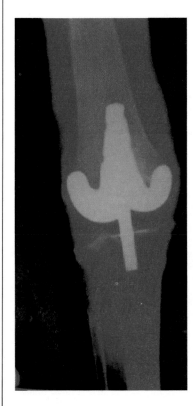

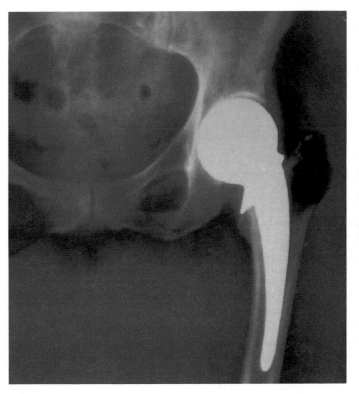

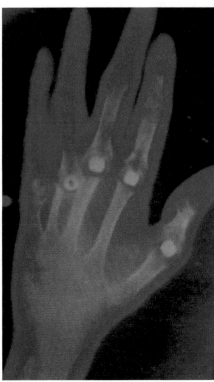

KNEE *The metal parts which replace the damaged bone of thigh and lower leg articulate on a plastic pad which cannot be seen on X-ray.*

HIP JOINT *The replacement joint at the head of the thigh bone is a special alloy ball, highly polished so that it will move smoothly in the hip socket. It is cast on the end of a peg which is inserted in the thigh bone. Often the hip socket is replaced too, either by plastic or metal.*

FINGERS *Replacement knuckle joints on the first three fingers include metal, which shows on X-ray. The little finger joint is plastic and cannot be seen.*

OSTEOCHONDRITIS

The softening of an area of bone. There is then the risk of the bone being pressed out of shape, causing deformity. The spine, hip and shin are the bones most likely to be affected. Children are the main victims of the disease.

Symptoms

• Osteochondritis can affect the hip in children in the five to ten age group, when it is known as PERTHES' DISEASE. The symptoms are a limp and pain. This early deformity of the spine may be overlooked in children who are shy about undressing in front of others.

• The backbone of children aged ten to 16 can be attacked. Unless treated early enough, the spine curves outwards, producing a hunched back and some pain.

• The disorder can also affect the top of the shinbone in children of ten to 16. The affected area of bone becomes tender and swollen. The pain is aggravated by exercise.

Duration

• The condition usually lasts about two years.

Causes

• The cause is unknown.

Treatment in the home

• None is advised.

When to consult the doctor

• Immediately the condition is suspected.

What the doctor may do

• He will have the affected bone X-rayed. If osteochondritis is suspected, the patient will be sent to hospital.

• Hospital treatment will aim to protect the affected bones from bearing weight. For some bones no treatment other than rest may be necessary.

• If pain in a bone is severe it will be put in plaster for a month to protect it.

Prevention

• Prevention is not possible.

Outlook

• Excellent, provided treatment is started early. After about two years the softened bone hardens of its own accord. However, if a major bone is pressed out of shape and hardening occurs before treatment is started, deformity and disability can result and may be followed by OSTEOARTHRITIS.

See SKELETAL SYSTEM *page 54*

OSTEOGENESIS IMPERFECTA

A rare hereditary condition in which the bones are unusually brittle and liable to fracture. In severe cases a child will be born with multiple fractures and may not survive. In less-severe cases fractures are caused by very slight knocks, and deformities can develop because the soft bones have been bent or have not joined properly. Patients with this condition often have a blue tinge to the whites of their eyes. They may be deaf from OTOSCLEROSIS and be very 'loose jointed'.

OSTEOMALACIA

The adult equivalent of RICKETS, in which the bones become softened because of insufficient vitamin D which is necessary for the uptake of calcium. This may be caused by an inadequate diet or by poor absorption of fats containing the vitamin in the bowel. The patient suffers from pain in the bones and often muscle weakness as well. The condition is diagnosed by blood tests and X-ray, and treated by increasing the intake of vitamin D and giving extra calcium.

OSTEOMYELITIS

Inflammation of the bone by bacterial infection. Osteomyelitis starts as an acute condition but if the infection is severe or gets established, it may be extremely difficult to eradicate, even with the appropriate antibiotic, and will become chronic. The sufferer is often a child or teenager.

ACUTE OSTEOMYELITIS

Symptoms

• Sudden onset of pain, tenderness and sometimes swelling in a bone—usually an arm or leg bone. The pain may begin after a knock on the bone.

• Difficulty in moving the affected part, due to pain.

• High temperature and shivering.

Duration

• If the condition is diagnosed and treated early, it should subside in a few days.

Causes

• Injuries in which a broken bone becomes infected through a wound.

• Infection carried in the bloodstream from infections, such as abscesses, elsewhere in the body.

• Often no obvious source of the infection is identified.

Complications

• Chronic osteomyelitis may develop, and spread to adjacent bones.

• SEPTICAEMIA.

• Retarded growth of the affected limb bone.

Treatment in the home

• Rest the affected part and seek early medical advice.

When to consult the doctor

• If there is unexplained pain in a limb, especially of a child.

• If the pain is severe, or if it is associated with fever, or lasts for more than eight hours, consult the doctor immediately.

What the doctor may do

• Arrange for immediate admission to hospital.

• Arrange blood tests to confirm diagnosis and identify the bacterial organism causing infection.

• Prescribe antibiotics. *See* MEDICINES, 25.

• Operate early to drain pus from the bones and shorten the course of the illness.

Prevention

• Adequate treatment of wounds and suspected fractures.

Outlook

• Good if the condition is diagnosed early and treated with the appropriate antibiotic.

CHRONIC OSTEOMYELITIS

Symptoms

• Previous attack of acute osteomyelitis.

• Intermittent discharge from an abscess connecting the infected bone to the skin.

• Small pieces of dead bone as well as pus may be discharged through the abscess.

Duration

• It is difficult to say how long the condition may last, even with treatment. Symptoms may subside for long periods. wrongly suggesting that the infection has been completely cured.

Causes

• Failure to eliminate acute osteomyelitis.

Complications

• Bone destruction and spread of infection to other bones.

• In children, failure of bone to grow.

Treatment in the home

• Rest.

When to consult the doctor

• As soon as any symptoms appear in someone who has had acute osteomyelitis.

What the doctor may do

• Take swabs and blood tests to determine which bacteria are causing the infection.

• Prescribe the appropriate antibiotic.

• Send the patient to a surgeon, who may operate to

remove the infected or dead bone.

Prevention
• Early treatment of acute osteomyelitis.

Outlook
• The outlook is unpredictable as the condition may clear up quickly, or there may be several recurrences of it.

See SKELETAL SYSTEM *page 54*

OSTEOPATHY

A system of treating mechanical disorders of the body, particularly the spine, through manipulation. It is not usually available under the National Health Service, but many doctors refer patients to qualified osteopaths for successful treatment of chronic SLIPPED DISC, a common cause of absence from work in industry; and for sporting injuries such as TENNIS ELBOW.

In the past osteopaths have made many claims for their manipulative treatment. Modern osteopaths do not claim to be able to cure infective or degenerative diseases, such as TUBERCULOSIS or CANCER.

Osteopathy is respected by many doctors as a potential cure for back pains and unexplained muscle and joint problems, which orthodox medicine can alleviate with painkillers, but not necessarily remove entirely. Some osteopathic principles have been incorporated into physiotherapy, which is carried out under the general direction of a doctor.

Registered osteopaths undergo an extensive and lengthy training. Their standards of practice and professional behaviour are controlled by the General Osteopathy Council (GOsC), set up by Act of Parliament in 1993. Most osteopaths have undergone four years of full-time instruction at a college such as the British School of Osteopathy.

OSTEOPOROSIS

Weakening of the bones. The disorder is most common in women past the MENOPAUSE, since they have a failure of oestrogen secretion.

Symptoms
• Often there are none. The condition is then discovered only if an X-ray is taken for another reason.
• Bones may be broken or compressed by only minor injuries or even normal activities.
• Persistent backache is common.

• The back may develop a curve, resulting in loss of height.

Duration
• The condition is permanent, and progressive unless treated.

Causes
• Most commonly, hormonal changes after the menopause. Lack of physical activity seems to play a part in bringing on the disorder.
• It can also occur after prolonged treatment with steroid drugs. *See* MEDICINES, 32.

Treatment in the home
• Rest in bed and painkillers. *See* MEDICINES, 22.

When to consult the doctor
• When symptoms occur.

What the doctor may do
• Arrange for the affected areas to be X-rayed.
• Carry out a blood test to check that no other disorder is causing the symptoms.
• Prescribe pain-relieving tablets, and perhaps calcium tablets and vitamin D tablets to replace calcium loss. *See* MEDICINES, 36.
• Arrange physiotherapy or remedial exercises.

Prevention
• Those over 40, particularly women past the menopause, should take regular exercise.
• Hormone replacement therapy prevents post-menopausal osteoporosis.

Outlook
• Once established, osteoporosis increases slowly with age.

OTITIS EXTERNA

An infection of the outer-ear canal that can occur at any age, especially among swimmers. It is sometimes known as 'swimmer's ear'. There may be general infection of the area, or small but painful boils within the canal, especially if it is scratched or damaged.

Symptoms
• Discharge or weeping from the infected ear, which can range from slight to profuse. Boils in the outer-ear canal do not discharge until they burst.
• Earache or pain in the outer-ear canal, which can be severe.
• An eczema-like rash may develop in the skin near the opening of the external ear canal and the ear hole. This is more likely in someone who has had eczema.

• Temporary deafness.

Duration
• With treatment, a few days.
• Without treatment, the condition may persist for many months.

Causes
• Bacteria or fungi.
• Swimming in chlorinated water.
• Severe infections may result from bathing in certain tropical waters or freshwater lakes.

Treatment in the home
• Clean any discharge from the opening of the outer-ear canal and ear lobe.
• Do not attempt to clean inside the outer-ear canal.
• Allow the discharge to drain out. At night place a piece of plastic between the pillow and pillowcase to prevent the pillow from being stained.
• If necessary, take painkillers in recommended doses to ease earache. *See* MEDICINES, 22.
• Make sure water does not enter the ear.

When to consult the doctor
• Within 48 hours of onset of symptoms.

What the doctor may do
• Gently clean some of the discharge from inside the ear.
• Prescribe drops or ointment to put in the ear, or pack the canal with a wick soaked in antibacterial/antifungal liquid. *See* MEDICINES, 40.
• Arrange for further cleaning of the ear.
• Arrange treatment by an ear, nose and throat specialist in severe or prolonged cases.

Prevention
• Do not poke inside the ears with cotton wool or any foreign body. Clean any wax from the outside with a tissue or handkerchief.
• Two or three drops of olive oil placed in each ear before swimming may give protection.

Outlook
• Although it is not dangerous, otitis externa tends to recur and can be persistent and troublesome.

See EAR *page 38*

OTITIS MEDIA

There are three variations of this infective inflammation of the middle ear: acute, chronic-secretory ('glue ear') and chronic-suppurative. According to which form it takes, the condition can cause deafness and severe earache.

ACUTE OTITIS MEDIA

The inflammation frequently affects babies and young children, particularly in the winter. However, it can occur at any age and at any time of year.

Symptoms
- Earache, which may come on suddenly. It often accompanies a COMMON COLD or cough.
- Babies may cry inconsolably and rub the lobe of the affected ear.
- Fever, with temperature becoming as high as 102°F (39°C) or more in infants.
- Vomiting may occur.
- Soft wax or pus may run out of the ear.
- Partial deafness in affected ear.

Duration
- One to four days.

Causes
- Bacteria or viruses.
- Mechanical causes such as coughing or nose-blowing which may force an infection from the throat into the ear. This may also happen in diving.
- Enlargement of the ADENOID.

Complications
- In rare cases PERFORATED EAR-DRUM may occur.
- Chronic otitis media may develop, with further discharge, deafness and pain.

Treatment in the home
- Reduce fever by giving cool drinks, removing surplus clothing and bedclothes, and by tepid sponging. Cooling is particularly important in babies and children, avoid overcooling by nursing the patient in a room that is comfortably warm and not cold. Give painkillers to ease discomfort and help reduce fever. *See* MEDICINES, 22.
- Give extra fluids such as water, milk or fruit-juice to replace liquid lost from the body because of fever. It does not matter if babies and small children do not eat.

When to consult the doctor
- If otitis media is suspected.
- If children are feverish and crying inconsolably despite cooling them down.
- If a baby's fontanelle (soft spot on the top of the head) is bulging or is very much depressed when not crying.

What the doctor may do
- Examine the ear-drums with an otoscope.
- Prescribe antibiotics or decongestant medicines and advise about pain and fever. *See* MEDICINES, 25, 40.
- Examine the patient after recovery, particularly if there have been previous attacks or if it is suspected that the hearing has been affected.

Prevention
- Do not overheat a child with a feverish illness. Keep him cool and do not wrap him up.

- Reduce the chance of spread of infection through coughing and nose-blowing by treating coughs and colds in the home.

Outlook
- With prompt treatment, recovery is usually complete.
- Most children grow out of the tendency to ear infection by the age of five or six and have normal hearing.

CHRONIC-SECRETORY OTITIS MEDIA

Many children suffer from a persistent blockage of the EUSTACHIAN TUBE, which causes a vacuum in the middle-ear cavity. This draws in the ear-drum and gathers unwanted fluid behind it. There is often no infection in the ear. The condition is also known as glue ear.

Symptoms
- Children between five and seven are most commonly affected. At this age the adenoid is largest and the Eustachian tube most likely to be blocked.
- Partial deafness in the affected ear following acute otitis media, colds or other causes of Eustachian tube blockage. The deafness may be only slight, but may be noticed at school.
- Sometimes there is a sensation of dullness in the ear. There is no discharge or pain.

Duration
- Without treatment, deafness may persist for months or years. This may result in poor progress at school and sometimes poor speech development.

Causes
- Persistent Eustachian tube blockage.
- Recurrent acute otitis media.

Treatment in the home
- None possible.

When to consult the doctor
- As soon as deafness is suspected.

What the doctor may do
- Test the hearing with a tuning fork. He may arrange more accurate testing by an audiometer (*see* DEAFNESS).
- Examine the ears, particularly the ear-drum.
- Prescribe medicine to open the Eustachian tube.
- If partial deafness persists for more than a few weeks, special tests may be made by an ear, nose and throat specialist. If necessary, small tubes called grommets are placed through the ear-drum, in hospital, under a general anaesthetic. These tubes equalise the pressure across the ear-drum so that fluid can drain away through the tube and hearing can return to normal. The tubes serve the function that should be performed by the Eustachian tube. The grommets may drop out or be removed after about six months.

Prevention
- Full treatment and follow up of acute otitis media.

Outlook
- The condition often resolves completely, without treatment, over a period of weeks.
- With treatment, recovery is complete without permanent hearing loss.
- If persistent and untreated, permanent deafness can result.

CHRONIC-SUPPURATIVE OTITIS MEDIA

A persistent infection of the middle ear affecting older children and adults. The infection gradually damages the small bones of the middle ear as well as the ear-drum. Children suffer from this form of otitis media if recurring attacks of acute otitis media are neglected or inadequately treated.

Symptoms
- Discharge from the ear, frequently intermittent and often offensive. The discharge comes from the middle ear through the hole in the ear-drum. *See* PERFORATED EAR-DRUM.
- Increasing deafness in the affected ear.
- Occasional earache.
- Severe pain is unusual, and suggests the possibility of complications.

Duration
- Months or years.

Causes
- Incomplete recovery from acute otitis media, together with perforated ear-drum.

Complications
- In rare cases, infection may spread to cause MASTOID-ITIS or LABYRINTHITIS.
- As the lining of the middle ear is shed, it may collect above the ear-drum forming an infected mass that puts pressure on surrounding structures. This is called cholesteatoma, and causes a foul discharge and sometimes pain.
- Sometimes small non-cancerous polyps appear in the infected middle-ear cavity.

Treatment in the home
- None possible.

When to consult the doctor
- If deafness, discharge or pain persists in one or both ears.

What the doctor may do
- Refer the patient to an ear, nose and throat specialist for treatment.
- The specialist will clean out the ear using viewing and suction devices with a general anaesthetic if necessary. Antibiotics may be prescribed. *See* MEDICINES, 25.
- Once infection is removed, the specialist may operate to repair the bones of the middle ear and the ear-drum.

• An operation may also be necessary if the specialist discovers mastoiditis, cholesteatoma, or a polyp in the ear.

Outlook

• Very good, provided expert medical attention is sought early and then followed.

See EAR *page 38*

OTOSCLEROSIS

Several members of the same family may be stricken with otosclerosis, which causes deafness. It occurs in the 20-40 age group and is more common in females.

The condition involves a thickening of the bone around the oval window through which sound is transmitted from the middle ear to the inner ear. The stapes—the innermost bone of hearing of the middle ear—becomes fused to the bone of the oval window, so that it can no longer vibrate and sound cannot be properly conducted to the inner ear.

Symptoms

• Increasing deafness in both ears.
• Ringing in the ears (TINNITUS).
• Giddiness.
• In the early stages hearing may be better in noisy surroundings.
• The patient often speaks with a soft voice, rather than shouting as do other deaf people.

Duration

• Permanent, unless treated.

Causes

• Probably inherited.

When to consult the doctor

• If deafness or tinnitus persists.

What the doctor may do

• Arrange for an operation to be performed on the ear that is most affected. If successful, the other ear may then be operated on. The surgeon may remove the stapes and fit an artificial replacement.
• Recommend a hearing-aid.

Prevention

• None.

Outlook

• An operation can bring about a dramatic improvement in the condition.

See EAR *page 38*

OVARIAN CYST

A swelling in the ovary which contains fluid and is usually only a few centimetres in diameter. Occasionally cysts may become cancerous and others may grow large enough to simulate pregnancy.

Symptoms

• There may be no symptoms, in which case the condition will be discovered only if the patient is examined for some other reason.
• Intermittent pain in the lower abdomen, often during menstruation or ovulation.
• Pain during sexual intercourse.
• Sometimes there is swelling in the lower abdomen.

Duration

• Small non-malignant cysts may persist for years without symptoms.
• Malignant cysts grow rapidly and may spread to other organs.

Causes

• Most ovarian cysts are caused by the retention of fluid within the ovarian glands.
• Some cysts are filled with blood and are caused by ENDOMETRIOSIS.
• In some women the cysts may occasionally be due to CANCER of the ovary.

Complications

• Ovarian cysts sometimes twist, rupture or bleed, causing severe pain in the abdomen.

Treatment in the home

• None advised. If a cyst is suspected, consult your doctor.

When to consult the doctor

• Immediately there is any pain or swelling in the lower abdomen.

What the doctor may do

• Feel the abdomen.
• Carry out an INTERNAL PELVIC EXAMINATION.
• If the presence of an ovarian cyst is confirmed, the doctor will arrange for the patient to be examined by a gynaecologist who may advise an operation.

Prevention

• Not possible.

Outlook

• Simple cysts may stay the same for years, whereas others may enlarge or develop complications. Cancerous cysts require urgent treatment.

See FEMALE GENITAL SYSTEM *page 48*

OVERBREATHING

This is known medically as hyperventilation, or may be called 'sighing respiration' or 'air hunger'. Many people suffering from ANXIETY always overbreathe slightly, causing enough change in the chemistry of the blood to produce persistent symptoms. It may be difficult for a patient to understand that hyperventilation is the cause of such symptoms, but the diagnosis can be confirmed by deliberately breathing hard and fast for several minutes. If the same symptoms are produced by this exercise, then their cause is obvious. Some individuals are especially liable. Symptoms may be started by pain, acute anxiety or sudden changes of mood—even laughter or watching television. A vicious circle is set up because the patient's anxiety is increased by the symptoms leading to further overbreathing. You should never overbreathe deliberately when you are alone, though experienced skin divers sometimes do so before going under water.

Symptoms

• Dizziness, light headedness and lack of concentration.
• Tiredness and listlessness.
• Tingling or numbness in the hands, feet and face. In severe cases muscles tighten automatically, particularly the muscles of the face, forearms and hands.
• An awareness of the heart beating, sometimes rapidly.
• Yawning, sighing and a dry mouth.
• A sensation of shortness of breath (air hunger), although the patient is actually overbreathing.
• If rapid overbreathing continues, the patient may collapse and look very ill.

Duration

• Longstanding anxiety may produce symptoms for months or years.

Causes

• Acute pain, especially BACK PAIN or period pain.
• Anxiety or a sudden shock.

Treatment in the home

• Try to calm the patient.
• Breathing in and out of a paper bag (not a plastic bag) will give relief.

When to consult the doctor

• If the symptoms are getting worse.

What the doctor may do

• Examine the heart and lungs to confirm that they are normal.
• Prescribe mild tranquillisers. These help prevent the anxiety and further overbreathing. *See* MEDICINES, 17.
• Try to discover the cause of the anxiety or pain that

brought on the overbreathing. If the cause is known, it may be possible to help relieve it. The patient should be encouraged to try out his own simple methods of breath control.

Outlook
- There are no long-term dangers from overbreathing. The patient should recover completely, but recovery may take some time, particularly if symptoms are longstanding.

See RESPIRATORY SYSTEM *page 42*

OVERDOSE
Intentional or unintentional consumption of a greater amount of a drug than is recommended. In adults an overdose is usually considered by doctors to be a cry for help or a deliberate attempt to commit SUICIDE.
See MENTAL SYSTEM *page 33*
DRUG ABUSE

OVULATION SYNDROME

Sometimes when the ovary discharges an egg into the Fallopian tube at ovulation time (the mid-point of each menstrual cycle), mild abdominal pain can be felt. The ovulation syndrome does not arise while taking the contraceptive pill because ovulation does not occur.

Symptoms
- Abdominal pain is felt on the right or left side of the lower abdomen 12-16 days after the start of the last period. Occasionally if this is marked and on the right side, confusion with APPENDICITIS occurs.
- There may be a low fever, tender breasts and a slight spotting of blood from the vagina.

Duration
- The pain usually settles with rest in three to six hours.
- Occasionally the pain persists for one to three days.

Causes
- Slight bleeding, at the point where the ovary discharges the egg, irritates the abdominal lining (peritoneum) and causes pain.

Complications
- None.

Treatment in the home
- Rest and take mild painkillers in recommended doses if the diagnosis is certain. *See* MEDICINES, 22.

When to consult the doctor
- If the pain is on the right side and does not settle after

four hours' rest.
- If there is any unexpected abdominal pain, even at ovulation time.

What the doctor may do
- Carry out an INTERNAL PELVIC EXAMINATION to exclude the possibility of serious disease.
- Admit the patient to hospital for observation if there is doubt about the diagnosis.
- Occasionally an operation has to be performed to be certain that the pain is not due to appendicitis.

Prevention
- None.

Outlook
- Apart from dangers of confusion with appendicitis, the disorder is harmless. Most sufferers cease to have symptoms after 35.

See FEMALE GENITAL SYSTEM *page 48*

PACEMAKER
The part of the heart that sets the rate of heartbeat, speeding it up during exertion and slowing it down during sleep. In cases of HEART BLOCK—when the natural stimulation is impaired and the heart's pumping action is slowed down—an artificial pacemaker is sometimes fitted, when drugs cannot control the condition.

ARTIFICIAL PACEMAKER *A tiny computerised electrical unit can be implanted in a patient's chest to regulate the heartbeat if the natural pacemaker fails.*

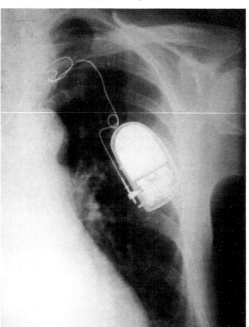

PAGET'S DISEASE OF THE BONES

A progressive thickening of the bones, mainly affecting the skull, spine, pelvis and the leg. It seldom develops before the age of 50.

Symptoms
- Dull, continuous bone pain that becomes worse on walking.
- Noticeable broadening of the skull.
- Often there are no symptoms and the condition is discovered during X-ray for another reason.

Duration
- The disorder is lifelong as it cannot be cured.

Causes
- The cause of the disease is unknown.

Treatment in the home
- Take painkillers in recommended doses. *See* MEDICINES, 22.

When to consult the doctor
- If painkillers do not relieve the pain.

What the doctor may do
- Take a blood sample to confirm the diagnosis and check that the symptoms are not caused by some other disease.
- Arrange X-rays.
- Prescribe pain-relieving tablets.
- If pain is severe, he may prescribe calcium, hormones and other drugs. *See* MEDICINES, 33, 36.

Prevention
- Prevention is not possible.

Outlook
- Treatment may slow down but cannot stop the progress of the disease.

See SKELETAL SYSTEM *page 54*

PAIN

The sensation of pain is known to every individual. Despite this, pain is often difficult to describe and misunderstandings may arise as a result. Pain is usually created by injury to body tissues. Different types of pain may be caused by different injuries. Thus swelling or inflammation in a confined space causes a continuous throbbing pain, as in a boil or in toothache; stretching a hollow tube such as the bowel or womb will cause severe stabbing pain that comes and goes; cutting down the blood supply to an organ, as in GANGRENE or ANGINA, will cause continuous severe pain; destruction of tissues by heat or chemicals will cause a burning pain; minor strains and muscle spasm usually cause a continuous ache.

Pain performs two important functions. Firstly, it forces the sufferer to stop doing whatever it is that causes the pain and to rest the affected tissue. Such enforced rest also allows the injured tissue to heal. Secondly, pain acts as an early warning system which allows individuals, especially doctors, to recognise (and follow) the presence of disease. The diagnostic significance and implications of pain of different types felt in different parts of the body are fully described in the SYMPTOM SORTER.

Three characteristics of pain need explanation: First, pain may spread or radiate to affect a wider area than that damaged by injury. Thus, pain from a damaged heart will spread down the arm, while pain from a slipped disc may radiate down the leg. These special characteristics help doctors recognise which disorder is causing the pain. Second, pain caused by injury at one point may sometimes be felt in a totally different place. Thus, pain felt in the shoulder may originate from inflammation of the lungs or gall-bladder. After a leg has been amputated, pain is sometimes still felt in the toes which have been removed. This type of pain is called referred pain.

Third, pain has what doctors call a threshold level or 'threshold of awareness'. If this level of awareness is raised, the pain felt is less or not noticed; if the level is lowered, trivial pain feels worse and previously non-painful sensations, such as touch or noise, may be felt as painful. These temporary variations often bear little relationship to the state of the damaged tissue.

The following influences, which are unrelated to the cause of pain, tend to raise thresholds and therefore reduce the amount of pain felt:
• Physical influences such as painkillers (see MEDICINES, 22), ACUPUNCTURE, heat applications, anaesthetics and alcohol.
• Psychological influences such as excitement, concentration of interest, self-confidence, confidence in a doctor or faith. Thus a footballer may be unaware of how an injury occurred during an exciting game.

By contrast, other influences tend to lower pain threshold and therefore increase the severity of pain felt. These include:
• Physical influences such as ill health, hunger, cold or pain from another source. Thus shaving or even touching

the skin near to a boil or aching tooth may be very painful.
• Psychological influences such as fear, worry, ANXIETY, fatigue, INSOMNIA, DEPRESSION, frustration and boredom. Thus, pain which is bearable during the day may become unbearable during the night.

The significance of these influences is often not appreciated, even by doctors. But full understanding is important, because faith, confidence in the doctor, friendship, affection and interesting activities are often more important than painkillers in helping to deal with pain.

Recent research suggests that substances called endorphins, produced in the body as a result of psychological as well as physical influences, may affect the way pain is felt, by raising and lowering pain thresholds.

PAINFUL ARC SYNDROME
A condition in which there is pain in the shoulder joint when the sufferer raises an arm sideways. At first the movement is painless, but as the arm gets further from the side, increasing pain is felt. This painful 'arc' of movement limits the sufferer's use of the shoulder. This symptom may arise in FROZEN SHOULDER or ROTATOR CUFF LESIONS.
See SKELETAL SYSTEM page 54

PALPITATIONS
Awareness of the heart beating. This is normal with fear and after heavy exercise, but it may sometimes be a symptom of heart disease.
See SYMPTOM SORTER—PALPITATIONS

PALSY
Palsy derives from an old French word and simply means PARALYSIS. It is still used in certain compound forms.
See BELL'S PALSY

PANCREAS, CANCER OF
Tumours of the pancreas are not common. The symptoms depend on the site of the tumour. About 70 per cent of all pancreative tumours occur in the 'head' of the pancreas; these block the pancreatic and bile ducts, causing nausea, loss of appetite and weight, and painless progressive JAUNDICE.
Cancer of the 'body' of the pancreas causes a gnawing pain which can be felt in the back; this may be worse after meals and when lying down.
See DIGESTIVE SYSTEM page 44

PANCREATITIS

An uncommon condition in which the pancreas (a gland near the stomach) becomes inflamed. Pancreatitis can be acute or chronic.

ACUTE PANCREATITIS
Symptoms
• Severe pain in the middle or left upper abdomen, which goes through to the back. It is worse on movement, and is occasionally colicky.
• Vomiting.
• The temperature rises to 100-102°F (38-39°C) in the first few days.
• In severe attacks the patient is in a state of shock, and is pale with clammy skin, rapid pulse and low blood pressure.
Duration
• Acute pancreatitis develops rapidly, then may remain constantly severe for several days or weeks, gradually settling over weeks.
Causes
• Disorders of the gall-bladder.
• ALCOHOLISM and morphine addiction.
• MUMPS, operations, and drugs such as diuretics, antibiotics or even the Pill may occasionally cause pancreatitis. In one-third of patients no cause is found.
Complications
• JAUNDICE may occur if the bile ducts are involved.
• Paralytic ileus (paralysis of the bowel) may occur in severe cases. See BOWEL OBSTRUCTION.
• Relapses may occur after apparent recovery.
Treatment in the home
• The symptoms are usually severe enough to require early medical help, so call your doctor as soon as possible.
What the doctor may do
• Give the patient an injection to relieve the pain.
• Admit the patient to hospital for investigation to exclude other disorders and for treatment with fluids intravenously.
• Surgery is sometimes vital to exclude a perforated DUODENAL ULCER or APPENDICITIS.

CHRONIC PANCREATITIS
Chronic inflammation of the pancreas, causing damage to the gland.
Symptoms
• Recurrent attacks of upper abdominal and back pain and vomiting, as in acute pancreatitis, usually worse

after food or alcohol and on lying down.

Duration

• Chronic pancreatitis may go on for years, with some attacks worse than others.

Causes

• These are many and include alcohol, abdominal surgery and CYSTIC FIBROSIS.

Complications

• Diabetes develops as pancreatic cells are destroyed. *See* DIABETES mellitus.

• The loss of digestive enzymes produced by the pancreas cause bulky, smelly stools. *See* STEATORRHOEA.

• Cancer of the pancreas is more common in people with chronic pancreatitis than in others.

Treatment in the home

• Alcohol must be avoided for life.

• Take a low-fat diet, with normal carbohydrate and protein to maintain nutrition.

When to consult the doctor

• If the pain keeps coming back.

What the doctor may do

• Send the patient to hospital to confirm the diagnosis.

• Give advice about diet and alcohol avoidance.

• Prescribe painkillers. *See* MEDICINES, 22.

• Prescribe pancreatic extracts to be taken with meals to help fat absorption, and drugs to reduce gastric acid production. *See* MEDICINES, 36.

• Prescribe calcium and vitamin D supplements.

• Diabetes usually needs insulin therapy.

See DIGESTIVE SYSTEM *page 44*

PAPILLOEDEMA

Swelling of the optic disc, the head of the optic nerve, which leads from the rear of the eyeball to the brain. Usually both eyes are affected. The condition is discovered by examination of the eyes with an ophthalmoscope.

Papilloedema is caused by pressure within the skull as the result of one of several serious disorders, among them extremely high blood pressure, meningitis, severe kidney disease or a brain tumour, brain abscess or brain haemorrhage. If the underlying cause is not remedied for some time and the pressure increases the victim may go blind.

PAPILLOMA

A usually benign (non-cancerous) tumour that develops either on the skin or on a mucous membrane, the moist tissue that lines most of the cavities and passages in the body. Any wart that becomes painful, changes in appearance or emits a discharge should be reported to a doctor.

Papilloma of the bladder may cause recurrent, painless attacks of blood in the urine. Although not cancerous, it can be difficult to eradicate and may cause ANAEMIA.

PARALYSIS

A muscle is said to be paralysed if it is unable to contract in the normal way. The condition occurs when muscular control is lost somewhere along the route from the brain, via the nerves, to the muscles. For example, a STROKE may affect the route at the brain. MOTOR NEURONE DISEASE may affect a nerve, and MYASTHENIA GRAVIS may affect the point where a nerve and muscle meet. When muscular control is only partially lost, the condition is known as paresis.

See NERVOUS SYSTEM *page 34*

PARANOIA

Sufferers from this mental illness or PSYCHOSIS hold the fixed but unfounded belief that they are being persecuted by someone or something. As a result, they can interpret any event irrationally so that it fits in with their delusions. It is usually a symptom of other mental illnesses, such as SCHIZOPHRENIA, DEMENTIA or occasionally DEPRESSION.

See MENTAL SYSTEM *page 33*

PARAPLEGIA

PARALYSIS of both legs. In most cases it is caused by injury or a disease of the spinal nerves, such as multiple sclerosis, or a tumour. There is usually loss of sensation in the paralysed area and urinary incontinence.

In quadriplegia (or tetraplegia) there is paralysis of all four limbs, usually following neck injuries. In monoplegia only one limb is paralysed: many different diseases could cause this.

PARATYPHOID

A highly infectious disease which is a serious cause of food poisoning. It is spread by food or water which has been contaminated by flies that carry the infection from human faeces. Some people carry the disease (often in the gallbladder) without having any symptoms, and infection can be passed on by food they handle. It is less severe than typhoid and the carrier state is less frequent.

Symptoms

• A rash of rose-coloured spots.

• Headache.

• Diarrhoea, which may be preceded by a period of constipation.

• The illness follows a few days after an attack of food poisoning.

Causes

• Bacteria called *Salmonella paratyphi*.

When to consult the doctor

• If there is persistent unexpected fever or diarrhoea.

• If you are a food handler and develop diarrhoea.

• If you have recently been in a foreign country or in contact with the disease.

What the doctor may do

• Take blood and faeces for laboratory examination.

• Prescribe antibiotics for carriers. Antibiotics may not help the acute illness and may prolong it. Replacement of fluids and nursing are the main treatment.

• Sometimes an operation to remove a carrier's gallbladder may be suggested.

Prevention

• Carriers who handle food should not return to work until they have been declared free from infection.

See INFECTIOUS DISEASES *page 32*

PARKINSON'S DISEASE

A disease of the nervous system, also known as paralysis agitans, in which muscular stiffness and tremors develop, becoming progressively worse with the passing of time. The condition is rare in people under the age of 50, and more common in men than in women. About two people in 1,000 develop Parkinson's disease every year. The onset of symptoms is gradual, and the first stages may pass unnoticed.

Symptoms

• The first symptoms include tremors in the hands, arms and legs. The head may nod rhythmically. The hands may tremble involuntarily, as if a pill were being rolled between thumb and fingers. Tremors are generally worse while the patient is resting than while he or she is moving about. They tend, however, to disappear during sleep.

• Gradually, the muscles of the face begin to stiffen up. Patients tend to stare with a blank, unblinking expression or develop a slight frown.

• The limbs become stiff and resist movement. Walking becomes more and more difficult. Patients tend to stoop and shuffle, taking only small steps. In severe cases, they may find it easier to walk backwards than forwards.

- Patients often become depressed, sometimes deeply.

Duration
- The condition generally deteriorates slowly, over many years. In severe cases, however, its progress is more rapid and may reduce the normal expected life-span.

Causes
- In Parkinson's disease parts of the base of the brain degenerate, leading to a deficiency of dopamine, a vital brain chemical.
- The cause of the damage is not known, but some cases have followed epidemics of ENCEPHALITIS.
- There may be links with smoking and heredity—smokers and relatives have a slightly higher risk.
- Similar symptoms (parkinsonism) may be triggered by certain medicines or, rarely, by trauma or TUBERCULOSIS.
- Parkinsonism is common in elderly people with ATHEROMA, but the parts of the brain involved differ.
- In a few cases other family members are afflicted.

Complications
- Death may occur if the muscles of respiration are seriously affected.

Treatment in the home
- None. Consult the doctor if symptoms suggest the condition.
- Symptoms of parkinsonism due to drugs usually stop when the medicine is stopped. Parkinsonism due to other factors is irreversible. However, a great deal can be done to lessen its effects and support the patient at home. Physical exercise and social contact should be encouraged. Doctors, nurses, occupational therapists and physiotherapists can all help, but the main burden of such support usually falls on relatives and friends.

When to consult the doctor
- If the symptoms described occur.

What the doctor may do
- Prescribe drugs to slow deterioration and relieve stiffness and tremors. See MEDICINES, 24.
- Recommend that relatives and friends give support and encouragement against depression. The doctor may also prescribe antidepressants. See MEDICINES, 19.
- Prescribe physical therapy and walking aids.
- In severe cases, where other courses of treatment fail, the doctor may recommend a brain operation.

Prevention
- Little can be done to prevent Parkinson's disease, though avoiding smoking reduces the risk slightly.

Outlook
- Although Parkinson's disease worsens over time, the treatments described above often slow down its progress and bring marked relief of the symptoms.

See NERVOUS SYSTEM page 34

PARONYCHIA

An infection of the fold of skin at the side of a finger or toe-nail which can occur in acute and chronic forms.

ACUTE PARONYCHIA
Symptoms
- Pain and throbbing in the nail fold.
- The skin is red and swollen.
- Pus develops and may be visible under the nail.
- Young babies sometimes develop small paronychia, which settle with simple cleansing.

Duration
- The condition becomes very painful within hours and subsides as soon as pus is released or the infection cured.

Causes
- Bacterial infection after a minor prick or other injury.
- COLD SORES virus may cause a very painful infection without pus formation.

Treatment in the home
- Bathe the finger in hot water and poultice with magnesium sulphate (Epsom salts) paste to bring the pus to a head.
- Do not use antiseptic creams as these will not get through the skin to the infection.

When to consult the doctor
- If the infection lasts for six hours and is getting worse.

What the doctor may do
- In the early stages, prescribe antibiotics to stop the infection developing. See MEDICINES, 25.
- Remove the finger-nail or lance the abscess under anaesthetic to let out the pus and relieve the pain.

Prevention
- No special precautions are possible except for nursing and medical personnel who should wear protective gloves wherever possible. See WHITLOW.

Outlook
- Complete recovery.

CHRONIC PARONYCHIA
The condition is mostly caused by a fungus infection and is particularly common in diabetics and those whose hands are often in water; for example, housewives, cleaners, barmen, fishworkers and chefs.

Symptoms
- The nail fold is swollen, rounded and red causing the space between the nail and nail fold to open up. Dirt easily accumulates in this space.
- The nail becomes ridged and furrowed.

- Green, yellow or black evidence of infection may develop below the nail.
- Several fingers are usually involved.
- Severe pain is unusual.

Duration
- Paronychia can persist for years unless treated.

Causes
- Cutting nails too short.
- Fungal or bacterial infection.

Complications
- Recurrences and deformity of the nail are common.

Treatment in the home
- Keep the hands dry as much as possible.
- If rubber gloves are worn they must be cotton-lined in order to absorb sweat.
- Do not rub softening creams into the nail folds.
- Soak the infected finger-nails in surgical spirit for five minutes every day.

When to consult the doctor
- As soon as possible. There is no medical substitute for keeping the hands dry, but the sooner treatment can be started, the sooner fungus infection will clear.

What the doctor may do
- Prescribe antifungal ointment or lotion.
- Prescribe antibiotics. See MEDICINES, 43.
- Test the urine to see whether DIABETES is the cause.
- Examine other sites that could be infected by fungus, such as the buttocks or the vagina.

Prevention
- Keep the hands dry.
- Do not cut the nails too short.

Outlook
- Healing is unpredictable and usually takes several weeks. Patience is required, but if the hands can be kept dry treatment will eventually succeed. However, the condition can recur.

See SKIN page 52

PAROXYSMAL TACHYCARDIA

Attacks of rapid beating of the heart which start and stop abruptly and usually occur in otherwise healthy adults; younger age groups are mostly affected.

Symptoms
- If the attack is short, the patient will be aware of the

heart beating rapidly, or fluttering.
- If the attack lasts longer, breathlessness, chest pain (ANGINA) and fainting may occur.

Duration
- From a few seconds to hours, or even days.

Causes
- Often no cause is found.
- Excess alcohol, caffeine or nicotine.
- Sensitivity to a wide variety of drugs.
- If an ELECTROCARDIOGRAM (ECG) is taken, various minor irregularities of little significance may be found.

Treatment in the home
- Avoid exertion. Sit while the attack lasts.

When to consult the doctor
- If the attack has lasted longer than ten to 15 minutes.
- If breathlessness is embarrassing.
- If chest pain (angina) or fainting occur.

What the doctor may do
- Attempt first to stop the attack by pressing the carotid artery in the neck. If this succeeds, he may teach this or similar techniques to the patient.
- Send the patient to hospital for an electrocardiogram.
- If simple cures do not work, he will prescribe drug therapy, usually by injection. If this does not work, he will send the patient to hospital. *See* MEDICINES, 5.

Prevention
- Coffee, alcohol and nicotine should be taken only in modest amounts by those subject to attacks.

Outlook
- Attacks often recur. Time intervals will vary with different people.
- Most attacks are not serious, and when over the patient can lead a normal life.

See CIRCULATORY SYSTEM *page 40*

PATENT DUCTUS ARTERIOSUS
A relatively rare congenital abnormality of the heart. In the fetus most of the circulating blood leaving the heart via the pulmonary artery is shunted through a short artery called the ductus arteriosus straight into the aorta, thus bypassing the lungs. At birth, as the lungs expand, the ductus arteriosus normally closes and blood circulates through the lungs, but if the duct remains open, high pressure in the aorta forces blood back from the aorta into the pulmonary artery and it is needlessly recirculated through the lungs. A baby with this condition is not blue, because blood is over-oxygenated, but the heart must do extra work and breathlessness should be reported to a doctor.

See CIRCULATORY SYSTEM *page 40*

PATTERN THERAPY
The use of various shapes and patterns to promote healing, based on the belief that they possess their own specific power or energy. The best-known example is the classical pyramid—constructed so that the height is equal to the radius of a circle which has a circumference that measures the same as the perimeter of the pyramid's square base. Sitting or sleeping under pyramids is claimed to benefit health, for example by reducing hyperactivity and menstrual cramps. The pyramid can be made of anything from brown paper to plywood. The important thing to the believer is the precision of the dimensions. The whole issue of pattern therapy is being studied by scientists in the United States and the Soviet Union, but no one has yet produced conclusive evidence that it works.

PELLAGRA
A disease caused by extreme deficiency of nicotinic acid (niacin), one of the vitamin B group found plentifully in meat, fish, whole-grain cereals and yeast extracts. The disorder is rare in Britain.

PEMPHIGOID

This is a rare condition, mainly affecting the over-60s, in which large blisters develop for no known cause.

Symptoms
- Large blisters, 1 in. (25 mm.) or more in diameter, suddenly appear. The abdomen, front of the thighs and the arms are the common sites, although blisters may form in the mouth.
- The blisters may be only on one site for months before spreading.

Duration
- Many months or years.

Causes
- Unknown.

Treatment in the home
- None. Consult the doctor.

What the doctor may do
- Send the patient for a BIOPSY (a scraping from the blister for examination under a microscope).
- Treatment may be successful with steroid creams, but more often corticosteroids by mouth or other drugs are necessary. *See* MEDICINES, 32, 43.

Prevention
- None is known.

Outlook
- The disease responds well to treatment, and even if not treated will eventually disappear over some years.

See SKIN *page 52*

PEMPHIGUS

This rare, often fatal, disease gives rise to blisters. It occurs in the 40-60 age range and most sufferers are Jewish.

Symptoms
- Large blisters develop, wherever there is friction on the skin, such as in the groin, between the buttocks, under the arms. The inside of the mouth, the eye, the anus and the vulva may also be affected.
- The blisters soon break, leaving raw areas which may increase in size.
- The blisters may be confined to one area for months before spreading.
- The patient soon becomes ill.

Duration
- Progress of the untreated disorder may be rapidly fatal or continue over many months, ending ultimately in death.

Causes
- Unknown.

Treatment in the home
- None. Consult the doctor.

What the doctor may do
- Send the patient to hospital for investigation, nursing and treatment with corticosteroids. *See* MEDICINES, 32.

Prevention
- None possible.

Outlook
- When untreated, pemphigus is usually fatal. Modern treatment may be successful but is never certain.

See SKIN *page 52*

PENIS
Symptoms affecting the penis and foreskin include pain, itching, discharge, deformities, and ulcers and lumps on the surface.

See SYMPTOM SORTER—PENIS, FORESKIN AND URETHRA

PERFORATED EAR-DRUM

A hole which may develop in the ear-drum due to injury or infection.

Symptoms
• Deafness in the affected ear following acute OTITIS MEDIA, or EAR INJURY.
• The pain of acute otitis media may be suddenly relieved by perforation of the drum.
• Possible ringing in the ears (TINNITUS) where injury is involved.
• Discharge as pus drains from the middle ear through the perforation and the outer-ear canal—so releasing pressure and easing pain.

Duration
• With children, healing is usually complete within two weeks. With adults, healing may take longer although most small perforations heal within weeks.

Causes
• Severe or untreated acute otitis media.
• Ear injury—particularly a sudden blast of noise, or a slap on the ear that produces a large pressure difference across the ear-drum .
• Diving, or the misuse of aqua-lung equipment.

Treatment in the home
• Protect the ear with cotton wool soaked in Vaseline when bathing, showering or washing the hair.

What the doctor may do
• Treat an infection with antibiotics. *See* MEDICINES, 25.
• Clean out any discharge.
• In the case of a persistent, large perforation, a 'patch' may be surgically placed on the drum to close it. The operation is performed under general anaesthetic.
• Advise against swimming until the perforation has closed.

Prevention
• Use ear protectors when working with guns, explosives or anything else that makes a loud noise.
• Make sure that any case of acute otitis media is properly treated and cleared up.
• Do not go diving without proper training and proper equipment.

Outlook
• Excellent, providing the injured or infected ear is medically treated. However, if an infection does not clear up in adults, chronic suppurative otitis media may develop.

See EAR *page 38*

PERICARDITIS

Inflammation of the pericardium, the sac that forms the outer covering of the heart. Occasionally the inflamed pericardium thickens and constricts the heart, a condition known as constrictive pericarditis. In some cases fluid may accumulate and swell the sac (pericardial effusion). Pericarditis sometimes occurs together with PLEURISY.

Symptoms
• Pain in the chest is often severe and may simulate pleurisy or CORONARY THROMBOSIS.
• Abnormal breathlessness.
• In constrictive pericarditis the abdomen and ankles may swell.
• In some cases there are no symptoms and the person is unaware that he has the condition.

Duration
• How long the disorder lasts depends on the cause. Some attacks last only a few days; others continue for months.

Causes
• Infections by many different micro-organisms.
• As a complication of: CORONARY THROMBOSIS, RHEUMATIC FEVER, CANCER, RHEUMATOID ARTHRITIS and many other diseases.

Treatment in the home
• None is possible.

When to consult the doctor
• If chest pain or breathlessness occur for no apparent reason.

What the doctor may do
• He will arrange for the patient to have X-rays, an ELECTROCARDIOGRAM (ECG) and blood tests, to discover the underlying cause of the disorder.
• Once the underlying cause is discovered, it will be treated as described in the entry for that condition.
• If tests reveal constrictive pericarditis, surgery may be needed to relieve the pressure on the heart.
• If tests show that the fluid in the pericardium is abnormal or interfering with the pumping heart, the fluid will be withdrawn from the pericardium.

Prevention
• For the preventive measures possible, see the entries for the conditions mentioned under **Causes**.

Outlook
• This depends on the underlying cause.

See CIRCULATORY SYSTEM *page 40*

PERIOD PROBLEMS

About 3 per cent of visits to an average family doctor are by women with menstruation problems. Most of the disorders have simple causes that can be treated and are nothing to worry about. Amenorrhoea (absence of periods) is most often caused by pregnancy. Dysmenorrhoea (painful periods) is very common in girls and young women and rarely indicates disease. In some women the pattern of menstrual periods may change (dysfunctional menstrual bleeding); sometimes periods become heavier (menorrhagia).

Cancer is a rare cause which can be treated if caught early, and it is important to report any unexpected bleeding either between periods, during PREGNANCY or after the MENOPAUSE.

AMENORRHOEA
Absence or stoppage of periods, or very slight periods (oligomenorrhoea). This is usually a normal consequence of pregnancy or the menopause.

Symptoms
• Absence or stoppage of periods.
• Very slight periods.

Duration
This depends on the cause:
• If the cause is ANOREXIA NERVOSA or serious physical disease, periods will eventually start again once weight has returned to normal.
• If the Pill is the cause, periods will start again when the Pill is stopped, but sometimes not for six to 12 months. *See* FAMILY PLANNING.
• With the end of the menopause, periods cease for good, but the process may take several years.

Causes
• PREGNANCY is the most common cause. Other signs of pregnancy will appear in a few days.
• The menopause usually occurs between the ages of 45 and 50, when periods become less heavy and less frequent.
• The Pill sometimes produces slight or absent periods.
• Anorexia nervosa.
• Certain chronic diseases such as ANAEMIA, MYXOEDEMA or TUBERCULOSIS.
• Major ANXIETY or worries.
• Congenital abnormalities of the genital organs are very unusual, but are a possible cause in a girl of 16 or 17 who has never had a period.

Complications
• In rare cases, INFERTILITY.

Treatment in the home
• None possible.

When to consult the doctor
• If periods stop without apparent explanation.
• If a girl over the age of 16 has never had a period.
• If pregnancy is likely.

What the doctor may do
• Carry out a general examination and an INTERNAL PELVIC EXAMINATION.
• Carry out a pregnancy test.
• Arrange blood tests for anaemia.
• Prescribe a short course of hormone tablets for excessive flushes due to the menopause. See MEDICINES, 33.

Prevention
• None.

Outlook
• Apart from stoppage due to the menopause, periods will return to normal once the underlying condition has been resolved.

DYSFUNCTIONAL MENSTRUAL BLEEDING
A name given to any change in the normal menstrual pattern, producing heavy or irregular periods for which no cause can be discovered. The condition, also known as dysfunctional uterine haemorrhage, is most likely to affect girls who have just started having periods, or women nearing the MENOPAUSE.

Symptoms
• Irregular periods. These may be more frequent, heavier or last longer than normal.
• Any other change in the normal menstrual pattern.

Duration
• The condition may clear up after a few months, or occur intermittently for several years.

Causes
• The cause is not known; hormonal imbalance is often suspected.

Complications
• ANAEMIA.

Treatment in the home
• None possible.

When to consult the doctor
• If there is a change in the menstrual pattern lasting more than three months.
• If pregnancy or serious disease is possible, it may be necessary to report before waiting three months.

What the doctor may do
• Exclude or arrange treatment for other more serious disease by INTERNAL PELVIC EXAMINATION, CERVICAL SMEAR, blood tests, or referral to a gynaecologist for dilatation and curettage (D & C).
• Try the effects of the Pill, or a similar course of hormone

tablets, if no clear cause is found. See MEDICINES, 33.

Prevention
• None possible.

Outlook
• This is usually a temporary problem which clears up without treatment.

DYSMENORRHOEA
Painful periods. There is pain in the lower abdomen at the beginning of a period. This condition is common in girls and young women. It often disappears after the birth of the first baby.

Symptoms
• Low abdominal pain, usually intermittent (colicky).
• Low backache.
• Sometimes nausea or vomiting.
• Feeling faint.

Duration
• The pain usually lasts for only one or two days at the beginning of the period.

Causes
• In teenage girls and young women it is possibly due to a tight cervix.
• In older women it may be caused by ENDOMETRIOSIS or chronic SALPINGITIS.
• Contraceptive coil (IUD). See FAMILY PLANNING.
• Anxiety and tension.

Complications
• None.

Treatment in the home
Every decision about home treatment depends on physical and personal factors (see PAIN), and there is always a compromise between 'carrying on' and taking action to deal with an upsetting, though harmless complaint.
    Steps which help are:
• Painkillers. See MEDICINES, 22.
• Rest in a chair or in bed.
• A hot bath or a hot-water bottle held over the site of the pain.
• The sufferer, parents, teachers and friends should aim for an attitude which is understanding and not too demanding.

When to consult the doctor
• If the pain interferes with daily life.
• If periods become painful when they have previously been pain free, or if they are becoming more painful.

What the doctor may do
• Carry out an INTERNAL PELVIC EXAMINATION.
• Prescribe a painkiller, hormone tablets or the Pill. See MEDICINES, 33.
• Arrange an examination by a gynaecologist if he is uncertain about the cause.

Prevention
• Sensible discussion with parents before a girl's period starts may help to prevent fears and worries which may aggravate pain.

Outlook
• The condition usually disappears after the birth of the first baby.

MENORRHAGIA
Excessively heavy periods, sometimes called 'flooding'. If no obvious cause is found, the complaint is sometimes included by doctors as another form of dysfunctional menstrual bleeding.

Symptoms
• Regular, heavy or prolonged periods.
• Periods that are heavier than usual.
• Fatigue.

Duration
• This condition may last for two or three months if it is caused by hormonal imbalance. If it is caused by uterine FIBROIDS, or missed ABORTION, the condition will persist until these are treated.

Causes
• Hormonal imbalance.
• Uterine fibroids.
• Missed abortion.
• Contraceptive coil (IUD). See FAMILY PLANNING.

Complications
• ANAEMIA.

Treatment in the home
• If bleeding is excessive lie down and rest.

When to consult the doctor
• If the periods have become heavier than usual, and the change persists for more than three periods.
• If there are signs of anaemia.

What the doctor may do
• Exclude or arrange treatment for other more serious disease by INTERNAL PELVIC EXAMINATION, CERVICAL SMEAR, blood tests, or referral to a gynaecologist for dilatation and curettage (D & C).
• Try the effects of a course on the Pill or other hormone tablets, if no clear cause is found. See MEDICINES, 33.

Prevention
• Often none possible.

Outlook
• This depends on the underlying cause.

POSTMENOPAUSAL BLEEDING
Any bleeding after periods have stopped with the MENOPAUSE. The menopause usually begins in the early or middle 40s and periods may end abruptly or gradually with increasing gaps in between. Although it may be

difficult to judge whether the menopause is over, it is very important to report to a doctor any postmenopausal bleeding even if it might prove to be a late period. In general any bleeding more than three to six months after the last period should be reported.

See FEMALE GENITAL SYSTEM *page 48*
SYMPTOM SORTER—BLEEDING FROM THE VAGINA

PERIOSTITIS

Inflammation of the periosteum, the thin layer of tissue surrounding a bone. It may be caused by injury, when it is treated with anti-inflammatory drugs; or by one of several diseases, including TUBERCULOSIS, when treatment is of the disease involved.

PERISTALSIS

Wave-like contractions of muscle in the walls of certain organs and passages, by which their contents are pushed along. Peristalsis is what conveys food through the whole digestive tract, from the gullet to the rectum. In women it causes egg cells to pass down the Fallopian tubes into the uterus (womb).

PERITONITIS

Inflammation of the peritoneum, the membrane that lines the abdominal cavity surrounding the stomach and other soft internal organs.

Peritonitis is an acute and always serious condition which follows inflammation of other abdominal organs. It can be a complication of a burst appendix abscess, a burst gastric or duodenal ulcer, a ruptured ectopic pregnancy, or any ulcer which perforates the wall of the bowel and allows the intestinal contents to escape into the surrounding abdominal cavity. The presence of infected material and pus outside the bowel paralyses all bowel movements (*see* ILEUS), and can cause death in 24-48 hours if not treated in hospital.
See DIGESTIVE SYSTEM *page 44*

PERSONALITY PROBLEMS

The term is usually reserved for those who have difficulty with personal relationships and therefore do not fit into normal society. If the misfit is aggressive, antisocial and disruptive, he may be labelled a sociopath or a psychopath. Milder forms of personality disorder can be coped with by the individual and by society in general.
See MENTAL SYSTEM *page 33*

PERTHES' DISEASE

A condition in which the growing part at the top of the femur (thigh bone) becomes inflamed and softened. The diseased part of the bone dies, but is completely replaced by living bone as the femur grows. The hip joint must be protected from weight-bearing during this healing phase, otherwise the head of the femur will become deformed. The condition occurs in children aged between four and ten years and usually affects only one hip.
Symptoms
• The child starts to limp.
• Mild pain, often felt in the hip but sometimes felt in the knee.
• Hip movement may be restricted.
Duration
• Two or three years.
Causes
• Lack of blood supply to the growing part of the head of the femur. The reason for this is not known.
Complications
• ARTHRITIS of the hip in later life.
Treatment in the home
• None advised. Seek medical advice.
When to consult the doctor
• Immediately the condition is suspected, or if a child limps for more than 48 hours.
What the doctor may do
• Send the child to hospital immediately for examination by an orthopaedic specialist.
• The specialist will either operate or, in some cases, put the hip in splints to prevent weight-bearing while the healing process is taking place.
Prevention
• None known.
Outlook
• If the disease is detected early, in young children, the outlook with treatment is excellent. The outlook is less good if treatment is delayed or if the disease occurs after the age of eight.

See SKELETAL SYSTEM *page 54*

PETIT MAL
One of the three main types of epilepsy. Petit mal mainly affects young people, occurring between four years and adolescence.
See EPILEPSY

PETS

Domestic pets in Britain transmit very few diseases to human beings, but they can cause allergic reactions ranging from minor rashes to severe attacks of asthma.

Some people develop asthma or hay fever when they inhale animal scurf (tiny flakes of dry skin) or fur. Others develop itchy hives or rashes within minutes of being licked by a cat or a dog. People who are particularly susceptible to cats can develop a swelling of the eyelids which may be severe enough to close both eyes within minutes of entering a cat-inhabited room.

Gerbils, rabbits, guinea pigs and other furry animals can also cause allergic reactions.

The trouble is mostly caused by an ALLERGY to protein in the animal's urine which contaminates its fur. The symptoms of allergy develop promptly after the animal is cuddled or handled closely.

The only effective prevention is to get rid of the animal and allow at least two or three months for all the fur and scurf to be cleared from the home. Desensitisation treatment is not generally available in the United Kingdom, and there is little evidence that it works.

DISEASE FROM CATS
A rare ailment that can be caused by cats is CAT-SCRATCH FEVER. The main symptom is a swelling of the glands in a part of the body that has been bitten, scratched or licked by a cat. The swelling is accompanied by a slight fever and 'flu-like' symptoms. The cause is thought to be a virus.

The disease almost invariably gets better by itself, and requires just a short course of painkillers in recommended doses to relieve the aches and pains. *See* MEDICINES, 22.

WHEN FLEAS BITE
Fleas are often brought into the home by pets. Dog and cat fleas live by feeding off the blood of the pets, and people usually get bitten only when an animal is no longer available—typically, when a home is vacated by a pet-owning family and inhabited by a family who do not have pets.

Most fleas spend only a proportion of their lives on an animal. They live for the rest of the time in its bedding, or in furniture near its favourite resting place.

Flea bites cause nothing more than itching in Western countries, although they can become infected if scratched. But in tropical countries, fleas can transmit dangerous disease such as bubonic PLAGUE.

To rid the home and the pet of fleas, use a flea powder, and then fit the pet with a flea collar. If that is not effective, take your animal to the vet and ask the local council to spray your home with insecticide.

PETS WITH WORMS

In Britain, domestic pets, especially dogs, can transmit two worm diseases to humans—hydatid cyst and TOXOCARIASIS. Both diseases are caused by swallowing the eggs of parasite worms which are found in the faeces of dogs and cats. People are infected either through direct contact with the animal, or by contaminating their hands in a public park where dogs are being exercised. Children who play in parks and playgrounds are particularly at risk and, partly because of this, many local authorities have banned dogs from some recreation areas.

Hydatid cyst is caused by the eggs hatching into larvae in the victim's intestine. The larvae penetrate the wall of the intestine and enter the blood system, lodging in places such as the liver and lungs where the blood is richer than elsewhere in the body. A cyst then begins to grow, sometimes taking as long as 20-30 years to develop fully. The cyst may reach the size of a grapefruit, and it is its sheer size which produces the symptoms of the disease—abdominal pain or discomfort, sweating, fever, malaise.

Hydatid disease is very rare except in sheep-rearing areas such as Wales, New Zealand and Australia, where it is passed backwards and forwards between dogs and sheep.

Infection with toxocariasis occurs in the same way as hydatid cyst—by swallowing the eggs. Once in the blood, the eggs hatch into larvae which are carried to the liver, lungs and brain, where the body sets up a vigorous defence reaction producing large quantities of white blood cells, known as eosinophils.

Toxocariasis is usually a mild disease, perhaps causing vague aches and pains but it may also spread to the back of the eye, particularly in children, whose vision may be damaged. To guard against it, dogs and cats should receive proper de-worming treatment (see box).

RABIES

This is a dangerous disease transmitted to humans in the saliva of infected animals, by a bite or lick or occasionally by the inhalation of drops of saliva. Animals which are known to transmit the disease include cats and dogs (most common), rats, bats, foxes, squirrels and cattle.

Rabies has not yet been discovered in the wild animal population of the United Kingdom, but it is endemic in the wild animal populations of Europe, North and South America, and the continents of Africa and India.

A newly developed vaccine now makes treatment against rabies much less unpleasant and more effective than it used to be.

PSITTACOSIS AND BIRD-FANCIER'S LUNG

Two diseases are caused by caged birds. Both are a result of close contact with live birds. They are not caused by eating poultry.

PSITTACOSIS is a virus-like germ which usually infects birds, especially the parrot family. Humans become infected by inhaling the germ from the dried droppings of infected birds. Symptoms range from those of mild influenza to a severe type of pneumonia, including aches and pains and a persistent dry cough. A chest X-ray may show signs of pneumonia.

A course of antibiotics destroys the germ that carries the disease, but will not provide immunity against re-infection. The bird usually dies; if it survives it will no longer be infectious.

Bird-fancier's lung is an allergic reaction to a protein in a bird's blood supply, which finds its way into the droppings. Symptoms of the allergy often develop within four to eight hours of cage-cleaning, when heavy doses of the protein are inhaled. They include breathlessness and aches and pains, together with a 'flu-like' illness.

Permanent damage can be done to the lungs unless an early diagnosis is made and the patient avoids exposure to birds. Uncaged birds provide no problem, since their droppings do not accumulate and so are not inhaled.

Keeping your pet free of disease

To prevent your pets from contracting diseases, which could also affect humans, you should take them to the vet for the following treatments:

CATS

☐ Worming of mother cat in the second half of pregnancy.

☐ Worming of kittens at five weeks of age and then again between eight and nine weeks.

☐ Vaccination against feline enteritis and cat flu at 12 weeks. Booster injections should be given every 12 months or two years, depending on which vaccine is used. Ask your vet for advice.

DOGS

☐ Worming of pregnant bitch.

☐ Worming of puppy between four and seven weeks of age, and again between 14 and 20 weeks. Thereafter, worming treatment should be repeated every six months of the dog's life.

☐ Vaccination against distemper, hardpad, infectious hepatitis and leptospirosis is all given by two injections, one two weeks after the other, when the puppy is between eight and 12 weeks old.

☐ Vaccination against canine parvovirus between ten and 12 weeks.

☐ Vaccination against kennel cough when pup is between six and 12 months old.

☐ Booster injections for all vaccinations should be given every 12 months.

OTHER PETS

☐ Rabbits should be vaccinated against myxomatosis at 12 weeks.

☐ Ferrets should be vaccinated against distemper at 12 weeks.

☐ Caged birds and rodents, such as gerbils, guinea-pigs, hamsters and mice, need no routine vaccinations.

PHAEOCHROMOCYTOMA

A usually benign (non-cancerous) tumour of certain body cells. In most cases it develops within one of the two adrenal glands, which lie on top of the kidneys, but it may occur in various other parts of the body, including the brain and urinary tract. The main feature of the disease is extremely high blood pressure. There are also any or all of the following symptoms: severe headache, vomiting, fast heart rate, palpitation, sweating, constipation, and impairment of vision. The treatment is surgical removal of the tumour.

PHANTOM LIMB PAIN

In almost every case where a limb is amputated, the patient feels at times as if it were still there. It often feels capable of movement or to have shape. As time passes the patient may even feel that the limb is changing shape.

The condition occurs because the nerve fibres cut through in the operation still send messages to the brain from the stump. The brain interprets them as meaning that the limb is still present. The sensations include tingling and pins and needles in the missing limb, a feeling that it is warm or cold, light or heavy.

About 35 per cent of patients also feel pain in the phantom limb. It may be triggered off by pressure on another part of the body, by urination or by an emotional upset. Sometimes, an overgrowth of nerve tissue (NEURO-FIBROMA) develops on the stump and exaggerates the sensation of pain.

Generally, phantom limb sensations are mild and fade away with the passing of time. However, in 5-10 per cent of cases, pain is severe and gets worse over the years. In these circumstances, patients may be treated with a local anaesthetic. The stump may be injected with a strong painkiller, phenol or a solution of salt in order to relieve the pain.

See NERVOUS SYSTEM *page 34*

PHARYNGITIS

Inflammation of the pharynx, the passage connecting the back of the nose with the back of the mouth and leading into the larynx and the oesophagus. Pharyngitis may be either acute or chronic.

ACUTE PHARYNGITIS

Inflammation of the pharynx because of infection by viruses or bacteria. At least 40 per cent of the population get acute pharyngitis each year. The symptoms are not usually severe and life need not necessarily be disrupted at all. If tonsils are present and inflamed the condition is called TONSILLITIS.

Symptoms
• Sore throat.
• Raised temperature, chills and headache.
• Swollen glands in the neck.
• Dry cough.
• CONJUNCTIVITIS (redness of the eyes) sometimes occurs.

Duration
• The incubation period (the time between coming into contact with the infection and the appearance of the first symptoms) is usually three to five days.
• In non-smokers and children the worst of the illness is over within 48 hours. Some soreness of the throat may persist for up to ten days, particularly if the patient is a smoker.

Causes
• Most cases are caused by respiratory viruses. Some are caused by bacteria (streptococci).
• Children in their first year at school are particularly vulnerable to pharyngitis because they come into contact with large numbers of viruses to which they have not built up resistance.
• Less-common causes include: MEASLES, GERMAN MEASLES, and INFLUENZA.

Complications
• RHEUMATIC FEVER and acute NEPHRITIS may follow pharyngitis, but these diseases are now uncommon.

Treatment in the home
• Drink plenty of fluids to relieve the soreness and prevent dehydration.
• Take painkillers in recommended doses to relieve the pain and lower the temperature. *See* MEDICINES, 22.
• Rest.
• If conjunctivitis is present, close the eyes and wipe away the discharge with cotton wool soaked in warm water.
• Stop or at least cut down SMOKING until the condition clears up.

When to consult the doctor
• If green or yellow phlegm is being coughed up from the lungs and there is a raised temperature.
• If earache develops.
• If a rash develops.

What the doctor may do
• Prescribe an antibiotic if there are bacterial complications. *See* MEDICINES, 25.
• Whether caused by bacteria or viruses, pharyngitis will clear up by itself in a few days. There is no advantage in routinely taking antibiotics such as penicillin. Unless there are special risks of complications the doctor can do no more than advise the measures outlined in treatment in the home.

Prevention
• None.

Outlook
• Recovery is complete, usually within ten days.

CHRONIC PHARYNGITIS
Persistent inflammation of the pharynx.

Symptoms
• Persistent sore throat.
• Redness of the throat.

Duration
• As long as there is exposure to an irritant.

Causes
• Exposure to dust or other irritants.
• Smoking. The smoke irritates the sensitive lining of the pharynx.
• Mouth breathing (due, for example, to SINUSITIS, NASAL POLYPS, or DEVIATED NASAL SEPTUM) can cause unfiltered, unwarmed air to irritate the pharynx.
• Persistent sore, red throat may sometimes be noted in cases of anxiety or depression. The reason for this is not understood.

Complications
• None.

Treatment in the home
• Mouthwashes and gargles may ease the symptoms. One soluble aspirin dissolved in warm water and gargled two or three times a day is a suitable mixture.
• Avoid irritants, particularly spicy foods, alcohol and tobacco.

When to consult the doctor
• If the condition appears to be caused by mouth breathing.
• If severe depression or anxiety is suspected.

What the doctor may do
• Examine the nose and throat.
• Treat any underlying cause.

Prevention
• Avoid smoking.

Outlook
• Chronic pharyngitis is not dangerous, but can be annoying and tends to recur, for example at times of emotional stress.

See RESPIRATORY SYSTEM *page 42*

PHARYNX, GROWTH IN

A growth in the pharynx, or any part of the throat, needs early medical attention. It can occur in both men and women, but rarely appears before the age of 30.
See LARYNX, GROWTH IN

PHIMOSIS

Tightness of the opening of the foreskin. A related condition, paraphimosis, occurs when the foreskin has been drawn back and constricts the tip, or glans, of the penis.

Symptoms
- The opening of the foreskin is very tight and the foreskin itself cannot be drawn back over the glans.
- Little boys may have difficulty with urination. The foreskin may balloon because the urine has only a minute opening from which to escape.
- Adults may experience sexual difficulties.
- Paraphimosis may cause pain and swelling in the glans.

Duration
- Both conditions last until treated.

Causes
- Phimosis may be present at birth.
- Infection, especially in the elderly.
- Paraphimosis is usually caused by a minor infection of the foreskin.

Complications
- Inflammation of the glans. *See* BALANITIS.

Treatment in the home
- With little boys gentle retraction of the foreskin may help the eventual stretching caused by normal erection and washing.

When to consult the doctor
- If the symptoms appear.

What the doctor may do
- Examine the penis.
- In some cases circumcision (surgical removal of the foreskin) may be necessary.
- Paraphimosis can normally be corrected by medical manipulation of the penis, but some cases may require emergency circumcision.

Prevention
- Guard against infection by strict personal hygiene.

Outlook
- With treatment both conditions are quickly cured.

See MALE GENITAL SYSTEM *page 50*

PHLEBITIS

Inflammation of the lining of a vein, occurring most commonly in the legs. If a blood clot forms the condition is known as THROMBOPHLEBITIS.

PHOBIA

A form of ANXIETY, similar to COMPULSIVE OBSESSIONAL BEHAVIOUR, in which intense anxiety and abnormal fear may be triggered off by a specific situation or object. Phobias caused by situations include agoraphobia (the fear of open spaces) and claustrophobia (the fear of crowded places, riding in lifts, being shut up in small spaces). Similar situational phobias include fear of social situations, particularly when the sufferer has to perform some function such as speaking in public. Meeting people and eating in public may also become phobias to some people.

Another type of phobia is related to an abnormal fear of objects, particularly animals including dogs, cats, spiders, snakes, birds and mice. Fear about illnesses such as cancer and heart disease also come into this category.

When placed in the feared situation, the sufferer experiences agitation, sweating, rapid pulse and all the symptoms common in anxiety. The frequency of the condition is difficult to measure because many sufferers manage to avoid the situation which makes them tense. Some sufferers are afflicted so severely that they cannot lead a normal life, and may even become housebound.

The phobia may be caused by a fear of something in the sufferer's unconscious life, or by repressed aggressive impulses.

The condition is treated with tranquillisers and attempts to modify behaviour to cope with the feared situation. Treatment sometimes takes the form of desensitisation by saturation therapy, which works by exposing the sufferer to the object of his fear for gradually increased periods of time.

See MENTAL SYSTEM *page 33*

PHOTOSENSITIVITY

A condition in which some people are abnormally sensitive to sunlight and develop 'sunburn' after short exposure to the sun. *See* SUNBURN.

Symptoms
- Skin develops sunburn out of proportion to the time spent in the sun. In minor cases sun-tan follows red skin, in more severe cases, painful, tender, swollen skin is followed by blistering.

Duration
- A few days if the patient is not exposed to further sunlight.

Causes
Drugs are the most common cause and include:
- Phenothiazines, used for nervous disorders and to control vomiting.
- Certain antibiotics of the tetracycline group.
- Sulphonamides.
- Griseofulvin, used to treat fungal infections.
- Nalidixic acid, used for urinary infections.
- Barbiturates.

Other causes include:
- Nicotinic acid deficiency, which occurs in countries with chronic malnutrition.
- Other rare medical disorders, for example PORPHYRIA and conditions where pigment is absent.

Treatment in the home
- Keep the skin cool by dabbing with calamine lotion or by applying cold compresses. Antihistamine creams have little effect.
- Leave blistered areas exposed to the air.
- Take painkilling tablets in recommended doses, if necessary. *See* MEDICINES, 22.
- Avoid clothes rubbing the sore area.
- Do not allow further exposure to sun.
- Tell the doctor about all drugs and medicaments being used.

When to consult the doctor
- If you have an unusual reaction to sun or to a sun-lamp.

What the doctor may do
- Arrange for the sufferer to be tested with sunlight applied to a limited area of skin. This will establish a firm diagnosis.

Prevention
- Use sun-filter creams if you are fair skinned.
- Stop the responsible drug unless there is no alternative.

Outlook
- Preventative measures are usually successful.

See SKIN *page 52*
DRUG RASH

PIGEON CHEST

An abnormally prominent breastbone, which may be present from birth. Occasionally pigeon chest may be a symptom of RICKETS. It is nearly always harmless and no cause for concern.

PIGEON TOES

Turning-in of the toes. Mild forms of this condition are normal and are first noticed when a child begins to walk.

The condition tends to start between the ages of two and six, but unless the deformity is excessive and persists into adult life, it does not require treatment.

See SKELETAL SYSTEM *page 54*

PIGMENTED NAEVUS

A harmless coloured birthmark. Pigmented naevuses may be pale or as heavily pigmented as to appear almost black. They start as blotches or firm nodules and occur anywhere on the body. Nearly every person will have one or more. Most people will average 20 or more. They usually become noticeable around puberty and grow slowly to up to 2 in. (50 mm.) in diameter during adult life. When occurring on the face, they may grow as the 'common mole' which is dome shaped, and often has strong hairs growing from it.

Duration
• Naevuses last for ever unless they are surgically removed.

Causes
• The abnormality is probably present at birth.

Treatment in the home
• Leave the naevus alone. Do not attempt home removal.
• It is safe to remove hairs growing from a mole.

When to consult the doctor
• If the naevus is causing anxiety or there is a wish to have it removed.
• If the naevus or its surrounding skin changes colour or size, bleeds, or gives pain over a period of two or three weeks.

What the doctor may do
• Reassure the patient that the naevus is harmless, and arrange for it to be removed if that is what the patient wants.
• If diagnosis is in any doubt, the doctor will arrange for the naevus to be surgically removed for examination under a microscope.

Prevention
• None is possible.

Outlook
• A dark-coloured naevus lightens and becomes less noticeable with age.
• The naevus that undergoes no changes remains harmless and will not become cancerous.

See SKIN *page 52*
MELANOMA

PILES

Varicose (swollen) veins outside or inside the anus, also known as haemorrhoids. Piles appear as lumps which frequently bleed. They are the commonest cause of bleeding at the anus.

EXTERNAL PILES
Symptoms
• Small, rounded, blue-purple lumps just outside the anus.
• They may develop rapidly after straining to pass a motion and are often painful for up to five days.
• If they are rubbed they may bleed, which releases the tension and relieves the pain. Sometimes the bleeding produces small dark clots of blood.

Duration
• External piles usually break through the skin and then heal within a week or two. They often leave skin 'tags'.

Causes
• A vein outside the anus bursts after straining. The bleeding that follows raises a swelling under the skin. Clots then form in the vein.

Treatment in the home
• Hot baths or hot compresses (a sponge or flannel squeezed out in hot water and pressed on to the anus) will help to relieve the pain.
• Soothing ointments can be obtained from a chemist.

When to consult the doctor
• If the pain is severe.

What the doctor may do
• Anaesthetise the area to incise and release the clot.
• Prescribe an anaesthetic ointment to apply temporarily. *See* MEDICINES, 4.

INTERNAL PILES
Varicose veins inside the anus.
Symptoms
• Soft, purplish lumps which may protrude during defecation, or even stay permanently outside.
• Bleeding, usually bright red, flecking the toilet paper or even dripping into the pan. Blood lies on the surface of the stool on defecating.
• Itching.
• Leaking of mucus may occur.
• A feeling of fullness in the rectum. This leads to continued straining, which may in turn lead to permanent prolapse with swelling, thrombosis and even strangulation if the pile twists on its stalk.

Duration
• Brief attacks may follow constipation, settling in a few days or two or three weeks.
• Recurrent bouts may occur over years.
• Prolapsed piles may stay down until treated.

Causes
• Increased pressure in internal veins of the rectum due to straining to pass a motion, chronic cough, OBESITY, PREGNANCY or abdominal tumours.
• Liver vein obstruction. *See* CIRRHOSIS OF THE LIVER.

Complications
• ANAEMIA from continued blood loss.

Treatment in the home
• If the piles are swollen or protruding, hot baths or compresses (as for external piles) will relieve pain. Pushing the piles back with the hot sponge will help.
• Keep the anus clean by carefully wiping with a damp tissue or sponge and patting dry.
• Suppositories, which you can buy at the chemist, may help to soothe pain. *See* MEDICINES, 4.
• Rest in bed helps to reduce both swelling and pain.

When to consult the doctor
• If you have severe pain or bleeding, or if the piles cannot be easily pushed back after defecation.

What the doctor may do
• Examine you to exclude other causes of bleeding.
• He will then either inject the piles (though they tend to recur), or send you to a surgeon for removal of large piles or treatment by 'anal stretch' under anaesthetic.

Prevention
• Avoid straining and chronic constipation.
• Take roughage or a bulk laxative, with fruit, vegetables, and adequate fluids. *See* MEDICINES, 4.

Outlook
• Good with proper treatment.

See DIGESTIVE SYSTEM *page 44*

PILONIDAL SINUS OR CYST
An opening, lined with hairs, that develops in the skin between the buttocks. From time to time it becomes infected and painful. The disorder mainly affects young adults. It is cured by surgical removal.

PIMPLE
A small, raised, inflamed spot on the skin that contains pus. It may occur as the result of grease from a sebaceous gland clogging a pore, which then becomes infected. Large numbers of pimples and blackheads, a condition known as ACNE, are common in adolescence.

PINS AND NEEDLES

A tingling feeling in a limb, caused by pinching of a nerve. People who experience frequent pins and needles should see a doctor, since the condition may indicate a nervous disease.

PINTA

An infectious skin disorder. Scaly patches appear on the face, neck, hands and feet. At first they are red or blue, but eventually they turn white. In addition, the skin on the hands and feet may harden. The disease, which is caught by bodily contact with an infected person, occurs mainly in tropical America. Penicillin cures it.

PITYRIASIS ROSEA

One of a group of diseases in which delicate, bran-like scales form on the skin. The most common forms of the condition are pityriasis rosea, which is normally seen in young adults, particularly women, especially in spring and autumn, and pityriasis capitis (see DANDRUFF).

Symptoms
• A single red patch $\frac{4}{5}$-4 in. (20-100 mm.) in diameter, usually on the torso, precedes the main rash by seven to ten days.
• About a week later there is a general outbreak of patches about $\frac{1}{5}$-$\frac{4}{5}$ in. (5-20 mm.) in diameter, on the torso and upper limbs. The area affected is often described as that covered by a short-sleeved T-shirt.
• The spots are usually round or slightly oval with scaly edges and are slightly itchy. In the beginning each spot is salmon-pink or rose-red in colour.
• After one to four weeks, the centres of the patches may lose their scales and turn light brown, while the outside of the patches are left as slightly raised red rings.

Duration
• The condition usually clears up after three or four weeks. Occasionally it persists for several months.

Causes
• Unknown. Possibly an infection.

Treatment in the home
• If the patches itch, a soothing lotion such as calamine may be helpful. No other treatment is required.

When to consult the doctor
• Although the condition does not normally require treatment, it is sensible to consult the doctor when the red patches first appear so that he can rule out other causes.
• If itching from the patches becomes severe.

What the doctor may do
• Examine the patches and possibly take a blood test to rule out other diseases and to confirm the diagnosis.
• Prescribe drugs or soothing lotions such as calamine to relieve any itching. See MEDICINES, 43.

Outlook
• Pityriasis clears up spontaneously and recovery is complete.

See SKIN page 52

PLACEBO

A preparation that has no medicinal powers. A placebo is prescribed when a doctor decides that a patient has no need of a drug but knows that the patient will not be satisfied unless he is given a prescription. In many cases the placebo relieves the patient's condition, simply because he believes it to be a medicine and therefore has faith in its powers.

PLACENTA PRAEVIA

An abnormal condition of pregnancy in which the placenta (the afterbirth) which nourishes the fetus, develops not in the upper part of the womb but in the lower. Its danger is that it may obstruct the passage of the fetus and cause heavy bleeding during labour.
See PREGNANCY

PLAGUE

A serious infectious disease of animals, principally rats, caused by a bacterium called *Yersinia pestis*. It is transmitted to humans by fleas from infected rats. The symptoms, which appear suddenly after an incubation period of two to four days, are high temperature and swollen lymph glands. There may also be severe headache, vomiting and delirium. The patient becomes extremely ill and may develop PNEUMONIA. The disease occurs where rats densely populate areas with inadequate sanitation.

In earlier centuries, major epidemics killed vast numbers of people throughout the world (25 million people died in Europe alone in the 14th century). Today epidemics are rare and a vaccine that gives protection is available to those at high risk of contracting the disease. Treatment is by antibiotics, and prevention is by controlling the rat population.
See INFECTIOUS DISEASES page 32

PLANTAR FASCIITIS AND CALCANEAL SPUR

Inflammation of the muscle sheaths in the sole of the foot (the plantar fascia) near the heel. This condition may be related to an abnormal sharp projection on the heel bone —calcaneal spur.

Symptoms
• Acute pain in the heel on standing or walking which may extend forwards into the sole. The pain usually affects only one foot.

Duration
• The condition lasts for one to six months.

Causes
• The exact cause of the disorder is unknown, but obesity, excessive standing or walking and badly fitting shoes may all play a part in its development.

Treatment in the home
• Wear a sponge-rubber cushion in the heel of the shoe to protect the heel from rubbing.
• Rest the foot.

When to consult the doctor
• If the pain is not relieved by home treatment.

What the doctor may do
• Arrange a blood test and an X-ray of the heel.
• Prescribe a cushion for the heel of the shoe.
• Inject hydrocortisone into the heel. This often brings rapid relief of the pain. See MEDICINES, 32.
• If the above treatment fails to work, the doctor may refer the patient to hospital for physiotherapy. In a few cases an operation may be necessary, to remove part of the bone.

Prevention
• Wear well-fitting shoes.
• Try to avoid becoming overweight.

Outlook
• Nearly all cases clear up of their own accord or respond to treatment, but the condition sometimes recurs.

See SKELETAL SYSTEM page 54

PLASTIC SURGERY

The branch of medicine that deals with surgical reconstruction of deformed, disfigured or injured parts of the body. When surgery is performed solely to improve the appearance it is called cosmetic surgery.
See COSMETIC SURGERY

PLEURISY

The lungs are separated from the inside of the chest wall by pleura—a delicate membrane which is lubricated by a thin film of fluid. This allows the lungs to expand and contract smoothly when breathing. Pleurisy can take one of two forms—dry, in which the membrane becomes inflamed; or wet, in which excess fluid is produced, separating the lungs from the chest wall. Both types have similar symptoms and usually occur as a complication of other diseases.

Symptoms
- Sharp, or stabbing pain in the chest clearly related to the movements of breathing.
- Pain is most severe in dry pleurisy.
- Dry cough.
- Fever is common. There may be other symptoms from the underlying disease.

Causes
- Infections due to viruses and bacteria.
- PNEUMONIA.
- CANCER.
- Injury to the chest wall, as in road accidents.
- Sometimes no cause is identified.

Treatment in the home
- Rest in bed and take painkillers in recommended doses. *See* MEDICINES, 22.

When to consult the doctor
- If you have any of the above symptoms.

What the doctor may do
- Examine the patient to identify the cause.

Outlook
- Depends on the underlying disease.

See RESPIRATORY SYSTEM *page 42*

PNEUMONIA

An acute inflammation of the lungs caused by either a bacterial or virus infection. Bacterial pneumonias may develop rapidly in healthy lung tissue or as a complication of an anaesthetic or previous infection such as BRONCHITIS.

Symptoms
- A persistent dry cough.
- A high fever with a very rapid rate of breathing.
- Chest pain often on one side only that is aggravated by breathing and coughing. Such pain usually indicates the presence of PLEURISY and is rarely present in pneumonias due to viruses.
- The sufferer quite suddenly becomes much more ill.
- There is little spit but what there is may contain reddish streaks of blood.
- In babies and toddlers the symptoms of pneumonia are not always obvious. Cough may be slight or absent. The only obvious signs may be high fever with rapid respirations and indrawing of the lower ribs. The baby is often grey, limp and obviously ill. Such a situation warrants an immediate medical opinion.

Duration
- Bacterial pneumonias treated with the appropriate antibiotic rarely last longer than seven to ten days.
- Viral pneumonias are less serious, unaffected by any treatment and rarely last longer than seven days.

Causes
- Bacteria such as the pneumococcus or staphylococcus.
- Q FEVER and PSITTACOSIS are typical examples of pneumonia caused by viruses.
- Spread to the lungs by bacterial infections in the upper respiratory tract.

Complications
- Since the advent of antibiotics complications are few. Recurrences and BRONCHIECTASIS may occur.

Treatment in the home
- Rest in bed and take plenty of fluids while waiting for the doctor.

When to consult the doctor
- If the above symptoms suggest the disease or if there is a sudden worsening in the general condition of a sufferer with any respiratory infection.

What the doctor may do
- Check the diagnosis by examination.
- Arrange a chest X-ray.
- Prescribe an antibiotic if a bacterial pneumonia is considered possible. *See* MEDICINES, 25.
- Arrange for close follow up with chest X-rays to check complete cure. This is vital in children who are more liable to complications and in patients over 40, in whom there is occasionally an underlying LUNG CANCER.

Prevention
- Pneumococcal vaccine gives some protection against one type of pneumonia. It may be recommended for people with diabetes or heart or lung disease, or if the spleen has been removed.

Outlook
- With treatment the outlook at all ages is good.

See RESPIRATORY SYSTEM *page 42*

PNEUMOCONIOSIS

A lung disease of coal miners caused by inhaling large quantities of coal dust. It is a prescribed industrial disease and sufferers may obtain state compensation.
See OCCUPATIONAL HAZARDS

PNEUMOTHORAX

Normally the membrane covering the lung is in close contact with that lining the inner surface of the chest wall: only a thin layer of moisture separates the two. In pneumothorax air gets between them, causing the lung to collapse.

Symptoms
- An extremely sudden onset of sharp pain in the chest, aggravated by deep breathing or coughing.
- Sometimes pain is also felt in the shoulder.
- Shortness of breath. In severe cases this may be extreme; in mild cases it is often absent.

Duration
- Symptoms subside over one to four weeks as the air outside the lungs is gradually absorbed.

Causes
- The formation and rupture—for no known reason—of a small bubble of tissue on the surface of the lung. This is a common cause that usually occurs in young adults, especially young men.
- A fractured rib piercing the lung.
- Any injury that penetrates the wall of the chest may cause pneumothorax.

Treatment in the home
- Pneumothorax is an emergency. If the condition is suspected the patient should be kept at complete rest until seen by a doctor.

When to consult the doctor
- Immediately pneumothorax is suspected.

What the doctor may do
- Arrange immediate X-ray or admission to hospital.
- The sufferer will be kept under observation until the danger of lung collapse is over.

Prevention
- None.

Outlook
- A few individuals are prone to recurrences.
- The outlook is good.

See RESPIRATORY SYSTEM *page 42*

POLIOMYELITIS

A virus infection occurring in epidemics. The disease has what is known as a prodromal stage; that is, early vague symptoms that come before the main severe symptoms. In 95 per cent of cases there is complete recovery at this stage. Patients do not even know that they have had polio, but will be immune from further attacks. The infection is spread by excretion of the virus in the faeces of an infected person. Careless sanitary habits in toddlers and people in overcrowded homes, in schools and changing-rooms encourage such spread. Since immunisation became available in the 1950s it has become possible to control outbreaks of the disease, but immunisation is not always accepted and the number of cases reported in Britain has been increasing since 1975.

Symptoms
• Early (or prodromal) symptoms are mild fever, or flu-like illness, with a sore throat and headache, lasting a few days.
• In a minority of cases the fever recurs in five to ten days and signs of ENCEPHALITIS may develop, causing severe headache and vomiting.
• The patient is conscious and alert.
• Fast pulse.
• Cramping muscle pains and spasms in large groups of muscles, for example a whole leg.
• Paralysis or weakness may develop in the painful limb. In children under five years, paralysis of one limb is common. The older the patient, the more muscles are usually affected.
• Paralysis is more likely to develop in muscles that have been greatly used during the prodromal period.
• Paralysis of the breathing or swallowing muscles, which may threaten life.

Incubation period
• Two to five days.

Duration
• Prodromal symptoms last only a few days.
• Duration of encephalitis symptoms or paralysis depends upon their severity. Paralysis may be permanent.

Causes
• Three polio viruses (types 1, 2 and 3).

Treatment in the home
• None. If you suspect polio call the doctor.

What the doctor may do
• Admit the patient to hospital to confirm the diagnosis.
• There is no specific treatment. Nursing care and, if necessary, artificial respiration on a breathing machine will support the patient until he recovers.

Prevention
• Control of polio depends on widespread immunisation, and parents should be encouraged to have their children immunised.
• Live polio vaccine given orally in three doses during the first year of life, together with the diphtheria, tetanus and whooping-cough injection, produces immunity in 90 per cent of cases.
• A booster dose is given on starting and leaving school.
• Travellers to countries outside northern Europe should seek advice about immunisation before they travel.

Outlook
• Paralysis is permanent, but disability depends upon the site and extent of the paralysis.

See INFECTIOUS DISEASES *page 32*

POLYMYALGIA RHEUMATICA

A rheumatic condition, usually affecting people over 50. It comes on suddenly and often prevents getting out of bed, and is easily disregarded by the sufferers who consider the symptoms are due to old age or vague rheumatism.

Symptoms
• Pain and stiffness in the muscles of the neck and shoulders. Other joints and muscles may also be affected.
• Muscle weakness.
• Mild fever or feeling of ill health.

Duration
• Six months to six years.

Complications
• TEMPORAL ARTERITIS, that is, inflammation of the temporal artery.

Treatment in the home
• None advised before medical advice.

When to consult the doctor
• Immediately the condition is suspected.

What the doctor may do
• Take blood tests to check the diagnosis.
• Tell the patient to rest.
• Prescribe painkillers. *See* MEDICINES, 22.
• If there is no improvement within a week to ten days or if the sufferer's condition deteriorates, the doctor may prescribe a four to six months' course of steroids. *See* MEDICINES, 32.

Prevention
• None known.

Outlook
• Good, if the condition is diagnosed and treated at an early stage.
• Recovery is usually complete but recurrences are common and are controlled by further courses of steroids.

See SKELETAL SYSTEM *page 54*

POLYNEUROPATHY

The condition is also known as neuritis, or polyneuritis. It is a collection of diseases affecting the peripheral nerves, that is, the nerves connecting the brain and spinal cord with all other parts of the body.

Symptoms
• The muscles feel weak and begin to waste. The symptoms are usually noticed first in the hands and feet, the muscles of which are the farthest from the brain and have the longest nerves leading to them.
• The skin feels numb and loses its sensitivity, a process also beginning in the hands and feet.
• The normal jerking reflexes do not work properly when tested by tapping the knee or ankle tendon, for example.

Duration
• The condition is often reversible but likely to persist until its cause is treated.

Causes
• A deficiency of vitamin B1 (thiamine).
• Lead, mercury or arsenic poisoning may result in polyneuropathy, as may excessive drinking of alcohol (the disease is a feature of ALCOHOLISM).
• Polyneuropathy may result from a wide variety of disorders including DIABETES, DIPHTHERIA, GUILLAIN-BARRÉ SYNDROME, LEPROSY and a number of virus infections.

Treatment in the home
• None. If symptoms suggest the condition, a doctor should be consulted.
• If paralysis of limbs persists, physiotherapy and help for the patient at home is crucial.

When to consult the doctor
• If symptoms occur.

What the doctor may do
• Examine the nervous system, including knee-jerk and ankle-jerk reflexes.

- Measure the speed at which nerves can carry messages by inserting needles under the skin.
- Take blood tests to find evidence of vitamin deficiency, poisoning, alcoholism or diabetes.
- Treatment will depend on the cause.

Prevention
- A diet including foods such as wholemeal bread and cereals reduces the risk of vitamin B1 deficiency. Avoiding excess drinking of alcohol will further limit the likelihood of polyneuropathy.

Outlook
- Polyneuropathy is often a feature of some other disorder, and will clear up if its cause can be treated.

See NERVOUS SYSTEM *page 34*

POLYPOSIS OF THE COLON

Polyps are non-malignant growths which form on a mucous membrane. When they occur on the lining of the large bowel, the condition is referred to as polyposis of the colon. The tumours may be single or multiple, flat in shape or with a stalk of variable length.

Symptoms
- Bleeding when the bowels are opened.
- Discharge of mucus from the rectum and anus.
- Mild diarrhoea.

Causes
- Single or small groups of polyps apparently occur because of a malfunction of gland cells in the bowel lining.
- One form of the condition, familial adenomatous polyposis, tends to run in families. The polyps develop during the teens but do not become evident until the 30s, when symptoms such as mucous discharge occur.
- Various inflammatory diseases such as ULCERATIVE COLITIS, Crohn's disease (regional ILEITIS) or AMOEBIASIS may result in polyps forming.

Complications
- On rare occasions, polyps may become cancerous, and an operation to remove a portion of bowel may be advised.

Treatment in the home
- None advised.

When to consult the doctor
- If there is a change of bowel habit or the passage of

blood or slime that persists for longer than two weeks.

What the doctor may do
- Advise specialist examination in hospital. X-rays may be taken, or ENDOSCOPY viewing instruments inserted into the colon to determine whether polyps are present, and to ascertain their extent. Polyps low down in the bowel can be removed by the doctor during the course of the examination.
- Polyps which are higher up, very widespread or numerous may require an operation to remove the affected bowel.
- Where familial polyposis is diagnosed, the doctor will recommend that blood relatives of the patient should be examined to see if the disease is present.

Outlook
- Full recovery can be expected as long as the possibility of a cancer forming has been averted by appropriate surgery.

See DIGESTIVE SYSTEM *page 44*

PORPHYRIA
A group of rare, inherited disorders caused by a disturbance of the metabolism of porphyrine, the breakdown products of the red blood pigment. The condition may be in the liver (hepatic porphyria) or in the bone marrow (erythropoietic porphyria) or both. Characteristic features of the defect are discoloration of the urine, which may turn dark brown if left standing for an hour or so, sensitivity to sunlight, which causes blistering skin rashes, bouts of abdominal pain, mental disturbances and NEURITIS. There is no specific treatment but sufferers should avoid certain drugs which may bring on an attack. These include some anaesthetics, barbiturates, chloroquine, the contraceptive pill and sulphonamides.

PORT-WINE STAIN

This is a flat patch of dark red staining in the skin. The stain can be very small or cover a large area. It is present at birth, but does not spread or grow except as the body grows. Port-wine stains are not passed on from parent to child.

Duration
- The 'stain' is permanent.

Causes
- An abnormality of the capillary blood vessels.

Treatment in the home
- There is not much that can be done for a port-wine stain. It cannot be cured with ointments or lotions, but a stain on the face can sometimes be hidden with cosmetics. Large lesions on the face can cause much self-consciousness in a growing child. Parents should provide understanding, yet encourage a matter-of-fact acceptance.

When to consult the doctor
- To consider the possibility of plastic surgery.

What the doctor may do
- Send the patient to a plastic surgeon.
- In a very few cases a plastic surgeon may be able to remove the stain by using a skin graft, but the scars from the operation may be worse than the original condition.
- Recently, laser treatment has proved effective.

Prevention
- None is available.

Outlook
- Port-wine stains do not cause skin problems and eventually people learn to live with them.

See SKIN *page 52*

POST-CONCUSSIONAL SYNDROME

Concussion is caused by head injury. It is recognised if the victim is knocked unconscious or has no memory of events just before or just after the injury. Post-concussional symptoms may then follow—although the victim may not know that concussion has caused his condition.

Symptoms
- Loss of memory for recent events just before or just after head injury.
- Unexplained headaches and irritability.
- Judgment may be upset, and the sufferer appears to be drunk for an hour or two after the injury.
- Easy fatigue. All symptoms tend to be aggravated by fatigue.
- DEPRESSION. This may be severe. Sufferers should always be warned that temporary depression is likely.
- The effects of alcohol (and sedatives) are increased.

Duration
- Symptoms usually persist for several days; if the initial period of unconsciousness lasts longer than a few seconds, the subsequent symptoms may persist for one or two weeks.

Causes
• The exact nature of the injury to the brain caused by concussion is not certain.

Complications
• Repeated incidents of concussion, as suffered by punch-drunk boxers or rugby players, may cause permanent brain damage.
• Sometimes concussion is associated with a skull FRACTURE or bleeding within the skull—SUBDURAL HAEMATOMA and EXTRADURAL HAEMATOMA.
• Sufferers often aggravate the effects of concussion by trying to carry on as usual or by taking alcohol.

Treatment in the home
• The sufferer should be stopped from doing anything physically active, including driving, and kept at complete rest until seen by a doctor.
• No alcohol should be taken for one or two weeks after any concussion.

When to consult the doctor
• At once, following any period of unconsciousness resulting from head injury.

What the doctor may do
• Check that there is no underlying fracture or internal bleeding.
• Order a period of complete bed-rest.
• See the sufferer again to check that symptoms, especially depression, have disappeared.

Prevention
• Wear protective head-gear when riding motor-cycles and horses.
• Avoid the sort of activity which is likely to lead to repeated blows to the head.

Outlook
• In the absence of complications, prolonged unconsciousness and repeated incidents, the outlook, with proper rest, is excellent.

POULTICE
A warm, moist, pulpy preparation applied to the skin to relieve pain, reduce inflammation or increase local blood circulation. Kaolin is a common constituent of modern proprietary poultices. The mustard plaster, an old-fashioned home-prepared poultice, is a mixture of mustard, flour and water.

PREGNANCY
The nine-month period from conception to labour is one in which the mother-to-be needs to take special care and requires special support from her husband, family and the medical services.
See HAVING A BABY *page 416*

SEEING BY SOUND
A mother's first sight of her baby

With the ultrasound scanner a mother can see her baby moving about in her womb even before she can feel it herself. By studying the pictures of the baby produced by the scanner a doctor can check that the pregnancy is progressing normally and be alerted to any problems. Ultrasound scanning is quite painless, it makes no intrusion into the body and doctors are convinced that, unlike X-rays, it is safe. Monitoring pregnancy is not the only use of the ultrasound scanner. It is also used for gynaecological and abdominal examinations, for examining the heart and for investigating the brain without interfering with the skull.

When sound meets an object some of it is reflected. With audible sound we can sometimes hear this reflection as an echo. Ultrasound is a very high-pitched sound—too high for the human ear to detect—and it can be directed very accurately at what the investigator wants to examine. Bats use ultrasound for navigation. By recording the echo, a picture can be built up of the object: where it is and how large it is, for example.

The ultrasound scanners have a scanning head—transducer—which produces the sound, picks up the echo and converts the sound into electric signals. These are passed to an analyser which turns the signals into a black-and-white picture on a screen. Some substances, such as bone and gas, reflect a lot of sound and will show up as white on the screen. Parts like the placenta, which do not reflect so well, appear grey. The amniotic fluid does not reflect any sound at all so it appears black. There are two types of scanner currently in use: the Real Time scanner which shows movement, and the Static B scanner which gives still pictures. Most pregnant mothers may be scanned as a routine matter. The first scanning is done at around three months to confirm the mother's forecast date for delivery. The size of the baby's head and abdomen are measured and compared with a chart which tells how large the baby should be at each stage of pregnancy. There may be a second scan at 16-17 weeks to check for abnormalities such as ANENCEPHALY, HYDROCEPHALUS and SPINA BIFIDA, and a third at 34 weeks to check that the baby is still growing normally.

If the mother has a history of difficult pregnancies or there is an emergency such as bleeding, then she may be scanned to determine the position of the placenta and check on the baby's condition. The ultrasound scanner is also used to check the possibility of a multiple birth.

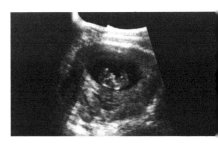

10 WEEKS *This baby is about 1½ in. long. His face, which is just beginning to develop, is tucked into his body. His limbs are growing. He floats in amniotic fluid—the black area around him.*

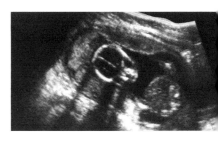

16 WEEKS *The baby has been growing rapidly and is now almost 7 in. long. He receives his nourishment from the placenta—the long grey area along the wall of the abdomen above him.*

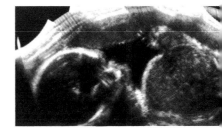

34 WEEKS *The baby is now too large to move about freely in the womb. He is lying with his head to the left; the outline of his forehead, nose and chin can be seen. His arms and legs are tucked in.*

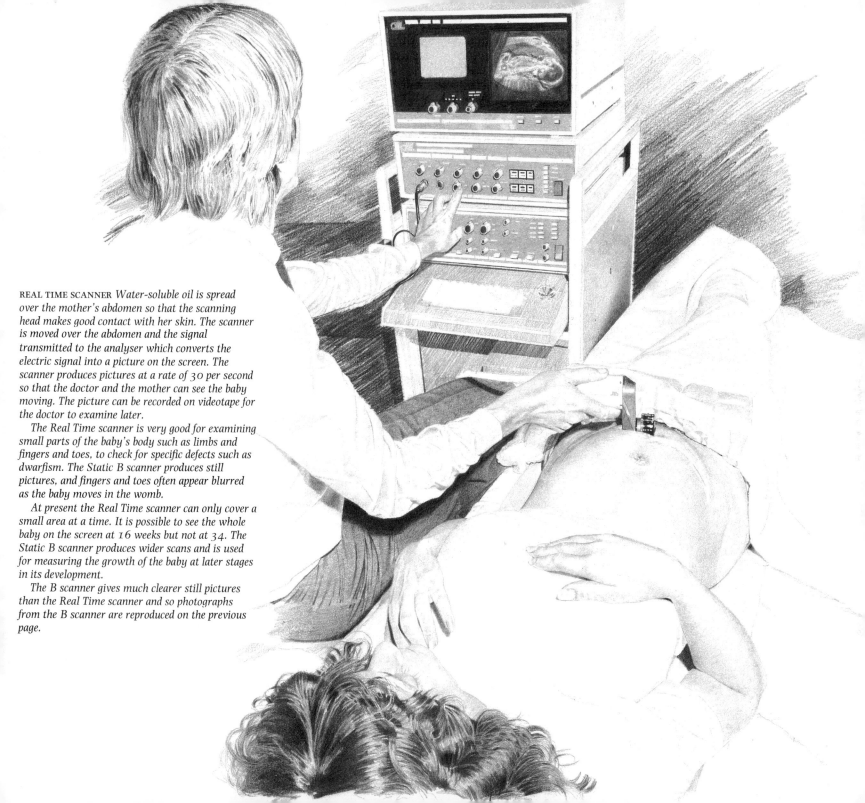

REAL TIME SCANNER *Water-soluble oil is spread over the mother's abdomen so that the scanning head makes good contact with her skin. The scanner is moved over the abdomen and the signal transmitted to the analyser which converts the electric signal into a picture on the screen. The scanner produces pictures at a rate of 30 per second so that the doctor and the mother can see the baby moving. The picture can be recorded on videotape for the doctor to examine later.*

The Real Time scanner is very good for examining small parts of the baby's body such as limbs and fingers and toes, to check for specific defects such as dwarfism. The Static B scanner produces still pictures, and fingers and toes often appear blurred as the baby moves in the womb.

At present the Real Time scanner can only cover a small area at a time. It is possible to see the whole baby on the screen at 16 weeks but not at 34. The Static B scanner produces wider scans and is used for measuring the growth of the baby at later stages in its development.

The B scanner gives much clearer still pictures than the Real Time scanner and so photographs from the B scanner are reproduced on the previous page.

Having a baby

FROM CONCEPTION TO CHILDBIRTH—A STEP-BY-STEP GUIDE TO HELP THE MOTHER-TO-BE UNDERSTAND AND ENJOY HER PREGNANCY

During pregnancy, a single microscopic cell develops into a full-grown baby containing more than 6 million million cells. It is the time of the most rapid growth in a human being's life, and it is not surprising that the changes in the growing baby are reflected in the mother. Hormones act as chemical messages from the unborn child to its mother, passing into her body where they affect her whole being—physically, emotionally and mentally.

Having a baby is one of the most exciting and rewarding events of a woman's life. Three-quarters of women in the western world have at least one child. And, as they are increasingly helped by medical advances, this brings into focus the unique relationship between the pregnant mother and those who aid and advise her, from the moment she discovers she is pregnant until after her baby is born—which is usually in hospital but sometimes at home.

THE DEVELOPMENT OF THE EMBRYO *The human being grows faster in the womb than at any other time in his life. The new individual starts as an embryo, formed by a fusion of a sperm (from the father) and an ovum (from the mother). In the next 38 weeks, that single cell multiplies to more than 6 million million cells. After settling in the womb, the embryo begins to develop and by eight weeks most of its organs are already appearing and the embryo begins to resemble a human being. By 14 weeks all the limbs and internal organs have been made and development is then by growth only. At this stage the embryo (or fetus) is a miniature human being.*

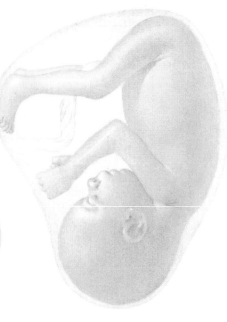

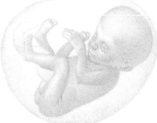

8 WEEK FETUS   14 WEEK FETUS   20 WEEK FETUS

How the baby's sex is decided

□ The sex of the baby is determined at the moment of conception by the man's sperm. The woman's egg always carries one female chromosome (known as the X chromosome), but the sperm can carry either a female or a male-making chromosome (the Y chromosome). The egg and sperm chromosomes join; if both chromosomes are female (XX), a girl is produced, if one is male a boy is made (XY).

□ For the first 28 days, there is little sexual difference in the outside of the embryo. But by the fifth week the effects of the sex chromosomes on the embryonic baby start to show. Either a penis and a prostate gland develop, or a pair of Fallopian tubes and a uterus.

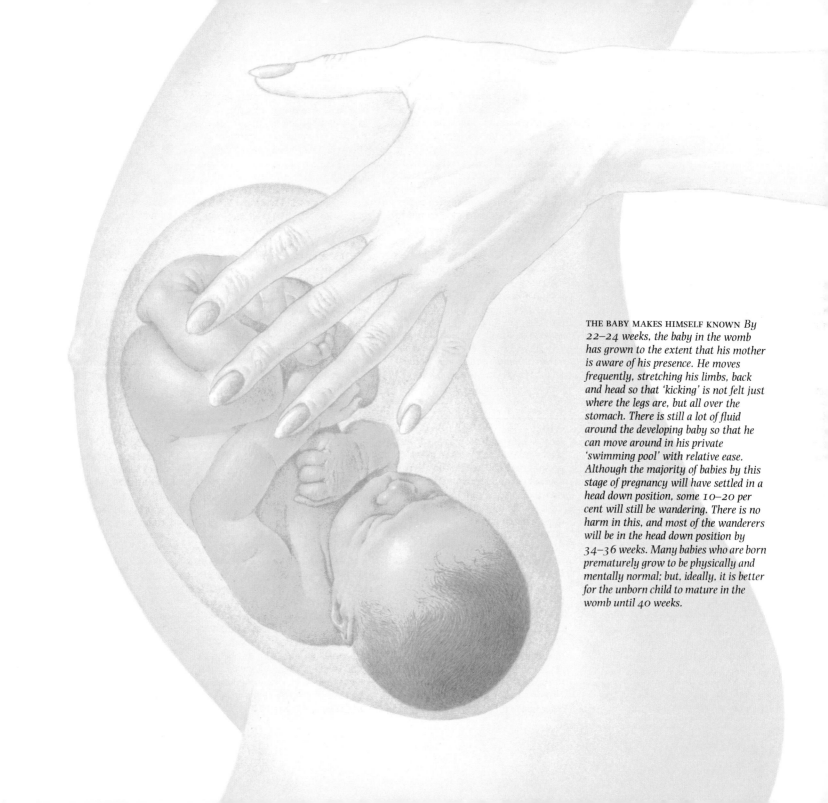

THE BABY MAKES HIMSELF KNOWN *By 22–24 weeks, the baby in the womb has grown to the extent that his mother is aware of his presence. He moves frequently, stretching his limbs, back and head so that 'kicking' is not felt just where the legs are, but all over the stomach. There is still a lot of fluid around the developing baby so that he can move around in his private 'swimming pool' with relative ease. Although the majority of babies by this stage of pregnancy will have settled in a head down position, some 10–20 per cent will still be wandering. There is no harm in this, and most of the wanderers will be in the head down position by 34–36 weeks. Many babies who are born prematurely grow to be physically and mentally normal; but, ideally, it is better for the unborn child to mature in the womb until 40 weeks.*

HOW A BABY IS CONCEIVED

To start a baby, an egg must be fertilised by a sperm. Eggs are produced by the woman's two ovaries which lie beside the womb. The eggs ripen, usually one each month, under the influence of hormones produced by the woman's pituitary gland, beneath her brain.

When it is released from the ovary, an egg passes straight into the funnel-shaped end of one of the Fallopian tubes connecting the ovary to the womb. This egg is too small to be seen by the naked eye. It has no powers of movement of its own and stays for about a day in the part of the tube nearest the ovary.

Whenever a couple have sexual intercourse, the man deposits between 600 and 1,000 million sperm at the upper end of the vagina. A tiny proportion of these pass into the woman's womb, known medically as the uterus. They swim in a rapid jerky fashion, like tadpoles, in the moisture on the surface of the uterus, and of the few thousand which pass into each Fallopian tube, only a few hundred will reach the end nearest the ovary.

If intercourse occurs in the right phase of the menstrual cycle, there will be an egg waiting there. The sperm will cluster around it and one of them will penetrate through the outer layers of the egg, allowing fusion of the father's and the mother's genetic material. Within 30 minutes the outer layers become impervious to other sperm.

Six to eight hours later the fertilised egg divides into two cells, then four and then many others, soon making a clump. During this process all the combined chromo-somal material from the sperm and the egg is being passed to every cell so that when the baby is born all cells have the genetic potential from father and mother.

The egg passes down the Fallopian tube towards the uterus—massaged along by the muscular activity of the walls of the tube and carried in the flow of fluid. Its journey through the tube usually takes about seven or eight days.

In this time, the lining of the uterus has become thicker, with an increased number of blood vessels, to receive the fertilised egg. When the egg arrives there, it moves into the lining where it can be supplied with oxygen and food. If no fertilised egg arrives within a few days, the blood vessels supplying the lining of the womb shrink and are shed with some blood—the menstrual period.

WHEN WILL THE BABY BE BORN?

Most doctors date pregnancy from the first day of the woman's last normal period. They do this even though conception will not have occurred until about 14 days later. This is a useful convention, because most women have no idea which act of intercourse actually made them pregnant. The first day of the last normal menstrual period is often better remembered. The baby will be born about 40 weeks (280 days) from that day.

THE BABY TAKES SHAPE

In the first four weeks the egg develops to $\frac{1}{8}$ in. (3 mm.) in length. In the next two weeks it grows to 1 in. (25 mm.), and the embryonic baby inside it becomes almost $\frac{3}{8}$ in.

(10 mm.) long. The head is formed and, with the use of ultrasound, the heart can be seen beating. In the following two weeks (eight weeks since the last menstrual period), the fetus grows to about $1\frac{1}{4}$ in. (30 mm.) in length. The limbs are formed and later the fingers and toes. After another month (12 weeks) the fetus is now about 2 in. (50 mm.) long, and all the organs have begun to develop.

The rapidly growing baby lies within the main cavity of the womb and is fed with food and oxygen through the umbilical cord. This is attached to the baby's navel at one end and to the placenta at the other.

WHAT ARE THE SYMPTOMS OF PREGNANCY?

The most obvious symptom of pregnancy is the lack of periods. However, often before this, the woman may notice changes in her body. The first of these may be an enlargement or tingling of the breasts. There is an urge to pass water more frequently and sometimes an irritation in the vagina or a slight fluid discharge.

Many women, particularly those who have had a child before, notice there is something different, but not easily defined, about them in early pregnancy. They may notice a craving for some particular food, loss of appetite or nausea; perhaps some slight dizziness or faintness, or a tendency to weep or irritability.

Lack of periods is a more recognisable symptom. If a woman who has had regular menstruation every four weeks for some years is exposed to unprotected intercourse and then has a gap in her periods,

she is probably pregnant and she should see her doctor for confirmation. This is best done soon after the first period is missed.

The doctor may conduct an internal (vaginal) examination and find a soft enlarged uterus. If he is in doubt, he will test her urine for traces of hormones from the developing baby.

Urine tests may also be arranged by family planning clinics, and kits are available from chemists for a woman to carry out her own test. Another test that can be used is ultrasound, a beam of high-pitched sound directed at the woman's abdomen. The beam is reflected by any solid object in its path, and the pattern of reflections creates a picture of the contents of the uterus. Ultrasound can picture the baby as early as six or seven weeks.

COPING WITH 'MORNING SICKNESS'

Nausea or vomiting may start soon after the first missed period. Occasionally it occurs even earlier and may be the first symptom a woman notices. It is commonly called 'morning sickness', but it does not always occur in the morning; often there is some evening sickness. It can best be overcome by avoiding hunger—by having a small snack or cup of tea and a biscuit every few hours. The husband can help each morning by bringing his wife tea and toast before she gets out of bed. It is not known what causes 'vomiting of pregnancy'. It is not entirely psychological in origin, although worry occasionally makes it worse. Nausea usually finishes by the 12th to 14th weeks of pregnancy.

GOING TO THE ANTENATAL CLINIC

When your pregnancy has been diagnosed, your doctor will probably send you to the antenatal clinic at your local hospital. There you will receive regular check-ups before the baby is born. These are designed to detect problems of the unborn baby before symptoms occur so that more help can be given. At the clinic you will also get to know the people who will attend the birth.

The clinics can be impersonal and rather frightening places, but the staff are usually friendly and receptive to questions, so try not to be too embarrassed to ask.

Hospital clinics can be difficult to get to and may involve expensive transport costs. Many family doctors therefore arrange a schedule of antenatal care in conjunction with the hospital. Visits may follow a pattern like this:

Weeks 6-8 Mother reports to her family doctor.

Week 12 She is referred to hospital clinic by her family doctor and booked there for delivery.

Weeks 16-32 She reports every four weeks to her family doctor.

Week 34 She is referred back to the hospital clinic by her doctor.

Weeks 36-40 She reports every week to her family doctor.

Week 40 (approximately) She goes to hospital for delivery when labour starts.

HEALTH CHECKS ON MOTHER AND BABY

The first visit to the clinic is the most thorough and the longest. A midwife will usually ask questions about your past medical history and previous pregnancies. A doctor may examine you, checking heart and lungs, spine, stomach and pelvis—all vital tests to ensure that you have no disease. At the same time, your urine will be checked for protein (to exclude kidney disease) and sugar (to exclude diabetes). A small blood sample will be taken from your arm to be examined for iron content and to check the blood group and Rhesus group. The blood group may be O, A, B, or AB. The hospital needs to know your group in case a transfusion is needed in an emergency.

The antibodies for German measles and other diseases which might be transmitted to the baby may also be checked in the mother's blood.

At some clinics a test for spina bifida is also done on the blood sample. You can ask for this test if it is not a routine at your clinic.

An ultrasound scan of the uterus may give a more precise measurement of the baby. It is quite safe and can detect twins as early as 16 weeks.

Financial help for expectant mothers

□ Pregnant women are entitled to financial help from the state and from their employers.

□ There is no longer a maternity grant, but women with low family incomes may be able to claim help from the social fund.

□ A working woman who becomes pregnant must be given reasonable time off on full pay to receive antenatal care.

□ Statutory maternity pay is a weekly payment from your employer. It replaced the former maternity allowance and maternity pay schemes. It can be paid for up to 18 weeks, starting 11 weeks before the week of the birth. Maternity allowance (£43.75 a week from April 1993, also for up to 18 weeks) is retained for those who do not qualify for statutory maternity pay.

□ The amount of statutory maternity pay due depends on how long a woman has worked for an employer. A woman who has worked for the same employer for at least 2 years will get 90 per cent of her average weekly earnings for 6 weeks, followed by payments at a lower rate for another 12 weeks. A woman employed for less than 2 years can get payments at a lower rate for up to 18 weeks. The lower rate (from April 1993) is £47.95 a week.

□ Women who have worked for the same employer for at least 2 years may also claim back their jobs, provided they return to work within 29 weeks of the birth.

□ Booklets giving full details are available at Jobcentres. The booklets advise on such subjects as what to do if your baby is born abroad, and whether an expectant mother is entitled to free milk and vitamins.

RHESUS-NEGATIVE MOTHERS

Fifteen per cent of women have blood which is classed as Rhesus negative (*see* RHESUS (RH) FACTOR). If their husbands are Rhesus positive and their baby is of the father's Rhesus group, the blood of the mother and baby will be incompatible.

At first this incompatibility does not matter because the baby's blood inside the womb is quite separate from the mother's blood which circulates outside the womb.

However, during the delivery of the baby, the blood of baby and mother may mix and the mother may then become immunised against the Rhesus-positive factor. If this occurs, the Rhesus-positive antibodies produced in the mother's blood would affect the blood of any subsequent Rhesus-positive baby— leading to anaemia, jaundice, or even death of the baby.

However, an injection of gamma globulin at the time of delivery or after miscarriage protects Rhesus-negative mothers from problems of this sort in future pregnancies.

LEARNING ABOUT WELFARE BENEFITS

At your first visit to the antenatal clinic, you should learn about the social welfare benefits that are available and how to apply for them (*see page 419*).

At most clinics advice will be given about visiting a dentist to check your teeth. Dental treatment during pregnancy is free.

You should also make arrangements to attend parentcraft or relaxation classes.

CHECKING FOR ABNORMALITIES IN THE BABY

Some women are more likely than most to have babies born with congenital abnormalities. They may be offered special tests in pregnancy, such as amniocentesis or chorionic villus sampling (CVS). The tests may detect DOWN'S SYNDROME (mongolism), SPINA BIFIDA, ANENCEPHALY and some other rare, inherited diseases. Some of these conditions may also be detected by ultrasound scans and blood tests.

The risk of having a Down's syndrome baby increases as the mother grows older. At age 25, the risk is only one in 1,500; at 35 it is one in 300; at 40, one in 100; and at 45, one in 30.

'Triple Testing'—a blood test between 15 and 23 weeks of pregnancy —may help to identify women who might benefit from amniocentesis or CVS.

Amniocentesis is performed by withdrawing fluid from the womb through a fine needle inserted through the abdominal wall at about 16 weeks of pregnancy. The results arrive four weeks later. From them, the baby's sex can be detected, as well as any abnormalities. One woman in about 100 may miscarry because of the test.

CVS is performed by passing a small tube through the abdomen or the neck of the womb at about eight weeks of

pregnancy and removing a tiny piece of placenta (afterbirth). The results come within two weeks. The test reveals the same abnormalities as amniocentesis except for spina bifida and anencephaly, for which a blood test can be carried out at 16 weeks. The risk of CVS causing a miscarriage is between one in 10 and one in 50. CVS may also cause physical abnormalities in the baby.

If an abnormality is revealed, termination of pregnancy can be discussed with doctors.

FEELING THE BABY MOVE

The baby, who has been moving its limbs from about six or seven weeks of pregnancy, eventually makes its presence felt. Women who have had a baby before feel this from about 16 weeks, while those to whom the sensation is unfamiliar may go until 20 or 22 weeks before they notice the baby's movements.

CHANGES IN THE MOTHER'S SKIN

After three or four months the abdomen and breasts will have become swollen, and there may be darkening of the skin of the nipples and the upper part of the cheeks and the forehead. In some women a line of pigmentation also appears in the middle of the stomach from the navel down to the pubic hair.

This darkening usually fades, but may not disappear completely after delivery.

Later, stretch of the stomach wall may lead to fine scars under the skin; stretch marks are found also on the buttocks, the thighs and the breasts. There is nothing that the woman can do to prevent stretch marks as

they are dependent on the elasticity of the skin. However, after the pregnancy they fade and may become inconspicuous.

THE PHYSICAL PROBLEMS OF PREGNANCY

Many women go right through pregnancy without any problems. Sometimes, however, there are troubles that may pass away of their own accord or can be cleared up.

Breathlessness As the mother's weight goes up, her heart has to work harder. Oxygen is also required by the growing baby, making even more demands on her heart. A healthy woman will usually adapt well, although she may notice palpitations or breathlessness on slight exertion. This is normal, as the growing uterus is pressing up on the underside of the lungs and there is less space to breathe.

Heartburn The expanding uterus forces some of the acid contents of the stomach into the gullet where it produces heartburn. Bending forward or lying flat makes the feeling worse. It is best treated with mild antacids obtained from the chemist. At night try propping yourself up with several pillows.

Piles Varicose veins (piles) form around the anus as a result of pressure inside the abdomen. Constipation makes the condition worse, so it is necessary to keep the motions soft by drinking more than usual and eating plenty of dietary fibre in the form of bran, salads and vegetables (*see page 380*). A doctor may recommend a mild laxative.

Urine The urinary tract is often stimulated by the increased flow of blood, and the woman needs to pass

urine more often. Later this is worsened because the growing uterus presses on her bladder.

Varicose veins Two sorts of varicose veins occur in pregnancy. The first are small, spidery groups of thin, blue lines on the thighs and are often accompanied by a discoloration of the skin of the lower legs. These varicose veins are due to hormone changes and usually disappear after the baby is born.

The larger varicose veins are soft knot-like swellings formed by enlarged veins under the skin. In the later stages of pregnancy these may occur inside the thighs, behind the knees and along both sides of the calves. The wearing of elastic tights or stockings will collapse the veins and remove some of the discomfort, but will not stop the veins forming. Put on the tights before getting up in the morning and do not remove them until going to bed.

After the birth most of the large varicose veins reduce considerably, but never disappear entirely unless treated by injection or operation.

HOW MUCH WEIGHT SHOULD YOU PUT ON?

During pregnancy an average-sized woman commonly puts on 20–28 lb. (9–12 kg.).

The increase in weight is due to the baby and changes in the essential organs:

Fetus (the developing baby) 7 lb. (3.2 kg.).

Placenta 1 lb. (453 g.).

Fluid around baby 2 lb. (907 g.).

Uterus 2 lb. (907 g.).

Increase in blood in body 2 lb. (907 g.).

Increase in breasts 2 lb. (907 g.).

Thus about 16 lb. (7.2 kg.) of extra weight arise directly from pregnancy. The other 4–12 lb. (1.8–5.4 kg.) are fat and water in the mother. Anything more than this is unnecessary and does not help the baby.

ADJUSTING TO THE EMOTIONAL CHANGES

Later in pregnancy some women become depressed. There may be a temporary feeling of wellbeing when they try to do much more. Then, finding that they cannot, they react with depression.

This is a critical time in a woman's life and she needs all the support she can get. If she lives a long distance from her own mother, she will rely to an even greater extent on her husband. If he is away at work, she may have difficulty in finding anyone with whom to relate. Pregnancy is the concern of both father and mother, and both should be together as much as possible during the months the baby is growing in the uterus. In many cases helpful friendships are made when attending the antenatal clinic.

ALTERATION IN A MARRIAGE

The emotional and physical changes during pregnancy may affect the mother's relationships with her husband and other children. The husband may feel resentment and even stronger feelings, but both partners should realise the change in marriage which pregnancy brings.

The woman naturally is concerned with the growing baby, and becomes more introspective. The man does not constantly have the reminder with him, and may sometimes forget his wife's preoccupation with her pregnancy. He should remember that pregnancy concerns them both, and involve himself as much as possible. He may attend the antenatal clinic with his wife occasionally, and some wives find it a great help if the husband is present during the labour—which can further strengthen the loving bond between them.

Fears of childbirth

☐ There are deep-rooted fears of childbirth based on the tendency of acquaintances, friends and relatives to exaggerate in retrospect their own unpleasant experiences of childbirth.

☐ Uncertainty about the actual date of delivery.

☐ Despite calculations performed, using the last menstrual period, there is often little precision about the expected date of delivery. The baby will come within two weeks of that date, and it is misleading for a woman to expect the baby to be born exactly on the day.

☐ That the baby will be born dead or abnormal. Today, very few babies die at childbirth—less than 15 out of every 1,000 in England and Wales, compared with 37 per 1,000 25 years ago and 62 per 1,000 50 years ago.

☐ Some women have an even greater fear of the baby being born malformed. Approximately 20 in every 1,000 births have some malformation, many of which can be corrected. Tests are available to check on certain malformations, including spina bifida and Down's syndrome (mongolism). They can be arranged by the antenatal clinic.

☐ Some women fear that giving birth will cause physical damage and that the womb will split as the baby is being pushed out. This very rarely happens—and only when the strong muscular wall has previously been weakened.

☐ The days when women died in childbirth are almost ended. Only one death of a mother occurs in every 10,000 births today, compared to four per 1,000 50 years ago.

SEXUAL INTERCOURSE DURING PREGNANCY

Some people fear intercourse in pregnancy. But, unless there has been bleeding, there is no reason why intercourse should not continue as usual. As the woman increases in size she may suffer discomfort if the man lies on top of her. Many couples adopt other positions, particularly lying on their sides, face to face. The woman raises her upper thigh, resting it on the man's upper thigh. This position involves little pressure on her stomach.

Many couples gradually lose interest in sex as the delivery date approaches. This is perfectly normal.

PERSONAL CARE DURING PREGNANCY

During pregnancy, normal hygiene should be practised, but douching or a bidet should be avoided.

The breasts should be washed normally, dried carefully, and massaged with a little cream. This will help later if breast-feeding is carried out. Put on a little powder afterwards. Some women whose nipples are flat may require the use of breast shields to help bring them out, from about the 25th week. A doctor will advise on this.

Clothing should be comfortable and reasonably loose. Brassières should support the breasts properly; specially designed maternity brassières should be used and a woman may need this earlier than she thinks. Her midwife will advise her. Right through pregnancy it is wise to wear flat heels rather than high heels, which tip the pelvis forwards and are more likely to cause falls.

EATING AND EXERCISE

During pregnancy, you should adjust your diet to help the growing baby. There is no need to 'eat for two'—the excess food will only make you fat. However, the growing baby does require protein and certain vitamins, so eat at least one meal a day with a good portion of protein—meat, fish,

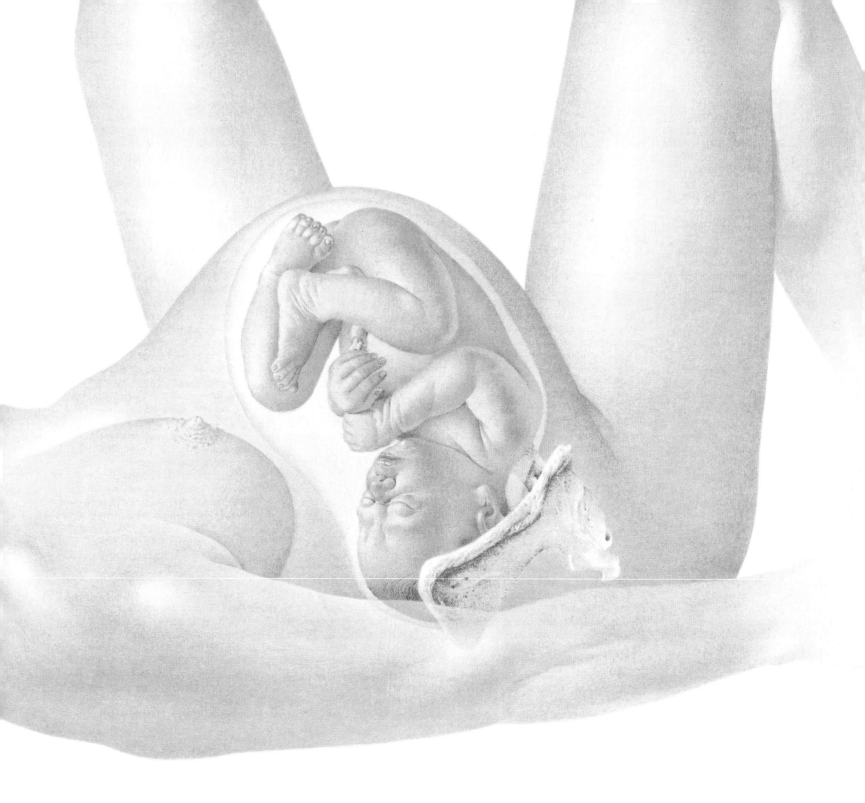

THE BABY MOVES DOWN THE WOMB *In the final weeks of pregnancy, the baby moves down the womb and often—at this stage—its head passes into the pelvic cavity. When this happens the head is said to have engaged. This means that the maximum diameter of the baby's head has passed down through the entrance of the mother's pelvis. The transition can be detected by a midwife or doctor by feeling the mother's stomach. If there is any doubt —as with a plump woman—an internal examination is also given to check the position of the head. Engagement of the head usually occurs a few weeks before labour among women expecting their first baby; but the process is often delayed in those who have had a baby before, and it may not occur until the labour contractions have started. However, doctors at the antenatal clinic can check by a simple test that the head will engage.*

eggs or cheese. Fresh fruit and vegetables are good, and one citrus fruit a day (orange or grapefruit) helps the baby to get vitamin C regularly. Vitamin C is not stored in the body and so should be taken daily.

A pint of milk a day is enough to provide all the calcium you need: more than this will make you put on weight.

Doctors recommend a diet high in folic acid (folate), beginning two months before becoming pregnant and continuing into the first three months of pregnancy—or else folic acid in tablet form—to reduce risk to the baby of SPINA BIFIDA and ANENCEPHALY.

Exercise in pregnancy will tone up your muscles and make you feel better. However, too much exercise can be harmful because it may dislodge the baby, and no new strenuous activities should be started. It is probably unwise to go horse riding, skiing or deep underwater swimming. Walking, social swimming and social tennis are all excellent in early and mid-pregnancy. As the rising bump in the stomach becomes larger, exercise gets harder, but walking and swimming can be done right up to the day that labour starts.

CAN SMOKING AND DRINKING AFFECT THE BABY?
The constituents of cigarette smoke pass across the placenta and may result in a smaller baby. As it grows into childhood it is likely to remain smaller than it would otherwise have been. If a woman can avoid cigarette smoking she should.

Drinking alcohol may also affect

the developing baby. Alcohol may possibly lead to a small baby, abnormalities in the foetus, and mental retardation. It is unwise to drink: the less alcohol taken in pregnancy the better it will be for the baby.

THE THREAT OF A MISCARRIAGE
Occasionally, during the first 14 weeks of pregnancy, a woman bleeds from the vagina. The blood may be bright red or dark red and may be accompanied by cramps in the abdomen. These signs indicate that she is threatening to miscarry. She should go to bed and ask the doctor to call. If the bleeding gets worse or clots of blood are produced, he may suggest moving her to hospital as a miscarriage may have become inevitable.

With proper care, most women who threaten to miscarry go on to carry their baby through pregnancy and produce a normal child.

THE RISKS OF HIGH BLOOD PRESSURE
Later in the pregnancy, usually after the 20th week, some women develop raised blood pressure. If this is accompanied by the passing of protein in the urine it is called toxaemia of pregnancy or pre-eclamptic toxaemia (PET). It is important to make the regular visits to the antenatal clinic suggested by your doctor so that your blood pressure, weight and urine can be checked. PET at its worst may reduce the blood supply to the baby and affect its growth and its ability to withstand contractions of the uterus during labour. If the blood pressure

is raised, the woman should rest; if the blood pressure persists despite bed-rest at home, she may be admitted to hospital for tests and further bed-rest. If the mother is near her expected date of delivery, labour may be induced.

WHERE WILL THE BABY BE BORN?
In the United Kingdom and in most other Western countries more than 95 per cent of babies are born in a hospital where staff and equipment are available for any sudden emergency.

Not all hospitals are large impersonal places. In the British Isles there are about 400 General Practitioner Hospitals, ranging in size from ten to 100 beds. Many of these hospitals have maternity units, in which family doctors supervise the births. Your own doctor will know if there is one in your district.

A few women want their babies delivered at home. The health authority has a legal obligation to ensure that a midwife is available, but it is often difficult to find a doctor willing to attend a home delivery. In many parts of the country there is not enough staff for home deliveries. If a woman is determined on a home delivery and has difficulty, she should get in touch with her district health authority.

THE BIRTH OF THE BABY
The process of childbirth (known as labour) is divided into three stages:
First stage The neck of the uterus dilates from being fully closed to being about 4 in. (100 mm.) open.
Second stage The baby is pushed from the uterus down through the

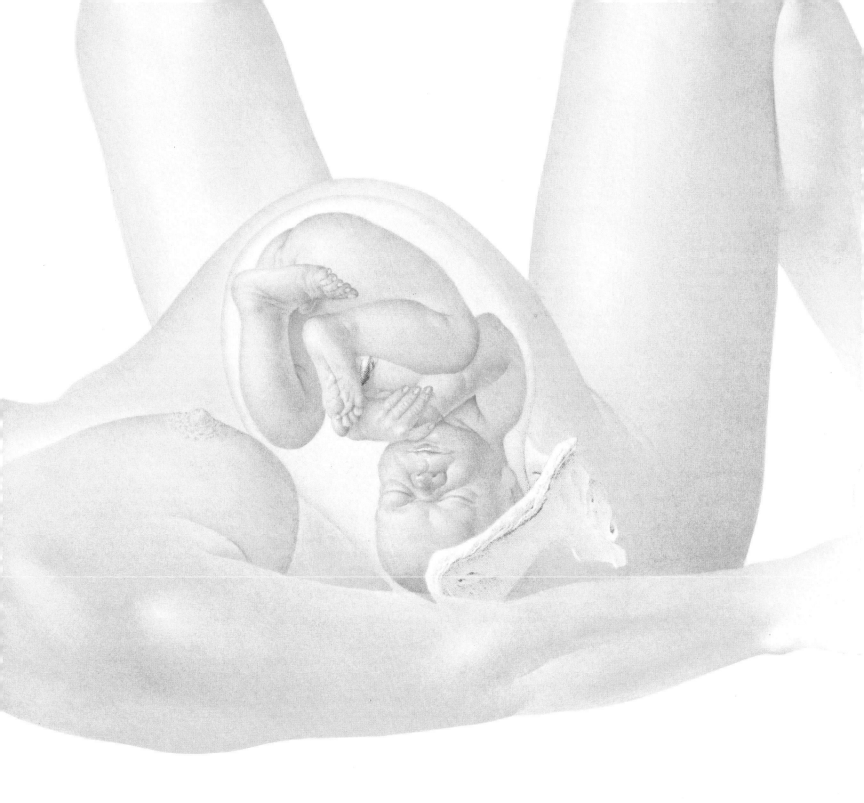

THE START OF LABOUR *As labour begins, the womb muscles contractions make the baby's head descend through the mother's pelvis. In order to negotiate the variations of the bony length of the pelvic canal, the baby's head rotates like a key turning in a lock. This happens naturally as the descending head presses against the pelvic floor muscles. The muscles—which form the pelvic floor's sloping 'gutter'—assist the rotation of the head so that its maximum diameter comes into line with the maximum diameter of the mother's pelvis. To ease the delivery, the baby's head folds against his chest so that the head presents the smallest possible diameter to the pelvic canal. If the womb muscles do not contract properly, or if the baby's head does not press well into his chest, the labour may be prolonged. However, most babies rotate their heads and descend without difficulty.*

pelvis and the vagina, aided by the mother's efforts, and is then born.
Third stage The placenta and membranes (the afterbirth) are delivered.

The length of these stages varies. The first stage is by far the longest, lasting many hours. The second stage lasts usually about an hour and rarely more than two hours. The third stage lasts only a few minutes, rarely longer than 20.

THE FIRST STAGE OF LABOUR
In the last months of pregnancy you will feel contractions of the womb as its muscles start limbering up for the delivery. These contractions are usually not painful, but they can be sharp enough to make you stop what you are doing. True labour contractions are more painful than the limbering-up spasms, and they occur at regular intervals.

Labour starts in one of three ways. Usually it is signalled by contractions starting in the small of the back and moving round to the front of the stomach just above the pubic bone. When you have had several contractions at regular 20 to 30 minute intervals, you can feel sure that you are in labour and should go to the hospital or obstetrical unit where you are to have your baby. At most hospitals husbands are able to stay. You can make sure well in advance at the parentcraft class.

Less often, labour can start by a show of blood or by 'the breaking of the waters', the release of a clear fluid that usually occurs at the end of the first stage of labour. In either event, it is advisable to lose no time in getting to hospital.

There is a big difference in the form of labour between a woman who is having a first baby and a mother who has had a baby before. A first-time mother may have uncomfortable contractions of the womb for several days before she feels sure that their frequency and regularity indicate that she is in labour. On the other hand, a mother who is expecting a second or

What to take to hospital

When the time approaches for the baby to be born, pack a small suitcase with the things you will need in hospital:

☐ Two nightdresses.

☐ Dressing-gown (preferably a short-sleeved, cotton type).

☐ Slippers.

☐ Bedjacket or cardigan.

☐ Two maternity brassières.

☐ Bath and hand towels.

☐ Handkerchiefs (preferably paper).

☐ Sanitary belt and pins, and two packets of maternity pads.

☐ Toiletries.

☐ Books or something else to pass the time.

subsequent baby will give birth more speedily than she did the first time.

When the mother is admitted to a hospital ward, a midwife may remove any excess hair from the entrance to the vagina by clipping or shaving. If her bowel is heavily loaded, she may be given a suppository. She may be given a warm bath to help her relax, and she will then be taken to the labour ward.

As the first stage of labour progresses, contractions will become more frequent, and if she has learned relaxation exercises she should begin to use them. Between contractions she should get as much rest as possible and when each contraction starts she should take deep breaths (*see page 432*). If her husband has also attended the relaxation classes he can now be a great help by talking to his wife, preventing boredom and helping her to relax between contractions.

As labour advances, the contractions become more frequent and shivering without feeling cold may occur. There is a great sensation to open the bowels and the bladder, caused by the pressure of the advancing baby's head. Often towards the end of the first stage, the desire arises to push out the baby with the abdominal muscles. This should be avoided until the midwife has announced that the cervix (the neck of the womb) is fully open and time has come for pushing the baby out.

THE SECOND STAGE OF LABOUR
In the second stage, many women find great relief, for they can now start doing something active—

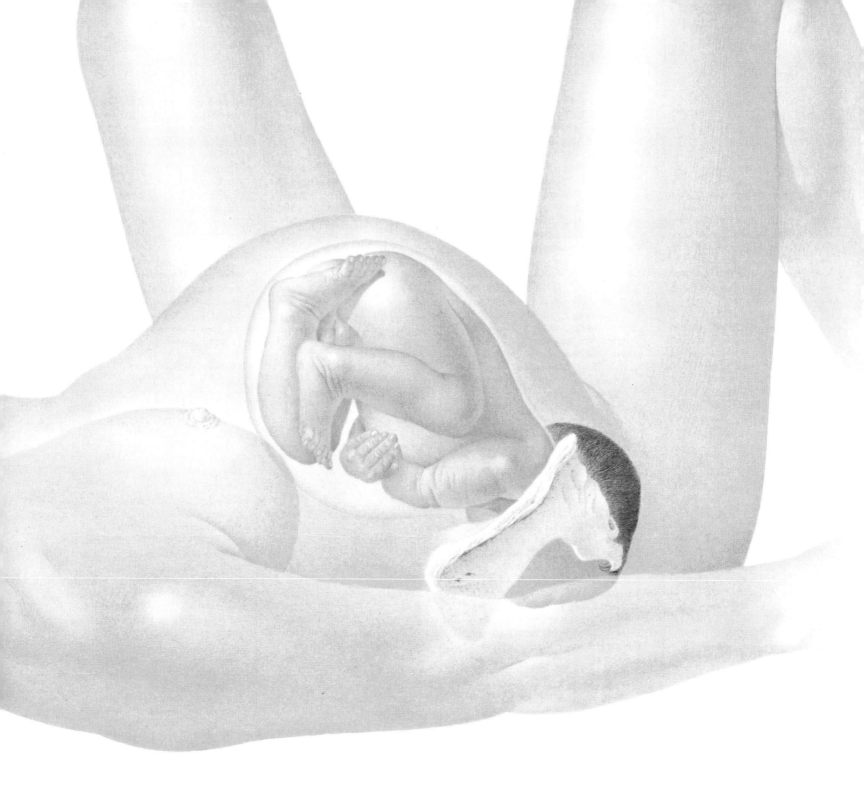

THE SECOND STAGE OF LABOUR BEGINS
As the womb contractions propel the baby's head downwards, the cervix at the neck of the womb opens rather like a closed rubber ring that expands by having a large, solid object pushed through it. Eventually, the cervix dilates to about 4 in. (100 mm.) so that the baby can pass from the womb to the vagina. The second stage of labour now begins and the mother can assist by pushing with each contraction of the womb. This helps to pass the baby head first down the vagina. With each contraction, the mother takes a deep breath, holds it and pushes down into the abdominal cavity. Before long, the baby's head emerges into the outside world.

helping in the delivery of their baby.

Regular waves of contractions pass from the top of the uterus to the bottom, propelling the baby down the birth canal. They increase in frequency until at the end of labour they come every other minute. With each contraction, the woman should take a deep breath and push steadily down into the lower pelvis, keeping up the pressure for ten to 15 seconds. Under the midwife's instruction this push can be repeated several times with each contraction, letting out the breath quickly and sucking in another deep breath between each push. Four or five pushes may be made with each contraction. Between the contractions it is again wise to have a rest. Many women find that it is a great support to have their husbands to talk to between contractions, and to share the excitement of the imminent arrival of the baby.

When the baby is almost ready for delivery, the woman may feel discomfort in the bottom of the vagina as it is stretched. She should not fight against this but allow the baby to stretch the area. When the midwife explains that the last few contractions are coming, the woman should push with the stomach muscles, relaxing the pelvic floor muscles. After the baby's head is delivered, she will be asked to stop pushing so that the midwife can deliver the shoulders and the rest of the baby. Now, she can see her child for the first time—one of the most rewarding experiences in a woman's life.

The umbilical cord is cut to separate the baby from the mother. The cord contains no nerves, so the cutting is painless.

THE BABY'S FIRST BREATH
Now, for the first time, the baby has to begin breathing air for itself. Until the moment of birth it received oxygen from its mother's blood, transferred across the placenta. But this oxygen supply has now stopped. Usually within 30 seconds, the lungs expand with the first breath and the baby will start to cry. Having lived in a virtually gravity-free, quiet, dark environment, he is now in a noisy, cool, light place and has to breathe to survive.

The baby is usually wrapped in a warm blanket, and is then handed to the mother to hold for the first time. Early close physical contact between mother and baby plays an important part in creating lasting bonds.

THE THIRD STAGE OF LABOUR
Even though the baby has been born, there is still a final stage of labour to come when the placenta and membranes are expelled. This is usually done by the midwife, who puts a hand on the woman's

What are the chances of having twins?

□ Twins occur in about one in 100 pregnancies in the United Kingdom. Triplets occur about once in 7,000 births and quadruplets about once in 250,000 births.

□ Four out of five pairs of twins are non-identical and need not be of the same sex. They are made from two separate eggs produced during one menstrual cycle and fertilised by two separate sperms.

□ Identical twins occur when a single egg fertilised by one sperm splits into two separate individuals soon after conception. Physically, the twins resemble each other closely. They are the same sex and have the same complexion and hair colour.

□ Twins are usually diagnosed at about 30 weeks, as the womb is larger than expected. If, however, there has been an ultra-sound examination, twins may be diagnosed as early as 16 weeks after conception.

□ Twins cause more stretch in the abdomen, and so the mother is more likely to have varicose veins or piles, urinary problems or stretch marks.

□ The mother is also more likely to have pre-eclampsia—raised blood pressure accompanied by pronounced swellings of the ankles and protein in the urine—and will probably go into an early labour one to three weeks before the expected time for a single child.

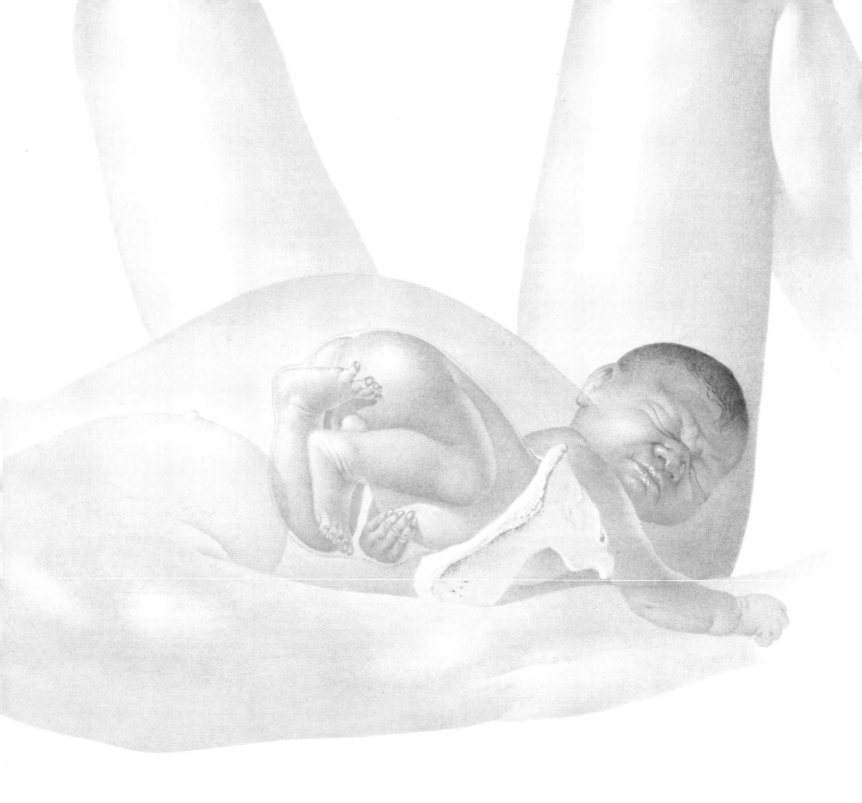

THE BABY'S FRONT SHOULDER APPEARS
After the head emerges, the most difficult part of labour is over. However, it is a delicate procedure to deliver the rest of the baby—and the help of a midwife or doctor is usually needed. The baby's head has passed through the pelvis by a corkscrew-like movement. Now the baby's shoulders must do the same. The baby rotates so that the widest shoulder diameter fits the longest diameter of the mother's pelvis. This means that the head, already outside, must rotate too—with the baby looking at one or other of his mother's thighs. This allows his shoulder to negotiate his mother's pelvis. Once the front shoulder has slipped under the mother's pubic arch, the delivery of the other shoulder—and the rest of the baby's body—is usually easy.

abdomen over the uterus and, when she feels the uterus contract, gently helps the placenta to be born.

EATING AND SLEEPING DURING LABOUR

During labour the mother should not eat, nor should she drink much. Food does not leave the stomach but just sits there. If a general anaesthetic should be required in the last stages of labour, it will be dangerous if she has food in her stomach. So most hospitals do not feed mothers in labour but suggest they take little sips of fluid or give fluid intravenously in certain conditions.

Labour is tiring. If it should go on through a night and delivery is not imminent, the mother may be given a mild sedative to help her to sleep, so that she wakes fresh to continue later.

RELIEVING THE PAIN OF LABOUR

Labour is a painful process for most women and there are several ways of giving relief. The simplest is an injection of the painkilling drug pethidine in the first stage of labour. It takes 20–30 minutes to work and so should be given before the pain is likely to become severe. A mother should not wait until the last minute before asking for this injection. It is always available, and a midwife can give it on her own authority without sending for a doctor. Two-thirds of women having a baby rely upon pethidine, and several injections can safely be used.

In some hospitals a stronger method of pain relief, called an epidural anaesthetic, is also available. A local anaesthetic is injected through the back into the area around the spine from where the nerves flow to the uterus. This is a low-risk anaesthetic and it blocks the pain in the uterus. It has a minor disadvantage in that a small number of women require a forceps delivery because the anaesthetic also removes other sensations which help her to 'push'. The obstetrician is consulted before the injection is given.

The third commonly used method of pain relief is the inhalation of nitrous oxide and oxygen. This is a good method for pain in the second stage of labour, but it is not so effective in the first stage. It is self-administered by the woman herself, so she should learn to use the mask at the parentcraft classes.

If the woman has learned a method of relaxation she should tell the labour ward staff so that they can help. For some it works well, but the mother must not feel let down if it does not carry her through the whole of labour. She should be prepared for other methods of pain relief to be used.

CHECKING THE BABY'S HEARTBEAT DURING BIRTH

Labour is the time of maximum risk to the baby, for the contractions of the uterus temporarily cut off the supply of blood with its oxygen. The baby is checked at intervals by a midwife listening to its heart. She will hear if it is showing the effects of lack of oxygen.

Most hospitals have equipment for the continuous recording of the baby's heart if there is any doubt about its condition. This is done either by recording the movements of blood in the baby's aorta by an ultrasound machine or by attaching an electrode directly to the baby's scalp through the vagina. The second method is more commonly used in labour and has few complications.

The continuous recording of the baby's heart may be supplemented by an examination of a small spot of blood removed from the baby's scalp. This test reveals the amount of oxygen in the blood. If the baby is in trouble a Caesarean or other operation may be indicated.

CUTTING THE VAGINA

The tissues at the bottom of the vagina are stretched considerably by the baby's head, which is often 4 in. (100 mm.) in its smallest diameter. They consequently may tear, and some obstetricians think it preferable for the woman to have a clean cut in the floor of the pelvis (called an episiotomy). It is easier to repair and may give a better long-term result.

Nobody does episiotomies routinely, and most doctors and midwives wait until they see tension on the lower tissues of the vagina. If the stretch will allow the baby's head to go through, nothing is needed; if not, they may do an episiotomy. After the baby has been born, the cut will be repaired with absorbable stitches that do not have to be removed.

WHEN LABOUR NEEDS TO BE INDUCED

Four-fifths of women go into spontaneous labour at about the right time. For the rest, the obstetrician may consider it wise that delivery should be induced. This may be because the mother's blood pressure is rising or because he thinks the

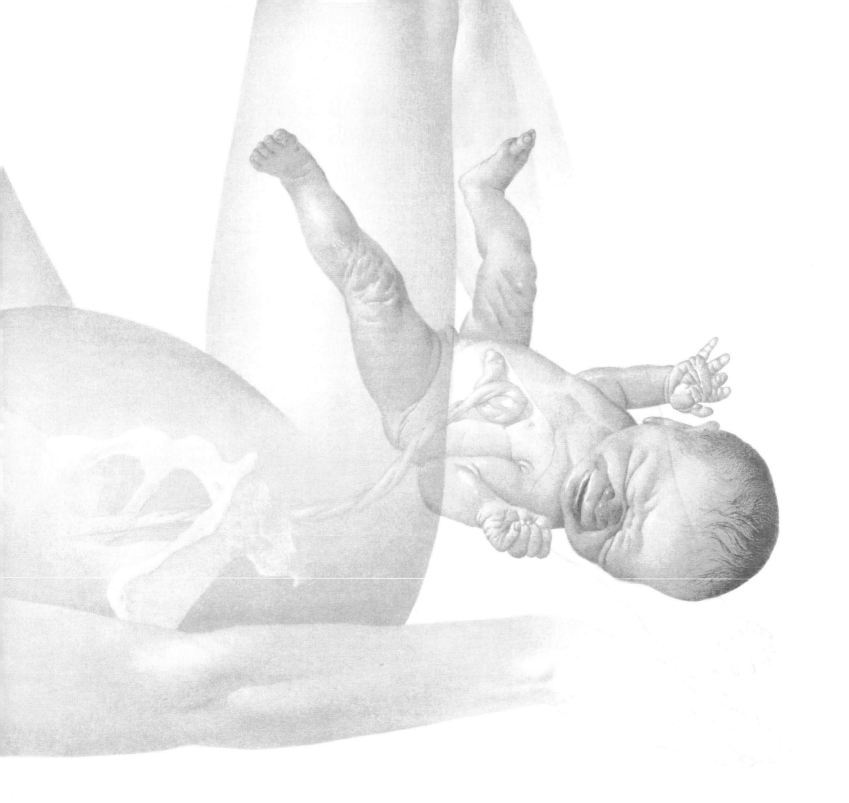

THE BABY STARTS TO BREATHE *Now that the baby is born he can no longer depend on the placenta for his oxygen supply and must seek another source of oxygen. Firstly, this is because the blood vessels in the umbilical cord— which connects the baby to the placenta —have cooled in the outside air and become contracted. Secondly, the placenta itself has become separated from the wall of the womb. Most babies start breathing within a few seconds of birth. The baby's diaphragm descends and sucks air into his lungs. Thus the infant becomes an air-breathing mammal like his mother. The umbilical cord may pulsate for a few minutes after birth, but the baby will be breathing by now so clamping and cutting the cord is quite safe.*

time for birth is overdue.

Labour can often be induced simply by puncturing the bag of waters around the baby. Usually in addition a prostaglandin pessary is inserted into the vagina, or hormones are given through an intravenous drip. These mimic the hormonal changes which occur during normal labour. Sometimes a drip will be given to speed up a labour which has already begun.

Induced uterine contractions may be stronger than natural ones, so labour may be shorter but more painful. And there is a slightly higher chance of needing other help during birth, though most induced women deliver normally.

ASSISTED DELIVERIES

Sometimes the second stage of labour is slow or difficult, and the obstetrician may decide that the baby needs to be helped out. Sometimes he judges that the baby needs to be delivered quickly, for example if its heartbeat becomes irregular. Assisted deliveries are carried out under local anaesthetic. The baby's head is gently helped out, either with obstetric forceps that slip around the sides of the head, or with a ventouse, a special suction cup that fits over the crown of the head.

THE NEED FOR CAESAREAN BIRTHS

Sometimes obstetricians may judge that the risk to the baby of a normal vaginal delivery is too great, and the baby is born by an operation through the mother's stomach wall. The mother may have a general anaesthetic putting her to sleep or an epidural anaesthetic so that the area of the abdomen is numbed and she is awake to see her child very soon after delivery. The layers of the stomach wall and uterus are opened and the baby eased out. After removal of the placenta, the layers are closed individually by stitches. The operation takes about 45 minutes,

HOW WILL YOU FEEL AFTERWARDS

In the few days after the baby's birth the remains of the uterine lining are shed like a heavy period. There is bright red loss at first, but this slowly fades to brown. Most women stop bleeding about two weeks after delivery; a few have occasional light bleeding for three or four weeks.

The tightening of the uterus after the delivery can be painful, and afterpains can be felt by women for some weeks, particularly while breast-feeding. They are worse if she has had a baby previously, for with each pregnancy a little more fibrous tissue is laid down in the uterus; this stops it stretching so easily. Soluble aspirin will give relief from the pain.

RETURNING HOME

Women often have a choice now of how long to stay in hospital after the birth—typically a couple of days, sometimes a week. Some areas even offer a 'domino' scheme, allowing a woman to return home a few hours after the birth.

The hospital will tell the health services about the birth, but when she gets home the mother should let her family doctor know too. Some GPs like to call; others will leave this to the mother.

At home, she will be visited in the first two or three days by the health visitor, who will help with the care

Getting back to your normal shape

☐ A woman who has had a normal delivery is not ill and therefore should not be kept in bed for long. The day after childbirth she should be up walking, to encourage the flow of blood in her legs to prevent clotting. However, she should avoid excessive activity, striking a balance between movement and adequate rest.

☐ In the weeks following delivery, her stomach becomes flatter but the muscles are not necessarily firmer, and she should take three to five minutes four or five times each day to do the postnatal exercises shown to her in hospital (*see also page 248*).

☐ Exercises done in the early days after delivery help in restoring her original shape, and in re-strengthening her stomach wall and pelvic floor.

of the child and his feeding.

If a mother has relatives or friends available to help her, the best time for them to do so is during the week after her return from hospital. A home help can also often be arranged through your midwife or doctor.

Arrangements will be made for the mother to attend the infant welfare clinic where further advice is given. The clinic may be run by her own family doctor or by community paediatricians who work outside the hospital.

It is important that the mother herself visits the hospital or her family doctor about six weeks after delivery for a check-up. This postnatal visit will probably include an examination of the stomach and pelvis to ensure that the pelvic organs have returned to their pre-pregnant state.

An important aspect of this visit is to discuss contraception and planning of the family in the future (*see also* FAMILY PLANNING).

Learning relaxation techniques and parentcraft

☐ Most maternity units conduct parentcraft classes which aim to increase confidence about pregnancy and childbirth by explaining what to expect and how to cope. Fathers are invited to participate, as the involvement encourages them to be more understanding and helpful to their wives during the pregnancy. Most parentcraft classes begin in the 32nd week of pregnancy and continue weekly until the birth.

☐ At the classes a doctor explains the medical management of pregnancy and childbirth. A midwife describes the three stages of labour, and methods available for relief of pain (by techniques of relaxation and by drugs). A physiotherapist explains the physical and emotional aspects of pregnancy. A health visitor discusses the practical aspects of both antenatal and postnatal care (for example, bathing the baby). A dietician advises on weight and nutrition.

☐ Gentle exercises are prescribed to prevent unpleasant side-effects of pregnancy, such as backache. The classes also give advice on problems caused by hormonal changes, such as constipation, varicose veins, indigestion and piles.

☐ Parentcraft classes place great emphasis on relaxation and breathing techniques which can be very helpful during labour. For many mothers having their first baby, labour can be a period of stress—largely due to lack of knowledge about exactly what will happen, and in some cases by listening to old wives tales and alarmist stories that are quite untrue.

☐ Apprehension may lead to muscle tension and an alteration in breathing, and this can cause exhaustion in the early stages of labour. An expectant mother who has learned how to relax and to control her breathing will be able to conserve her energy for the moment of birth.

☐ During labour, breathing should be easy and comfortable, with any emphasis on the outward rather than the inward breath. When the contractions become more severe, breathing tends to become more rapid and more shallow, and as the contractions build up to their peak, the mother sometimes reacts by overbreathing. As this may impair the contractions, she is taught a gentle sighing technique to control this tendency, again with the emphasis on the outward breath.

☐ Parentcraft classes do not only deal with the physical problems of pregnancy. A woman expecting her first baby may feel a sense of isolation before the birth, particularly if she has recently given up work. The classes provide an opportunity for companionship and mutual support, from women in the same situation who live in the same area.

MOTHER AND BABY REUNITED *Once the baby is breathing regularly and effortlessly, the mucus in his nose and the back of his throat is gently sucked out through a soft plastic tube by the midwife or doctor. The infant should then be returned to his mother as soon as possible. There is no need to keep him in a cot or an incubator unless there is some difficulty with his breathing—which is rare. But the baby should not be reunited with his mother until the umbilical cord has been cut. Otherwise, if the infant is put at a higher level than the placenta, blood will drain from him, through the cord and into the placenta. This could be dangerous because it is the baby—not the placenta—who needs the blood. Skin-to-skin contact with the mother is comforting for the baby and helps to establish an early mother-infant relationship. The couple will next be covered with a loose blanket or woollen sheet.*

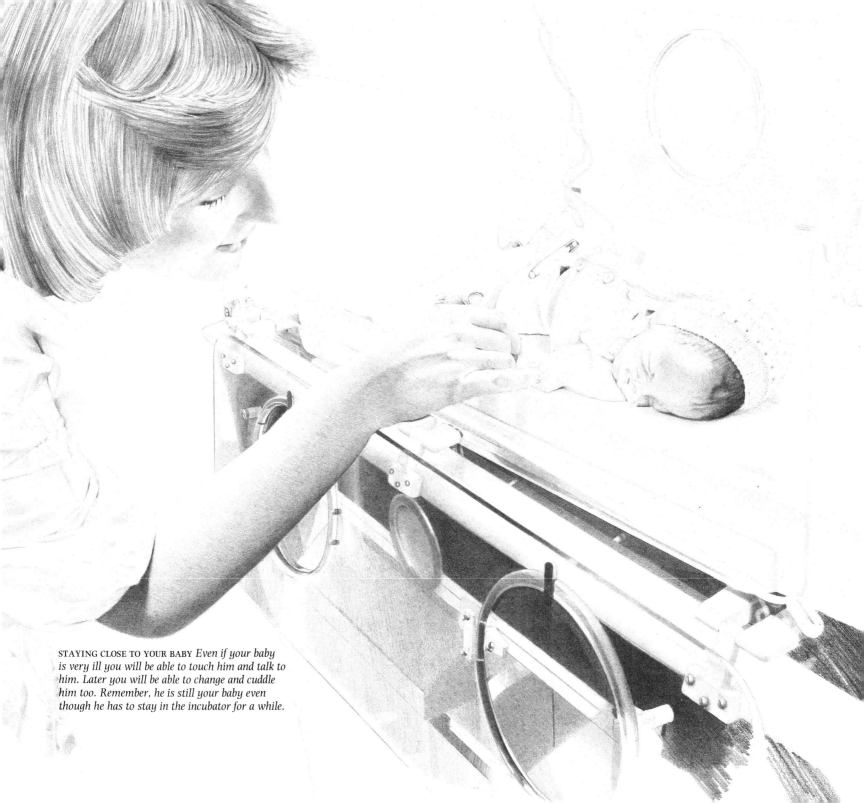

STAYING CLOSE TO YOUR BABY *Even if your baby
is very ill you will be able to touch him and talk to
him. Later you will be able to change and cuddle
him too. Remember, he is still your baby even
though he has to stay in the incubator for a while.*

THE SECURITY OF AN ARTIFICIAL WOMB
Caring for the premature baby in a neonatal unit

A premature baby is perfectly formed when born, but his body systems may not be fully developed. Because of this he may face major problems including difficulties in feeding and breathing. In addition he has little or no resistance to disease and gets cold very quickly because he lacks the layer of fat under his skin which helps a normal infant to retain body heat. The neonatal (from the word 'neonate', meaning new-born child) unit is specially designed to look after babies with these problems. Most babies needing the support of the neonatal unit are under-developed because they have been born before the normal nine months of pregnancy are up, and have missed several days or weeks of support from the womb. Others, however, although full-term, may not have been properly nourished in the womb, or may be suffering from some congenital abnormality or illness.

The most important items of equipment in the neonatal unit are the incubators—cots with clear covers to keep heat in and infection out. For severely ill babies there may be cots with overhead heating instead of covers so that the baby is kept warm but the nursing and medical staff can get to him quickly if necessary. The whole unit is kept very warm so that babies do not get cold when they are taken out of the incubator to be cuddled or changed.

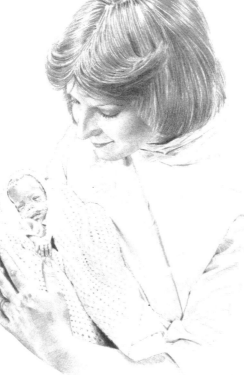

SEEING TO EVERY NEED *In the incubator the baby lies on a special pad which triggers an alarm if he stops breathing. If he finds it difficult to breathe, extra oxygen may be added to the air in the incubator or he may be put on a ventilator which does his breathing for him. If he cannot suck or swallow, he may be fed through a little tube that goes down the back of his nose into his stomach, or by special nutrients passed straight into his bloodstream. Electrodes fixed to the baby's skin check that his heart rate, blood pressure and temperature are all normal.*

PREGNANCY, DISEASES OF

Some disorders occur only during pregnancy. Routine tests during visits to the antenatal clinic are designed to identify them and, if necessary, treatment will be provided. Hyperemesis gravidarum (excessive vomiting in pregnancy) and a group of three disorders—pregnancy-induced hypertension, pre-eclampsia, and eclampsia—are covered in full below.

Disorders identified through blood tests are ANAEMIA, due to iron and folic acid deficiency, and RHESUS INCOMPATIBILITY. ANTEPARTUM HAEMORRHAGE is another disorder that is watched for.

A variety of tests (including ultrasound scans) are carried out to locate the position of the baby and the placenta in the womb. The baby's normal, head down, position may be reversed, it may face forwards instead of backwards, a shoulder, arm, foot or face may present instead of the top of the head. If necessary the baby's position may be corrected during antenatal visits.

If the tests show that a normal birth will not be possible, the doctor or midwife will be prepared for a Caesarean operation. Normal birth may be difficult if the baby's head is too big, or the bones of the mother's birth canal too narrow. Birth may also be difficult if the placenta is attached to the lower part of the womb rather than the upper (PLACENTA PRAEVIA), because it may hinder the passage of the baby through the neck of the womb.

Multiple pregnancies such as twins or triplets are identified at the antenatal clinic.

Excess amniotic fluid (hydramnios) in the womb may be a sign of a multiple pregnancy or abnormalities. If the doctor or midwife suspects abnormalities then a sample of the amniotic fluid may be tested (amniocentesis).

Pregnancy may also aggravate existing diseases or increase the likelihood of others. Diseases occurring during pregnancy include CYSTITIS and other urinary infections (which may only be identified during routine analysis of the urine sample), and vaginal thrush (see VAGINITIS). Dental decay is often aggravated by pregnancy and regular visits to the dentist are important (see TEETH). If the mother has DIABETES the insulin dosage may have to be altered. The mother is also examined for heart and lung diseases such as MITRAL STENOSIS, ASTHMA and TUBERCULOSIS, VENEREAL DISEASE, raised blood pressure (HYPERTENSION) which is not caused by pre-eclampsia, and OVARIAN CYSTS, FIBROIDS and other pelvic tumours.

HYPEREMESIS GRAVIDARUM

Persistent, severe vomiting which is an extreme form of 'morning sickness'. *See* PREGNANCY.

Symptoms
- Frequent vomiting at any time of day or night.
- Loss of weight.
- Little or no preceding nausea.

Duration
- Vomiting in pregnancy usually starts after the 4th week of pregnancy and has cleared by the 14th-16th week.

Causes
- The exact cause is not known, but vomiting may be due to the changes in the levels of hormones or the effects of the growth of the uterus. Fears and worries may then aggravate the tendency to vomit.

Complications
- The patient may become very short of body fluids, minerals and vitamins.

Treatment in the home
- Frequent small sips of water.
- Continue with normal activities if possible.

When to consult the doctor
- If vomiting is extreme or preventing normal activities.

What the doctor may do
- Exclude other causes of vomiting.
- Give fluids, extra food supplements and encourage normal activities.
- Prescribe sedatives and antivomiting drugs (*see* MEDICINES, 17, 21).
- Send the patient to hospital for rest and isolation if the above measures are ineffective.

Prevention
- None.

Outlook
- Vomiting clears by the 16th week of pregnancy. Severe vomiting is usually controlled with treatment.

PREGNANCY-INDUCED HYPERTENSION, PRE-ECLAMPSIA, ECLAMPSIA

Despite being relatively common, these three disorders are not clearly understood. Each condition tends to merge into the others. Some women have raised blood pressure in the first 20 weeks of pregnancy, often because their blood pressure is raised even when they are not pregnant. Pregnancy-induced hypertension (PIH) is higher blood pressure in late rather than early pregnancy. If there is also protein in the urine, the condition is called pre-eclampsia. If pre-eclampsia is severe or inadequately treated then the pregnant mother may occasionally become severely ill with a tendency to develop fits—eclampsia. Hospital treatment is then necessary.

Symptoms
- Raised blood pressure.
- Headaches.
- Marked swelling of the ankles. (Slight ankle swelling occurs in the last three months of many normal pregnancies.)
- Unexplained gain in weight.

Duration
- These three conditions may start any time after the 24th week of pregnancy. They tend to get worse as the pregnancy progresses but are cured within a matter of hours after the birth of the baby.

Causes
- The cause is not known, but the three conditions are more likely to arise in first pregnancies, in older mothers, if there is OBESITY, if there was previous hypertension, if the mother has DIABETES, if there are twins or RHESUS INCOMPATIBILITY.

Complications
- Fully developed eclampsia is rare, but is dangerous for both mother and baby.
- If symptoms of early pre-eclampsia are ignored or inadequately treated there are risks of ANTEPARTUM HAEMORRHAGE, STROKE and kidney damage. The baby is also at risk and may be small or premature. Occasionally severe pre-eclampsia may cause a still birth.

Treatment in the home
- Follow the doctor's routine advice about rest, diet and sedatives during pregnancy.

When to consult the doctor
- If there are any unusual symptoms at any time.

What the doctor may do
- Test blood pressure, weight and urine regularly.
- Advise rest, diet, sedatives and regular aspirin.
- Admit the patient to hospital if treatment at home is ineffective.

Prevention
- Close co-operation with the doctor or midwife, following all their instructions conscientiously will prevent most, if not all, of these conditions.

Outlook
- Excellent if antenatal care is followed conscientiously.

PREMENSTRUAL TENSION

Troublesome but harmless symptoms that affect women before a period. Most women have premenstrual tension at some time during their fertile years and accept it as an inevitable part of their life.

Symptoms
- Moodiness, irritability, tearfulness, listlessness, headache and fatigue, which often cause upsets and arguments with other people.
- Painful breasts, backache and abdominal discomfort.
- A slight gain in weight.
- Symptoms begin during the ten days before a period and disappear soon after it starts.

Duration
- Premenstrual tension usually lasts for about two to seven days.

Causes
- The condition is caused by natural changes in the balance of the female hormones. The changes lead to a build-up of fluids in the body.

Treatment in the home
- If family, friends or colleagues fail to appreciate that the symptoms are not within the woman's control, she should explain to them the nature of premenstrual tension so that they will be more understanding, and will provide her with the support that she needs.
- The sufferer should try to adjust her daily routine so that she is not under special stress in the ten days or so leading up to a period.
- Some women find that taking EXERCISE or doing YOGA makes them feel generally fitter and more relaxed, which helps with feelings of tension.

When to consult the doctor
- If the symptoms are intolerable or are interfering with normal activities.

What the doctor may do
- Prescribe diuretic tablets to make the patient pass more urine and so release the build-up of body fluids. *See* MEDICINES, 6.
- Prescribe synthetic hormones to be taken as tablets or as vaginal suppositories. *See* MEDICINES, 33.

Prevention
- There is no prevention.

Outlook
- The condition may disappear after a few years or a pregnancy.

See FEMALE GENITAL SYSTEM *page 48*

PRIAPISM

A prolonged erection of the penis, usually painful and often unrelated to sexual activity. Priapism during sleep is normal, but if it is causing pain, anxiety or occurs at other times a doctor should be consulted.

See MALE GENITAL SYSTEM *page 50*

PRICKLY HEAT

An intensely irritating skin rash, which may develop in hot, humid weather. The condition may be just a minor nuisance or a severe disability. Infants and the obese are especially liable. It is known medically as miliaria rubra.

Symptoms
- Small pimples or blisters appear, particularly in the skin creases and wherever clothing has been tight. In infants the skin around the neck, chest, groin and armpits is involved.

Duration
- This can persist until cooler weather or until the patient moves to a cooler climate.

Causes
- Swollen skin cells, caused by excessive sweating in hot, humid conditions.
- Blocked sweat ducts due to the swollen skin cells.

Treatment in the home
- Wear loose clothing.
- Breaking the hot-sweat cycle by lying under a fan in the middle of the day may help.
- Bath frequently in cool water using little soap.
- Apply calamine lotion or spirit with 0.4 per cent phenol to the affected area.
- There is no simple, effective, quick remedy.

When to consult the doctor
- If the irritation is too bad to bear.
- If there is lethargy and weakness.

What the doctor may do
- Send the patient to hospital for cooling treatment if there is much weakness and symptoms are severe.

Prevention
- Avoid tight clothing in hot climates.
- Susceptible people should keep to cool conditions or achieve a cool non-sweating rest-break in the middle of each day.

Outlook
- On moving to a cooler climate the skin rapidly returns to normal.

See SKIN *page 52*

PRIMAL THERAPY
A technique based on the assumption that neurotic behaviour is the result of a traumatic experience before or immediately after birth, or in early childhood. The patient is first isolated for three weeks, and then brought into group psychotherapy where, under the guidance of a psychotherapist, he or she is encouraged to 'relive' the traumatic experience and undo the neurotic pattern it has created. The process is often accompanied by a substantial discharge of emotion, characterised by the so-called primal scream of anguish.

PROCTITIS

Inflammation of the lining of the rectum.

Symptoms
- Discomfort is felt in the rectum.
- A repeated and often unsuccessful urge to empty the bowels. This is known as tenesmus.
- Diarrhoea, in which blood, mucus (or slime) and pus may be present.
- Pain while passing the loose motion, which may be followed by a more severe and involuntary painful muscular contraction, with the urge to empty the bowels again.

Duration
- Depends on the underlying cause.

Causes
- Proctitis may complicate both ULCERATIVE COLITIS and Crohn's disease (regional ILEITIS).
- Infections such as AMOEBIASIS and GONORRHOEA which may affect the rectum.
- Radiation treatment (for cancers of nearby organs, for example) may cause similar symptoms, as may certain drugs or injury.

Complications
- Narrowing (stricture) of the rectum.
- Splits (fissures) may occur in the rectal wall.
- Openings (fistulae) may occur in the rectal wall, issuing into the bladder or vagina.
- PILES.

Treatment in the home
- Antidiarrhoeal and antispasmodic medicines may be taken to relieve mild symptoms. *See* MEDICINES, 1, 2.
- A bulk-forming laxative may ease the passing of motions. *See* MEDICINES, 3.

When to consult the doctor
- If any prolonged bout of diarrhoea occurs.
- If blood, pus or mucus are present in stools.

What the doctor may do
- Investigate and treat any underlying cause.
- Prescribe suppositories or enemas containing steroids, to be placed in the rectum overnight. *See* MEDICINES, 32.
- Prescribe an antispasmodic.
- Prescribe a sulphonamide antibiotic. *See* MEDICINES, 25.

Prevention
- Once the underlying cause has been identified, it may be possible to prevent proctitis recurring.

Outlook
- Depends on the underlying cause.

See DIGESTIVE SYSTEM *page 44*

PROLAPSE
The forward or downward displacement of part of the body. The most common prolapses are of a spinal disc (SLIPPED DISC) and, in women, of the UTERUS, bladder or RECTUM.

PROPHYLAXIS
Treatment aimed at preventing illness. Examples are immunisations against diphtheria, poliomyelitis and other diseases, and the dental removal of the hard deposit calculus from the teeth to prevent possible gum disorders.

PROSTAGLANDINS
Substances which are contained in various body tissues and fluids—including the brain, womb and semen—and which have a variety of functions. For example, they affect the flow of blood through the kidneys and stimulate contractions of the womb during menstruation. Doctors use prostaglandins in drug form to induce abortion or labour.

PROSTATE GLAND, ENLARGED

Part of a man's semen is produced by the prostate gland, an organ the size of a plum which lies just below the bladder. The urethra runs through the middle of it. In men over the age of 50, the prostate gland often becomes enlarged, growing to the size of an apple and obstructing the flow of urine. It may also develop malignant growths.

Symptoms
- Hesitant attempts to pass urine.
- Small amounts of urine passed.
- Frequent passing of urine, especially during the night.

• The feeling, after urinating, that the bladder has not been completely emptied.
• Prolonged and painful erections of the penis.
• Total stoppage of urine.

Duration
• The condition may persist for years, giving only occasional mild symptoms.

Causes
• In older men the prostate gland slowly grows, exerting pressure on the bladder and the urethra.
• Cancer of the prostate.
• Infection of the bladder.
• Alcohol may aggravate the condition.

Treatment in the home
• Dribbling of urine from the penis after urination may cause underclothes to smell and so create an annoying social problem. The dribbling can be avoided or reduced if, after urination, the urethral tube is pressed firmly upwards and forwards from a point 2-3 in. (50-75 mm.) behind the scrotum with one hand, and the last drops of urine are 'milked' out of the penis with the other hand.
• In emergencies, difficulty in passing urine may be reduced if the sufferer sits in a hot bath and urinates.

When to consult the doctor
• If the symptoms are mild, make a routine appointment.
• If incontinent, visit the doctor within 24 hours.
• Immediately, if there is a total stoppage of urine.

What the doctor may do
• Test urine and blood.
• Examine the rectum.
• Send the patient to hospital for an operation to 'rebore' the prostate, usually aided by ENDOSCOPY.

Prevention
• Do not drink too much alcohol.
• Never let the bladder become too full.

Outlook
• Some cases persist for years, giving only occasional mild symptoms. More severe cases may require an operation or may be controlled by hormone treatment.

See MALE GENITAL SYSTEM *page 50*

PROSTATITIS

Inflammation of the prostate gland, which can be either acute or chronic. Symptoms and treatment are the same for both forms. The chronic form lasts longer and is more resistant to treatment.

Symptoms
• Pain (often burning) in the genitals on passing urine.
• Pain may also be felt in the lower abdomen while passing urine and often for some time afterwards.
• Urine is passed more often than normal, day and night. The urge to urinate is usually sudden, and it may be difficult to hold on before a lavatory can be reached.
• Urine may be cloudy, bloody, and have a fishy smell.
• High temperature.
• Painful swelling or feeling of heaviness just in front of the anus behind the scrotum.
• There may be no symptoms, the infection being discovered only after routine examination of the urine.
• Poor general health.

Duration
• Untreated, acute prostatitis often lasts a week or longer.
• The chronic condition lasts for weeks or months.

Causes
• The usual cause is a germ that lives in the bowel entering the urethra (the channel through which urine is passed) and reaching the bladder.
• A more recently described cause is jogging with a full bladder. This forces urine into the urethra and prostate, causing irritation.
• CONSTIPATION.
• The chronic condition usually follows the acute form, the use of a catheter or an abnormality in the urinary tract—for example, a STONE, or STRICTURE or a deformity present from birth.

Complications
• If left untreated the infection can spread to the testes and epididymis, causing inflammation.
• Cystitis can occur.
• A rare complication is PYELONEPHRITIS.

Treatment in the home
• Go to bed and rest.
• Drink plenty of non-alcoholic fluids.

When to consult the doctor
• If the symptoms described occur. When symptoms are severe, and if blood or other changes are noticed in the urine, the doctor should be seen immediately.

What the doctor may do
• Ask for a specimen of urine, to test for germs and pus.
• Perform a rectal examination.
• Prescribe antibiotics. *See* MEDICINES, 25.
• Send cases resistant to treatment to a specialist.

Prevention
• Avoid constipation and long periods without fluids.
• Do not jog with a full bladder.

Outlook
• With treatment, acute prostatitis usually clears up within five days.
• The outlook for the chronic condition even with treatment is less good and recurrences are common.

See MALE GENITAL SYSTEM *page 50*

PSIONIC MEDICINE
A technique that combines orthodox treatment with aspects of RADIESTHESIA and HOMEOPATHY, and is based on the assumption that disease results from the disruption of vital forces within the body. Diagnosis relies heavily on the use of 'dowsing', in which a pendulum is held over the body, or over hair or a blood sample.

Exponents assert that certain ailments—for example, measles—create 'miasms', or predispositions towards other diseases. According to psionic theory, a sufferer from tuberculosis—a hereditary 'miasm'—can impart to his descendants a tendency towards asthma, hay fever, diabetes and leukaemia.

PSITTACOSIS
An infectious disease of birds, particularly parrots, caused by bacteria called *Chlamydia psittaci*. Human beings may develop the disease, usually by breathing in germs from infected droppings or feather dust rather than by a bite from the bird. Although humans most likely to be affected are those working with birds, it can be contracted from even brief association with an infected bird or its environment. Symptoms closely resemble those of PNEUMONIA and develop after an incubation period of seven to 14 days. Treatment is by tetracycline antibiotics (*see* MEDICINES, 25). The disease is difficult to identify and is probably commoner than is realised because cases are treated as pneumonia, given antibiotics and then recover without tests being made.

See INFECTIOUS DISEASES *page 32.*

PSORIASIS

A recurring scaly eruption of the skin. Psoriasis usually begins between the ages of five and 25. It is not infectious and sufferers can learn to live with it.

Symptoms
• A red spot slowly develops, covered by a scale. About one-third of patients complain of slight itching.
• Several spots merge together to form patches which

may be 2-3 in. (50-75 mm.) across.
• The patch is deep red, covered with silvery scaling which can be scraped off. The centre of the patch may revert to normal skin, leaving an oddly shaped rash.
• Sometimes, especially in children, the onset of the rash is sudden, involving the trunk and limbs, with many small circular patches. The face is rarely involved. Such an attack (called guttate psoriasis) may follow any general illness.
• Pitting and destruction of the nails.
• The scalp may be affected with severe crusting and some hair loss.
• ARTHRITIS may develop.
• Psoriasis may develop in scars or recent wounds.
Duration
• Although the skin may heal, it is common for psoriasis to recur throughout life.
Causes
• Unknown, but in some people the condition is hereditary.
• Surgery to skin, streptococcal infections, worry and some drugs may precipitate or aggravate an attack.
Complications
• Arthritis usually affecting hands may arise in 5 per cent of sufferers. The arthritis is similar to RHEUMATOID ARTHRITIS but less severe.
Treatment in the home
• There is no effective treatment for psoriasis without medical advice.
When to consult the doctor
• At the first sign of an eruption.
• If there is a recurrence of the condition which does not respond to previous treatment.
• If there is soreness, discomfort or moistness when using dithranol ointment.
What the doctor may do
• Explain the condition and treatment so that the patient can manage his own condition.
• Prescribe coal tar or dithranol ointment. These are the most effective treatments, but they are messy and stain clothes and bedding. *See* MEDICINES, 43.
• Treatment using steroid creams under a polythene outer cover is undoubtedly effective and less messy. The disease tends to recur after treatment, and side-effects make it essential that such treatment is used under careful medical supervision.
• Arrange admission to hospital for the regular treatment of large skin areas.
• Arrange ultra-violet light treatment which is beneficial but carries the risk of skin cancers in later years.
Prevention
• None is known.

Outlook
• Although one or two patches of psoriasis may persist, most patients come to terms with their condition and seldom see the doctor.

See SKIN *page 52*

PSYCHOPATHY
Individuals who behave in persistently antisocial ways are often loosely described as psychopaths. Doctors often do not understand the causes and cure is rare. The abnormal behaviour of a heroin addict is an example of psychopathy in which the cause is clear.
See MENTAL SYSTEM *page 33*

PSYCHOSIS
A term used to describe the group of serious mental illnesses that includes SCHIZOPHRENIA, DEMENTIA, MANIC DEPRESSION, ALCOHOLISM and DRUG ABUSE. A psychosis is characterised by the fact that the sufferer has no insight into his condition, not realising that he is ill at all. He loses contact with reality, having previously led a comparatively normal life.
   Although psychoses account for only 1 per cent of all consultations for mental illness, most of the beds in mental hospitals are occupied by sufferers from psychotic illnesses.
See MENTAL SYSTEM *page 33*

PULLED ELBOW OF CHILDREN
Pain and restricted movement in a child's arm. The condition usually follows injury especially when the child has been pulled along by a faster-walking adult. The condition is due to a partial dislocation of the head of the radius (one of the bones in the forearm) which is not fully developed in a child. The problem can usually be dealt with by the doctor by manipulation and without anaesthetic. An audible click can sometimes be heard as the radial head is felt to slip into position.

PULMONARY EMBOLISM

Blockage of blood vessels in the lung, usually caused by a clot of blood. Occasionally the cause is fat (after a bone fracture) or air (after a diving accident or an error in injecting into a vein). Whatever the cause the blockage is called an embolus.
Symptoms
• Abnormal shortness of breath.
• A cough that comes on suddenly.
• Pain in the chest. In mild attacks the pain is often in the side of the chest and the victim catches his breath. If the embolism is large the pain may be severe and constricting, locating over the front of the chest.
• The lips may turn blue.
• Spitting of blood may occur.
• Signs of shock or unconsciousness, in very severe attacks.
• Fever usually follows.
Duration
• The clot and the damaged lung usually heal in a few weeks.
Causes
• The clot of blood develops in a segment of inflamed vein (THROMBOPHLEBITIS) elsewhere in the body, becomes detached, and is then carried up the veins, through the heart and into the lungs. Thrombophlebitis most commonly occurs in the veins of the leg when the patient has been immobilised after injury, operations or childbirth. The pelvic veins are another common site of thrombophlebitis after abdominal operations. Some people and families are especially prone to attacks.
Treatment in the home
• Remain at complete rest in the position of greatest comfort until seen by the doctor.
When to consult the doctor
• Seek medical advice at once if symptoms appear.
• If respiratory symptoms (cough, chest pain, shortness of breath, spitting blood) develop in the course of other illnesses or after childbirth and operations. The symptoms may begin some days or weeks afterwards.
What the doctor may do
In mild cases:
• X-ray the chest.
• Prescribe anticoagulant drugs, and other drugs which influence the clotting of blood, to prevent further emboli. *See* MEDICINES, 10.
In severe cases:
• Send the patient to hospital for oxygen, anticoagulants, and possible surgery to remove the embolus.
Prevention
• Move about (both in bed and out of bed) as much as possible after operations, injuries and childbirth.
• Anticoagulants are prescribed before certain operations which carry a high risk of thrombophlebitis.
• People who have had more than one attack may have to take anticoagulants on a long-term basis.

Outlook

- Large emboli can cause sudden death.
- Lesser emboli heal on their own without leaving any permanent disability.
- Very small emboli are harmless and often heal without being recognised.

See CIRCULATORY SYSTEM *page 40*

PUS

A yellowish liquid that forms when the body fights a bacterial infection. It consists of white blood cells, which combat bacteria; dead and living bacteria; fragments of tissue destroyed by the bacteria; and serum, the watery fluid that remains after blood has clotted. Pus may form inside or on the surface of the body.
See ABSCESS

PYELONEPHRITIS

Inflammation of one or both kidneys due to infection. There are two types of pyelonephritis: acute, lasting a few days; and chronic, which may, if untreated, last for many years and occasionally cause kidney failure and death.

The infections may be precipitated by the presence of other disorders, for example cystitis or congenital abnormalities.

ACUTE PYELONEPHRITIS

Symptoms

- A sudden onset of pain in the back and sides, in the region of the waist, and sometimes in the lower abdomen.
- A need to pass urine often.
- Often a high temperature, which may start with violent shivering.
- Babies and young children may just be pale and ill with fever.
- Adults may have associated symptoms of CYSTITIS.
- Pregnant women may have no symptoms at all—the disease is then discovered at routine antenatal visits.

Duration

- Antibiotics clear up most cases within 14 days.

Causes

- Infection by bacteria, usually the result of another condition—for example, enlargement of the PROSTATE GLAND or cystitis or an abnormality of the urinary tract

that is present from birth.

Treatment in the home

- Drink plenty of fluids.
- Rest in bed.
- Take painkillers in recommended doses to relieve pain (*see* MEDICINES, 22). Raising the foot of the bed by about 6 in. (150 mm.) will also help to relieve severe pain.

When to consult the doctor

- If there are the symptoms described.

What the doctor may do

- Examine a specimen of urine.
- Prescribe antibiotics. *See* MEDICINES, 25.
- Arrange for the patient to have X-rays and send him to a specialist if there is evidence of other diseases.

Prevention

- Treat cystitis or other causes of pyelonephritis.

Outlook

- Antibiotic treatment clears up most cases within days. When the bacteria prove resistant to antibiotics or when there is an abnormality of the urinary tract the disease occasionally becomes chronic. The urine should always be checked after treatment until free of bacteria.

CHRONIC PYELONEPHRITIS

Symptoms

- As in acute pyelonephritis.
- Sometimes raised blood pressure or kidney failure.
- Babies and young children may look generally unwell and fail to put on weight.

Duration

- The condition is liable to persist unless treated.

Causes

- As for acute pyelonephritis.
- Acute pyelonephritis is especially liable to become chronic in the elderly.

Complications

- Kidney damage in the young.
- STONES (calculi) may form.

Treatment in the home

- As for acute pyelonephritis.

When to consult the doctor

- If symptoms recur (or persist after treatment) for longer than two or three weeks.

What the doctor may do

- Check the patient's blood pressure and urine.
- Arrange for the patient to have X-rays and send him to a specialist for investigation and treatment if indicated.
- Put the patient on a low-protein diet.

Prevention

- Always ensure that your urine is checked for 'cure' on the completion of any course of antibiotic treatment for CYSTITIS or acute pyelonephritis.

Outlook

- This is usually good, provided patients are conscientious about taking treatment and checking urine. The outlook is less good if the patient is elderly, if the infecting organisms are resistant to antibiotics, if there is extensive damage to one or both kidneys, or if there are congenital abnormalities.

See URINARY SYSTEM *page 46*

PYLORIC STENOSIS

The pylorus is a strong muscle valve at the outlet of the stomach. It controls movement of food down into the duodenum and small intestine. Pyloric stenosis is an obstruction of this muscular ring. One form of the condition is specifically associated with babies.

Symptoms

- Spasms of pain in the abdomen.
- A severe spasm, with vomiting. The vomit may be copious and projectile, that is, thrown upwards and some distance away from the body.
- Remnants of partially digested food, eaten hours or even days beforehand, may be found in the vomit.
- Weight loss and dehydration.
- A previous history of DUODENAL ULCER.

Duration

- Pyloric stenosis among adults is usually found among those suffering from duodenal ulcer, and may persist after the ulcer heals.

Causes

- Inflammation around an active duodenal ulcer affecting the pylorus. A long-standing ulcer which has become scarred is particularly likely to have this result.

Complications

- Loss of acid through vomiting may result in tetany, a calcium deficiency in the blood.

Treatment in the home

- Eat small, frequent meals of foods without fatty, spicy or acid content. Bread or dry biscuits with warm milk are particularly soothing.
- Antacids will also help to heal the ulcer and so reduce inflammation. *See* MEDICINES, 1.

When to consult the doctor

- If persistent or projectile forceful vomiting occurs.
- If any recurrent stomach pain occurs.

What the doctor may do

- Prescribe antacids and antispasmodics. *See* MEDICINES, 1.

- Advise X-rays. You will be asked to swallow a liquid compound of barium beforehand. This blocks the X-rays, so that the pylorus shows up in silhouette.
- You may also be examined with a gastroscope, an instrument for inspecting the stomach visually. It is inserted, with little discomfort, through the mouth.
- An operation may be recommended in severe cases of pyloric stenosis.

Prevention
- Adequate treatment of duodenal ulcer stops the development of scarring that causes pyloric stenosis.

Outlook
- Good with treatment.

PYLORIC STENOSIS IN BABIES
Males, particularly first-born, are affected four times as often as females. *See* CHILD CARE—CHILDHOOD ILLS *page 151*.

Symptoms
- Vomiting begins between the second and sixth week after birth.
- It increases, and becomes projectile (like a spout) after every feed.
- The vomit is never stained with the yellowish-green of normal bile.
- Failure to gain weight follows.
- The child tends to be constipated and to cry from hunger.

Duration
- Until treated.

Causes
- Overdevelopment of the stomach outlet (pylorus). The condition tends to run in families, for reasons that are unknown.

Complications
- If not treated, the baby may suffer serious effects from starvation and fluid loss.

Treatment in the home
- Not advised.

When to consult the doctor
- If recurrent vomiting develops or becomes projectile.

What the doctor may do
- Feel below the right rib margin for evidence of abnormal pyloric growth. This is most easily achieved if the child is feeding quietly.
- On the slightest suspicion of pyloric stenosis, the doctor will advise that the child be admitted to hospital for continued observation. An operation may be recommended if pyloric stenosis is diagnosed.

Prevention
- None.

Outlook
- Mild cases may cure themselves or only require medicine and observation. Severe cases will need an operation, which will result in a complete cure.

See DIGESTIVE SYSTEM *page 44*

Q FEVER
An infectious disease of sheep, goats and cows, caused by rickettsia—a minute organism between a bacterium and a virus. The infection can be passed on to human beings by contact with the animal's excretions or drinking its milk, but it cannot be passed from one human being to another. Symptoms, which develop after an incubation period of about 19 days, are fever, headache and general weakness. Pneumonia follows a few days later and the patient may lose weight, but then recovers completely. Treatment is by antibiotics (*see* MEDICINES, 25). Protective vaccines are available for people at great risk, such as some slaughterhouse, tannery and dairy workers.
See INFECTIOUS DISEASES *page 32*

QUARANTINE
The isolation of a person who has, or has been exposed to, a contagious disease—such as DIPHTHERIA or TYPHOID—to prevent the disease from spreading. The person is kept under observation in hospital for a period that varies according to the disease.

QUINSY

An abscess under the mucous membrane which surrounds the tonsils.

Symptoms
- Difficulty in swallowing, speaking and opening the mouth.
- Pain, mostly on one side of the throat, may spread to the ear.
- Spasm of the jaw muscles.
- High temperature.

Duration
- If untreated, the abscess bursts within four to ten days.
- With treatment, recovery is quicker.

Causes
- TONSILLITIS. In an attack of tonsillitis, the bacteria may spread and cause quinsy within a week.

Complications
- Recurrences may occur.

Treatment in the home
- Drink extra fluids.
- Take painkillers. *See* MEDICINES, 22.
- Go to bed while the condition is acute.

When to consult the doctor
- Within 24 hours.

What the doctor may do
- Prescribe a course of antibiotics. *See* MEDICINES, 25.
- Open the abscess to release the pus and relieve the symptoms. The opening and draining of the abscess is usually performed under local anaesthetic.

Prevention
- Subsequent attacks of tonsillitis, the underlying cause of quinsy, should be treated with an antibiotic.
- Many doctors recommend the removal of the tonsils after the inflammation has cleared.

Outlook
- Excellent with treatment.
- Recurrences may occur if the tonsils are not removed.

See DIGESTIVE SYSTEM *page 44*

RABIES

A dangerous infectious disease caused by the rabies virus which is carried by animals, particularly dogs and foxes. It is also known as hydrophobia (literally, fear of water) because this fear is one of its more spectacular symptoms. The disease is transmitted to man through an open wound, such as the bite of an infected animal. The virus travels straight from the wound to the brain where it causes ENCEPHALITIS. The nearer the wound is to the brain (on the face or neck, for instance) the less far the virus has to travel and the quicker the treatment must be to prevent the disease. Before symptoms begin, the wound usually heals but remains red and inflamed. Once the symptoms have developed, treatment is ineffective and the patient usually dies within four days. Rabies occurs in most parts of the world, except Britain, Scandinavia, Australia, Japan and Antarctica, and about 15,000 cases are reported each year.

Symptoms
- Fever, headache, sore throat and muscle pains are followed by pain or numbness at the site of the wound.
- One to four days later the patient becomes restless and agitated.
- Confusion and hallucinations develop.
- Muscle spasms, stiffness of the neck and back,

convulsions and areas of paralysis may also develop.
- Excess saliva and difficulty in swallowing produce foaming at the mouth.
- Painful throat spasm with a reaction of terror on trying to swallow liquids develops.

Incubation period
- Ten days to over a year, but usually 20-90 days.
- Shortest in children injured on the face.

Causes
- The rabies virus.

When to consult the doctor
- Immediately if you think you have been infected by a rabid animal.

What the doctor may do
- Treatment depends upon the risk of rabies. If the disease is known to occur in an area, any human who is injured by an animal should check the correct position for that area with a doctor or veterinary surgeon.
- A series of injections will be necessary if the risk of rabies is confirmed. They must be given before symptoms develop.

Prevention
- Stopping rabid animals from reaching disease-free areas such as Britain is the only prevention. This may involve strict checks on animals at sea and airports.
- People at risk from rabies, such as veterinary surgeons, or those going to live where rabies is a high risk, should consider immunisation.

See INFECTIOUS DISEASES *page 32*

RADIESTHESIA

The art of divining or dowsing—using hazel twigs or branches to detect underground deposits of water—has been practised for centuries, although no one has yet explained exactly how it works. Radiesthesia, developed in France in the early 1900s, attempts to apply dowsing to the diagnosis of disease.

Practitioners use a pendulum, rather than a hazel rod, held over a sample of hair, nail parings or blood taken from the patient. The movements of the pendulum are said to show the nature and site of the disease, and to suggest possible remedies.

Some practitioners of radiesthesia also hold orthodox medical qualifications, but many do not, and the technique is generally disapproved of by doctors. It forms part of PSIONIC MEDICINE, and also the basis of RADIONICS.

RADIONICS

A technique evolved from RADIESTHESIA, in which machines are used to diagnose illness from a sample of the patient's blood, hair or nail parings. Practitioners claim that it also involves an element of extra-sensory perception. The technique is illegal in many American states and its claims have never been substantiated.

RASH

A temporary eruption on the skin consisting of red patches or spots. Most rashes are a reaction to physical or allergic irritation, but they may also be a symptom of disease.

See SYMPTOM SORTER—RASH

RAT-BITE FEVER

A disease caused by the bite of an infected rat or mouse. Fever develops one to 28 days after the bite and is accompanied either by swelling of the lymph nodes or by joint pains, headache and vomiting. Sometimes there is also a rash. Treatment is with antibiotics. The disease is most prevalent in parts of Asia.

RAYNAUD'S SYNDROME

A condition of the hands, fingers and feet which affects people who are unduly sensitive to cold.

Symptoms
- The hands, fingers and sometimes the feet turn white and then blue. As the circulation returns, the skin becomes red.
- Numbness.

Duration
- About 15-30 minutes—provided the cause is removed.

Causes
- Contraction of the arteries supplying blood to the hands. Sometimes pressure, such as gripping or carrying objects, may precipitate an attack.
- Occasionally, underlying disorders are found—such as extra ribs which press on arteries in the neck; arteries inflamed by other diseases; nerve paralysis; vibration from using power tools; drugs used for other purposes; cigarette SMOKING.

Complications
- In the event of underlying disease, the ends of the fingers may alter in appearance and, in extreme cases, GANGRENE may set in.

Treatment in the home
- Warm the hands and body.

- Keep hands in a low position.

When to consult the doctor
- If the symptoms are extreme or do not respond to warming.

What the doctor may do
- Prescribe drugs to help circulation. *See* MEDICINES, 8.
- Arrange X-rays and blood tests to exclude any underlying disease.

Prevention
- When possible avoid conditions and activities which start attacks, such as extremities of cold, excessive use of power tools and smoking.

Outlook
- If there is no underlying disease the condition is harmless but will continue to be troublesome.

See CIRCULATORY SYSTEM *page 40*

RECTUM, PROLAPSE OF

A prolapse is the displacement of an organ from its normal position. A rectal prolapse occurs when part of the bowel lining is forced downwards and protrudes from the anus. In adults, prolapse of the whole rectal wall may occur.

Symptoms
- A ring of pink or red, moist and swollen tissue protruding uncomfortably through the anus.

Duration
- The condition is liable to continue unless treated.

Causes
- The mucous membrane which lines the rectum may be forced down by straining too long to empty the bowels. This is the common cause of prolapse in children.
- In children, prolonged bouts of coughing.
- In adults, rectal prolapse is often associated with internal PILES. The rectal lining may be displaced when the piles are forced out.

Treatment in the home
- Lie down and relax.
- The prolapsed tissue, and any piles also protruding, may be gently eased back into place with the fingers, or with a warm, moist sponge.

When to consult the doctor
- If you are unable to push the prolapse back, even after several hours of rest.

What the doctor may do
- Manipulate the tissue to reduce the prolapse.

- Prescribe suppositories. *See* MEDICINES, 4.
- In children the condition may settle in a week or so at home.
- In severe or recurrent cases and in adults where piles are associated, surgery may be advised to restore the displaced tissue.

Prevention
- Avoid overstraining and CONSTIPATION.
- Never require children to strain too long or hard to empty their bowels, during toilet training for example.

Outlook
- In cases where simple treatment fails, surgery will generally restore the prolapsed tissue.

See DIGESTIVE SYSTEM *page 44*

REFLEXOLOGY

The ancient Chinese believed that areas of the feet and lower legs correspond to other parts of the body—for example, the tip of the left big toe is associated with the head. As a result, they believed that deep massage—the application of enough pressure to stimulate the muscles—of the appropriate region of the foot can cure functional disorders such as MIGRAINE, SINUSITIS, ASTHMA and stress. The technique, which is also sometimes called zone therapy, was popularised in the United States in the first half of this century and is now widely followed, although there is no convincing scientific explanation that reflexology works.

REFRACTIVE ERRORS

Refraction is the process whereby the light from outside the eye is focused on to the retina (the screen of nerve cells inside the eye). The image formed on these nerve cells is conveyed back to the brain by the optic nerve, and there interpreted into the sensation we call sight.

Symptoms
- Difficulty in focusing clearly and blurring of vision.
- Refractive errors may cause the eyes to ache. Less commonly they cause headaches.

Causes
There are four main types of refractive error:
- Myopia (short-sightedness). Short-sighted people have difficulty in seeing objects at a distance, but can see well for close work. A short-sighted child, for instance, will have difficulty in seeing the blackboard if he sits at the back of the class, but he will be able to read a book quite easily.
- Hypermetropia (long-sightedness). Long-sighted people have difficulty in focusing on near objects. Objects at a distance can be seen quite clearly by younger long-sighted people—and when the condition is relatively slight.
- Presbyopia (a form of long-sightedness which comes with middle age). After the age of about 40 or 45 the lens of the eye begins to harden. The muscles which pull on

Patterns of imperfect vision

People suffering from various eye disorders—such as tunnel vision or cataracts—have individual problems when reading the page of a book. The following eight examples show how their vision can be affected. The black areas indicate that the sufferers have problems seeing in those particular areas—*not* that they actually see black. In the case of presbyopia, or long-sightedness, there is no problem in reading the page—as long as it is held sufficiently far away from the eyes, or if the correct spectacles are worn.

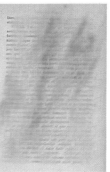
PRESBYOPIA

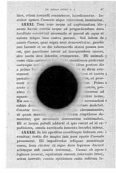
CORNEAL DYSTROPHY

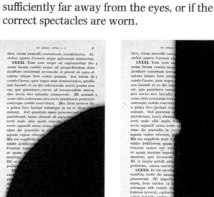
DETACHED RETINA

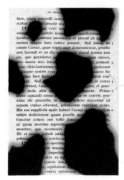
HEMIANOPIA

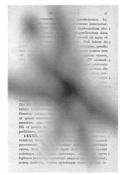
CATARACT

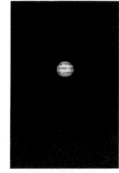
MACULAR DEGENERATION

TUNNEL VISION

DIABETIC RETINOPATHY

the lens to alter its shape and so bring the images of near objects into focus have less effect as the lens itself gets harder. Reading small print is increasingly difficult and books and papers have to be held further away to be seen clearly.

• Astigmatism (distortion of the vision). This is a fairly common condition where the curvature of the cornea (the front of the eye) is of a different diameter to the horizontal curvature. This may cause some distortion of vision, particularly if the differences in curvature are marked.

Treatment in the home

• Minor difficulties in seeing can sometimes be helped by ensuring that any really close work, such as reading, is done in a good light, preferably coming from above the left shoulder.

• If you are over the age of about 40 or 45, it is wise to have regular eye check-ups at an optician's or medical eye centre, as the correction of refractive errors is important for comfort. Regular check-ups will also detect the early presence of eye disorders such as GLAUCOMA, MACULAR DEGENERATION, CATARACTS and so on—which, if undetected, may lead to severe disability.

When to consult the doctor

• If there are difficulties with seeing and focusing, not associated with any other symptoms, it is reasonable to consult an optician before consulting a doctor.

• Eye pain, redness of the eyes, headaches and loss of vision should be referred to a doctor.

What the doctor may do

• The doctor or optician is likely to test the vision in each eye by means of a chart with letters of varying size, and he may then re-check by getting the patient to look again at the chart through a pin-hole disc, which concentrates the light. If the vision improves on looking through the pin-hole the problem is likely to be due to a refractive error. As a result of this, the doctor may advise the patient to consult an ophthalmic optician or a medical eye centre.

• The optician will do more detailed eye tests and is then likely to prescribe spectacles. With hypermetropia or presbyopia convex lenses are prescribed, while concave lenses are needed for myopia. If there is astigmatism, a cylindrical correction will be made in the lens.

Prevention

• As most errors of refraction are due to hereditary variations in the length of the eyeball or to developments in the lens and the cornea, nothing can be done to prevent them.

• If spectacles help they should be worn.

• The eyes cannot be strengthened by using them without the aids which make seeing more comfortable.

• Never wear other people's glasses.

Outlook

• Most refractive errors can be corrected, so bringing comfort and clearer sight to the majority of patients.

• Contact lenses can be used instead of spectacles in many cases.

• A new operation—radial keratotomy—may correct myopia. Most patients are pleased with the result, but the long-term effects are not yet fully known.

See EYE *page* 36

REITER'S DISEASE

A disease mostly affecting men, which causes ARTHRITIS, CONJUNCTIVITIS and URETHRITIS.

Symptoms

• Discharge from the urethra, which starts soon after exposure to infection.

• Painful joints, usually the ankle, knee, wrist or those of the foot. Joint pains usually start four to 30 days after the urethral discharge.

• Backache. The sacroiliac joints (those between the spine and the hip) may be involved, or there may be tenderness in the heel.

• A transient painful redness of the eyes.

• Small ulcers may develop in the mouth or on the heels.

Duration

• Usually one to six months.

Causes

• Reiter's disease follows an infection, usually of the bowel or genitourinary tract, often a SEXUALLY TRANSMITTED DISEASE. It occurs particularly in genetically susceptible young males, and seems to be due to an abnormal body reaction to the infection.

Complications

• The condition can become chronic and relapsing.

Treatment in the home

• None advised.

When to consult the doctor

• If the condition is suspected.

• If the above symptoms are present.

What the doctor may do

• Send the patient to hospital immediately for X-rays and blood tests to confirm the diagnosis.

• If the condition is at an acute stage, admission to hospital may be necessary. The patient will be given an anti-inflammatory drug to relieve the pain, and an antibiotic if the cause is identified. *See* MEDICINES, 37, 25.

• The joints affected may be splinted during the acute phase.

Prevention

• Avoid SEXUALLY TRANSMITTED DISEASE.

Outlook

• Most cases respond to treatment if they are detected early and the appropriate treatment is given, although there may be recurrence in about one-third of cases.

RELAPSING FEVER

Alternating periods of high fever and normal temperature caused by infection with bacteria carried by body lice and ticks. The bouts of fever, which last for up to ten days, are accompanied by pain in the joints and muscles, headache, rapid heartbeat, vomiting and sometimes a widespread rash. Antibiotics are usually prescribed to clear up the disorder.

RESPIRATORY INFECTION

Infection of the upper air passages—nose, nasal sinuses (cavities around the nasal passages), throat (pharynx), voice-box (larynx), windpipe (trachea) and upper bronchi (the two tubes formed from the division of the windpipe).

Upper respiratory infections are very common, particularly in children, and in most cases are relatively mild. They account for 25 per cent of all diseases reported to the doctor.

There are more than 200 different micro-organisms (bacteria and viruses) that can cause infection (for example, the INFLUENZA group of viruses), and it is often impractical or even impossible for a doctor to identify the specific cause in each individual case.

Symptoms

The symptoms vary according to the part of the respiratory tract that is affected. For example, the influenza A virus may affect the nose, causing catarrh; the pharynx, causing a sore throat; the windpipe, causing a painful cough; or even lower parts of the respiratory tract.

Below are the main symptoms of different infections according to the site of infection, together with the infection and the possible cause.

SITE: Nose

Main symptoms: Nasal blockage; catarrh; nasal discharge.

Infection: Acute RHINITIS or acute nasopharyngitis.

Possible causes: COMMON COLD viruses; other respiratory

viruses, including influenza A and B.
SITE: Nasal sinuses
Main symptoms: Headache, facial pain over affected sinus; nasal blockage; high temperature; chills.
Infection: Acute SINUSITIS.
Possible causes: Common cold viruses; some other respiratory viruses; common bacterial infections.
SITE: Throat (pharynx)
Main symptoms: Sore throat; pain on swallowing.
Infection: Acute PHARYNGITIS or acute TONSILLITIS.
Possible causes: Any respiratory virus; one of several common bacteria.
SITE: Voice-box (larynx)
Main symptoms: Sore throat; hoarseness; loss of voice.
Infection: Acute LARYNGITIS.
Possible causes: Any respiratory virus; common bacteria.
SITE: Windpipe (trachea)

Main symptoms: Hoarse, painful cough.
Infection: Acute tracheitis.
Possible causes: Respiratory viruses; bacteria.

In addition to the main symptoms described, an acute upper respiratory infection may occasionally cause spitting or coughing of blood; chest pains related to breathing or wheezy, laboured breathing, which is often accompanied by tightness across the chest. If any of these less-common symptoms occur, a doctor should be consulted as soon as possible.

Duration
• Rarely longer than four or five days.
Complications
• The infection may descend into the lungs and cause PNEUMONIA.
Treatment in the home
• The aim of treatment is to prevent the spread of

infection down the respiratory tract. The patient should rest, preferably in bed in a warm room; overactivity may encourage the spread of infection.
• Meals should be light and easily digestible.
• SMOKING should be avoided.
• Regular steam inhalations may help a blocked nose.
What the doctor may do
• Prescribe mild painkillers and a soothing mixture for a cough or sore throat. *See* MEDICINES, 22, 16.
Prevention
• None. Antibiotics may be given to protect babies and the elderly from pneumonia. *See* MEDICINES, 25.
Outlook
• With simple measures the symptoms usually disappear in one to five days.

See RESPIRATORY SYSTEM *page 42*

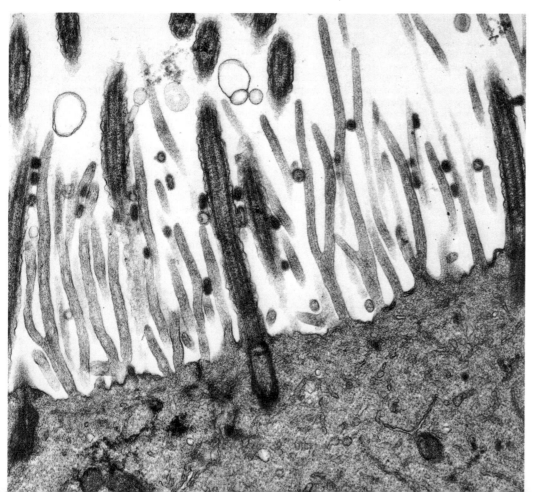

INFLUENZA UNDER THE MICROSCOPE   *The small dark blots in this cross-section of the surface of the windpipe are influenza viruses. The threadlike structures are cilia, tiny hairs which line the windpipe, moving to and fro to sweep the area clean of germs and dust. However, some of the influenza viruses attach themselves to the hairs, causing them to stick in clumps. As this happens gaps are created which allow more viruses to travel down between the clumps to the surface of the windpipe. Once there, they can start to multiply and set about their deadly business of penetrating the body's tissues and setting up infection. The viruses are seen here magnified 35,000 times by an electron scanning microscope.*

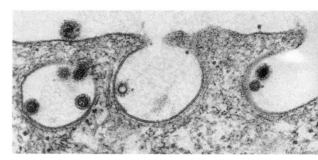

CELL DESTRUCTION   *As the viruses reach the surface of the windpipe they attach themselves to the cell membranes. The membranes then form 'pockets' and try to smother the viruses. However, the viruses penetrate the cells, where they multiply and kill the cells off.*

RHESUS (Rh) INCOMPATIBILITY

A number of substances were first discovered in human blood as a result of experiments carried out with Rhesus monkeys in 1940. One of these substances, Rhesus-factor D, is found in the red blood cells of 85 per cent of all people—these people are Rhesus (Rh) positive. The remaining 15 per cent who lack factor D are Rh-negative. The presence or absence of the Rh factor is inherited and is important in blood transfusions and pregnancy.

An Rh-negative person who receives Rh-positive blood in a transfusion may form antibodies in his blood. Should he then receive more Rh-positive blood the antibodies will destroy the red cells in the Rh-positive blood. To guard against this, the patient's Rh factor is determined before transfusion.

In pregnancy, an Rh-negative woman who is carrying a child with Rh-positive blood, inherited from the father, may pick up some of her baby's red cells in the bleeding which takes place at birth—if this happens, antibodies against the Rh-positive factor will be formed in her blood. There is usually no problem with the first pregnancy, but in subsequent pregnancies antibodies may enter the bloodstream of the unborn child and destroy its red cells. Treatment during pregnancy can prevent the antibodies forming, but in a very few cases the baby will be born dead. In other cases a total blood transfusion can be given to the baby—if necessary before it is born.

RHEUMATIC FEVER

Inflammation of the heart, which sometimes follows an attack of tonsillitis. Rheumatic fever, which occurs most commonly in children, is often associated with poor social conditions. Many attacks are probably mild and pass unrecognised. The disease is less common than it was, but damaged heart valves following unrecognised infections are not infrequent.

Symptoms
- Fever.
- General illness.
- Painful swelling of the joints. More than one joint is usually affected, though not necessarily at the same time.
- There may be a rash on trunk and limbs, and nodules (hard swellings) near to the joints.
- ST VITUS'S DANCE (involuntary writhing movements of face, arms and body) may develop in children at a later stage.

Duration
- Rheumatic fever usually lasts about two to four weeks, but its duration varies and it may persist for several months.

Causes
- Attacks follow a week or two after a throat infection caused by streptococcal bacteria. Rheumatic fever occurs only in about one in 100 of those suffering from sore throats from this cause.

Complications
- Recurrent attacks and long-term damage to the heart valves may occur.

Treatment in the home
- If the disease is suspected, keep the patient at rest until a medical opinion is obtained.

When to consult the doctor
- If a child (or adult) becomes ill following an attack of TONSILLITIS or other infection in the nose and throat, especially if there are painful joints or a rash.

What the doctor may do
- Keep the patient in bed.
- Prescribe painkillers. *See* MEDICINES, 22.
- Take throat swabs and blood for examination.
- Regularly examine the heart.

Prevention
- Avoid overcrowding. Those in schools, barracks, prisons and in poor areas are especially at risk.
- Anybody who has had rheumatic fever should mention this to the dentist before any kind of dental treatment. He will give antibiotics to reduce the risk of damaged heart valves becoming infected. *See* MEDICINES, 25.
- Do not ignore painful joints in children.
- Do not believe in growing pains.

Outlook
- An attack usually passes quickly, without appearing to leave any damage.
- Damage to heart valves often develops, but it may not become apparent until much later in life.
- Recurrences are common and long-term antibiotics may be advised.

See CIRCULATORY SYSTEM *page 40*

RHEUMATISM
A general term for pain, with or without stiffness, affecting the muscles and joints, used more by the lay public than the medical profession. Problems of this kind are rare in children but by the age of 75 most people suffer from them. Rheumatism covers many conditions including OSTEOARTHRITIS, RHEUMATOID ARTHRITIS, FIBROSITIS, and CERVICAL SPONDYLOSIS.

RHEUMATOID ARTHRITIS

A progressive, slowly destructive swelling of the joints. At first, the disease particularly affects the joints of the fingers and feet. It then spreads to include the wrists, knees, shoulders, ankles and elbows. Once the disease is established, it progresses by repeated attacks. It can affect any age group; most cases start between the ages of 25 and 55. More than twice as many women as men are affected.

Symptoms
- Swollen joints.
- Stiffness and pain in the affected joints, often worse first thing in the morning.
- Red, shiny skin over the affected joints.
- General stiffness in joints and muscles.
- Limited movement.
- Sometimes CARPAL TUNNEL SYNDROME is an early symptom.
- Occasionally, weight loss, fever, a general feeling of ill health and loss of appetite also occur.
- Eventually the affected joints, particularly those of the hands, become destroyed and deformed and lose their function.

Duration
- The disease usually lasts for many years.

Causes
- The cause is unknown.

Complications
- ANAEMIA commonly develops.
- Occasionally the functioning of the eyes and lungs becomes slightly impaired.

Treatment in the home
- Take painkillers in recommended doses for relief of pain. *See* MEDICINES, 22.

When to consult the doctor
- Immediately the disease is suspected.

What the doctor may do
- Arrange a blood test to confirm the diagnosis and to check that the symptoms are not caused by another disorder.
- Arrange for the affected joints to be X-rayed to determine the severity of the disease.
- Prescribe anti-inflammatory drugs to relieve pain and slow the progress of the disease. *See* MEDICINES, 32, 37.
- Arrange for the affected joints to be put into splints to minimise damage.
- Arrange for physiotherapy.
- If a joint is severely deformed, the doctor may send the

patient to hospital for an operation to replace the joint with an artificial one.

• In cases of severe disablement, the doctor will arrange for the patient to receive help concerning his or her occupation, accommodation and transport, and to be supplied with any necessary aids and appliances in the home.

Prevention

• Prevention is not possible.

Outlook

• Most cases of rheumatoid arthritis run a long course of alternating attacks and remissions and eventually cause destruction and deformity of the affected joints. However, badly deformed joints can be replaced and this generally leads to much increased mobility for the patient.

• After many years, attacks may die out altogether.

See SKELETAL SYSTEM *page 54*

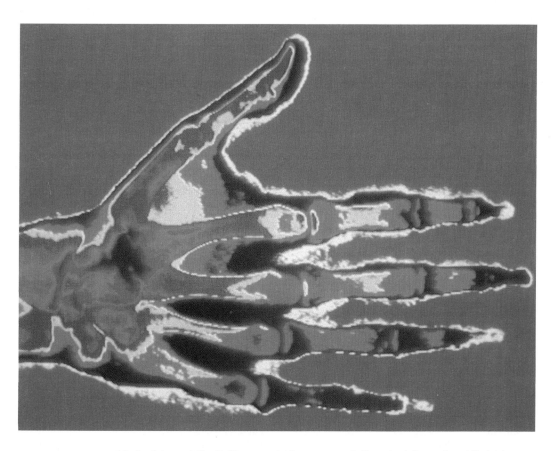

ARTHRITIS IN ACTION   *Attacks of rheumatoid arthritis can persist for years on and off, causing inflammation at the joints. The inflammation gives rise to swelling and eventually destroys the affected joints. In this computer-enhanced heat image of an arthritic hand the colours—red, orange, yellow, green, blue and violet—represent the varying degrees of heat caused by the arthritic inflammation. There is 1°F ($\frac{1}{2}$°C) difference between each colour, ranging from the hottest and most affected parts (red) down to the coolest and least affected parts (violet).*

RHINITIS

Inflammation of the lining of the nose. This lining helps to moisturise the air breathed in, so that dry air does not irritate the throat, trachea (windpipe) and small lung passages. Small hairs in the front part of the nose act as a mechanical filter, blocking dust and dirt particles from the atmosphere. How much dust and dirt that has been trapped can be seen when the nose is blown into a handkerchief. The inflammation blocks the nose and makes it run and feel stuffy. Excess mucus is produced which not only runs from the nose, but may also drip into the throat and cause soreness and coughing. Rhinitis occurs in three forms: acute (*see* COMMON COLD), chronic and allergic—commonly known as hay fever.

CHRONIC RHINITIS

The inflammation is usually caused by irritants such as dust and smoke.

Symptoms

• Frequent attacks of catarrh.

• Recurring runny nose. The discharge, which is usually clear, causes frequent nose-blowing.

• Blocked nose. To begin with, this is intermittent and is worse in certain positions, such as in the lower nostril when lying on one side.

• Headache, or a feeling of fullness at the front of the head.

• Mouth breathing and snoring.

• Loss of the sense of smell.

• Frequent sneezing.

• A cough.

Duration

• The condition lasts until the irritant is removed.

Causes

• Alcohol, even in small quantities.

• Certain nose drops.

• Exposure to dust, pollen, chemical vapours in the atmosphere, certain cosmetics, fumes, especially tobacco fumes.

• A very dry atmosphere.

Complications

• Chronic SINUSITIS often develops.

Treatment in the home

• Steam inhalations using a proprietary preparation, crystals of menthol and eucalyptus, friar's balsam or Vick, may help to ease the symptoms.

• Alcohol may aggravate the condition and should also be avoided.

● Do not use nose drops. Many contain drugs which, although they may appear to be beneficial at first, usually make matters worse in the long run.

● Take painkillers in recommended doses. *See* MEDICINES, 22.

When to consult the doctor

● If the headache is not relieved by treatment with painkillers.

● If symptoms persist when you are not in contact with irritants, or if you are unable to go to work.

● If only one nostril is repeatedly blocked, as this could mean a polyp or other obstruction.

● If deafness develops.

What the doctor may do

● Examine the nose, ears and mouth, and possibly recommend a sensitivity test in case the cause is an allergy.

● If a NASAL POLYP or other complication is suspected, send you to be examined by an ear, nose and throat specialist.

● Prescribe antihistamine tablets or other medicines containing steroids or cromoglycate. These can be taken only under medical supervision and are not beneficial in every case. *See* MEDICINES, 12, 13, 14, 41.

Prevention

● If you have to come into contact with known irritants, wear a face mask.

● Avoid places and fumes known to cause sneezing and a running or blocked nose.

● Do not smoke and avoid tobacco fumes.

Outlook

● Although chronic rhinitis is not serious it can be extremely troublesome and persistent. Often symptoms come and go over periods of months or years. There may be long symptom-free periods.

● The symptoms often improve from middle age onwards.

● Relief from emotional strain is frequently followed by a marked improvement in symptoms.

● Symptoms caused by irritants often improve quickly once the patient is able to avoid them.

ALLERGIC RHINITIS

In spite of its common name, hay fever, this condition is neither caused by hay, nor associated with fever.

Symptoms

● Mostly similar to those for chronic rhinitis, though they are often seasonal (spring and summer). In addition there may be:

● Sneezing.

● Sore, watering eyes.

● Sore throat.

● Other associated allergic conditions such as ECZEMA or ASTHMA.

● Symptoms may worsen at night because of mattress dust.

Duration

● First symptoms often appear during the teens.

● Seasonal allergic rhinitis occurs during the same season each year.

● Where the substance to which the patient is allergic is present all the year round, the symptoms are present all the time.

Causes

● Allergic rhinitis can run in families.

● Certain grasses, weeds and trees, which depend upon wind for cross-pollination, release their pollen into the air. Allergy to pollens produces symptoms during the pollen season—spring and early summer.

● Allergy to house dust or house-dust mites—small insects present in every home—produces symptoms all the year round.

● Animals, birds, moulds, plants or chemicals can all affect certain individuals.

● In many cases no cause can be found for symptoms.

● Emotional tension or unhappiness may make symptoms worse.

Treatment in the home

● Antihistamine preparations, bought from the chemist, may give relief. *See* MEDICINES, 14.

● Soothing proprietary eye baths may ease eye discomfort.

When to consult the doctor

● If symptoms are severe or interfering with school, examinations or work.

● If only one nostril is blocked.

What the doctor may do

● He may prescribe antihistamines or other medicines to give relief. These can cause drowsiness.

● He may prescribe cromoglycate by nasal spray, inhaler or eye drops to try to prevent symptoms occurring.

● In certain circumstances, he may arrange skin tests to determine the cause of the allergy.

● Sometimes steroid drugs by nasal spray or inhaler may be prescribed. *See* MEDICINES, 14, 41.

Prevention

● Avoid exposure to the pollen or offending substance (if known).

● Remove old, musty dust-collecting furniture.

● Vacuum-clean furniture and mattresses frequently.

● Keep pets out of the house.

● Avoid fresh flowers during the pollen season.

● Avoid toys that collect dust and cannot be washed.

● Avoid tobacco fumes.

● In the bedroom: use foam pillows; damp dust every second day; use a minimum amount of furniture.

Outlook

● With care taken to avoid the cause of the allergy, if known, symptoms can be avoided.

● Symptoms often get less severe as the patient gets older (after about age 20).

See RESPIRATORY SYSTEM *page 42*
ALLERGY

RHINOPHYMA

Permanent lumpy, red swelling of the nose, often occurring together with the intermittent flushed skin condition ROSACEA. It mainly affects men. Those with marked disfigurement can have PLASTIC SURGERY to correct the condition.

RICKETS

A children's disease, in which the growing bones soften, bend and are malformed. It is caused by a deficiency of vitamin D which results in not enough calcium salts being deposited in the bones to make them rigid. Although the condition is no longer common in Britain due to improvements in diet, it is prevalent in some developing countries.

Symptoms

● The child is miserable, with pains in the bones affected.

● Prominent forehead.

● Bow legs and knock knees.

● Swelling and deformity of bones at wrists, knees and ankles.

● A row of knobs appears at the front of the ribs where they join the breastbone.

● Hunchback.

● Distorted pelvic bones.

Duration

● The condition lasts until the vitamin deficiency is corrected. But many of the deformities cannot be reversed unless treatment is early.

Causes

● A deficiency of vitamin D in the diet due to lack of milk and other foods containing the vitamin.

● Lack of sunshine (ultra-violet light), which converts skin fats into vitamin D.

● Difficulty in absorbing foods containing vitamin D as in conditions such as COELIAC DISEASE.

Complications
• Permanent bone deformities such as bow legs, knock knees, hunchback and deformities of the chest.
• In females deformities of the pelvis will lead, in adult life, to difficulties in childbirth, as the baby may be unable to pass through the narrowed pelvis.

Treatment in the home
• None. If you suspect rickets, consult your doctor.

When to consult the doctor
• If the bones of the wrist, knees and ankles swell and are painful.
• If bow legs or knock knees are noticed; usually these conditions are not caused by rickets but are a normal phase of growing up.

What the doctor may do
• Arrange for X-rays of the bones and blood tests to check the diagnosis.
• Prescribe extra supplements of vitamin D.
• Advise on a better diet.
• Refer the patient to hospital if corrective measures or appliances are required.

Prevention
• Ensure vitamin supplements are given to all children.
• Give children foods, such as milk, which contain vitamin D.
• Pregnant women and children who move from hot countries with plenty of sunlight to northern, temperate climates with less sun are at special risk and need extra supplements of vitamin D.

Outlook
• Good—if the condition is diagnosed early and the vitamin D deficiency is corrected before deformities develop.

See DIGESTIVE SYSTEM *page 44*
NUTRITION

RINGWORM

A highly contagious fungus infection known medically as tinea. Although no worm is involved, which makes the name ringworm misleading, a ring is formed because, as the infection spreads, the inflamed patches extend at their edges while their centres revert to a normal skin appearance.

Ringworm can affect any part of the body as the fungus lives on the dead, horny outer layer of the skin. But the sites most commonly attacked are the moist warm areas such as the groins, armpits, beneath the breasts and the feet.

The Latin names used to describe the disease in different areas of the body are: tinea capitis—affecting the scalp; tinea corporis—the body; tinea cruris—the groins: and tinea pedis—the feet (*see* ATHLETE'S FOOT).

TINEA CAPITIS
This type is most common in children although, if the infection is caught from pets, adults may also be affected.
Symptoms
• There may be no symptoms apart from mild irritation.
• A patch of inflammation with some scaling and hair loss. The patch enlarges for a few weeks. When it stops growing, another patch begins in another part of the head.
• The hairs break off, leaving stumps about ⅛ in. (3 mm.) long, giving the hair a moth-eaten appearance.
• The scaly inflamed areas may become infected with bacteria, producing impetigo.
Duration
• With treatment the condition clears in a few weeks.
• Without treatment it can last until puberty, when the fungus automatically dies off.
Causes
• Various types of fungi. Some attack hair and others invade the rest of the skin also.
• Depending on the type of fungus, tinea capitis may be acquired from other infected children, from animals, particularly dogs and cats, and from the soil.
Treatment in the home
• Once medical treatment has been started it is necessary to avoid reinfection. Bed linen should be boiled, pillow cases changed frequently, and combs and hair brushes replaced as disinfectants and antiseptics do not kill all fungi.
When to consult the doctor
• If patches of baldness and scaling develop on a child's head.
What the doctor may do
• Take a scraping from the infected patch for examination under a microscope to identify the type of fungus.
• Prescribe griseofulvin tablets. This antibiotic has replaced all other treatment and should be continued for one or two months. *See* MEDICINES, 26, 43.
Prevention
• Avoid pets or cattle that have not been treated for tinea capitis. Avoid overcrowded sleeping conditions, as proximity encourages the disease to spread.
Outlook
• The hair and scalp will return to normal once the fungus dies off.

TINEA CORPORIS
Symptoms
• The infection starts as a red pimple, which spreads at the edges with clearing in the middle. There may be just one pimple or a number.
• Itching with mild scaling of the skin is common.
• The patches of inflammation may be small or large, and may affect any part of the body.
• A distinctive infection is found in the beard area of men (*Tinea barbae*). Abscesses can form on the inflammation, especially when the infection is contracted from cattle.
Duration
• Spread continues for several weeks or months until a static phase is reached. If left alone it usually clears after some months or years.
Causes
• Various types of fungus infection. These can spread from the patient's own feet or hair, or from other people, or domestic animals or cattle.
• The condition is commoner in warm humid climates.
Treatment in the home
• Apply an antifungal preparation, such as Whitfield's ointment which contains benzoic and salicylic acid, or magenta paint. You can buy these at the chemist.
• If you have a patch of ringworm always look for other patches in other parts of the body and in other members of the household, and treat them also.
When to consult the doctor
• If you suspect you have ringworm.
What the doctor may do
• Take a scraping of infected skin for examination under a microscope, to confirm the diagnosis.
• Prescribe an antifungal cream, ointment or griseofulvin (antibiotic) tablets. *See* MEDICINES, 26, 43.
Outlook
• Complete cure is normal.

TINEA CRURIS
This type, which affects the groin, is usually found in men, and is extremely common. It is also known as dhobie itch.
Symptoms
• Inflamed pimples develop on the inside of the upper thigh. They soon merge to form a scaly red patch with a distinct edge.
• The rash is often in both groins and spreads down the thighs, into the genital area and the cleft between the buttocks.
• Intense itching is very troublesome.
Duration
• The condition may last indefinitely unless treated.

Causes
- Various fungus infections.
- The infection is encouraged by hot, humid climates and by tight clothing.
- Infection from domestic pets is unlikely.

Treatment in the home
- Wash the affected area frequently, and dry it thoroughly.
- Apply magenta paint or salicylic-benzoic acid ointment. These are effective but messy.

When to consult the doctor
- If you suspect you have the infection.

What the doctor may do
- Take a skin scraping from the infection to identify the fungus under a microscope.
- Prescribe antifungal cream, ointment, or griseofulvin (antibiotic) tablets. *See* MEDICINES, 26, 43.

Prevention
- Frequent washing of the groins and powdering with talcum, avoiding tight clothing, and regular clean clothing are the best preventive measures.
- Do not use other people's towels in communal changing-rooms.
- Do not share clothing or bedding with infected people.

Outlook
- Complete cure is to be expected with the proper treatment.

See SKIN *page 52*
ATHLETE'S FOOT

ROCKY MOUNTAIN SPOTTED FEVER

An infectious disease caused by a rickettsia—a minute organism. It occurs mostly in the southern and western states of America and is transmitted to human beings by tick bites. After an incubation period of three to 12 days severe headache and fever develop. There may also be muscle, joint and abdominal pains and the patient may be extremely ill. A rash of pink, flat spots may develop, appearing first on the wrists and ankles. Treatment is by antibiotics, and should be given early in the course of the disease, which is sometimes fatal.
See INFECTIOUS DISEASES *page 32*

RODENT ULCER

A type of skin cancer, known as basal cell carcinoma, that occurs on the face and neck. Unlike other cancers it is never fatal because it does not spread to other parts of the body.
See SKIN CANCER

ROSACEA

This is a common disorder in which there is reddening of the skin on the face. In women it occurs most frequently in middle age. Men are affected at a younger age and more severely.

Symptoms
- Recurring redness of the nose and cheeks is an early sign. This is followed by dilation of minute blood vessels in the skin and permanent redness.
- Pimples and pus-filled blisters develop over the red areas of skin.
- In severe cases, usually in men, the nose becomes nodular, knobbly and gross (a condition known as RHINOPHYMA).
- In younger women, red pimples sometimes form around the mouth (perioral dermatitis).

Duration
- After an initial bout of clearing and recurring, the condition gradually becomes permanent.

Causes
- The cause is unknown, but rosacea more often occurs in highly nervous people, especially those with dark hair and oily skins.
- Alcohol is not a direct cause, but may make facial flushing and nasal redness worse.

Complications
- CONJUNCTIVITIS (inflammation of the cornea in the eye).

Treatment in the home
- Avoid anything which aggravates facial flushing, for example, strong spices, curried foods, alcohol, exposure of the face to wind, cold and sun.
- Do not use hydrocortisone or other steroid creams unless under regular medical supervision.
- Do not use preparations containing sulphur. These do not help and may aggravate the redness.
- Aqueous cream B.P. is safe to apply. *See* MEDICINES, 43.

When to consult the doctor
- If the condition is causing embarrassment.
- If pus-filled blisters develop.
- If the eyes become inflamed.

What the doctor may do
- Prescribe antibiotics. *See* MEDICINES, 25.
- Prescribe tranquillisers for anxiety, to help reduce facial blushing. *See* MEDICINES, 17.
- Send the patient to a plastic surgeon if rhinophyma has developed.
- Send the patient to an eye specialist if there are eye complications requiring expert attention.

Prevention
- No effective measures are known.

Outlook
- The tendency is lifelong, but during severe eruptions remissions are to be expected.
- About one-third of patients with rosacea can expect some inflammation around the eyes at some time.

See SKIN *page 52*

ROSEOLA (ROSEOLA INFANTUM)

A mild disorder that affects children under three. It is marked by the sudden onset of high fever, 103-105°F (39.5-41°C), which lasts for about four days. Convulsions—involuntary contortions of the body or limbs—may occur. As the child's temperature returns to normal a widespread pink rash appears. The probable cause of roseola is a virus. Symptoms should be reported to a doctor, who will suggest rest and possibly drugs such as paracetamol to reduce the fever. Recovery is rapid and complete.

ROTATOR CUFF LESION

The shoulder is capable of a very wide range of movements and is therefore a complex joint. The rotator cuff is a ring of muscles and tendons which hold the rounded top of the arm bone against the shoulder bone to make the shoulder joint. This cuff of tendons can be injured and torn by accident. Also, as an individual ages, it degenerates and may develop spontaneous disorders. These include FROZEN SHOULDER, PAINFUL ARC SYNDROME, SHOULDER HAND SYNDROME and supraspinatus tendinitis. With the exception of frozen shoulder these conditions have similar causes, symptoms, treatment and outlook.

Symptoms
- Pain in the shoulder made worse by movement involving the joint.
- The upper arm and shoulder are moved together. Muscle spasms produced by pain 'freeze' the shoulder joint itself, and sufferers compensate by moving the shoulder-blade and humerus (upper-arm bone) frozen together as one bone.
- Pain may be a dull ache or a sharp pain occurring with movements of the humerus on the shoulder-blade.

Duration

• This depends on the cause. A severe injury may weaken the shoulder permanently.

• Most degenerative or spontaneous lesions take about three months of rest to heal.

• Frozen shoulder, which affects the whole joint capsule, takes up to two years.

Causes

• Injury.

• In older age groups previous minor injuries, excessive use of the joint, DIABETES and chronic ALCOHOLISM, all render rotator cuff lesions more likely.

Complications

• Permanent weakness of the shoulder joint.

Treatment in the home

• None is advised.

When to consult the doctor

• Immediately the symptoms occur.

What the doctor may do

• Arrange an X-ray of the shoulder to check that the symptoms are not the result of a fracture.

• When pain is severe, arrange physiotherapy.

• He may inject hydrocortisone and a local anaesthetic. *See* MEDICINES, 32.

• Patients who are not elderly may be sent to hospital for an operation to sew together the torn tendons.

• Afterwards the arm is rested in plaster for three weeks and then shoulder exercises are practised.

• In elderly patients the degeneration of the tendon usually makes an operation impracticable, and the torn tendons are allowed to heal of their own accord. The doctor will then arrange physiotherapy to help the patient regain full use of the arm.

Outlook

• In patients who are not elderly, treatment usually restores the arm to normal.

• In most elderly patients, some of the arm's mobility is permanently lost.

See SKELETAL SYSTEM *page 54*

ROUNDWORMS

These worms are usually found in children. Infections occur in developed communities, but are particularly common in Africa and the Far East. They are among the largest parasites, 4-12 in. (100-300 mm.) long, and look rather like earthworms. The disease, known medically as ascariasis, is caused by swallowing the worm's eggs in contaminated water or food or, with toddlers, soil. The eggs develop into worms in the intestines. The worms lay eggs which are excreted in the faeces. If sanitary conditions are poor, food and water become infected by egg-ridden soil and the cycle of infection begins again.

Symptoms

• Stunted growth.

• Malnutrition.

• A worm in the stools.

Causes

• Egg-infested food or water.

Treatment

• Cure is by the drug piperazine, taken by mouth (*see* MEDICINES, 29). It paralyses the worms, which can then be expelled in the faeces with the help of laxatives. Once children are cleared of worms they put on weight and their general health improves.

See INFECTIOUS DISEASES *page 32*

RUBELLA *See* GERMAN MEASLES

RUPTURE

1. The popular term for an inguinal HERNIA, in which a segment of intestine protrudes through a break in the wall of the lower abdomen.

2. Any tearing of tissue through injury or disease.

SAFETY IN THE HOME

More accidents happen every year in Britain's homes than on the roads—and most of them could be avoided by taking a few simple precautions. *See* SAFETY IN THE HOME *page 454*

ST VITUS'S DANCE

A jerky, involuntary twitching condition, also known as Sydenham's chorea, and related to RHEUMATIC FEVER.

Symptoms

• Irregular twitches affect one part of the body, then another. The face, for example, may suddenly adopt a peculiar expression, or the arms may jerk uncontrollably. Attacks tend to be worse when the patient is excited, and to disappear while the patient is asleep.

• There is weakness and loss of co-ordination in the muscles. The patient tends to drop things, and in severe cases may be unable to stand.

• The patient is confused and emotionally upset, suffering periods of elation and depression.

Duration

• Symptoms generally persist for about two months.

Causes

• The precise cause is unknown.

Complications

• Carditis, or heart disease, as in RHEUMATIC FEVER.

Treatment in the home

• Keep the patient in bed until the movements cease.

• Aspirin may be taken.

When to consult the doctor

• If symptoms occur.

What the doctor may do

• Prescribe sedatives. Aspirin and steroids may be given. *See* MEDICINES, 22, 32.

Prevention

• Rheumatic fever (and hence St Vitus's Dance) can be prevented by treating bacterial tonsillitis with penicillin.

Outlook

• St Vitus's Dance is becoming increasingly rare, as is rheumatic fever. Symptoms may cause alarm but have no lasting effect on the body unless there is carditis.

See NERVOUS SYSTEM *page 34*

SALIVARY GLANDS— INFECTIONS, STONES AND TUMOURS

The salivary glands control the flow of saliva to the mouth. There are three pairs. The largest are the parotids, just below and in front of the ear, with ducts issuing into the mouth near the upper back teeth. The two smaller pairs lie under the tongue and the jaw. Their ducts empty below the tongue.

Stones and non-cancerous tumours may form in a gland and may block the duct to the mouth. Stones are sharp stony masses, generally formed from calcium salts present in the body's fluids.

Symptoms

• Swelling or discomfort may occur in any of the glands,

though it is most common in the parotids. Infection is rare, except in the case of infectious parotitis, a virus disease better known under its household name of MUMPS.
• Stones exhibit no symptoms unless they move from the gland to block the duct. The gland may swell visibly and uncomfortably as saliva is produced but cannot drain into the mouth.
• A tumour appears as a solitary, hard lump, with similar symptoms.

Duration
• Both stones and tumours are likely to persist unless treated.

Causes
• Not known, in either case.

Complications
• There are not usually any complications.

Treatment in the home
• Avoid sharp, acid food and drinks such as those containing lemon or vinegar. These stimulate saliva production which will increase the swelling and discomfort.
• Clean the teeth and rinse the mouth thoroughly to avoid bacterial infection of the glands.

When to consult the doctor
• Whenever swelling of the glands occurs.

What the doctor may do
• If the swelling is caused by a stone, the doctor may be able to manipulate it with his finger and 'milk' it out of the duct.
• If this fails, the doctor may advise surgical treatment to release it. A small incision will be made, in hospital, to release the stone.
• If the swelling is caused by a tumour, surgery may also be advised.

Prevention
• None.

Outlook
• A stone is easily removed by surgery; healing is rapid and recovery complete.
• Generally, removing a tumour will also be a very minor operation, though the tumour may recur if any of the affected tissue is left in the gland.

See DIGESTIVE SYSTEM *page 44*

SALK VACCINE

A preparation that provides immunisation against poliomyelitis (polio). The injectable vaccine—containing living but weakened viruses which stimulate the body to produce antibodies against the disease—was devised in 1954 by the American virologist Jonas Salk (1914–   ).
See POLIOMYELITIS

SALPINGITIS

An infection of the Fallopian tube that links ovary and womb, which are often also infected. Infections may be acute or chronic. The condition is also known as pelvic inflammatory disease.

ACUTE SALPINGITIS

Symptoms
• Pain in the lower abdomen, can be severe and may be either colicky or continuous.
• Vaginal discharge.
• High temperature.
• Vomiting.

Duration
• The condition lasts only a few days if treated correctly.

Causes
• The infection may be caused by many different bacteria, including, sometimes, a venereal bacteria, the gonococcus, which causes gonorrhoea.
• Occasionally follows pregnancy or ABORTION.

Complications
• The infections may become chronic and cause scarring which can block the Fallopian tube causing infertility.

Treatment in the home
• Rest in bed.
• Take a simple painkiller in recommended doses.
• Avoid intercourse, as this may be painful or spread the infection.

When to consult the doctor
• If the symptoms described occur.
• If the right tube is affected the condition requires early advice to distinguish it from acute APPENDICITIS.

What the doctor may do
• Examine the abdomen by pressing it with his hands.
• Carry out an INTERNAL PELVIC EXAMINATION.
• Take a swab of vaginal discharge to discover which bacteria is causing the infection.
• Prescribe antibiotics. *See* MEDICINES, 25.
• Admit to hospital for observation if there is doubt about the diagnosis.

Prevention
• Avoid promiscuity.

Outlook
• Good if treated early.

CHRONIC SALPINGITIS

Symptoms
• Persistent or recurring pain in the lower abdomen.

• Persistent vaginal discharge.
• Pain during sexual intercourse.
• Heavy, and sometimes irregular periods.

Duration
• The condition can last for months and is difficult to diagnose.

Causes
• An acute infection that has not been treated correctly.
• Tuberculosis.
• In many cases no obvious cause is found. Contraceptive coils (IUD) may increase the chance of developing the disease.

Complications
• Infertility if both tubes are affected.

Treatment in the home
• As for acute salpingitis.

When to consult the doctor
• If the symptoms described occur.

What the doctor may do
• As for acute salpingitis. He is, however, more likely to refer the patient to a gynaecologist.

Outlook
• Even with full treatment, symptoms occasionally persist for several months.

See FEMALE GENITAL SYSTEM *page 48*

SANDFLY FEVER

A virus disease, known medically as phlebotomus fever, occurring in the Middle East and Central Asia during the hot, dry months of summer and autumn. It is transmitted by infected female sandflies which usually bite during the night. The flies are small and can easily pass through protective insect screens. Symptoms are headache, fever and muscle pains, which develop about three days after the bite, but most bites are painless and so go unnoticed.

The fever persists for about three days, then the patient gradually recovers, although he may be left feeling weak and depressed and suffer a second attack between two and 12 weeks later. There is no specific treatment, but rest in bed, plenty of drinks and painkillers in doses recommended on the container will help recovery, which is always complete.
See INFECTIOUS DISEASES *page 32*

SARCOMA

A malignant (cancerous) tumour of connective tissue, which includes bones, cartilage, muscles, tendons and ligaments.
See CANCER

SCABIES

Commonly known as 'the itch', scabies is a highly contagious skin disease due to infestation by the mite *Sarcoptes scabiei* which burrows into the skin. The sites usually attacked are between the fingers, the insides of the wrist, the palms of the hands, the soles of the feet and the penis.

Symptoms
- Very itchy pimples which appear anywhere on the body about three or four weeks after the burrows have been made. Itching is usually severe and worse at night.
- Sores develop where the itching pimples are scratched.
- Skin-coloured or greyish ridges $\frac{1}{8}$-$\frac{3}{8}$ in. (3-10 mm.) long, where the mite burrows in.

Duration
- If untreated the condition becomes chronic with persistent scratching, producing inflammation and coarsening of the skin.
- The itch may take ten days to settle after treatment.

Causes
- A parasite (the scabies mite) which lives only on human skin. The female mite is fertilised on the skin surface and then burrows into the skin to lay eggs. The eggs hatch in four days and the mature mite emerges on to the skin surface ten days later.
- The itching and pimples are due to an allergy to the mite, the eggs and the larvae.
- Close bodily contact, sharing of beds or clothing.

Treatment in the home
- Anti-scabies lotions are available from chemists.
- Calamine lotion will ease itching.

When to consult the doctor
- If there is a persisting skin irritation and rash.

What the doctor may do
- Take a scraping from a burrow to confirm the diagnosis under a microscope.
- Prescribe a course of treatment using benzyl benzoate emulsion or gamma benzene hexachloride not only for the patient but for all members of the household or community. This is necessary since scabies is highly contagious and quickly spreads by direct contact from person to person. *See* MEDICINES, 43.
- Prescribe an antibacterial cream for the infected pimples when the parasite has been killed.

Prevention
- Avoid overcrowding, especially sharing a bed with a sufferer.
- To prevent reinfection, kill the mites and larvae by laundering all clothes and bedding, and treat all the sufferers in a single household at the same time.

Outlook
- Scabies is easily cured, but recurrences may be difficult to prevent, particularly in overcrowded conditions.

See SKIN *page 52*

SCALP
The layer of skin and muscle protecting the skull. Symptoms affecting the scalp include ITCHING, scaling, loss of hair (*see* BALDNESS) and lumps.
See SYMPTOM SORTER—SCALP

SCARLET FEVER

A highly infectious disease caused by bacteria called *Streptococcus pyogenes*—the same germ that causes tonsillitis, pharyngitis and impetigo. The infection is spread by close physical contact and germ-laden air breathed out by patients. The main danger of the disease is its complications, but most patients recover from scarlet fever without any trouble. Patients should be kept isolated for seven days from the onset of the disease.

Symptoms
- Sore throat.
- A rash of tiny spots, which feels like sandpaper and turns white when pressed, begins on the neck and chest and spreads over the whole body, two days after the onset of the sore throat. The rash is worse along skin folds.
- Fever.
- Vomiting.
- The face is flushed, but the area round the lips may be pale.
- The tongue may be coated white, with patches of red (strawberry tongue).
- The skin may peel when the rash clears.

Incubation period
- Two to four days—sometimes longer.

Duration
- One or two weeks.
- The rash usually lasts four or five days.

Causes
- Bacteria.

Complications
- RHEUMATIC FEVER (acute rheumatism).
- OTITIS MEDIA.
- NEPHRITIS (inflammation of the kidneys).

Treatment in the home
- Keep the patient in bed.
- Give plenty of cool drinks.
- Give fever-reducing tablets in doses recommended on the container.

When to consult the doctor
- Within a day or two if you suspect scarlet fever.

What the doctor may do
- Prescribe a course of antibiotics to help prevent complications. The course should start within nine days of the onset of the sore throat. The antibiotics may not make much difference to the progress of the scarlet fever itself, as this gets better on its own. *See* MEDICINES, 25.

Prevention
- There is no effective immunisation against scarlet fever.

Outlook
- Most people recover from scarlet fever without complications.
- One attack of scarlet fever does not make the patient immune to further infections by the streptococcus.

See INFECTIOUS DISEASES *page 32*

SCHISTOSOMIASIS
A parasitic disease, also known as bilharziasis, caused by flukes (flatworms) called schistosomas, which live in the blood of human beings and animals in tropical and subtropical countries. The flukes, which are about $\frac{1}{2}$ in. (13 mm.) long, lay eggs which are excreted in the urine or faeces of the infected person. When the eggs reach water they hatch and the undeveloped larvae find their way into snails living in the contaminated water. When the developed larvae are released from the snails they can penetrate the skin of humans or animals bathing or wading in the water, and the cycle begins again.

Over 200 million people in more than 70 countries suffer from the disease. The blood vessels of the bowel, bladder, spleen, liver, lungs and brain may all be involved, producing a variety of symptoms which include diarrhoea, abdominal pain on passing water and blood in the urine and bowels.

Treatment, which is effective, is with antimony-containing drugs, but careful hygiene and separation of sewage from irrigation ditches are necessary to prevent the disease. Attempts to destroy the infection by using chemicals in the water and by mass-treatment of the population have not proved entirely successful.
See INFECTIOUS DISEASES *page 32*

Safety in the home

A ROOM-BY-ROOM GUIDE TO ELIMINATING ACCIDENT BLACK-SPOTS AND POTENTIAL HEALTH HAZARDS AROUND THE HOUSE

A million people go to hospital in Britain every year because of accidents in the home. And over 6,000 victims of home accidents die—about the same number as die on the roads. Non-fatal accidents can mean confinement to hospital, or permanent scarring or disability. Even the most minor accidents can cause a great deal of pain. Home accidents have an enormous number of causes, and not everyone faces the same risks. Types of accidents depend on the age of the person involved and the layout of the home.

Safety symbols to look for

☐ Many household products are manufactured to standards set by the British Standards Institution. Some items will have the letters BS followed by a number. Others will bear the British Standards kitemark or safety mark.

☐ Electrical products may also be tested by the British Electrotechnical Approvals Board.

☐ The symbols below signify that any new products bearing them have been made to safe standards.

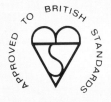

BRITISH
STANDARDS INSTITUTION
KITEMARK

BRITISH
STANDARDS INSTITUTION
SAFETY MARK

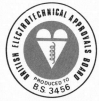

B.E.A.B. APPROVAL SEAL
(BRITISH ELECTROTECHNICAL
APPROVALS BOARD)

BABIES AND TODDLERS

Small babies are in special danger of choking on something they have swallowed. So they must never be left alone when feeding, and small objects such as buttons and peanuts must be kept out of their reach.

Toddlers must be protected from hazards such as playing with matches, pulling unstable furniture or a hanging table-cloth down on themselves, and poisoning—the commonest accident in this age group. Medicines and household cleaners must be kept out of reach.

SOCKET SAFETY PLUGS *Electricity sockets should have safety plugs to stop small children electrocuting themselves.*

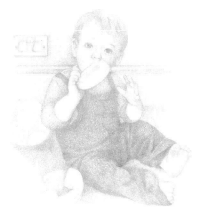

SECURE ALL WINDOWS
Catches should be fitted to windows and replaced if faulty. Chains stop pivoting windows from opening and wooden blocks secure sash windows.

Scalding is another hazard for the toddler. Be very careful when handling hot liquids or food near them, and never pass hot liquids over their heads. A cup of hot tea can scar a child for life. Make sure that a toddler cannot reach the flex of an electric kettle, and keep teapots well away from the edge of the table.

Keep power-driven electrical appliances such as drills, food mixers and hair dryers away from toddlers— carelessly handled, they can cause physical injury and electric shocks.

A toddler's balance is not very good, and as they fall, they may grab or push anything left low enough—a heavy vase, or a pot of coffee.

SCHOOL-AGE CHILDREN

Children over the age of five are likely to rush about, perhaps falling against glass doors. Ordinary glass in doors can be dangerous at any age, because it breaks into sharp shards. If you can afford it, replace ordinary glass with safety glass (toughened or laminated). Or cover it with a DIY plastic film which stops the glass from scattering.

Closed glass doors can be difficult to see, so mark them with coloured adhesive tape or transfers.

Do not let children run about with scissors or knives, or with pencils in

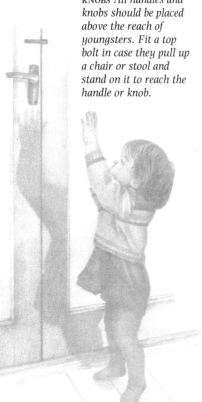

DOOR HANDLES AND KNOBS All handles and knobs should be placed above the reach of youngsters. Fit a top bolt in case they pull up a chair or stool and stand on it to reach the handle or knob.

their mouths. Discourage them from carrying bottles and other glass articles. Wrap broken glass in newspaper and put it in the dustbin.

ADULTHOOD

The years from young adulthood to late middle age are those in which most people run a home and become involved with mains electricity.

Electrical appliances are major labour-saving aids, but unless maintained and handled with care, they can be dangerous. High-speed power tools may be particularly hazardous, causing injury and electric shocks.

If possible, buy appliances with the plugs already attached. This reduces the possibility of incorrect wiring or the wrong fuse being fitted.

Always unplug an appliance before cleaning it or doing any maintenance work.

Never plug appliances into lighting sockets. They can overload the wiring system and cause a fire.

When lengthening a lead or mending a damaged flex, use a proper connector.

Before changing a fuse in the main fuse box, switch off the electricity at the mains, and use wire of the gauge recommended for the circuit.

Gas installations, repairs and maintenance should all be carried out by a Gas Board engineer, or by a firm registered with the Confederation of Registered Gas Installers (CORGI).

Many of the products used in 'do-it-yourself' jobs are hazards. Turpentine, methylated spirit, caustic soda and cyanoacrylate glues, for example, are all poisonous. If there are children about, such materials—as well as tools—must be locked away.

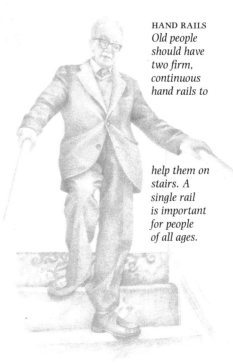

STEP LADDERS If you have to climb when working about the house—for instance, when changing a light bulb—use a firm pair of ladders, not a chair or stool. Use step ladders if you have to climb when working in the garden.

HAZARDS OF OLD AGE

With a failing sense of smell, an elderly person is less likely to detect a fire or gas leak. With failing eyesight, stairs become a special hazard. With forgetfulness, old people may leave articles such as shoes where they or others can trip over them, or turn on the gas and fail to light it. Such problems are made worse when rheumatism makes an old person clumsy, or when he is taking drugs.

Falls happen to everyone—they are the second most common cause of home accidents—but elderly

people are particularly vulnerable. Install sufficient electricity points to avoid trailing flexes and make sure that there is adequate lighting. Carpet should be held down with metal strips where it ends or meets with another carpet, as in doorways. Or at least, if the edges of carpet or linoleum become frayed, trim them so that they do not cause people to trip. Make sure that floor tiles are glued down firmly.

Elderly people living on their own may urgently need help if they have an accident. Even a minor injury may have serious consequences if it is not treated. To avoid hazards, old people should have regular visitors, a telephone or an alarm system connected to a neighbour's home.

HAND RAILS Old people should have two firm, continuous hand rails to help them on stairs. A single rail is important for people of all ages.

WHERE ACCIDENTS HAPPEN

The most dangerous parts of the house are the living-room and dining area (often the same), the kitchen and the garden. Nearly half of all home accidents occur in these places.

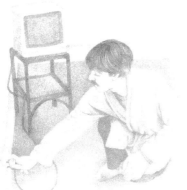

TV SET *At bedtime, switch off and unplug your television set. Otherwise, if faulty, it may catch fire.*

THE LIVING-ROOM AND DINING AREA

Table-cloths are tempting to toddlers and small children. As they tug, they may bring down hot liquids or heavy objects on top of themselves.

Do not hang mirrors over fireplaces. The clothes of a person leaning forward to look in the mirror could catch fire.

If possible, buy furniture that is upholstered with traditional horsehair and springs. Most modern upholstery is made of polyurethane foam, which is cheaper. When it burns, the fumes can overcome a victim in two or three minutes. New furniture must now either pass a test to prove it can resist a burning cigarette, or it must carry a warning label.

THE KITCHEN

Cooking is potentially the most dangerous activity in the house as it involves heat and is attractive to children.

Some electric rings stay black when hot, and children should be warned of this. When the oven is on, even the outside of a cooker can burn a baby's tender skin.

Do not fit wall cupboards or shelves over a cooker—reaching up to them while you are cooking can cause your clothes to catch fire.

Do not dry tea-towels over the cooker, where they may start to smoulder.

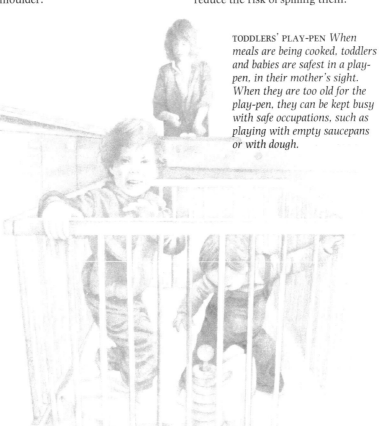

TODDLERS' PLAY-PEN *When meals are being cooked, toddlers and babies are safest in a play-pen, in their mother's sight. When they are too old for the play-pen, they can be kept busy with safe occupations, such as playing with empty saucepans or with dough.*

Chip-pan fires are the most common kitchen fire. Never fill the pan more than one-third full of fat. Always turn off the heat when you have finished cooking.

Try not to position the cooker next to a window. If it is unavoidable, make sure that the curtains are not made of flammable material. Do not place a gas cooker near a door. The pilot light or a burner may be blown out by a sudden draught.

Arrange your work surfaces as close as possible to the cooker. By reducing the distances over which hot food and liquids are carried, you reduce the risk of spilling them.

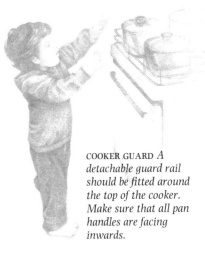

COOKER GUARD *A detachable guard rail should be fitted around the top of the cooker. Make sure that all pan handles are facing inwards.*

More electrical appliances are used in the kitchen than anywhere else. Make sure that the flex of an electric kettle is out of a toddler's reach.

Never leave the iron on when you are called away. When the ironing is finished, unplug the iron and leave it to cool out of the reach of children.

Do not operate electric switches with wet hands—this can cause a severe shock, since moisture is an excellent conductor of electricity. Position switches and sockets away from wet areas such as the sink.

Do not position sockets so that flexes trail over the cooker.

Keep plastic bags safely away from small children. They are likely to put them over their heads, and run the risk of suffocation.

Never put a baby's bouncing cradle on a work-top or table. It may shift as the baby bounces, and fall on the floor.

Many accidents involve household cleaners. Never keep bleach, oven cleaner, caustic soda, turpentine or methylated spirit under the sink. Most are poisonous, some can damage the skin or eyes, and others are highly flammable. They should be stored in a lockable cupboard out of the reach of children.

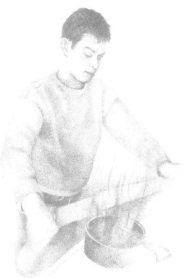

PAN FIRE *If a pan catches fire, do not try to move it. Turn off the heat and cover the pan with a damp cloth.*

Never keep cleaners with food, or in food containers such as jam-jars and squash bottles. Children may assume that they still contain food or drink, and swallow the contents.

When using an aerosol, be careful to spray in the direction indicated by the pointer. People with poor sight should be especially careful.

Never throw an empty aerosol on a fire, where it may explode.

Never mix bleach with other toilet cleaners, as a poisonous gas may be given off.

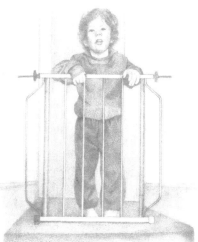

SAFETY GATES *To prevent babies of crawling age and toddlers from climbing stairs, safety gates should be put at the top and bottom.*

THE STAIRCASE

Teach toddlers to climb down stairs safely—backwards, on all fours.

Make sure that staircases, and even single steps, are well lit. Shadows and dark areas can lead elderly people into a misjudgment, and a bad fall.

Keep stairs free of toys and other articles. Check for loose or fraying carpet, to prevent tripping.

Do not have a glass door at the bottom of a staircase—anyone falling downstairs and crashing into it could break it, and suffer cuts as well as other injuries.

If you have young children in the house, avoid horizontal banister (or balcony) rails. They are inviting 'ladders'. Children's heads can also get stuck between them, and babies can crawl underneath and fall.

Staircases with open, ladder-type steps can be dangerous. Young children may slip down between the treads, and old people, feeling insecure, may stumble.

BATHROOM AND TOILET

If you have a modern gas water-heater, it will have a balanced flue through an external wall, but many older types are still in use. Both need regular checking by a Gas Board engineer or registered gas installer. The advantage of the balanced flue is that it gets its air from outside, and does not, like older heaters, use the air from the bathroom itself. With older heaters a door or window should be open when you draw off hot water. This will prevent a build-up of poisonous carbon-monoxide gas if the flue gets blocked and waste gases stay in the room. If you have an airbrick or any other kind of ventilation let into the wall or window-pane make sure that it is kept clear of dirt and obstruction.

Never bring a portable electrical appliance, such as a heater or hair dryer, into a bathroom. As moisture is an excellent conductor of electricity, wet bodies are especially vulnerable to electric shock. Electric shavers are the only exception as

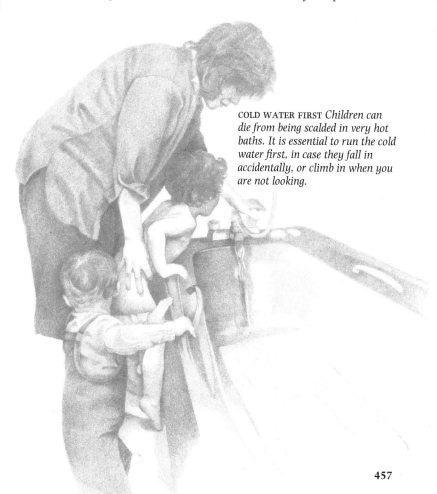

COLD WATER FIRST *Children can die from being scalded in very hot baths. It is essential to run the cold water first, in case they fall in accidentally, or climb in when you are not looking.*

they use a special socket with an isolating transformer.

Electric bathroom heaters must be wired-in, and have a cord pull-switch—as should the light switch—so that there is no direct contact between the hand and the switch.

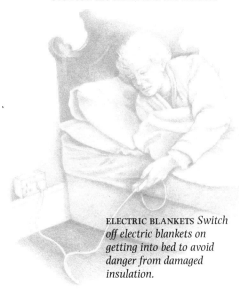

ELECTRIC BLANKETS *Switch off electric blankets on getting into bed to avoid danger from damaged insulation.*

If there are small children in the house, medicines must be locked up at all times.

Most medicines are now in containers with child-resistant closures. Do not transfer medicines to an easily opened container.

Dispose of old, left-over medicines, particularly if they have lost their labels and are unidentifiable. Either flush them down the lavatory or return them to the chemist.

Children can drown in very little water. Never leave a baby or toddler alone in the bathroom. If the telephone or the doorbell rings, take the baby with you, wrapped in a towel to protect it from draughts.

To prevent children and old people slipping, the bath should have a non-slip interior finish or a rubber bathmat in the bottom. A grab rail fixed to the bath or to the wall is a welcome aid to old people. Many local authorities have an occupational therapist who can advise old or disabled people about such aids.

If there are small children in the house, bolts on the inside of toilet and bathroom doors should be fitted high out of reach, and keys should be removed. Otherwise children may lock themselves in.

THE BEDROOM

Do not put babies to bed or to sleep with anything that can catch round their necks, such as ribbon on a cardigan, or a string on a dummy. They could be strangled.

To avoid scalds, never leave a hot-water bottle in the bed after putting young children or old people to sleep.

When using electric under-blankets follow the maker's instructions. Fold electric blankets loosely, and do not place anything on them, otherwise the insulation may crack. Have electric blankets checked by the maker every two years. Do not buy a second-hand electric blanket unless the maker has checked it.

A radiant heater in a child's or old person's bedroom should be fixed to the wall. People of all ages should avoid flowing nightwear if there are radiant fires in the bedroom. Pyjamas are safer than nightdresses. Nightwear should be made of fire-resistant fabrics.

Smoking in bed is dangerous for everyone in the house—especially if it is done by forgetful elderly people, and anyone who has taken alcohol or sleeping-pills before going to bed.

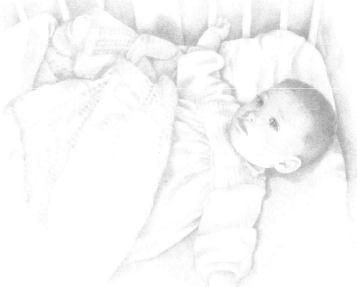

AVOIDING COT SUFFOCATION *Young babies in their cots are in danger of suffocating because they cannot easily turn over. So no baby under 12 months should be given a pillow. For older babies, specially designed safety pillows are available from baby equipment shops.*

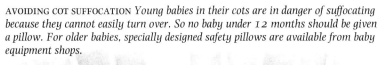

CAT NET *Fit a cat net over a pram or cot in the garden so that a cat cannot lie on the baby's face and smother it.*

OUTSIDE THE HOUSE

Shallow water is as dangerous to toddlers in the garden as it is in the bathroom. If you have a garden pool, turn it into a sand-pit, or cover it with strong mesh so that small children cannot accidentally fall in and drown.

All sharp garden tools can be dangerous, particularly to children. After use, store them in a locked shed or cupboard.

The most common accident with electric mowers happens when the user forgets that the blades continue to rotate for some time after the power has been switched off.

Power tools for the garden are often used in wet conditions, so they must be even more carefully maintained than power tools used indoors. Always unplug electrically powered tools before making adjustments to them.

COPING WITH HOME INJURIES

For advice on how to deal with injuries in the home, *see* FIRST AID page 540.

GETTING HELP WITH PARTICULAR PROBLEMS

If you have specific questions about making your home safe that are not answered on these pages, your local council might employ a Home Safety Officer who will help. Or one of the council's Environmental Health Inspectors might also give advice. The council's Trading Standards Officer will want to know of any products which you find unsafe in use.

The Health Education Officer with your District Health Authority will have safety information on alcohol and smoking in the home.

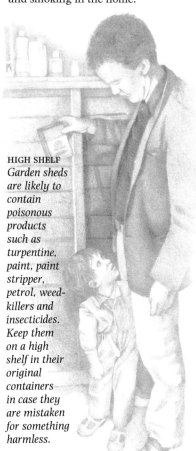

HIGH SHELF *Garden sheds are likely to contain poisonous products such as turpentine, paint, paint stripper, petrol, weed-killers and insecticides. Keep them on a high shelf in their original containers in case they are mistaken for something harmless.*

How to avoid fire in the home

☐ Always store matches well out of the reach of children, preferably in a locked cupboard. Remember that a determined child will drag a chair to a cupboard and climb up.

☐ Always use ashtrays to dispose of cigarettes—never waste-paper baskets that might contain flammable materials.

☐ Remember that smoking in bed is dangerous, particularly if the smoker has had an alcoholic drink or has taken sleeping-pills.

☐ Keep electrical wiring and appliances in good order. If you have sockets that take plugs with round pins, your wiring is old and should be checked.

☐ Do not overload power points with multi-way adaptors; it can cause fire in the wiring. Install more power points instead.

☐ If you buy a second-hand electrical or gas heater have it checked by a service engineer before it is installed.

FIXED FIREGUARD Fit a fireguard around all open or radiant fires. The guard should cover the entire fireplace, not just the fire. It should be fixed to the wall with secure fastenings that a child cannot undo. It should stand at a sufficient distance from the fire to prevent bits of paper poked through by children from catching alight.

☐ Never leave a young child alone in a room with a fire.

☐ Do not air or dry clothes round a convector heater or radiant fire, or put them on a storage heater.

☐ Never store rags or old newspapers near a fire or heater.

☐ Keep furniture, curtains and bedding well away from fires and heaters.

☐ Keep paraffin heaters away from doors, where they may be upset.

☐ Never move paraffin heaters when they are alight, and turn them off before filling them.

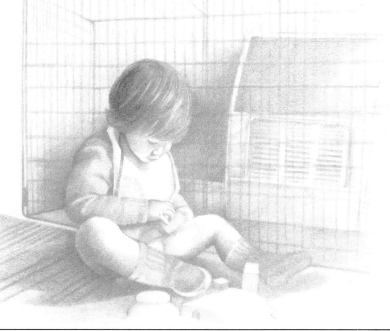

☐ Store paraffin out of doors.

☐ Ensure that gas appliances are checked by the Gas Board every year. The greatest danger is from carbon-monoxide poisoning if the flues are blocked.

☐ Do not leave keys in gas taps if there are children about.

☐ If you use solid fuel, have the chimney swept every year.

☐ Do not bank solid-fuel fires too high, in case soot catches fire or burning fuel falls out.

☐ Finally, close internal doors at night, just in case of fire.

SCHIZOPHRENIA

A serious mental illness or psychosis in which the sufferer lives in a dream world and feels threatened when faced by real people and real decisions of everyday life.

It has four sub groups, called hebephrenia, catatonic, paranoid and simple schizophrenia, which differ slightly from each other.

The sufferer has no insight into his own condition and therefore may require compulsory hospital treatment. It affects about one person in 1,000 and usually occurs for the first time between the ages of 18 and 30. Schizophrenic behaviour may be thought grossly abnormal by others, but will be considered perfectly acceptable by the sufferer.

Symptoms
- The sufferer's conversation may be unreal and disturbing to the listener.
- Thoughts and perceptions are odd and distorted and often imply persecution of the patient.
- The sufferer may hear voices, see visions, have irrational beliefs and delusions.
- Inappropriate emotional responses to situations. Sufferers may show no response or laugh at bad news.

WATCHING THE BRAIN AT WORK
The PETT scan gives new insight into the mind

The PETT III scanner shows the brain at work, unlike surgery and the CT scanner which can only show what it looks like. The brain gets its energy from glucose, and the harder it works the more it consumes. By feeding the brain with mildly radioactive glucose, then recording the different levels of consumption in each part of the brain, a picture of the brain working is created. This is done by the PETT III (Positron Emission Transaxial Tomography), which detects the radioactivity and registers it on a screen. Different conditions of the brain show different patterns of activity.

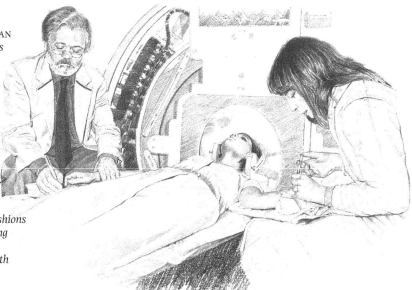

PREPARING FOR A SCAN
Radioactive glucose is injected into the patient's arm and given time to travel through to the brain. Anyone having a scan is exposed to very little radiation because the mixture is only radioactive for a very short time. The patient lies on a couch with her head held still by foam cushions in the circular opening of the scanner—a large disc covered with radiation detectors.

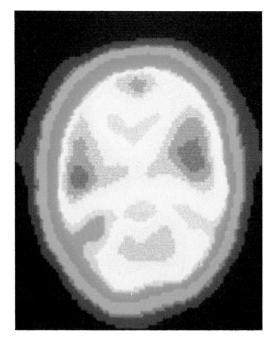

THE NORMAL BRAIN *The PETT III scans the brain in horizontal sections. These four scans show the same section in four different people. The picture is colour coded to show the rate at which brain tissue is consuming glucose. Blues are the areas of lowest activity, then the scale goes through green and yellow to white—the area of highest activity. In a normal brain, activity is roughly symmetrical.*

- Behaviour may be bizarre.
- The sufferer may be agitated and may behave in an antisocial or even violent way.

Duration
- Acute episodes can last a few weeks or longer.
- Some people have only a single attack but often there is a tendency for the condition to recur after a long normal period.
- The condition may become permanent or progress slowly over the years with distressing results.

Causes
- No cause is known; chemical factors and inheritance may play a part.

Treatment in the home
- None. Seek early medical advice if symptoms of schizophrenia are suspected.
- Delusions and hallucinations appear real to sufferers. Attempts to persuade them otherwise tend to upset them.

When to consult the doctor
- If the condition is suspected.
- If abnormal behaviour is disturbing the family.

What the doctor may do
- Confirm the diagnosis and prescribe drugs.
- If the patient is disturbed the doctor may arrange for the patient to see a specialist or be admitted to hospital.

See MENTAL SYSTEM *page 33*

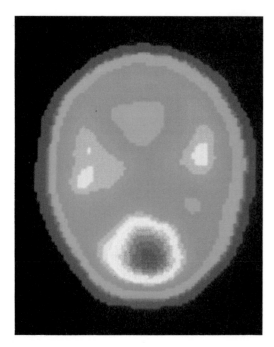

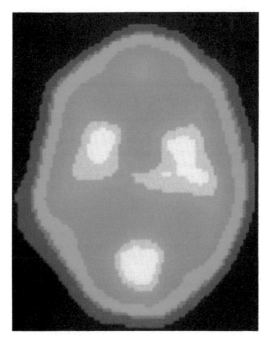

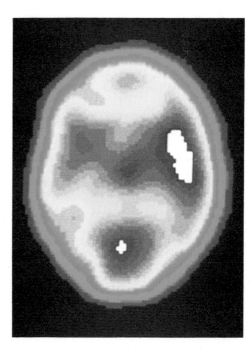

DEMENTIA *Patients suffering from dementia show a characteristic picture when scanned. The pattern of activity remains roughly symmetrical, but there is an overall reduction in activity compared to the normal brain pattern—much more green and blue. The more advanced the state of dementia, the lower the activity. Dementia usually strikes the elderly and patients show forgetfulness, confusion and delusions.*

SCHIZOPHRENIA *The brain scan of a schizophrenic patient shows a reduced level of activity overall compared with normal. The front of the brain (top), thought to be one of the areas involved in control of the emotions, consumes glucose at a particularly low rate. The outward signs of schizophrenia may sometimes be confusing. The PETT system makes diagnosis much simpler and less liable to error.*

MANIC DEPRESSION *So far it has only been possible to obtain a scan for the manic phase of manic depression, but that is very distinctive, especially when compared with a scan of schizophrenia with which it is sometimes confused. The pattern is asymmetrical, with the whole brain showing a much higher rate of activity than normal. This coincides with periods of wild elation and action.*

SCIATICA

One of the many common forms of back trouble. It may result from any abnormal pressure on any part of the sciatic nerve, which runs down the legs from its roots in the lower back. Such pressure usually arises in the spine itself from a SLIPPED DISC. The pain may start suddenly after lifting something heavy, or straightening up after bending. Sometimes the onset is more gradual and follows a series of worsening attacks in which there is no apparent cause.

See BACK PAIN

SCOLIOSIS

Sideways curvature of the spine. Scoliosis may be structural, beginning in childhood or adolescence and increasing until growth stops; or the result of an attempt to relieve pain in the spine, caused for example by a SLIPPED DISC; or present from birth; or the result of disease such as POLIOMYELITIS. Most cases improve by themselves, but the more severe may require plaster jackets and operations.

SCURVY

A vitamin deficiency disease. Scurvy is the result of a lack of vitamin C (ascorbic acid) in the diet. Vitamin C is present in fresh fruit, especially oranges, grapefruit and lemons, and also in vegetables such as cabbages and potatoes, overcooking destroys it. An ordinary mixed diet contains adequate supplies of vitamin C. Those who are most likely to suffer from a deficiency include the homeless, alcoholics, lonely housebound women, and bottle-fed babies.

Vitamin C is essential to maintain the connecting tissue in the skin, muscles and the lining of the blood vessels. Without it, the blood vessels are weakened and cause general bruising under the skin of the legs and arms, and severe infection of the gums in children and adults. Anaemia eventually develops and without treatment the outlook is poor.

Scurvy is prevented by keeping to a balanced diet with plenty of fresh fruit and lightly cooked vegetables. At one time sailors were particularly prone to the disease because of weeks and months spent without fresh fruit and vegetables. The disease was prevented when the navy issued rations of lime juice to all sailors.

Established scurvy is treated with large doses of vitamin C tablets, but once the deficiency has been corrected arrangements must be made to ensure a continuing supply of the vitamin.

SEA-SICKNESS

Nausea and vomiting suffered by some people when travelling by sea, caused by a disturbance of the inner ear.

See MOTION SICKNESS

SEASONAL AFFECTIVE DISORDER

Recurrent cyclic bouts of depression during the winter months. Sufferers, 80 per cent of whom are women, complain of tiredness, a craving for carbohydrates, and weight gain. SAD is associated with seasonal changes in day length. Exposure to bright light for several hours daily to simulate natural sunlight may help in alleviating symptoms. Appetite suppressants or stimulants may also be helpful.

SEBACEOUS CYST

Cysts are common in the sebaceous (oil-bearing) glands of the skin. There are two kinds: the epidermal cyst, which can appear anywhere on the body and easily becomes infected, and the pilar cyst, which usually appears on the scalp and is not generally infected.

EPIDERMAL CYST
Symptoms
- A small painless lump 1-2 in. (25-50 mm.) across usually starts in young adults where there has been severe acne, but it may occur anywhere.
- The lump enlarges over a period of years to form a dome-shaped swelling 2-3 in. (50-75 mm.) in diameter.
- The cysts may become painful, inflamed and infected, containing much pus.

Duration
- The cyst will last for ever unless it is removed.

Causes
- This is not known, but any damage to the skin, such as acne or an accident, may cause cysts to form.

Treatment in the home
- If the cyst is infected, apply a hot compress of magnesium sulphate (Epsom salts). One heaped teaspoon to 10 fl. oz. (300 ml.) of water, about every hour, to bring the infection to a head.
- When the cyst bursts, cover it with a clean dry dressing. Be sure to change the dressing frequently.
- Do not attempt to remove the cyst by squeezing. This will only encourage infection.

When to consult the doctor
- If it is not certain what caused the lump.
- If there is repeated infection.
- If the sufferer wishes to have the cyst removed.

What the doctor may do
- Treat any infection.
- Send the patient to hospital to have the cyst removed surgically. Successful removal requires all the wall to be taken away. This is usually not difficult, but it is better to do it when the cyst is not infected.

Prevention
- None is known.

Outlook
- The cyst will not disappear on its own, but it may never enlarge. If it is completely removed surgically it will not recur.
- An infected cyst may shrink as the infection clears, but it is likely to erupt again.

PILAR CYST
Symptoms
- Little painless lumps appear, usually on the scalp, and gradually enlarge to dome-shaped swellings, which cause embarrassment and easily catch in a comb.

Duration
- The cyst will last until it is surgically removed.

Causes
- Not really known, but pilar cysts tend to run in families.

Treatment in the home
- No action is necessary apart from a suitable hair-style to hide the cyst.

When to consult the doctor
- To seek advice about removal.

What the doctor may do
- Send the patient to hospital to have the cyst surgically removed.

Prevention
- None is known.

Outlook
- Pilar cysts very gradually enlarge over many years, but once removed, they do not recur.

See SKIN *page 52*

SEBORRHOEA

Excessively greasy skin. The condition by itself needs no

medical treatment but it may lead to ACNE or ECZEMA. It is often accompanied by DANDRUFF.

Symptoms
- The skin becomes very greasy at puberty.

Duration
- Seborrhoea is generally a lifelong condition.

Causes
- The cause is unknown, but the skin changes are thought to follow increases in the secretion of the sex hormones.

Treatment in the home
- The skin should be washed often with a mild soap. A skin-drying lotion may also be used.
- Oily or creamy cosmetics aggravate the condition and should be avoided.

When to consult the doctor
- There is no need to see a doctor unless acne or eczema develops.

Prevention
- The greasiness can often be reduced by not eating dairy produce or sweetstuffs, particularly chocolate.

See SKIN *page 52*

SEBORRHOEIC WARTS

These are brown or black with a rough, greasy surface which makes them look as though they are stuck on to the skin. They occur after middle age and usually start as a brown thickening of the skin—anything from $\frac{1}{8}$-1 in. (3-25 mm.) across—which can be scraped off at first with a finger-nail, but then gets thicker. They develop on any part of the body, except the palms of the hands and soles of the feet, and gradually increase in size and number with age. It is not known what causes them, but they tend to run in families. They are not painful or itchy and never cancerous. If they catch on clothing cover them with a plaster.
See WARTS

SEROLOGY

The study of blood serum and its components for use in diagnosing infectious diseases and in providing protection for the body against them.

SERUM SICKNESS

An allergic reaction to an injection of serum. It usually occurs 7-12 days after the injection and is marked by nettlerash, joint pains, swollen lymph glands and often mild fever. The condition normally clears up on its own.

SEX PROBLEMS

Society's attitude towards sex has undergone a revolution since the end of the 1950s. Once, it was almost forbidden to discuss the subject. Now, it is relentlessly examined by newspapers, books, radio and television.

Modern methods of birth control mean that for many people the fear of an unwanted pregnancy is no longer a deterrent to sexual intercourse and, partly for that reason, sex before marriage has become the norm for many young people. Even extra-marital sex no longer attracts the disapproval it did.

In all ages and classes, expectations of what sex has to offer are higher than they were a generation ago, particularly among women. Their pursuit of equality in society at large has been mirrored by the feeling that, in love-making, they are no longer man's chattel to do with as he will. They expect to get as much from sex as he does.

But although the changes have brought benefits by lifting some undesirable taboos, they have produced ill-effects, too.

First, publishers and broadcasters, aware of the sales potential of sex-related subjects, have fostered an image of sexual expression and fulfilment which implies that 'good' sex is the right of everyone and is entirely a matter of performance, like an athletic achievement.

Their misleading message is that failure to achieve an orgasm means there is something wrong with one of the partners or with the way they are making love—an emphasis on the purely physical side of sex which has undermined the confidence of many people and caused much distress.

Secondly, the shift from regarding all sexual intercourse outside wedlock as something to be condemned to a situation in which those who do not indulge in it may be looked upon as freaks has created intolerable pressures for some. They feel obliged to indulge, in order to maintain status with friends or colleagues, or because it is fashionable, even though they do not really want to break their own moral code.

Thirdly, the new frankness about sex has encouraged people to discuss their problems and anxieties, which they would formerly have kept secret. That is often beneficial, but it can be harmful if the person's fears are exaggerated by unrealistic expectations from sex. Nearly everybody has occasional worries about sexual performance. The majority are transitory and not significant but a small proportion are enduring and disabling.

SEXUAL AROUSAL

Although men and women are different, and never more so than in their sexual make-up, the bodily events that occur in both sexes during arousal in love play are strikingly similar. They develop in two stages.

Stage one There is a greatly increased flow of blood to the sexual organs—most importantly to the penis in the man and the vaginal areas of the woman. The penis is inside an inelastic capsule, and as the enormous inflow of blood fills the available space, the organ becomes enlarged, lifts, and hardens into an erection.

The vagina swells, but remains soft, because it has no limiting membrane. The clitoris, the rudimentary female penis, becomes erect and acutely sensitive, and so does the surface of the vulva which surrounds it. The walls of the vagina lengthen and bulge and then pour out a clear, lubricating fluid over the internal surfaces and at the opening.

In both sexes, skin around the genitals and often the anus becomes highly sensitive. The heartbeat and breathing quicken, and the pupils of the eyes dilate. The woman's breasts may become sensitive—usually pleasantly, but not always so—and enlarged.

This stage is described as the 'vasocongestive phase' and it is operated by the same control mechanisms in the nervous and endocrine systems of both sexes.

Stage two The natural conclusion of the sex act is the climax or orgasm, but it does not necessarily always follow stage one.

In both men and women, there is an increasing level of arousal which leads to a series of spontaneous, muscular contractions occurring at regular intervals of 0.8 seconds in the penis or the vagina, accompanied by extremely pleasurable erotic sensations.

In the man, the contractions provide the driving force for ejaculation—the emission through the head of the penis of sperm in a series of bursts into the vagina.

The sperm are deposited near the neck of the womb, making fertilisation possible if the couple have taken no contraceptive measures.

There is no similar emission in the woman.

Orgasm is followed in the man by a recovery period, during which the penis loses erection. The length of time before another erection is possible varies from minutes to hours and even days, and from person to person, and from occasion to occasion.

The woman may remain fully aroused after orgasm, and may be capable of a series of orgasms.

PSYCHOLOGICAL INFLUENCE

Sexual arousal is heightened by body contact and deliberate physical stimulation of the sexual organs, but its roots are in the mind. Psychological components arouse desire and affect sexual appetites.

Sexual tastes vary widely. There can be no fixed view of who is an attractive man and who is a desirable woman. Sexual arousal can be affected by a whole range of factors such as: personality, appearance, intelligence, dress, cleanliness, education, cultural background and physical response. Smell can play an important role as a stimulant. Man has created a vast industry to create pleasant smells, partly as a potential for sexual arousal—even blanking out the natural aromas of man and woman which, perhaps, are the most arousing smells of all.

Sexual tastes and frequency of intercourse also depend on the nature and depth of relationship between two people.

SEX DRIVE

This age of the liberated woman has helped to discount one myth, that of the male/female stereotypes. The myth portrays lascivious man in a permanent state of sexual readiness, with exploited woman, suffering under brutish man, but occasionally cajoled to respond.

In fact, there is an enormous variation between individuals, both men and women, in their desire for sex. This libido, or sex drive, is greatly heightened or lessened by the physical, social and psychological factors.

A person's bodily or mental well-being will affect sexual desire and performance. Libido will be excited by the availability of the desired person, and by the opportunity for sex and the setting in which the opportunity arises. Soft lights and sweet music really do stimulate love and set the scene for love-making.

Satisfactory sex and sexual arousal feed on themselves: desire fulfilled stimulates more desire. Similarly, disappointment diminishes desire.

Despite the wide difference in libido and in sexual tastes, vast numbers of couples reach a happy compromise and a level of sexual activity which suits them both. They discover how to arouse each other, what is an acceptable setting for sexual activity and the type of sexual activity acceptable to them both. These balances serve to adjust libido and to make happy sexual relationships possible.

TYPES OF SEXUAL FAILURE

Erection Sexual arousal normally leads to erection in the male, but this natural progression is sometimes interrupted. Failure to achieve erection or to maintain it is a common cause of sexual failure.

Failure may cause anxiety and fear, sometimes amounting to panic. This has a disastrous and repetitive effect, through the fear that failure will occur next time. And it often does, because anxiety has a harmful effect on the mechanism of erection.

The problem worsens and love-making ceases to be a delightful and emotional experience. Erotic and bodily feelings are replaced by fears of failure. As catastrophe follows catastrophe, the unhappy man finds that the very prospect of sexual involvement causes panic, and so it becomes something to avoid. He becomes impotent.

Erection problems can start off as a result of one or two disappointing performances in a man who has previously enjoyed satisfactory sex. Poor performances can occur if there have been stresses between the couple, if the man is over-tired, if he has been drinking heavily, or for many other minor reasons. Deep-seated physical causes are rare. Occasional sexual failures are common among couples and most people can shrug them off or ignore them.

Why then do they lead to long-lasting problems in a few men? The answer probably lies either in the man's personality or in the relationship between the couple.

Some men see every encounter as a trial of physique and any failure as intolerable weakness. A fundamental need to succeed can make a man vulnerable to any erection failure, and can aggravate the damaging effects of anxiety.

If the couple are antagonistic to each other in their daily lives, and he is hoping that improved sexual performance may overcome the hostility, or if her exposure to his problem is to put greater pressure on him and thus increase his feelings of inadequacy, his erection failures may also become habitual.

Often the problem of erection failure is worsened by the reaction of the partner who may feel, in some ill-defined way, to be partly to blame. Is she not attractive enough? Does he no longer find her desirable? Can she not arouse him? This can lead to the woman feeling undesired and rejected. Resentment and hostility can follow. Eventually sex between the couple becomes difficult, or even impossible.

Lubrication The body mechanisms involved in lubrication of the vagina are similar to those which control erection. There are, however, some very important differences. First, erection of the penis, without which intercourse does not happen, is not matched by any such obvious sign in the female.

Secondly, although anxiety about sexual competence and adequacy may affect men and women equally, men with sexual problems tend to worry about trouble with their penises, whereas women do not give their sexual difficulties such a precise focus.

Worries about the way they are made, or about the way they have been damaged, for instance by childbirth, certainly concern women. But female anxieties are less-clearly defined and more subtle than those of men. They are compounded of a mixture of fantasies about what they are like inside—the size, shape, direction or texture of their vagina, or whether it is blocked—and concern about whether their sex drive is too high, too low, or abnormal.

Failure to lubricate is not the 'shop window' of female sexual difficulty, but one of the signs of not being sexually aroused, or of losing arousal. Invariably it is a minor component of a bigger problem. Even if a woman does not lubricate, she can still have sexual intercourse, though it is uncomfortable, or even painful. Non-lubrication is the most common cause of painful intercourse (dyspareunia). Occasionally, it can be accompanied by a more serious condition—vaginal spasm or vaginismus—which may be a complete barrier to intercourse. Any attempt by the male partner to penetrate the vagina is met by an automatic constriction of the vagina. This is usually a response to a fear of being hurt, or, more subtly, to a form of sexual guilt.

Rarely a woman may have a vaginal barrier, such as an unusually tough hymen (the membrane at the opening of the vagina), which needs to be removed surgically. More commonly 'vaginal barriers' are the result of vaginal spasm.

Ejaculation By far the commonest reason for failure of a man to reach a satisfactory climax with his partner is premature ejaculation. This affects, at some time in their lives, a great number of men.

Ejaculation occurs almost immediately after penetration, or even before. In extreme cases there may be erection followed instantly by ejaculation. It is not a physical abnormality, but it can have a demoralising effect on the man and his partner.

The problem may occasionally be self-perpetuating, through a fear of recurrence and through loss of confidence. In the majority of cases, premature ejaculation is not a lasting problem. It commonly occurs in times of stress, in relationships where the couple do not know each other very well, and in sexual intercourse when the man is a beginner.

Making a habit of having sex hurriedly can also lead to premature ejaculation. This can happen after having irregular sex with prostitutes or where a relationship has been exploited solely to relieve sexual tension. In these cases a growing and maturing relationship may be all that is needed to correct the problem.

Non-ejaculation is a much less common complaint, but it does occur. In some men ejaculation is achieved only by masturbation or in foreplay, but not during sexual intercourse. The relationship can often be a happy one, initially, giving satisfactory orgasms to the woman. Problems may not begin until the couple want to start a family and the woman begins to resent what she sees as a withholding by the man. This can lead to a deterioration in sexual activities, and can create anxiety in the man, leading to erection failure.

Sometimes the practice of deliberately withholding ejaculation during intercourse as a means of birth control becomes so habitual that eventually it becomes difficult to allow it to happen.

Non-ejaculation can also be the result of personality defects. The man is unable to abandon himself to emotions which for some reason are very threatening to him. This may be the result of a pattern of behaviour learned in childhood, or it may be that he cannot allow feelings to take over for fear of damaging his partner. In an extreme state, non-ejaculation can lead to marriage breakdown.

Female orgasm A great deal of discussion about the female orgasm has taken place in recent years. This has arisen partly because frequency of orgasm varies greatly between individual women. There has been a growing concern among women and their partners that orgasm should be the right of all.

In the female climax there is no equivalent of a man's sensation of ejaculation, but there is a more widespread involvement of the whole body, not just the genital area. For some women, one orgasm may be followed immediately by another. This varies from person to person, and even for the same individual from occasion to occasion. Some women only rarely achieve orgasm and do not repeat the process for a long time.

The drive to attain climax is greatest in men in their late teens, and then gradually diminishes. In women, orgasm is sometimes not achieved at all until the teens have passed and may not occur easily until they are in their thirties.

Failure to achieve orgasm can have a number of explanations. Some women are unable to abandon themselves to highly charged emotional commitments. Sexual intercourse does not arouse sufficiently the erotic sensations. Some fail because of poor love-making technique, or because they have an unsatisfactory relationship. Some may simply have a low or abnormal sexuality. Some women can climax only in the non-threatening, but potentially physically more stimulating, context of masturbation.

Many women never experience orgasm, yet they enjoy their sexual experiences. Others lack sexual experiences, but have self-induced orgasms that give them happy and fulfilling sex lives.

REASONS FOR SEXUAL FAILURE

Anxiety Some people are born worriers; but worriers do not inevitably have problems with their sex lives. It is when things go wrong between them and their partners that anxiety, always hovering in the background, appears and sex problems begin.

Some people have more specific anxieties. Men worry that their penises are too small or their erections are not hard enough. Women worry that their vaginas are obstructed. Others worry that they are not very good at sex, or not as good as they used to be, or not as good as someone else. They regard sexuality as a form of athletic performance; if they have not been doing well they should strive harder. Nothing could be more damaging to sexual expression than this type of anxiety.

Some situations are likely to induce anxieties—the fear of pregnancy, the possibility of being overheard, or the fear of being discovered in compromising circumstances.

The most damaging feature of sexual anxiety is the way it feeds on itself. What begins as a fleeting difficulty, may become a major or even complete barrier to sex.

Upbringing We are all fashioned by the twin influences of heredity and environment. Upbringing plays its part in a person's attitude both towards sex and towards emotional commitment in relationships.

Parents' own attitudes to sexuality, especially when strongly expressed or negatively inferred, influence the outlook of the child. A person brought up in a family in which sex is something secret or disapproved of, may grow to find it a subject of fear or even shame. It is something not to be talked about. This approach can leave a young person suffering from ignorance of and anxiety about sex before they have any sexual experience. A deliberate parental policy of 'not in front of the children' leads to a corresponding children's reaction of 'not in front of the parents'.

Emotional anxieties are aggravated by a background of insecurity. Drunken, aggressive parents who fight and threaten to separate, not only set a bad example, but also damage the developing personalities of their children. Where there is no love or emotional commitment from the parents, a child's ability to feel warmth, or to express it, can be undermined. Feelings of love and emotion go unrewarded and become painful, even intolerable. A barrier may be erected against such feelings, so that the person actually shies away from any emotional entanglement, and this in itself leads to sexual problems later.

Ignorance The permissive society has stripped away the secrecy from sex. Today a knowledge of the sex organs and their functions is commonplace. Most children are fully acquainted with the facts well before they reach their teens. Yet ignorance still leads to sexual problems and causes anxiety and unhappiness for many people.

A simple factual knowledge of the sexual functions does nothing to explain the emotions that are involved. Uncertainty leads to anxiety and anxiety leads to sexual problems.

Some people have a fear of sexuality itself. It has, for them, frightening undertones which they cannot explain. They have an inability to come to terms with feelings that cannot always be kept under control.

Some people believe that it is unnatural and even harmful not to have an orgasm. It may be disappointing to members of both sexes, but it needs to be kept in proportion. Orgasm will not always happen, and its absence should not be allowed to wreck an otherwise good relationship.

People mistakenly think that their sex drive should always be the same. It is not. It fluctuates for all sorts of reasons, such as health, fatigue, worry, and, not least, the simple fact of availability of a partner. When there is little opportunity for sex a person—man or woman—is less likely to become aroused than when it is regularly present.

Some people do have a natural, if unexplained, cyclical ebb and flow of sexual desire. It is more marked in some than in others and there is no cause for alarm when sex drive falls off. In most cases this will be only temporary.

Age, too, plays its part—though it is wrong to believe that middle-aged people are over the hill or that they are burned-out sexually. There is less pressure for sex in the mature than there is in the young. It may have ceased to be a new and exciting adventure, a challenge to the vigour of youth. But it should—and in most cases has—become a joyful part of a deeper and lasting relationship. Older people are wrong to compare their sex drive with the performances of their youth. It can be a cause of anxiety that can ruin their chances of a happy sex life as they get older. To accept this modification of the sex drive is part of a natural progression to a happy relationship in later life.

There is one other major area of ignorance that damages sex relations for many men: that the quality of sexuality should be measured in terms of size or hardness of a man's erection. There are, of course, certain basic physical requirements; beyond these it is the relationship between the couple which matters.

Conflict When arguments and disagreements enter a relationship, the couple are unlikely to have a good sex life.

The conflict sometimes takes a subtle form, a sort of sexual sabotage. One partner makes himself or herself as unattractive as possible, then blames the other one for avoiding sex. Another form of 'negative aggression' is to

465

alternately entice and then reject the partner. Just as love-making is about to begin, one or other remembers some mundane task—such as switching off the oven or locking up the car. This ploy can soon deter the other partner, who is then blamed for cooling off.

Lack of communication, too, is in a sense a conflict in marriage. It leads to neither partner appreciating nor considering the other's feelings or attitudes to sex. The period when a couple set up home together involves changes in their roles. If these changes are not understood and perhaps discussed, stresses can result.

Responsibility replaces a carefree existence. The sexual relationship can change from being a joyful, shared experience to an obligation, a subsidiary of the marriage contract. Open discussion of each partner's hopes and intentions is the best way to eliminate the chances of sexual conflict. A man who continues his bachelor habit of a 'night out with the boys' without first resolving any resentments by his wife, can be heading for conflict.

Couples, particularly the woman, face a new challenge with parenthood. Conflict will arise where a man fails to understand his wife's natural close involvement with their children. The woman may also be torn between a desire to have more babies and a fear of pregnancy because of lack of money. The couple need to talk about the problem.

Another type of conflict is individual and internal. It is a conflict of drive and instinct, a battle between a person's natural and uninhibited pleasure-seeking desires and the same person's feelings of sexual guilt and shame. For some people this makes sexuality and fertility inextricably intertwined. Intercourse without the chance of conception becomes unacceptable. Others are unable to have sex except in the dark, or until they have suppressed their inhibitions with alcohol. At its worst, this internal guilt manifests itself as a revulsion against all things sexual, and love-making is impossible.

TREATMENT OF SEX PROBLEMS

Communication Lack of discussion between couples is the root of many sex problems. 'If only I had been told'; 'I didn't know'—countless relationships have collapsed because of those simple failings. Apparently insuperable difficulties can vanish when each partner understands the other's needs and feelings.

Simply talking about it is the best way to remove a person's anxiety about sex. Striving to do better sexually does not help; striving to have a better relationship can help a great deal. And a better relationship comes from having a better understanding of each other.

A man with erection problems, growing more and more anxious, less and less certain, may react by avoiding love-making, leaving his partner with fears of rejection. Anger and criticism follow until marital disharmony aggravates loss of potency. Communication can solve the problem. The woman should be led to realise that she has not become undesirable to her husband.

A newly wed girl resenting the dramatic changes in early married life and, perhaps, resenting her husband's carefree continuation of his old habits can quickly go off sex. Communication with the husband could clear up the problem and restore a happy relationship.

The same is true of a wife struggling with her natural desires for motherhood against economic necessities. Her needs and disappointments need to be shared, and the husband should try to understand the subconscious drives of his wife.

Some couples are unable to communicate with each other without outside help. They may need to turn for help to a doctor or a specially trained counsellor.

Therapy Often therapy is needed to remove the anxieties that underlie sexual failure. The cure can involve making more love but having less sex—less, that is, in the sense of striving for more coitus.

This therapy is the basis for treatment formulated by Masters and Johnson, the American doctors who pioneered the modern investigation and treatment of sex problems. The therapy begins by prohibiting for a few weeks full sexual activity. This removes the pressures to perform that lie at the root of the anxiety.

The couple are encouraged to rediscover erotic feelings. The Masters and Johnson 'sensate focus therapy' involves the caressing and exploring by the couple of each other's bodies at a gradually increasing level of intimacy. It begins with an exploration of the body in general, and proceeds, by stages, to the sex organs. With no requirement to achieve sexual intercourse, the therapy usually leads to normal sexual arousal.

This form of therapy can be highly successful, but usually needs to be carried out after consultation with a doctor or a behavioural psychologist who is able to supervise the relationship as a whole, and to identify any resistances which may emerge.

A more specific form of therapy that is successfully used to overcome premature ejaculation is the squeeze technique. This involves squeezing firmly the end of the erect penis, adjacent to the glans, immediately before ejaculation becomes inevitable. By repeating this exercise over several weeks there is a gradual increase in the time between arousal and climax. It is wise to seek expert medical advice before trying to use this method.

Vaginismus, the vaginal spasms in women that can become a complete blockage to intercourse, can be treated by self-examination of the vagina. This is best carried out under the supervision of a doctor, so that vaginal fantasies can be shown to be unfounded.

Sex aids There are all manner of sex aids to assist erection and to stimulate the vagina. They produce large profits for the makers and little benefit to the buyers.

Many drugs and extracts of herbs are sold as aphrodisiacs, but they have no effect. The only drugs useful in restoring sexual drive must be prescribed by a doctor.

Lubricant jelly can partially solve the problem of painful intercourse resulting from difficulties of penetration and lack of lubrication. In making intercourse possible and not painful it can help to remove the anxieties which are a major cause of failure.

Further advice may be obtained from *The Family Planning Association* (see p. 255), and from *Relate Marriage Guidance*, Herbert Gray College, Little Church Street, Rugby, Warwickshire CV21 3AP (0788-573241).

HOMOSEXUALITY AND OTHER SEXUAL VARIATIONS

Everyone is different—as much so sexually as in appearance. There is an infinite variation in the complex elements that make up the sexual orientation of people. Perhaps it is impossible to say that any one human is 100 per cent male or female. But, most people are at one or other end of the scale that defines for all practical purposes a man or a woman.

Most people are heterosexual—that is, they have an unquestioned physical desire for the opposite sex. Even so, many adolescents, who later become heterosexuals, go through a passing phase of homosexuality—that is, physical desire for people of the same sex. A few do not emerge from this phase, but become passive or active homosexuals for the rest of their lives. Others are destined, from before birth, to become homosexual, not that this necessarily will become apparent until after childhood.

There are degrees of homosexuality. There are some people, both men and women, whose sexual interest remains permanently and only with people of the same sex. Others have their homosexuality finely balanced. They can be bisexual, moving from one sex to the other. Married men and women, capable of heterosexual relationships, can sometimes have sexual affairs with people of their own gender. Some adults, in situations where their only sexual opportunities are homosexual ones, adapt to homosexual relationships. This happens among seamen and prisoners.

There are many theories about the causes of homosexuality. Dominant mothers have been blamed for creating homosexual sons. So have absent or uninvolved fathers. But, distorted parental relationships are likely, at most, to be only a minor factor. The way one is put together as an individual almost certainly has far more to do with sexual orientation than family influences, although influences at the adolescent stage may be critical in many cases.

Society's attitudes to homosexuality are not constant. At present the trend is towards more liberality and more acceptance of homosexuals. There are still many people who recoil instinctively at the thought of love-making between people of the same sex, but, even so, there is comparatively little stigma attached to being what is now commonly known as gay. Legally this has been accepted, and it is no longer unlawful for consenting adults, over the age of 21, to practise homosexuality in private.

Homosexuality is the most widespread sexual variation. Two other variations which can cause great concern to both individuals and family are transvestism and transexualism.

Transvestism is dressing up in the clothes usually worn by the opposite sex, and it is most common among male adolescents. Often it is nothing more than a minor compulsion during growing up. Help is rarely sought unless the relationship is under strain. There is no specific treatment. Counselling and behaviour therapy offer the best chance of success.

Transexualism is an absolute conviction by a person that he or she has been born in the wrong gender. There is a striving to put this right, which can become an obsession. In extreme cases this leads to the person seeking a sex-change operation. This is an avenue which should be avoided until all other therapy has been exhausted.

SEX—WHAT TO TELL YOUR CHILD

How can parents show children that sex is a normal part of family life? The first thing to remember is that children copy their parents, and if sex is not discussed with them they are unlikely to bring up the subject. So if they are to be given a positive approach to sex they must be taught the good things about it. If parents suggest that it is wrong or dirty, the children will develop a similar outlook and become inhibited. A child needs to learn that sex is part of a loving, happy relationship which is something to look forward to.

EARLY AWARENESS
Children become aware of sex at a very early age. While changing a baby boy, a mother will notice that he enjoys having an erection and holding his penis. She will also see that her little girl may sit holding herself between her legs. Pleasure from stimulation of the sex organs is obvious at two or three years of age when children are often chastised for playing with themselves. They may then come to believe that touching their genital organs is wrong or dirty.

The best approach is to ignore what the child is doing, and distract it to occupy its hands in some other way. This early phase of sexual stimulation is often a comfort as well as a pleasure, and is usually over by the time the child is four or five.

WANTING TO KNOW
In these early years a child will become extremely interested in its body and the fact that it is so different from its brothers or sisters. It will want to know where it came from and exactly how babies are born.

A boy will also want to know what his genital organs are for and why girls do not have the same. He will wonder why he doesn't have breasts like his mother. This time of self-examination is an ideal one to tell children exactly what they want to know. Stories invented to avoid embarrassment—such as babies being brought by storks—will only confuse children later on when they start hearing different versions from teachers and friends.

A good time to have an anatomy lesson is in the bath, and it is even better if others, including parents, are bathing too. Similarities and differences can be explained. A boy will discover that he has one little hole through which he passes water, and another one behind for his waste food. He may see little point in owning testes, as he does not seem to need them. He could be told that they contain seeds so that when he grows up he can help to make babies. It is not wise to fabricate stories such as calling them 'men's milk sacs' similar to his mother's breasts. It may take many years for him to disbelieve such a tale.

Little girls may not realise that they have more than two holes in their bottoms. They will find out that it is women who have babies, and that one day they may have one too. They can then discover the purpose of the middle hole—a place for babies to come out from the mummy's tummy. Having discovered her vagina, a girl may well explore herself and push things into it. This can lead to infection and should be discouraged.

Both small boys and girls may think it very silly that a penis has to go into the vagina for a seed to get inside and grow into a baby. They may find the whole idea ridiculous. One boy asked his mother: 'Did it make you laugh?'

'WHERE DID I COME FROM?'
Children find it difficult to believe that the world existed before they did. But faced with family conversations about events that occurred before they were born they may ask the puzzled question: 'Where did I come from?'

It may be helpful to introduce them at an early age to a pregnant friend or to a new baby. It is even easier if their mother becomes pregnant herself. Children enjoy attending antenatal clinics with their mother to help the doctor feel the new baby. Some little girls insist that they are going to have a baby too, and want their own tummies to be felt. When the baby is born they can delight in seeing a smaller version of themselves; they also see that their mother has suddenly become much thinner.

Country children have the advantage of being surrounded by the seasons and animals giving birth. They have every opportunity to watch puppies and kittens being born. They can see the chickens and butterflies mount their mates and know that the bull is put into a field with cows for a reason.

City children need to have these things pointed out to them during trips to the country. They will also learn a great deal from keeping pets such as guinea pigs or hamsters. Growing flowers from seed in a pot on the window-sill is an ideal example of how a plant can grow from something small and then produce seeds itself so that more plants can grow.

Most schools will have a biology class where reproduction is discussed. Many parents feel that they can leave all discussion of sex to the school. The disadvantage is that children will turn to their teacher rather than to their parents when they need advice. Sex, too, becomes confined to a biological setting and is not seen as part of family life with the accompanying emotions.

Children will be eager to discuss sex with their friends at school. They will exchange information and ask each other if it really is true. They will often embroider what they hear to make it sound more fantastic. Myths then start and are passed around. If they find their parents receptive they will come home and talk about them. Parents can then take the opportunity to dispel any fears, and discover their children's attitude to sex.

Sex education is never over. One important milestone to prepare for in a girl is menstruation.

THE FIRST PERIOD
Puberty can begin in girls as early as nine or as late as 16. The first sign is the beginning of breast development and the appearance of pubic and underarm hair.

Menstruation usually begins about a year after these early signs. It is a terrible shock for a girl to find she is bleeding if she is not expecting it. She must be told about it at the first signs of physical maturity.

Many girls look forward to their first period as a sign of maturity. For others, even if prepared, a first period can produce tears and mixed feelings. When entering adulthood a girl ought to be at her best. Instead she is probably tubby and spotty, blushes every time a boy talks to her and is ready to burst into tears at the slightest provocation. Her clothes are changing in type, but they do not fit and she is trying to get used to wearing a bra. She is awkward with herself and with other people, and when she has a period she may have stomach pains and worry about leaking.

The family needs to make a bit of a fuss of her without turning her into an invalid. Mother should help her to buy the different types of pads and tampons, as she may be too embarrassed to buy them herself. Father often tries to keep out of the way on this occasion, but it could do nothing but good for him to buy her flowers or some little gift to mark the important event.

WHY DO GIRLS MENSTRUATE?
Some women believe that menstruating is getting rid of 'the poisons' or 'bad blood' and that if they do not bleed much the blood will stay inside and cause problems. This is not so. Menstruation takes place because each month a girl produces an egg as a first step towards producing a baby. The egg moves from the ovary to the womb, but in order to develop into a baby it has to be fertilised by male sperm. If fertilisation does not take place, the egg does not settle in the womb. Instead, the lining of the womb thickens, and is shed as soft lumps along with blood. This is the bleeding that takes place at a period.

The womb is made up of muscle so that it can stretch when accommodating a growing baby. Because it is muscle it can become congested and have painful spasms or cramps just like any other muscle.

Just before her period starts, a girl may put on weight. This means that her breasts get bigger and feel tender, the abdomen may become distended, and her ankles swell. At the same time she may feel generally irritable. All this is known as PREMENSTRUAL TENSION.

An adult woman has periods about every 28 days. However, the cycle is seldom regular to start with. Periods may only occur three or four times a year before a set pattern is established. Even then, the cycle is easily disrupted. A change of environment, travel or an emotional crisis can delay the next period.

PADS OR TAMPONS?
Many mothers wonder whether they should let their daughters use tampons before they get married. There is

no reason why they should not be used if they are comfortable as an alternative to the different types of pads so that the girl can decide which she prefers. Tampons are a great advantage when playing sports, and may be preferred by girls who wear tight jeans. Mothers are sometimes worried that inserting tampons may hurt or affect a girl's virginity in some way. If a girl finds that she cannot insert a tampon because she has a tight hymen, or that they make her uncomfortable, she can abandon them for the time being.

If a mother does not show her daughter the alternatives she may be thought of as old-fashioned or lacking in understanding, as girls are bound to find out these things from their friends.

LITTLE BLOOD IS LOST
Girls may be frightened at first by the amount of blood they see. They also may worry that it will not stop. It is not unusual to pass clots during the first two days of the period, but even so the amount of blood lost during a period is quite small. Some women pass as little as a dessertspoonful and others as much as a small cupful. The average amount is less than half a cupful, only one-tenth of the amount given by a blood donor at one session. Most women think that they bleed a lot and worry that the loss of blood will cause anaemia. In fact, bleeding stimulates the body to make more blood and unless the periods are very heavy there should be no ill effects, provided a normal balanced diet is eaten (see NUTRITION).

PERIOD PAINS
Many teenagers dread their periods because they get so much pain, and often have to stay away from school if they get diarrhoea and vomiting at the same time. It is little consolation to be told that the pains will get better as they get older, and that they will disappear after childbirth.

Probably the best way of preventing period pains is to take exercise in the week before the period is due.

Few girls feel up to playing sport on the first day of a period, but they should be encouraged to move around, either by walking or by doing exercises lying down, rather than going to bed with a hot-water bottle. There are many effective painkilling tablets for period pains which do not have unpleasant side-effects. The teenager should take these rather than retiring to bed as if she were ill.

OLD WIVES' TALES
It used to be said that a woman should not bath or swim or wash her hair during a period, but there is no reason

against any of these. Bathing should be encouraged and those households with a bidet will find it especially useful at this time. Hair washing cannot possibly cause harm just because it is done during a period. Swimming depends on how much she is bleeding and whether she uses tampons—in which case no blood will escape, provided they are changed regularly.

Girls should be helped to accept their periods as a physical function which carries with it the privilege of being able to bear children. They also need to accept their bodies, whatever their size and shape, and to be aware that very few people look like models. Pride in their bodies will help them to develop pride in themselves.

BOYS' PROBLEMS
Boys, too, have their problems during puberty. They may be fully mature sexually in their teens, but they suffer terribly from shyness, acne, squeaky voices and ungainly gait. Adolescent boys often withdraw to their bedrooms for hours, seemingly doing nothing. This privacy is essential for all teenagers.

Boys start sexual maturity at about 13, and focus their attention on their genital organs, unlike girls who think about sex in more general, romantic terms.

Boys become concerned about the size of their penis, especially on erection, and may become preoccupied with it. They easily have an erection and may do so several times a day, but worry that others might notice the bulge under their trousers. They have wet dreams and talk to their friends about the act of sexual intercourse itself, rather than romance. They find it difficult to understand why girls are not also preoccupied with the act of sex as much as they are.

Girls invite them to parties, wear sexy clothes, entice them to kiss and then send them packing. This erratic behaviour can be very puzzling. A boy can become excited quickly and easily, and is keen to find his goal. Girls are more concerned with the game.

MASTURBATION
One way of relieving the build-up of sexual tension is masturbation (producing an orgasm by stimulating the sex organs). Despite the myths that abound about the consequences of masturbating (for example, that it causes blindness), masturbation does not harm the body in any way. Not only does it release sexual tensions, it also helps boys and girls to understand their bodily responses. Lovemaking will be made easier by knowing the sensitive areas of their bodies and by being able to anticipate their own reactions. Many people may never wish to indulge in such an activity and some people believe that is wrong, but others find that it helps their enjoyment of sex.

HOMOSEXUALITY

Homosexual urges are not uncommon around puberty, and boys, especially those in boarding schools, may receive homosexual advances. This is something that their fathers need to discuss with them.

For many boys a homosexual experience is the first sexual encounter they have. Usually it is a passing tendency, and once heterosexual relationships are possible they tend to take over.

Girls seldom experience physical homosexuality, but may have a crush on an older girl at school.

Teenagers who have experienced homosexuality may have difficulty in understanding their sexuality as they mature, and may be unsure whether they prefer their own or the opposite sex. But some teenagers may not find the opposite sex at all attractive. The subject should be discussed openly within the family and possibly with the family doctor. Guilt feelings about homosexuality are very destructive, and an important part of growing up is coming to terms with sexuality whatever it may be.

There is ample opportunity to talk to children and teenagers about their sexuality. As they get older they watch plays and films on television, and read books and magazines—all with some sexual content. Families who discuss their attitudes to what they read and see are better able to talk about specific problems.

SEX HORMONES

People's sexual development and reproductive functions are controlled by the sex hormones, which are produced largely by the testes or ovaries. Androgens are the male sex hormones and oestrogens and progesterones the female.
See STEROIDS

SEXUALLY TRANSMITTED DISEASES

Diseases acquired by sexual contact. They were formerly called venereal diseases, and are now widely known as STDs. GONORRHOEA, SYPHILIS, non-specific URETHRITIS, genital WARTS and GENITAL HERPES are almost always sexually transmitted. AIDS, CHLAMYDIA INFECTIONS, REITER'S DISEASE, HEPATITIS B, THRUSH, trichomonal VAGINITIS, CRAB LICE and SCABIES can all be caught through sexual contact as well as by other means. Each of these diseases has its own entry.

In addition, chancroid, a tropical STD, may occur among travellers or their contacts. It causes small, painful pimples which ulcerate, accompanied by enlarged lymph glands in the groin. It is readily treatable.

Most large towns run special clinics giving confidential advice and treatment for STDs. The address of your nearest clinic can be obtained from the telephone directory or local hospital.

SHIATSU

A form of massage developed in Japan and based on the same principles as ACUPUNCTURE. It is sometimes called acupressure, and involves the stimulation of certain areas of the skin with the fingers and thumb.

SHINGLES

A blistered, localised skin eruption over an area of skin supplied by a particular nerve. It is known medically as herpes zoster. Older adults are commonly affected, but it may occur in a younger person who has had chickenpox.

Symptoms
- Severe pain, without any apparent reason and normally only on one side of the body, followed by blisters over the painful area two to four days later.
- Mild fever and general upset.
- The pain may persist long after the rash has healed.
- The chest is affected in about half the cases.

Duration
- Scales form after a week and the rash disappears in two or three weeks leaving some scarring.
- The pain may persist for months after the rash has cleared (post-herpetic neuralgia).

Causes
- The chickenpox virus which lies dormant in nerve cells. Only people who have had chickenpox develop herpes zoster although some cannot recall the original infection.
- Radiotherapy as well as age may reactivate the virus.
- Chickenpox may follow contact with shingles, and shingles may be activated by contact with chickenpox.

Treatment in the home
- Wear loosely fitting clothes, to ease pressure or rubbing on the affected area.
- Painkillers are helpful.
- Cool bathing may help. Avoid powdery lotions as these irritate the areas where blisters have broken.
- Avoid contact with women in late pregnancy or others to whom chickenpox could be dangerous. *See* CHICKENPOX.

When to consult the doctor
- For diagnosis and strong painkillers.
- For any eruption near the eye as this could damage the sight unless treated early.
- Rarely ENCEPHALITIS follows, so any change in general health, for example, headache or loss of alertness, should be reported to the doctor.

What the doctor may do
- Prescribe an antiviral drug. If applied early to the blisters, this will reduce the length of an attack and help prevent post-herpetic neuralgia. *See* MEDICINES, 27.

Prevention
- None known.

Outlook
- If eye complications can be prevented, healing of other skin lesions is uncomplicated.
- At the area of infection there may be permanent damage to the nerves with numbness of the skin.
See SKIN *page 52*

SHORT-SIGHTEDNESS

A focusing problem, known medically as myopia. Short-sighted people have difficulty in seeing objects at a distance, but can see clearly for close work.
See REFRACTIVE ERRORS

SHOULDER

Pain or stiffness in the shoulder is usually caused by injury, but may be due to a general disorder.
See SYMPTOM SORTER—SHOULDER

SHOULDER-HAND SYNDROME

Pain and restricted movement in the shoulder, with a swollen hand, stiff fingers and shiny stretched skin. The condition comes on gradually and may follow a heart attack or a stroke. The cause is unknown.

SILICOSIS

An occupational lung disease caused by breathing in dust from rock, such as quartz or silica. Particularly at risk are those who blast hard rock in mines or quarries.
See OCCUPATIONAL HAZARDS

SINUSITIS

Inflammation of the mucous membrane of the sinuses— bony cavities leading from the nose. Many people get sinus discomfort from time to time, particularly during a COMMON COLD or chronic RHINITIS. The pain is caused by temporary blockage and congestion of the small openings to the sinuses. If the sinuses actually become infected, symptoms are more severe and the condition is then called sinusitis. The sinuses in the forehead and cheeks are most commonly affected. Although small children can develop inflammation in the maxillary sinuses (those in the cheeks), the frontal sinuses (in the forehead) do not develop until the age of four or five and therefore cannot be affected.

Sinusitis may be either acute or chronic.

ACUTE SINUSITIS
Inflammation of the sinuses, usually occurring three to ten days after a common cold or if chronic rhinitis becomes exacerbated.

Symptoms
• Persistent pain in the front of the head or cheeks made worse by stooping, lying down, coughing, or pressure changes during flying or diving.
• Discharge from the nose which may be streaked with blood and continues to be green and yellow more than ten days after a common cold.
• A blocked nose on the affected side and a diminished sense of smell and taste.
• Raised temperature.
• Heaviness and watering of the eyes.
• Redness or swelling of the face over the affected sinus.
• Soreness when the bone over the affected sinus is pressed.
• Painful teeth.

Duration
• Acute sinusitis usually clears up within three weeks even without antibiotics.

Causes
• Infection from a common cold passing through the tiny connecting holes between the nose and the sinuses.
• Infection from diseased upper teeth may spread into the maxillary sinuses.

Complications
• Chronic infection of the sinus.

Treatment in the home
• Rest if you have a raised temperature and feel ill.
• Take painkillers in recommended doses to relieve the pain.
• The inhalation of steam, especially with the addition of crystals of menthol and eucalyptus, or proprietary inhalants, helps recovery. The steam humidifies the air and the heat may loosen the mucus, allowing it to drain more freely. *Be careful not to expose children to danger of scalding if boiling water is used.*
• Decongestant medicines from the chemist may ease symptoms and help recovery.

When to consult the doctor
• If treatment in the home has been tried for 48 hours and the patient is still feverish and in pain.

What the doctor may do
• Feel for tenderness over the sinuses by pressing on the forehead and cheeks.

• Shine a light through the skin to see if the sinus cavities are clear—transillumination.
• Recommend dental treatment if infection has spread from or to the teeth.
• Prescribe a course of antibiotics, together with the recommendation that the treatment in the home should be continued. *See* MEDICINES, 25.
• Arrange for X-rays of the sinuses if there is any doubt about the diagnosis, or if he suspects that chronic sinusitis is developing.
• Sometimes it is necessary to wash out the sinus and make a new hole for it to drain into the nose. This is done by passing a needle through the nose using local anaesthetic. This can produce dramatic relief of symptoms.

Prevention
• Avoid tobacco smoke, which irritates the lining of the nose and sinus.
• Do not blow the nose too vigorously during a COMMON COLD. This may push infections into the sinuses.

Outlook
• Sinusitis responds well to treatment but recurrences are fairly common, although by no means inevitable.

CHRONIC SINUSITIS
Long-standing inflammation of the sinuses. Many people suffer recurrent congestion of the sinuses, without actually developing the chronic inflammation of chronic sinusitis.

Symptoms
• Persistent blockage of the nose and discharge from one or both nostrils.
• Persistent pain in the front of the head or face, worse on stooping, lying down or coughing.
• Poor sense of taste and smell.

Duration
• Sinusitis may recur at the same time of the year on exposure to certain allergens or irritants. It may persist for years, or it may clear up spontaneously.

Causes
• Chronic RHINITIS (inflammation of the mucous membranes lining the nose).
• Exposure to dust or irritants, particularly tobacco smoke, over long periods.

Complications
• The constant discharge down the back of the nose may cause infection and damage to the lungs in children.

Treatment in the home
• Avoid any known causes, particularly irritants or substances to which the patient is allergic.
• Treat acute episodes as for acute sinusitis.
• Do not use any drops or sprays unless prescribed by the doctor. Some can make the condition worse.

When to consult the doctor
• If chronic sinusitis is suspected and troublesome.
• If fever and severe pain develop, call the doctor within 48 hours. A course of antibiotics may be necessary.

What the doctor may do
• Order X-rays of the sinuses to confirm the diagnosis.
• Prescribe a course of antibiotics. The course must be completed to prevent a recurrence. *See* MEDICINES, 25.
• Sometimes an operation is necessary to make a hole from an infected sinus into the nose or mouth. This allows drainage of pus and relief of symptoms.

Prevention
• Do not smoke.
• Avoid exposure to dust or irritants.

Outlook
• Symptoms may persist on and off for years, particularly if the advice on prevention is not followed.

See RESPIRATORY SYSTEM *page 42*

SKIN
Tough, resilient and constantly renewing itself, the skin nevertheless needs a certain amount of care and attention.
See SKIN CARE *page 472*

SKIN ABNORMALITIES
Problems with the skin include rashes, roughness, colour changes, and many different types of lumps, cysts, moles, warts and birthmarks.
See SYMPTOM SORTER—SKIN ABNORMALITIES

SKIN CANCER

There are three kinds of skin cancer: RODENT ULCER, which is quite common, attacks the face or neck and is only serious if left untreated; malignant melanoma, which is uncommon, but can occur anywhere on the body; and the rare SQUAMOUS CELL CARCINOMA (epithelioma) which may evolve from warts on the hands, head, ears, face (including lips) or neck of the elderly.

SQUAMOUS CELL CARCINOMA
This type of cancer develops on its own or forms in the hard, corn-like growths that sometimes appear on the back of the hands, top of the head, face, ears, lips and neck, usually in elderly people.

Symptoms

• After several weeks, sometimes months, the lump enlarges and an ulcer forms.

• They are not usually painful.

Causes

• This is not really known, but this cancer does seem to be related to age, prolonged (that is, several years) exposure to strong sunlight, radiation and certain chemicals.

Treatment in the home

• None.

When to consult the doctor

• If any wart-like growth develops in the skin and lasts longer than a month.

• If the lump enlarges quickly, becomes ulcerated or bleeds, consult the doctor immediately.

What the doctor may do

• Send the patient to have the growth removed surgically and examined.

Prevention

• Avoid prolonged direct exposure of the skin to strong sunlight, especially if spending many years in a hot climate.

Outlook

• This is usually excellent if treatment is early.

MALIGNANT MELANOMA

This is an increasingly common cancer of the pigment-containing cells of the skin. Many malignant melanomas develop in existing pigmented spots or nodules.

Symptoms

• Change in the size, colour or shape of an established, or newly developed, pigmented spot or nodule on or under the skin.

• Bleeding, itching, inflammation or crusting in a long-established, or newly developed, mole.

• Moles with a notched edge or multicoloured surface are especially suspect.

Duration

• The cancers grow fairly rapidly over weeks and months and spread through the body.

Causes

• Exposure to ultraviolet light, mainly sunlight, seems to play a major role.

Treatment in the home

• Do not attempt home treatment.

When to consult the doctor

• If a pigmented spot has any of the above features.

• If you have a pigmented mole larger than $\frac{1}{4}$ in. (7 mm.) across.

What the doctor may do

• Have the nodule removed surgically and examined. A

wide margin of surrounding skin and underlying tissue will need to be removed at the same time.

Prevention

• Avoid excessive exposure to sunlight.

• Use high-factor sun block lotions.

• Wear a wide-brimmed hat in bright sunlight.

Outlook

• The prospects after early surgery are good.

• The growth can spread rapidly through lymph vessels and if this happens the prospects are not good.

RODENT ULCER

A common, slow-growing tumour of the skin, properly known as basal-cell carcinoma. The tumour does not spread to the other parts of the body. The usual sites for rodent ulcers are the face, neck, eyelids, nose and ears.

Symptoms

• A small, waxy, pearl-like pimple appears first. This enlarges over months or years to a pale, shiny nodule.

• Later an ulcer appears in the nodule. This scabs over, appears to heal, but breaks down again.

• The edge of the ulcer is raised and shiny.

• Sometimes the nodule grows slowly over months or years into the surrounding skin.

Duration

• Until the ulcer is removed.

• Ulcers do not disappear. If left untreated they grow and spread for years, even invading underlying bone.

Causes

• These are not known. Prolonged sunlight may be a cause, although rodent ulcers appear in shaded skin.

• The condition rarely occurs among people with dark skins.

Treatment in the home

• Do not attempt 'home remedies'.

When to consult the doctor

• As soon as possible if you suspect that a pimple or ulcer might be a rodent ulcer.

What the doctor may do

• Send the patient to hospital to have the ulcer removed by curetting (scooping the ulcer out of the skin), surgical excision or radiotherapy.

• Treatment will depend on both the site and the size of the ulcer.

Prevention

• Wear a broad-brimmed hat to protect the face and neck from prolonged exposure to sunlight.

Outlook

• With treatment, cure is always expected. The cancer does not spread to other parts of the body.

See SKIN *page 52*

SKIN TAGS

These are tiny, loose, painless growths of skin, about $\frac{1}{8}$ in. (3 mm.) long, which sometimes develop in the groin, armpits, trunk and the side of the neck. They can occur at any age, but are very common in elderly women.

Duration

• They last for ever unless surgically removed.

Causes

• This is not known.

Treatment in the home

• None. The tags should be left alone.

When to consult the doctor

• If there is a wish to have the tag removed.

What the doctor may do

• Cauterise it. That is, cut it off with an electrically heated wire.

• Send the patient to a specialist to have the tag cut out under a local anaesthetic.

Prevention

• None is known.

Outlook

• The skin tags do not grow to any great size if left alone.

See SKIN *page 52*

SLEEPING SICKNESS

A disease known medically as trypanosomiasis, caused by a minute parasite called a trypanosome which is carried by the tsetse fly in tropical Africa. The infection is transmitted by a bite from the fly. Symptoms are a lump which forms at the site of the bite, followed two weeks later by fever and swollen glands. Eventually, chronic inflammation of the brain causes lack of concentration, a vacant facial expression, tremors, convulsions, coma and death. The whole process may take many more years. Early treatment by chemotherapy is effective, but this must be started before the brain is damaged. Personal protection is best achieved by wearing protective clothing, using insect repellents and by taking antitrypanosome drugs.

See INFECTIOUS DISEASES *page 32*

SLEEP-WALKING

This is almost exclusively confined to children and is rarely a cause for concern.

See CHILD CARE—CHILDHOOD ILLS

Skin care

YOUR SKIN NEEDS DAILY CARE AND ATTENTION—HERE IS A PLAN OF ACTION

The skin continually regenerates itself during life, though the process becomes slower as we grow older. The fine surface scales being repeatedly shed, and the thin layer of natural grease being constantly removed, give the skin a new surface each day and, in ordinary circumstances, make it almost impervious to the elements. So the skin can take care of itself in most situations. However, we should protect normal skin from such things as sunburn and chemical irritants.

A routine for face care:
1. Cleansing

Women who wear make-up should carry out a routine of cleansing, toning and moisturising each evening, as well as washing the face in the morning. Cleansing will remove old make-up and the grime and grease that have been accumulated during the day.

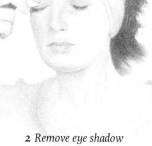

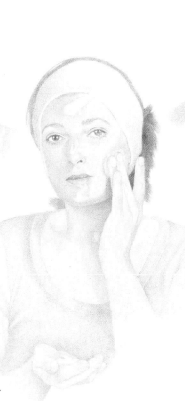

1 Remove mascara with a cotton bud dipped in eye-cleansing lotion. To make the job easier, keep your hair off your face.

2 Remove eye shadow by gently wiping it off with a pad of clean cotton wool moistened with eye-cleansing lotion.

3 Pour a little face-cleansing cream into the palm of one hand and dab it generously over the nose, chin, forehead and cheeks— using two fingers of the other hand.

4 Massage the cream into the skin, starting under the throat, using a gentle, upward motion.

EXPOSURE

In temperate regions of the world, where much of the skin is covered by clothing, these harmful influences mostly affect the exposed areas of the face and hands. Skin care applies equally to men and to women, whatever their race or colour; although the darker a skin is, the greater is its inbuilt protection against strong sunlight.

The colour and, to a lesser extent, the texture of the skin reflect the general state of a person's health (especially in childhood and youth), and a sensible, well-planned life-style should help to keep the skin healthy. Fresh air, regular exercise, a balanced diet and sufficient sleep all help people to look and feel their best. And the results of this will show in the skin.

For external care of the skin, regular washing with soap remains a first principle. Soap emulsifies grease so that it can be washed off by water. Soap and water also remove dirt, dead skin scales, and some of the bacteria which normally live on the skin. The skin usually replaces the removed grease within hours.

WHICH SOAP IS BEST?

All soap contains alkalis which break up the horny top layer of skin, allowing water to penetrate more—as well as to escape. Although normal skin quickly renews the horny layer, repeated use of soap may weaken the repair process. This can cause extreme scaling and dryness known as chapping. Washing the hands

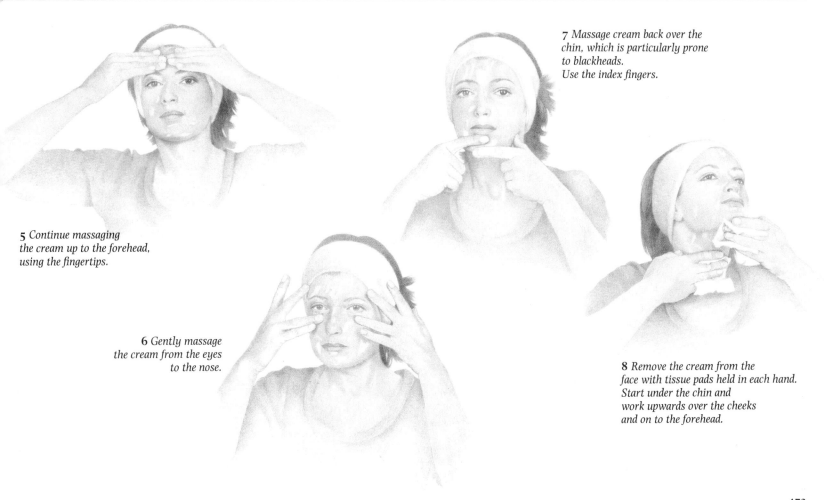

5 Continue massaging the cream up to the forehead, using the fingertips.

6 Gently massage the cream from the eyes to the nose.

7 Massage cream back over the chin, which is particularly prone to blackheads. Use the index fingers.

8 Remove the cream from the face with tissue pads held in each hand. Start under the chin and work upwards over the cheeks and on to the forehead.

more than six to eight times a day tends to have this effect on most people. Inadequate drying also seems to aggravate chapping.

Perfume added to soap makes it much more fragrant to use, but has no other virtue. Medicated soap (for example, one to which an antiseptic has been added) has no advantages on a normal skin. Medicated soaps are helpful in treating septic skin diseases such as BOILS. The usual bacteria on the skin cause little trouble and can be removed with ordinary soap. Attempting to remove them too vigorously with antiseptics can allow more virulent organisms to take their place.

The addition of any chemical colouring, perfume or antiseptic to soap increases the possibility, however remote, of irritation. The safest soap to use is the simplest sort without added disinfectant, and containing no perfume. Detergents, which are synthetic chemical compounds, will remove grease from the skin more effectively than soap. But their actions are too harsh for regular use and they easily cause chapping.

CREAMS FOR DRY SKIN
When the skin is dry and scaly, it can be eased by applying a cream. There are two kinds of skin cream: oil-in-water mixtures, which are easily washed off ('vanishing cream'); and water-in-oil mixtures, which are more oily and less easily washed off ('cold cream').

Because of their water content, all creams moisturise the skin slightly. Lanolin, an oil obtained from wool fat, used to be used for dry skin but many people are allergic to it.

People who need to wash their hands very frequently, because of their jobs, are particularly susceptible to chapping and irritation. The risk can be lessened by applying a barrier cream at the start of the day.

People with very dry skin, such as those with ICHTHYOSIS (an inborn, inherited dryness) or ECZEMA (an inflammation), may not be able to tolerate soap and water at all. If so, they should use an emulsifying cream when washing.

EFFECTS OF CLIMATE AND AIR CONDITIONING
Cold winds, extremes of temperature and raised barometric pressure cause increased dryness and scaling of the skin, which may need treatment with a cold cream.

The very low humidity in air-conditioned houses and offices can dry and irritate the skin. The best remedy is to keep the humidity level at 40–50 per cent by using humidifiers.

THE HAZARDS OF SUNBATHING
Exposure to the sun's rays can also harm the skin. Acute SUNBURN is painful if short-lasting, and the discomfort can be eased by calamine lotion, or a similar application.

More serious effects on the skin are caused by continual exposure to the sun over many years.

White skin is more susceptible to sunlight than dark skin, and prolonged sunbathing can prematurely age white skin, causing loss of elasticity, thinning and wrinkling. It is also implicated in causing skin cancers. *See* SKIN CANCER *page 471*.

This effect of the sun has been a long-standing problem for the white-skinned population of Australia and the sunnier parts of the USA. The modern fashion for holidays in the sun increases the hazard for Britons, as does the increasing use of sunlamps at home. People who work out of doors for much of the time are more likely to develop problems.

Sun-tan creams or lotions should be used regularly when sunbathing in order to limit the amount of radiation reaching the skin.

COSMETICS AND ALLERGIES
Many facial cosmetics have a greasy or oily base. Women usually use them to improve their appearance—and not for any protection they may give to the skin.

There are also many cleansing and solvent agents available. These will

---

A routine for face care: 2. Toning

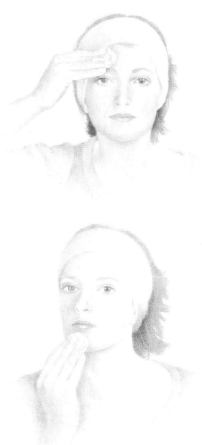

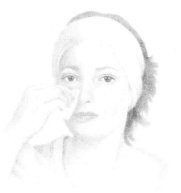

Toners remove all traces of dirt, make-up or cleanser that remain after cleansing.

1 *Immediately after cleansing, apply toner to the forehead and cheeks on a pad of cotton wool.*

2 *Apply the toner to the crevices around the nose.*

3 *Apply the toner to the crevices around the chin.*

remove the natural grease from the skin—but their principal purpose is to remove previously applied cosmetics.

Most cosmetics are perfectly harmless. But some contain chemicals which, when applied to the skin, can occasionally cause irritation or set up an allergy. The first sign of such an allergy is itching, and later redness occurs where the cosmetic has been applied. This might be followed by the development of ECZEMA.

If an allergy develops, it is essential to stop using a suspected product. If the particular cosmetic proves hard to trace, or the allergic reaction persists, seek medical advice.

AGEING AND ALCOHOL

Ageing of the skin—whether or not accelerated by prolonged sunlight exposure—is irreversible. The skin loses its elasticity and becomes thinner and dry. Creases and wrinkles become deeper and more numerous, and the slightest injury may cause bruising. The clever use of make-up may disguise the condition.

Dilated veins on the cheeks and nose are probably due to individual susceptibility, as well as to ageing and weathering. The veins can be disguised by using covering cream. Despite popular belief, they are not usually caused by the excessive consumption of alcohol.

BAGS UNDER THE EYES

Bags under the eyes—which often run in families—are again not related to heavy drinking, or to late nights. They occur in people who have loose skin around the eyelids.

Some people have a permanent flush on their cheeks and nose, which is also wrongly associated with too much drink. In fact, they are likely to be suffering from ROSACEA.

ACNE AND YOUNG SKIN

In adolescence the skin produces much more grease than at other times, mostly on the face and upper trunk. In many young people this is so excessive that it leads to blocking of the pores. *See* ACNE.

Three types of facial cosmetics

Cosmetics are usually labelled for three main types of skin. These are:

□ **Oily skin** Generally has a thick texture and noticeable pores, and may have blackheads and spots.

□ **Dry skin** Tends to be fine in texture, to flake and feel tight—and to develop lines earlier than other skins.

□ **Normal skin** In between these two extremes.

A routine for face care: 3. Moisturising

Without moisture, the skin will not remain smooth and supple. The face is exposed to the drying effect of the weather, so moisturisers—which form a film over the skin— contain and augment the natural moisture.

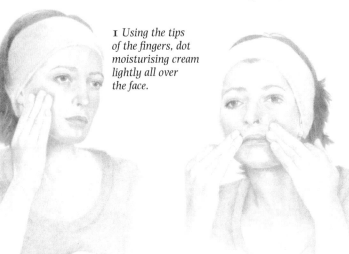

2 Press the fingers of both hands into the centre of the forehead and work the cream slowly outwards. Pat the cream gently around the eyes.

1 Using the tips of the fingers, dot moisturising cream lightly all over the face.

3 Work the cream around the jawline, chin and mouth with the middle fingers of both hands.

4 Massage the cream over the throat with alternating hands, using upward strokes from collar-bone to chin.

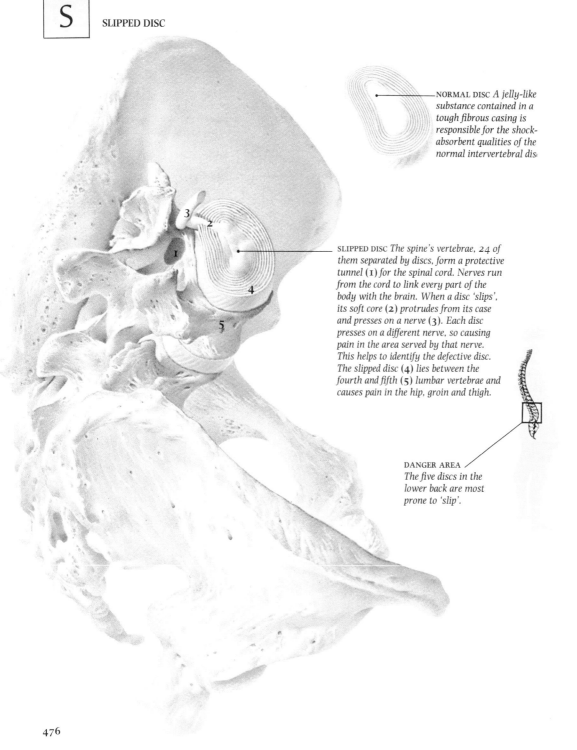

NORMAL DISC *A jelly-like substance contained in a tough fibrous casing is responsible for the shock-absorbent qualities of the normal intervertebral disc*

SLIPPED DISC *The spine's vertebrae, 24 of them separated by discs, form a protective tunnel (1) for the spinal cord. Nerves run from the cord to link every part of the body with the brain. When a disc 'slips', its soft core (2) protrudes from its case and presses on a nerve (3). Each disc presses on a different nerve, so causing pain in the area served by that nerve. This helps to identify the defective disc. The slipped disc (4) lies between the fourth and fifth (5) lumbar vertebrae and causes pain in the hip, groin and thigh.*

DANGER AREA *The five discs in the lower back are most prone to 'slip'.*

SLIPPED DISC

A bulging of one of the rubbery, shock-absorbing, discs that lie between most vertebrae in the spine. The bulge presses on the adjacent nerves causing pain and sometimes muscle weakness. The bulging occurs between the vertebrae in the neck (cervical) and waist (lumbar) regions. This condition is also known as a 'prolapsed intervertebral disc'. A slipped disc in the neck arises as a part of CERVICAL SPONDYLOSIS. A slipped lumbar disc is the main cause of the symptoms of sciatica and lumbago.

Symptoms
- A severe pain in the lower back which spreads down one or both legs.
- The pain may be made worse by bending, getting up after sitting, coughing or straining and is easier when lying flat, standing or walking.
- The pain often starts suddenly after lifting something heavy or straightening up after bending. Sometimes the onset of pain is gradual or only gets worse after several mild attacks; in severe cases it is often impossible to identify a causal injury.
- The lower leg and outer foot may become numb.

Duration
- Most attacks take two to six weeks to clear up.

Causes
- After the age of 25 intervertebral discs gradually start to degenerate and soften. Any sudden lifting or strain may precipitate a prolapse.

Complications
- OSTEOARTHRITIS of the spine and muscle wasting.
- In rare cases the leg muscles may become weak or wasted, and FLAT FOOT may develop.

Treatment in the home
- Rest, preferably on a firm flat bed without sag. In emergencies place a thin mattress or layer of foam—2-4 in. (50-100 mm.) thick—on the floor.
- Take painkillers in recommended doses.
- A hot-water bottle or heat lamp applied to the area of pain may give relief.

When to consult the doctor
- If pain is severe or getting worse and not relieved in a day or so by the above measures.
- If there have been previous attacks.
- If the injury occurred at work.

What the doctor may do
- Confirm by examination, X-ray or CT scan.
- Prescribe strong painkillers.
- Insist on complete rest on a firm bed or one with

boards under the mattress if it is too soft.
- Arrange physiotherapy.
- Some cases may require immobilisation in a plaster jacket or corset.
- Manipulation may help but can be dangerous, and should be considered only after an X-ray and discussion with the doctor.
- Recommend an operation, either micro-surgery to remove the disc or, in extreme cases, a major operation on the spine.

Prevention
- The risk can be reduced by keeping the back straight and bending at the knees when lifting. Avoid lifting and twisting at the same time, especially. These precautions are vital in people who have already suffered a slipped disc.

Outlook
- Many mild attacks get better in a few days and never recur. About 75 per cent of more severe attacks recur within five years but may then get better.

See SKELETAL SYSTEM *page 54*

SLIPPED FEMORAL EPIPHYSIS

The epiphysis is the knobbly growing end of a long bone which fits into another bone to form a joint, such as at the hip or elbow. In adults the epiphysis is fused to the shaft, forming a single bone, but in children and adolescents the growing bone is in two parts, the knobbly head and the shaft, which are separated by cartilage. This cartilage area is a potential weak spot and normal physical stress in an active child can cause partial or complete separation of the knobbly head from the cartilage. If separation occurs at the head of the femur (thigh bone) it is known as a slipped femoral epiphysis, and this condition can cause serious disability. It affects boys more than girls, mainly in the age group ten to 20, and half the children affected are overweight. Both hips may be affected.

Symptoms
- A limp develops. In some cases an injury is clearly the cause.
- Pain, which may strike suddenly or come on gradually. It tends to be felt in the knee, though the actual site of the disorder is the hip.

Duration
- Untreated, the displacement is permanent and a varying degree of disability in the affected hip follows.

Causes
- Slipping of the epiphysis after injury to the potentially weak cartilage area between the epiphysis and the shaft of the bone.

Complications
- A permanent limp.
- Degenerative ARTHRITIS in the hip in later life especially if early diagnosis is not made.

Treatment in the home
- None possible. Consult the doctor.

When to consult the doctor
- Immediately the condition is suspected.
- If a child or young person develops a limp which persists for more than 48 hours.

What the doctor may do
- Send the patient immediately to an orthopaedic specialist.
- The specialist will check the diagnosis by X-ray.
- If a small slip is revealed, it can be remedied by an operation.
- In the case of a more severe slip, traction (that is, controlled stretching of the leg) may be necessary before an operation.

Prevention
- Do not let children or adolescents become overweight.

Outlook
- Excellent if detected and treated early.

See SKELETAL SYSTEM *page 54*

SMALLPOX
For centuries smallpox was one of mankind's most dreaded killer diseases. But after a ten year campaign by the World Health Organisation it was officially declared to have been eradicated in October 1979—two years after the last-recorded natural case which occurred in Somalia.

The virus that causes smallpox was preserved in a few laboratories around the world and in 1978 a woman laboratory worker in Birmingham, England, died from the disease. There have been no cases since. The remaining virus stocks will be destroyed, and there is no longer any call for vaccination.

The main characteristic of the disease was a rash that left permanent pitted scars in the skin of those who recovered. There was no specific treatment, but vaccination with cowpox virus conferred immunity.

See INFECTIOUS DISEASES *page 32*

SMOKING

Britain's Royal College of Physicians says that 'cigarette smoking is still as important a cause of death as were the great epidemic diseases of the past'. The US Surgeon-General calls it 'the largest preventable cause of death in America'. Without doubt, smoking is one of the most dangerous habits we now indulge in. Nearly 100,000 deaths a year are estimated to be caused by smoking in Britain alone, and over 300,000 in the USA. It has been calculated that a male cigarette smoker who dies as a result of his smoking loses an average of 15 years of life. The male smoker who dies of coronary heart disease will lose an average of nearly 20 years—the difference between dying at 50 and dying at 70.

In Britain, 25 per cent of all deaths from coronary heart disease are estimated to be caused by smoking, and 90 per cent of all deaths from lung cancer and chronic bronchitis. An objection occasionally made to these statistics is that they suggest a connection between smoking and illness but do not prove it. But the connection is too close for coincidence. Lung cancer, for instance, is extremely rare in non-smokers and was virtually unknown at the beginning of this century before cigarette smoking had become widespread.

In addition, experiments have shown that the tarry residue of burned cigarette tobacco can produce skin cancer. Even more convincing, examination of lung tissue from smokers, non-smokers and ex-smokers shows progressive changes in the cells, which reverse when a person stops smoking.

Other statistics—taken from a study made of smoking and non-smoking British doctors—show up the relative risks of dying of lung cancer, bronchitis or heart disease run by smokers and by non-smokers. Since lung cancer is rare in non-smokers, the risk is more than ten times as great. The risk is less for heart disease, because it has many causes other than smoking; but more people actually die from smoking-related heart disease than of lung cancer (41,000 from heart disease and 29,000 from lung cancer in Britain each year). On the other hand, smokers are nearly 17 times more likely to die of bronchitis than non-smokers. The reason is that bronchitis is fairly rare among non-smokers, and smoking is one of its major causes.

Heavy cigarette smokers are at greatest risk. Pipe and cigar smokers occasionally get lip and mouth cancer, but their risk of getting lung cancer, bronchitis or coronary heart disease is only about half that of cigarette smokers.

This is thought to be because people who smoke only pipes or cigars do not inhale as much as cigarette smokers. If this is true, it still cannot be said that pipe and cigar smoking is safe. It would depend on how the pipe or cigars are smoked.

Heavy smokers are more likely to die of lung cancer, bronchitis or heart disease than light smokers. People who smoke one to 14 cigarettes a day run eight times the risk of dying of lung cancer as non-smokers. Medium smokers (15-24 a day) run 13 times the risk, and heavy smokers (25 or more a day) 25 times the risk.

Unfortunately, it does not follow that you can reduce your risk by cutting down. The important factor is the amount of smoke that goes into the lungs. Recent research in Britain shows that when they cut down, some smokers tend to compensate by inhaling more smoke from each cigarette. To the lungs, ten cigarettes a day at 20 puffs per cigarette is the same as 20 cigarettes a day at ten puffs per cigarette.

Research also suggests that low tar cigarettes are less dangerous than medium tar cigarettes, and that high tar cigarettes are the most dangerous. However, switching from high to low tar cigarettes will not necessarily help if you smoke more low tar cigarettes than you used to smoke high tar. One study shows a higher death rate from lung cancer for low tar smokers on 20-40 cigarettes a day than for high tar smokers on one to 20 a day.

Perhaps the most unfair effect of smoking is that it puts the unborn child at risk. Smoking by mothers produces smaller babies and shorter children, and the babies have an increased risk of dying at birth or during the first week of life. The effects of smoking during pregnancy are greatest after the fourth month. So it is still not too late for women to stop during the first four months of pregnancy.

The risks of incurring lung cancer, bronchitis and heart disease decrease progressively after a smoker gives up. After ten years as a non-smoker, he runs no more risks of contracting these diseases than someone who has never smoked. Some of the benefits of giving up appear immediately—for instance, there is more oxygen and less carbon monoxide in the bloodstream.

METHODS OF GIVING UP

Hundreds of different methods of giving up smoking have been tried. In 17th-century Persia and Russia, tobacco smoking could be punished by decapitation. This century, more humane methods have been employed, including HYPNOSIS. Success rates claimed for hypnosis range from 96 per cent to 13 per cent. The high rates are usually claimed by private clinics whose clients pay for treatment, and where the method was not compared with any other. The studies that have used non-paying clients and compared hypnosis with other methods have found it to be no more successful than others. The only recommendation that can be made about hypnosis is that it does work for some people. It may be worth trying, but you should first check with your doctor that the hypnotist is properly qualified.

Numerous kinds of aversion therapy have been used to help people stop smoking. One of the methods formerly most favoured by therapists was electric aversion therapy. The client starts smoking a cigarette, and is then jolted by an electric shock, usually through electrodes strapped to the forearm. He then extinguishes the cigarette. This procedure is repeated until the very act of lighting-up evokes fear of an electric shock.

Although tough methods like this can achieve quite high success rates in the short term, they are now regarded by some therapists as unethical. Also many people go back to smoking later.

The same applies to satiation, in which the aversion is produced by chain smoking for ten or 20 hours continuously, and to rapid smoking, with an inhaled puff every six seconds for about half an hour. Some people might find this approach useful as part of a more comprehensive plan to stop smoking. It does put people off smoking for a while, and to smoke twice your usual quantity the evening before giving up can provide a helpful start. By itself, however, aversion is not an effective way of helping people to give up smoking.

Another treatment is with a nicotine substitute. Lobeline is a substance derived from the leaves of an Indian tobacco plant (*Lobelia inflata*); but there is no evidence that it is an effective stimulant.

A third form of therapy involves nicotine by itself. It is addictive, but less dangerous than tar and carbon monoxide, which are linked to heart disease and cancer. Nicotine alone can be absorbed into the body through a chewing-gum which contains nicotine and gets it into the bloodstream in smoking-sized doses when the gum is chewed. It is available in Britain on private prescription. A study published in the *British Medical Journal* in 1980 reported that one year after treatment with the gum 38 per cent of smokers were still not smoking. Alternatively, nicotine skin patches (available without a doctor's prescription, or stronger ones on prescription) provide a more gradual release of nicotine into the body. However, nicotine replacement may only be necessary with heavily addicted smokers, so gum or skin patches are probably not needed by all smokers.

Many smokers may only need more motivation to stop smoking. Motivation and support could be provided by the smoker's own family doctor, and there is increasing awareness among doctors that they have a role to play. Research in Britain has shown that simple but firm advice from a doctor to stop smoking, backed up by leaflets and a warning that he will keep a check on his patient's efforts, has helped 5 per cent of a sample group of people to stop smoking for at least a year. Five per cent does not sound many, but it represents half a million smokers in Britain.

Many antismoking aids are available over the counter. They include dummy cigarettes, filters that progressively reduce the tar and nicotine dose of the cigarette, tablets intended as nicotine substitutes, and tablets designed to make cigarettes taste horrible. To these aids could be added therapies that can l e paid for privately, like acupuncture and psychotherapy. Few of these aids and methods have been tested scientifically. All that can be said about them is that they may help some individuals to give up.

DO YOU REALLY WANT TO STOP?

How, then, can you give up smoking without going to costly clinics or taking unproven drugs?

Before you decide to try, it is essential to ask yourself: 'Do I really want to stop smoking?' If you have not clarified your motives for stopping, you will find it difficult to keep trying when the going gets tough.

Step one: Making the decision Do you only want to stop smoking if it will be easy and painless? If so, you may not want to stop enough. The important thing to do at this stage is to decide why you want to stop smoking, and how much you want to stop.

There is no easy way. Smoking has probably been part of your life for years, and such an ingrained habit is not wiped out easily. It will take months of effort. Are you prepared for this? Does it matter enough to you to stop?

When you are considering these questions, think about your own health now, and what it may be like in ten, 20 or 30 years' time. Think how many years of life you may be putting at risk, and what your physical health may be like, even if you are lucky enough to escape serious disease or premature death.

Think also about other people who may be affected by your decision—relatives, family, children, unborn babies. But don't forget to consider the reasons for continuing to smoke, including the pleasure you get out of smoking. Your decision to stop smoking should be realistic, not based solely on optimism. If, after thinking about all these questions, you still want to stop, decide finally that you are *going* to stop. Once you have made this decision, fix a date and commit yourself to stopping.

Step two: Stopping Different treatment methods and antismoking aids only play a small part once you have decided to stop. Your decision to stop is the most important part of the whole process, because your motivation and will-power is your most powerful aid. At this stage, you must decide for yourself what sort of programme you will follow. The first is to use common sense. Don't try to stop smoking if your marriage has just broken up, your car been stolen, or you have lost your job. If possible, choose a relatively stress-free period. Think ahead and anticipate stressful situations that are going to arise in the coming weeks or months.

Write these down if necessary and decide how you are going to handle them. If you simply wait for them to happen, it may be too late.

Aim to stop smoking *completely* from the first day. Gradual reduction is probably not a good idea. You may find it helpful to smoke all your remaining cigarettes the evening before you stop. This should get rid of the desire to smoke for a while. If you can, get instructions on how to relax from an expert—a physiotherapist, or a teacher of YOGA, for example. If you feel you will need encouragement to maintain your determination arrange mutual support with a friend or colleague who also wants to stop. If you think you will need more help than that, go to a clinic or 'stop-smoking' group. Ask your doctor if he can help, or ask Action on Smoking and Health (ASH) for the address of a group near your home. If you think some particular antismoking aid may be helpful, try it. But if it doesn't seem to help, don't give up the struggle. Remember that no aid can be a substitute for strong motivation or will-power.

If after several days you are feeling tense and irritable, have an intolerable craving for cigarettes and cannot concentrate, you may need a substitute such as nicotine chewing-gum. Ask your doctor about this, too. It is at this difficult stage (about one to three weeks) that you must remind yourself how important it is to stop smoking. If you do not really want to stop smoking you may abandon the effort. The worst part should be over in four to six weeks, even earlier for many people. But you must be careful and sensible for at least six months.

One final warning. Do not try a cigarette after several months, just to see what it is like, or to prove to yourself that you don't need it, or because someone says 'just have the one'. A lot of people relapse by doing just that, and it is remarkable how many friends will keep offering you cigarettes.

If you want to stop smoking enough, and if you can stick to these general principles, you will succeed. Although nearly 100,000 million cigarettes were bought in Britain in 1984, this was more than 23 per cent fewer than in 1972. In 1972, 52 per cent of men smoked, and 41 per cent of women. By 1984, these proportions had dropped to 36 per cent and 32 per cent. Millions of people have stopped smoking—including most British doctors, who saw the risks run by their smoking colleagues.

WHO CAN HELP?
Your family doctor.
Your local District or Regional Health Authority.
Your Health Education Department.
Each of these will know of any local 'stop-smoking' group or clinic.
Action on Smoking and Health, 109 Gloucester Place, London W1H 3PH (Tel. 071-935 3519).
ASH will put you in touch with your nearest 'stop-smoking' group or clinic.
Health Education Authority, Hamilton House, Mabledon Place, London WC1H 9TX (Tel. 071-383 3833).
The council offers booklets listing the most effective ways of how to stop smoking.

SNEEZING
An involuntary expulsion of air from the nose and mouth due to irritation or inflammation of the nasal passages. The most usual causes of inflammation are the COMMON COLD and HAY FEVER.

SOUND THERAPY
All molecules, and the atoms within them, are in a permanent state of vibration, the speed of which can be altered by exposing them to sound-waves. Sound therapists believe that illness is accompanied by a change in the vibration rate within molecules in part or all of the body, and that if the vibrations can be returned to normal, the illness can be cured.

Although much research still needs to be carried out, ultrasonic techniques, using machines that produce sounds above the frequency of 20,000 cycles a second—that of the highest notes most humans can hear—already have several applications in orthodox medicine.

Ultrasonic waves of relatively low frequency are used to help in diagnosis. The echo they produce when directed at the affected part of the body is fed back into a machine known as an echogram, which shows up any abnormalities.

Higher intensity ultrasonic waves, produced by an electronic applicator, are applied directly to the body to help in the treatment of muscular and bone disorders—for example, ARTHRITIS and FIBROSITIS. Ultrasound treatment can claim some spectacular results in the treatment of sporting injuries. Waves of even higher intensity are used to destroy cancerous body cells.

SPEECH DISORDERS

A child starts learning to speak long before he says his first word. While still a baby he listens to people speaking, and practises babbling sounds. He learns to communicate when he finds that crying or shouting draws his mother's attention.

Before his first birthday he is able to understand several words, and soon afterwards he begins to use a few words meaningfully.

Speech is a skill that children acquire at widely different ages. One child may speak fluently at the age of 18 months, while others, particularly boys, have only a few words at the age of two. Both are completely normal, so it is unrealistic to compare one child's progress with another's.

Most children make sudden spurts, then appear to make no progress for several weeks while they absorb new information and develop different skills.

While they are learning to talk, children's ideas come faster than the words they need to express them. They may therefore go through a phase of hesitating and repeating sounds or words while they search for the right one. This is not a problem—it is a normal stage of speech development.

HOW SPEECH IS FORMED
The first stage of putting a thought into words takes place in the brain, where words are selected and arranged into sentences. The voice is made by breath from the lungs passing over the vocal cords in the larynx, causing them to vibrate and produce sound. The sound is amplified in the chest, neck and head and shaped into speech by the palate, tongue and lips. The brain and nervous system control all the movements; hearing is used automatically to check that the words sound correct and have the appropriate rhythm and intonation.

Hearing is vital for normal speech development because children learn to talk by imitating speech they hear. It should be checked regularly either by your doctor or Child Health Centre, and later by the school health staff. The doctor can arrange for further testing if doubt arises.

ARE YOU WORRIED ABOUT YOUR CHILD'S SPEECH?
If at 18 months a child shows little sign of trying to use words, or if at two and a half he has not put two words together, or if a three year old speaks unintelligibly, you could prevent problems from developing by seeking

advice. Take the child to your doctor, or to the Child Health Centre. Ask to be referred to a speech therapist.

CHILDREN'S SPEECH PROBLEMS
Speech problems may occur in children who are otherwise quite normal. The most common problem is a difficulty in learning to say sounds clearly. The child may substitute the sound 't' for 'k' as in 'tup of tea' or 'l' for 'y' as in 'lellow', or he may leave out sounds altogether—'ca' (cat), 'do-ie' (doggie). The substitutions are normal in very young children and they gradually learn to say the right sound without any help, but some children find the process difficult and need extra help. One of the most difficult sounds to produce is 's', and many children lisp words with this sound, substituting 'th'. If the child has not got it right by the age of six or seven, he can be helped to correct it.

Another problem is slowness in learning how to use language. The child may have difficulty in understanding the more complex parts of speech, such as the words referring to where an object is—in front of, behind, on top of, and above. Or he may fail to use small words such as is, are, the, and a.

Any of these problems may be due to a temporary loss of hearing caused by colds or ear infections. Whether the problem corrects itself when the hearing loss clears up depends on how long and at what age the ear infections or colds occurred. Some children are plagued by heavy colds or ear infections throughout early childhood. If the hearing deficiency is not prolonged the child can catch up, but if hearing is frequently inadequate at this age, which is crucial for learning speech, the child will need extra help. If the mother realises this she can encourage her toddler to speak (see opposite).

A child with normal hearing may have difficulty recognising speech sounds and remembering the order in which they occur. Emotional problems can sometimes hold back speech development or cause a child to regress to an earlier stage of development. There may also be slow development of the co-ordination of the speech muscles or more permanent minor problems of muscle control.

The doctor or health visitor will refer children with these problems to a speech therapist. For children who have difficulty in saying sounds, exercises may be given to improve the ability to distinguish and remember sounds, or to develop muscle control. Children with language problems need help in learning to understand and use longer, and more complicated, sentences, and in learning the meanings of words.

Treatment takes place at speech clinics, or hospitals, or in some schools. It may consist of a session once or twice a week or a block of several days in the school holidays. Parents are usually asked to follow up treatment with work at home. For young children most of the work is carried out in the form of games.

CLEFT PALATE is a condition in which the two sides of the roof of the mouth fail to knit together before birth. It is usually detected at birth and artificial palates are made to help with feeding and speech until the baby is old enough for an operation. With modern operating techniques, very good results are obtained, and speech therapy can help achieve a good standard of speech.

If excessively nasal speech is evident in a child, investigation may reveal a small, undetected cleft. The problem may otherwise be due to a palate which is too short to make firm contact with the back wall of the throat to block off the nasal cavities, or to a palate which has poor movement due to weakness or lack of co-ordination in the palate muscles. Speech therapy will alleviate the speech problem, and surgery can help compensate for physical deficiencies.

DEALING WITH A STAMMER
Four per cent of the population stammer, and about four times as many men as women. The person who stammers is generally of normal intelligence, and psychologically as well-adjusted as everyone else. The disorder is not inherited, though stammering sometimes runs in families. The words 'stammer' and 'stutter' are synonymous.

Stammering may be due to delay in the brain's mechanism for checking what it has heard; or to slow development of the co-ordination of palate, tongue and lips required for speech. In childhood, stammering is sometimes triggered by a distressing experience such as a severe illness, a feeling of rejection caused by the birth of a brother or sister, or insecurities caused by the pressure of parents' ambitions for their children.

There is no truth in the popular belief that stammering can be caused specifically by forcing left-handed children to become right-handed, although the process could cause the sort of emotional pressure that gives rise to stammering.

When a child between the ages of two and five is learning to talk, he may go through a phase of repeating and hesitating which can sound as if he is starting to stammer. This is a normal stage of development, and so long as everyone around him remains relaxed, he will become fluent as his ability to express himself matures. Over-anxious relatives can make a child feel that something is wrong when he is stuck for words. If he then becomes anxious about his speech, he is in danger of developing a stammer.

There is no single cure for stammering, but there are many different aids and techniques which improve fluency. A person who stammers may be referred by his family doctor to a speech therapist, who will choose a method that is suited to the individual personality. These include headphones which prevent the stammerer from hearing the sound of his own voice, systems of reward and punishment, techniques for relaxation, and speech exercises.

Residential courses in speech-therapy units attached to hospitals or clinics can be helpful in offering a concentrated period of therapy to establish new speaking skills. Referral to these and other courses should be obtained through a family doctor or a speech therapist.

Some stammerers find that their speech is fluent when they sing or act in a play. Such activities can provide a relief from the strains of stammering, and also give a boost to the confidence. But be wary of the 'cures' sometimes advertised which, after a seemingly rapid improvement, can leave the stammerer worse off.

Initiative on Communication Aids for Children, 336 Brixton Road, London sw9 7AA (Tel. 071-274 4029) is an umbrella organisation for a number of bodies that provide support for people with communication problems, including stammerers.

DISORDERS CAUSED BY INJURY, DISEASE OR STRESS
A number of speech disorders—more common in adults than children—can be brought about by injury to the brain or nerves, through disease, or even by emotional stress.

Breakdown of language When someone suffers brain injury—for example from a STROKE or a road accident—the parts of the brain which control the use of language may be damaged. Breakdown of language—or dysphasia—results. It may be impossible to recall the words for even the most common objects: the person may see a cup, and know it is for drinking, but the word 'cup' is forgotten.

If the damage occurred in an area of the brain where speech is interpreted, the ability to understand language is impaired. The person may be able to speak freely, but the words emerge as nonsense because he has lost his ability to monitor his speech to ensure that it makes sense. Because writing, gesture and mime are other forms of language they, too, are impaired.

Even when a dysphasic person appears to understand little or nothing, it is important not to damage his self-respect by ignoring him, or talking about him as if he were not there. He may glean a great deal from the tone of voices around him and the occasional understood word, and much distress can be caused by under-estimating this.

As soon as a dysphasic person is well enough to co-operate he can be encouraged to remember the words for common objects, to say them, point to the object when it is named, and recognise the written word. The speech therapist will suggest a programme to meet the individual needs. Re-learning language is an exhausting process, and the motto for helpers should be 'little and often'. In many towns, mutual aid can be found at stroke clubs, where people who share the same problems can get together. Information about such clubs can be obtained from the speech therapist at the nearest hospital or clinic.

The rate and degree of recovery from brain damage depends on the extent of the original damage and the persistence of the individual. The most rapid recovery is made in the first six months; thereafter the rate of progress slows, but many people continue to improve for years.

POOR SPEECH FORMATION

Impaired speech formation—or dysarthria—is due to damage to the brain or to the nerves activating muscles that control breathing, lips, tongue, or palate. The muscles may be either too slack or too stiff, and their movements lack co-ordination. Speech becomes slurred, its rhythm and intonation are faulty, or its volume is uncontrolled. Dysarthria may be a symptom of a nervous disorder such as PARKINSON'S DISEASE, or it may be due to brain damage from an accident or a stroke. Because the same muscles are affected, eating and drinking may also be difficult.

Specialist advice is needed from a speech therapist, who will devise exercises suited to the particular type of dysarthria.

For people who cannot speak at all, an electronic communicator can be a valuable aid. Letters or whole words are typed out and displayed on a screen which can vary in size from a television screen to one that is worn on the wrist.

Using a communicator requires the ability to use language, so it has limited value for some people with brain damage. But the machine, though slow, may offer a means of communication to people who are otherwise unable to express themselves.

Electronic communicators are expensive, and it is important to establish which, if any, would be suitable. The Assisted Communication Centre at the Speech Therapy Department, Frenchay Hospital, Bristol BS16 ILE (0272 701212), offers opportunities to experiment with electronic aids, so that the needs of each individual can be met.

POOR VOICE PRODUCTION

In poor voice production—or dysphonia—the voice may alter in quality in various ways. It may become weak and hoarse, it may change uncontrollably in pitch or volume, or it may become nasal in tone. There are several possible causes:

Misuse of the voice Putting too much strain on the voice by raising it constantly is an occupational hazard of teachers, clergymen, singers and others who use their voices professionally. It can cause chronic LARYNGITIS. If the misuse continues, small swellings, or nodes, may occur on the edges of the vocal cords. These can be removed surgically, but they will recur unless a speech therapist teaches the sufferer how to put less strain on his voice.

Emotional problems A person's normal voice closely mirrors emotional states. It becomes 'high-pitched with fear', 'hoarse with excitement', 'tremulous with uncertainty'.

In periods of emotional tension or depression, such as may follow a bereavement or coping with family problems, temporary hoarseness or complete loss of voice may result. Tension may cause a feeling of a lump in the throat, which increases the burden of worry with unnecessary fears of cancer.

Conditions such as these are temporary, and usually disappear with the cause of stress. If they persist, the advice of the doctor should be sought to exclude any physical cause, and, if necessary, for referral to a speech therapist.

Benign or malignant growths Benign (harmless) growths

How to encourage a toddler to speak

□ Chewing, licking and swallowing all exercise the muscles used for speech, so as soon as the child is old enough, give him rusks or pieces of apple to chew, and encourage him to keep his mouth closed when he is eating.

□ Speaking is harder for a child if he is trying to breathe through his mouth at the same time, so make sure that his nose is clear, and that he can breathe comfortably through it when his mouth is closed. Teach him to blow his nose properly whenever it gets blocked for any reason.

□ Do not meet all his needs before he has a chance to ask for them, or he will never have any incentive to speak for himself.

□ Talk to your child, tell him stories and nursery rhymes, sing songs, and get him to repeat them back to you. Play whispering games so that speech becomes fun. When you are feeding or dressing your child or doing the housework, talk about what you are doing, and everything you can see, feel or hear. You are giving your child valuable experience of conversation and the use of speech.

□ Show with smiles or words of encouragement that you enjoy hearing him speak. Be patient when 'speaking' involves imitating a train all afternoon.

□ Turn the television and radio off sometimes so that he is not trying to hear speech against constant, confusing background noise. If there are other children in the family, make sure he has a chance to speak without interruption.

□ If he makes a mistake, correct him unobtrusively, but in an encouraging way: 'Daddy goed to work in the tar'—'Yes, that's right, Daddy went to work in the car.'

□ Don't say 'Take it slowly', or 'Start again' when he hesitates and repeats himself. Have patience and wait quietly for him to get the words out.

□ Never associate speech, or the absence of speech, with punishment—never say: 'I won't speak to you if you do that.'

□ Make sure he has plenty to talk about. Outings to the zoo are excellent, but trips to the supermarket or visits to play with friends are all extra experiences for the developing child and provide just as many opportunities for him to learn new words.

□ Encourage imaginative play such as dressing-up. Wearing your old clothes, the child will automatically imitate the way that you and your friends chat when you meet.

can be removed surgically. The presence of malignant (cancerous) growths may call for laryngectomy—removal of the larynx, with its vocal cords. Afterwards, the patient can learn to speak again by drawing air through the mouth and making it vibrate at the back of the throat, producing a sound which can be shaped into speech in the normal way. There are also mechanical vibrators, which are held near the throat. They produce a sound which passes up into the mouth for articulation into speech. The National Association of Laryngectomee Clubs will provide further information, support and advice.

Paralysis of the vocal cords This may be congenital, or caused by accident or disease.

If both the vocal cords are paralysed the person will lose his voice completely (a condition known as aphonia) and will only be able to produce a faint whisper. The result of paralysis of one cord can vary from a relatively good voice to aphonia. Speech therapy or surgery will make the most of whatever potential voice is available to the sufferer.

Abnormalities of the resonators Conditions such as paralysis of the palate allow too much air to escape through the nose, resulting in very nasal speech. A similar, but temporary, effect may follow the removal of ADENOIDS. A speech therapist will recommend exercises to strengthen the palate.

If you or your child suffer a prolonged period of hoarseness or other change in the voice quality, you should consult your doctor. He may refer you to an ear, nose and throat specialist, who may recommend training by a speech therapist.

USEFUL ADDRESSES

The Association For All Speech Impaired Children, 347 Central Market, Smithfield, London EC1A 9NH (Tel. 071-236 6487). The association aims to improve the facilities for speech-impaired children and has local branches where parents can meet to discuss problems.

The Council for Handicapped Children, National Children's Bureau, 8 Wakley Street, London EC1V 7QE (Tel. 071-278 9441). The council's booklet *Help starts here* is a source of reference and addresses for parents of children with special needs.

Action for Dysphasic Adults, Canterbury House, 1 Royal Street, London SE1 7LN (Tel. 071-261 9572).

The National Association of Laryngectomee Clubs, 39 Eccleston Square, London SW1V 1PB (Tel. 071-581 3023).

Chest, Heart and Stroke Association, 123-7 White Cross Street, London EC1Y 8JJ (Tel. 071-490 7999).

College of Speech and Language Therapists, 7 Bath Place, Rivington Street, London EC2A 3DR (Tel. 071-613 3855).

SPHINCTER

A ring of muscular fibres that by relaxing or contracting opens or closes a passage in the body. Some sphincters are under conscious control—for example, those of the bladder and rectum. Others act automatically; an example is the sphincter at the base of the stomach, which relaxes spontaneously to allow food into the intestine.

SPHYGMOMANOMETER

An instrument for measuring BLOOD PRESSURE. A wide, flat, rubber cuff is placed around the upper arm and inflated, stopping the blood flow in the large artery. Air is then slowly released from the cuff and the renewed pumping of blood passes impulses down a tube connecting the cuff to a mercury scale. The scale measures pressure in the artery when the heart pumps blood (systolic pressure) and when the heart relaxes (diastolic pressure).

SPIDER NAEVUS

A small, painless, bright red spot on the face, body and legs with thin red 'legs' (blood vessels) coming from it, making it look rather like a spider. If the centre of the spot is pressed with a fine point, the blood vessels empty and the legs disappear. Spider naevuses are painless.

Duration
• They may last weeks, months or years.

Causes
• The spot is a little-understood development from superficial blood vessels (capillaries).
• The spots may develop in pregnancy.
• They may occur as part of a general liver disorder.

Treatment in the home
• None.

When to consult the doctor
• If the spots cause anxiety.

What the doctor may do
• Send the patient for blood tests if a liver disorder is suspected.

Prevention
• Not possible.

Outlook
• Spider naevuses do not cause disfigurement.
• They disappear after pregnancy.

See SKIN *page 52*

SPINA BIFIDA

The literal meaning of spina bifida is 'split spine'. Doctors call it a neural tube defect, meaning that the bones and other tissues surrounding the spinal column do not form properly, leaving nerve fibres and membranes exposed. The condition develops in the womb and is present at birth. It may occur in every grade of severity. Spina bifida occulta, for example, is a mild defect of the bones which has no practical significance. Severe forms, however, may result in physical or mental handicap, even when treated immediately.

Symptoms
• Mild cases of spina bifida occulta produce no symptoms, though bone defects may be revealed by X-rays.
• In the most severe forms of spina bifida, a sac may protrude from the middle of the back, containing the membranes and nerve fibres of the spinal cord.
• Muscular paralysis and deficient control over bladder and bowels may occur in severe forms of spina bifida.
• Brain damage and an associated HYDROCEPHALUS may cause a child to be mentally handicapped, unless it is treated soon after birth.

Duration
• Spina bifida is present from birth. Without treatment, its symptoms will persist throughout life.
• Severe cases may be fatal.

Causes
• Exactly why the bones of the spine fail to develop properly is not known. However, a tendency to spina bifida appears to run in families. If a mother gives birth to one spina bifida child, there is a one in 20 chance of another child being born with the same condition.

Complications
• Without treatment, a child with severe spina bifida will probably contract MENINGITIS.

Treatment in the home
• None.

When to consult the doctor
• Spina bifida will normally be detected at or before birth.

What the doctor may do
• In the milder forms of spina bifida, no treatment is necessary.
• In more severe forms, an operation to protect the spinal cord may be performed soon after birth. Surgery may save the child's life, but physical or mental handicap may ensue from damage already done.
• A child handicapped by spina bifida usually requires

special schooling. The doctor may arrange for admission to a special centre or school. A spina bifida society exists to give help and advice. Contact:
Association for Spina Bifida and Hydrocephalus. ASBAH House, 42 Park Road, Peterborough PE1 2UQ (Tel. 0733-555 988).

Prevention
• Taking vitamin supplements around the time of conception may reduce the risk of spina bifida developing in an unborn child. A blood test may be carried out during the 14th to 16th weeks of pregnancy, which generally reveals whether a severe form of the condition is present. Alternatively, a needle is inserted into the amniotic fluid which surrounds the fetus, and a sample removed for analysis. In severe cases, there will usually be an abnormally high level of a particular protein (alphafetoprotein).

Amniocentesis may also reveal other diseases such as DOWN'S SYNDROME, but does itself carry certain risks. However, it is often performed if the mother has already had one spina bifida child, so that she can be offered a termination of the pregnancy if the child is affected.

Outlook
• Spina bifida can be a very serious condition, but surgical treatment carried out soon after birth may arrest any further damage.

See NERVOUS SYSTEM *page 34*

SPORTS INJURIES

One of the main reasons why adults play sport is to maintain their health and fitness, but an injury on the playing field can easily put them in a hospital bed.

The risk of injury in sport depends largely on the sport itself and whether the player has properly prepared himself to play.

The most dangerous sport widely played in Britain is rugby. It has a higher rate of injury than soccer, and a greater number of broken bones and injuries to the face. Soccer injuries usually affect the legs.

In cricket and hockey a major cause of injury is the hard ball hitting a player in the head.

Squash, tennis and badminton—with soft balls and little physical contact between the players—have a lower injury rate. Pulled muscles and sprains are the most common cause of trouble, but eye injuries are common in squash.

When death occurs in sport it usually results from injuries to the head and spine—possibly caused by being thrown from a motor-cycle or falling while rock-climbing or mountaineering.

Unorganised swimming in sea, lakes and rivers causes far more deaths than any other sporting activity. About 2,000 people are drowned every year in Britain and the United States (200 of them in Britain), but swimming in supervised pools is one of the safest of all sports.

Total deaths at various sports per year in Great Britain and the USA

Swimming, diving, underwater swimming	2,000.0
Canoeing	34.0
Mountaineering	13.5
Rock-climbing	12.0
Rugby	11.0
Motor-cycle racing	9.0
Soccer	7.0
Cricket	6.0
Horse racing	0.9
Gliding	0.5
Professional boxing	0.3
Running	0.25

Sports injury rate per 100 players per year

Rugby	4.9
Skiing	4.9
Soccer	3.2
Gymnastics	2.9
Hockey	2.9
Cricket	2.4
Judo	2.1
Rowing	2.1
Squash	2.0
Tennis	2.0
Fencing	1.8
Badminton	1.4
Cycling	1.4
Basketball	1.4
Golf	0.5
Swimming	0.3

Many sports accidents can be prevented. Rules which are designed to protect the players must be vigorously enforced, either by the referee, as in soccer, or by self-discipline, as in rock-climbing.

Anyone taking up a sport for the first time should obtain coaching to learn the correct techniques. Riding a horse without proper instruction, for example, can result in serious injuries from a fall. An instructor will not only teach a learner to ride but he will introduce him to the riding hat that protects riders from head injuries.

Proper instruction is essential for any underwater or airborne sport, such as scuba diving or hang-gliding. Accidents from incorrectly used equipment or from 'fooling around' can lead, with very little warning, to serious injury or death.

Fooling around accidents can occur in almost any sport. People have died after being pushed off a high-diving board, and after performing dare-devil acrobatics on a trampoline and falling on the floor.

Some sports injuries cannot be avoided, because they depend on factors which the individual cannot control—icy ground, for example, or an unforeseen break in equipment. But many injuries can be reduced in severity or prevented altogether by careful preparation; and prompt treatment will promote faster healing.

Prevention has two stages. First, there is long-term prevention through proper training, and second there is preparation immediately before a match is played or exercise is started.

PREVENTION THROUGH TRAINING
Fitness is a combination of four factors: strength, stamina, skill and suppleness. The fitter someone becomes the less likely he is to injure himself. *See* EXERCISE.

Training can strengthen muscles and probably tendons as well. Strong muscles and tendons can tolerate greater strains without tearing. They will also protect vulnerable parts of the body, such as the back, against pulls and tears. It is important to balance the muscle development on both sides of the body, and it is important to develop the muscles which will actually be used and under stress. There is no point in lifting heavy weights to strengthen shoulders and arms if you are training for cross-country running. The easiest way to make sure that the correct muscles are being strengthened is to play a modified version of your sport as training. Although occasionally it may be necessary to vary a routine to prevent boredom, in general, runners should run, swimmers should swim, and cyclists should cycle.

Weight-training is useful as a means of strengthening muscles, but it should never be attempted without the advice of a trained instructor.

Stamina is the capacity to sustain one's performance over a long period of time. It is affected by the capacity of the heart and lungs to transport oxygen to the muscle cells and by the blood's ability to take glucose to the muscles. The greater the stamina, the longer a person is able to swim, run, cycle or play tennis without a marked drop in the standard of play. Stamina also prevents injury because many injuries take place when people are tired and become careless.

The skilled sportsman runs a lower risk of injury than the unskilled beginner. In the first place he is able to control and co-ordinate his actions more carefully and does not put unnecessary strains on his muscles and joints; and secondly he is experienced. The skilled skier not only turns and stops more safely, he is also better at looking ahead and identifying changes in the texture of the snow which may throw him off balance.

Take lessons to learn the correct way of doing things from the very beginning. Faults in technique which may cause injury, such as an awkward golf swing, only get more difficult to eradicate as time goes on. Remember too that skills acquired in the training arena—a gymnasium or an artificial ski slope—may not be enough to prevent injury when they are put into practice. Only when playing does the individual approach the limits of his strength and ability. Beginners should always be ready to practise their skills in a real situation even though they may have learned it in the gym.

Improving suppleness is the aspect of training that is most frequently neglected, and yet is often a crucial factor in preventing injury. Many people concentrate on strength, stamina and skill, but do not work to keep their joints and muscles as supple as they were in childhood. Some stiffening inevitably takes place with age, but much of this is probably due to life-styles, and not just to the ageing process. Adults have to keep moving, otherwise they stiffen up. This is one of the reasons why exercise should be taken regularly and not in one burst on a Saturday afternoon.

Yoga is the best means of staying supple, and many people who are strong and skilled and have stamina could reduce their risk of injury still further by concentrating on joint mobility through the practice of yoga. *See* YOGA.

PREVENTION OF INJURY BY CORRECT PREPARATION

Using the right kit and equipment cuts down the risk of injury. In some sports inadequate equipment can be more dangerous than in others. It is more important that care be taken over choice of ski equipment, particularly bindings, than of golf equipment. But, in almost every form of exercise foot problems are reduced if you wear the right shoes—broad enough tennis shoes, for example, or jogging shoes with heels which prevent you jarring the spine. When choosing equipment or kit with safety in mind, take advice from someone with experience.

Sportsmen have differing ideas about 'warming up', but any routine which prepares the muscles properly will reduce risk of injury.

If the muscles which are being used are made more elastic by being stretched very slowly and gently ten or 20 times before being put under strain, there will be less chance that the fibres in the muscle will tear.

The muscles which are most commonly injured are the hamstring at the back of the thigh, the quadriceps above the knee, the calf muscles and muscles in the groin. These are often torn when running.

To stretch the hamstring muscles: put one foot on a table about waist height. Now keep the knee straight and very slowly, and very gently, reach forward with the opposite hand towards the toe of the foot which is on the table. You will feel the hamstring muscles at the back of the thigh stretch. Slacken off by straightening up and then repeat ten times. This can also be done by slow and gentle touching of the toes. Keep the back absolutely straight, bend from the hips, and bend only until you can feel your hamstring stretch: there is no need actually to touch your toes.

To loosen the quadriceps muscle: bend one leg until the foot is near the buttock. Hold the foot with one hand and pull it up and back, slowly and gently, until you can feel tension in the muscle. Slowly pull a little further, and then relax.

To loosen calf muscles: stand and place one foot well in front of the other. Keeping the rear foot flat on the ground, gently bend the knee of the front foot until you can feel a tension in the calf muscles of the rear foot. Bend a little further and then relax.

To loosen the groin muscles, sit with the knees bent so that the buttocks rest on the heels and bend the trunk and head backwards.

PRINCIPLES OF TREATMENT

There are many types of sports injury from tennis elbow to a torn ligament, but they fall into two main groups: those caused by over-use (chronic injuries), and those caused by a blow or a sudden unexpected movement (traumatic injuries).

Over-use injuries Regular exercise often involves the repeated use of the same part of the body, and this can lead to the gradual development of painful injuries such as tennis elbow, golfer's shoulder and footballer's ankle. To begin with, one part of the body, the knee or elbow for example, aches for a short time towards the end of exercise and for a little while afterwards. Then, as the damage increases, the pain lasts longer after exercise and may occur at other times, perhaps when in bed or driving the car.

This type of injury needs expert attention. The first step is a period of rest, but if that does not help, see a doctor. Qualified physiotherapists are skilled in treating chronic aches in joints and muscles. If the chronic pain is in the back or neck, consult a qualified osteopath or chiropractor if the doctor says the problem is not serious but is unable to cure it. Similarly, a qualified chiropodist should be approached for aching feet and heels. If the condition does not respond, go back to your doctor.

Many people who have not been properly trained nevertheless call themselves chiropodists, chiropractors, osteopaths or physiotherapists. To make sure that the person you consult is properly qualified, check that physiotherapists have the letters MCSP, SRP or ACPSM (for therapists dealing specially in sports medicine) after their name; chiropodists, SR Ch; osteopaths, MRO, MBNOA or LLCO; and chiropractors, MBCA.

Traumatic injuries Two types of traumatic injury are more common in exercise than in daily life—pulled muscles and joint injuries.

In both muscle and joint injuries the damage is the same. The tissue is torn, and bleeding takes place because blood vessels are torn, together with the muscle fibres and ligaments. The bleeding causes swelling and pain, and pushes the injured tissue still further apart.

If such an injury occurs, stop playing immediately. If the player can use the injured part within five minutes without any pain then it is safe to play on. If the pain persists then the injured part should not be used.

A FRACTURE should be suspected and an injured person taken to see a doctor when:

- The swollen part cannot be used.
- The swelling becomes pronounced very quickly.
- The pain continues to be severe.

If the pain is not too severe and the swelling develops slowly it is usually safe to treat the injury without expert help. The four principles of home treatment can easily be remembered using the word ICER.

- Ice.
- Compression.
- Elevation.
- Rest.

Cool the injured part by using ice-cubes in polythene bags, a hot-water bottle of crushed ice, or an ice-pack. This causes the blood vessels to narrow and reduces the rate of bleeding. Ice can burn the skin, so it should never be used without protective covering such as a towel. Limit ice therapy to 20-30 minutes.

Compression also closes the blood vessels and slows the rate of bleeding. Enough force is gained by pressing the ice-pack, or a pad soaked in cold water, to the injured part. It is dangerous to bind the part too tight.

Elevation slows the rate of bleeding by emptying the blood vessels. This is the best means of reducing bleeding in the first 24 hours after an injury.

Cold and pressure should be applied, and the injured part raised above the level of the heart for 30 minutes to an hour, and then elevation should be continued for 24 hours.

It may be necessary to take painkillers in recommended doses to help sleep the first night after an injury, but painkillers should never be used to allow exercise to be taken. Pain is a valuable warning sign which should not be ignored.

When the injured part has been free of pain for ten days, exercise can be started, but only very light exercise to begin with. Hard exercise should only be taken once there is the full range of pain-free movement, and the limb is as strong as it was before the injury. If recovery is very slow, or if the problem recurs frequently, seek the advice of a doctor or a physiotherapist.

Stiffness No one is quite sure what happens when muscles stiffen, but it is probable that one of the causes is very minor small tears. Also during exercise, pressure builds up inside the blood vessels in the muscles. Some of the fluid in which the blood cells-are carried seeps out into the muscle fibres and builds up the pressure there. This causes stiffness. The best treatment is gentle exercise, easy swimming for example, which helps reabsorption of the fluid, but prevention is better than cure.

Stiffness is one of the results of unfitness and so one of the best preventive measures is to become fit. Careful warming up reduces stiffness and so does 'windingdown'. After hard exercise do not stop immediately; have a period of gentle exercise. Avoid wallowing in a hot bath after exercise. A quick shower, either hot or cold, and a brisk rub down are much better.

The message is clear—it is important to take exercise to enjoy fitness, but it is also important to become fit to enjoy exercise.

SPOTS

Small patches of discoloured skin which may appear as single pimples containing pus (*see* ACNE), or as a rash affecting all or part of the body.

See SYMPTOM SORTER—SKIN ABNORMALITIES

SPRAIN

The sudden stretching or tearing of a ligament, the strong flexible tissue that links the bones at a joint. The ankle is the joint most commonly affected.

Symptoms
• Pain and tenderness in the affected joint, becoming worse if it is moved.
• Swelling of the joint.

Duration
• A sprain can last for up to 14 days, depending on its severity.

Causes
• A sprain is usually caused by a fall.

Treatment in the home
• Rest the affected joint.
• Apply to the joint a pad of cloth wrung out in cold water and wrap the joint firmly with bandage. This will reduce the swelling.
• Many proprietary sprays, ointments and other applications for easing pain are also available.
• Take painkillers in recommended doses to relieve pain.

Do's and don'ts about sports injuries

□ *Do* roll a player who becomes unconscious on to his front immediately, in the unconscious position (*see* FIRST AID *page 612*).

□ *Do* remove foreign material (chewing-gum, broken dentures, broken teeth, grass) from the mouth to prevent inhalation in an unconscious player.

□ *Don't* lay an unconscious person flat on the face.

□ *Do* support the injured area with a splint or bandage.

□ *Don't* attempt to manipulate a fractured bone or dislocation.

□ *Do* sit upright and press a cold pad to a black eye—which results from bleeding into the soft tissue around the eyeball.

□ *Don't* waste time and money on applying a raw steak to a black eye. This is no more effective than using a cold pad.

□ *Do* treat nose bleeding by squeezing the soft part of the nose between finger and thumb and breathing through your mouth for 15 minutes.

□ *Don't* continue with the treatment if the nose bleeding lasts for more than 30 minutes. Either contact your doctor or go to a hospital accident department.

□ *Do* splash water with your hand on your eye if you get dirt or mud in it.

□ *Don't* add antiseptic to the water used on the affected eye.

□ *Do* thoroughly clean and disinfect an abrasion caused by the skin being scraped along a hard surface, such as the ground.

□ *Don't* use old creams, pastes or harsh disinfectants on wounds, they can infect the cut or destroy the tissues.

□ *Do* see a doctor if particles of dirt remain in the abrasion after cleaning. A partly cleaned abrasion can result in an ugly scar—especially if the face is affected.

□ *Do* make sure that you are protected against tetanus (lockjaw)—which can arise from a simple scratch—by an antitetanus injection. Booster injections should be given every ten years in order to ensure total protection.

□ *Do* wash and carefully dry your feet immediately after sport to prevent ATHLETE'S FOOT—a fungus that affects sweaty skin.

□ *Don't* soak your feet in very hot water.

□ *Do* take a quick warm shower or bath—followed by a cold shower or dip—to ease stiffness. Gentle exercise also helps.

□ *Don't* wallow in hot water after sport or exercise.

□ *Don't* sit around 'resting'.

When to consult the doctor

- If painkillers and rest fail to relieve pain.
- If the pain and swelling have not subsided after three or four days.

What the doctor may do

- Arrange an X-ray to check that the symptoms are not due to a fracture.
- Put an elastic strapping round the joint to support it.
- Prescribe pain-relieving tablets.

Outlook

- After the sprain has healed, the joint will almost always return to normal.

See SKELETAL SYSTEM *page 54*

SPRUE

A disease, also known as psilosis, in which food and essential nutrients are inadequately absorbed from the intestines and the lining of the small intestine becomes inflamed. Victims suffer flatulence after meals, abdominal pain and distension and diarrhoea. There may be various conditions associated with vitamin deficiencies. The condition is common in the tropics, but often clears up without treatment after the sufferer has left the tropics. Otherwise treatment with antibiotics and vitamin supplements is usually effective.

SQUINT

A squint or 'cast in the eye' is more than an unsightly blemish or embarrassment, and needs to be taken seriously because it can cause permanent loss of vision in one eye.

Symptoms

- Double vision (seeing two images in place of one) when looking in certain directions. The image from one eye is then suppressed by the brain which (in the absence of medical treatment) leads to loss of vision in this eye (lazy eye).
- In babies or toddlers, who cannot explain what they see, a squint can be recognised by the fact that in certain positions the baby's eyes appear to face in different directions.

Causes

- In babies and young children the cause is usually due to some failure in the development of proper vision with both eyes together. This is quite often due to long sight,

which makes focusing for near vision difficult. In such cases a squint may become apparent only at the age of three or four or even later, when the child is beginning to look at pictures and books for more concentrated spells than he does as a baby.

- In older children and adults a squint can be caused by injuries, severe infections, circulation problems or pressure on the nerves supplying the muscles which move the eye.

Treatment in the home

- None. Any suspicion of a squint in anyone over the age of six months should be reported to the doctor. Up to the age of six months many babies squint, as focusing properly takes time. Older babies may also squint for the same reason or because the bridge of the nose is particularly wide, but it is not worth taking any risks; because if there is a true squint, which can only be discovered by special tests, the child will not grow out of it and one eye may have its vision suppressed and become permanently blind.

What the doctor may do

- The doctor will test the eye movements by watching both eyes as they look at some object (such as a rattle) as it is moved from side to side or up and down. He will also ask the patient to look at an object with one eye while the other eye is covered and then, when the vision is fixed, uncover the previously masked eye to see if that second eye is looking in the same direction as the first.
- If the doctor is unsure about the diagnosis, he may ask to see the patient again after a period of time to reassess the situation. But in most instances if there is reasonable suspicion of squint (and it is often not easy to detect squint by simple tests) the doctor will send the patient to an eye specialist.
- The specialist will probably arrange a number of tests including examination of the inside of the eyes with an ophthalmoscope after dilating the pupils with eye drops.
- If a squint is confirmed he will arrange treatment by an orthoptist (a specialist in eye exercises) and the child may have to wear special spectacles and/or an eye patch. It is often difficult to get young children to co-operate fully in the rather tedious treatment that is involved, but persistence is important to save full vision.
- In older children and adults there may have to be a series of tests including blood tests and X-rays to establish the cause of the squint, and an operation may be necessary.

Prevention

- Although it is not possible to prevent a squint from developing, it is possible to be alert and report to the doctor any suspicion of frequent or persistent squinting after the age of six months.

- Once a squint has been diagnosed, permanent damage to the sight of one eye can only be prevented by strictly following the treatment advised. This may be tedious and difficult for the child and his parents, but the effort is well worth making.

Outlook

- Provided squints are tackled early enough—that is before four years of age and certainly before six—the outlook is good in terms of correcting vision and avoiding permanent damage. The sight in the 'lazy' eye cannot be restored, if it is left too late, although operations can be done for cosmetic reasons to improve the appearance.
- The outlook for squints arising from causes other than incorrect binocular vision will depend largely on the underlying causes.

See EYE *page 36*

STAMMER

A speech disorder in which there is interruption to the normal flow of speech and repetition of the first letters or syllables of words. It is another name for stutter.
See SPEECH DISORDERS

STEATORRHOEA

The passing of large, pale, foul-smelling fatty stools, which may float and be difficult to flush away. Consult the doctor if the condition lasts for more than two weeks.

The main causes of steatorrhoea are COELIAC DISEASE and SPRUE, but it can also be due to obstructive JAUNDICE, chronic PANCREATITIS and some stomach operations, such as GASTRECTOMY, which limit the body's absorption of fat and vitamins from the intestines.
See DIGESTIVE SYSTEM *page 44*

STENOSIS

The narrowing of a blood vessel, heart valve, duct or any other channel in the body. Marked stenosis causes illness. For example, AORTIC VALVE STENOSIS constricts the flow of blood from the heart and PYLORIC STENOSIS obstructs the passage of stomach contents into the intestine.

STERILITY

Inability in a man or woman to have children. Sterility may be due to natural infertility or the result of an operation such as vasectomy or hysterectomy.
See INFERTILITY
FAMILY PLANNING

STEROIDS

The steroids are a group of chemical compounds that can occur naturally in the body, and may also be man-made. Those used in medicine include:
• Corticosteroids, cortisone and related steroids, that stimulate the action of HORMONES produced by the adrenal gland. They may be used on the skin and orally to treat ASTHMA and RHEUMATOID ARTHRITIS, in transplants, and to reduce the effects of inflammation.
• Female sex hormones—oestrogens and progestogens, produced by the ovaries, and used for contraception.
• Male sex hormones—androgens—used in medicine on rare occasions to treat retarded sexual development in boys, and breast cancer in women.
• Anabolic steroids, a group of synthetic steroids similar to androgens. Originally thought to build up the body, their use has been abandoned by doctors because they have dangerous, permanent side-effects and their muscle-building properties are uncertain. Their use in sport is both foolish and dangerous to the individual.

STEROID SKIN CHANGES

Steroid preparations are often used in the treatment of skin disorders, but while they are helpful in combating many diseases the stronger preparations may cause changes in the texture of the skin. If the corticosteroids are used for long periods, that is, many months or years, the skin changes are likely to become permanent.

These alterations may develop more quickly if the steroid preparations are being applied under a polythene cover. See PSORIASIS.
Symptoms
• The skin is thin and red with many visible tiny blood vessels.
• Fine hair often grows on the affected skin.
Duration
• The hair growth disappears when the corticosteroid applications are stopped, and the skin becomes thicker over a period of months.
• The little blood vessels will lessen, but may never disappear.
Treatment in the home
• Do not use corticosteroid skin preparations on condi-

tions other than those for which they are prescribed.
• Do not continue treatment for long periods without having the skin examined by a doctor.
• Do not be tempted by any initial benefit to go on applying corticosteroids to the face.
• Never use preparations prescribed for other people.
When to consult the doctor
• Regularly (every three to eight weeks), if you are using corticosteroids over many months.
• If you are having corticosteroid treatment and notice signs of skin changes.
What the doctor may do
• Change the treatment if skin changes are occurring. The original skin condition may return or be difficult to manage at first, until it responds to the new treatment.
Outlook
• Once the corticosteroid treatment is stopped the skin usually partially recovers in time.
See SKIN page 52

STITCH
A sharp pain in the abdomen that occurs during strenuous exercise, usually running and generally soon after a meal. The pain, which is most commonly felt on the left-hand side, is caused by the sudden contraction of a muscle. The condition is harmless and passes naturally.

STOMACH CANCER

A malignant disease usually occurring after the age of 40. It is more common in men, and may run in families. The number of cases of stomach cancer has been falling in many countries over the past few decades.
Symptoms
• Pain in the upper abdomen.
• Loss of appetite and loss of weight.
• Swollen stomach.
• Vomiting.
• Bleeding from the stomach and vomiting up blood.
• Anaemia.
Duration
• Because early symptoms are often slight or non-existent in the potentially curable stage, the outlook is not good and the duration a question of one to four years.
Causes
• Unknown, but smoking, excess alcohol, pernicious ANAEMIA, atrophic GASTRITIS, POLYPOSIS and GASTRIC ULCERS

appear to increase the risk.
• There is some hereditary influence—people with blood group A are at higher risk.
• The role of diet remains disputed.
Complications
• Ulceration and bleeding of the stomach.
• Obstruction to swallowing or to the outlet of the stomach.
• Spread to other organs, especially the liver and glands.
Treatment in the home
• None advised. Consult the doctor.
When to consult the doctor
• If any of the above symptoms occur.
What the doctor may do
• Send the patient to hospital for X-rays or a gastroscopy (examination of the stomach with a long illuminated tube).
• If cancer is diagnosed an operation will be necessary.
Prevention
• None known, except avoid smoking.
Outlook
• Not good; even with treatment the five-year survival rate is low.
See DIGESTIVE SYSTEM page 44

STONES IN THE URINARY TRACT

Every year, about one person in 2,000 develops stones in the urinary tract—usually in the kidney in developed countries, and in the bladder in underdeveloped countries.

The stones, which are known medically as calculi, may be formed by an excess of salts in the bloodstream which then crystallise in the urine. Alternatively, they may be the result of an infection of the urinary tract, especially if this causes some obstruction to the flow of urine.

Stones in the kidney and bladder may grow to a very large size and can remain unnoticed as long as they stay in place. On the other hand, a tiny stone may cause excruciating pain if it leaves the kidney and tears the lining of the urinary tract on its way to the bladder.
Symptoms
• An excruciating pain starts in the back over one kidney and spreads to the front of the abdomen down in the scrotum, penis or vulva.

- The pain builds to a climax, lasts about a minute before it eases and then returns again in a few minutes.
- Often there is pain on passing water.
- Blood in the urine.
- There may be no symptoms.

Duration
- Large stones may take years to develop, but others may form within a week or two.

Causes
- An excess of salts in the bloodstream, caused by gout or hormone disorders.
- Infections of the urinary tract, especially if these obstruct the flow of urine.
- Not drinking enough fluids.
- Prolonged bed-rest.
- The condition is more common in certain geographical areas, such as Holland, and stones are probably also caused by minerals in the water supply.

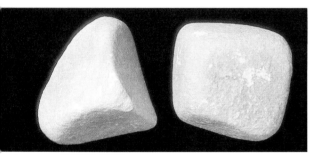

BLADDER STONES

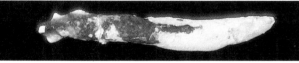

URETER STONES

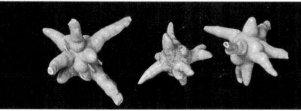

BRANCHED KIDNEY STONES

Complications
- Kidney disease.

Treatment in the home
- Drink plenty of fluids.
- If the pain is acute, raise the foot of the bed and lie down.

When to consult the doctor
- Immediately the pain becomes severe.

What the doctor may do
- Test urine
- Give a pain-relieving injection.
- Refer the patient to hospital for X-rays and specialist examination.
- Treat the underlying causes, such as gout or infections of the urinary tract.

Prevention
- Drink plenty of fluids, which will prevent minerals being concentrated in the urine.

Outlook
- This varies according to the size and nature of the stone. Small stones are passed as gravel in the urine.
- Large ones can be removed surgically, often with the help of ENDOSCOPY, or, sometimes, disintegrated by powerful sound waves (lithotripsy). In some cases, the kidney is damaged and may need to be removed.

See URINARY SYSTEM *page 46*

STRAWBERRY NAEVUS

A bright red 'birthmark' only rarely present at birth, which usually appears in the first week of life.

Symptoms
- Commonest on the head and neck. It varies from a

STONES THAT GROW IN THE BODY *Salts in the body's fluids sometimes separate out to create hard pebble-like objects in various parts of the urinary system. They form like stalactites in a cave—only more quickly. Those that form in the kidney (bottom) range in size from tiny particles that pass unnoticed in the urine, to large, often branched formations up to 2 in. (50 mm.) across. Stones in the bladder (top) are either formed there by obstruction or infection, or are passed from the kidney. Bladder stones can develop into masses weighing up to 3 lb. (1.4 kg.). Ureter stones (centre) are passed into the ureter from the kidney or bladder.*

small spot to a swollen, irregular, dome-shaped nodule 4 in. (100 mm) across. It is not painful.

Duration
- The naevus grows for a year or so, then becomes pale, slowly shrinks, and generally disappears without treatment by the age of five years.

Treatment in the home
- None. Leave the naevus alone.

When to consult the doctor
- For diagnosis and regular checks.

What the doctor may do
- If a naevus is fast-growing, in a very inconvenient place, or persists after the age of six, the doctor may consider treatment with surgery or radiotherapy.

See SKIN *page 52*

STRETCH MARKS

Lines of discoloration on the skin, due to stretching. The marks, which are harmless, are mainly found at puberty—in two-thirds of girls and more than a third of boys—and on pregnant women.

Symptoms
- Smooth, purplish shallow lines on the skin commonly occurring on the abdomen, buttocks, thighs, upper arms and breasts.
- The marks may itch slightly.

Duration
- The marks fade or disappear. This process may take several years.

Causes
- Most stretch marks are thought to be due to the change in hormones that takes place at puberty and during pregnancy.
- The marks are sometimes produced in people taking corticosteroids, drugs used to treat inflammation or to regulate the balance of salt and water in the body.

Treatment in the home
- No self-treatment is possible.

When to consult the doctor
- There is no need to see a doctor.

Prevention
- Not possible.

Outlook
- In most young people, stretch marks fade, then disappear.
- Following pregnancy, they fade and usually become inconspicuous.

STROKE

A sudden loss of function on one side of the body, due to an interruption of the blood supply to part of the brain. Strokes, also known as apoplexy, are uncommon before 50; after that they become more common with age.

There are two main types described below: a complete stroke, which is a serious loss of function that clears up only slowly and partially; and a TRANSIENT ISCHAEMIC ATTACK, which results in a mild loss of function that disappears within a few minutes but that keeps recurring.

Symptoms

Symptoms vary according to which part of the brain is affected. In nearly all cases they consist of one of the three following groups:

- Paralysis or weakness of the right side of the face and arm and right leg. The paralysis is often accompanied by an inability to speak, write, read or understand speech.
- Paralysis or weakness of the left side of the face, left arm and left leg. Often the left half of the person's awareness in space is lost, including awareness of the left half of his own body.
- Difficulty in swallowing and speaking with only slight weakness of the limbs.
- In all three groups, confusion, drowsiness, depression and involuntary urination may be present at the outset and the sufferer will lose consciousness in a severe attack.

Duration

- Some cases of stroke clear up within a few days or weeks; others continue for many months.

Causes

- A blood clot or haemorrhage in the brain, in most cases due to high blood pressure, hardening of the cerebral arteries, or heart disease.

Complications

- Recurrences are not uncommon.
- Varying degrees of residual weakness are permanent.

Treatment in the home

- Do not try to move the patient unless you have at least two helpers.
- If the patient is unconscious, put him to bed. Conscious patients do not need bed-rest.
- Only if swallowing is normal should normal amounts of food and drink be given to the victim of a stroke.
- Support a paralysed arm with pillows, keeping it stretched out from the body, with the hand fully opened.
- When lifting a patient with a paralysed arm, place the hand under the armpit on the paralysed side.
- Never pull on a paralysed arm.

When to consult the doctor

- Immediately any of the symptoms described occur.

What the doctor may do

- Severe cases need hospital care for investigation, nursing and rehabilitation. In a few special cases an

---

Living with a stroke

☐ Stroke victims can frequently overcome their disabilities by their own efforts, courage and determination and the help of family and friends.

☐ In the early days, at home, your relatives or helpers should learn how to exercise the affected limbs to prevent muscle and joint stiffness.

☐ As recovery progresses, you can take over the exercises yourself.

☐ Be patient. Rehabilitation cannot be rushed.

☐ Help of various sorts is available, including HOME NURSING, chiropody, meals-on-wheels, and in some areas even laundry services and holidays. Technical aids are also available, including special beds, hoists and walking frames. Your doctor, health visitor or social service department can advise you.

☐ To reduce the risk of further strokes, stop smoking, watch your weight and follow any treatment prescribed for high blood pressure.

☐ If your speech is affected, try to use gestures, writing or drawing. Try printing if your writing is affected, or if you have to change hands.

☐ Relatives and friends can help by speaking slowly or repeating things that seem not to be understood. They should listen carefully if speech is poor, and spend time talking, looking at pictures or photographs and encouraging former interests.

☐ Advice is available from *The Chest, Heart & Stroke Association*, 123-7 White Cross Street, London EC1 (Tel. 071-490 7999).

---

operation may be necessary to improve the blood flow.

- As soon as the immediate problems of the stroke have been dealt with, the hospital will arrange a course of physiotherapy aimed at restoring the patient to as much activity as possible as soon as possible in his own home. Relatives, with the help of their family doctor, district nurses and hospital out-patient treatment, can make a large contribution to recovery. Many areas have day hospitals which the patient can attend to ease the burden on relatives and at the same time receive additional professional help.
- Hospitals and local authorities can provide aids for use in the home by stroke patients. *See* DISABILITY.

Prevention

- Many strokes would be prevented if all middle-aged people with high blood pressure were properly treated.

Outlook

- The long-term prospects for the victim of a complete stroke depend on the extent of brain damage sustained and also on the physical and mental condition of the person before the stroke. Recovery can be complete, with little risk of recurrence; but more usually—especially in elderly patients—the arm and, to a lesser extent, the leg remain disabled. The aim is to restore confidence in, at the very least, the basic activities of independent living. A massive stroke, especially in an older patient, is grave, but if patients survive the first month the subsequent mortality is not high and a surprising degree of activity can often be restored.

See NERVOUS SYSTEM *page 34*

STUTTER

Another name for stammer, a speech disorder in which there is interruption to the normal flow of speech and repetition of the first letters or syllables of words.

See SPEECH DISORDERS

STYES

A stye (sometimes called a hordeolum) is a small boil in the glands at the root of the eyelashes. It is a common, unsightly and uncomfortable condition but can often be treated without medical help.

A meibomian abscess behaves in the same way as a stye and is treated in the same way: the only difference is that meibomian abscesses 'point' and discharge on the inner surface of the eyelid, while styes discharge on the margin of the lid.

Symptoms
• Pain and swelling on the eyelid.
• There will be pointing and discharge from the swelling at a later stage.

Duration
• A stye will often last for a week or ten days without treatment.

Causes
• A stye is caused by infection with bacteria. The infection can be caught from the nose or skin of the patient or by direct contact with boils or styes on other people.

Treatment in the home
• Once a stye is discovered it should be encouraged to come to a head and point, and so discharge. To do this, cover the bowl of a wooden spoon with cotton wool secured by a strip of bandage and immerse it in water as hot as can be borne. Apply the hot compress repeatedly to the affected eye for about ten minutes every two or three hours.

When to consult the doctor
• If the stye has not pointed after two or three days.

What the doctor may do
• After examining the eyelids the doctor may recommend further hot bathing.
• The doctor may also prescribe antibiotic ointment to put in the eye to prevent the infection spreading. *See* MEDICINES, 38.
• If styes have been recurrent, the doctor may recommend ointment for use in the nose, as this may be a source of the bacteria which causes styes.

Prevention
• Styes cannot usually be prevented, but you can help to stop them spreading by washing your hands after touching the stye.
• Use only your own towel and face-cloth and do not let anybody else use them.

Outlook
• Occasionally styes come in crops or in fairly rapid succession, but they invariably resolve either on their own or with simple treatment, and the infection causing them vanishes with time.

See EYE *page 36*

SUBACUTE

A term used to describe a disease that progresses more quickly than a chronic condition, yet does not become acute.

SUBARACHNOID HAEMORRHAGE

Bleeding into the fluid-filled space around the brain, as the result of a rupture in weak blood vessels on the surface of the brain. The disorder occurs mainly in young adults.

Symptoms
• Sudden instantaneous onset of severe headache and drowsiness.
• Stiff neck.
• Intolerance of bright light, and sometimes a squint.
• In some cases, paralysis of the arms and legs.
• Unconsciousness—if the bleeding is heavy.

Duration
• Symptoms often persist for four weeks or more.

Causes
• A weakness in the blood vessels on the surface of the brain, sometimes present from birth.
• Usually the vessels rupture for no apparent reason. Occasionally a subarachnoid haemorrhage is brought on by exertion.

Complications
• After a small haemorrhage, recovery is usually complete but recurrences are then likely.
• After a large haemorrhage, coma may be followed by death or recovery with residual weakness as in a STROKE.

Treatment in the home
• Lie the patient down flat in a quiet, darkened room. He should be disturbed only to be given food and drink and to have his toilet needs attended to.

When to consult the doctor
• Immediately the attack occurs. Subarachnoid haemorrhage is an emergency.

What the doctor may do
• Arrange immediate hospital admission. In hospital diagnosis will be confirmed by special X-rays and a lumbar puncture.
• Treatment involves rest and 'life support' measures.
• Once the patient has recovered, an operation may be necessary to seal off the ruptured vessels and any vessels that are considered likely to rupture in future.

Prevention
• There is no means of discovering who is liable to have a subarachnoid haemorrhage.
• Once an attack has occurred and been treated, there is nothing apart from an operation that will lessen the risk of a further attack.

Outlook
• If the bleeding stops and the source is sealed off by an operation, recurrent bleeding can be avoided. Nevertheless, without surgery the risk of recurrent haemorrhage remains.

See NERVOUS SYSTEM *page 34*

SUBCONJUNCTIVAL HAEMORRHAGE

A painless, bright red collection of blood on the surface of the white of one eye. It may occur spontaneously, particularly in middle-aged or elderly people, or it may follow a blow to the eye. It is caused by bleeding from a tiny blood vessel, and is of no serious significance. There is no need to consult a doctor, provided there is no obvious injury and the redness is not accompanied by pain, irritation, discharge or disturbances of vision. No treatment is necessary. Over two or three weeks the redness will gradually turn brown and clear spontaneously. The outlook is excellent and the condition will not usually recur. If subconjunctival haemorrhages occur frequently, however, it is advisable to consult a doctor, who may wish to do some tests to check for a bleeding disorder.
See EYE *page 36.*

SUBDURAL HAEMATOMA

The subdural veins run across the surface of the brain, inside the skull. A subdural haematoma is a mass of clotted or fluid blood which may build up if one of these veins is ruptured by head injury. If bleeding is severe, symptoms develop rapidly, resembling those of EXTRADURAL HAEMATOMA. Bleeding can also be very slow and symptoms develop over several weeks; a condition known as chronic subdural haematoma.

Symptoms
• Immediately after the head injury, the patient may not be aware of any ill effect. Gradually, however, over days or weeks, headache and drowsiness begin to develop, and the memory begins to fail.
• The patient becomes increasingly confused and may finally lapse into a coma.

Duration
• In severe cases, the patient may lapse into a coma within hours of the initial injury. In less-severe cases, the development of symptoms may occur over days or even weeks.

Causes

• Road accidents are the most common cause of head injuries in healthy people.

• Even a relatively minor blow to the head may cause a subdural haematoma. The very young and the elderly are particularly vulnerable because the veins are fragile. Patients on anticoagulant medicines are also prone to the condition, as are alcoholics.

Treatment in the home

• None is advisable. If a patient lapses into a coma, make sure the airway is clear. If breathing has stopped, give ARTIFICIAL RESPIRATION until the doctor or ambulance arrives.

When to consult the doctor

• Immediately symptoms develop or for any reason the condition is suspected.

What the doctor may do

• Arrange for X-rays or a scan of the head to find out whether a haematoma is present.

• The doctor may have the patient sent straight to hospital. An operation may be necessary to remove the pressure of blood on the brain. Holes are drilled into the skull under anaesthetic to release the blood.

Prevention

• Seat belts should be worn in cars, and protective helmets on motor-cycles.

• Protective helmets should be worn in any industry or situation where head injury is possible.

Outlook

• If a patient is taken to hospital in good time, an operation usually releases the pressure on the brain, producing complete recovery.

See NERVOUS SYSTEM *page 34*

SUDDEN INFANT DEATH SYNDROME

During the first year of life (generally between the ages of two and six months) one in 500 babies dies suddenly and unexpectedly while asleep. The death is usually peaceful.

A cause, such as congenital malformation or 'silent' pneumonia, may be detected after death, but it may not have produced any symptoms before death. Other babies may have had symptoms such as unusual drowsiness, irritability, altered crying or being off their feeds in the hours before death. In many cases, no cause can be found: the baby may simply have failed to breathe because of reduced brain activity during sleep.

The risk of sudden infant death is reduced if babies are not exposed to tobacco smoke, are not allowed to sleep face down, and are not wrapped in too many clothes or blankets. A baby's bedroom should not be too hot or too cold, but comfortable for lightly clothed adults: 61-68°F (16-20°C).

Apart from bringing grief, sudden infant death syndrome (cot death) can produce in the parents unjustified feelings of guilt. Parents who have suffered the tragedy of a cot death may find it helpful to discuss the event—and the future—with their GP, a paediatrician or the *Foundation for the Study of Infant Death*, 35 Belgrave Square, London SW1X 8QB (Tel. 071-235 1721/0965).

See CHILD CARE

SUICIDE

A desire to kill oneself is relatively rare. It has been found that nearly all attempted suicides are relieved to fail.

Suicide rates are always highest in prosperous well-developed countries. The rate falls in times of war. In underdeveloped countries it appears to be extremely rare.

The reasons for suicide are linked with lack of success, feelings of failure, and loneliness. Those at risk include people who feel they are failures, and those who live very isolated lives, like a student in a bed-sitting-room, a man living on his own while working away from home, a housewife who is on her own a lot, a woman who may have lost her husband and feels she has nothing to live for, and elderly people suffering from incurable illnesses.

It is a risk to be kept in mind for anyone who has been suffering from depression.

Genuine suicide attempts occur more in men than in women and most often in those of middle age onwards. Three out of four men who try to commit suicide succeed, whereas only one woman in four does. Two-thirds of all attempts are made with drugs.

An overdose is often a case of parasuicide (another form of attempted suicide). In these cases, the person does not really wish to die, but needs to escape temporarily from a difficult situation, or tries to attract attention with a 'cry for help'. It may also be a threat, or a form of emotional blackmail.

Another cause may be 'disappointed love' in adolescents, and some women, because reality did not live up to their idea of romantic love. Overdoses of drugs, or alcohol, are usually taken on the spur of the moment, and of course, some of the parasuicidal attempts succeed by accident. These parasuicidal attempts are usually made by the younger age groups, and women attempt this three times more often than men.

Each year about two people in every 1,000 may attempt parasuicide but only one in 10,000 succeeds in killing himself. Suicide rates fell by 36 per cent during 1963-75, and this could be connected with the expansion during that period of the Samaritans into a nation-wide service. They offer a 24 hour telephone service to 'befriend the suicidal' and their telephone numbers can be found in every telephone directory.

Always listen carefully when anyone talks of suicide, and do not dismiss a 'cry for help'. In a group of deaths by suicide recently investigated, it was discovered that two out of three of the people had told someone of their intention beforehand.

If one attempt fails, the person may make a second attempt and succeed in killing himself.

Where to turn for help

• Ring the Samaritans.

• Talk to someone, family, friends or the doctor.

If you find someone who has attempted to end his or her life:

• If by hanging, try to cut him down while supporting the body. Dial 999 and get an ambulance quickly.

• If by a drug or alcohol overdose, immediate hospital treatment is often life-saving. Send for an ambulance or doctor to take him to hospital if he is conscious. Make an assessment of the nature and likely quality of alcohol or drug swallowed. Send with the patient all drug capsules and written details of quantities and likely time of swallowing.

See MENTAL SYSTEM *page 33*

SUNBURN

Inflammation of the skin after exposure to the sun. Fair-skinned people have little protection from pigment in the skin and burn easily.

Symptoms

• Minor sunburn produces a red skin. The mild inflammation causes little discomfort, lasts for three or four days and is followed by increased pigmentation (a suntan).

• More severe sunburn starts with painful, tender,

swollen skin a few hours after the first exposure. This may blister and crust.
- The 'burn' develops for one or two days after exposure.
- Peeling and irritation of the skin a few days later.

Duration
- This depends on the severity of the burn, but the condition is at its worst about 48 hours after exposure.

Causes
- Ultra-violet rays from the sun.

Treatment in the home
- Keep the skin cool with calamine lotion or cold compresses. Antihistamine creams have little effect.
- Leave blistered areas exposed to the air.
- Take painkillers. *See* MEDICINES, 22.
- Avoid clothes rubbing the sore area.
- Do not allow further exposure to the sun.

Do's and don'ts about sunbathing

☐ *Do* avoid the sun if you have very fair skin.

☐ *Do* limit exposure to the sun to 30 minutes the first day, increasing by 30 minutes as each day goes by.

☐ *Do* use a sun-tan preparation and keep applying it.

☐ *Do* keep small children covered. They do not care if they miss out on a sun-tan.

☐ *Do* protect your skin when skiing.

☐ *Don't* assume that because it is cloudy you cannot be burned. Eighty per cent of ultra-violet rays get through cloud.

☐ *Don't* forget you can be burned even while feeling cool because you are in the sea.

☐ *Don't* use aftershave lotion.

☐ *Don't* expect artificial skin-tanning creams to protect you.

When to consult the doctor
- If the sunburn is very severe and distressing.
- If the skin has burned out of all proportion to the time exposed to the sun.
- If there is headache, nausea or fever.

What the doctor may do
- Prescribe corticosteroid creams to give relief. *See* MEDICINES, 32, 43.

Prevention
- Avoid over-exposure to the sun on the first day of a holiday, particularly if you are fair skinned. Expose the skin to the sun in gradually increasing stages. This will stimulate a tan which protects against burning.
- Remember that light cloud does not stop burning sun rays. Sun reflected from snow or water can burn.
- Use a protective sun-tan lotion or cream. Most of these are all easily washed off and need to be applied at least every one or two hours in hot sun. Filter-type sunscreens may contain anaesthetic substances. These can cause skin reactions, so be sure to follow the instructions on the container.

Outlook
- Complete recovery from sunburn is usual.

See SKIN *page* 52

SWEATING

Excessive sweating is an annoying but harmless condition which affects adults. It may occur on any part of the body, but is most common on the palms, soles and in the armpits. Occasionally it is a symptom of illness—for example, of THYROTOXICOSIS.

Symptoms
- Clothing becomes saturated with sweat—especially under the arms.
- Unpleasant odours are common.

Duration
- Excessive sweating may last for life or a few years.

Causes
- It is not known why some people sweat excessively, but the condition can be inherited. Minor exercise, heat, emotional states and obesity all aggravate the sweating.

Treatment in the home
- Frequent washing, changes of clothing and use of antiperspirants usually keep the problem under control.

When to consult the doctor
- If the simple measures above do not work.

What the doctor may do
- The doctor will exclude the possibility of thyrotoxicosis.
- Advise about clothing, diet and antiperspirants.

Prevention
- Not possible.

Outlook
- The problem usually improves with age.

See SKIN *page* 52

SYNDROME

A collection of signs and symptoms that combine to make up a particular disease or condition such as CUSHING'S SYNDROME and RAYNAUD'S SYNDROME.

SYNOVITIS

Inflammation of a joint, usually the knee or ankle, that most commonly occurs after an injury.

Symptoms
- Swelling and redness of the joint.
- Pain when the joint is moved.

Duration
- The condition normally lasts for only three to 14 days.

Causes
- Injury to the joint.

Treatment in the home
- Rest the joint.
- Take painkillers. *See* MEDICINES, 22.

When to consult the doctor
- If the inflammation and pain do not subside with rest.

What the doctor may do
- Arrange for the joint to be X-rayed to check that the continued inflammation is not due to a fracture.

Outlook
- Most cases clear up within 14 days.

See SKELETAL SYSTEM *page* 54

SYPHILIS

A venereal, sexually transmitted disease—which can cause serious damage to many organs throughout the body in later life. Early treatment with penicillin prevents many of the serious effects of the disease, and since 1940 there has been a 90 per cent drop in the frequency of these late effects. Unfortunately, such treatment has not affected the numbers of people initially infected; these have increased recently in most civilised countries.

Symptoms

There are three clear stages of the disease. After each stage the symptoms may clear up, and the sufferer may fail to seek treatment because of the mistaken belief that he is cured.

• First stage: This is confined to the site of the infection. Two to four weeks after sexual relations with an infected person, a small, hard, painless pimple or nodule forms on or near the penis, in the vagina or some similar point of close sexual contact such as arms, lips or fingers. This pea-size nodule then breaks down to form a small painless primary ulcer or chancre $\frac{3}{8}$-$\frac{3}{4}$ in. (10-20 mm.) across. Occasionally, and especially in women, this ulcer may go unnoticed. The lymph glands supplying the area (normally in the groin) also become swollen and tender. The open ulcer is highly infectious and usually heals in two to four weeks. At this stage there are no other symptoms.

• Second stage: This affects the whole body and starts one to 12 months after the primary ulcer has healed. A skin rash like that due to drugs or measles appears all over the body and inside the mouth. The rash does not itch and may vary considerably in both appearance and extent. At this point there is often fever and the sufferer is highly infectious, and may be unaware of the serious nature of the rash. The rash disappears within a week or two after which the condition becomes less infectious.

• Third or late stage: After a symptom-free period of one to 30 years, during which the disease lies dormant in the body with low infectivity, the organism without warning becomes active again and attacks any part of the body to produce a wide variety of serious disorders. These include any or all of the following:

• Slow-growing abscesses called gumma (very rare).

• Disorders of the large arteries and heart (*see* ANEURYSM and AORTIC INCOMPETENCE).

• Disorders of the brain (*see* GENERAL PARALYSIS OF THE INSANE below).

• Disorders of the spinal cord (*see* TABES DORSALIS below).

• Disorders of the sufferer's unborn babies (*see* CONGENITAL SYPHILIS below).

Duration

• Lifelong if not treated.

Causes

• A corkscrew shaped bacterium called *Spirochaeta pallida*

which is transmitted by sexual intercourse or close physical contact (including kissing) with an infected person.

Complications

• Any or all of the late stage effects described below.

Treatment in the home

• None is advised.

When to consult the doctor

• If the possibility of any sexually transmitted disease is feared or suspected.

• If any unexplained nodule or open ulcer appears on or near the penis, vagina, lips, anus or breasts.

• The presence of other sexually transmitted disorders such as urethral discharge, GONORRHOEA, URETHRITIS, CRAB LICE or SCABIES.

• Any unexplained rashes in an adult, especially if the sufferer is aware of a possible source of infection.

What the doctor may do

• Take blood tests, which usually become (and remain) positive four to eight weeks after infection.

• Refer the patient to a specialist or special clinic for further checks and treatment if the disease is suspected or tests are positive.

Prevention

• Avoid promiscuity.

• Use of a condom may help to prevent infection.

• Complete treatment until blood tests are negative will prevent the serious late complications. Sufferers should be conscientious about all courses of treatment.

• Testing and treatment of sexual contacts is vital to prevent re-infection and spread of the disease.

Outlook

• Excellent if the disease is diagnosed early and the patient follows treatment conscientiously. The treatment of the disease in its third and quiescent stage is often ineffective. Irreversible damage to vital organs may occur, possibly followed by death.

GENERAL PARALYSIS OF THE INSANE

Sometimes known as GPI, this complication of syphilis which affects the brain and personality of the sufferer is now fortunately rare.

Symptoms

• Steady, progressive, irreversible mental deterioration. This is associated with loss of memory and the capacity for self care.

• Changes of personality. Emotional responses to loved ones and near relatives may change considerably.

• Delusions of grandeur and megalomania may develop.

• There may be other symptoms associated with the late stage (see below).

Duration

• Symptoms may develop slowly over several years or in

a matter of weeks.

Complications

• Physical deterioration and death may follow.

Treatment in the home

• None advised.

When to consult the doctor

• If the condition is suspected by relatives.

What the doctor may do

• Refer to hospital for full investigation and treatment.

Prevention

• As for syphilis.

Outlook

• Once symptoms have developed, treatment of any kind is often ineffective.

TABES DORSALIS

Sometimes called locomotor ataxia, this disorder is caused by the syphilis organism destroying the dorsal nerves of the spinal cord.

Symptoms

• Shooting pains in the legs; as if a red hot needle has been pushed in.

• ATAXIA occurs. There is unsteadiness in walking which is much worse in the dark or if the sufferer closes his eyes. The sufferer walks with a high stamping gait and legs wider apart than normal.

• Muscles, especially of limbs, may feel weak and eyelids may droop.

• Impotence, difficulty in passing urine, and abdominal pains may occur.

• Other symptoms associated with late syphilis may arise.

Duration

• Symptoms, once present, persist and progress slowly over several months or years, despite treatment.

Complications

• Kidney infections and chronic ill health are not uncommon. ARTHRITIS often marked, may affect the large limb joints.

Treatment in the home

• Considerable support in the home may be required once the diagnosis has been made.

What the doctor may do

• Refer the sufferer for full investigation and treatment.

Prevention

• As for syphilis.

Outlook

• Once symptoms have developed, treatment with antibiotics is often ineffective.

CONGENITAL SYPHILIS

If any woman with untreated or inadequately treated

syphilis becomes pregnant, the unborn child may be affected in many serious ways. For this reason in developed countries every blood test on any pregnant woman is routinely tested for syphilis. This allows antibiotic treatment to be started early enough to prevent infection of the unborn baby.

Symptoms

• Recurrent miscarriages. With modern preventive methods, syphilis of the mother is rarely responsible for repeated miscarriages.

• After several miscarriages there may be a still birth.

• If a live baby is eventually born to an untreated mother, the baby may have many developmental defects of bones, skin, eyes, hair, teeth and other organs.

Prevention

• Regular routine blood testing of all pregnant women, followed where necessary by treatment, has virtually eliminated syphilis as a cause of either repeated miscarriages or congenital defects of babies in Britain and most other Western countries.

SYSTOLE

The period of muscular contraction in a heartbeat. It alternates with a period of rest, called DIASTOLE. Each contraction, which lasts about two-fifths of a second, pumps blood through the circulatory system.

See EXTRA SYSTOLES

T'AI CHICH'UAN

A technique of dances and exercises developed in ancient China. The basic principles are found in the T'ai-Chi classics, three small volumes written in the 13th century AD. T'ai-Chi is also called 'moving meditation', and is said to improve health and the general feeling of well-being by releasing untapped reserves of energy, or chi. Adepts claim it takes at least ten years to perfect and that it can be used for self-defence.

TAMPON, RETAINED

A tampon that has been forgotten at the end of a period and left in the vagina.

Symptoms

• An unpleasant-smelling, sometimes bloodstained discharge from the vagina. It starts one to three weeks after insertion of the tampon.

Treatment in the home

• Try to remove the tampon by probing with your fingers. If you are successful, take plenty of baths over the next few days to keep the vagina clean.

When to consult the doctor

• If you cannot remove the tampon or have a discharge as described.

What the doctor may do

• Locate the tampon and remove it.

Outlook

• There are no complications or after-effects provided the tampon is removed soon after symptoms begin.

See FEMALE GENITAL SYSTEM *page 48*

TAPEWORM

A parasitic worm, up to 11 ft (3.3 m.) long, that lives in the human intestine, where it absorbs food and grows and produces eggs that are excreted in the faeces. There are three main kinds of tapeworm: the pork tapeworm (*Taenia solium*); the beef tapeworm (*Taenia saginata*); and the fish tapeworm (*Diphyllobothrium latum*). The eggs of most tapeworms are not infectious to human beings unless they develop into cysts in their intermediate hosts, that is, cattle, pigs or fish.

If meat is well cooked before eating, any cysts present will be killed. But they will survive in rare or undercooked meat, and tapeworm infection may follow.

Many people with a tapeworm have no symptoms, but others develop abdominal pain or discomfort, diarrhoea, anaemia or loss of weight.

A human being can act as an intermediate host for the pork tapeworm. If the eggs excreted in his faeces come into contact with his mouth, he may swallow them and they may form cysts in his muscles, eyes and brain.

The illness caused may resemble a brain tumour or produce convulsions. Tapeworm infection can be treated with drugs and prevention is by good hygiene and the adequate cooking of raw meat.

See DIGESTIVE SYSTEM *page 44*

TATTOO

A tattoo may not only be made deliberately by injecting pigment under the skin, but may be the result of an accident in which dirt or coal dust, for example, has lodged beneath the skin. A type of scar known as KELOID

may develop in a tattoo, especially in dark-skinned people.

Duration

• A tattoo is permanent unless medically removed.

Treatment in the home

• A person with a tattoo should not try to remove it himself. As well as being ineffective, the attempt is likely to cause a disfiguring scar.

When to consult the doctor

• If the tattoo is regarded as a disfigurement and there is a strong wish to have it removed. However, removal may leave scarring and the prospect of having this in place of a tattoo should be considered before seeking treatment.

What the doctor may do

• Arrange for the patient to undergo laser treatment. If available, this gives very good results.

• He will generally refer the patient to a hospital outpatients' clinic. There, after a local anaesthetic has been given, the tattoo is removed by abrasion, either by hand or with a high-speed rotary drill.

• In some cases of accidental tattooing, plastic surgery may be necessary.

Prevention

• No young person should be tattooed, since regret in later life is common.

See SKIN *page 52*

TEAR-DUCT, BLOCKED

A tear-duct is situated at the inner corner of each lower eyelid and its function is to drain tears (which are being secreted all the time—not only when we cry) down into the nose. Blocked tear-ducts are not uncommon in babies, but are fairly rare in adult life.

Symptoms

• The eye appears to be 'watering' continuously. Sometimes the eye lining becomes infected and there is sticky discharge which makes the eyes difficult to open after sleep. *See* CONJUNCTIVITIS.

Duration

• The symptoms will persist until the blockage is relieved, either naturally in two or three weeks, or by an operation to open up the duct.

Causes

• In newborn babies the duct is not always fully open, or being very small may become blocked. In adult life the duct sometimes becomes blocked after injury or infection.

Treatment in the home
- If an infant (usually aged between one and four months) has a persistently watering eye, the mother should gently massage the corner of the eye beside the nose, every two or three hours. This may help to dislodge any debris that has collected and eventually relieve the obstruction. Massaging is less likely to succeed in an adult with a blocked duct, but it does no harm to try.

When to consult the doctor
- If the symptoms of watering persist for more than three or four weeks.
- If there is any sign of infection, redness of the eyes, stickiness or discharge.

What the doctor may do
- Prescribe some drops and/or ointment to combat any infection. If the blockage does not clear he will probably refer the patient to an eye specialist, who may recommend an operation—in the case of a baby to probe the tear-duct in order to clear it, or in the case of an adult, to bypass or remove the duct.

Prevention
- There is no way that you can prevent a tear-duct becoming blocked.

Outlook
- Without medical treatment an infant's blocked tear-duct may continue to cause symptoms or may clear spontaneously.

See EYE *page 36*

TEETH
The commonest diseases of Western man are those affecting the teeth and gums. Yet for most of us a simple routine of cleaning, started in childhood, would preserve our teeth throughout life.
See CARE OF THE TEETH *page 496*

TEMPERATURE
Raised temperature, or fever, is usually associated with the presence of infection. Temperature below normal (HYPOTHERMIA) is also a symptom of disorder.
See SYMPTOM SORTER—TEMPERATURE
HOME NURSING—TAKING TEMPERATURE

TENDINITIS
Inflammation of a tendon, the fibrous end of a muscle that attaches it to a bone. Usually it occurs together with TENOSYNOVITIS, inflammation of the sheath surrounding the tendon.

TENDON, RUPTURE OF

A tendon is a tough tissue that attaches a muscle to a bone, and the means by which the pull of the muscle can move the bone. Although they are very strong, tendons can be ruptured if the contraction of the muscle is greater than the strength of the tendon. Rupture can also take place with less tension if the tendon is weakened by disease, such as RHEUMATOID ARTHRITIS, or by old age. A tendon can also be divided or injured by an open wound. The tendons of the shoulder and arm are the ones most often injured or ruptured.

Symptoms
- When any tendon ruptures, a sudden pain is felt at the site of rupture and there is often a sensation that a muscle has suddenly given way.
- Weakness, swelling and tenderness may be felt at the site of the pain.
- The affected muscle feels weak.
- Laceration of the skin, especially of the hand and wrist, may suggest that a tendon has been cut.

Duration
- Several weeks to several months.

Causes
- Injury.
- Over-exertion of a muscle.

Complications
- Permanent loss of normal function of the muscle, caused by lengthening of the tendon as it heals. For example, if the ACHILLES TENDON in the heel is ruptured, it can cause loss of spring in the step.

Treatment in the home
- Keep an open wound clean and cover it with a dressing.
- Rest until medical advice is obtained.

When to consult the doctor
- Immediately the condition is suspected.

What the doctor may do
- Examine the muscle weakness to confirm the diagnosis.
- Send the patient to hospital, where X-rays may be carried out to exclude a fractured bone.
- If there is an open wound, the injured tendon will probably be stitched or clamped together immediately.
- After repair the limb will be splinted in a position of relaxation. Arms are usually kept in splints for at least three weeks. In the case of a leg the splints will be retained for up to six weeks.
- If there is no open wound, the ruptured tendon may

require only surgical repair or may be kept in plaster to immobilise it, depending on the site and extent of the rupture.

Prevention
- Unfit people and those with rheumatoid arthritis are especially liable and should not exercise their muscles excessively.

Outlook
- Good if detected and treated early.

See SKELETAL SYSTEM *page 54*

TENNIS ELBOW

Inflammation of the tendons that attach the muscles of the forearm to the elbow, following sudden excessive use of the forearm.

Symptoms
- A gradual onset of pain on the outside of the elbow, often extending down the forearm.

Duration
- The condition persists for anything from one to 12 months.

Causes
- Unaccustomed over-use of the forearm muscles during any activity. Tennis is only one of many activities that can create the problem.

Treatment in the home
- Do not use the arm in any way that aggravates the pain.

When to consult the doctor
- If the pain interferes with normal activities.

What the doctor may do
- Arrange an X-ray of the elbow to check that the trouble is not due to injury.
- Prescribe painkilling tablets.
- Inject hydrocortisone and a local anaesthetic at the point of greatest tenderness in order to reduce the inflammation. *See* MEDICINES, 22, 39.
- Arrange physiotherapy.
- In cases of severe pain he will refer the patient to hospital. The arm may then be put in plaster above the elbow for six weeks.

Outlook
- No matter how painful a case of tennis elbow may be, it will almost always clear up without side-effects.

See SKELETAL SYSTEM *page 54*

Care of the teeth

TOOTH DECAY AND GUM DISEASE CAN BE PREVENTED BY FOLLOWING A SIMPLE DAILY ROUTINE OF CLEANING AND CARING

The two most prevalent diseases in Western man are dental decay and a gum disease called gingivitis. It is only within the last ten years that research has shown not only what causes these diseases, but how we can prevent them and keep our natural teeth for life.

From birth, the mouth contains many kinds of bacteria. Only a few are harmful—those that constantly form a sticky film called plaque on the teeth and gums. Plaque harms the teeth most when it is combined with sugar, but it is also harmful by itself if allowed to remain on the teeth for more than 24 hours. When sugar is taken into the mouth in either food or drink, it is immediately absorbed by saliva, which then attaches itself to the sticky film of plaque.

Within 12 minutes of any sugar entering the mouth the dissolved sugar and plaque combine to increase dramatically the level of acid, always present in small quantities. The acid eats into the tooth enamel and so starts the process of dental decay. The acid level does not return to normal until at least 25 minutes later.

The vital factor in acid formation is how often sugar is consumed rather than how much. If sugar is consumed throughout the day, the acid in the mouth is continually rising to a high level and exposing teeth to attack.

Dental decay can start when a child is only one year old and can continue throughout life. But decay and gingivitis can be prevented by cleaning the teeth regularly and thoroughly, cutting down on sweetstuffs and visiting the dentist regularly.

Brushing

Teeth should be brushed at least once a day to remove plaque—an almost invisible film of bacteria that forms on the surface of the teeth—particularly between the teeth and just below the gum line. Plaque is a major cause of dental disease, and it should be removed by using a medium-soft nylon toothbrush and a fluoride toothpaste. Brushing should be firm, but do not scrub. Spend three minutes cleaning your teeth carefully and thoroughly.

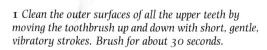

1 Clean the outer surfaces of all the upper teeth by moving the toothbrush up and down with short, gentle, vibratory strokes. Brush for about 30 seconds.

GINGIVITIS

If dental plaque is not removed effectively every 24 hours, it accumulates around and underneath the gum margin (where the tooth meets the gum) and gradually forms a hard, rough substance called calculus, or tartar, which collects plaque more easily and leads to inflammation of the gums. The many fibres that attach the tooth to the jawbone and act as a 'cushion' against shocks are also destroyed. Eventually, the teeth become loose and have to be removed, or else fall out of their own accord.

The main symptom of gingivitis is bright pink gums which bleed on brushing. The disease can start at a very young age—often under five years. If it is not corrected with careful oral hygiene, the damage eventually becomes irreversible to the extent that teeth may be lost.

CLEANING THE TEETH

The teeth should be brushed really thoroughly with a fluoride toothpaste at least once a day, preferably immediately before going to bed.

Ordinary toothpastes and powders are not essential, as they do little to improve cleaning. However, products containing fluoride have been shown to reduce decay by about 25 per cent when used regularly. The best kind of toothbrush is one with a small, flat head of medium-soft nylon tufts. The brush needs replacing as soon as the tufts have become splayed; for

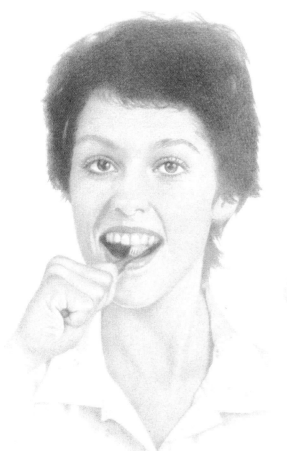

2 Use a similar up-and-down stroke to clean the inner surfaces of the upper teeth, only this time tilt the brush to make access easier.

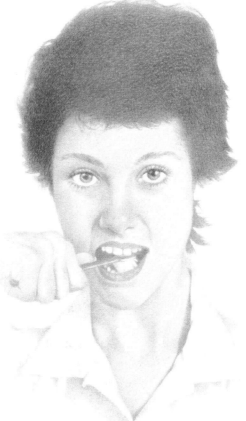

3 Clean the lower teeth by repeating the appropriate brushing procedure on the outer and inner surfaces in turn, spending about 30 seconds on each.

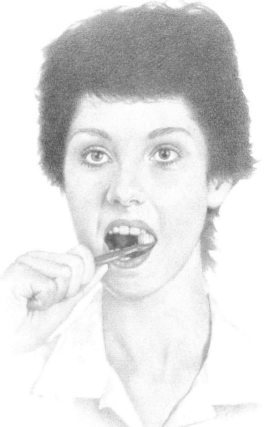

4 Brush along the biting surfaces of the upper teeth using firm, horizontal strokes. Repeat the brushing technique to clean the biting surfaces of the lower teeth.

most people, that means at least four times a year.

You should start brushing at a different place every time you clean your teeth. Otherwise you may find yourself cleaning the same areas over and over again, while leaving other areas uncleaned.

Anyone who cannot use his hands properly may find an electric toothbrush useful. Invalids or severely handicapped people need their teeth cleaned daily for them. *See* HOME NURSING.

An inter-space brush—one with a very tiny head—is useful for cleaning any large gaps in the teeth, and essential for anyone wearing a fixed brace, because it can reach under the delicate wires without damaging them. It is also useful for cleaning behind the back teeth, if an ordinary brush fails to reach.

When brushing your teeth, do not wet the brush first. Put a small dab of paste—the amounts shown in

toothpaste advertisements are too large— on to a dry brush. The saliva in your mouth will provide all the moisture needed; a lot of paste creates a lot of frothing which actually hampers cleaning.

There is no single, correct way of brushing. Any method that removes all the plaque from the backs, fronts and biting surfaces of all the teeth and the gum margins, and as much as possible from between the teeth, is suitable. You can find the way that suits you best by using a disclosing tablet—a harmless dye which, when chewed, colours the plaque on teeth and gums, making it show up. Until all the stained plaque has been brushed off, the teeth are not clean. Disclosing tablets, disclosing solutions and food dyes are available from a chemist's, and the whole family should use one or other of them once a week.

Even regular brushing will not remove all the plaque from between

the teeth. Supplement it by using dental floss or—for people with clear gaps—wooden points. Both are available from a chemist's, but get your dentist's advice before trying either, because used incorrectly they can damage the gums.

Dental floss is a strong, unspun, nylon thread specially made for its purpose. Never use ordinary spun thread, as that can harm the mouth.

If the gums bleed after flossing, either the floss was used incorrectly or the user has gingivitis. In the second case, thorough daily brushing and flossing once a week will clear up the trouble.

TOOTH CARE IN YOUNG CHILDREN

A baby produces his first tooth at about six months. It is easier to clean this with a cotton-wool bud or a piece of gauze than with a baby toothbrush. However, introduce a toothbrush into the hygiene routine of young children as soon as they will accept it in their mouths, even if at first they treat it as a plaything. It helps to get them used to the idea of brushing. Do not use toothpaste until the child is old enough to rinse his mouth.

Once a baby can support himself in a highchair, the best way of cleaning his teeth is from behind, with his head facing the light and resting comfortably against the mother's arm and chest.

Until the age of seven or eight, a child does not have the manual dexterity to clean his own teeth properly. During these early years, an adult must do most of the cleaning.

DIET

Keep sweet foods to a minimum in the diet. In particular, do not take

sweet snacks. If snacks are needed, they should consist of cheese, savoury biscuits or fresh fruit. These can also be substituted for a sweet pudding after dinner. If you buy convenience foods, choose those that contain the lowest amount of sugar or glucose.

A baby is not born with a 'sweet tooth'; he acquires one. Help him not to do so by not giving him a dummy coated with sweetstuff and by not adding sugar to his food and drinks. When the child becomes older, sweets become a problem. Ideally, they should be limited to a small amount given one day each week as a treat.

Many patent medicines for childhood illnesses contain a high percentage of sugar. If medicines, fruit or cola drinks are given just before bedtime, the child's teeth should be cleaned afterwards or, at the least, his mouth should be rinsed with water.

FLUORIDE

Extensive research has proved that fluoride strengthens the enamel on the teeth and makes it more resistant to decay. Its greater strengthening effect is on the enamel of a baby's permanent teeth when these are forming high up in the jaw soon after birth.

The fluoride level in drinking water varies from area to area. The dentists in each area know if the level is high enough to provide maximum protection to the teeth. If it is not, then a child should be given fluoride drops (not exceeding the amount recommended by the dentist) from six months until all the permanent teeth other than the wisdom teeth have appeared—which is usually by about the age of 14.

Alternatively, fluoride can be given

Types of toothbrush

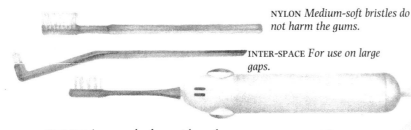

NYLON *Medium-soft bristles do not harm the gums.*

INTER-SPACE *For use on large gaps.*

ELECTRIC *Anyone who does not have the full use of his hands will find an electric toothbrush a boon. Those that are mains-operated are cheaper and more convenient to use than those requiring batteries which need to be changed.*

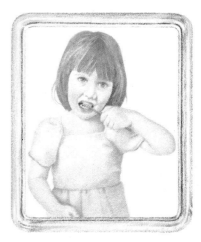

2 *Tell the child to swallow any saliva and to brush her teeth, trying to remove the dye. One good brushing a day, using colouring, is better than several hasty and inadequate brushings.*

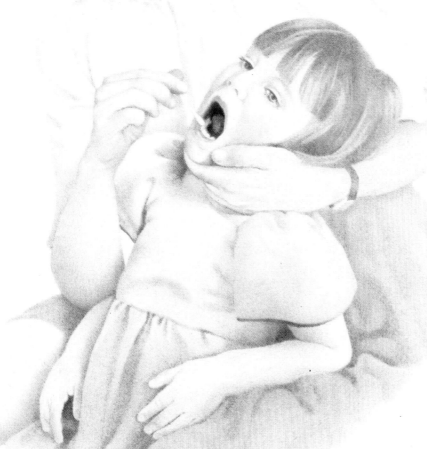

Colouring and brushing

To help prevent dental problems, the plaque on a child's teeth can be identified by being coloured with a harmless, vegetable dye. The child can then see the plaque and appreciate why her teeth need to be regularly cleaned. The colouring and brushing should start as early as possible since, by the age of three, 90 per cent of British children have suffered dental decay and early gum disease. By the time they are aged 12, 20 per cent of their teeth are either decayed, missing or filled.

1 *Using a cotton bud, the mother rubs plaque-revealing dye firmly on her child's teeth. All the teeth must be coloured, including those at the back.*

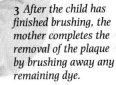

3 *After the child has finished brushing, the mother completes the removal of the plaque by brushing away any remaining dye.*

Glossary of dentistry

Anaesthetics
A local anaesthetic—most commonly lignacaine—is injected into the tissues around the teeth to cause complete loss of sensation in one or more teeth and the surrounding tissues.

A general anaesthetic is used to produce either unconsciousness or complete or partial loss of sensation throughout the body. The most commonly used is nitrous oxide gas, given by mask. Intravenous anaesthetic agents—often Valium or sodium brietal—are injected into a vein.

Bridges
A bridge consists of one or more false teeth set on to a small metal plate. The natural tooth on either side of the gap where the bridge is to go is prepared for a covering crown. The crowns are fixed on to the plate on either side of the false tooth or teeth, and then cemented over the adjoining natural teeth. Once fitted, a bridge can only be removed by a dentist.

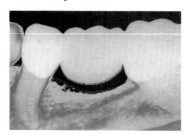

DENTAL BRIDGE

Crowns
A crown is a covering made to fit over a tooth that is broken down through decay, misshapen or badly discoloured. Porcelain is generally used for front teeth. Gold or gold covered with porcelain is used

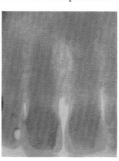

for back teeth. A post crown is a crown which is built on to a metal post fitted into the root of the tooth.

CROWNS

Extractions
Teeth are extracted for various reasons: among them are bad decay, faulty development, loosening due to gum disease, and an abscess on the root of the tooth. Most extractions are executed by a dentist using a local anaesthetic. Difficult extractions, needing a general anaesthetic, may be executed in hospital.

Fillings
A filling is a replacement for an area of tooth that has decayed and been drilled away. Amalgam (a dark, silvery alloy of various metals) is generally used to fill back teeth because of its strength. Composite (a white substance with a ceramic or glass basis) is used for front teeth.

Impacted teeth
An impacted tooth is one which is unable to properly emerge as it is wedged against another tooth below the gum. The teeth most vulnerable to impaction are the third molars, or wisdom teeth, which usually emerge when the person is about 18 years old. An impacted wisdom tooth will probably be removed in hospital under a general anaesthetic. The hospital stay will be about 24 hours.

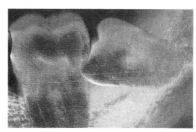

IMPACTED WISDOM TOOTH

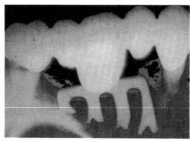

IMPLANT

Implant
The relatively new technique of 'implantation'—permanently attaching false teeth to the jaw-bone by means of a metal framework—has still to be proved effective. Usually implants are inserted as a last resort when no other satisfactory way of replacing missing teeth can be found.

Root-canal fillings
In many cases when an abscess has severely infected the pulp of a tooth (the living tissue at its centre), the tooth need not be extracted. Instead, the pulp and nerve can be removed, the roots and abscess drained and the root canals and interior of the tooth filled.

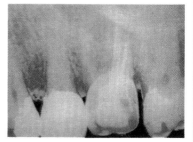

ROOT-CANAL FILLINGS

X-rays
Dentists often need an X-ray of the teeth and jaws to diagnose a dental problem. Most dental surgeries use a bite-wing, in which the film is held inside the mouth and exposed by radium released from outside. A pregnant woman should tell the dentist of her condition before having an X-ray.

to the child by the dentist or hygienist in the form of a gel every six months (the gel is a thick fluid in which the child immerses his teeth for several minutes at the dental surgery). Fluoride can also be obtained in liquid form to be used regularly as a mouth rinse at home.

There is another process that strengthens children's teeth against decay. The back teeth have pits in their biting surface and it is almost impossible to remove plaque from these pits. However, the dentist can seal them with plastic, applied like paint, as soon as each permanent back tooth appears. The process is known as fissure sealing.

CARE OF DENTURES

Unfortunately, preventive dentistry is often too late to stop people losing their teeth. Nearly 2 million sets of dentures are supplied in Britain each year. When natural teeth have been extracted, the gums shrink—quite rapidly for the first six months, then more slowly. Anyone wearing new dentures, therefore, may find that they become loose and may need to return to the dentist to have minor adjustments made to them. Full and partial dentures should be checked for fit by a dentist if they become uncomfortable, and a full set should be examined once every five years.

Unclean dentures are unattractive to look at and uncomfortable to wear. Once a day they should be removed and thoroughly cleaned.

The best way to clean dentures is to brush them with a medium-texture brush and a proprietary brand of denture paste. Rinse the paste off

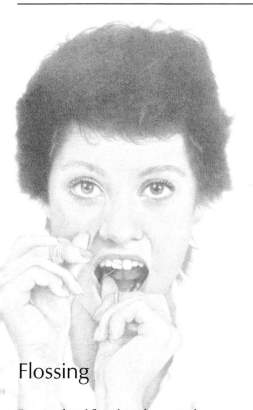

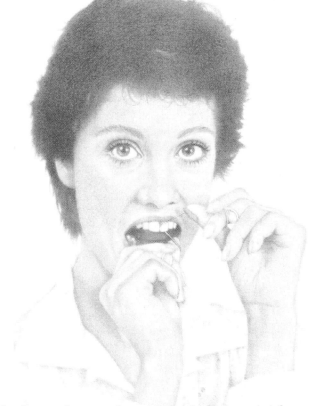

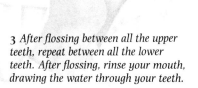

Flossing

Running dental floss through your teeth once a day removes food particles and helps prevent the build-up of plaque. An 18 in. (450 mm.) length of floss is wound around the middle fingers of each hand and controlled with the thumbs and forefingers.

1 Guide the floss between the centre of the two upper front teeth. Slide the floss firmly down the side of each tooth, taking care at the gum line.

2 Repeat the flossing against the adjacent teeth. As you proceed, wind the floss from one middle finger to the other to gain a clean, strong piece of floss.

3 After flossing between all the upper teeth, repeat between all the lower teeth. After flossing, rinse your mouth, drawing the water through your teeth.

in lukewarm water and continue brushing until the dentures are meticulously clean. Soaking dentures in a cleanser may only bleach them.

Dentures should be removed before the wearer goes to sleep and put in water to help keep them fresh.

VISITING THE DENTIST
Everyone, especially children, should visit the dentist every six months. Apart from examining the teeth for any decay, the dentist will check whether developing permanent teeth are growing correctly or will need straightening by an orthodontist. All patients visiting the dentist should tell him if they are taking any course of medicine, or suffering from a weak heart.

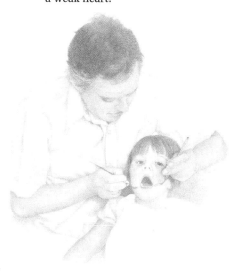

GOING TO THE DENTIST *A sympathetic and skilful dentist can put a child at ease and make 'going to the dentist' a rewarding experience. Dental disease is easy to prevent and should be prevented, as it can cause a child great suffering and distress.*

ORTHODONTICS
The art of correcting faultily positioned teeth and improving facial appearance and profile

Orthodontics is a branch of dentistry that corrects badly positioned teeth, both to improve appearance and to lessen the risk of tooth decay and gum disease presented by the faulty aligned teeth. It is usually carried out while the teeth are still developing, but in some cases adults can be treated.

Successful orthodontic treatment does not depend solely on the skill of the orthodontist, but also on the co-operation of the patient, and if the patient is a child, his parents. Perfectly 'straight' teeth are seldom achieved—indeed this is not usually the aim. The orthodontist's objective is to create a healthy mouth combined with an improved appearance.

What faults can be treated by orthodontics?
Orthodontic treatment is used to correct projecting upper teeth (buck teeth) or lower teeth (Hapsburg jaw); to reposition crowded teeth and teeth that have twisted round (rotated teeth), and to close up gaps caused by missing teeth—whether lost by extraction or accident or missing naturally—or to open up such gaps so that they can take false teeth.

Children with a cleft palate usually need orthodontic treatment to correct missing, rotated or misplaced teeth that occur together with the defective palate.

Who carries out orthodontic treatment?
Most treatment is carried out by general dental practitioners (GDPs), but these are referring an increasing number of their patients to orthodontists,

specialists in orthodontics. A GDP or orthodontist will sometimes refer a patient to a hospital specialist in orthodontics for a second opinion. Cleft-palate treatment is generally carried out in hospital since surgery is usually required.

When should treatment be carried out?
Most orthodontists believe that a child with badly positioned teeth should first be seen at the age of nine or ten. Whether treatment is started at that age depends on what is wrong and on the stage of development of the teeth and jaws.

Treatment is best carried out before the age of 14, but it can be performed much later, provided that the teeth and their supporting structure are healthy.

How long does treatment take?
Treatment usually lasts for 18 months to two years, and generally entails a visit to the orthodontist every three or four weeks.

What does treatment involve?
Often some permanent teeth have to be extracted, usually to make room for other, crowded teeth to grow; for some patients extraction is the only treatment needed. For others, whether teeth have been removed or not, braces may be required on the teeth in order to move their position.

A brace is an appliance that is attached to faultily aligned teeth and by pressure on them gradually forces them into the correct position; it may be removable or fixed. A removable brace is taken off the teeth after meals to be cleaned. It consists of a plastic base-plate which holds the wires and springs or screws that regulate the pressure on the teeth. Some removable braces use the muscles of the jaws to help move the teeth; others prevent unwanted pressure by cheek, lip and tongue muscles on the teeth.

Fixed braces are used to rotate teeth and to achieve 'bodily movement in any direction' or to alter the position of the root of the tooth or the crown of the tooth (the part above the gum). An adjustable wire across the front or back of the teeth exerts pressure on them. It is kept firmly in position by being attached to a small bracket on each tooth. Each bracket may be cemented directly on to the tooth or may be part of a metal band surrounding the tooth and cemented on to it.

In some cases, wire on the upper set of teeth is connected to wire on the lower set by elastic to help move the teeth in the required direction.

Sometimes the braces have to be connected to special equipment worn outside the mouth in order to exert the necessary pressures on the teeth. This equipment, in the form of collars or headcaps, has to be worn for about 14 hours a day in order to be effective.

In a few cases, where faulty positioning of the teeth is due to the structure of the jaw, surgery on the jaw will be required.

Getting used to wearing a removable brace is like becoming accustomed to wearing a set of dentures. Sometimes, for about three days, it feels as if it is filling the mouth. A fixed brace feels less of a mouthful. Even so, it will take a few days for the tongue, lips and cheeks to get used to the appliance. Either type of brace may hurt for three or four days after being fitted and after each adjustment.

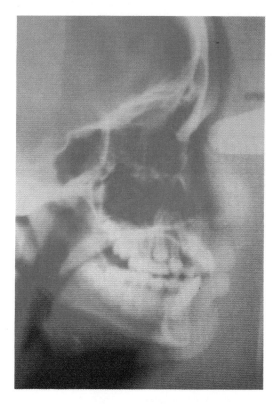

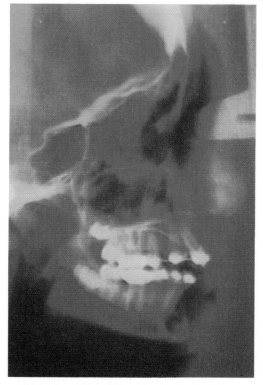

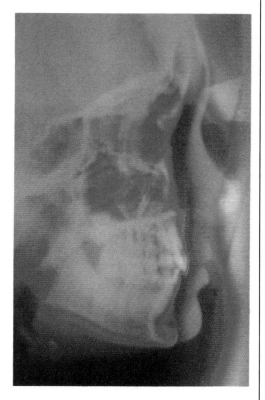

CASE HISTORY: JUDITH AGED 10 *Judith suffered from protruding upper incisors, or biting teeth, which made her mouth bulge outwards. As her first permanent upper side teeth emerged, two of them were extracted to make room to reposition the faulty teeth. To balance her teeth, and relieve crowding, two of her bottom side teeth were also removed.*

CASE HISTORY: JUDITH AGED 11 *A year later Judith is wearing a fixed upper brace to correct the protruding teeth and adjust her biting position. The faulty teeth are gradually being moved back into the spaces provided by the extracted upper teeth. A fixed lower brace closes the spaces where the bottom two side teeth were.*

CASE HISTORY: JUDITH AGED 13 *The braces on Judith's teeth were removed when she was 12 and now—a year later—all her teeth are in their proper position. Her bite is now correct and her mouth no longer bulges. She must see her orthodontist for some years to come to make sure her teeth remain stable.*

TENOSYNOVITIS

Inflammation of the sheath of tissue around a tendon, a fibrous cord that attaches muscle to bone. The inflammation usually occurs where a tendon passes over a joint, as, for example, at the wrist, ankle and shoulder.

When tenosynovitis is caused by repetitive movement, it may be called repetitive strain injury (RSI).

Symptoms
- The tendon is painful to use.
- It is felt to creak when used.

Duration
- The disorder may last for up to two years.

Causes
- Overuse of the affected tendon.
- RHEUMATOID ARTHRITIS
- Repetitive movements, as when operating keyboards.

Treatment in the home
- Rest the affected limb.
- Take painkillers in recommended doses to relieve pain.

When to consult the doctor
- If the symptoms do not subside with rest, or interfere with normal activity.

What the doctor may do
- Advise persisting with rest.
- Inject a steroid into the affected area. *See* MEDICINES, 32, 37.
- Arrange physiotherapy.
- Send the patient to hospital, where the affected limb may be put in plaster for four to six weeks.

Prevention
- Adopt a proper working position, and use ergonomically designed furniture.

Outlook
- Tenosynovitis invariably clears up with rest but tends to recur.

See SKELETAL SYSTEM *page 54*

TENSION HEADACHE

This is the most common type of headache. There is rarely any nausea, vomiting or disturbance of vision (*see* MIGRAINE). The headache does not persistently affect one side of the head alone, nor is it likely to wake the sufferer from sleep. *See* CLUSTER HEADACHE.

Symptoms
- A tension headache tends to come on towards evening, when the sufferer is tired. There is a sensation of tension or pain, generally felt towards the back of the head, though sometimes it is located at the front.
- The muscles at the back of the neck feel tense and sensitive.

Duration
- Severe pain does not usually last more than a couple of hours, though the sensation of tension may persist over much longer periods. In a person prone to the condition, headaches may recur for days, months or years on end.

Causes
- The headache is caused by persistent contraction of the scalp muscles which may result from any prolonged period of concentration.
- People who need but do not use spectacles are particularly susceptible.
- Emotional stress is a common cause. People suffering from DEPRESSION or ANXIETY are prone to recurrent tension headaches.
- Many patients have difficulty identifying (or admitting to themselves) a cause for tension headaches.

Complications
- None.

Treatment in the home
- The most important thing is to avoid, or come to terms with, the stresses and strains that precipitate tension headaches.
- A period of sleep, a rest or friendly chat over a cup of tea may relax tense muscles.
- Warmth or massage on the neck and scalp.
- Mild painkillers in recommended doses may ease the headache. *See* MEDICINES, 22.

When to consult the doctor
- If headaches are severe or frequent.
- If they occur with other symptoms such as nausea, vomiting or visual disturbance.
- If the sufferer for any reason is worried by fears of more serious, progressive disease.
- If a sufferer is becoming confused or drowsy, or there is a noticeable change in his or her emotional state.
- If there is any noticeable deterioration of eyesight with persistent or recurrent headaches.

What the doctor may do
- Ask whether there is any special cause, such as emotional stress or overwork. He may ask quite broad questions about life-style, since sufferers may not be able to identify the cause, or alternatively may be subconsciously concealing it from themselves.
- In severe cases, the doctor may arrange investigations to exclude the possibility of more serious disease.
- He may recommend treatment by a psychiatrist or clinical psychologist.

Prevention
- If the headache results from anxiety or overwork, minor alterations to life-style may prevent recurrent tension headaches.
- Adequate fresh air and physical exercise reduce the risks of headaches occurring, by relaxing the scalp muscles and toning up the circulation.

Outlook
- Occasional, mild tension headaches are a common hazard of modern life. Almost everybody experiences them from time to time. The problem lies in discovering the cause and finding ways to cope with it.

See NERVOUS SYSTEM *page 34*

TESTICLE, TORSION OF

Twisting of the testicle, the vas deferens (the duct which carries sperm from the testicle) and its arteries. The torsion cuts off the blood supply to the testicle. It is a rare condition that occurs most often just before or at the beginning of puberty. It is particularly likely to occur in an undescended TESTICLE.

Symptoms
- Severe pain, tenderness and swelling in the affected testicle. If the testicle is undescended, the pain and tenderness may be felt in the abdomen and confused with the symptoms of some other disorder.

Duration
- The condition lasts until treated.

Causes
- What causes torsion is not known.

Treatment in the home
- None is possible.

When to consult the doctor
- Immediately the condition is suspected.

What the doctor may do
- If the condition is treated early enough he may be able to manipulate the testicle back to its normal position.
- If manipulation is not possible, an emergency operation will be carried out to restore the testicle to normal.

Prevention
- Not possible.

Outlook
• Good if treatment is carried out within a few hours. Otherwise there is a possibility that the testicle will later shrink and cease to manufacture sperm, thus reducing fertility.

See MALE GENITAL SYSTEM *page 50*

TESTICLE, UNDESCENDED

Failure of one or both testicles to descend from the abdomen to the scrotum before birth. The testicles need to be in the scrotum because there they are at the right temperature for the normal production of sperm. If they remain too long in the abdomen, this will result in reduced sperm production or complete INFERTILITY but may not affect sexual potency.

Symptoms
• One or both testicles are absent from the scrotum.
Duration
• Unless treated, the condition is permanent.
Causes
• The condition is caused by an unknown fault in the development of the fetus in the womb.
Treatment in the home
• No attempt should be made to treat the condition at home.
When to consult the doctor
• The fault is usually discovered at a routine examination of the baby after birth.
• Parents who have any worry that their baby's testicles are incorrectly positioned, should see their doctor right away.
What the doctor may do
• Wait to see if the testicle descends normally, as it sometimes does after birth (within four weeks in half of the cases).
• If the testicle is not far above its correct position in the scrotum, hormone injections are sometimes all that is necessary to produce descent.
• If the testicle does not descend, an operation to lower it will be carried out before the child is five.
Prevention
• Not possible.
Outlook
• If the condition is corrected early, fertility will be unaffected.
• Delaying treatment increases the risk of reduced or

total infertility, malignant tumour of the testicle and torsion of the testicle.

See MALE GENITAL SYSTEM *page 50*

TESTICLES
Problems that may arise with the testicles or scrotum include the absence of one or both in baby boys, pain, swellings or deformities.
See SYMPTOM SORTER—TESTICLES AND SCROTUM, PROBLEMS OF

TETANUS

An infectious disease causing acute muscle contractions, particularly of the jaw and neck. The characteristic spasm of the jaw muscles gives the disease its common name of lockjaw. The symptoms are produced by the powerful poison from bacteria called *Clostridium tetani*. The bacteria exists as spores in soil and animal faeces, which develop only in tissue without oxygen—that is in damaged flesh. They lie dormant, ready to germinate if they find their way to a suitable breeding ground, such as a skin wound. Puncture wounds, burns, animal bites, road and agricultural accidents all produce a risk of tetanus.

The disease can also follow a non-medical abortion or the practice, in some countries, of putting dirt on the umbilical cord of newborn babies. Throughout the world about 1 million people die each year from tetanus. In Britain there are only ten to 20 cases each year, very few of which are fatal. Even so, all suspect wounds and injuries should receive medical attention.
Symptoms
• Early symptoms are vague. The patient feels unwell and there may be stiffness and pain in the jaw, difficulty in swallowing, and raised temperature, with headache and sweating.
• Stiffness of other muscles may occur, in which case there may be painful arching of the back and drawing down of the neck.
• Sudden muscle contractions may be brought on by noise or touching the patient.
Incubation period
• Usually six to 15 days, but can range from one day to several months.
• A short incubation period indicates the presence of a severe disease.

Duration
• Muscle contractions usually subside by the end of the second or third week.
• Some muscle stiffness may last for over a month after the infection.
Causes
• Bacteria.
Complications
• Choking.
• Pneumonia.
Treatment in the home
• None. Hospital treatment is necessary.
• If you suspect that a wound, even one several weeks old, may lead to a tetanus infection, go to the nearest hospital casualty department at once.
What the doctor may do
• Thoroughly cleanse an infected wound.
• Give an injection to neutralise the poison produced by the tetanus bacteria.
• Prescribe drugs, to control muscle contractions and stiffness.
• If breathing is difficult, it may be necessary to make an opening into the windpipe to insert a breathing tube. *See* TRACHEOTOMY.
Prevention
• Immunisation is the surest prevention. For children antitetanus is included in the three routine injections in the first year of life, with boosters on starting and leaving school. Older people who have not been immunised should have a full course of three injections, at intervals of six weeks and six months.
• A booster immunisation is usually given after an injury if it is more than five years since the last injection. Otherwise a routine booster is recommended every ten years.
• An injection to neutralise tetanus poison may be given after a major injury.
• Reactions to immunisation are usually mild and not dangerous. The injection site may be sore for a day or so.
Outlook
• The disease is frequently fatal in people who have not been immunised.

See INFECTIOUS DISEASES *page 32*

TETANY
A condition in which an abnormally low level of calcium in the blood causes muscle spasms and twitchings, mainly in the hands, feet and face, and sometimes CONVULSIONS. It is distinct from TETANUS, which has some similar symptoms.

THALASSAEMIA MAJOR

This disease is a form of ANAEMIA, which occurs in people from Mediterranean countries, or of Mediterranean origin. It is passed on from parent to child and affects both sexes equally.

Symptoms
- Slight yellow discoloration of the skin and whites of the eyes. *See* JAUNDICE.
- Feverishness, weakness and other symptoms of ANAEMIA recur throughout childhood.

Duration
- The condition is chronic, and attacks are likely to occur throughout a patient's life.

Causes
- An inherited abnormality in haemoglobin, the red pigment present in blood which carries oxygen from the lungs to the tissues. This abnormality causes the red blood cells to break down too easily.

Complications
- Without treatment, thalassaemia major often results in death during childhood.

Treatment in the home
- None advised.

When to consult the doctor
- As soon as any symptoms of jaundice with feverishness, weakness or anaemia occur.

What the doctor may do
- Take blood tests to find out whether any abnormalities are present.
- If thalassaemia major is diagnosed the doctor will arrange for an immediate blood transfusion, and for transfusions to be given regularly afterwards.
- In some cases, an operation to remove the spleen may be advised. This may help to reduce the need for repeated transfusions.

Prevention
- Not possible.
- If you suffer from the condition, it may be helpful to talk to your doctor if you are thinking of starting a family.

Outlook
- No cure for thalassaemia major has yet been discovered, and transfusions are the only form of treatment available at present. However, promising research into the condition and its treatment is currently under way, and a cure may be forthcoming.

See ANAEMIA

THERMOGRAPHY
The measurement of heat emitted by different parts of the body. It is carried out by photographing the body with film sensitive to infra-red rays. Thermography is used to detect CYSTS and tumours at an early stage.

THREADWORMS

Infection by threadworms is extremely common and can occur in people of all social groups, even in the cleanest of homes. Also known as pinworm, seat worm and enterobiasis, it is one of the oldest known of human infections, threadworm eggs having been found in fossils 100,000 years old. The worm lives in the intestines and during sleep the female crawls into the anus and lays up to 10,000 eggs which cause severe itching. Patients scratch the anus, the eggs get under the fingernails and eventually into the mouth, then down into the intestines where they hatch and the cycle begins all over again. Eggs may also contaminate nightclothes and bed linen, where the infection can lie for two or three weeks. The worms, which are like little strands of white cotton less than $\frac{1}{2}$ in. (13 mm.) in length, can be seen wriggling in the faeces.

Symptoms
- Itching around the anus.
- In young girls, vaginal irritation sometimes with slight bloody discharge.
- In children, abdominal pain.

Duration
- May be lifelong if not treated.

Causes
- The worm *Enterobius vermicularis*.

Treatment in the home
- None. If you see threadworms consult your doctor.

What the doctor may do
- Prescribe an anti-infestive drug to eradicate the infection. The whole household should be treated to stop the infection spreading. *See* MEDICINES, 29.

Outlook
- There is no danger in threadworms. Treatment is usually completely effective, although it does not prevent reinfection at a later stage.
- Adults who have had the infection for a long time may require prolonged treatment.

See INFECTIOUS DISEASES *page 32*

THROAT, LUMP IN

It is not unusual to feel a 'lump in the throat' at times of emotional stress. It is a sign of anxiety and may last only a few minutes. If it persists it is called 'globus'. It occurs mostly in middle-aged women, although it can occur in men or women at any age.

Symptoms
- The only symptom is a persistent feeling of a lump in the throat which is more noticeable when swallowing saliva. However, there is no blockage or difficulty when swallowing food.

Duration
- The feeling may persist for months or years. Until the patient has come to terms with her own feelings, it may be difficult to accept that there is not a physical lump in the throat.

Causes
- Anxiety, unhappiness or grief, may all interfere with the smooth working of the muscles of swallowing in the throat and oesophagus (food pipe).
- Indigestion can also accompany the false impression that there is a lump in the throat.

When to consult the doctor
- If the symptoms persist for longer than two weeks, so that the doctor can confirm that they are harmless and put the sufferer's mind at rest.
- If there are symptoms which suggest other diseases. Such symptoms include painful swallowing, a sensation that food is sticking in the food pipe and an unexplained hoarseness.

What the doctor may do
- Take a history of the symptoms and examine the throat. If physical causes are eliminated, the doctor may be able to help with the emotional problems if the patient is frank and co-operative.
- Send the sufferer to an ear, nose and throat specialist for more extensive tests if there is any doubt about the diagnosis.

Outlook
- There is no danger in globus, but it can recur at times of stress.
- Some sufferers are not easily reassured by the absence of physical causes, because the sensation of a lump is so real. But in time (sometimes months or years) the sufferer is able to ignore the symptoms, which then gradually disappear.

See RESPIRATORY SYSTEM *page 42*

THROAT, SORE

A sore, painful or red throat is very common among both children and adults, and is usually a symptom of infection such as a COMMON COLD or TONSILITIS.
See SYMPTOM SORTER—THROAT, SORE, PAINFUL (and) RED

THROMBOPHLEBITIS

Inflammation of a length of vein, usually in the leg. It is associated with THROMBOSIS, a blood clot which blocks the vein. It often accompanies VARICOSE VEINS.

Symptoms
• Painful swelling of a length of vein.
• In a surface vein, the overlying skin may also be red and swollen.
• In deep veins, there may be pain when pressed, but there is nothing to see on the surface. The ankle may swell.
• In extreme cases, the leg may become very pale and swollen. *See* WHITE LEG.

Duration
• One to four weeks.

Causes
• Varicose veins.
• Injury to vein.
• Constriction of vein.
• Immobility after operations.
• Immobility after childbirth.
• Some contraceptive pills.

Complications
• If part of a large clot in an inflamed vein becomes detached and moves to the lungs, it can cause PULMONARY EMBOLISM.

Treatment in the home
• Lift the leg to relieve pain, making sure the feet are higher than the buttocks.
• Avoid any pressure on the veins which will restrict the blood flow.
• Do not be more mobile than is necessary.
• Do not apply tight bandages, which will aggravate the condition.

When to consult the doctor
• As soon as the symptoms described occur.

What the doctor may do
• Try to determine the cause of the thrombophlebitis.
• Prescribe drugs to relieve the pain and to alter the tendency of the blood to clot. *See* MEDICINES, 10.

Prevention
• Seek treatment for any VARICOSE VEINS.
• Do not constrict the limbs with garters, tight straps or bandages.
• Avoid direct and sustained pressure on veins—especially during long car or air journeys.
• Become mobile as soon as possible after operations and childbirth.

Outlook
• The inflammation usually dies down within two weeks of treatment. However, if the patient has varicose veins then the trouble often recurs.
• If a deep vein remains blocked, swelling of the legs may persist.

See CIRCULATORY SYSTEM *page 40*

THROMBOSIS
The blocking of a blood vessel by a blood clot, or thrombus, which has formed in an artery. Thrombosis of the veins usually occurs in the legs and pelvis. But it may also take place in the portal vein that carries blood to the liver. When it occurs in the coronary artery it is one of the main causes of death in developed countries.
See CORONARY THROMBOSIS

THRUSH

A fungus, known medically as candidiasis or moniliasis. The organism normally lives on the skin and in the bowel, and at times it causes chronic infection of the skin, mouth or vagina (*see* VAGINITIS). Some groups of people are more prone to thrush than others. These include fat people, who have deep skin clefts where sweat encourages the fungus to grow; babies, especially those who suck dummies; people with dentures; diabetics; people who are weak or ill, or who are taking steroid or antibiotic drugs.

Symptoms
• A mildly itching area of skin which is shiny, moist and red. It has an irregular but clearly defined edge, commonest under the breasts, in the groin, the armpits, navel, between the buttocks and around the genitals.
• Chronic infection of the finger-nails (*see* PARONYCHIA) is found in those whose hands are frequently in water for long periods (for example, housewives or young mothers).

• Napkin dermatitis in babies may be due to thrush.
• Painful cracks in the skin around the angles of the mouth. *See* MOUTH ULCERS.
• Soreness and white flecks inside the mouth.

Duration
• The condition often lasts only a few days.

Causes
• A yeast-like fungus called *Candida albicans*.
• It is not clear why the infection should develop in some people more than others. But prolonged use of antibiotics, which destroy bacteria but not fungus organisms, makes thrush more likely. With no bacteria in its way, the organism rapidly multiplies.

Complications
• None.

Treatment in the home
• Do not take more baths than necessary; but keep the body folds well washed, powdered and dry to reduce the chance of infection. Proprietary powders against thrush can be bought at any chemist, who will give advice on the choice available.
• Do not wear tight clothing.
• If overweight, lose weight.

When to consult the doctor
• If the symptoms described occur.
• If the itching skin rash does not respond to washing and powdering.

What the doctor may do
• Take a scraping or swab from the infected area for examination with a microscope to confirm the initial diagnosis.
• Prescribe a cream or lotion for the skin.
• Test the patient's urine for sugar to see if DIABETES is present.
• Prescribe tablets to be taken by mouth to control thrush infection in the bowel.
• Prescribe tablets or a mouthwash to control infection in the mouth. *See* MEDICINES, 26, 43.

Prevention
• Keep diabetes under control.
• Regularly clean the mouth of a very ill patient. *See* HOME NURSING.
• Clean dentures regularly.
• Sterilise dummies.
• In patients with chronic infection of the nails, any possible thrush infection elsewhere on the body should be treated at the same time.

Outlook
• Skin and mouth infections can always be controlled and symptoms removed.

See SKIN *page 52*

THYROTOXICOSIS

Over-activity of the thyroid gland (hyperthyroidism) due to over-stimulation by the pituitary gland at the base of the brain. It causes toxic reactions in the body. The condition is also known as Graves' disease.

Symptoms
- Nervous over-activity, anxiety and tension.
- Sweating.
- Feelings of heat.
- Loss of weight despite large appetite.
- Slightly shaking hands, tremor.
- Bulging eyes.
- Loose motions and diarrhoea.
- Rapid heartbeat and pulse rate with palpitations.
- Enlargement of thyroid gland in the neck.

Duration
- With treatment, all symptoms can be controlled. In two-thirds of all cases treatment must be continued throughout life.

Causes
- The precise causes are uncertain, but the symptoms are due to an increase of the normal secretion of the thyroid gland.

Complications
If untreated, the condition may lead to:
- Irregularities of heart rhythm and heart failure.
- Body overheating and collapse.
- Eye infections.
- Being run-down and liable to serious infections.
- Nervous breakdown.

Treatment in the home
- None advised. Consult your doctor if you suspect the condition.

When to consult the doctor
- If the symptoms described appear.

What the doctor may do
- Since it is difficult to differentiate between the symptoms of natural nervousness and ANXIETY and those of thyrotoxicosis, the doctor will arrange for thyroid-function tests. If they are positive these tests will show high levels of thyroxine (the hormone secreted by the thyroid gland) in the blood.
- If the diagnosis is confirmed, the choice of treatment depends on age, general health, state of heart and lungs, and size of thyroid gland.
- Prescribe antithyroid drugs to control the secretion of the thyroid hormone. These drugs may need to be taken for many years and in some cases relapse may occur when

they are finally stopped. *See* MEDICINES, 31.
- Arrange for the surgical removal of three-quarters of the thyroid gland. The remaining quarter usually produces enough thyroxine, but as the person becomes older, some extra thyroid-hormone supplements may become necessary.
- Prescribe radioactive iodine to be taken as a drink. This inactivates many of the tissues of a thyroid gland and, if the right dose is given, should result in a stable normal production of hormones. But sometimes too much of the gland is inactivated, and thyroxine supplements may have to be given to make up the deficiency.

Prevention
- There is no known prevention.

Outlook
- Good: over-activity of the thyroid gland can almost always be controlled with drugs, surgery or radioactive iodine.

TIC
A twitch of the muscles, or any other seemingly purposeless movement, which may become a nervous habit. It is also known as a habit spasm. A person may tend to blink one eye or clear the throat repeatedly, for example. An arm may jerk, or a shoulder shrug for no apparent reason.

Tics are very common complaints. They may develop at any age, and children are especially susceptible to them. They are found particularly in families where a child (or the parents) are insecure or very anxious. But they also occur in the most balanced children.

Anxiety and insecurity tend to make the tic worse, so there is no point in scolding or drawing attention to it. Childhood tics often develop at the same time as other habits such as nail-biting or a tendency to nightmares. A tic usually disappears after a few months. The best policy is to ignore it; this will probably make it disappear all the more quickly.

There is generally no need to consult the doctor, unless more serious symptoms of psychological disturbance are present. In these cases the doctor may recommend psychiatric advice for the family.
See NERVOUS SYSTEM *page 34*

TICK FEVER
Any infectious disease transmitted by a blood-sucking parasite called a tick. *See* INFECTIOUS DISEASES *page 32*
ROCKY MOUNTAIN SPOTTED FEVER
TULARAEMIA
TYPHUS

TINNITUS

A condition in which the sufferer is conscious of a ringing, buzzing or tinkling noise in the ears that has no external source.

There are a large number of causes: EAR WAX, OTITIS MEDIA, MÉNIÈRE'S DISEASE, DEAFNESS, OTOSCLEROSIS, HYPERTENSION, or an overdose of drugs such as aspirin or quinine. Very occasionally, the condition is caused by an ACOUSTIC NEUROMA. Sometimes tinnitus is aggravated by psychological causes such as ANXIETY or DEPRESSION. Tinnitus may also be the forerunner of an attack of epilepsy or fainting. In old people, the problem is often the result of deafness due to ageing.

Unless there is a simple cause, such as wax in the ear, there is little that can be done. But if the symptoms could be due to anxiety they should be reported to the doctor as soon as possible. Firstly, because they may be caused by a serious disease and not by anxiety at all. And secondly, because if a doctor can reassure the sufferer about the cause of the symptoms, it will help to prevent the vicious circle of chronic anxiety from developing. The doctor will explain that tinnitus always has a physical cause and will help the sufferer to learn to live with it.

In some cases, with Ménière's disease, for instance, the intensity of the ringing noises can be controlled by the use of drugs.

In Britain, sufferers from tinnitus can keep in touch with the latest research into the problem through the British Tinnitus Association. The association publishes a newsletter and runs a network of groups throughout the country at which sufferers can obtain information, advice and support.
The British Tinnitus Association, 14-18 West Bar Green, Sheffield, Yorks S1 2DA. Helpline: 0345 090210.

TIREDNESS
Frequently caused by boredom or depression, tiredness is also a symptom of many diseases both trivial and serious. It is a vague term and difficult to interpret.
See SYMPTOM SORTER—APATHY

TOILET TRAINING
Training a child to use a pot so as to eventually do away with napkins. The age at which this should begin depends upon the temperament of the child.
See CHILD CARE—FIRST MONTHS

TONGUE PROBLEMS

Variations in the texture of the tongue include fissures, cracks, furring and the development of a smooth red surface. Most of these variations have no great medical significance.

FISSURES AND CRACKS
Irregular formations on the surface of the tongue, which may be either painful or painless. *See* MOUTH ULCERS.
Symptoms
• Fissures are round-edged, painless and appear as irregular channels on the surface of the tongue.
• Cracks are indentations, splits or tears which may become inflamed, painful and form an ulcer.
Duration
• Fissures are usually present from birth and will persist throughout life.
• Cracks rarely persist for more than a few days before healing.
Causes
• Cracks are almost always caused by the tongue being bitten, stretched or irritated in some other way.
• In rare cases, a fissure or crack may result from cancer or infection elsewhere.
Complications
• Very occasionally, a tumour may form; it can be either harmless or malignant.
Treatment in the home
• Practise normal dental hygiene, and keep the mouth clean by rinsing with water or a mouthwash after eating.
• Apply a drop of glycerin to a very sore crack, dabbing it on with the finger.
When to consult the doctor
• Any hard lump, ulcer, large, sore crack or smooth grey area which appears on the tongue should be reported if it persists for more than a couple of weeks.
What the doctor may do
• If the doctor suspects any serious condition he may advise an investigation by biopsy. This involves removing a tiny section of the affected tissue for examination. The biopsy is usually carried out in hospital, under anaesthetic.
Prevention
• Normal oral hygiene will reduce the risk of a crack becoming inflamed.
• Any persistent cause of irritation to the tongue (such as ill-fitting dentures) should be attended to before any sores can develop.

Outlook
• Fissures and cracks hardly ever present a health hazard, and a sore on the tongue usually heals rapidly without treatment.

FURRY TONGUE
It is often popularly believed that any furring of the tongue is a sign of ill health (indicating constipation, 'liverishness', and so on). This is not the case. A certain amount of furring is quite natural. It is produced by cast-off cells on the surface of the tongue, in which particles of food, of tobacco smoke and other substances taken in the mouth may accumulate.
Symptoms
• In normal furring, the coating may be grey, yellowish or brown.
• Excessive furring is a thick coating which may be mildly uncomfortable and dull the sense of taste.
• A dry tongue often accompanies thick furring.
• 'Black hairy tongue' is a particularly dark furring, almost black, which makes food taste unpleasant.
Duration
• Without treatment, excessive furring may last anything from an hour or so to an indefinite period.
Causes
• Thick furring often occurs if a person's diet is restricted to soft, milky foods lacking the abrasive action required to clear away excess particles.
• Dry furring is characteristic of feverish or dehydrated patients who are not producing enough saliva to cleanse the tongue. It is common in the chronically ill, the elderly and after alcoholic excess, it may also follow a course of antibiotics.
• 'Black hairy tongue' often results from heavy smoking or a course of antibiotics.
Complications
• None.
Treatment in the home
• Excess furring can be cleaned away with a toothbrush and water.
• For a dry tongue, ensure that adequate fluids are being taken.
• The dark furring of 'black hairy tongue' can be removed and usually cured in a few days by regular brushing with a concentrated solution of bicarbonate of soda. Place two 5 ml. spoons of water in an egg-cup and stir in bicarbonate until no more will dissolve.
When to consult the doctor
• This will rarely be necessary, unless more serious symptoms of feverishness or dehydration are present.
What the doctor may do
• Advise treatment as above.

Prevention
• Simple oral hygiene and a balanced diet will prevent excessive furring in a healthy person.
• Giving up smoking will often prevent 'black hairy tongue'.
Outlook
• Furring of the tongue has no significance in itself and will clear up with simple treatment.

SMOOTH RED TONGUE
A condition common among anaemic people and those suffering from iron deficiency.
Symptoms
• The tongue becomes red and smooth, losing its normal abrasive texture.
• It becomes uncomfortably sensitive to hot or highly flavoured food and drink.
• Symptoms should not be confused with patchy or 'geographical' tongue, in which smooth pinkish patches may appear on an otherwise healthy and normal tongue. This painless condition has no significance and will recover on its own.
Duration
• Smooth red tongue may clear up on its own, or persist indefinitely unless its cause is treated.
Causes
• A deficiency of iron or vitamin B.
Complications
• None.
Treatment in the home
• Take a short course of iron and vitamin B tablets.
When to consult the doctor
• If symptoms persist for several months or recur after treatment.
What the doctor may do
• Take samples of blood to check the iron level and test for anaemia.
• Question and examine you for any cause of iron deficiency such as poor diet, poor iron absorption or blood loss (through heavy menstruation or haemorrhage, for example).
Prevention
• A balanced diet including iron-rich foods such as liver, eggs and leafy green vegetables will prevent the condition occurring in a healthy person.
Outlook
• Smooth red tongue is a symptom of a deficiency rather than a disease in its own right. Once the deficiency has been diagnosed and treated accordingly, the condition will clear up.

See DIGESTIVE SYSTEM *page 44*

Removing tonsils—true or false

☐ *True* Tonsils are part of the body's system of protection from infection.

☐ *True* Tonsils can themselves become infected by viruses and bacteria. This is called tonsillitis.

☐ *True* Frequently tonsillitis clears up without treatment. An antibiotic is only effective if the cause is bacterial. Antibiotics have no effect on viruses.

☐ *True* Taking out tonsils may reduce the number of sore throats suffered.

☐ *True* Sore throats usually get less frequent after the age of seven.

☐ *True* Tonsillitis can occur without a sore throat being present.

☐ *True* Removing tonsils is usually safe and straightforward, especially in children over five.

☐ *True* A hospital stay and operation can be deeply upsetting for a small child, and symptoms such as bedwetting, clinging, headaches and stomach upsets may result.

☐ *False* Tonsils are a useless part of the body like the appendix.

☐ *False* Abnormal tonsils are a cause of frequent colds and coughs, allergy, asthma, general ill health, small size, poor eating.

☐ *False* Tonsillitis should always be treated with an antibiotic.

☐ *False* Taking out tonsils will prevent coughs and colds.

☐ *False* Removing tonsils is always safe and there are never complications.

TONSILLECTOMY

An operation to remove the tonsils, performed in hospital under a general anaesthetic. A tube is passed down the patient's windpipe, or trachea, to allow him to breathe during the operation. The mouth is held open and the tonsils are cut away from the throat. The ADENOIDS are often removed at the same time if they are enlarged.

Since tonsils are part of the body's defence against infection, their removal is controversial. Many patients still suffer from attacks of PHARYNGITIS or sore throats after a tonsillectomy. Most surgeons, therefore, remove the tonsils only of those patients who have severe problems. These include: QUINSY after tonsillitis has subsided, recurrent OTITIS MEDIA, difficulty in breathing or swallowing between infections due to enlarged tonsils, repeated tonsillitis and a failure to grow properly on account of recurrent sore throats.

See RESPIRATORY SYSTEM *page 42*

TONSILLITIS

An inflammation of the tonsils, which is most common in children. It is usually associated with a general inflammation of the throat. *See* acute PHARYNGITIS. The condition, which has an incubation period of three to five days, is most infectious at the beginning, even before the symptoms, which strike suddenly, have appeared. Children in their first year at school are particularly vulnerable because they come into contact with large numbers of viruses to which they have not had time to build up a resistance.

Symptoms
• Sore throat. Young children may not be able to localise the pain and may therefore complain of stomach ache. Infants just cry.
• The tonsils and back of the throat look inflamed, being deep red and often covered with white flecks of pus or exudate.
• High temperature.
• Swollen glands in the neck.
• The tongue is white coated and the breath may smell unpleasant.
• There may be a fine red rash which first appears at the neck. This may be caused by bacteria (SCARLET FEVER) or by a virus.
• Dry cough.
• Mild CONJUNCTIVITIS.

Duration
• The worst of the illness is usually over within 48 hours.
Causes
• Respiratory viruses or bacteria.
• Less-common causes include: MEASLES, GERMAN MEASLES, INFLUENZA, GLANDULAR FEVER and, very rarely, GONORRHOEA.
Complications
• An attack of tonsillitis may be followed by QUINSY, RHEUMATIC FEVER, or NEPHRITIS.
Treatment in the home
• Drink extra fluids. Do not worry about not eating.
• Take painkillers in recommended doses.
• Go to bed while the symptoms are at their worst.
When to consult the doctor
• After three days if the symptoms, including the high temperature, persist.
• If the phlegm coughed up is green or yellow.
• If a child becomes pale and listless, or does not drink enough to pass urine.
• If there is a rash which lasts for more than 24 hours.
• If the symptoms appear in an adult over the age of 40.
What the doctor may do
• Advise on home treatment, as above.
• Take a swab from the throat.
• Prescribe an antibiotic if a bacterial cause is considered likely. Antibiotics will not cure tonsillitis, if the disease is caused by a virus. *See* MEDICINES, 25.
Prevention
• Not practical.
Outlook
• Complete recovery, if there are no complications.

See RESPIRATORY SYSTEM *page 42*

TORN LIGAMENT

A ligament is a short band of flexible tissue binding two bones at a joint. If the joint is sprained or strained the ligament can be torn. The most likely sites for this to happen are the knees and ankles, especially if there is a history of previous injury.
Symptoms
• Pain in the injured area.
• Swelling.
• Bruising.
• If the tear is complete, especially in the knee, there

may be abnormal movement or instability of the joint.

Duration
• In an incomplete tear or sprain, symptoms usually settle in seven to ten days.
• A complete tear even when treated can take many weeks to heal.

Causes
• Usually injury.

Complications
• If a complete tear is not treated, or treated inadequately, the ligament can lengthen. The joint is then permanently weak and subject to further injury, and ARTHRITIS in later years.

Treatment in the home
• A cold compress followed by a firm crêpe bandage reduces swelling and limits movement during the first few days.
• Give painkillers in recommended doses if necessary to relieve pain.

When to consult the doctor
• If there is excessive swelling, pain or bruising.
• If a complete tear is suspected.
• If you suspect injury to a bone.

What the doctor may do
• Examine the joint and arrange an X-ray if necessary.
• Send the casualty to hospital if a complete tear is suspected.
• If the ligament is completely torn, the limb will need to be immobilised, sometimes in plaster, for several weeks.
• Surgical repair of the ligament may be necessary.

Prevention
• Take care when walking in the dark, or on slippery or uneven surfaces.
• If possible, wear shoes or boots suited to the conditions underfoot.
• Special care and supporting bandages may be needed to protect previously damaged joints.

Outlook
• Most torn ligaments are slow to heal.
• Those which require surgical repair usually have a good result.
• However good the treatment, where there has been a complete tear of ligaments and joints, they are liable to remain permanently weakened.

See SKELETAL SYSTEM *page 54*

TORTICOLLIS
A deformity in which the head is tilted to one side while the face is turned to the other. It is commonly known as wryneck. A muscle on one side of the neck is over-stretched, probably during birth; later the scar tissue contracts to cause torticollis in children between the age of six months and three years. The condition responds to physiotherapy or surgery.

TOXIC SHOCK SYNDROME

This is a newly recognised, rare condition, usually among women using tampons during menstruation. It is thought to be caused by a build-up of staphylococcal bacteria in the body. The risk of toxic shock occurring is very slight, but if it happens immediate medical treatment is vital. Symptoms develop rapidly in a few hours.

Symptoms
• Sudden high temperature, vomiting and diarrhoea.
• Fluid loss, pallor, rapid pulse and other signs of shock may be severe.
• During convalescence a red skin rash and peeling of the skin of the hands and feet may develop.

Causes
• A poison (toxin) released by bacteria.

Treatment in the home
• None. Call the doctor immediately if you suspect toxic shock.

What the doctor may do
• Send the patient to hospital.
• Give fluids intravenously.
• Prescribe antibiotic injections or tablets. *See* MEDICINES, 25.

Prevention
• Change tampons at least every 3–4 hours.

See INFECTIOUS DISEASES *page 32*

TOXOCARIASIS

An infection by worms of the nematode (or ROUNDWORM) family, which can be passed to human beings by dogs or cats. The worms, *Toxocara canis* carried by dogs, and *Toxocara cati* carried by cats, release their eggs in the faeces of the animal, and the eggs incubate in the soil. If the well-incubated eggs are later picked up on the hands of a human being, particularly a child, they may get into the mouth, hatch into larvae and spread throughout the body via the bloodstream. Young children playing in public parks are particularly at risk from the infection. In a recent survey of public parks in Britain, eggs were found in 25 per cent of soil samples. Toxocariasis is usually only a mild illness. Often there are no symptoms and the illness goes unrecognised. It is estimated that 4 per cent of the children who play in public parks will have been infected, often without knowing it. Very occasionally, toxocariasis can cause serious eye disease possibly leading to blindness.

Symptoms
• Often there are no symptoms.
• As it is usually impossible to distinguish the disease from the much commoner infections of childhood, the diagnosis may have to be considered in children with persistent unexplained fever, skin rashes, respiratory symptoms or blindness and who play in public parks.

Causes
• A parasitic worm.

When to consult the doctor
• If a child develops any of the unexplained symptoms mentioned above.

What the doctor may do
• Take blood tests to check the diagnosis.

Prevention
• Discourage children from playing near soil contaminated by dogs' or cats' faeces.
• Prevention lies chiefly in deworming animals and preventing the animals from fouling areas where children play. Dogs and cats should be treated for worms monthly until the age of six months and then at three-monthly intervals.

Outlook
• Most cases of toxocariasis recover without problems.

See INFECTIOUS DISEASES *page 32*

TOXOPLASMOSIS
A serious disease of mammals, birds and reptiles, caused by a parasite known as *Toxoplasma gondii*. Humans can be infected by eating under-cooked meat, or through contact with the faeces of animals, particularly cats. The disease affects the central nervous system, lymph nodes, spleen and eyes. Sometimes there are no symptoms and the disease remains harmless and unrecognised. In more severe cases symptoms are similar to those in GLANDULAR FEVER, with enlargement of the lymph nodes.

If the disease occurs during pregnancy, the baby may be miscarried or born prematurely and it may be ill at

birth with fever, jaundice, convulsions and eye and brain disease. Most cases of toxoplasmosis, even in pregnant women, respond to treatment with antibiotics.
See INFECTIOUS DISEASES *page 32*

TRACHEOTOMY

An operation which allows air to reach the lungs without first passing through the upper airways, that is the nose, mouth, pharynx or larynx. A vertical cut is made in the front of the neck below the Adam's apple, through which a small tube, or air pipe, is passed.

The operation is performed, sometimes in an emergency, if the patient's upper airways are obstructed by severe facial injuries, by a foreign body in the pharynx, by paralysis of the vocal chords, by cancer of the larynx or by a swelling of the throat. A tracheotomy may also be performed if the patient has difficulty in breathing after a head injury, a chest injury, a drug overdose or a stroke.

Once he has recovered the tube is removed, the wound is closed and the patient reverts to normal breathing.
See RESPIRATORY SYSTEM *page 42*

TRACHOMA

A contagious and serious disease of the eyes common in the Mediterranean area and the Far East. It is caused by a virus that is easily spread by contaminated hands or towels. The eyelids, usually of both eyes, swell, become inflamed and discharge pus, and the eyes cannot tolerate bright light.

If the disorder is not treated at this stage, the conjunctiva, the delicate membrane that lines the eyelids and covers the front of the eye, becomes covered with tiny grey swellings beneath the upper lids. The cornea, the transparent area at the front of the eye beneath the conjunctiva, may thicken. Scarring of the lids, and sometimes of the cornea, takes place. The lids often turn inwards, so that the eyelashes scratch the cornea, making it prone to bacterial infection.

If treatment with antibiotics is started early, recovery is usually complete. If the disease is neglected, blindness can result.

TRACTION

When a bone breaks, the surrounding tissues contract, making it difficult to set the bone—particularly in the leg. Traction is a force applied to counteract the tension and allow setting of the bone. It is usually applied with pulleys, ropes and weights.

TRANSIENT ISCHAEMIC ATTACK

The rate of recurrence of this mild form of stroke varies considerably from case to case; some sufferers have several attacks each day, others only one attack. People who suffer from attacks should not drive vehicles or operate potentially dangerous machinery.
Symptoms
• A sudden onset of weakness on one side of the face, or in one arm or leg.
• The weakness may be accompanied by tingling in the affected arm or leg.
• There may be loss or impairment of speech, or disturbance of vision in one or both eyes.
Duration
• Complete recovery usually takes place within an hour.
Causes
• Minute fragments of blood or cholesterol that clot in the brain and disperse of their own accord.
• Similar symptoms can be caused by nipping of the arteries in the spine in the neck. *See* VERTEBRO-BASILAR INSUFFICIENCY.
Complications
• In one-fifth of sufferers these attacks may be followed by a full STROKE.
Treatment in the home
• Rest when an attack begins.
When to consult the doctor
• Immediately after the first attack occurs. It is important to seek treatment since some sufferers are at risk of having a completed stroke.
What the doctor may do
• Check the patient's heart, blood pressure and large blood vessels in the neck that carry blood to the brain.
• Examine the eyes and test the nervous system for evidence of damage.
• Arrange blood tests and possibly X-rays.
• In many cases the doctor will prescribe tablets and may advise an operation.
Prevention
• As for completed stroke.
Outlook
• With treatment, attacks stop.
• Without treatment, attacks may cease or continue indefinitely.

See NERVOUS SYSTEM *page 34*

TRAVEL AND HOLIDAYS

All too often holidays and business trips abroad are spoiled by people failing to take the necessary health and comfort precautions. Travelling itself can cause various illnesses, including MOTION SICKNESS (travel sickness) and jet lag, which can impair your powers of reasoning and quick thinking. At the destination unfamiliar local conditions and living standards can create ailments ranging from the minor (such as fatigue) to the major (such as MALARIA or YELLOW FEVER).

Whether you are travelling for pleasure or for work there are some basic guidelines to follow that reduce the risk of illness, and lessen the strain of long journeys.

PREPARE YOURSELF BEFOREHAND
Find out about the conditions at your destination. You need to know about the climate, the food, any locally prevalent diseases that require immunisation, and the availability and cost of medical treatment. The best sources of information are your travel agent, the airline if you are flying, and the embassy or tourist office of the country you are visiting.

For foreign trips, take out medical insurance against sickness or accident. Although some countries offer special medical concessions to British visitors, they do not always cover the full cost of treatment—which can be expensive, particularly in the USA. British travellers to Common Market countries are entitled to medical help at the same charges as for local people. But generally you will have to produce form E111 and your passport to prove your entitlement; and even then you may have to pay in full at first and reclaim part of the cost later. Form E111 is available from any office of the Department of Health. Ask for leaflet SA30 which gives further details and shows you how to apply.

TAKE THE RIGHT CLOTHING
Whether you are travelling at home or overseas, the clothes you wear can help to make the journey more comfortable. You should be adequately warm, without being over-hot. Take a top-coat, gloves, scarf and hat if you are likely to have to break your journey in a cold, damp or draughty place—for example, a railway station—and remember that all forms of transport are capable of failing in harsh weather conditions.

When you are travelling, do not wear non-absorbent materials—particularly nylon and polyester—next to the skin, as they do not soak up perspiration and can quickly make you feel hot and clammy. Cotton underwear and socks are more pleasant. Outer clothing should be loose-fitting and light. Again, natural fibres are more comfortable than artificial ones, but they crease more easily. The best solution is a blend, for example, of polyester and cotton or wool—which does not require much ironing.

Shoes should be well broken-in and not too tight, as some people's feet swell slightly when they have been sitting for a long time in a train, car, bus or aeroplane. Avoid tight-fitting undergarments, belts and ties that impede the flow of blood and the circulation of air around the body. Seasoned travellers loosen ties and belts—and, where possible, take off their shoes and jackets and put on slippers and a sweater or cardigan.

If you are heading for a hot climate, your clothes should be lightweight, heat-reflecting (light colours reflect heat; dark colours retain it) and able to absorb perspiration. If the clothes next to your skin do not soak up sweat you may contract PRICKLY HEAT and, possibly, ATHLETE'S FOOT.

It is preferable in hot, dry areas to wear a lightweight, light-coloured hat when in the open as protection against sunstroke. But if the climate is hot and humid, a hat is not normally necessary, and hinders the evaporation of perspiration from the neck and scalp.

For cold climates, take normal indoor clothing (which is totally adequate if you are spending much of your time in well-heated buildings) and suitable outdoor wear. You can be chilled in just a few minutes outdoors in severe cold. To guard against this, you need a long warm overcoat, gloves, scarf and a warm hat that covers your ears and prevents the possibility of FROSTBITE.

Take a pair of stout shoes or boots for walking on icy or snowy surfaces. Those with moulded and contoured soles, or with cleats, give the best grip. To protect business shoes in snow or ice, wear overshoes or galoshes. A pair of thick woollen socks to slip over your normal socks or tights when out of doors gives added protection against the cold.

SUNBURN

One of the greatest risks of holidays in hot countries is SUNBURN. Even when the sky is overcast, the tropical sun burns with a ferocity unknown in more temperate climates. Reflection off the sea and sand can also be intense. The safest thing is to take sunbathing gradually. In tropical climates, 15 minutes' exposure is enough the first day, 30 minutes' on the second day, one hour on the third and so on. If there is any redness or blistering of the skin do not increase the exposure time.

Good quality sun screens which stop penetration by ultra-violet light should be liberally applied to the skin before exposing it to the sun, and remember that once you enter the water they tend to be washed off—so re-apply on coming out. If you do get burned, apply calamine lotion liberally and avoid further exposure.

PROTECTION AGAINST MALARIA

Nearly 2,000 cases of malaria are reported annually in the United Kingdom—all imported from abroad and nearly all affecting travellers who had not taken the appropriate precautions.

Although malaria has been largely eradicated in Europe, it is still prevalent in tropical and sub-tropical areas. It is common on the west coast of Africa and throughout Central Africa, the Middle East, Pakistan and India, Thailand, Malaysia and Indonesia—and in Central and South America.

The type of malaria varies in different regions of the world, as does the sensitivity of the malaria parasites to preventive drugs. The most common agents used are proguanil (Paludrine), taken daily, and chloroquine, taken weekly, which may be prescribed separately or together. In some areas, malaria is resistant to proguanil, and maloprim, taken weekly, is advised instead. The patterns of malaria change rapidly, so tables listing the recommended preventive drugs for different countries are regularly updated. Your doctor or travel agent will advise on the best current combination. All tablets should be taken from seven days before entering an infected area until 28 days after return home, to ensure that any parasites in the bloodstream are killed. If after returning you develop symptoms such as a high fever or a headache be sure to consult your doctor.

The malaria-carrying mosquito (the female anopheline mosquito) only bites between dusk and dawn. So, to avoid being bitten, keep yourself well-covered after dark—wear long-sleeved dresses or shirts; tuck trouser bottoms into your socks. Apply mosquito-repellent creams to exposed parts of the skin—face, neck and hands. Air-conditioning keeps mosquitoes away; without it, mosquito netting should be used over doors and windows to the bedroom and over the bed itself. It is also advisable to spray the room with an insecticide.

PROTECTION AGAINST DIARRHOEA AND DYSENTERY

One of the commonest maladies experienced in tropical or sub-tropical countries is traveller's DIARRHOEA. The majority of attacks last only from one to three days, but they can cause great discomfort and embarrassment. The complaint is given different names in different parts of the world, including: Malta Dog, Basra Belly, Delhi Belly, Rangoon Runs, Hong Kong Dog, Ho Chi Minhs, Tokyo Trots, Montezuma's Revenge, Aztec Two-Step and, in Mexico, Turista—as it usually strikes at tourists.

The diarrhoea is caused by bacteria found in contaminated water, milk and food. To avoid the condition, boil all milk and water—even water used for cleaning your teeth. Where this is not possible, add water-sterilising tablets to suspect water. The tablets, such as Halozone and Sterotabs, are sold by most chemists at home and abroad. In an emergency, a few drops of tincture of iodine in a glass of water can be an effective method of sterilisation.

Many people who take adequate precautions with their drinking water make the mistake of placing ice-cubes in their drinks. If the ice has not been made from boiled water it, too, can be unhygienic. When in doubt, it is best to drink spirits neat or to stick to reputable brands of mineral water.

A more serious form of diarrhoea is DYSENTERY, which comes in two forms—bacterial and amoebic. Bacterial dysentery causes violent bowel movements and is accompanied by abdominal pain, vomiting and fever. There is also extreme dehydration coupled with rapid loss of weight. Symptoms start six to 48 hours after eating infected food.

Amoebic dysentery, on the other hand, develops more slowly, is much more serious and more difficult to cure. Symptoms include watery motions, fever, pain and general ill health. Among the complications that can set in are abscesses of the liver and of the brain, which can be fatal. See AMOEBIASIS.

To remain healthy in tropical or sub-tropical zones, it is advisable to avoid all doubtful water, milk, ice and high-risk foods. These include shellfish, raw or underdone meat, raw seafood, egg products, cream, mayonnaise, uncooked fruits, vegetables, salad ingredients and desserts. Ice cream should also be treated with caution and should never be bought from a street vendor.

Restaurants often display dishes in outside buffets, which are infested by disease-carrying flies. If a restaurant itself is fly-infested it is a sure sign that the kitchen will contain even more of the insects.

Always remember: food should be well and recently cooked, and re-heated food should never be eaten. Uncooked fruit and vegetables are best avoided if possible. Thorough washing with chlorinated water may help but does not prevent infection that originates from human disease carriers during cultivation.

As well as these basic precautions, you can take prophylactic tablets which guard against stomach upsets. These can be obtained from your doctor and the dosage is one tablet taken twice a day while you are abroad.

TIME ZONES AND BODY RHYTHMS

The world is divided into 24 different time zones, and travelling through these from east to west, or west to east, can upset your natural body rhythms, or circadian rhythms—from the Latin *circa*, meaning 'around', and *dies*, meaning 'day'. Jet aircraft can pass through more than eight time zones in 24 hours. Rapid arrival in a new time zone can cause severe disruptions in the body rhythms or jet lag. The most drastic disruption is usually to sleep. *See* INSOMNIA. In addition, judgment, short-term memory and the ability to do simple arithmetic can be impaired. If you have business affairs to conduct, it is wise to wait for at least 24 hours before starting work.

It can take up to nine days for your body rhythms to adjust to the time zone and light/dark cycles of your ultimate destination. However, with north-to-south, or south-to-north, flights the circadian rhythms are not upset, as the time of day does not change—and you only have to contend with the normal fatigue of travel.

The best way to avoid jet lag is to plan to arrive at your new environment in the evening (local time). Go to bed early and take a mild sedative or sleeping-pill—possibly Valium 5 mg.—and do not touch any alcohol. The golden rule is never to mix drink and drugs. For the first few nights your sleep will be shortened; do not repeat the sleeping-pill, and after five to ten days your circadian rhythms will have adjusted to the new time zone and the jet-lag symptoms will have disappeared.

EATING AND DRINKING WHILE IN THE AIR

Airlines tend to be lavish with their hospitality, and unwary travellers may be served rich meals that they do not need or want. Eating out of boredom or anxiety can have disastrous results on the digestive system—which closes down between 2 and 4 a.m. in the morning *your time*.

It is asking for trouble to eat large meals during what is normally your night—even if it is lunchtime in the particular time zone you have entered. The solution is to eat sparingly at such times, or else do without food until it is once again *your* meal time—and not that of the recently joined passenger sitting next to you.

Remember that the air in aircraft cabins at high altitudes is very dry—the higher the aircraft, the drier the air. It makes the nails and hair dry and brittle; it reduces the output of urine; and it dries the mucous membranes of the nose, throat, mouth and breathing passages, causing a certain amount of discomfort.

To combat this dehydration it is necessary to drink 4 or 5 pints (2.2 or 2.8 litres) of fluid a day while flying. However, alcoholic drinks—particularly spirits—and strong coffee and tea produce further dehydration. Alcohol draws fluid into the gastrointestinal tract; tea and coffee stimulate the kidneys to produce more urine. They should be cut down as much as possible—or totally avoided.

Water and fruit squashes are the best drinks to take; fizzy, carbonated drinks should also be left alone as they can cause stomach discomfort and flatulence.

ACCLIMATISATION

Air travel can take you from a temperate climate to the tropics or sub-tropics in a few hours. The body is faced with a sudden increase in temperature, and it responds with a marked increase in sweating. The sweat evaporates and so helps to cool the skin.

To aid this process you should drink a pint of fluid a day for every ten degrees of Fahrenheit temperature. If the temperature is in the 90s you should therefore drink 9 pints of fluid between rising one morning and getting up the next. (Where the temperature is measured in centigrade, drink 2 litres plus 1 litre for every ten degrees, so at a temperature of 20°C, drink 4 litres; at 30°C, drink 5 litres.)

The drawback of excessive sweating is that it reduces the body's stock of salt. In a temperate climate your average daily salt need is ½ oz. (15 g.), and in a tropical climate ½-1 oz. (15-25 g.). The most effective way to maintain this is by adding extra salt to your food—as soluble salt tablets may cause nausea, and the type that dissolve in the intestine may be passed unabsorbed if you have diarrhoea.

Acclimatisation to temperature change mostly occurs within the first week, and by the end of the second week it is 80-90 per cent complete. The final 10-20 per cent takes place within six weeks. Travel to high altitudes may also cause nausea and require several days' acclimatisation by not being too energetic physically.

TRAVELLING BY ROAD

Unless unavoidable, long road journeys should be started early in the morning after a good night's sleep. Once on the motorway, high-speed driving should be limited to periods of two hours. Regular stops should be made for non-alcoholic drinks, high-carbohydrate foods such as chocolate, and exercise.

WHEN VACCINATION IS NEEDED

Before setting out on a foreign journey, check whether you should be vaccinated against any disease. The situation is constantly changing, and each week the World Health Organisation issues a vaccination chart listing countries where immunisation for yellow fever, cholera and typhoid are currently recommended.

The chart can be seen at British Airways and Thomas Cook vaccination centres. Your family doctor is also likely to have a copy.

YELLOW FEVER vaccination, which is needed for equatorial parts of Africa and South America, can only be given at special centres, lists of which are held by travel agents, airlines and embassies. Before taking the injection, any previous strong reactions to any injection or immunisation should be reported to the doctor giving the injection, and checked. This also applies to anyone who is allergic to eggs, because yellow fever vaccinations contain an egg base.

CHOLERA vaccine is rarely given—it provides little protection and may itself cause symptons, but a few countries still ask for it. Hygienic precautions give better protection—avoid drinking untreated water or milk, or eating uncooked fruit or vegetables.

TYPHOID inoculation is not obligatory under international health regulations, but it is recommended for many parts of the world, including some European countries. Your doctor will advise on this.

TETANUS serum is recommended for all countries, and is especially advisable for those travelling in agricultural areas of the world. The serum is given in a series of three injections, and a booster injection is given at intervals of ten years thereafter.

MENINGITIS vaccine is now available for travellers to high-risk areas, mainly in India and Africa.

HEPATITIS A epidemics periodically occur in parts of the world—notably India, Nepal, Kashmir and south-east Asia. Two doses of vaccine give protection for journeys lasting up to a year. A booster dose after 6 to 12 months gives much longer protection. HEPATITIS B vaccination is sometimes given when medical treatment in an emergency could pose a risk.

POLIOMYELITIS vaccine is given by mouth, and provides protection for five years.

TYPHUS, transmitted by the body louse, is still found in India, Pakistan and south-east Asia—particularly after natural disasters or during wars. Immunisation is effective ten days after injection and lasts for a year.

RABIES vaccination is recommended only for animal-handlers and those in other high-risk occupations, usually when they are travelling to rabies-endemic areas and have a high risk of contact with wild animals. After possible exposure to a wild or rabid animal, or every one to three years if staying in high-risk areas—such as India, Pakistan, the Middle East or the Far East—a booster should be taken.

SMALLPOX has been declared eradicated by the World Health Organisation, and vaccination is no longer required.

TRICHINOSIS

An infection caused by tiny worms, usually caught from inadequately cooked pork or other meat. Although most infected people do not have any symptoms, some will develop diarrhoea and abdominal pain within two days of eating uncooked or undercooked meat. A week later fever, CONJUNCTIVITIS, swollen eyes, muscle pains and weakness may appear. Infections can be treated by drugs, but prevention by heating meat in its entirety to at least 60°C before eating it is much more important.

TRIGEMINAL NEURALGIA

The trigeminal nerve links the face and front of the head to the brain. Trigeminal neuralgia is a recurrent pain experienced when abnormal electrical discharges arise in the nerve (see NEURALGIA).

Symptoms
• Excruciating attacks of pain are felt in one side of the lips, gums, chin, cheek or temple.
Duration
• Attacks are brief, lasting only a few seconds. However, bouts of repeated attacks may persist for weeks or months, separated by periods when no pain is felt.
Causes
• Pain may be triggered off by a certain facial movement, or by pressure or cold on an area over the nerve. The exact cause is not known, but ATHEROMA in late middle age may play a part.
• In some cases, dental trouble may cause trigeminal neuralgia by pressing on or inflaming a nerve.
Complications
• There are no physical complications, though the pain may cause sleeplessness and acute distress.
Treatment in the home
• Painkillers may be taken to relieve repeated attacks.
When to consult the doctor
• If symptoms occur.
What the doctor may do
• Prescribe regular doses of a drug such as carbamaze-pine which will prevent attacks. See MEDICINES, 22.
• The nerve may have to be destroyed by injection or operation.
Prevention
• Patients prone to the condition may be able to identify certain incidents which have triggered off attacks: going out in a cold wind, for example. These may then be avoided.
• Regular dental check-ups should eliminate dental trouble as a cause.
Outlook
• Trigeminal neuralgia may persist for years without treatment. However, injection, or the prescription of drugs, often results in a complete cure. In other cases the condition may clear up of its own accord.
See NERVOUS SYSTEM *page 34*

TUBERCULOSIS

An infectious disease in which nodules—tubercles— form in body tissue and destroy it. Until the introduction of safe and effective treatment, tuberculosis, or TB, was widespread. Now it is rare in Britain and similar developed countries but is still common in less well-developed countries. Important factors in the spread of tuberculosis appear to be poverty and overcrowding. As the standards of living in a country rise so the incidence of tuberculosis falls.

Tuberculosis can affect all parts of the body. The most common site of infection is the lungs—pulmonary tuberculosis or consumption. Other relatively common sites are the lymph glands and the membranes covering the brain (tuberculous meningitis). In some cases tuberculosis may spread through the body when a large number of small tubercles form (miliary tuberculosis).

Every individual has to develop immunity to tuberculosis, which can be helped by immunisation; malnutrition and close contact with a sufferer may break down this immunity. Occasionally individuals fail to develop any natural immunity; in these cases infection is severe or even fatal.

There are certain general symptoms of tuberculosis; others vary according to the site of the disease.
General symptoms
• Feeling ill and weakness.
• Loss of appetite.
• Loss of weight.
• Fever.
• Night sweats.
Lung symptoms
• Persistent cough, producing yellowish spit.
• Blood-stained sputum.
• Loss of weight and unexplained ill health.
• Chest pain.
• Breathlessness.
• In young people there may be fever, swelling of lymph glands in the neck or painful red lumps on the shins.
Lymph gland symptoms
• Swelling and tenderness of the glands, often in the neck, which may discharge through the skin.
Bone symptoms
• Softening and collapse of the bones leads to deformity and usually pain in the area affected. If the spine is affected (Pott's disease) the disease may cause hunchback.
Kidneys
• Destruction of kidneys and subsequent inflammation of the bladder cause symptoms of a continuous, steadily progressive chronic CYSTITIS.
Genital symptoms
• In women infection may cause an otherwise symptom-less INFERTILITY.
• In men there is painless, persistent swelling of one or both testes.
Generalised infections
These include tuberculous meningitis, and may arise in individuals, especially babies, with low or absent immunity.
• Fever with obvious rapidly progressing severe symptoms, including headache and coma, leads in one to three weeks to a dangerous illness, with a high mortality rate.
Duration
• Depends on the immunity of the individual, the part of the body infected and the delay before start of treatment. Some individuals may overcome an infection without any symptoms, others may be disabled for years.
Causes
• Infection by the bacillus *Mycobacterium tuberculosis*. There are two strains of tubercle bacillus—human and bovine (present in cattle). The human strain is spread through inhaling infected droplets. This usually causes pulmonary tuberculosis. The bovine strain is spread through the milk of cows with infected udders. This type of tuberculosis is rapidly disappearing because of the elimination of infected cattle, pasteurisation and improved public hygiene.
Complications
• Tuberculosis originally infecting one part of the body may spread to other parts. For example, pulmonary tuberculosis may lead to tuberculosis of the lymph glands, tuberculous meningitis, or miliary tuberculosis.

• Tuberculosis not treated in the early stages may cause scarring even when healed and this may lead to sterility and other residual defects.

Treatment in the home

• None possible.

When to consult the doctor

• As soon as tuberculosis is suspected, especially if the patient has at any stage been in contact with the disease.

• Anyone who has been in contact with a sufferer should immediately consult their doctor and have regular chest X-rays.

What the doctor may do

• Send specimens (sputum, urine, etc.) for laboratory analysis to check whether tuberculosis is present.

• Check possible sources of infection in contacts, friends and relatives.

• Send the patient to a mass X-ray unit or hospital for X-ray of lungs, kidneys or bones.

• Refer the patient to a specialist who will prescribe drugs that destroy the tubercle bacilli. Drug treatment usually lasts six to 24 months depending on response. General care of tuberculosis no longer requires automatic admission to a hospital or a sanatorium. Hospital admission is only necessary for those living alone or those unable or unwilling to co-operate.

• If a case is identified, all contacts will be referred for X-ray.

Prevention

• Immunisation with BCG (Bacillus Calmette-Guérin), a weak type of tubercle bacillus which confers immunity. In Britain it is given to 12 to 13-year-old children after a tuberculin test has identified those lacking natural immunity. Babies and children at risk may be immunised earlier.

• Mass X-ray screening increases the likelihood of early identification of the disease and identifies carriers.

• Vigorous public health measures are the best method of prevention, including control of overcrowding and malnutrition and search for, and treatment of, contacts.

Outlook

• Very good if the disease is detected early. Modern drugs can halt the infection and avoid serious damage.

See INFECTIOUS DISEASES *page 32*

TULARAEMIA

An infectious disease of wild animals, particularly rabbits, caused by a bacterium called *Francisella tularensis*. The infection can be transmitted to humans either by direct contact with an infected animal or by ticks or flies carrying the disease. Symptoms, which develop after an incubation period of three to seven days, are a small itchy lump on the skin, which later develops into an ulcer with swollen lymph glands in the area of the infection. Pneumonia, diarrhoea or eye symptoms may follow. The disease is diagnosed by blood tests, and treatment is by antibiotic drugs, such as streptomycin. An effective vaccine is available for people such as rabbit hunters or butchers, who are at high risk of catching the disease during an epidemic. Tularaemia is also known as rabbit fever, deer-fly fever and Ohara's disease.

See INFECTIOUS DISEASES *page 32*

TUMOURS OF THE MALE GENITAL SYSTEM

Abnormal growths of tissue that most commonly affect the prostate gland, the testicles and the penis. There are two types of tumour: benign (non-cancerous), which remains localised; and malignant (cancerous), which spreads, sometimes uncontrollably. Since malignant tumours of the male genital tract are easily diagnosed, they are often treated at an early stage when a total cure is possible.

BENIGN TUMOUR OF THE PROSTATE GLAND

The prostate gland, which produces a fluid that forms part of the semen, lies beneath the bladder. If a tumour develops, the gland enlarges and often the passage of urine from the bladder is obstructed. A benign tumour of the gland is the most common of the benign tumours that affect the male genital system. By the age of 60 most men suffer from it to some degree—but in most cases with only minor inconvenience.

Symptoms

• Urinating more often than usual; having to get up at night to do so.

• A reduction in the size and force of the jet of urine.

• Difficulty in starting and then stopping urination.

• Rarely, complete inability to pass urine, blood in the urine or pain on passing urine.

Duration

• Indefinite unless the tumour is removed.

Causes

• What causes the tumour is not known.

Treatment in the home

• Dribbling of urine from the penis after urination may cause underclothes to smell and so create an annoying social problem. The dribbling can be avoided or reduced if, after urination, the urethral tube is pressed firmly upwards and forwards from a point 2-3 in. (50-75 mm.) behind the scrotum with one hand, and the last drops of urine are 'milked' out of the penis with the other hand.

• In emergencies, difficulty in passing urine may be reduced if the sufferer sits in a hot bath—into which he can then urinate.

When to consult the doctor

• As soon as the symptoms described begin to occur. Complete inability to pass urine, blood in the urine or pain on passing urine require immediate medical attention.

What the doctor may do

• Feel through the rectum for an enlarged prostate gland.

• Take samples of blood and urine for analysis and arrange X-rays.

• If the symptoms suggest that the prostate gland is obstructing the outflow of urine from the bladder, the doctor will refer the patient to a specialist in urinary surgery.

• The specialist will decide whether an operation is needed to remove the obstructing part of the gland. Drinking alcohol can bring on complete obstruction, and the patient may be advised to abstain.

Prevention

• No preventive measures are possible.

Outlook

• Modern surgery produces excellent results.

MALIGNANT TUMOUR OF THE TESTICLE

This tumour varies considerably in malignancy from case to case. It occurs at any age—often during the most sexually active years, and even during childhood. There is a higher than average risk of the tumour developing in an undescended TESTICLE.

Symptoms

• A painless swelling of one testicle.

Causes

• The cause of the tumour is unknown.

When to consult the doctor

• Immediately any lump in a testicle is noticed. The earlier the treatment, the more likely is a successful outcome.

What the doctor may do

• If he suspects the lump is a malignant tumour, he will refer the patient immediately to a specialist for investigation.

• If the diagnosis is confirmed, treatment will be either radiation therapy or removal of the testicle together with radiation therapy.

Prevention
- There is no way of preventing the disorder, but if a male periodically examines his testicles any swelling can be detected at an early stage.

Outlook
- This varies according to the age of the patient at the onset of the tumour, the type of tumour and how long it was present before treatment.
- The removal of one testicle has no effect on sexual potency or fertility.

MALIGNANT TUMOUR OF THE PENIS
A rare tumour that affects the tip of the penis. Its incidence is lower in circumcised men.

Symptoms
- A warty, painless growth appears on the foreskin or glans (tip) of the penis.
- Later the growth may become infected. It may bleed or be painful and discharge pus.

Causes
- Unknown, but the tumour has been linked with genital WARTS.

Treatment in the home
- None is possible.

When to consult the doctor
- As soon as any abnormality of the penis is noticed.

What the doctor may do
- If the tumour is reported at an early stage, it can be treated by being removed surgically or by X-ray therapy or radium therapy.

Prevention
- The penis should always be kept clean, particularly by uncircumcised men and boys.

MALIGNANT TUMOUR OF THE PROSTATE GLAND
The prostate gland, which helps to produce semen, lies underneath the bladder. A tumour causes the gland to enlarge and often obstructs outflow of urine from the bladder. Malignant tumours of the gland are rare before 50 but become increasingly common in old age.

In most cases, even when the disease spreads, it can be controlled by drugs.

Symptoms
- As for benign tumour of the prostate gland.
- If the disease spreads, there may also be a general feeling of ill-health and loss of appetite and weight.

Causes
- The cause of the tumour is unknown.

Treatment in the home
- None is possible.

When to consult the doctor
- As for benign tumour of the prostate gland.

What the doctor may do
- Arrange for the patient to have blood tests and for part of the prostate gland to be removed for analysis.
- Treatment is with drugs chemically similar to female sex hormones. In a few cases this treatment may produce some enlargement of the breasts.

Prevention
- Prevention is not possible.

Outlook
- Often extremely good.
- This is one of the few cancers that can be controlled completely with drugs alone.

See MALE GENITAL SYSTEM *page 50*

TYPHOID FEVER

A highly infectious disease most often contracted in Asia or the Mediterranean countries. Like PARATYPHOID it is an enteric fever—that is it affects the intestines. Typhoid is caused by bacteria that live in human faeces. The infection is spread by food, particularly shellfish, and water, contaminated by flies. About 3 per cent of patients become carriers after they have recovered from the disease. They probably harbour the infection in the gall-bladder and continue to excrete the bacteria in their faeces. They do not have any symptoms and so do not know that they are still infectious. The only way of detecting a carrier is by identifying the organism in the faeces. Carriers can start an epidemic, particularly if they are food handlers, without knowing that they are responsible. The possibility of infection is usually raised because the patient has been in contact with the disease or in a community with poor sanitation.

Symptoms
- Prolonged fever. Often the first indication of serious disease is when the fever is rising on the fifth day and after.
- Headache.
- Mental confusion.
- Abdominal pain.
- A rash of rose-coloured spots beginning in the second week of the disease.
- Constipation, which may be followed by diarrhoea.

Incubation period
- Ten to 14 days.

Duration
- One to eight weeks, depending upon the severity of the

infection and treatment.
- There may be a relapse (recurrence of symptoms) about two weeks after apparent recovery.

Causes
- A bacillus called *Salmonella typhi*.

Treatment in the home
- None. Consult the doctor if you suspect typhoid, particularly after returning from abroad.

What the doctor may do
- Send the patient to hospital.
- Test specimens of blood, urine and faeces to confirm the diagnosis.
- If typhoid is confirmed, prescribe antibiotics. *See* MEDICINES, 25.
- Isolate the patient.
- Good nursing care and replacement of lost fluids by frequent drinks are the main treatment.

Prevention
- Immunisation against typhoid, which gives some protection for about three years, is not compulsory, but is recommended for travellers going outside North America or northern Europe. Any travellers would be wise to ask if tetanus immunisation is also necessary.

See INFECTIOUS DISEASES *page 32*

TYPHUS
A serious, acute infectious disease caused by a rickettsia—a minute organism between a bacterium and a virus. There are various types of typhus, most of which are transmitted by lice in conditions of poverty, overcrowding and close contact. Fleas, ticks and mites (scabies) may also spread some forms of the disease; symptoms, which occur after an incubation period of seven to ten days, are headache, fever and weakness, followed by a rash that appears first at the armpits. Treatment by antibiotics such as tetracycline or chloramphenicol is extremely effective.

Prevention is by the control of lice with DDT or other insecticides. There is also an effective vaccine available for those at high risk. Although still serious, typhus is no longer the dreaded disease it once was. At the end of the First World War it spread through eastern Europe attacking 30 million people, 3 million of whom died.

See INFECTIOUS DISEASES *page 32*

ULCER
An inflamed break in the skin or in the mucous membrane lining the alimentary tract. There are many different kinds of ulcer, ranging from the small ulcers

that appear inside the mouth, to the more serious gastric, duodenal and malignant ulcers. See DUODENAL ULCER, GASTRIC ULCER, MOUTH ULCERS, VARICOSE ULCERS.

UNCONSCIOUSNESS

Temporary loss of consciousness may last only a few seconds or several minutes and has many causes. Deep unconsciousness is COMA.
See SYMPTOM SORTER—CONSCIOUSNESS, DISTURBANCES OF FIRST AID *page 611*

UNDULANT FEVER

A disease of cattle, pigs and goats, also known as brucellosis. It is sometimes caught by people such as farmers or vets who are in contact with infected animals.
See BRUCELLOSIS

URETHRITIS

Inflammation of the urethra, the channel through which urine is emptied from the bladder. There are two types: acute, which usually lasts for only a few days, and chronic, which may last for months or years. The symptoms for both types are the same. As there are many causes of both types, it is often difficult for the doctor to decide whether the patient has urethritis.

URETHRITIS IN MEN

In men urethritis may be caused by one of a number of infections. The most common are the sexually transmitted diseases, especially GONORRHOEA. Other common infections are caused by inflammation of the urinary tract. In some cases, infection results from THRUSH or trichomonas VAGINITIS in a sexual partner. Often, however, the germs responsible for urethritis cannot be determined by routine laboratory analysis. Research suggests that most are transmitted through promiscuity, but they may also be contracted in a faithful sexual partnership, from a woman who has a non-venereal infection. Urethritis of unknown origin is called non-specific urethritis (NSU).

Symptoms
- The penis discharges a slight, clear, sticky fluid which may contain pus.
- There may be a burning sensation in the penis when urine is passed. In some cases this may feel as though

broken glass is being passed down through the penis.
Duration
- Acute non-specific urethritis usually lasts for one to three weeks.
Causes
- The germs responsible for NSU generally cannot be identified by available laboratory tests.
Treatment in the home
- No home treatment is advised.
When to consult the doctor
- As soon as the symptoms described are noticed. There should be no delay simply because the symptoms are slight.
What the doctor may do
- He will take a swab of the discharge for analysis and arrange a blood test. The patient's sexual partner will also be examined. These measures are to exclude sexually transmitted diseases (SYPHILIS, GONORRHOEA) and if possible identify other infecting organisms. The patient will be discouraged from looking for a discharge by milking the penis, because this may perpetuate the discharge.
- A course of antibiotics or a second medical opinion may be advised. *See* MEDICINES, 25.
Prevention
- Avoid promiscuity.
- Condoms are often used to prevent contagion.
Outlook
- NSU eventually clears up with treatment.

ACUTE URETHRITIS IN WOMEN

The disorder is common in women. The short female urethra is liable to become infected from the bladder above, or from the vagina below. It may be acute or chronic.
Symptoms
- A burning pain on passing urine, and a need to pass urine often, both usually coming on within 24 hours of sexual intercourse.
- Pain during intercourse.
- In some cases, there may be a white or yellow vaginal discharge. Often it is slight and passes unnoticed.
Duration
- Most cases clear with treatment in three to ten days.
Causes
- Infecting organisms may enter the urethra from the bladder, vagina or bowel. Infection may arise by chance (as in other parts of the body) or be introduced by a sexual partner.
- Thrush and a number of different bacteria and virus can all cause such infection.
- Bruising after sexual intercourse or surgical operations

and the deficiency of female sexual hormones that occurs after the menopause all render the female urethra vulnerable to infection.
Treatment in the home
- Drink extra fluids.
- Take painkillers in recommended doses.
When to consult the doctor
- If symptoms are severe.
- If they last for more than 48 hours.
- If a sexual partner is involved.
- If symptoms keep recurring.
What the doctor may do
- Exclude serious or sexually transmitted disease.
- Ask for a sample of urine, to be tested.
- Carry out an internal vaginal examination.
- Prescribe antibiotics. *See* MEDICINES, 25.
Prevention
- Newly wed women should use lubricating jelly when first having intercourse.
Outlook
- The disorder clears with treatment but may recur.

CHRONIC URETHRITIS IN WOMEN

Symptoms
- As in acute urethritis, but recurring or persisting over long periods.
Duration
- If not treated, urethritis can persist for years.
Causes
- As for acute urethritis but often uncertain. Venereal disease rarely causes chronic urethritis.
- Allergy to contraceptive foam or a sheath is a possible cause.
Treatment in the home
- Drink extra fluids.
- Women are advised to wear cotton panties, which are absorbent; especially when wearing tights, which are non-absorbent.
- Use a lubricating jelly for intercourse.
- Experiment with different positions at intercourse to find which is the most comfortable.
- Empty the bladder as soon after intercourse as possible.
When to consult the doctor
- As for acute urethritis.
What the doctor may do
- Test urine for possible causes.
- Carry out an internal vaginal examination.
- Prescribe antibiotics or hormonal vaginal cream. *See* MEDICINES, 25, 33.
- Refer the patient to a specialist for further investigations if there is doubt about the cause. Stretching the urethra may relieve symptoms.

Prevention
- Always use a lubricating jelly before intercourse.
- Treat vaginal discharge.
- Avoid bubble baths.

Outlook
- Chronic urethritis usually clears up with treatment, but in some cases it resists treatment and can persist for years.

See URINARY SYSTEM *page 46*

URINATION

Problems with urination include pain, frequent urination, lack of control (incontinence), and failure to urinate. Urine itself may be discoloured (*see* JAUNDICE for dark urine), cloudy, or smell offensive.

See SYMPTOM SORTER—URINE AND URINATION PROBLEMS; BLEEDING

URTICARIA

In this skin disorder, fluid passes out of the skin's blood vessels and collects in the skin and its underlying tissues, causing them to swell. The resulting eruptions resemble a sting from a nettle, and this gives urticaria one of its common names, nettlerash.

The other common name is hives.

Symptoms
- A swollen area of pale skin surrounded by a red wheal. The wheals may occur anywhere on the body, and vary in size from a tiny pimple to a large patch several inches across.
- Intense irritation.
- Wheals may form along scratch or pressure lines so that patterns may be drawn on sensitive skins.

Duration
- The individual wheals last only a few hours, but others may erupt at different sites.
- In an acute attack eruption of wheals may continue for several days, or even two or three weeks, after the cause has been removed.
- Where no irritant can be found, chronic urticaria with recurrent eruptions may last for years.

Causes
- An allergic reaction to certain foods, for example eggs, nuts, chocolate, cheese, fish, or drugs (such as aspirin, penicillin and other antibiotics). Allergy to a food, drug or anything else may develop at any age for no known reason. For instance, a person who has eaten strawberries or fish for years may suddenly develop urticarial reactions.
- Some foods, for example shellfish and strawberries, and some drugs, such as aspirin and codeine, act directly on the skin and produce urticaria.
- Some eruptions have no known cause.
- There is no clear link between urticaria and nervous causes or stress.
- In sensitised people firm stroking of the skin produces a wheal. The reaction comes on three or four hours after pressure and lasts up to 24 hours.

Complications
- Swelling of the mouth, tongue or throat may occasionally obstruct breathing.
- Urticaria of the face, hands and feet may be particularly severe causing ANGIONEUROTIC OEDEMA.

Treatment in the home
- None. Local applications of ointments or lotions will not make any difference.
- Keep a careful note of any food or drugs taken before an attack. If there is a recurrence, this record may give you a clue to the cause.

When to consult the doctor
- If there is unbearably intense irritation or severe swelling.
- If there is swelling of the mouth or tongue, or tightness of the chest.

What the doctor may do
- Prescribe antihistamine tablets. Different people are suited by different antihistamine preparations, so there needs to be persistence in trying various types in order to find the most suitable one. *See* MEDICINES, 14.
- Give an injection of adrenalin if there is difficulty in breathing.
- Possibly also prescribe corticosteroid tablets. *See* MEDICINES, 32.

Prevention
- Unless a cause can be found and avoided, prevention is not possible.

Outlook
- The condition recurs whenever a person is exposed to the cause of the eruption.
- Once sensitised to something this sensitivity will last for life.
- When no cause is found, intermittent urticaria may continue for years.

See SKIN *page 52*
DRUG RASH
CHILD CARE—CHILDHOOD ILLS

UTERUS, CANCER OF

A malignant growth of the body of the uterus (womb) which, unlike cancer of the neck of the uterus, CERVICAL CANCER, is more common after the menopause. Most cases arise after the age of 50 in women who have stopped menstruating. Women at higher risk are those who are childless, those whose menopause was late, those whose periods have been irregular and those suffering from DIABETES or HYPERTENSION.

Symptoms
- Unexpected bleeding or a brown (sometimes offensive-smelling) discharge from the vagina, either before or after the menopause.

Duration
- The cancer may remain within the uterus, without spreading, for several months.

Causes
- The cause of the cancer is not known.

Treatment in the home
- None is possible.

When to consult the doctor
- Immediately there is any unexpected bleeding or discharge from the vagina, either before or after the menopause.

What the doctor may do
- Arrange for the lining of the uterus to be scraped to provide a sample of tissue for testing. *See* D AND C.
- If cancer is revealed, surgery or radiation treatment will be carried out.

Prevention
- There is no means of preventing the cancer from developing. Routine CERVICAL SMEARS may not reveal it, and it is therefore essential that any unexpected bleeding or discharge, at any age, is reported to the doctor immediately.

Outlook
- If the condition is treated early the outlook is good.

See FEMALE GENITAL SYSTEM *page 48*

UTERUS, PROLAPSE OF

The uterus drops out of position because the ligaments holding the uterus, bladder and rectum become over-stretched. The bladder may push back into the vagina creating a soft lump (cystocele) and causing incontinence of the urine, or the rectum may push forwards creating a soft rectocele. In severe cases the uterus descends into the vagina.

Symptoms
- A sensation that the contents of the uterus are dropping down or falling out of the vagina.
- Dragging pain is felt in the pelvis (backache is rare).
- Incontinence of urine on coughing.
- The hard uterus in severe cases appears between the lips of the vulva.

Duration
- Prolapses tend to progress unless treated.

Causes
- Repeated or difficult childbirth.

Complications
- Few, apart from urinary incontinence.

Treatment in the home
- Prolapse, however severe, is always temporarily helped by lying flat.

When to consult the doctor
- If there is discomfort or incontinence of urine.
- If a prolapse is interfering with daily living.

What the doctor may do
- Confirm the diagnosis by vaginal examination.
- Fit a pessary which occasionally helps older patients.
- Refer the patient to hospital for surgical treatment, which is usually required.

Prevention
- Careful repair of any vaginal tears after childbirth.
- Exercises conscientiously performed after childbirth.

Outlook
- Excellent with treatment.

See FEMALE GENITAL SYSTEM *page 48*

UTERUS, RETROVERSION OF

A uterus (womb) that slopes backwards instead of forwards. The condition is common (it occurs in one-fifth of women), is usually present from birth and generally needs no treatment. Rarely, it may cause INFERTILITY.

During the first three months of a pregnancy, a retroverted uterus that has been present from birth may become lodged in the pelvis as the baby grows.

Symptoms
- Usually there are no symptoms.
- Occasionally there is low backache that is worse during a period.
- In some pregnancies an inability to pass urine may develop.

Duration
- The condition persists throughout life, except in the few cases that need correction.

Causes
- In the majority of cases—those present from birth—it is not known what causes the abnormality to develop.
- In a few cases retroversion of the uterus develops after a pregnancy.

Treatment in the home
- None is possible.

When to consult the doctor
- If there is low backache that is worse during a menstrual period.
- If, during pregnancy, there is an inability to pass urine. In this case, a doctor should be seen immediately.

What the doctor may do
- Carry out an INTERNAL PELVIC EXAMINATION and try to tilt the uterus forward manually.
- If he is unable to tilt the uterus or if, as is usual, a tilted uterus fails to stay in its new position, the doctor may send the patient to a gynaecologist.
- If the gynaecologist considers that the retroversion is causing backache or infertility, an operation may be performed.

Outlook
- Most women with the condition experience no symptoms and need no treatment.

See FEMALE GENITAL SYSTEM *page 48*

VAGINA AND VULVA
The most common vaginal symptom is discharge, other symptoms of the vagina and vulva include ITCHING, or pain on intercourse, and swellings and sores.
See SYMPTOM SORTER—VAGINA AND VULVA

VAGINISMUS
Painful contraction of the vagina, making sexual intercourse difficult or impossible. The cause is usually psychological—for example, fear of pregnancy, intercourse, or aversion to the sexual partner. In some cases, however, there is a physical cause, such as VAGINITIS, PROLAPSE of the uterus, or extreme dryness of the vagina after the menopause.

VAGINITIS AND VULVITIS

Inflammation of the vagina and vulva involving discharge, itching and soreness which may arise from many different causes. In addition to an outline of the general condition, three separate types, classified by cause, are described. They are: thrush, trichomonas vaginitis, and atrophic vaginitis.

Symptoms
- Itching—often worse at night.
- Soreness.
- Discharge which may be colourless, white, yellow, green, offensive or frothy, depending on the cause of the infection.

Duration
- Unless treated, the inflammation may persist indefinitely.

Causes
- Simple skin irritation due to excessive perspiration, scratching, or sensitivity to deodorants, perfume, soaps, powders or sanitary pads.
- Any of the many causes of excessive vaginal discharge which include thrush, trichomonas vaginitis, atrophic vaginitis, and infection by bacteria.
- Retained TAMPON.
- Rarely, DIABETES.
- Long-standing itching and scratching can lead to thickening of the tissues of the vulva—leukoplakia.
- Ulceration of the vulva may be caused by simple inflammation, or, rarely, by SKIN CANCER.

Treatment in the home
- Normal hygiene.

When to consult the doctor
- If the symptoms develop.

What the doctor may do
- Examine and take specimens to identify possible causes.
- Exclude less-common causes for the discharge such as diabetes, sexually transmitted diseases, cancer of the UTERUS and CERVICAL CANCER.
- Treat according to the cause.

Prevention and outlook
- Depends on the underlying cause.

THRUSH
An infection of the vagina that can affect females of any age. Most will have one or two attacks in the course of their lives. Thrush affecting the vagina is also known as candidiasis and monilial vaginal infection.

Symptoms
- A vaginal discharge which is much heavier than the discharge many women normally have from time to time, particularly those on the oral contraceptive pill.
- The discharge is usually white, and thick, like curds.
- There is itching in the vagina and around the vulva.
- The woman's sexual partner may have itching of the penis.

Duration
- The condition often lasts only a few days.

Causes
- A fungus from the bowel entering the vagina; this is more likely to happen if the woman wears tight pants, tights or jeans.
- The oral contraceptive.
- Certain antibiotics.
- DIABETES.
- Pregnancy.
- Infection by the woman's sexual partner.
- Vaginal deodorants.

Treatment in the home
- Stop wearing clothing of the kind described.
- Make sure that a sexual partner known to have, or suspected of having, a sexual infection sees a doctor.
- Do not take more baths than necessary.

When to consult the doctor
- If the symptoms described occur.

What the doctor may do
- Carry out an internal examination of the vagina.
- Take a swab of the discharge for laboratory analysis.
- Prescribe antifungal pessaries to be inserted in the vagina to clear the infection. *See* MEDICINES, 26.
- Test the patient's urine for sugar, to see whether she may have diabetes.
- Examine and treat any sexual partner.

Prevention
- Avoid tight clothing of the kind described and vaginal deodorants.
- After a bowel action, always wipe the anus from front to back.
- Try to ensure that any sexual partner is free of a sexual infection.

Outlook
- Most attacks clear up with treatment; but reinfection may occur.

TRICHOMONAS VAGINITIS
Infection of the vagina, less common than thrush.
Symptoms
- Discharge which may be yellow or green and tends to be frothy.
- Soreness of the vulva.

Duration
- As for thrush.

Causes
- Infection by a parasitic organism.

Treatment in the home
- As for thrush.

When to consult the doctor
- As for thrush.

What the doctor may do
- Carry out an internal examination of the vagina.
- Take a swab of the vaginal discharge for laboratory analysis.
- Prescribe antiparasitic drugs. *See* MEDICINES, 28.
- Test the patient's urine for sugar to see whether she may have DIABETES.
- Examine and treat any sexual partner.

Prevention
- As for thrush.

Outlook
- As for thrush.

ATROPHIC VAGINITIS
Shrinkage and dryness of the vulva (the external female genitals) and the vagina in elderly women.
Symptoms
- Discharge from the vagina.
- Soreness around the vulva and in the vagina.
- Painful sexual intercourse.
- The symptoms occur in many elderly women but are distressing in only a few.

Duration
- Indefinite, unless the condition is treated.

Causes
- A fall in the level of the female hormone oestrogen after the menopause.

Treatment in the home
- Take regular baths.

When to consult the doctor
- If there are the symptoms described.

What the doctor may do
- Carry out an internal pelvic examination.
- Prescribe a vaginal cream or a short course of oestrogen tablets. *See* MEDICINES, 33.

Prevention
- Hormone replacement therapy (HRT) may be helpful. *See* MENOPAUSE.

Outlook
- Treatment is usually effective within a few weeks, but in some cases it is necessary to use the vaginal cream on and off for a year or more.

See FEMALE GENITAL SYSTEM *page 48*

VARICOCELE

A harmless swelling of the veins in the spermatic cord, which connects the testicle with the abdomen. It is usually the left cord that is affected. In some cases varicocele is associated with reduced sperm production.
Symptoms
- A painless, irregular, soft swelling within the scrotum, usually on the left side.
- Occasionally, the swelling causes discomfort after standing.
- Often the scrotum hangs lower than normal.

Duration
- Unless treated, the condition is permanent.

Causes
- Unknown.

Treatment in the home
- None is needed.

When to consult the doctor
- If any swelling develops in the scrotum.

What the doctor may do
- In most cases no treatment is necessary.
- If there is discomfort or it is discovered medically that sperm production is reduced, surgery may be considered.

Prevention
- There is no way of preventing the condition.

Outlook
- Varicocele presents no risk to health. The result of surgery is excellent.

See MALE GENITAL SYSTEM *page 50*

VARICOSE ULCERS

Ulceration of the lower leg, usually just above the ankle. The ulcers usually occur together with varicose veins.
Symptoms
- Ulcers, or open sores, that are usually painless and vary in size from that of a pinhead to several inches across.
- A discharge of fluid from the ulcers.
- Often, infection of the ulcers, which then become painful.

Duration
- With treatment, the ulcers usually heal within several

weeks. If neglected, they may continue indefinitely.

Causes
- Defective functioning of the veins in the leg—with or without varicose veins being present—makes the skin become devitalised and it readily ulcerates.

Treatment in the home
- Rest the affected leg in a raised position.

When to consult the doctor
- If there is discoloration of, or pain in, the lower leg.

What the doctor may do
- He will advise the patient to rest the leg in a raised position and to stand and walk as little as possible.
- If an ulcer fails to heal, a skin graft and the removal of any varicose veins may be required.

Prevention
- If varicose veins are present, wear support stockings.
- Avoid injury to lower leg and prolonged standing.
- See also VARICOSE VEINS.

Outlook
- Ulcers usually heal with treatment but often recur.

See CIRCULATORY SYSTEM *page 40*

VARICOSE VEINS

Veins in the legs become swollen and twisted. The condition is increasingly common from the late teens onwards and, in women, it often begins at the time of pregnancy.

The whole leg may be stricken, or only a short length of vein.

Symptoms
- Prominent knotted veins on the surface of the legs, particularly the calves.
- Fatigue when walking.
- Aching, particularly after standing.
- Swelling of the ankles.

Duration
- If the swollen veins are associated with pregnancy they may die down after childbirth. Otherwise, the condition can persist indefinitely.

Causes
- Defective valves in the veins allow gravity and back pressure to impede the blood flow and cause distension of the veins.
- Constipation increases pressure on abdominal veins, preventing them from taking blood away from the veins in the legs.

Do's and don'ts about varicose veins

□ *Do* walk rather than ride whenever possible.

□ *Do* keep moving, or at least flex your calf muscles, if you have to spend long periods on your feet.

□ *Do* get up and walk about whenever possible. Flex your calf muscles from time to time if you have a sedentary job.

□ *Do* try to lie down and raise your legs above heart level whenever possible.

□ *Do* wear support stockings, especially during pregnancy. These need not be unsightly, and they are available for men as well as women.

□ *Don't* remain motionless in one position—standing or sitting—for any length of time.

□ *Don't* become overweight.

□ *Don't* become constipated.

Complications
- If the underlying cause persists, then more veins will become varicose.
- Varicose veins may become inflamed, causing THROMBOPHLEBITIS.
- Ulceration may occur. *See* VARICOSE ULCER.

Treatment in the home
- Avoid standing whenever possible.
- Sit while ironing, cooking and so on.
- Raise legs whenever possible.

When to consult the doctor
- As soon as the condition is noticed.

What the doctor may do
- Prescribe support stockings.
- Inject veins so that they shrink and close.
- Arrange for the surgical removal of affected veins.

Prevention
- Avoid standing still as much as possible.

- Have a high fibre diet, which prevents constipation.

Outlook
- Once the swollen veins have taken hold, surgery is the only certain cure.

See CIRCULATORY SYSTEM *page 40*

VASECTOMY
A simple operation to sterilise the male by cutting and tying the tubes which carry sperm from the testes to the penis.
See FAMILY PLANNING

VEGETARIANISM
Vegetarians justify their dietary beliefs on one or both of two grounds—that it is morally wrong to eat animal flesh because that involves cruelty to other living creatures; and that meat does not form part of man's 'natural' diet, and can therefore be harmful.

The second argument has some support among those anthropologists who contend that, during most of the time it took for man to evolve, his staple food was fruit and vegetables. *See* MEGAVITAMIN THERAPY.

It is also partly borne out by modern scientific research. This links heart disease to high levels of cholesterol—present in animal fat—in the blood, and many disorders of the digestive system, particularly of the bowel, to lack of vegetable fibre, or roughage, in modern diets. Balanced vegetarian meals are low in cholesterol and high in roughage.

Most vegetarians abstain only from meat and fish, but allow themselves to eat other animal products—eggs, milk, cheese and butter. These contain protein, calcium and the B vitamins, and contribute towards a balanced diet.

However, vegans—stricter adherents of vegetarianism—forgo any food that comes from animals, and their meals may lack essential vitamins and minerals unless they regularly include nuts, wholegrain cereals and a broad selection of vegetables.
See NUTRITION

VENEREAL DISEASE
A general term for infections acquired during sexual contact or intercourse. The term is commonly abbreviated to VD, but doctors usually refer to such infections as sexually transmitted diseases (STDs).

See SEXUALLY TRANSMITTED DISEASES

VENTRICULAR FIBRILLATION

A serious disturbance of the normal heart rhythm. The main pumping chambers (ventricles) beat very fast, irregularly and inefficiently. The condition leads to sudden death unless treated immediately.
Symptoms
• Sudden collapse followed by unconsciousness.
• Absent heartbeat.
• Often there are no warning signs. Sometimes these symptoms develop unexpectedly in someone who already has symptoms of ischaemic heart disease.
Duration
• A few minutes.
Causes
• Myocardial infarction, due to CORONARY THROMBOSIS.
• Ischaemic heart disease.
Treatment in the home
• The patient needs immediate external massage of the heart, and artificial respiration if not breathing. *See* FIRST AID *pages 542-3.*
When to consult the doctor
• Call doctor or ambulance immediately, describing symptoms.
What the doctor or paramedic may do
• Continue heart massage and artificial respiration, and, using an electric defibrillator, administer controlled electric shocks to restore normal heart rhythm.
Outlook
• If the condition persists for more than a few minutes, death is inevitable.
• With external cardiac massage, survival time is lengthened and some attacks may stop. External cardiac massage may keep the patient alive until electrical defibrillation is possible.
• The recovery rate for those who survive is similar to that for people who have had heart attacks.
• The risk of recurrence is reduced by taking regular aspirin and beta-blockers. *See* MEDICINES (5).

VENTRICULAR SEPTAL DEFECT
A gap in the strong muscular wall (septum) that divides the ventricles, the main chambers of the heart. It is a form of congenital heart disease. Babies showing no symptoms at birth may develop heart failure in infancy.

The defect can be closed by surgery once the condition is detected. Sometimes the gap closes spontaneously later in childhood. If not, the heart may enlarge to compensate, but heart failure may occur as a result of respiratory infection or, in adulthood, pregnancy.

VERRUCA
A small solid growth on the skin, also known as a wart. There are five main types, usually appearing on different parts of the body.
See WART

VERTEBRO-BASILAR INSUFFICIENCY

This condition results when the flow of blood to the base of the brain is impeded. The vertebral arteries which run up the spine to the neck are obstructed.
Symptoms
• The patient experiences brief dizzy spells, vertigo or unconsciousness when moving the neck (to look upwards, for example).
• There may be double vision, and weakness or numbness in a limb.
Duration
• The condition tends to get worse with the passing of time. A dizzy spell, however, lasts only as long as the position of the neck is maintained.
Causes
• ATHEROMA (hardening of the arteries). This tends to develop in late middle age, or in the elderly, making the blood vessels more vulnerable to obstruction.
• CERVICAL SPONDYLOSIS. This is a degenerative disease affecting the bones of the neck, and may develop in adults of any age.
Complications
• None.
Treatment in the home
• After any severe dizzy spell the sufferer should rest, avoiding any awkward neck movements which could cause a second attack.
When to consult the doctor
• If symptoms occur.
What the doctor may do
• Ask you to move your neck around to see if symptoms result.

• If cervical spondylosis is present, the patient will find it hard to bend the neck from side to side, or to turn the chin towards the shoulder. The doctor may recommend X-rays to confirm the condition.
• The doctor may prescribe medication to ease symptoms.
• He will advise the patient to avoid awkward neck movements, and may arrange for a soft supportive collar to be provided. This limits neck movement and reduces the likelihood of attacks.
Prevention
• None.
Outlook
• There is no cure for the condition, but with treatment and care the symptoms need not be too troublesome.

See NERVOUS SYSTEM *page 34*

VERTIGO

The patient feels that his head is moving even when it is still. This produces an unpleasant sensation of giddiness.
Symptoms
• A feeling that the head or body is spinning.
• Deafness.
• Nystagmus, or flickering of eyes—usually from side to side. This may persist even after the vertigo has worn off.
Duration
• Repeated attacks can last from seconds to hours. They may occur daily or once or twice a year.
Causes
• Head injury.
• MÉNIÈRE'S DISEASE and LABYRINTHITIS, both of which disturb the hearing and balance of the inner ear.
• High blood pressure (*see* HYPERTENSION).
• A blockage of the blood vessels leading to the brain.
• Motion sickness.
• OVERBREATHING.
Treatment in the home
• During an attack, lie down quietly.
When to consult the doctor
• If attacks keep recurring.
• If there is severe vomiting.
• If deafness develops.
What the doctor may do
• Examine the ears, eyes and neck.
• Take the blood pressure.
• Test for nystagmus.

- Prescribe drugs which relieve the symptoms.

Prevention
- None.

Outlook
- Even without treatment, many patients recover spontaneously after several months. The elderly may suffer from vertigo without a treatable cause being found.
- Positional vertigo, felt when the head is in certain positions, may be recurrent.

See NERVOUS SYSTEM *page 34*

VIRILISM

The development in a woman of secondary male characteristics, such as increased facial and body hair, baldness, enlarged muscles and a deep voice. In addition, menstruation may stop and the sexual organs and breasts may become smaller.

The disorder is due to over-production by the adrenal glands of male hormones, which every woman possesses to some degree. The excess production is usually caused either by a tumour (in most cases non-cancerous) on the glands or the enlargement of them. But occasionally it is the result of receiving hormone drugs for some other disorder.

Treatment consists of stopping the drugs or replacing them with others. Despite successful treatment, the voice may remain permanently deep.

The development of excess hair alone is known as HIRSUTISM and may have a different cause.

VITILIGO

A loss of pigment from patches of skin which become permanently white. It is common, affecting about one person in 100. The onset may be at any age, but half the cases start before the age of 20. It is not painful, but disfigurement can be very marked if the patch is large or occurs on the face. It can be especially annoying for dark-skinned people.

Symptoms
- Well defined, round, oval or irregular white blotches develop in otherwise normal skin. The blotches slowly expand and join with others to form large patches.
- Any part of the skin may be affected and usually on both sides of the body at the same time.
- Hairs growing from affected skin become white.

- The pale blotches easily burn in the sun.

Duration
- After a few months the blotches stop enlarging and may even shrink a little. They rarely disappear completely.

Causes
- Unknown.

Treatment in the home
- Any patches which cause severe embarrassment can be covered with cosmetic dyes.

When to consult the doctor
- If the condition is causing anxiety.

What the doctor may do
- Try to re-pigment the skin using ultra-violet light and a drug which stimulates pigment-producing cells.
- If very large areas are involved it may be better to de-pigment unaffected areas.

Prevention
- None is available.

Outlook
- Cure is unlikely, but the combination of careful cosmetics and treatment usually enables a person to live a normal social life.

See SKIN *page 52*

VOMITING

A common symptom in adults and older children with a wide variety of causes, both trivial and serious.
See SYMPTOM SORTER—VOMITING
CHILD CARE—CHILDHOOD ILLS

VULVA, CANCER OF

An extremely rare malignant tumour that develops on the external genitals of elderly women.

Symptoms
- An ulcer, usually painless, develops on the lips of the vulva. The ulcer may bleed.

Causes
- It is not known what causes the cancer.

Treatment in the home
- None is possible.

When to consult the doctor
- If a painless ulcer on the vulva bleeds or does not heal.
- Some women will be too embarrassed to consult the doctor and will need to be persuaded to do so.

What the doctor may do
- Carry out an internal pelvic examination.
- Send the patient to a gynaecologist for surgery and radiotherapy.

Prevention
- No means of prevention is known.

Outlook
- The prospects are reasonably good if treatment is started early and the cancer does not spread rapidly.

See FEMALE GENITAL SYSTEM *page 48*

VULVITIS

Inflammation of the vulva, involving discharge, itching and soreness. The condition may be caused by infection or irritation.
See VAGINITIS AND VULVITIS

WARTS

These are small solid growths on the skin, also known as verrucas. There are five types, usually occurring on different parts of the body. All are caused by viruses and are slightly contagious.

COMMON WART
This is skin-coloured or brownish with a rough, horny surface. It is the biggest type $\frac{1}{8}$-1 in. (3-25 mm.), and one wart may join another. It can occur at any age, but is commonest in children, especially on the hands. It is painless, unless under a nail or at a site of pressure, such as where a shoe rubs. If left alone it may disappear but, very rarely, may last more than ten years.

PLANE WARTS
These are smooth, skin-coloured or light brown, and very small. They generally grow in clusters, often along the line of a scratch. Children are usually affected; the face, neck, arms and legs being common sites. The warts may disappear on their own.

PLANTAR WARTS
These are firm and round with a rough surface, and the base is embedded deep in the soles of the feet or the toes. They may be single or multiple and are often painful. When the top is pared off, dark spots can be seen. These are blood vessels supplying the wart and are not found in calluses or corns. Plantar warts may disappear spontaneously in a few months, but in some cases they can persist for years.

FILIFORM WARTS

These are thin strips of skin (filaments), up to ⅛ in. (3 mm.) in length with a hard tip. They usually grow on the face, neck, chin and eyelids and may be solitary or in clusters. They will disappear spontaneously if left, but because of their site, they are usually treated.

ANOGENITAL WARTS

These are multiple, small cauliflower-like growths on the vulva, penis and skin around the anus. They often grow quickly and irritate. They are usually, but not always, acquired from a sexual partner. They may disappear spontaneously, but reinfection may occur.

Anogenital warts are caused by the human papilloma virus.

Duration

• Most contagious warts persist or spread unless treated. Occasionally they disappear for no apparent reason.

Treatment in the home

• Suggestion therapy, whether performed by a lay or medical person is undoubtedly successful. Not recommended for smooth, skin-coloured warts or for facial, seborrhoeic or anogenital warts.

• Proprietary paints and pastes can be bought at the chemist. Apply paints daily and allow to dry. If using paste, cover the wart with a dressing. *See* MEDICINES, 43.

• Always follow the instructions on the container.

• *Do not* apply the pastes and paints to normal skin.

• When using pastes protect the surrounding skin with an adhesive 'corn-pad' or strapping.

• *Do not* continue treatment if the wart becomes painful.

• Pare off dead surface skin as treatment progresses, using a sharp, sterile blade. Never attempt this with elderly or diabetic patients.

Complications

• Most warts do not become cancerous. However, anogenital warts can cause cervical cancer.

When to consult the doctor

• For diagnosis of the less well-known warts.

• For treatment of persisting warts when simple paints and pastes have failed.

• For treatment of facial and anogenital warts.

What the doctor may do

• Freeze the wart off with dry ice (solid carbon dioxide) or liquid nitrogen.

• Burn it off with strong acid or an electrically heated platinum needle.

• Dig it out with a curette (a spoon-shaped instrument).

• Prescribe a paint for anogenital warts.

Prevention

• *Do not* go barefoot in places such as gymnasiums, public showers, wash-rooms and swimming-pools.

• Avoid physical contact with people who are known to suffer from contagious warts.

• *Do not* scratch warts, as this will encourage spread to the damaged skin.

• The risk of spreading anogenital warts and therefore cervical cancer is reduced by the use of condoms.

Outlook

• With treatment, most warts can be cured.

See SKIN *page 52*
SEBORRHOEIC WART

WEIGHT

Weight can be an important indicator of the individual's state of health. In particular, sudden changes in weight—either up or down—which are not related to an obvious cause, such as pregnancy or dieting, may be due to disease and should be reported to the doctor. But in Western

Desirable weights for men and women

The weights in pounds are given according to height and frame for men and women aged 25 and over. Women's heights include 2 in. heels and men's heights 1 in. heels. Weights include indoor clothing. For nude weights, deduct 5–7 lb. for men and 2–4 lb. for women. In addition, women aged 18–25 should deduct 1 lb. for each year under 25.

MEN

| HEIGHT | | WEIGHT | | |
ft	in.	Small frame	Medium frame	Large frame
5	2	112–120	118–129	126–141
5	3	115–123	121–133	129–144
5	4	118–126	124–136	132–148
5	5	121–129	127–139	135–152
5	6	124–133	130–143	138–156
5	7	128–137	134–147	142–161
5	8	132–141	138–152	147–166
5	9	136–145	142–156	151–170
5	10	140–150	146–160	155–174
5	11	144–154	150–165	159–179
6	0	148–158	154–170	164–184
6	1	152–162	158–175	168–189
6	2	156–167	162–180	173–194
6	3	160–171	167–185	178–199
6	4	164–175	172–190	182–204

WOMEN

| HEIGHT | | WEIGHT | | |
ft	in.	Small frame	Medium frame	Large frame
4	10	92–98	96–107	104–119
4	11	94–101	98–110	106–122
5	0	96–104	101–113	109–125
5	1	99–107	104–116	112–128
5	2	102–110	107–119	115–131
5	3	105–113	110–122	118–134
5	4	108–116	113–126	121–138
5	5	111–119	116–130	125–142
5	6	114–123	120–135	129–146
5	7	118–127	124–139	133–150
5	8	122–131	128–143	137–154
5	9	126–135	132–147	141–158
5	10	130–140	136–151	145–163
5	11	134–144	140–155	149–168
6	0	138–148	144–159	153–173

society, where one in three adults is overweight, the main weight-related problems are those due to excess weight.

Each of us has an ideal weight which offers the best opportunity for good health and physical fitness. Body build, height and sex are all factors in determining ideal weight, which can vary considerably between apparently similar individuals. As the tables on page 525 show, there can be an acceptable variation of more than 2 stones between women who are 5 ft 6 in. tall.

To work out your own ideal weight, try to remember what you weighed and what you looked like—unclothed —in your late teens. This is the age at which most people reach their ideal weight. If you were overweight in your teens and many people are or were—be guided by what you see, standing unclothed in front of a mirror. Most of us recognise fat at a glance. A further check can be made by grasping a fold of flesh on the abdomen or upper arm— if the fold is more than an inch thick, you are carrying excess weight.

People who are overweight are more likely to contract certain disorders, including DIABETES, HYPERTENSION and ARTHRITIS. They also run the risk of exacerbating other conditions, particularly heart disease. On the other hand, to be drastically underweight can be just as dangerous. The over-thin often have little resistance to infection, and may be less able to stand up to chemotherapy or surgery.

Ideal weight is a fairly broad path lying between the extremes of obesity and excessive thinness. It is maintained by a balanced diet in which surplus food is not available for laying down as fat on the body or in the arteries.

See ATHEROMA
NUTRITION
OBESITY

WEIGHT LOSS
Loss of weight that is not the result of a deliberate attempt to slim should always be taken seriously, especially if other symptoms suggest the possibility of serious disease.
See SYMPTOM SORTER—WEIGHT LOSS

WHIPLASH INJURY

A whiplash injury occurs when the neck is jerked forwards then backwards, rather like the movement made when a whip is cracked. It usually happens when a stationary car is struck from behind by another vehicle. The occupants in the stationary car, taken unawares, are propelled forwards.

The whiplash effect can cause damage to the bones of the neck, even fracturing them; to discs between the bones (slipping or displacement); to the nerves within the cervical spinal column, or to the nerves that emerge from between the cervical vertebrae on their way down the arms.

Symptoms
These may include:
- Headache.
- Pain and stiffness in neck.
- Weakness or paralysis of arms or shoulders.
- Pins and needles and changes in feeling in arms and hands.
- General depression and anxiety.

Such symptoms may occur at the time of the accident or may not become apparent until some time later.

Treatment in the home
- Rest and take painkillers if necessary.

When to consult the doctor
- If the symptoms persist.

What the doctor may do
- Provide a collar to restrict movements and provide support.
- Arrange for physiotherapy and possibly prescribe anti-inflammatory drugs.

See SKELETAL SYSTEM *page 54*

WHIPWORM

The infection caused by the whipworm is widespread throughout tropical Africa and the Far East, especially in areas with inadequate sewage disposal. Humans become infected by eating food contaminated by the eggs. The eggs develop into adult worms, up to 2 in. (50 mm.) long, in the gut and quickly produce eggs that are excreted in the faeces. If infected faeces contaminate food or water (particularly if defecation occurs in the open) the cycle of infection begins again.

Symptoms
- Often there are no symptoms.
- Persistent diarrhoea, which may contain blood.
- Abdominal pain.
- In chronic infections there may be anaemia and malnutrition.

Causes
- A parasite called *Trichuris trichiura*, or whipworm (since it looks like a whip), which lives in the intestines.

Treatment
- Antiworm drugs. *See* MEDICINES, 29.
- In areas where infection is common, sanitary conditions should be improved.

See INFECTIOUS DISEASES *page 32*

WHITE LEG
A pale, swollen leg caused by extensive thrombosis (blockage due to blood-clotting) of deep veins in a leg. It usually occurs one to four weeks after operations or childbirth (*see* THROMBOPHLEBITIS). Severe blood loss increases the risk of this complication.
See CIRCULATORY SYSTEM *page 40*

WHITES
A whitish or yellowish discharge of mucus from the vagina, also known as leucorrhoea. In most cases it is a natural occurrence and does not signify any disorder; it tends to increase before menstruation and after repeated use of a DOUCHE. However, if leucorrhoea is copious, and particularly if there is also irritation and an unpleasant smell, the discharge may be a symptom of a vaginal infection, most commonly trichomonal VAGINITIS.

A woman who has any abnormal discharge should see her doctor.

WHITLOW

An infection, usually staphylococcal, of the soft pad at the tip of a finger or thumb. Often confused with the less painful acute PARONYCHIA.

Symptoms
- Tenderness and throbbing pain in a soft, sensitive finger pad.
- Pain is severe and reaches a peak after one or two days.
- The 'pad' becomes tense but cannot swell or form a boil because the skin is thick and hence the pain. The pus cannot escape.
- Fever and shivering sometimes occur.

Duration
- Until the abscess in the pad is drained.

Complications
- An untreated whitlow can damage the bone at the top of the affected finger.

Treatment in the home
- Rest the affected hand.
- Painkillers will be needed.

When to consult the doctor
- As soon as the diagnosis is suspected or the pain gets bad.

What the doctor may do
- Prescribe antibiotics to try to stop the whitlow developing—rarely effective. *See* MEDICINES, 25.
- Arrange for the abscess to be drained under an anaesthetic.

Prevention
- Some individuals and households are especially liable to develop staphylococcal infections of all kinds, such as boils, whitlows and paronychia. Preventive measures should be considered and discussed with a doctor.

See SKIN *page 52*

WHOOPING COUGH

A severe infectious disease of childhood (known medically as pertussis). It is spread by droplets in the air breathed out by an infected child. Because of immunisation the number of cases in Britain fell considerably from 1957 until 1974. But publicity linking immunisation with the very rare chance of ENCEPHALITIS later discouraged parents from having their children immunised, and in 1977-9, when fewer than one child in three was being immunised, the largest outbreak of whooping cough since the mid-fifties took place.

Symptoms
- A cold with a runny nose and bouts of excessive coughing.
- The cough becomes worse, mainly at night. A few days after onset, the 'whoop' develops as a sudden noisy indrawing of breath at the end of a coughing spasm.
- Vomiting after coughing.
- Whooping may recur for some months afterwards if the child develops another cough.
- In severe cases, vomiting can lead to considerable loss of fluid, weight and sleep.

Incubation period
- Seven to 14 days.

Quarantine period
- Twenty-one days from onset of whoop.

Duration
- Three weeks to four months.

Causes
- Bacteria called *Haemophilus pertussis*.

Complications
- Pneumonia.
- Death occasionally occurs if fluid loss and vomiting are not controlled.

Treatment in the home
- Give extra fluids to the child.
- Proprietary cough medicines from the chemist may help. *See* MEDICINES, 16.
- Do not expose the child to cigarette smoke, as it will make his cough worse.

When to consult the doctor.
- When the symptoms described occur.

What the doctor may do
- Prescribe antibiotics to help early in the disease, and if pneumonia or another secondary infection develops.
- Give other children in the family a course of antibiotics.
- In severe cases the doctor will send the child to hospital for treatment.

Prevention
- As whooping cough is more dangerous than immunisation, all children should have a course of three injections (usually with diphtheria and tetanus vaccine) in the first year of life.
- But immunisation should not be given if the child has fits or epilepsy, or if there is a family history of the disorder; or if the child has a disorder of the nervous system, or if there is feverish illness at the time of the proposed injection; or if there has been a severe reaction to a previous dose of the vaccine. In all these cases your doctor should be consulted before the child is immunised.
- Eczema need not necessarily prevent immunisation, but if there is a severe allergy a doctor should be consulted before the injection is given.

See INFECTIOUS DISEASES *page 32*

WIND

Belching, rumblings in the abdomen, passing wind and a bloated feeling are all signs of gas in the digestive system. Rarely, wind is a symptom of disease: the main problems it causes are social rather than medical.

Gas is sometimes produced by swallowing air while eating, in which case it can be controlled by eating slowly; or it may be produced by fizzy drinks, which can be avoided. It is also produced as a by-product of digestion—particularly of foods which are not fully broken down by the digestive juices and therefore leave a residue which ferments in the bowel. Beans are the best known of these foods. Anyone who is embarrassed by a wind problem should try to discover which foods cause the trouble and avoid them.

See SYMPTOM SORTER—INDIGESTION

WORMS

Parasites such as HOOKWORM and WHIPWORM, present also in TOXACARIASIS and SCHISTOSOMIASIS. Other worms occur in many tropical areas.

See SYMPTOM SORTER—MOTIONS, ABNORMAL

WRIST

Problems that may affect the wrist include pain, swelling and injury. It is a common site for injury and diseases affecting other joints in the body.

See SYMPTOM SORTER—HAND, FINGERS AND WRIST

YAWS

A tropical disease of young children. It is spread by direct contact, particularly where hygiene is poor and clothing scanty. The first sign of the disease is a skin lump, known as the mother yaw, often on the leg. This heals within six months, but a more extensive skin eruption develops, mostly on the exposed surfaces of the body. The glands may be swollen and the child may have bone pains.

Treatment by penicillin is effective, but prevention is difficult.

See INFECTIOUS DISEASES *page 32*

YELLOW FEVER

An acute infectious disease of tropical Africa and northern regions of South America. It is caused by a virus and spread by mosquitoes. When an outbreak occurs it may affect thousands of people, but one attack gives a person immunity for life. The symptoms, which appear after an incubation period of three to six days, develop suddenly and vary in severity. They include headache and fever lasting for only two or three days in mild cases. More severe cases develop conjunctivitis, haemorrhage, jaundice and kidney failure. In very severe cases the patient can sink into a coma and die. There is no specific treatment, but immunisation is effective in preventing the disease, although it should not be given to infants under the age of nine months (*see* TRAVEL AND HOLIDAYS). International certificates of vaccination against yellow fever are valid for ten years.

See INFECTIOUS DISEASES *page 32*

Yoga

A PROGRAMME TO ENHANCE YOUR PHYSICAL WELL-BEING, AND TO RELAX YOUR BODY AND MIND

Although many people in Western countries regard yoga simply as a form of relaxation and an aid to keeping the body supple, in India—where the principles of yoga were laid down some 2,000 years ago—its followers regard it as a complete philosophy of life. Experienced practitioners, called yogis, believe that yoga can improve people's physical and mental health by helping them to become 'at one' with the universe. This, claim the yogis, will help those who are nervous or who suffer from lack of concentration.

Do's and don'ts about yoga

□ *Do* get instruction from a qualified yoga teacher.

□ *Do* ensure that your bowels and bladder are not full.

□ *Do* plan your mealtimes so that you always eat *after* completing the exercises. If this is not possible, wait for at least three hours after a heavy meal—and an hour after a light snack—before doing yoga.

□ *Do* take a shower or bath before and after doing yoga. This will refresh your body and stimulate your mind.

□ *Don't* begin yoga if you have any physical symptoms, any disabilities or if you are under medical treatment. Discuss the advisability with your doctor and the teacher.

□ *Don't* overstrain yourself when assuming yoga postures.

□ *Don't* do yoga after exposure to strong sunlight for several hours, otherwise you may feel sick and dizzy and the benefits will be destroyed.

□ *Don't* regard doing yoga as a substitute for medical care.

SOUND HEALTH
Several different types of yoga have evolved over the centuries. The one most widely practised in the West, and which lays greatest emphasis on health, is Hatha yoga. The word yoga means 'union', and Hatha refers to the self-discipline used in forming the various postures—which range from sitting cross-legged to extreme contortions which only yogis can do.

Yogis emphasise that there is no value in any posture if it requires excessive physical strain. However, physical effort is necessary.

Yoga need take up no more than 10–15 minutes once or twice a day. It can be safely practised by youngsters of four and grandparents of 84—provided their health is sound.

If you are suffering from any physical complaint you should check with your doctor before embarking on yoga.

Although you can perform Hatha yoga on your own, it is advisable to start with a fully trained and sympathetic teacher—possibly one who conducts a local authority night class. Find a teacher who deals with you as an individual and who regularly walks around the class observing and helping.

Preparing to do yoga

The nine postures on the following pages are suitable for beginners, but do not expect to do them perfectly at first. It may take weeks or even months to attain them. Follow the instructions to the best of your ability without straining your body.

The postures are not necessarily meant to be done in sequence every day. You can do just one or two of them once or twice a day. When you have more time, you might like to carry out the full sequence.

Yoga should be practised in a quiet, moderately warm, airy room in which you have space to fully stretch your body. Coldness makes it difficult to relax, so the floor should be carpeted—or else you should lie on a rug.

Clothing should be unrestricting and feet should be bare.

Hero posture

EXERCISE I

Some beginners will achieve this posture with little discomfort, but others—particularly those with weak knees—will find that they cannot kneel or sit right down on the floor at first. In some cases, their feet will splay out, whereas the big toes should turn slightly inwards. It will help to use a rolled blanket to support the arches, and a pile of magazines, cushions or folded blankets to sit on.

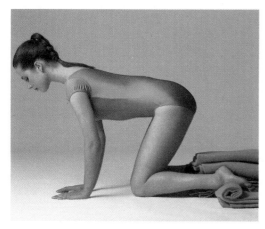

1 Kneel on the floor, preferably on a thick carpet or rubber mat, and support yourself with your hands. Keep your knees together and spread your feet about 18 in. (450 mm.) apart.

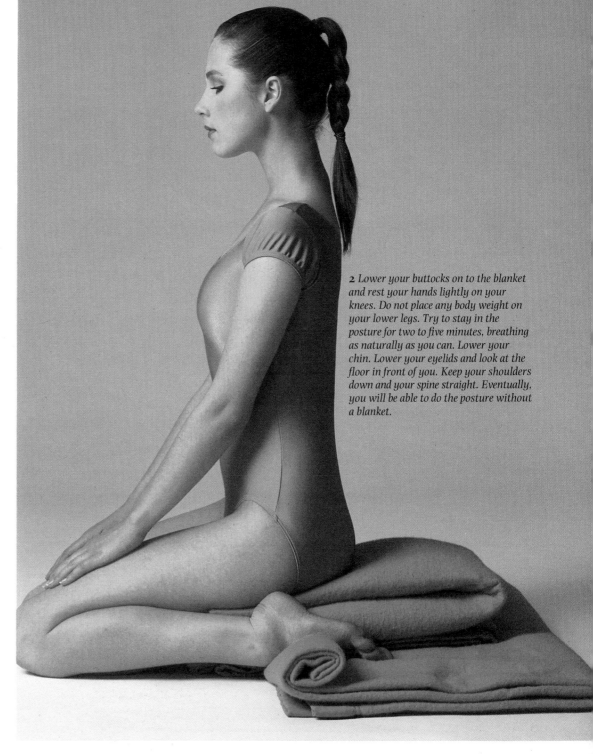

2 Lower your buttocks on to the blanket and rest your hands lightly on your knees. Do not place any body weight on your lower legs. Try to stay in the posture for two to five minutes, breathing as naturally as you can. Lower your chin. Lower your eyelids and look at the floor in front of you. Keep your shoulders down and your spine straight. Eventually, you will be able to do the posture without a blanket.

Lying-down hero posture

EXERCISE 2

Once you have mastered the hero posture, you might like to try the lying-down hero posture. Before starting the exercise, place the folded blanket—or blankets—to support the upper part of your back.

If your thighs lift too much during the exercise, you should put more folded blankets or firm cushions under your back and head and then part your knees. Yogis say that the posture relieves aching legs and is especially helpful for people who have to stand or walk for hours. It is also recommended by yogis for athletes and it can be performed shortly before going to bed, so that tired legs can be rejuvenated in the night.

Some people may experience backache during or on completing the exercise. To counteract this, sit up and stretch your knees as far apart as possible, with your feet held sideways so that your big toes and soles touch. Stretch your arms and trunk forwards along the floor, keeping your heels as near as possible to your buttocks. Then slowly stretch out your legs and get up.

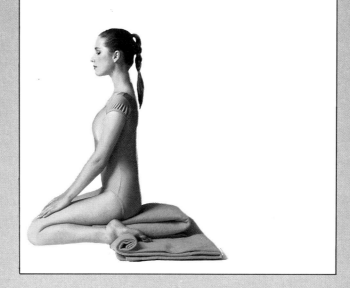

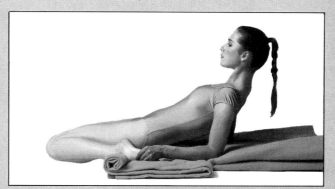

1 This posture follows on naturally from the hero posture and you begin by kneeling on the floor in the hero posture and breathing in.

2 As you breathe out, lean against the blanket and rest your elbows one by one on the blanket. Continue to breathe naturally.

3 Move your hands down along your body one after the other and straighten your arms. Gradually lower your back and then the back of your head on to the blanket. Your back should be flat in this posture. If your thighs lift too much, correct them by parting your knees. Hold the posture for two to five minutes. To get up, roll gently on to one side.

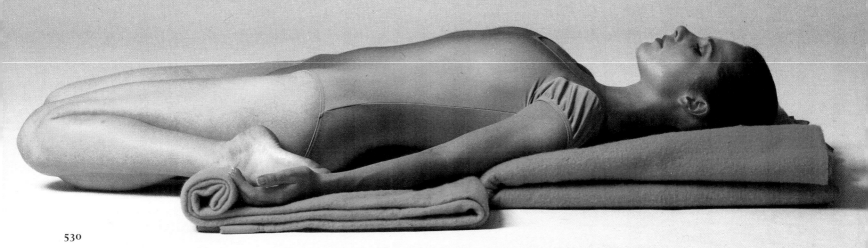

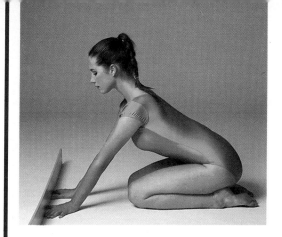

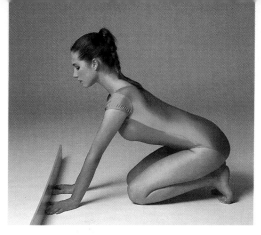

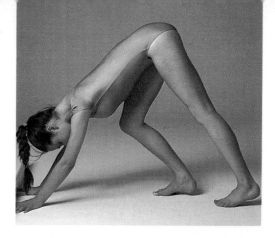

1 Kneel facing a wall, buttocks near your heels, and stretch out your hands on the floor. Press the thumbs, about 6 in. (150 mm.) apart, against the wall or skirting-board for support.

2 Slowly start to raise yourself. Your arms must become in line with the sides of your shoulders, and your feet in line with your hips. Turn your toes in slightly. This will stretch your arches.

3 To fully raise your body, keep your arms straight—flexing the insides of your elbows—and raise your body. Then pull your shoulder-blades into the body.

Head down dog posture

EXERCISE 3

This posture is an imitation of a dog stretching itself with its head and forelegs down and its hind legs up. It will be easier if it is performed against a facing wall.

At first, stay in the posture for one minute. As you become more expert, remain in the posture for up to five minutes.

The posture may be extended by doing the four stages in reverse—turning your back to the wall and placing the palms of your hands, with the fingers spread, where your feet were.

4 Push your heels gently down towards the floor. As the Achilles tendons strengthen, your heels may reach the floor. Keep your toes turned inwards and stretch the backs of your knees so that you feel a 'pull'.

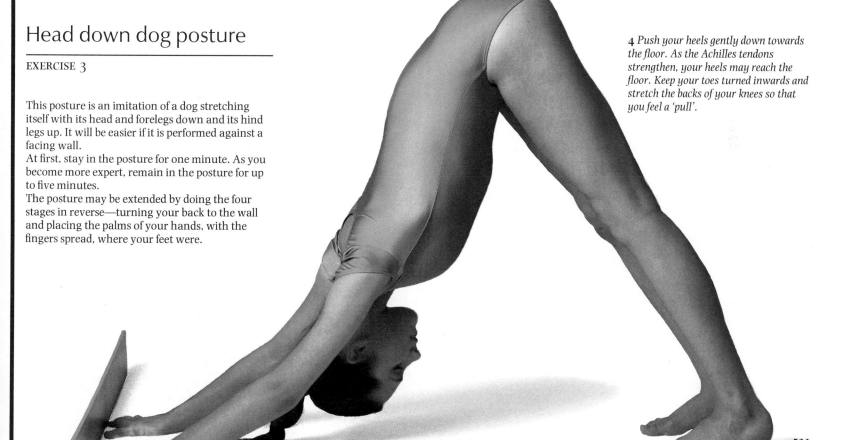

531

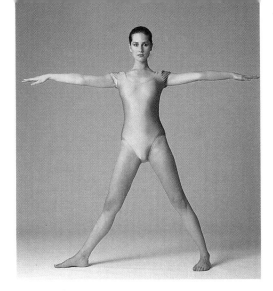

1 *Stand with your back against a wall and spread your legs 3 ft (90 cm.) apart. Stretch your arms at shoulder level with the palms of the hands down. Your shoulders, hips, little fingers and as much of your spine as possible should be touching the wall. Turn your right foot 90 degrees to the right and your left foot 45 degrees in the same direction.*

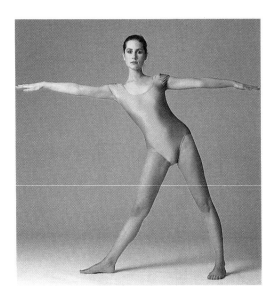

2 *As you breathe out, extend your right arm and trunk to the right.*

Extended triangle posture

EXERCISE 4

First complete the three stages of this pose, then repeat the posture in the other direction. You will probably find it harder working to one side than to the other. But this will balance out if you work harder on the 'difficult' side. Even so, it may take some months before you reach the fully stretched position.

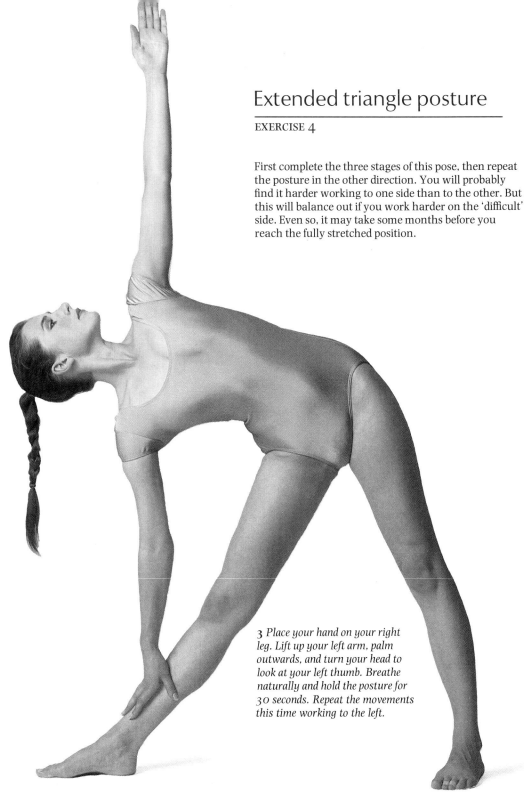

3 *Place your hand on your right leg. Lift up your left arm, palm outwards, and turn your head to look at your left thumb. Breathe naturally and hold the posture for 30 seconds. Repeat the movements this time working to the left.*

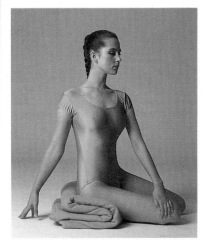

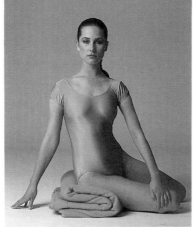

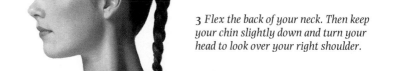

3 Flex the back of your neck. Then keep your chin slightly down and turn your head to look over your right shoulder.

1 Sit on a folded blanket with your knees bent and your legs pointing to the left. Put your left hand just above your right knee. Turning, place your right hand in line with your spine and touch the floor with the fingertips.

2 Pull at your right knee with your left hand; at the same time, push on the floor with your right fingertips. Twist your hips until your chest is in line with your forward leg. Make sure you are breathing evenly and quietly.

Sitting spine twist

EXERCISE 5

Beginners may find this posture easier if they sit sideways on a chair and use the back of the chair to pull themselves round.

When you have performed the posture in one direction, change position and do it to the other side.

Hold the posture for two minutes.

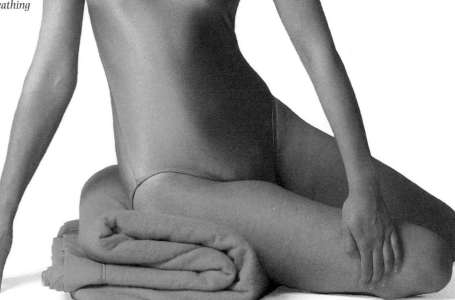

Bridge posture

EXERCISE 6

As well as two folded blankets, a solid wooden box about 12 in. (300 mm.) high is needed as a support while performing this posture. If such a box is not available, you can use a low stool or coffee-table. However, you must ensure that they are placed firmly on the floor and will not slip or slide. If they are too high for the posture you can place extra cushions or blankets—or even magazines or books—under your head.

In this posture, the body is stretched and arched like a bridge—with the shoulders, buttocks and heels acting as supports. With practice, you should be able to hold the posture for five minutes, gradually working up to ten.

Do not attempt to sit straight up from the posture. Slide backwards off the box or alternative support and lie with your knees bent for a few moments. Then roll gently on to your side and get up.

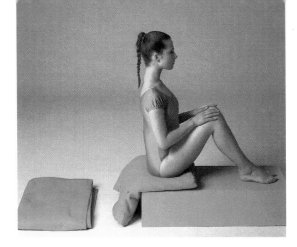

1 Place one of the blankets on the ground and the other on the near end of the box. Sit on the box blanket with your knees bent.

2 Slide your body towards the floor, keeping your lower spine supported by the box blanket. If you are unable to reach the floor, place more blankets there until your shoulders are supported.

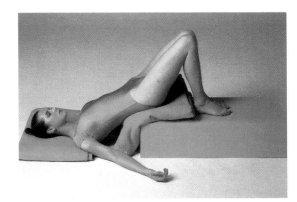

3 Stretch your arms overhead along the floor. If the shoulders are stiff, the arms will not reach the floor at first.

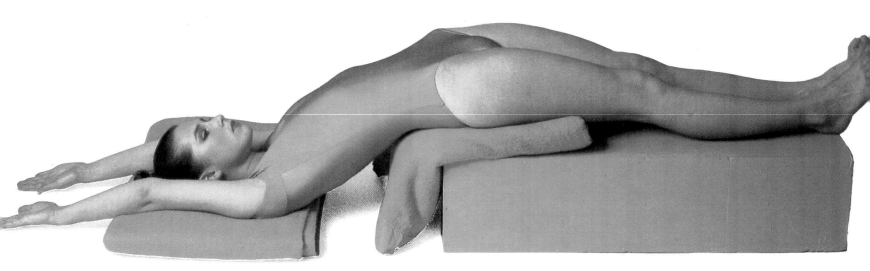

Plough posture

EXERCISE 7

In this posture, beginners should use a chair to support their feet. When you are lying down, the chair should be about 2 ft (60 cm.) behind your head. With practice, you may be able to dispense with the chair.

Use at least one or more folded blankets as a base on which to rest your neck, shoulders and elbows. Make sure the blanket is *not* placed under your head, otherwise your chin will touch your breastbone and hamper your breathing.

With practice, you should be able to hold the posture for three minutes, possibly building up to ten minutes as you become more skilled.

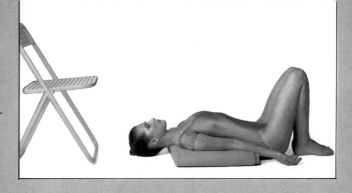

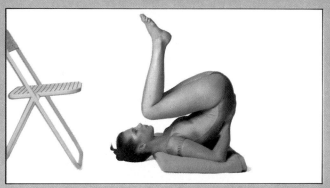

1 Lie with the back of your head on the floor and your neck and shoulders on the blanket. Place your arms by your sides, with the palms facing upwards.

2 Bend your knees and bring them as close as possible to your chest. Exhaling, lift your buttocks and back off the floor and immediately place your hands at the back of your waist. Fit people should have no trouble in doing this. Otherwise you can place your feet on the shoulders of a helper and push yourself up.

3 Rest your toes on the chair. If you feel uncomfortable, have your helper move the chair forward until your thighs are resting on it.

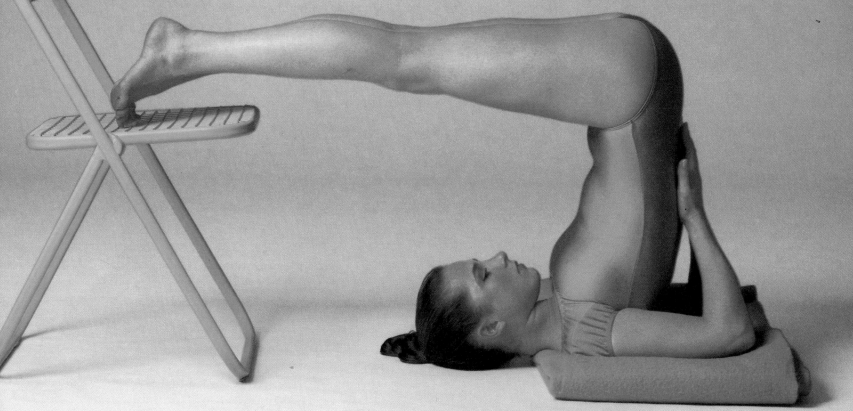

Shoulder stand

EXERCISE 8

The shoulder stand—or neck balance—posture follows naturally on from the plough position. Once you are in the 'up' position, you should not look at your feet except to check that they are level. Keep your eyes trained on a spot about 4 in. (100 mm.) above your navel. If you are not breathing evenly and easily, you should come down from the position.

To do so, bend your knees and lower your back to the floor vertebra by vertebra, at the same time taking your hands away from your back. With practice you should be able to hold the position for three minutes.

At the end of the exercise, relax on the floor, breathing naturally, and get ready to perform the final posture.

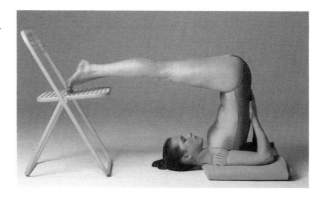

1 *This posture follows on naturally from the plough position. Starting from that position, place your hands firmly on your lower ribs, with your elbows well tucked in.*

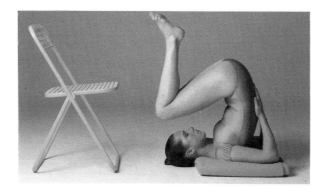

2 *Bring your knees away from the chair and near to your forehead. Keep on supporting your back and keep your elbows in place.*

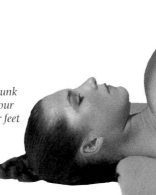

3 *Stretch your legs right up. Keep your hands where they are and bring your trunk closer to your face. Place the joints of your big toes together. Push the soles of your feet as far as possible towards the ceiling.*

Corpse posture

EXERCISE 9

The aim of this final posture is to completely relax your body and your mind. Although it is easy to keep your body still, it is much more difficult to still your mind. It may help you to relax by putting a folded blanket under your head—*not* the back of your neck. This will lower your chin.

On reaching this last exercise you may find that your back is aching. If so, place a firm cushion under the small of the back.

Yogis state that this posture forms the basis of the various relaxation therapies in use today throughout the world. The corpse posture should be held for about 15 minutes. You may find yourself falling asleep at the first few attempts, but eventually you will be able to stay awake—with your brain passive. If necessary, use a timer to wake yourself up.

To complete the posture, lift your eyelids and look up at the ceiling, while breathing deeply. Bring your knees up to your chest and roll gently over to the right. Swing your left arm over and release your right arm from under you. Your right hand will now touch the floor near your spine. You will feel totally relaxed and at peace with the world. When ready, raise your head and sit up gently.

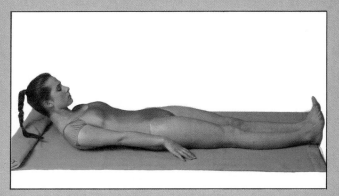

1 Lie flat with a folded blanket under your head. Keep your feet together with your toes pointing upwards. Raise your head and look along your body to make sure it is straight.

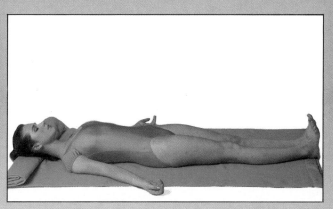

2 Spread your arms about 18 in. (450 mm.) away from your body with the palms up. Roll back your shoulders and lift the shoulder-blades just off the floor. Gently close your eyes. Push your feet away from you to extend your spine.

3 Relax your feet to the side. Open your mouth slightly then close your lips and breathe through your nose. Make sure your tongue is relaxed and resting on the floor of your mouth. Relax your face muscles and forehead. Be aware of the sound of your breath.

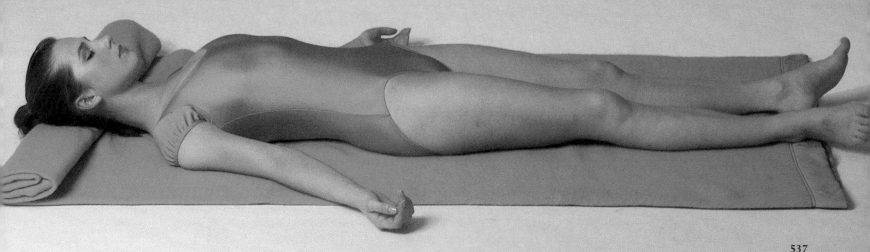

PART 4 FIRST AID

A guide to life-saving techniques and instant action in emergencies

Introduction

When someone is injured or suddenly falls ill, every second counts. Study the following pages on first aid NOW—before finding yourself called upon to treat a casualty. The information could save vital moments in an emergency—and a life.

In an emergency, ensure that the casualty cannot come to any more harm and treat those injuries which threaten his life. Then call medical help. Do not leave the casualty unattended, and be ready to give further first aid if he needs it.

Most first aid is practical common sense, which you can teach yourself. But one life-saving technique—artificial respiration combined with chest compression—should be studied under a qualified instructor, such as a member of the Red Cross.

Portable first-aid kit

A portable first-aid kit for your car or rucksack should fit into a container about 8 in. (200 mm.) long, 5 in. (130 mm.) wide and 2 in. (50 mm.) deep. It should be well sealed, securely fastened and easy to open. You can buy a container, complete with kit, from most chemists—or make your own from a plastic box lined with foam padding or quilting to protect the contents.

In an emergency, rescuers must be able to find the container immediately. It should therefore be clearly marked FIRST AID. A card giving medical details—such as blood groups and physical descriptions—of you and your family should be taped inside the lid.

Foil or 'space' blankets fold neatly into small packets and, when opened out, can be wrapped around a casualty to preserve his body heat in freezing temperatures. In hot weather they can be used as shelters, with the silver side uppermost, reflecting the sun's rays.

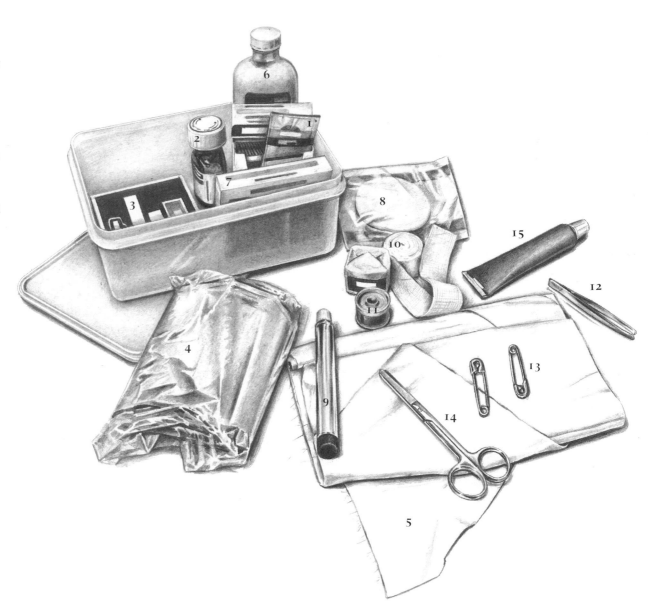

1 *Waterproof plasters*
2 *Soluble painkiller*
3 *Absorbent gauze*
4 *Foil or 'space' blanket*
5 *Triangular bandage*
6 *Calamine lotion*
7 *Antiseptic wipes*
8 *Eye pad*
9 *Pen torch*
10 *Open-weave bandage*
11 *Roll of 1 in. (25 mm.) plaster*
12 *Round-ended tweezers*
13 *Safety pins*
14 *Snub-nosed scissors*
15 *Antiseptic cream*

Casualty unconscious and not breathing

PRIORITY CHECK-LIST ONLY

1 Act quickly Check for danger

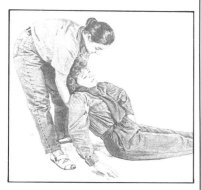

- Assess situation to make sure it is safe for you to approach.

- Do not move the casualty more than is necessary for treatment.

- Drag a casualty who cannot move out of any immediate danger—for example, traffic or fire.

2 Check casualty's breathing

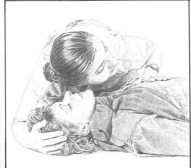

- Lay the casualty flat on her back, tilt her chin up so her neck is not constricted.

- Put your ear to the casualty's mouth to feel and listen for breathing. Put your hand on her chest to check for rise and fall.

- Check for five seconds before deciding if breathing is absent.

3 Clear mouth of any debris

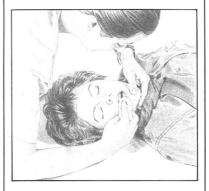

- Use fingers to clear the casualty's mouth. Pull her chin up so her neck is fully extended. Remove any dentures.

4 Feel for pulse at neck

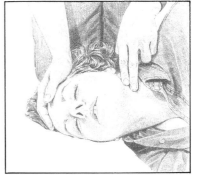

- Tilt head back, feel for Adam's apple with two fingers and slide them into hollow between apple and muscle beside it. Feel for pulse for at least five seconds.

5 Start mouth-to-mouth respiration

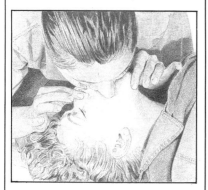

• If pulse is present, give artificial respiration to restart natural breathing.

6 Apply chest compression

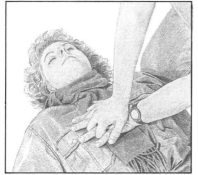

• If the casualty is not breathing, check her pulse for heartbeat. If there is no pulse, give two mouth-to-mouth inflations, then begin chest compression.

7 Recovery position

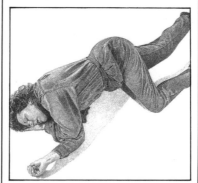

• When the casualty has begun to breathe naturally, arrange her in the recovery position, if possible with her head lower than the rest of her body.

• NEVER put pillows or coats under the casualty's head.

• Cover the casualty with one blanket only.

8 Send for help. Dial 999

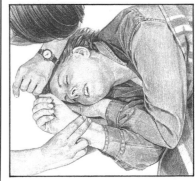

• Immediately call the emergency services if you can do so.

• Watch constantly for any changes in the casualty's condition and be ready to give further emergency first aid if necessary.

EMERGENCY

DIAGNOSIS
AND TREATMENT
CHECK-LIST

Casualty unconscious but breathing

PRIORITY CHECK-LIST ONLY

1 Act quickly Check for danger

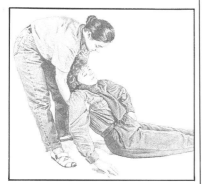

- Assess situation to make sure it is safe for you to approach.

- Do not move the casualty more than is necessary for treatment.

- Drag a casualty who cannot move out of any immediate danger—for example, traffic or fire.

2 Check casualty's breathing

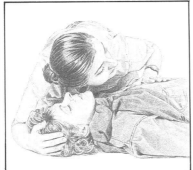

- Lay the casualty flat on her back, tilt her chin up so her neck is not constricted.

- Put your ear to the casualty's mouth for at least five seconds to feel and hear her breathing. Put your hand on her chest to check its rise and fall.

3 Clear mouth of any debris

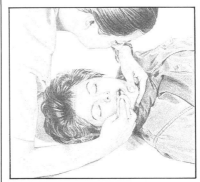

- Use fingers to clear the casualty's mouth. Pull her chin up so her neck is fully extended. Remove any dentures.

- If her breathing stops, start artificial respiration. Begin to treat any severe bleeding. Leave other injuries until later.

4 Turn casualty

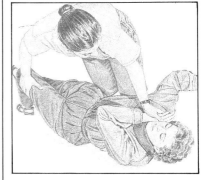

- If breathing is regular and you do not suspect fractures, straighten casualty's legs and put nearer arm at right-angles to body, elbow bent, palm up. Fold the other arm across chest and put that hand under cheek, palm down.

- With your other hand, raise casualty's knee and roll her towards you, supporting head.

5 Recovery position

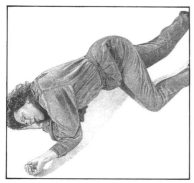

- Arrange the casualty in the recovery position, if possible with her head lower than the rest of her body.

- NEVER put pillows or coats under the casualty's head.

6 Loosen tight clothing

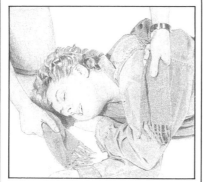

- Check that the casualty's neck remains fully extended.

- Loosen tight clothing at her neck, chest and waist.

- Gently ensure that the casualty stays in the recovery position, and is breathing freely.

7 Treat other injuries

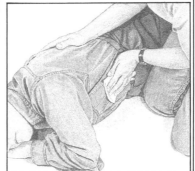

- Staunch bleeding and dress wounds not previously dealt with.

- Cover the casualty with one blanket only.

8 Send for help. Dial 999

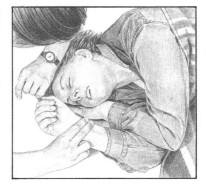

- Call the emergency services if you can do so without leaving the casualty unattended for more than a minute or two.

- Watch constantly for changes in the casualty's condition and be ready to give further emergency first aid if necessary.

EMERGENCY

DIAGNOSIS
AND TREATMENT
CHECK-LIST

Severe external bleeding

PRIORITY CHECK-LIST ONLY

1 Act quickly Check for danger

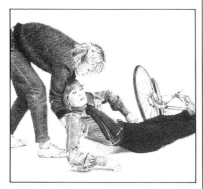

- Assess situation to make sure it is safe for you to approach.

- Do not move the casualty more than is necessary for treatment.

- Drag a casualty who cannot move out of any immediate danger—for example, traffic or fire.

2 Staunch flow of blood

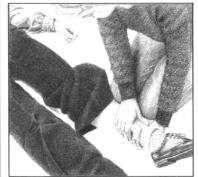

- Quickly press down with your hands on a bleeding wound. If you have a clean cloth or other suitable material put that on the wound before pressing. But do not waste time searching.

- Keep pressure on the wound until the bleeding stops.

- NEVER use a tourniquet.

3 Raise the injured limb

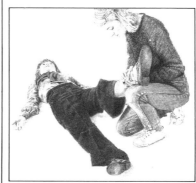

- If the wound is to a leg, arm or head, raise it while treating, unless there is a fracture.

- Treat stomach, leg or back wounds with the casualty lying down.

- Treat chest wounds with the casualty sitting up and inclined towards the injured side.

4 Clear loose debris

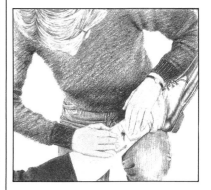

- With a clean cloth or clean handkerchief, wipe away any loose grit, glass or other material from AROUND the wound. Do not disturb the wound.

- Do not touch any foreign object that is firmly embedded in a wound. NEVER pull out an object that has created a puncture wound, for example, a knife.

5 Dress the wound

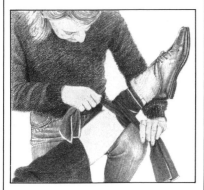

- When the bleeding stops, dress the wound. Use plenty of padding—gauze if available—or any clean material.

- Fix padding in place with a firm, but not over-tight, bandage. In an emergency, any absorbent material will do. If blood comes through the bandage, put another one on top.

6 Rest the casualty

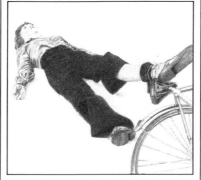

- Arrange the casualty with the wound above the level of her heart, unless movement would make other serious injuries worse.

- If the wound is in the foot or leg, keep the casualty lying down and prop her leg at an angle of 45 degrees. For an arm, improvise a sling.

7 Cover the casualty

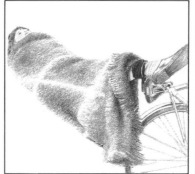

- Once the bleeding has been staunched and the wound bandaged, treat any less-severe injuries and lightly cover the casualty with a coat or single blanket, leaving the bandaged area visible.

- Severe bleeding can lead to shock.

8 Send for help. Dial 999

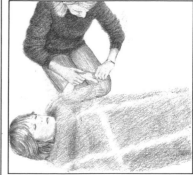

- Call emergency services if you can do so without leaving the casualty unattended for more than a minute or two.

- Watch constantly for changes in the casualty's condition and be ready to give further emergency first aid if necessary.

EMERGENCY

DIAGNOSIS AND TREATMENT CHECK-LIST

Road traffic accidents

PRIORITY CHECK-LIST ONLY

1 Stop, observe and act

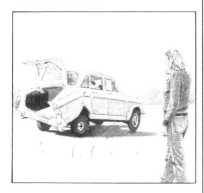

• Park your car at a safe distance behind the accident. Turn on your hazard warning lights.

• If the crashed vehicle is on fire, keep clear.

• Take charge of the accident scene if no one else has done so. If someone is already in charge, make yourself useful to him.

2 Immobilise crashed vehicle

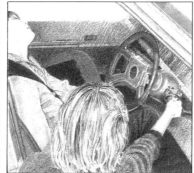

• Turn off the ignition. Remove the ignition key and drop it on the car floor.

• Count the casualties and check their condition.

• Do not smoke, and immediately put out any lighted cigarettes, cigars or pipes.

3 Ring the police. Dial 999

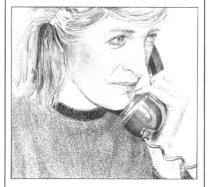

• Send someone to a telephone to call the police. If no one else is available, do this yourself.

• Give the police the location of the accident and the number and condition of the casualties. State if anyone is trapped in the vehicle. The police will notify the ambulance service and the fire brigade.

4 Warn other traffic

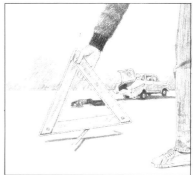

• Take your red warning triangle, if available, and place it on the ground about 100 yds (90 m.) behind the accident scene.

• Flag down any oncoming traffic.

• Return to the crashed vehicle and see if anyone has been thrown clear.

5 Do not move casualties

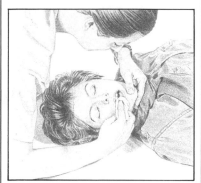

• Whatever position the casualties are in, leave them there.

• Do not pick out any glass from the flesh.

• Clear the mouth with your index finger, removing any dentures.

• Make sure the casualty can breathe freely. Loosen tight neck clothing.

6 Start self-help treatment

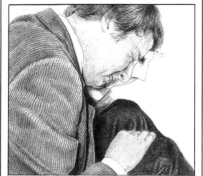

• See if the casualty can treat himself and show him what to do.

• He can stem blood coming from an arm or leg injury by gripping the wound with his hand. Alternatively, he can use a clean handkerchief or tissue to stem the blood.

7 Treatment priorities

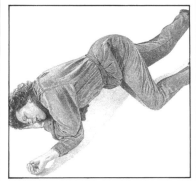

• Treat the casualties in the following order:
1 Unconscious and not breathing.
2 Severely bleeding.
3 Unconscious but breathing.

• Then search the scene in case someone has left the crashed vehicle and is wandering around in shock—or has collapsed at a distance.

8 Reassure the casualties

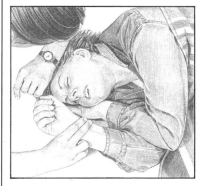

• Cover the casualty lightly with a car rug or overcoat.

• Tell her the ambulance is on its way.

• Tell her that any missing adult, child or animal is being taken care of.

• Do not give her anything by mouth.

EMERGENCY

DIAGNOSIS
AND TREATMENT
CHECK-LIST

Abdominal injuries

The abdomen—the lower two-thirds of the trunk—contains many vital organs which are richly supplied with blood. They include the bladder, uterus and intestines. A car accident, a fall, or a stab or bullet wound can cause serious damage to those organs, or to the blood vessels connected to them.

OPEN WOUNDS

Often, the injury is clearly visible. Sometimes an internal organ may protrude through the wound: do not attempt to push it back.

Warning signs

• Paleness, cold clammy skin and sometimes sweat on forehead.
• Faintness and/or nausea.

INTERNAL INJURIES

In other accidents, there may be little or no external sign of injury. However, the victim may be suffering from internal bleeding. All suspected abdominal injuries should be examined by a doctor as soon as possible.

Warning signs

• Pain or tenderness in the abdomen.
• Tightening of the abdomen.
• Bruises and abrasions.
• Nausea and vomiting.
• Muscular spasms.
• Paleness, cold clammy skin and sometimes sweat on forehead.
• Faintness and/or nausea.

VERTICAL OPEN WOUNDS/*ACTION*

1

In the case of a vertical wound, lay the casualty flat on her back with legs outstretched and feet slightly raised. That position helps to keep the wound closed. Do not put any coats or blankets under the casualty's head.

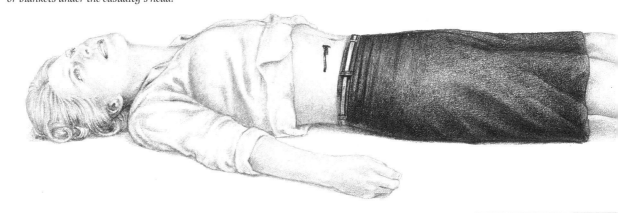

HORIZONTAL OPEN WOUNDS/*ACTION*

1

In the case of a horizontal wound, lay the casualty on his back with coats or blankets under his shoulders and under his bent knees. That position helps to keep the wound closed.

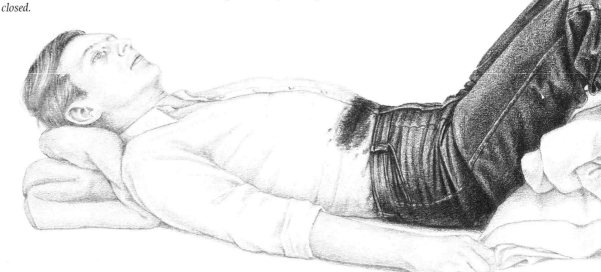

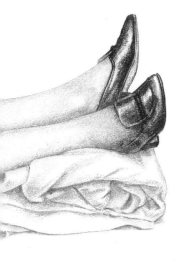

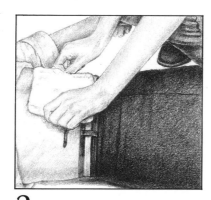

2
Expose the wound by gently removing the clothing from around it, and put a clean dressing over it. This will staunch the bleeding.

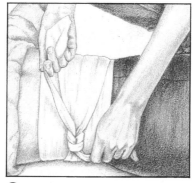

3
Tie the dressing in place firmly, but not too tightly, with a bandage or other suitable material. The knot should not be directly over the wound.

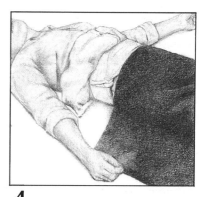

4
Cover the casualty with a coat or blanket, leaving her arms outside. Get medical attention as quickly as possible, but do not leave the casualty alone.

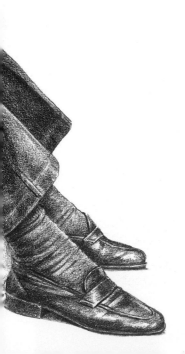

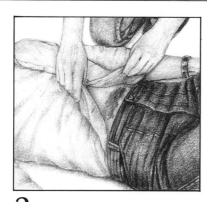

2
Gently remove the casualty's clothing from around the wound to expose it for treatment. Do not cough, sneeze or breathe on the wound, as that may cause it to become infected.

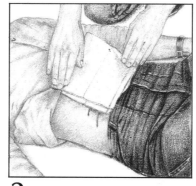

3
Cover the wound and any protruding organs lightly with a large dressing or fresh linen. Fix the dressing in place with a bandage, so that it covers, but does not press down on, the wound.

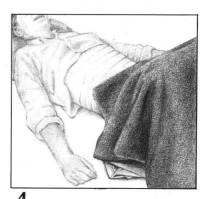

4
Cover casualty with a coat or blanket, leaving his arms outside. Get medical attention as soon as possible, but do not leave casualty alone. Check pulse and breathing rate frequently.

Artificial respiration/1

A casualty who has stopped breathing can live for only four to six minutes. After as little as three minutes, his brain suffers irreversible damage. Artificial respiration—applied without delay—puts air into the lungs until the victim can breathe for himself.

Look for blue-grey lips, cheeks or ear-lobes and for any movement of the chest or upper abdomen. Put your ear close to the casualty's nose and mouth to listen for breathing.

If it is feeble or non-existent, his heart may have stopped. Feel with two fingers for the victim's carotid pulse beside his windpipe. If there is none after five seconds, you must combine artificial respiration with chest compression.

Once the casualty is breathing normally, turn him on to his stomach and arrange him in the recovery position, unless you suspect his back or neck may be broken. Treat any bleeding or injuries. *See* UNCONSCIOUSNESS *pages 611-12.*

Watch his breathing carefully, and if it falters be ready to restart artificial respiration.

INFANTS AND SMALL CHILDREN
Resuscitation is performed more gently, just enough to make the chest rise.

INFANTS AND SMALL CHILDREN/*ACTION*
Clear the airway and hold the child with his head tilted slightly back. Cover his nose and mouth with your mouth and puff gently into his lungs, making his chest rise. Remove your mouth and turn your head to watch his chest fall. Continue until he is breathing regularly, then put him in the recovery position.

MOUTH-TO-NOSE ARTIFICIAL RESPIRATION
The most successful, and easiest, form of artificial respiration is the mouth-to-nose method. It reduces the danger of inflating the stomach and causing vomiting.

MOUTH-TO-MOUTH ARTIFICIAL RESPIRATION
If the nose is damaged or the nasal passage is blocked, use mouth-to-mouth artificial respiration—the kiss of life.

Mouth-to-nose and mouth-to-mouth artificial respiration can be given through a clean handkerchief.

In either method provide breaths at the rate of 10 inflations a minute.

HOLGER NIELSEN, REVISED METHOD
If the victim has severe facial injuries or is trapped face down, you can use the Holger Nielsen method which inflates the lungs by firm, controlled pressure on the casualty's back.

SILVESTER METHOD
This method, involving pressure to the casualty's chest, can be combined with heart massage. In other cases, it is best avoided.

Whichever method of artificial respiration you employ, the priorities are the same: get the casualty out of danger; check for breathing; clear the mouth; then start resuscitation.

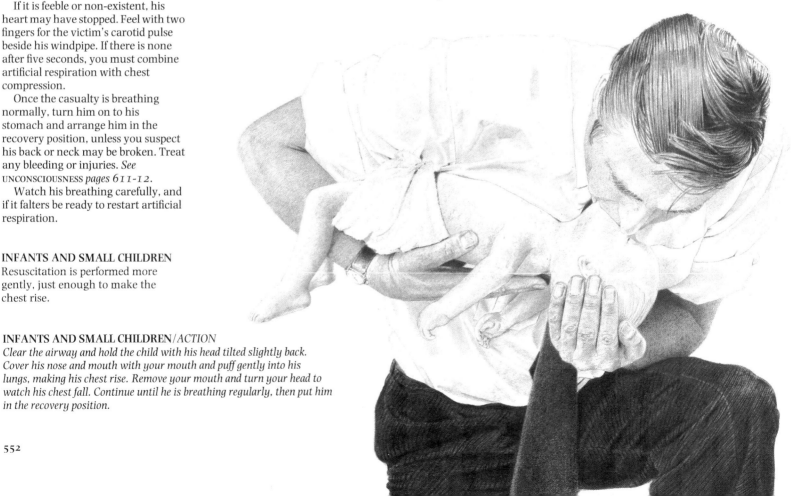

MOUTH-TO-NOSE ARTIFICIAL RESPIRATION/*ACTION*

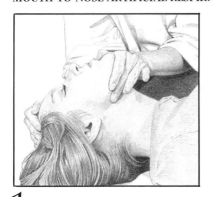

1

Put casualty face up, head to one side. Clear mouth with finger. Make sure there is pulse at neck. Tilt head up, mouth closed, hand on forehead.

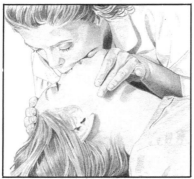

2

Raise casualty's chin and hold her mouth shut. Seal your lips around nose, using your cheek to seal the mouth, and breathe into her.

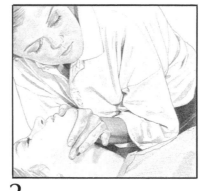

3

Remove your mouth and turn your head to watch chest fall. Breathe into nose again. Give breaths at rate of ten a minute.

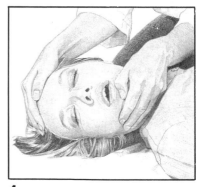

4

If the casualty vomits during resuscitation, turn the head to one side, and clear the mouth with your finger. Tilt head again and resume resuscitation.

MOUTH-TO-MOUTH ARTIFICIAL RESPIRATION—THE KISS OF LIFE/*ACTION*

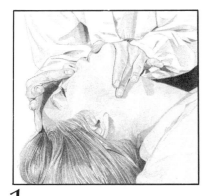

1

Clear the casualty's mouth of blood or vomit. Make sure there is pulse at neck. Straighten the head and tilt it up, with the chin well up. Pinch the casualty's nose shut with your fingers.

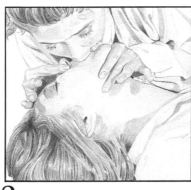

2

Seal lips around casualty's open mouth. Keep the nose pinched shut with one hand. Draw a full breath and breathe into casualty's mouth until chest rises. Then remove your mouth.

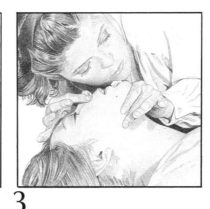

3

Turn your head to watch the casualty's chest fall. Replace your mouth and breathe into the casualty again. Continue at breathing rate of ten inflations a minute.

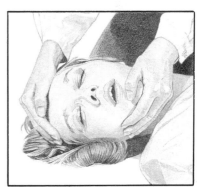

4

If the casualty vomits during resuscitation, turn the head to one side, and clear the mouth with your finger. Tilt the casualty's head again and resume artificial respiration.

553

Artificial respiration/2

HOLGER NIELSEN, REVISED METHOD/*ACTION*

1

Check the casualty's breathing and clear his airway. Do not use this technique if the victim has serious arm or chest injuries. If not, turn him face down. Arrange the arms, with elbows flexed and pointing outwards, slightly above shoulder level. Rest the hands side by side. Turn the head to one side with the neck extended. Kneel in a comfortable position at the casualty's head. Put your hands just below the casualty's shoulder-blades, with your thumbs together and your fingers in a 'butterfly'. Rock forward on your hands until your shoulders, arms and wrists are in a straight vertical line, and exert firm pressure.

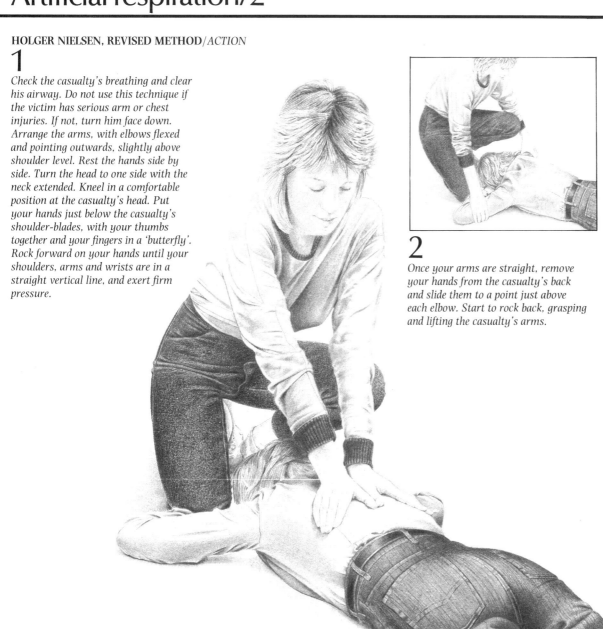

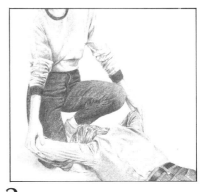

2

Once your arms are straight, remove your hands from the casualty's back and slide them to a point just above each elbow. Start to rock back, grasping and lifting the casualty's arms.

3

Keep lifting the casualty's arms as you rock back, until you can feel the resistance from the shoulder muscles. Then, still grasping the arms lower them slowly to the ground.

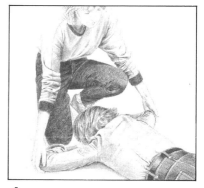

4

Slide your hands down to below the shoulder-blades, back to the 'butterfly' position. Then restart the cycle. Repeat the procedure 12 times a minute until recovery occurs.

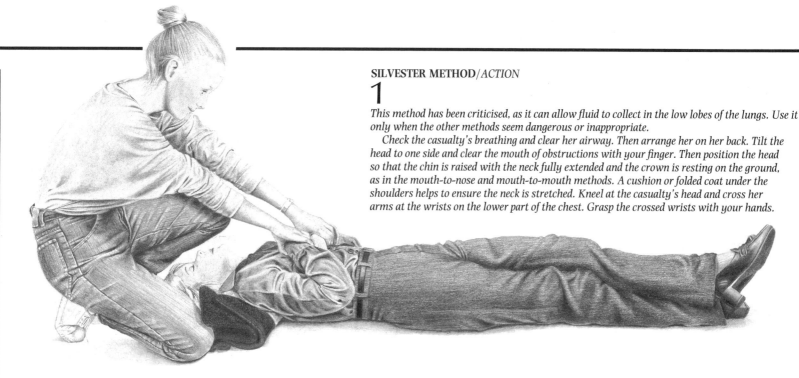

SILVESTER METHOD/*ACTION*

1

This method has been criticised, as it can allow fluid to collect in the low lobes of the lungs. Use it only when the other methods seem dangerous or inappropriate.

Check the casualty's breathing and clear her airway. Then arrange her on her back. Tilt the head to one side and clear the mouth of obstructions with your finger. Then position the head so that the chin is raised with the neck fully extended and the crown is resting on the ground, as in the mouth-to-nose and mouth-to-mouth methods. A cushion or folded coat under the shoulders helps to ensure the neck is stretched. Kneel at the casualty's head and cross her arms at the wrists on the lower part of the chest. Grasp the crossed wrists with your hands.

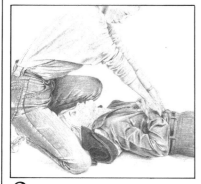

2

Rock your body forwards, pressing the casualty's arms and wrists firmly into her chest. Continue until your shoulders, arms and wrists are in a vertical straight line.

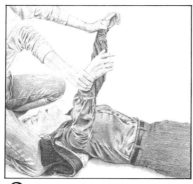

3

Release the pressure and rock your body back, still holding the wrists, to draw the casualty's arms up and outwards as far as they will go, using a sweeping movement of your arms.

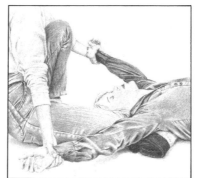

4

At the full extent of the movement, the casualty's arms should be almost touching the ground. Refold the arms on the chest and repeat the cycle 12 times a minute until the casualty recovers.

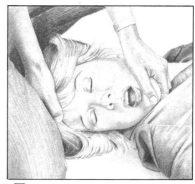

5

If the casualty vomits during resuscitation, turn the head to one side to clear the mouth with your finger. Return the head to the Silvester position and resume artificial respiration.

Artificial respiration/3

EXTERNAL CHEST COMPRESSION
This technique squeezes the heart and main blood vessels inside the chest. You thereby provide the casualty with an artificial pump for the blood.

In all cases, the pressure should depress the chest to $1\frac{1}{2}$–2 in. (4–5 cm.). If necessary, the resuscitation should be continued until medical aid arrives.

Adults Repeat the pressure at the casualty's normal pulse-rate—80 times a minute.

Children Lightly repeat the pressure 100 times a minute for a child below school age.

Infants Use two fingers to very lightly repeat the pressure 100 times a minute.

When you can detect a neck pulse, and the casualty's complexion appears to be returning from blue-grey to normal, discontinue the massage. Otherwise, the heart may stop again.

Chest compression and artificial respiration should be learned from a qualified instructor and should never be practised on a conscious, healthy person.

ADULTS/ACTION

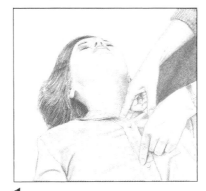

1
If you cannot detect a neck pulse and if the complexion is blue-grey, ensure the casualty is on a firm surface and feel for the breastbone. Give two inflations of the lungs.

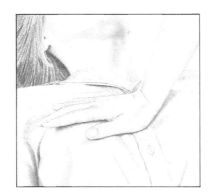

2
Place the heel of one hand on the casualty's chest, two fingers up from the bottom of the breastbone. Keep your thumb and fingers raised, so that they do not rest on the chest.

3
Keep the heel of your hand in place and place your other hand over it, fingers interlocked, thumb and fingers raised. Press down $1\frac{1}{2}$–2 in. (4–5 cm.). Let the chest rise.

4
Give 15 presses, then inflate lungs twice by artificial respiration. Check neck pulse after one minute. Repeat sequence until pulse beats on its own. Continue artificial respiration if necessary.

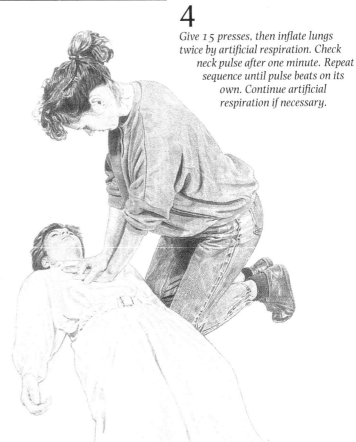

Asphyxiation

CHILDREN/ACTION

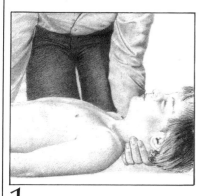

1

If the victim of a heart stoppage is a child below school age, lay him out flat. Prepare to press lightly with the heel of one hand on the lower part of the breastbone.

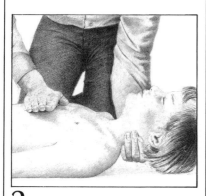

2

After pressing the breastbone down 1–1½ in. (25–35 mm.), let it rise. Give five presses, then one lung inflation. Repeat sequence until the pulse beats unaided. Continue if necessary.

INFANTS/ACTION

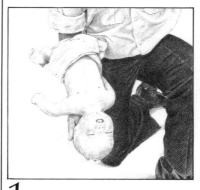

1

If the casualty is a young baby, support it along one arm with your hand cradling its head, which should be slightly tilted down. You can also give artificial respiration in this position.

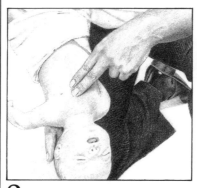

2

Press middle of breastbone down ½–1 in. (13–25 mm.), using two fingers, and let it rise. Give five presses, then one lung inflation. Repeat until the pulse beats on its own.

Someone suffering from asphyxiation (lack of oxygen in the blood) may die unless first aid is given promptly.

Among the most common causes are: contraction of the airway brought about by food, liquid or conditions such as asthma or bronchitis; blockage of the airway by food, blood, vomit or broken teeth, or by the tongue falling to the back of the throat; compression of the chest or damage to the lungs; gas poisoning or electrical accidents; diseases such as poliomyelitis; suffocation; and strangulation.

In most cases of suffocation, the victim's mouth and nose have been blocked and he cannot breathe. Remove the object causing the blockage—if, for instance, it is a polythene bag, by tearing it—and treat.

Warning signs
• Breathing is difficult. It may become noisy and, eventually, stop altogether.
• The face turns blue and is visibly congested with blood. The nail beds may become blue.
• The casualty gradually loses consciousness and may have fits.

ASPHYXIATION/ACTION

1

Check for danger to yourself and to the casualty. If there is a continuing threat —for example, from escaped gas— reduce it either by stopping it at the source or by dragging the victim clear. Check that the casualty is breathing.

2

If the victim has been strangled, cut or untie the cord or other material around his neck. If possible, keep the knot intact as possible evidence for the police.

3

Clear the casualty's airway by lying him on his back, turning his head to one side and removing blood, vomit or other debris from his mouth with your finger.

4

Check breathing and pulse. If necessary, give artificial respiration and chest compression. If you suspect the airway is blocked by food, treat for choking. Once breathing is normal, turn the victim on his stomach in the unconscious position. Get medical attention immediately, if you can do so without leaving the casualty unattended. Keep a careful watch on his breathing, and give artificial respiration again if it falters.

Asthmatic attack

Severe asthma, in which the victim suffers extreme difficulty in breathing, can be fatal if not quickly treated, although most attacks, while distressing, do not threaten life. During an asthmatic attack, the muscles around the air-tubes go into a spasm, impeding breathing. At the same time, the walls of the air-tubes swell, and the tubes are further blocked by thick, tenacious mucus.

Most asthmatic attacks take place at night, often when the sufferer is in bed. If this is the case, you should open the bedroom window to provide plenty of fresh air and prop the sufferer up in bed with a pillow.

Warning signs
- Noisy, wheezy breathing.
- Pale or bluish-grey complexion.
- Beads of sweat on the forehead.
- An anxious expression.
- In a prolonged attack, mental confusion because of lack of oxygen.
- The victim struggles for breath, and is often found sitting hunched up grasping chair arms, a table-top or similar object.

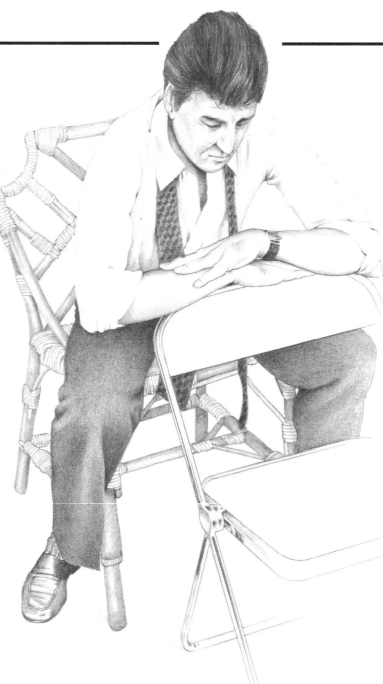

ASTHMATIC ATTACK/*ACTION*

1

If possible, sit the sufferer in an upright chair drawn close to a table or the back of another chair on which he can rest his forearms. His back should be fairly straight and his elbows spread out so that there is no pressure on the chest muscles. Open the windows, but keep the room warm. Moisten the air by pouring boiling water into a large pan, to make plenty of steam. Call the doctor for all but the briefest and mildest of attacks. Reassure the sufferer, telling him that expert help is on the way. If you have to take someone suffering from an asthmatic attack to hospital for treatment, it is better to transport him sitting up in the front passenger seat rather than lying down in the back.

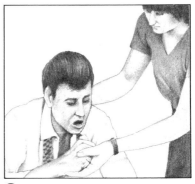

2

If the sufferer regularly gets asthma, he may have an inhalant spray for attacks. Help him use it. If he has an oxygen cylinder at home, give him oxygen only if you have been taught how to do so.

Back and neck injuries

Mishandling a casualty with broken bones in the back (spine) or neck may cause permanent paralysis and even death.

All too often the untrained layman treats a casualty for more obvious injuries—and overlooks a back or neck injury.

A casualty with a suspected broken back or neck should only be moved if he is in immediate danger —say from a burning building. Otherwise, any moving should be left to ambulancemen who have the right equipment.

Before you even touch an injured person look for possible clues. For instance, if he is lying at the foot of a ladder or a flight of stairs it is possible that he has sustained a neck or back injury.

Warning signs
• Loss of feeling and movement below the injured area, or a sensation of having been cut in half.
• Pain at the site of injury.
• A tingling sensation or pins and needles in the hands and feet (denotes neck injury).
• Inability to move fingers, wrists, toes or ankles when asked to do so, with no symptoms of a broken arm or leg.
• Inability to feel pain when the skin is gently nipped.
• Difficulty in breathing.

BACK AND NECK INJURIES/*ACTION*

1

Tell the casualty to lie still. Do not move him unless you have had proper first-aid training and have the necessary equipment, or can improvise it.

2

Cover him with a blanket and comfort him as much as possible. Do not raise his head or try to rest it on anything. Get trained medical help at once if you can.

3

If the casualty is unconscious keep him face upwards. Clear his mouth of any obstructions to breathing with your fingers.

4

Watch his breathing carefully. If it stops, begin mouth-to-nose or mouth-to-mouth artificial respiration immediately —even though tilting the head up risks further damage to the spine. Be as careful and gentle as you can.

Bandages/1

In first aid, bandages are used to keep a dressing in place, preventing germs or dirt entering the wound; maintain pressure over a dressing on a wound to control and absorb bleeding; support an injured part of the body, or immobilise it.

See SPLINTS *pages 605-7.*

Ready-made bandages are usually of calico or gauze. In an emergency, they can be improvised from sheets, pillowcases, stockings, scarves or any other suitable material; or a dressing can be secured with sticky plaster.

The two most widely used types are the triangular bandage—with three sides about 3 ft (90 cm.) long—and the roller bandage, which varies in width from 1 to 6 in. (25 to 150 mm.). Many first-aid kits contain combined bandage-dressings, which consist of a sterile pad attached to a roller bandage.

TRIANGULAR BANDAGES

The triangular bandage is among the most versatile pieces of first-aid equipment. Unfolded, it can quickly be turned into a sling, or a bandage for the scalp, shoulder, elbow, hand, chest, back or foot. It can be converted into a broad bandage— suitable, for example, for strapping one leg to the other to immobilise it.

When not in use, triangular bandages should be packed by folding them narrow, with the ends turned over towards the middle.

RAISED PAD

A raised pad dressing can be made from curved pads to hold the bandage away from a wound which has a foreign object buried in it.

ROLLER BANDAGE

Traditional roller bandages are made from non-stretch, open-weave gauze and are difficult to apply. Crêpe, elasticated, adhesive or conforming strip bandages are easier to put on, and, because they follow the contours of the body, the pressure they exert on the wound is more evenly distributed.

For fingers or toes, a 1 in. (25 mm.) bandage is wide enough; a 2 in. (50 mm.) bandage should be used for hands and a 2½ in. (65 mm.) bandage for arms. A 3 or 3½ in. (75 or 90 mm.) bandage is suitable for the leg; and body injuries require a width of 4 or 6 in. (100 or 150 mm.).

TUBULAR GAUZE BANDAGES

Seamless tubular gauze bandages are easier to apply than conventional bandages, as they do not need to be tied. They resemble stockings without feet, and are available from chemists in various sizes to fit different parts of the body. All these bandages are supplied with special applicators to slip them on.

Elastic netting bandages are similar, but of much wider mesh.

Other types of bandage include field dressings, the pad of these dressings is sterile, so do not touch or breathe on the inside of it, and do not allow the casualty to do so. Pull the dressing open by holding both ends of the bandage, apply it to the wound and fix it in place by holding the short end of the bandage and winding the long end around the limb or trunk. Tie the ends together with a reef bow or knot.

Bandages/2

IMPROVISING A TRIANGULAR BANDAGE/*ACTION*

1

Lay out the bandage on a clean, flat surface, ready for use.

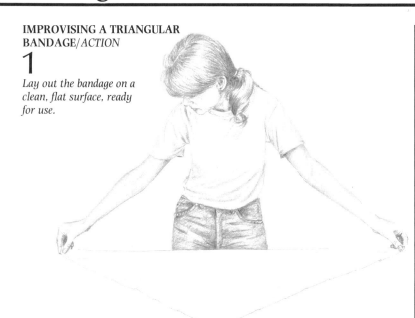

2

To make a broad bandage for emergencies, fold the top point of the triangle to the middle of the base and then fold it once more in the same direction.

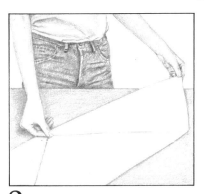

3

To turn a broad bandage into a narrow one, fold it a third time in the same direction. It is then the equivalent of a roller bandage and can be used to bind hands, arms and legs.

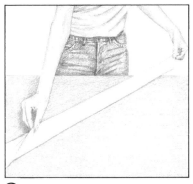

RAISED PADS/*ACTION*

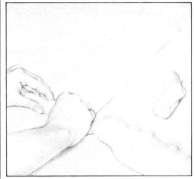

1

Put a clean cloth over the wound. Make at least two curved pads by rolling cotton wool or other material in clean cloth, if possible making the pads higher than the foreign body in the wound.

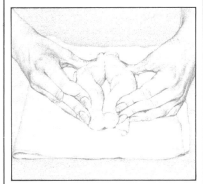

2

Place the pads around the foreign body, and bandage them on with diagonal strips of material. If the foreign body is higher than the pads, do not cross the bandage over it.

USING A ROLLER BANDAGE/*ACTION*

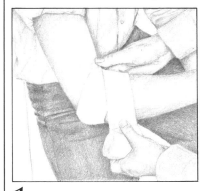

1

Support the injured part. Bandage a limb in the position in which it is to remain. Hold the bandage with the head uppermost and apply the outer surface to the body.

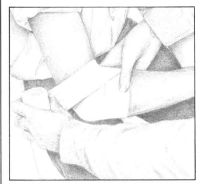

2

Bandage outwards from the body, maintaining even pressure. Start two or three turns below the wound, and finish two or three turns above it. Cut the end, tuck it in and pin.

TYING A BANDAGE/*ACTION*

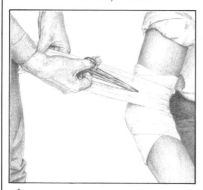

1

If you do not have a safety-pin or adhesive tape, leave an extra 9-12 in. (230-305 mm.) of bandage free. Cut this in half lengthways to tie above the wound.

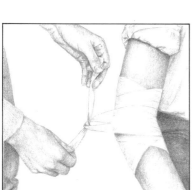

2

Tie the two cut ends together with a single loop knot, pulled fairly tight at the bottom of the cut. This prevents the bandage fraying or tearing—and helps control the bleeding.

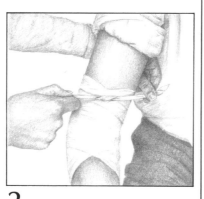

3

Take both ends round to the side of the limb opposite the knot, and secure them in a reef knot. Bring the left-hand end over the right-hand end and loop it underneath.

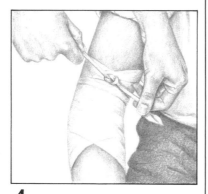

4

Loop the same end, which is now on the right, under the left-hand end, and pull both ends tight. Make sure that the knot does not press on the wound, causing discomfort to the victim.

USING TUBULAR GAUZE/*ACTION*

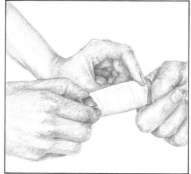

1

Cut a length of tubular gauze bandage more than twice as long as the injured finger. Place the applicator tongs over the finger and slip the whole of the bandage over the finger and tongs.

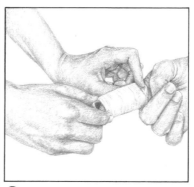

2

Hold one end of the bandage in place at the base of the injured finger with the finger and thumb of one hand. With the other hand retract the applicator, along with the other end of the bandage.

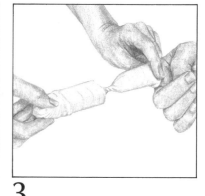

3

Once you have pulled the applicator tongs clear of the finger, turn them so that the length of bandage between the tip of the finger and the end of the tongs is slightly twisted.

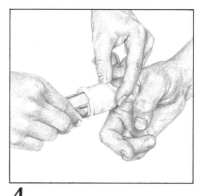

4

Replace the applicator tongs over the finger. Roll the bandage off the tongs and down to the base of the finger. As a result, the finger will now be covered by two layers of bandage.

Bites and stings

There are two types of bites—those from non-poisonous creatures, such as dogs, cats, ticks and people, and those from venomous creatures, chiefly snakes and insects.

Stings can be caused by insects, some fish, jellyfish and plants. The result in each case is localised pain, reddening and swelling, or in severe instances a general reaction including nausea, vomiting and a rash over the body. In the case of nettle stings, the pain is eased by rubbing dock leaves on the affected area.

ANIMAL BITES
Although the bites themselves are not poisonous, the wounds may become infected if not treated.

TICK BITES
Most tick bites occur when the adult ticks are most active, between May and September. Farm-workers and people who work and play in tick-infested areas are susceptible.

SNAKE BITES
The bites of some snakes can be serious and need immediate emergency action. But provided prompt treatment is given, such bites are rarely fatal in Great Britain.

INSECT STINGS
If the casualty suffers a strong reaction from a bee or a wasp sting, or if the sting appears to have become infected, get medical attention. In rare cases, where the casualty is allergic to such stings, they can be fatal unless immediate specialist treatment is given.

ANIMAL BITES/*ACTION*

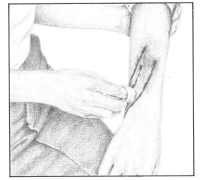

1

Wash the area thoroughly with soap and warm water, or a mild antiseptic. Dry gently, wiping down and away from the wound. Cover it with a clean dressing.

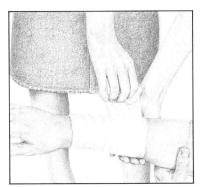

2

Fix the dressing with a sterile bandage or plaster. If the skin is broken, take the casualty to hospital. He may need injections against tetanus, or a course of antibiotics.

TICK BITES/*ACTION*

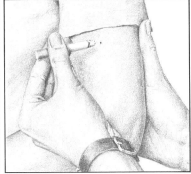

1

If the tick is attached to the skin, apply the glowing end of a cigarette to its body; this will make it fall off. Do not try to pull it off.

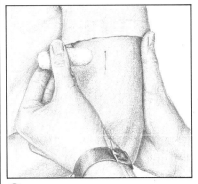

2

Swab the area thoroughly with soap and warm water and rinse well. Dry gently, wiping down and away. Gently rub in antihistamine cream—if available —to reduce any pain and swelling.

SNAKE BITES/*ACTION*

1

Rest the casualty in a comfortable position and reassure her. Do not let her move about if agitated.

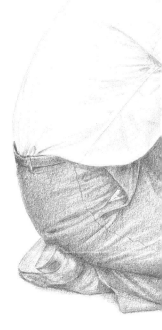

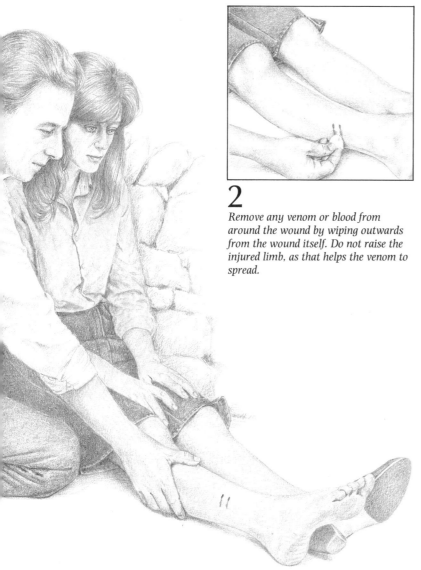

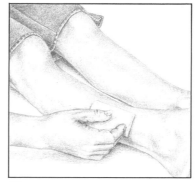

2

Remove any venom or blood from around the wound by wiping outwards from the wound itself. Do not raise the injured limb, as that helps the venom to spread.

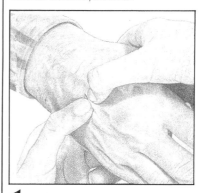

3

Apply a pad or sterile dressing to the wound. Never cut the side of the bite, or try to cauterise it. These 'remedies' simply make the condition worse. Immobilise the limb.

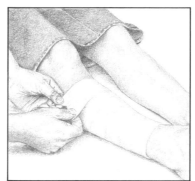

1

Scrape out a bee sting and poison bag with a fingernail, or any blunt edge. Take care not to squeeze the poison bag, as this will just pump more poison into the skin.

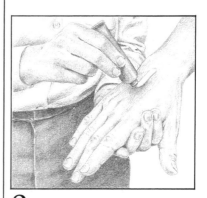

4

Bandage the wound firmly—if possible, with a crêpe or two-way stretch bandage. Call the emergency services, if you can do so without leaving the casualty.

2

For wasp, ant and bee stings, apply antihistamine cream or a dab of a solution of bicarbonate of soda. A cold compress will reduce swelling and pain.

Black eye

Bruising of the eye socket and lids produces internal bleeding which colours the skin dark blue or black and causes swelling. Do not apply a piece of raw steak to a black eye as it is ineffective.

BLACK EYE/*ACTION*

1

In the early stages, put an ice-pack or cold compress over the injured eye to try to prevent swelling.

2

If the lids are already swollen and closed, ice or a cold compress will relieve pain.

3

Take the casualty to a doctor as soon as possible to check that there is no serious damage to the eye or a fracture of the skull. A blow violent enough to blacken the eye may cause either.

Bleeding/1

Although external bleeding can be alarming and dramatic, most cases are not fatal provided the injury is treated promptly. Internal bleeding is always serious, and the casualty may die unless his condition is quickly recognised and he receives immediate hospital treatment.

EXTERNAL BLEEDING
Usually the bleeding is clearly visible. But after an accident, particularly in darkness, the casualty's position may conceal a serious wound.

Look for the other warning signs and feel all over and under the body for patches of sticky dampness. Assume they are blood until you are sure they are not.
Warning signs
• Escaping blood.
• Pale skin which is clammy and cold to touch.
• Profuse sweating.
• Fast but weak pulse.
• Anxiety and faintness or restlessness.

VARICOSE VEINS, BURST
A form of external bleeding. The abnormally swollen veins are usually found on the legs.

PRESSURE POINTS
When an artery can be pressed against an underlying bone to prevent blood flowing beyond that point, the site is known as a pressure point. If severe bleeding cannot be stopped by direct pressure on the wound, or if direct pressure cannot be successfully applied, it may be possible to control the bleeding by indirect pressure on the appropriate

pressure point.
Use a pressure point *only* to reduce severe blood loss while a dressing is being prepared for the wound. *Never* keep the pressure up for more than 10 minutes, otherwise the tissues may be permanently damaged and the limb may have to be amputated.

CONCEALED INTERNAL BLEEDING
Concealed internal bleeding may be the result of a fracture, and can show itself in a swelling containing several pints of blood. But sometimes when an internal organ is damaged there are no outward signs other than bruising.

VISIBLE INTERNAL BLEEDING
Visible internal bleeding—which shows itself later—is associated with injuries to the chest or digestive system.
Warning signs
• Coughing or vomiting frothy, bright red blood or brown blood.
• Swelling.
• Pale skin which is cold and clammy to the touch.
• Profuse sweating.
• Coldness and blue appearance of the tips of the hands and feet.
• Fast but weak pulse.
• Anxiety and faintness or restlessness.

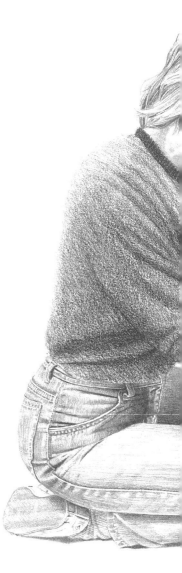

EXTERNAL BLEEDING/*ACTION*

1

Lay the casualty down. Remove clothing from around the wound if you can, without wasting time or distressing the casualty. Press down hard on the wound with any absorbent material or your bare hands, unless there is a foreign object in the wound.

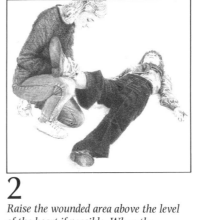

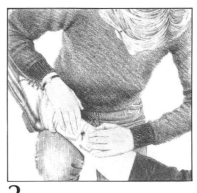

2

Raise the wounded area above the level of the heart if possible. When the bleeding stops, put on a sterile gauze or absorbent dressing. Calm and reassure the casualty.

3

If the blood seeps through the dressing, do not remove it, but put another on top. Keep the casualty's leg as steady as possible on your knee. Make sure the blood has stopped leaking.

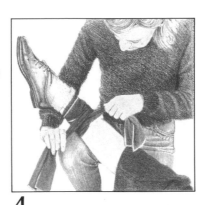

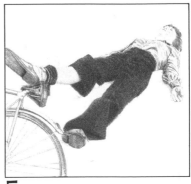

4

Tie the dressing in place with a bandage, scarf or other suitable material. Keep the casualty as still as possible. Do not give anything to eat or drink, even if it is asked for.

5

Get medical attention quickly, if you can do so without leaving the casualty for more than a moment. Regularly check the pulse and breathing and make sure the casualty is comfortable.

Bleeding/2

There are two main pressure points. One is on the inner side of the region where the brachial artery can be pressed against the bone. The other is high inside the thigh, where the femoral artery can be pressed against the pelvis.

PRESSURE POINTS

The only time to use pressure points is if bleeding cannot be controlled, or when the wound dressing is being prepared. It is vital that the pressure is applied for *no more than 10 minutes*. If it is kept up for any longer the limb tissues may be damaged beyond repair, and amputation may be necessary.

FEMORAL PRESSURE POINT/*ACTION*

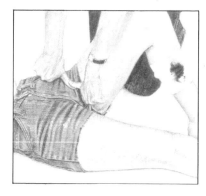

Lay the casualty down and bend the injured leg at the knee. Grasp the thigh with both hands. Press firmly downwards in the centre of the fold of the groin with both thumbs, one on top of the other, against the rim of the pelvis.

BRACHIAL PRESSURE POINT/*ACTION*

To find the pressure point, hold the casualty's arm out at right-angles to her body, palm upwards. The brachial artery runs along the inner side of the muscles of the upper arm. To control bleeding from the lower arm, wrist or hand, raise the injured limb so that it is roughly level with the casualty's shoulder. Place one hand under her upper arm and press your fingers firmly against the bone.

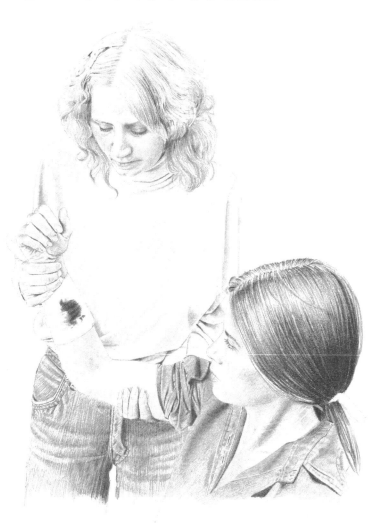

VARICOSE VEINS, BURST/*ACTION*

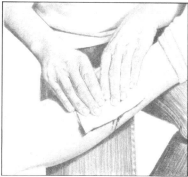

1

Press with a clean gauze pad on the area from which the blood is coming. Lay the victim down and raise the affected leg on to your thigh, maintaining the pressure on the wound.

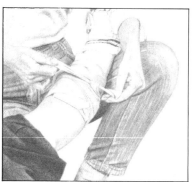

2

Keeping the leg raised, put on a gauze dressing and tie it in place with a bandage. Tell the victim to rest, and prop the leg up with pillows or on a chair seat. Get medical attention.

Blisters

Never prick a blister unless the taut skin is causing acute discomfort, as that will expose the tissue underneath to infection. Cover a blister with a clean dressing. *See* BURNS AND SCALDS *pages 568 -9.*

BLISTERS/*ACTION*

1

Remove shoes and socks. Gently wipe the blister with cotton wool soaked in methylated spirit, or wash it with soap and water or an antiseptic wipe.

2

Pass a sewing needle once or twice through a flame. Let it cool for a second or two but do not wipe off any soot, or touch the point.

3

Hold the needle flat on the skin, and press the point gently but firmly into the blister, just enough to burst it. Remove the needle and make a second puncture in the blister, opposite the first.

4

Remove the needle and press gently on the blister with a clean swab. Wipe and apply an adhesive dressing.

Bruises

The discoloration and swelling associated with bruising are the result of blood seeping into the tissues through damaged vessels. To begin with, the bruise is usually red or pink, turning bluish and then greenish-yellow.

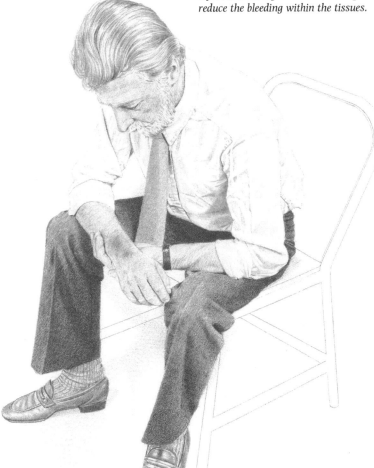

BRUISES/*ACTION*

1

Check that there are no other injuries. Look particularly for a fracture accompanying the bruise. Get the casualty into a comfortable position and make him support the injured part before and during treatment, to help to reduce the bleeding within the tissues.

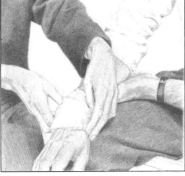

2

Apply an ice-pack or a cold compress to help reduce the swelling. If necessary, fix the compress in place with a stretch bandage, winding from below the injury to above it.

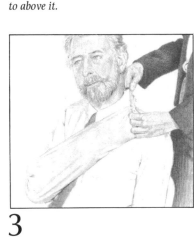

3

Support a bruised arm with a sling. If the leg is bruised, lie the casualty down and prop his leg up on a pillow. For bruises on the trunk, lie him down with pillows below his head and shoulders.

Burns and scalds

Dry heat, from fire or other sources, friction, electricity and chemicals can cause burns. Scalds are caused by moist heat, from boiling liquids or steam. The first-aid treatment is the same.

All but minor burns and scalds are potentially serious. Remove watches, rings and tight clothing. Hold the burnt area under cold running water for at least 10 minutes. Cover with a clean, non-fluffy dressing; never apply ointments or fats. If in any doubt as to the seriousness of a casualty's wound, take him straight to hospital.

Burns can be placed in two categories:

SUPERFICIAL BURNS AND SCALDS
Only the outer layers of skin are damaged.
Warning signs
• The skin is red and may look scorched, blackened and blistered.
• The area is painful.

DEEP BURNS AND SCALDS
The entire thickness of skin is destroyed.
Warning signs
• The skin may be dark red, charred or blistered.
• The area is less painful as the nerve ends have been destroyed.

CLOTHING ON FIRE
When a casualty's clothing catches fire, immediately quench the flames to stop combustion. If there is no water or other non-flammable liquid available, use an item of thick, non-synthetic material—such as a coat, rug or blanket—to smother the flames.

BURNS
Remove the casualty from the source of heat. Often, that will be a reflex action as the casualty pulls himself away from the heat source. But old people, or sufferers from epilepsy, may need help.

If the cause of the burn is electrical, pull out the plug or switch off the power source, taking care not to electrocute yourself.

When the burn is caused by a dry chemical, brush away as much as you can with a duster or soft brush, taking care to protect your own hands. Remove any contaminated clothing. Check that the casualty is not lying on any of the chemical.

Check the casualty's breathing. If it has stopped, give artificial respiration and chest compression. If he is breathing but unconscious, treat as for any unconscious person. Never give anyone who is unconscious anything to drink. *See* UNCONSCIOUSNESS *pages 611-12.*

For burns—and scalds—in the mouth or throat, give the casualty sips of cold water or ice-cubes to suck, to reduce swelling.

Get medical attention for all but minor burns and scalds.

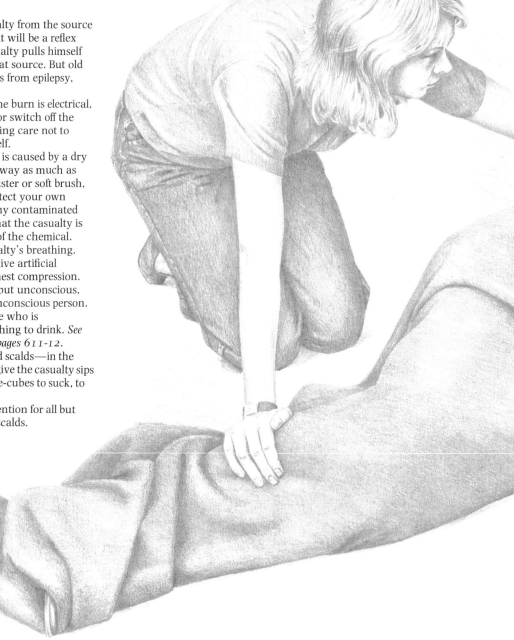

BURNS/*ACTION*

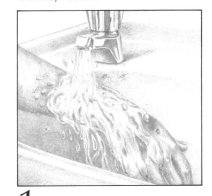

1

With superficial and minor burns, cool the burned area by flooding it with cold water for at least ten minutes. Never apply water if the casualty is in contact with a source of electricity.

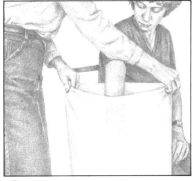

2

Prevent infection by covering the burned area with a clean dressing—freshly laundered handkerchiefs or pillowcases. Put a soft towel over the dressing to reduce the risk of further damage.

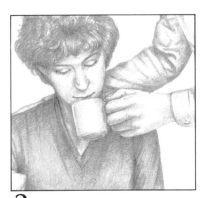

3

Reassure the casualty. If her mouth and throat are burned or scalded, give sips of cold water or ice cubes to suck in order to reduce swelling. Ensure the airway is not obstructed.

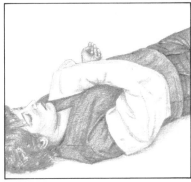

4

If the burning is extensive, lie the casualty down and treat for shock. Raise the legs above the level of the trunk. If the head, chest or abdomen is burned, put a blanket under shoulders.

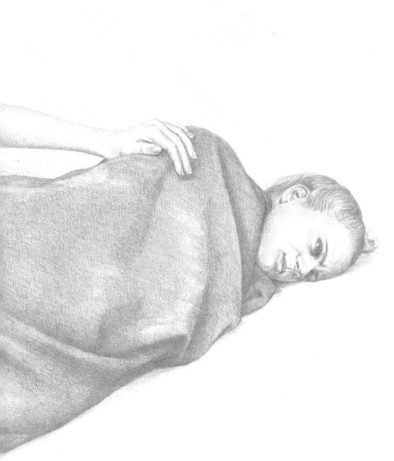

CLOTHING ON FIRE/*ACTION*

When approaching the casualty, fold a blanket, rug or coat in front of you for protection. Then wrap the material around the casualty and lie her on the floor, burned side uppermost, to smother the flames. If you use water, do not throw it, since the impact spreads the flames and creates scalding steam. More skin will be burned if the victim is allowed to run or walk about. Remove any hot clothing that can be taken off easily. Leave any fragments of clothing which have become seared to the skin. They form a sterile cover.

Chest injuries

Car accidents are the most common cause of chest injuries. Drivers and passengers not wearing their seat-belts are particularly prone to such injuries. The other main causes are stab wounds and crushing. *See* CRUSH INJURIES *page 575.*

'SUCKING' WOUNDS
If the chest wall has been penetrated by a sharp instrument or if a fractured rib protrudes through the outer wall, the wound is known as a 'sucking' wound. As the casualty breathes, air is sucked into his chest causing an injured lung to collapse. Blood will bubble from the wound.

CLOSED WOUNDS
If a rib has been fractured and enters a lung without penetrating the chest wall, the wound is known as 'closed'. The casualty will cough up bright red, frothy blood.

In both types of wound a triangular sling is applied to the casualty's arm on his injured side. This will give added support to any fractured ribs—especially if there is likely to be a bumpy journey to hospital. *See* SLINGS *pages 601-3.*

Warning signs
• Bruising or bleeding from the chest.
• Pain and tenderness, which often becomes worse if the casualty coughs or breathes deeply.
• Shallow breathing, indicating a fractured rib.
• A tight feeling in the chest, which may be accompanied by a distinctly heard crackling movement of the tissues below the skin.

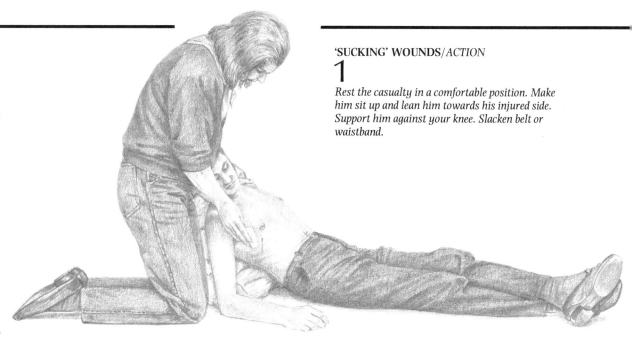

'SUCKING' WOUNDS/*ACTION*

1
Rest the casualty in a comfortable position. Make him sit up and lean him towards his injured side. Support him against your knee. Slacken belt or waistband.

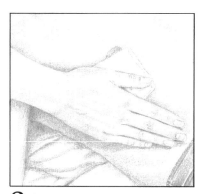

2
Staunch bleeding, first with your hand over the wound—start when casualty breathes out—and then with a bandage or dressing. Do not press down on the wound if you suspect fractured ribs.

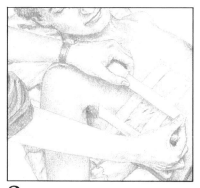

3
If air is entering or leaving the lung through a puncture wound, seal it rapidly, first with your hand and then with a dressing secured with adhesive plaster. Make sure it is air-proof.

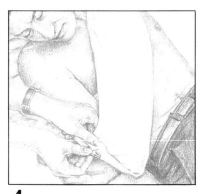

4
Place the arm on the injured side diagonally across the victim's chest. Support it with a triangular sling. Make sure he is still comfortable, then get medical help at once.

'CLOSED' WOUNDS/*ACTION*

1

Rest the casualty in a comfortable position. Make him sit up and lean him towards his injured side. Move the arm on the injured side diagonally across the casualty's chest, so that his hand rests on his opposite shoulder. The arm is now ready for a triangular sling—which is placed higher than an arm sling.

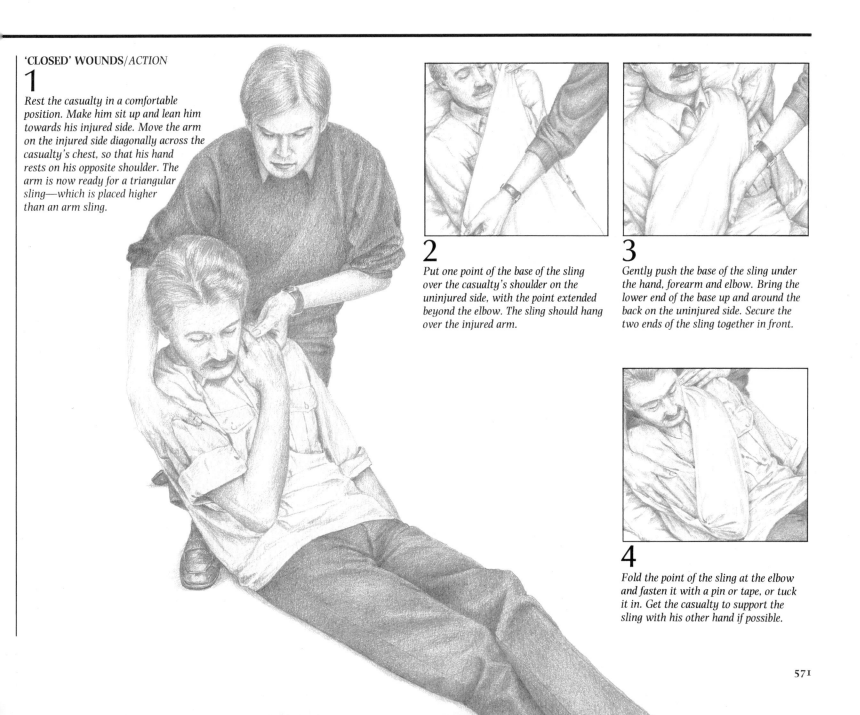

2

Put one point of the base of the sling over the casualty's shoulder on the uninjured side, with the point extended beyond the elbow. The sling should hang over the injured arm.

3

Gently push the base of the sling under the hand, forearm and elbow. Bring the lower end of the base up and around the back on the uninjured side. Secure the two ends of the sling together in front.

4

Fold the point of the sling at the elbow and fasten it with a pin or tape, or tuck it in. Get the casualty to support the sling with his other hand if possible.

Choking/1

A piece of food or some other substance stuck in the airway will cause choking. In severe cases the victim cannot breathe at all, and, if left untreated, will die.

It is vital to act promptly as—with a complete obstruction of the airway —asphyxiation quickly occurs.

Suspect choking if a casualty who is unconscious and not breathing is found anywhere near an eating area. However, a victim could have choked on sweets, chewing-gum or peanuts *away* from an eating area. Children can choke on toys which they put in their mouths, and adults can choke on dislodged false teeth.

Peanuts should not be given to young children—they are a common cause of choking in infants. When choking occurs, the child may have a fit of coughing and his face and neck will become congested.

He will make violent efforts to breathe. But the harder he tries to breathe in, the more firmly fixed the obstruction becomes.

Instant action is vital.

SLAPS ON THE BACK

Try to remove any obvious obstruction—for example, a piece of food—thought to be in the windpipe by giving the victim several hard slaps on the back between the shoulders, with his head lower than his chest. The slaps should dislodge the obstruction.

ABDOMINAL THRUST

A more recent method of removing an obstruction in the windpipe is the abdominal thrust, in America called the Heimlich Manoeuvre.

If an obstruction is hard to move, and slaps on the back do not work, then the abdominal thrust should be used. The abdominal thrust, with its lower and more sustained pressure, may help dislodge the obstruction altogether.

Children

The abdominal thrust can be successfully given to children (but not babies). Less pressure is used on them than on adults. Artificial respiration should also be given if necessary.

Adults—conscious

If an adult is conscious and choking, the abdominal thrust should be applied when he is either standing or seated.

Adult—unconscious

If an adult is unconscious and choking, the abdominal thrust should be applied with him lying on his back.

Treating yourself

Someone who is choking can apply the abdominal thrust to himself— either with his hands or by applying pressure against the edge of a firm table or the back of a heavy chair.

SLAPS ON THE BACK/*ACTION*

1

Giving up to five sharp, flat blows between the shoulder blades may clear the obstruction from the airway of someone who is choking. Use the palm of your hand. An adult can be treated standing, sitting or lying on his stomach or side. If the casualty is a baby, use much less force. Hold him upside down while giving the slaps.

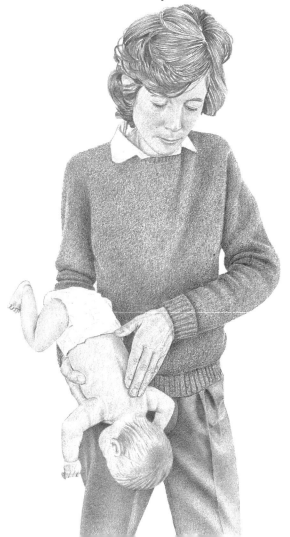

SLAPS ON THE BACK/*ACTION*

2

Encourage a child to cough up the obstruction. If this fails, lay the child face down across your thighs, with his head lower than his chest. Support his chest with one hand while you slap him hard between the shoulder blades with the heel of your other hand. The slaps should dislodge the obstruction. If they do not, sit the child on your knee and—if you have been trained to do so on a child—apply abdominal thrust. Use only one hand, and less force than for an adult.

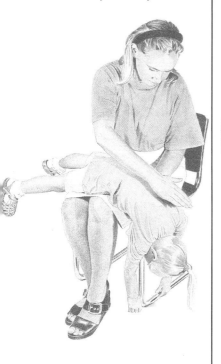

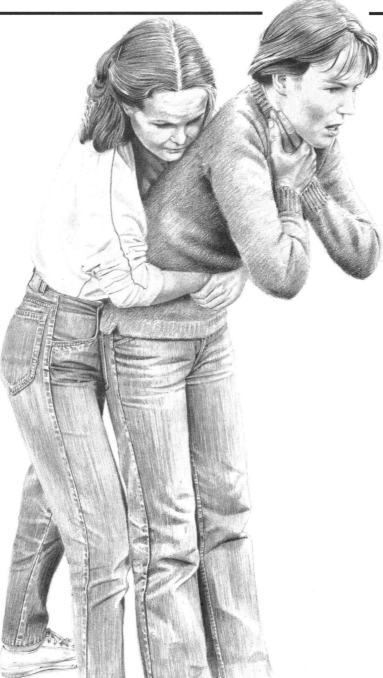

ABDOMINAL THRUST—conscious adult

1

Stand behind the casualty. Put your arms around her waist, making a fist with one hand. Place the thumb side slightly above the casualty's navel and well below her rib-cage. Hold the fist with your other hand and give up to five quick, strong pulls diagonally upwards and towards you. Use your hands to create the pressure; do not just squeeze with your arms.

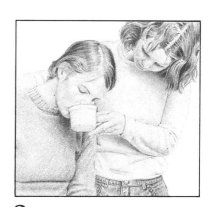

2

Reassure the casualty. Rest her in a comfortable position and give her frequent sips of water. Adults should sip half a cup of water over ten minutes to help them recover.

573

Choking/2

Concussion

ABDOMINAL THRUST—unconscious adult/*ACTION*

1

Turn the victim face up, kneel astride her hips and put your hand just above her navel. Push on it with your other hand, thrusting at an angle downwards and towards the casualty's head up to five times.

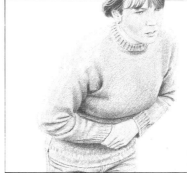

ABDOMINAL THRUST–self-help

1

Clench a fist and place it, thumb side against the abdomen, slightly above the navel. With the other hand, jerk it firmly inwards and upwards several times.

Alternative method

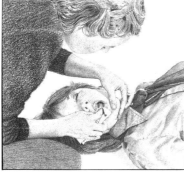

2

With your finger, clear the casualty's mouth of any expelled object, taking care not to push it back down the throat. If necessary, give artificial respiration.

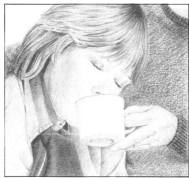

3

Once the casualty's breathing is normal, turn her into the unconscious position and get medical aid. Give her something to drink when she is fully conscious but not before.

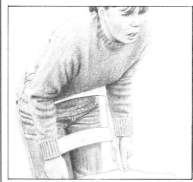

2

Use the back of a chair or table edge. Lean over the edge supported by your hands on either side. Thrust inwards and upwards just above the navel three or four times.

A blow to the head, or a heavy fall on to the feet, can shake and disturb the brain, causing concussion. The casualty's breathing becomes shallow and he may lapse into unconsciousness, or suffer shock, with loss of memory. On recovery, he may suffer from nausea and vomiting.

Any pressure on the brain—either from blood or fluid or from a fracture of the skull—can result in compression, when the casualty's alertness and level of consciousness fall. Compression can cause twitching of the limbs or even convulsions. The casualty's breathing may become noisy. His face may become flushed and his pulse may become slow. The pupils of his eyes may be unequal in size, dilated or they may not react to light. Usually, most of these symptoms occur, but the absence of any of them does not mean compression is not present.

Compression may develop immediately after an injury, or more slowly after the casualty has apparently recovered from concussion. In either case, *urgent* medical attention is needed.
See HEAD AND FACIAL INJURIES *pages 591-3.*

Cramp

A sudden, involuntary contraction of a muscle or muscles is known as cramp. It may be the result of poor muscular co-ordination, over-exertion or chilling—for example, while swimming. If cramp occurs when the casualty is in water, get him out quickly and cover him with a coat, towel or blanket.

CALF OR FOOT CRAMP
The sufferer can treat himself by straightening his leg, standing up and bearing down on his heel and toes so that the affected muscle is stretched.

THIGH CRAMP
Sit the casualty down, straighten his knee so it is as rigid as possible and lift his heel with one hand. Press down on the knee with the other hand.

HAND CRAMP
Straighten the fingers, gently using force. Get the casualty to spread his fingers and press down on the outstretched tips.

If cramp persists—with heavy sweating, vomiting or diarrhoea—get the casualty to drink plenty of slightly salted water, half a teaspoon of salt in each pint.

CRAMP/*ACTION*

To treat calf or foot cramp lie the casualty down, straighten her knee and toes and lever her foot firmly up towards her shin. Alternatively, straighten the toes and get the casualty to stand with her leg straight, pushing down on her heel and toes to stretch the affected muscle.

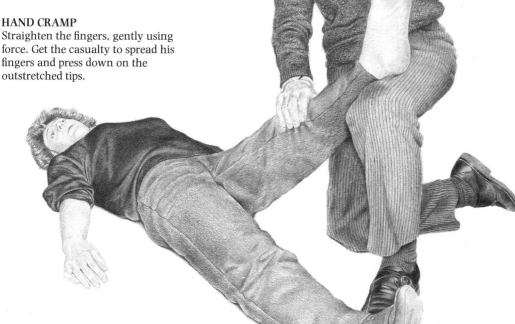

Crush injuries

Someone who has been trapped for more than a few minutes under a heavy weight—for example, fallen rocks or masonry—may suffer severe damage to the muscles or skin tissue.

At first, he may appear simply to have swelling or bruising. But the body tissues may continue to swell and harden, producing shock, a drop in blood pressure, and if medical treatment is not given, kidney failure and death.

Warning signs
• Redness, swelling, bruising or blistering of the trapped part.
• Numbness or tingling.
• Continued swelling and hardening of the injured tissue.

CRUSH INJURIES/*ACTION*

1
Try to establish how long the casualty has been trapped. If less than an hour, try to release him. If more, do not release him. And if the injuries look severe, treat them as best you can before considering releasing him.

2
Once he is released, keep the casualty on his back with his head low and his lower limbs raised if possible. Do not let him move. If he is unconscious, place in unconscious position.

3
Get medical attention as quickly as possible. Make sure that the doctor or ambulance attendant is told that there may be crush injuries. .

Cuts

Minor cuts and grazes do not need medical attention unless infection has set in or the wound was caused by a dirty or rusty object.

In general, the amount of blood lost and the extent of the injury show whether it is serious. But puncture or stab wounds are deceptive, because the surface damage may appear small. Get medical help after giving first aid.

When treating a minor cut make sure to clean the skin around it, using gauze or cotton swabs and lukewarm water with soap or a mild antiseptic. Wipe outwards and away from the injury and make sure the water you are using does not run into it. As each swab becomes soiled, change to a fresh one.

If the bleeding is severe, see BLEEDING *page 564.*

Cuts and grazes usually heal well if kept clean and dry.

CUTS/*ACTION*

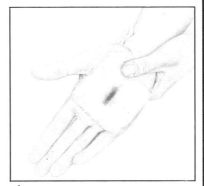

1

Take a clean piece of cloth and press it on the cut, or around the edges if a foreign body is in it. When bleeding stops, take the pad away and remove any foreign bodies that come out easily.

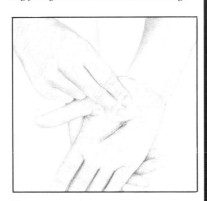

2

Gently wipe the wound outwards with a swab soaked in warm, soapy water. Use a fresh swab for each wipe. Gently dry around the wound with a clean swab and apply a plaster or bandage.

Diabetic coma

Someone suffering from diabetes who takes insulin to maintain his blood sugar at the normal level may become unwell, either because there is too much insulin in his body or because there is too little.

Warning signs
Excessive insulin
• Pale appearance, with sweating, rapid pulse, shallow breathing and possible trembling.
• Confused state, sometimes resembling drunkenness.
• Faintness, leading rapidly to unconsciousness.
• The breath is odourless.
Insufficient insulin
• Dry skin and flushed appearance.
• Deep, sighing breathing. The breath smells of nail varnish.
• Eventually, unconsciousness.

DIABETIC COMA/*ACTION*

1

If the victim is already unconscious, arrange him in the unconscious position and get immediate medical attention.

2

When the victim is conscious, he can tell you what kind of diabetic he is. In either case, give him sugar lumps, a non-alcoholic drink sweetened with two teaspoons of sugar or honey or jam. If he improves dramatically it is a sign of too much insulin, in which case give him more sugar in case he should lapse into unconsciousness.

Dislocation

A bone that is wrenched out of place at a joint is said to be dislocated. The injury is usually accompanied by torn ligaments—a sprain—and sometimes by a fracture.

The symptoms may include severe pain, swelling and bruising, and difficulty in moving the joint. Never try to push a dislocated bone back into place, but treat it as though it were broken.

In a case of dislocation, always assume there is a suspected fracture, as the symptoms are similar. *See* FRACTURES *page 588.*

Drowning/1

Death by drowning occurs because as the victim struggles for breath, water enters the airway and causes spasm of the epiglottis—a cartilage flap at the back of the tongue, which blocks the air supply. Quick action can still save the victim's life.

Each year in Britain there are nearly 1,000 deaths from drowning. Two-thirds occur in fresh water—because it is impossible to provide the same rescue facilities on rivers, lakes and canals as are available on holiday beaches. Most of the victims are able to swim and most drown within 10 yds (9.1 m.) of land.

Assume that anyone you see in the water fully clothed is a potential victim and be ready to help. But a swimmer who develops cramp or becomes exhausted is less easy to recognise. If he is having breathing problems, he may be unable to draw attention by shouting, and if he raises an arm to wave, then he will sink.

Warning signs
- As he gets more tired, the victim's body tends to sink until it is vertical and only his head shows.
- The victim's strokes become erratic and his movement through the water appears jerky or simply stops.
- The victim's face—particularly his lips and ears—become congested and may turn bluish-purple.

REVIVING A DROWNING PERSON/*ACTION*

1

If the drowning person has stopped breathing, start mouth-to-mouth artificial respiration. A strong swimmer trained in life-saving can begin while treading water. The technique can be easier in the sea than in rivers or lakes because the salt gives added buoyancy, but the victim's head and upper chest must be held clear of the water.

Remove any debris from her mouth with your index finger, tilt her head back over the crook of one of your arms and then breathe into her mouth—pressing your cheek against her nose to stop air escaping from there. Watch for the chest to rise and then remove your mouth. Breathe into the victim's mouth again once the air has escaped. Move towards dry land between breaths. Once the victim is out of the water, continue artificial respiration. If you cannot detect a pulse, give chest compression, too.

In shallow water the rescuer can begin immediate treatment.

Do not become discouraged too soon by lack of response. Children, in particular, have been revived 40 minutes after breathing has ceased.

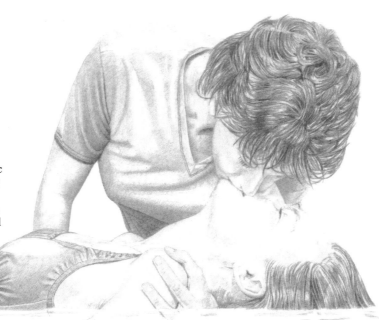

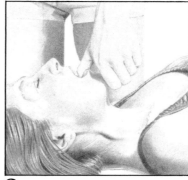

2

Victims of drowning often swallow large amounts of water, which is brought up during artificial respiration. Turn the victim's head to one side and clear her mouth frequently.

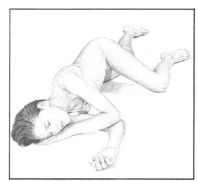

3

Once breathing has re-started, turn the victim into the recovery position. Cover her with blankets or towels and treat any injuries. Then get medical aid as soon as possible.

Drowning/2

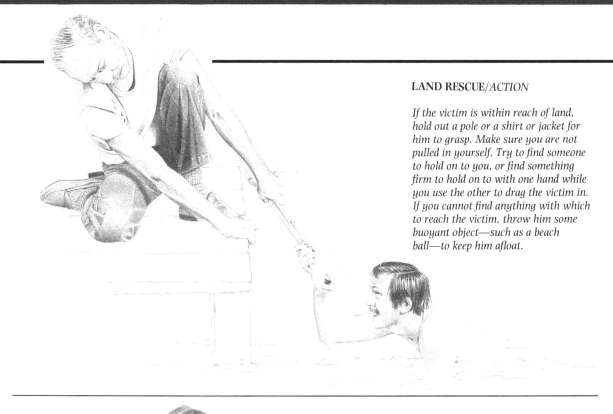

RESCUE TECHNIQUES

Swimming rescues should not be attempted by anyone who is not a strong and experienced swimmer. It is preferable that the rescuer has a working—or theoretical—knowledge of first aid. In an emergency, knowledge of first aid is as valuable as the ability to swim, as there are ways of rescuing a victim from water without swimming.

Land rescues can be the safest for a poor swimmer or for someone who does not swim at all.

Boat rescues should not be attempted if the sea is particularly rough, or if there is some other potential danger—such as a fast-running weir.

Ice rescues are perhaps the most difficult to perform. Always test the ice as much as possible, to make sure that it will bear your weight—and that of the victim. Any other people near by should be asked to assist, both to hold on to the rescuer and to send for help.

LAND RESCUE/*ACTION*

If the victim is within reach of land, hold out a pole or a shirt or jacket for him to grasp. Make sure you are not pulled in yourself. Try to find someone to hold on to you, or find something firm to hold on to with one hand while you use the other to drag the victim in. If you cannot find anything with which to reach the victim, throw him some buoyant object—such as a beach ball—to keep him afloat.

BOAT RESCUE/*ACTION*

If you go to the rescue in a small boat, reach for the victim over the bow or stern, rather than the side, to reduce the risk of capsizing. Lie down and wedge your feet under a fixed seat, or get someone to hold them. Put your head and shoulders over the bow or stern, grasp the victim's wrists with your hands and get him to grasp yours.

Ear injury

ICE RESCUE/ACTION

1

Tell the victim to stretch her arms forward and to kick back in the water to prevent being dragged under. Hold out a pole, branch, rope or scarf for her to grasp. Lie down to pull her in.

The most serious ear injury is a perforated ear-drum, which can result from a blow to the side of the head, blast from an explosion, a sudden change in the atmospheric pressure, or an inflammation of the middle ear.

If blood or cerebrospinal fluid (a straw coloured, watery fluid surrounding the brain and the spinal cord) is escaping from inside the ear it may be the sign of a fractured base of skull. Blood on its own, or pus, can also indicate that an ear-drum or ear canal is damaged. If the casualty is unconscious, place in the unconscious position with the injured ear down and a clean pad placed underneath it. *See* UNCONSCIOUSNESS *pages 611-12.*

Warning signs
- The escape of blood or cerebrospinal fluid.
- Violent earache.
- Dizziness and loss of balance.

EAR INJURY/ACTION

1

Stop the casualty from hitting himself on the side of the head to try to restore his hearing—as this may cause further damage to the inner ear.

2

Once the victim is on the ice, tell her to stay lying down, arms and legs spread to distribute her weight. Drag her in by the wrists to the safety of the bank or on to safe ice.

2

Put a small piece of cotton or gauze against the ear canal as protection, and bandage it lightly in place. Then get medical attention.

Electrical accidents

Electricity can kill or produce a wide range of injuries, including severe burns and asphyxiation. Most electrical accidents involve household appliances such as irons or electric fires, or contact with power sources such as supply cables or railway lines. Lightning—naturally generated electricity—has the same effect as high-voltage current.

The extent of the injuries depends upon three main factors: the strength of the current or electric charge; how long the victim was exposed to it; and how well he was insulated—for example, by wearing rubber-soled shoes and standing on a dry, bare wood surface.

Never approach the victim of an electrical accident until you are certain that you are not risking a shock—or worse—yourself. If the casualty is still in contact with the source of the electricity, cut off the power first.

In accidents involving a relatively low voltage—that is normally used in homes, or for heat and light in offices, shops and factories—turn off the supply at the nearest switch and, if the cause is a plug-in appliance such as an iron, pull out the plug as well.

High-voltage sources—power lines and some industrial equipment—can travel through the ground and give a fatal shock even at a distance of up to 20 yds (18 m.). Stay away until you can get an expert to cut the power; railway stations and many pylons and sub-stations display an emergency telephone number.

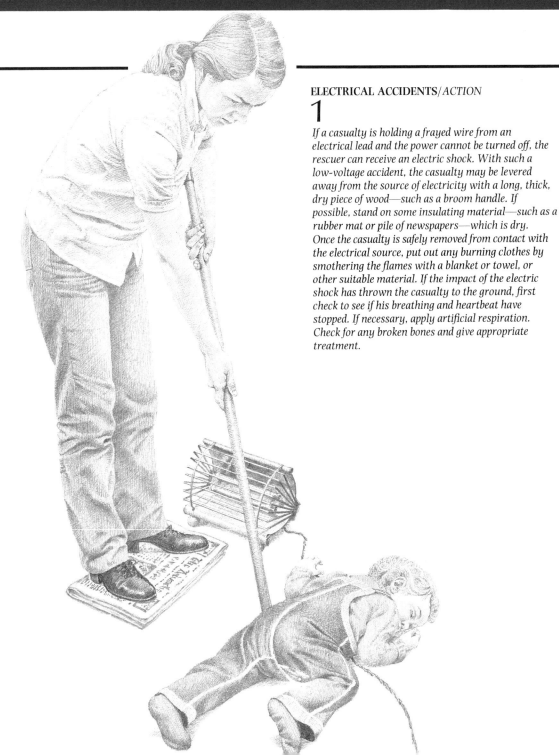

ELECTRICAL ACCIDENTS/*ACTION*

1

If a casualty is holding a frayed wire from an electrical lead and the power cannot be turned off, the rescuer can receive an electric shock. With such a low-voltage accident, the casualty may be levered away from the source of electricity with a long, thick, dry piece of wood—such as a broom handle. If possible, stand on some insulating material—such as a rubber mat or pile of newspapers—which is dry. Once the casualty is safely removed from contact with the electrical source, put out any burning clothes by smothering the flames with a blanket or towel, or other suitable material. If the impact of the electric shock has thrown the casualty to the ground, first check to see if his breathing and heartbeat have stopped. If necessary, apply artificial respiration. Check for any broken bones and give appropriate treatment.

Emergency childbirth/1

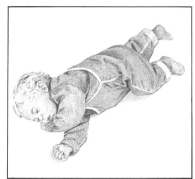

2
Once the casualty is breathing naturally, place him in the recovery position. Check his heartbeat by feeling his pulse. Look for any burns—they may be deeper than their size suggests.

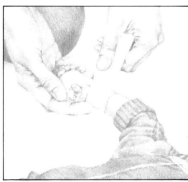

3
Treat any burns by cooling them with cold water and covering them against the air with dressings or suitable material such as linen. Call the ambulance service as soon as you can.

Most babies are born without difficulty. If you have to cope with an emergency delivery, a major part of your task is to keep calm and to reassure the mother and any others present.

In Great Britain, it is normally a legal offence for anyone other than a doctor or midwife to supervise childbirth, but in an emergency an unqualified person may have to take responsibility, and the law recognises that. Every effort should be made to contact a doctor or midwife.

Cleanliness is essential. Wash your hands and scrub your nails under running water before assisting and as often as necessary during the birth. Do not dry them. Keep people with open cuts or infections away from the mother and baby. Make sure that as far as possible all bedding, towels, cloths and swabs are clean.

Line the bottom of a cot with a folded blanket, shawl or towel. Fold another one ready to cover the baby when it is born. Do not use a pillow. If a cot is not available use a large basket, box or drawer.

Prepare a bed, or a clean surface such as a table, for the mother to lie on. Place a plastic sheet, or newspaper if you do not have any sheeting, over the surface and cover it with a clean towel or sheet. Collect pillows or cushions for the mother to lean on, and a blanket or warm garment in case she feels cold.

Have a large bowl (such as a washing-up bowl) ready for her to sit on to deliver the placenta, a small bowl to put it in, and another in case she vomits.

Keep the room comfortably warm. Fold a blanket into three from top to bottom and wrap it in a clean sheet. Use it to cover the mother's top during delivery. Collect three or four clean towels and pieces of cloth and sheeting, a sanitary towel for the mother and a nappy for the baby.

Labour lasts for some hours, there are three stages.

The first stage lasts several hours —up to 14 in a first pregnancy but less in subsequent births. The muscles of the body of the uterus begin to contract to open its neck for the baby's head to pass through.

The second stage, during which the baby is actually born, takes from 15 minutes to two hours. The contractions become stronger and the mother wants to bear down.

The third stage occurs after the baby is born and is vital to the health of the mother. The placenta, or afterbirth, to which the other end of the umbilical cord is attached, is expelled by further contractions.

Signs that labour is beginning
• Pains develop in the small of the back and move round to the lower abdomen as contractions begin. They usually occur about every 30 minutes, gradually becoming more frequent and painful.
• Watery fluid may run from the vagina (the 'breaking of the waters').
• Blood may seep from the vagina as labour begins.

How to help the mother during labour
• Encourage the mother to move about as much as she wants, to make herself comfortable.
• If the waters break, or as the contractions become more frequent, tell her to lie on a bed. Improvise one, if there is no bed available.
• Instruct her to relax and not to bear down.
• Encourage her to visit the lavatory whenever she wants to.
• If the pains are bad it may help if she breathes deeply, in and out, with each contraction and does not hold her breath.
• Give her occasional small drinks of milk, but nothing to eat.
• When the contractions become stronger the second stage of labour is beginning, and she will feel the need to bear down. Encourage her to lie in whatever position is more comfortable. With each contraction tell her to hold her breath and bear down, and relax between contractions.
• When the contractions are coming every two or three minutes, tell her to grasp her thighs behind her knees and pull up on her legs at the same time as she is pushing down.
• Do not touch the baby's head as it emerges. Tell the mother to stop bearing down, and to pant in quick breaths to prevent the baby being thrust out too forcefully.
• The majority of babies are born without problems. Very rarely, artificial respiration may be needed if the baby does not breathe immediately. In a very small number of cases the baby may appear with the umbilical cord round its neck, or bottom first (breech birth). Neither should cause difficulties; the main thing is not to panic.

Emergency childbirth/2

DELIVERING THE BABY/*ACTION*

1

Tell the mother to lie in whatever position is the most comfortable, with her knees bent. Support her shoulders with pillows and cushions. When the baby's head first appears, put a clean towel or cloth under the mother's buttocks and a clean towel or sheet on the bed between her legs.

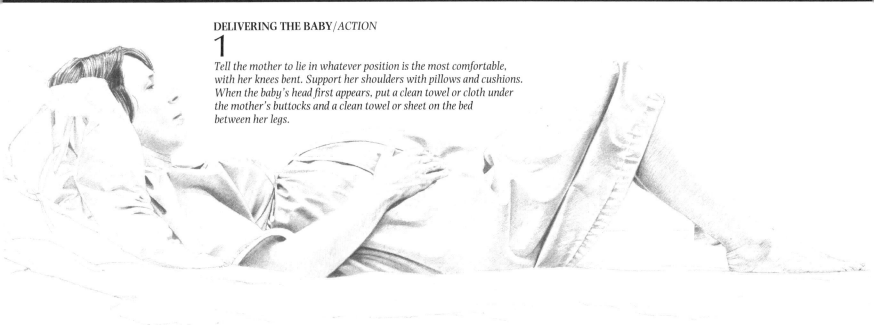

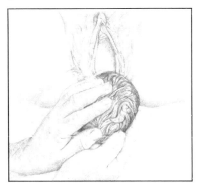

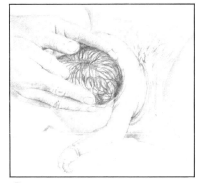

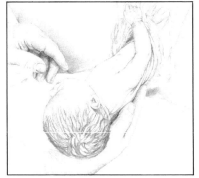

2

Control the baby's head with one hand on its way out. Do not let it just 'pop out'. If there is a caul, or membrane, over the baby's face remove it gently, but quickly.

3

As the shoulders emerge support them gently but do not pull. One shoulder appears first; the second will follow easily if you gently raise the baby's head.

4

The rest of the baby will be born without difficulty. Support the baby's body with one hand. When he is fully born, wipe away any mucus or blood from his mouth with a clean cloth.

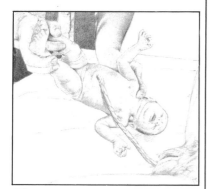

5

If the baby does not breathe immediately, hold him carefully with his head lower than his body to drain any mucus. Do not slap him on the back. If necessary, blow hard on his chest.

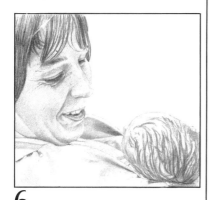

6

Wrap the baby warmly; otherwise he will lose heat quickly, especially from the top of his head. Give the baby to the mother, wrap her warmly with blankets and wait for the placenta to appear.

CORD AROUND THE NECK/*ACTION*

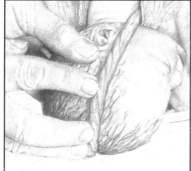

If the baby appears with the cord loosely around his neck, do not worry. Hook a finger round the cord and ease it gently over the baby's head. Do not pull the baby or the cord.

BREECH BIRTH/*ACTION*

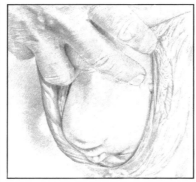

If the baby's bottom appears first, do not worry. Support the baby as he emerges, do not pull him. When the shoulders are out, hold the baby under his shoulders and ease his body up so that his mouth is clear to breathe.

AFTER DELIVERY/*ACTION*

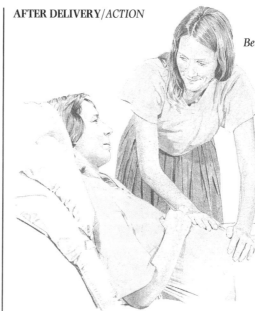

Between five and 15 minutes after the baby has been born, the placenta will be delivered naturally. Encourage the mother during contractions. When the placenta arrives, keep it intact. Slight bleeding is normal. If bleeding is more profuse, call for medical help. Gentle massage of the abdomen should stop the bleeding, and help the uterus contract and harden. Clean the mother, and make her comfortable.

After the baby has been born
Once the baby has been born and while you are waiting for the placenta to appear wrap a clean warm towel or blanket round the baby, being especially careful to cover the top of his head where much heat is lost. Being careful not to pull on the cord, give the baby to the mother, but if she becomes too tired to hold him, then lay him on his side with his head low, close to the mother. If she wants to put him to the breast let her do so, but do not leave the child uncovered. Do not wash the baby.

Wrap the mother warmly in blankets. After a pause of five to 15 minutes the uterus will contract to expel the placenta. When the uterus begins to contract place a bowl between the mother's legs; it will take between five and 20 minutes for the placenta to be pushed out. Do not cut the cord: the doctor or midwife will do this later. Put the placenta aside to show the doctor or midwife. Wash the mother, fix a sanitary pad or improvised pad in position and give her fresh clothes if possible. Make everything tidy around her. If she wants something to eat and drink she may now have it.

If the placenta has not been expelled, or looks as though only part of it has been expelled, get the mother to hospital or get medical help *as soon as possible.*

After the placenta has been expelled, put the baby to the mother's breast if she wants to feed him. If the mother is asleep, lie the baby in a cot on his side with his head low.

Exposure

Anyone who is exposed to the cold without adequate protection may suffer from a drop in the body's natural temperature, which can be fatal if left untreated. The most widely known form of the condition is cold exhaustion—also called wet-cold chilling.

Over-exertion out of doors in bad weather may bring on cold exhaustion, and anxiety—about being lost, for example—makes it worse. Although it develops more quickly in extremes of cold, it can occur at temperatures well above freezing—particularly if there is a biting wind or rain, or both.

The onset of cold exhaustion is insidious and may pass unnoticed. The severity of the condition varies with the victim's age and general health. But if precautions are not taken to prevent further loss of body heat, the victim will fall asleep. His temperature will drop to about 77°F (25°C) and if it falls to about 68°F (20°C) then death will occur.

Anyone who has been exposed to the cold for more than three or four hours will suffer from chronic hypothermia—a dangerous lowering of the body's temperature. He should be rewarmed gradually, to avoid drawing blood to the body surface and away from deeper organs. The condition may develop from cold exhaustion or immersion chilling, or may evolve gradually. It can be made worse if the sufferer has been taking alcohol or drugs, or if he has another illness—for example, diabetes.

Babies and old people are most at risk to chronic hypothermia or to chilling. Their bodies are less able than those of other age groups to regulate their own heat. Even if they are warm and well-wrapped, they can die from breathing freezing or near-freezing air over several hours—for example, if a window is left open in winter. Poor diet often contributes to the condition.

Part of the body only may be affected by severe cold—often hands and feet—while the rest of the body remains warm. In extreme cases this can lead to FROSTBITE. *See page 589.*

Warning signs
- Increasing physical and mental slowness.
- Stumbling, shivering and cramps.
- Slurring of speech and impeded vision.
- Erratic behaviour or irritability.
- If part of the body is affected it will become painful and stiff and the skin will become white and numb.

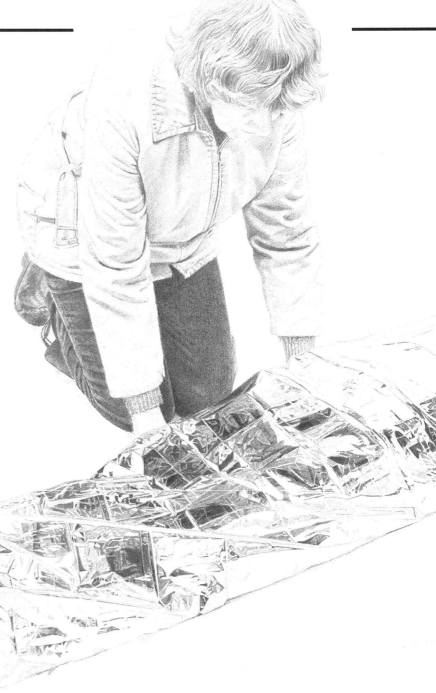

Eye injuries/1

EXPOSURE/*ACTION*

1

Wrap the casualty in spare, dry clothes, blankets or sleeping-bags over her own clothes and get her to a tent or other spot sheltered from wind and rain. Lie her on a blanket or groundsheet to prevent further heat loss. Remove wet clothes and put her into a sleeping-bag, or cover her with blankets or spare clothes. If you have any windproof material—such as polythene or aluminium foil—wrap this on top of the clothes for extra protection.

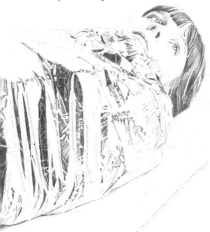

If the casualty has lost consciousness, put her in the unconscious position. Get help if you can, but do not leave her alone.

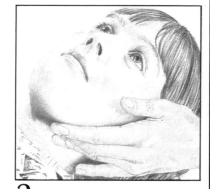

2

Watch her breathing and pulse and be ready to give artificial respiration with chest compression if necessary. The pulse can be felt in the carotid artery, beside the windpipe, below the chin.

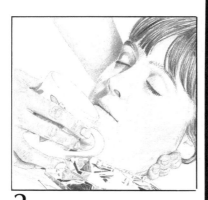

3

Give her a warm, sweet, non-alcoholic drink and chocolate or biscuits if you have any. Give her a warm (not hot) bath as soon as possible and get her into a warm bed.

Any injury to the eye is potentially serious and should receive expert medical attention, as well as on-the-spot first aid. The casualty should never rub or touch an injured eye, eyelid or eyebrow.

CHEMICAL BURNS
Any chemical which enters the eye is extremely dangerous. If it is a strong acid or alkali, act quickly to prevent serious damage.

**FOREIGN BODIES
UNDER AN EYELID**
A speck of dust, a tiny piece of metal, an eyelash or an insect under an eyelid irritates the eye, causing pain and, sometimes, swelling. The same treatment principle is used for upper and lower eyelids.

IMPALED OBJECTS IN THE EYE
Any object that impales or pierces the eye should be removed only by a doctor. Until medical help is available, cover the injured eye with a soft pad or makeshift article that protects the eye without pressing on it. This will stop the object from being accidentally moved. Both eyes should be bandaged to prevent eye movement.

CUT EYEBROWS
Small children are liable to cut their eyebrows if they bang their heads against sharp objects such as the corners of tables. Broken spectacles, shattered glass and flying debris from explosions can also wound the eyebrows. Sports injuries often take the form of cut eyebrows.

CHEMICAL BURNS/*ACTION*

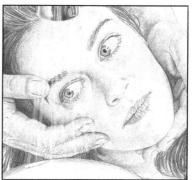

1

Tilt the casualty's head with the injured eye down. Flood the eye with gently running cold or lukewarm water. The chemical can also be washed away by splashing water from a basin.

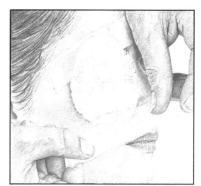

2

When you have thoroughly flushed the injured eye of the chemical, dry the area. Lightly put a clean dressing on it, and get the casualty to hospital as soon as possible.

Eye injuries/2

FOREIGN BODIES UNDER UPPER EYELID/*ACTION*

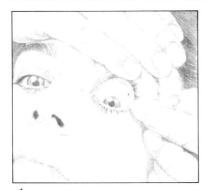

1

Tilt the casualty's head fully backwards. Then gently grasp the lashes of the upper lid. Try to dislodge the object with a piece of clean gauze.

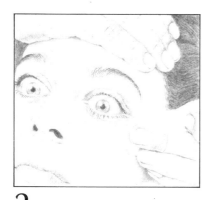

2

Release the upper eyelid and make the casualty blink. Prepare to wipe away any tears with another piece of clean gauze.

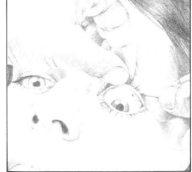
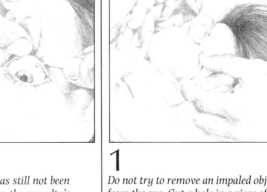

3

If the foreign body has still not been dislodged, press down the casualty's upper lid with a matchstick or similar object and pull up the eyelid with your fingers against the matchstick.

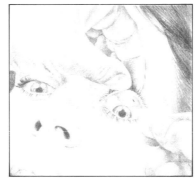

4

Remove the foreign body with the corner of a clean handkerchief and take away the matchstick. Replace the lid by pulling down gently on the lashes.

IMPALED OBJECTS IN EYE/*ACTION*

1

Do not try to remove an impaled object from the eye. Cut a hole in a piece of gauze and put it over the injured eye. Place a soft pad, paper cup or similar object over the gauze.

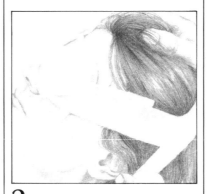

2

The pad or cup keeps the gauze in place and should be secured by a bandage. Cover the uninjured eye as well. Reassure the casualty and seek immediate medical help.

CUT EYEBROW/*ACTION*

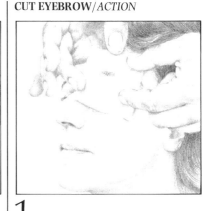

1

Make the casualty sit down with her head erect. This will stop the blood rushing to her head and becoming difficult to control. Gently place a gauze pad directly on the cut.

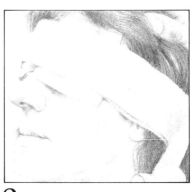

2

Once the bleeding is controlled, leave the pad in place and put a retaining bandage over it. Be careful not to put pressure on the eye. Arrange for immediate medical aid.

Fainting

If the blood supply to the brain is suddenly and temporarily reduced a person may faint. Fainting is usually the result of the victim being in a hot, stuffy atmosphere. But an emotional stimulus, such as an unpleasant sight, a fright or bad news, can also cause fainting. So can a drop in blood sugar due to missed meals or dieting, or standing still for long periods of time. Sometimes there may be a more serious cause, such as illness or injury—in which case a doctor should be consulted.

Someone who is standing still for a long time can reduce the risk of fainting by rocking gently from the heels to the balls of the feet. If someone is about to faint he should sit down. You should loosen tight clothing at the neck and waist and put his head down to his knees.

Warning signs
- The casualty's face becomes pale or greenish-white. He may yawn frequently, showing he is lacking air.
- His skin is cold and clammy.
- Beads of sweat appear on his face, neck and hands.

FAINTING/*ACTION*

If the casualty has passed out, but is breathing normally, lay her on her back with her legs raised as high as possible above the level of her head. Hold the legs up, or prop them on a chair or anything else suitable. Loosen clothing at the neck, chest and waist, and ensure that the casualty gets plenty of fresh air. If she is indoors, open the windows. If out of doors, use the same treatment and protect the casualty from the sun. She should remain lying down for a few minutes after recovering, before attempting to rise.

Fits

Usually, fits are caused by a sudden, uncontrolled surge of electrochemical energy in the brain. They may be a sign of brain damage or other serious disorders. In children, they may simply indicate a high temperature, sore throat, ear infection or even teething.

Whether the casualty is an adult or a child, always seek medical advice, particularly if there is a previous history of fits.

FITS/*ACTION*

1
Do not use force to restrain the casualty's movements. Rough handling may bring on another fit.

2
Remove all furniture and any objects which the casualty may bump into and hurt himself.

3
As soon as the fit is over, clear any blood, mucus or vomit from the mouth. If the casualty is breathing normally, turn him into the unconscious position and get medical help. If he is not breathing, start artificial respiration at once.

Fractures

A fracture is a cracked or broken bone. There are two main causes of fractures: direct force, when the bone breaks at the force point from a kick or blow; indirect force, when the bone breaks at some distance from the force point—for example, a collar-bone being fractured as the result of a fall on an outstretched hand.

There are three main kinds of fractures.

Closed fractures, in which the skin is unbroken, although it may be heavily bruised. Closed fractures can be *complicated*, when blood vessels, nerves or organs near the break are also severely damaged (such as when a broken rib penetrates a lung); or they can be *simple*, when there is little damage to the surrounding body tissues.

Compound or open fractures, in which a bone protrudes through the skin or there is a deep gash leading down to the break, allowing germs to enter.

The third type are greenstick fractures, in which the bone bends and half breaks. It is most common in children.

All doubtful cases of injured bones should be considered as fractures and expert diagnosis sought. However, the principles of treatment are the same in every case.

When treating fractures be sure to handle the casualty with care as careless handling can cause pain— and pain increases shock.

Warning signs
• Often, the casualty will have heard or felt the bone break. There may be crepitus—the feeling of broken bone ends grating, which can sometimes be heard.
• The casualty may not be able to use the injured part of the body, and will feel pain when he does.
• The area around the break may be tender to the touch, swollen or bruised.
• A limb may be in an unnatural position or deformed when compared to the uninjured side.

If you expect an ambulance soon:
Support the limb with the suspected fracture carefully, and ease it gently into its natural position. Steady and support it in this position until the ambulance arrives.
If you do not expect an ambulance soon, or if the casualty has to be moved:
Take the action shown here.

FRACTURES/*ACTION*

1

Treat the suspected fracture carefully and move the affected area as little as possible while making the casualty comfortable. Gently remove clothing from any open wound over the break.

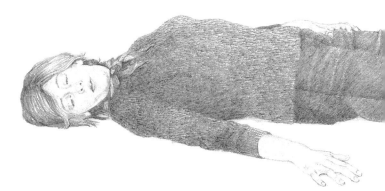

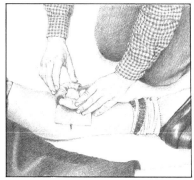

2

Cover the wound with a clean piece of lint and place raised pads over the protruding bone. Alternatively, pack over the wound using a matchbox or cigarette packet.

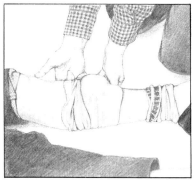

3

Bandage the wound, supporting the injured part carefully. The pads or packing will reduce the pressure on an open fracture. If applied too tightly, the bandage will interfere with circulation.

Frostbite

In freezing weather, exposed parts of the body—such as the nose tip, ear lobes, cheeks and chin—may develop frostbite as the skin on them cools and the blood vessels become constricted, cutting off the blood supply to the area. The hands and feet can also be affected, even when they are enclosed in gloves and boots. In severe cases, gangrene may develop unless the affected part is rewarmed.

Wherever possible, try to shelter or protect the victim from the freezing conditions.

Do *not* apply any form of direct heat to the frostbitten skin.

Do *not* rub the affected area.

Warning signs
- The affected part of the body feels cold, painful and stiff at first.
- The skin becomes hard and turns blue or white. Usually, it also goes numb, so that the feeling of cold and pain disappears.
- Frostbite that has partly thawed is a blue colour, and there may be blood-filled blisters in the affected area.

FROSTBITE/*ACTION*

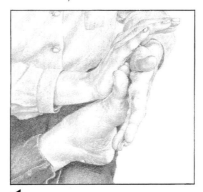

1

Warm the affected area slowly with your hands until the circulation returns. In the case of a frostbitten foot, remove the shoe and sock and cover the foot with a linen pad.

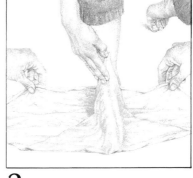

2

Put padding between the affected fingers or toes and secure with triangular bandage. Put the base of the bandage behind wrist or heel and bring the top point over hand or foot.

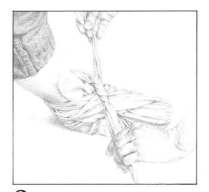

3

Pass the ends of the bandage around the wrist or ankle. Cross them over the top point and fasten with a reef knot, but not so tight that the circulation is impeded.

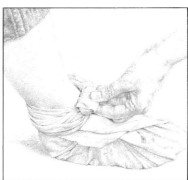

4

Bring top point down over knot and fasten. Cover foot with blanket or sleeping-bag and keep elevated. Put coats or blankets around the casualty and give him hot, sweet drinks.

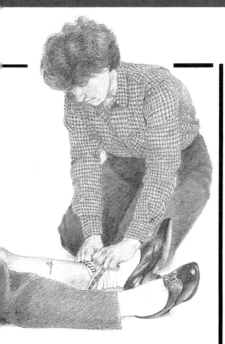

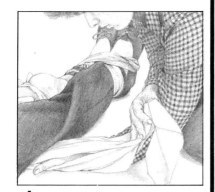

4

If the break is in a leg, tie the uninjured leg to the other leg with bandages at the knees and ankles and around the feet, and above and below the fracture. Pad between the legs.

Gassing

The use of natural, non-toxic gas in the home has greatly reduced the number of deaths from accidental gassing. But there are many other danger sources, including industrial gases such as propane and butane; ammonia, used in refrigeration plants; and the fumes given off by burning polyurethane foam—widely used in furniture—which contains hydrogen cyanide and carbon monoxide. Carbon monoxide is also present in car exhaust fumes.

Whatever the cause of gassing, the treatment is always the same.

If possible, before attempting a rescue tell someone else to call expert help. Do not attempt a rescue if you are likely to become a casualty yourself.

Warning signs
• The casualty may suffer from unsound judgment and be difficult and unco-operative.
• The casualty may be confused, stupefied or unconscious.

GASSING/*ACTION*

1

Mask your nose and mouth with a wet handkerchief. Pass your arms under the victim's armpits and link them across her chest, grasping one of your wrists. Drag the victim into the open air.

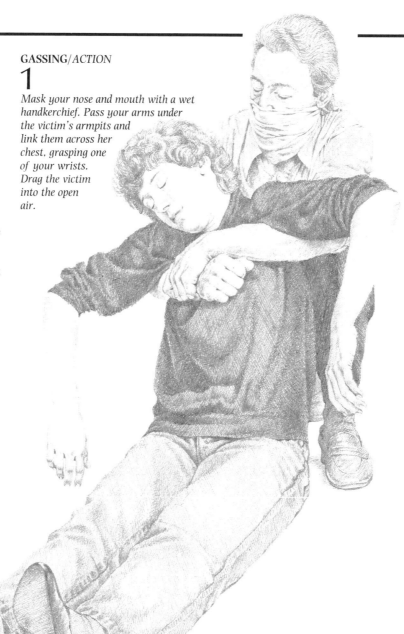

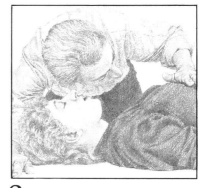

2

Put your ear close to the victim's nose and mouth to check her breathing. Check the rise and fall of her chest. If she is not breathing, then give artificial respiration.

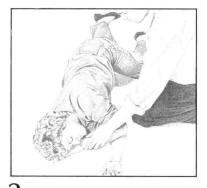

3

Once normal breathing has resumed, turn the victim stomach down into the recovery position. Call medical aid at once. Continue to check her breathing until help arrives.

Gunshot wounds

Most gunshot wounds are caused by shotguns, which are widely used in field sports. But all types of firearms —from pellet-firing airguns to small-bore weapons—are potentially dangerous.

In all types of gunshot accidents the bullet may leave two wounds— one at the point of entry into the body, and another and larger one at the point of exit.

When treating a gunshot wound, check both the point of entry and the other side of the casualty's body for an exit wound. The victim may only be aware of the entry wound.

If there is no exit wound, the bullet has either been deflected off the body—leaving a wound similar in appearance to an entry wound— or it is lodged inside.

The bullet will cause a great deal of tissue damage and it may hit and splinter a bone. All gunshot wounds require expert medical attention.

GUNSHOT WOUNDS/*ACTION*

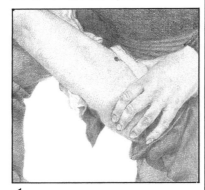

1

Unless you suspect there is a fracture, cover the wound with a clean pad or your bare hands to stop the bleeding. If there are entry and exit wounds, cover both.

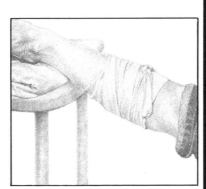

2

Once the bleeding has slowed, dress and bandage the wound and gently elevate it. Do not attempt to remove a bullet that is left in the wound. Then get medical help.

Head and facial injuries/1

Many of the casualties admitted to the emergency departments of hospitals have head injuries. Some are the victims of road accidents, but head injuries also occur frequently in sports accidents or as the result of a fall. They range from relatively minor bruises and cuts to fractures and damage to the brain.

With head injuries, there may be no obvious outward signs of brain damage except perhaps for brief unconsciousness. In old people, any slight knock to the head may cause internal bleeding which, if it is not recognised, can result in permanent damage.

Every casualty who has been even briefly unconscious after an accident, and all elderly people with head injuries, should be sent to hospital for examination.

If a casualty with a head injury is unconscious, make sure, when you put him in the unconscious position, that his head is level with the rest of his body. But if you are on sloping ground, his head should be up the slope. *See* UNCONSCIOUSNESS *pages 611-12.*

SCALP INJURIES
Although scalp wounds may cause severe and alarming bleeding, they are often less serious than they look. But however superficial the wounds may be, there is always the possibility of an underlying fracture—or of a foreign body being present.

BROKEN JAW
Usually, only one side of the jaw is affected and there is often a wound inside the mouth. The casualty may have difficulty in speaking and there may be an excessive flow of saliva— which is often blood-stained.

BLEEDING FACE
Again, a bleeding face often looks far worse than it is and needs little more than cleaning and bandaging.

Warning signs
• Cuts, bruises and swellings on the scalp, face or jaw.
• Headache.
• Confusion or drowsiness, which may be followed by unconsciousness.
• Loss of memory of events before or at the time of the accident.
• The eye pupils may be unequal, and the victim may have double vision.
• Weak pulse and shallow breathing.

Head and facial injuries/2

SCALP INJURIES/*ACTION*

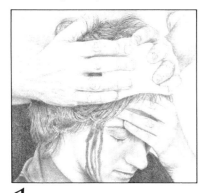

1

Gently feel the skull around the wound. If part of it seems to move, suspect a fracture and do not press on it. Otherwise, place a clean pad or your hands on the wound to stop bleeding.

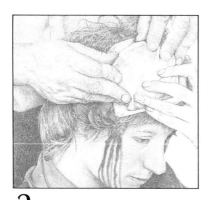

2

Cover the wound with a clean dressing. If there is a foreign object present, or if you suspect a fracture, put the dressing on lightly, with a pad on top of it to lessen any pressure.

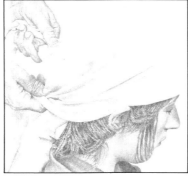

3

Fix the dressing or pad in place with a triangular bandage. Put the long edge across the forehead and the point at the nape. Bring the other two ends around to the nape and cross them.

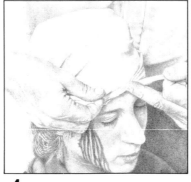

4

Next, bring the points forward again around the sides of the head to the forehead and tie them in a reef knot, securing the bandage. Keep the casualty's head as steady as possible.

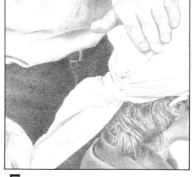

5

Gently place one hand on the bandage to stop it slipping. With the other, pull the point downwards, parallel with the back of the neck, ensuring that the bandage is drawn tautly over the scalp.

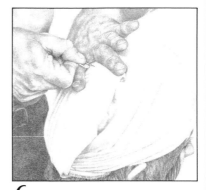

6

Bring the point of the bandage up to the crown and fix it lightly in place with a safety-pin or adhesive tape. Failing these, tuck the point into the edge of the bandage at the front.

BROKEN JAW/*ACTION*

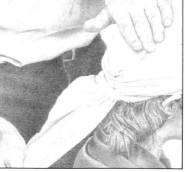

1

If the jaw is broken or dislocated, make sure the mouth is clear of any blood or debris. Then put a makeshift pad under the point of the chin. Put a narrow bandage or scarf under the chin.

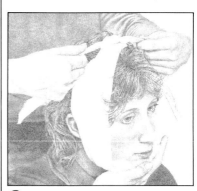

2

Tie the ends of the bandage on top of the head in a reef knot. The bandage should be tight enough to support the jaw, but not so tight that the casualty's teeth are clenched.

Heart attack

Heart stoppage

Heat stroke/1

BLEEDING FACE/*ACTION*

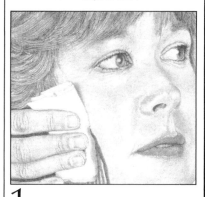

1

Press a sterile pad or clean handkerchief against the wound to stem bleeding.

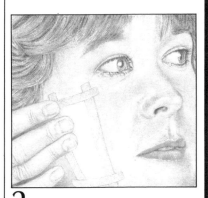

2

Tape the sterile pad or clean handkerchief in position.

A reduction of the blood supply to the heart causes a heart attack. It may be the result of a narrowing of the arteries, or the blockage of an artery by a blood clot.

Warning signs
- Shock.
- Severe and constricting pain in the chest—sometimes radiating down the left arm and up into the left side of the neck.
- Shortness of breath.
- Weak or irregular pulse.
- The victim may collapse and lapse into unconsciousness.

HEART ATTACK/*ACTION*

1

Check the victim's breathing and pulse. If necessary, give artificial respiration and chest compression.

2

Put the victim in the most comfortable position, perhaps half-sitting, and loosen his clothing at the neck, chest and waist. Encourage him to breathe deeply.

3

Get medical attention immediately. Give aspirin to chew slowly. Comfort the victim and keep onlookers from overcrowding him. Take and record his pulse-rate every ten minutes, and note the time at which it was taken.

The heart may stop beating as the result of a serious injury—for example, asphyxiation, choking, drowning, electrical accidents, or overdose—or because of a heart attack.

Warning signs
- The victim collapses into unconsciousness and stops breathing.
- There is no pulse at the wrist or in the carotid (neck) artery.

HEART STOPPAGE/*ACTION*

Turn the victim on to his back and administer artificial respiration and chest compression until breathing and pulse resume. See ARTIFICIAL RESPIRATION *page 556.*

Two distinct conditions arise from excessive heat: heat exhaustion and, more seriously, heat stroke.

HEAT STROKE
A very hot, humid atmosphere stops the body from controlling its temperature by sweating. Heat stroke (possibly preceded by heat exhaustion) may then rapidly occur. If the casualty is not treated quickly he may die. Babies and old people are particularly at risk.

Always get medical aid as soon as possible.

Warning signs
- The skin is hot and may feel dry.
- The casualty may complain of a headache, thirst, nausea and drowsiness. He may become dizzy and breathe noisily.
- His temperature will rise to $104\,°\text{F}$ ($40\,°\text{C}$) and beyond.
- As the condition worsens, he may become confused and lapse into unconsciousness.

HEAT EXHAUSTION
Profuse sweating—usually caused by hard physical activity in the sun—leads to the loss of excessive amounts of salt from the body. This causes muscle cramps and general weakening, but the sweating stops the temperature from rising. Without treatment, the condition slowly worsens until the casualty eventually may collapse.

Warning signs
- General exhaustion, restlessness, headaches and dizziness.
- The skin is cold, pale and clammy.
- Rapid pulse.
- Vomiting.

Heat stroke/2

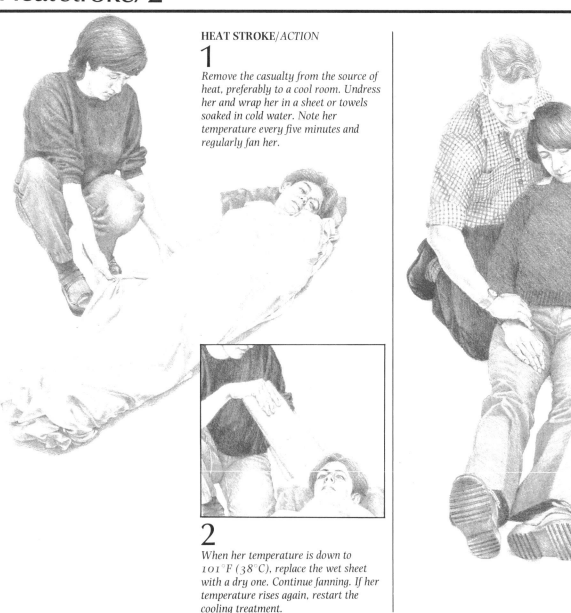

HEAT STROKE/ACTION

1

Remove the casualty from the source of heat, preferably to a cool room. Undress her and wrap her in a sheet or towels soaked in cold water. Note her temperature every five minutes and regularly fan her.

2

When her temperature is down to 101°F (38°C), replace the wet sheet with a dry one. Continue fanning. If her temperature rises again, restart the cooling treatment.

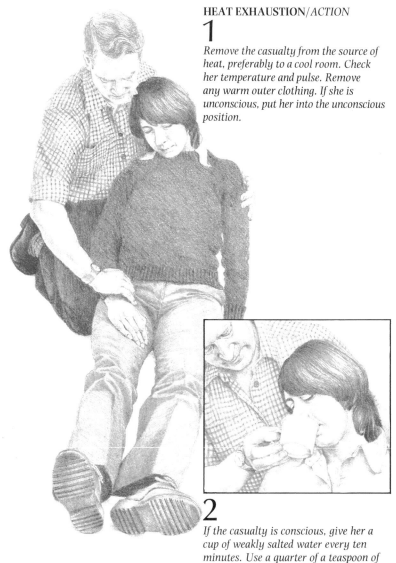

HEAT EXHAUSTION/ACTION

1

Remove the casualty from the source of heat, preferably to a cool room. Check her temperature and pulse. Remove any warm outer clothing. If she is unconscious, put her into the unconscious position.

2

If the casualty is conscious, give her a cup of weakly salted water every ten minutes. Use a quarter of a teaspoon of salt to each pint of water. Add fruit juice to improve the taste.

Hiccups

Eating or drinking too much or too fast can produce hiccups—involuntary spasms of the diaphragm. Sometimes, attacks are brought on by nervousness or, occasionally, by disorders of the digestive system or the lungs.

If an attack lasts for more than two or three hours, or if an attack is persistent, the casualty should see a doctor.

HICCUPS/ACTION

1

Tell the casualty to hold his breath several times, or to clasp his hands over his mouth and breathe in and out of them. Both procedures increase the amount of carbon dioxide in the body, which calms the spasms.

2

Sit the casualty quietly, and give him water to sip or ice or sugar to suck.

3

If this does not work, place a paper bag (not plastic) over the casualty's mouth and nose, and get him to breathe in and out. If the condition continues for two or three hours or more, seek medical advice.

Hysteria

A fit of hysterics is usually caused by an emotional upset or mental stress. The attack may resemble an epileptic fit but is more dramatised and is 'staged' to gain sympathy and attention. It will continue as long as there is an audience.

In an adult, hysterics take longer to develop than an epileptic fit and may vary from temporary loss of control, when the person shouts or screams, to a noisy display of arm waving, tearing at hair and clothes, and rolling on the ground in an apparent frenzy.

Although genuinely distressed, the person will take care not to cause self-harm. Do not slap a hysterical person on the face as this can cause psychological harm. In the case of someone with a weak heart, the shock could even kill him. Get medical aid. *See* FITS *page 587*.

Warning signs
• The casualty makes a lot of noise, trying to draw attention, and may 'collapse' into a fairly safe position, flail about wildly, or move weakly to suggest illness.

HYSTERIA/ACTION

1

Be firm but gentle. Reassure and try to calm the person down.

2

Clear relatives and onlookers from the scene.

Moving an injured person/1

An injured person should only be moved if he is in immediate danger—for example, from leaking gas or an unsafe building. There are several main methods that can be used to move a casualty to safety so that treatment can be given to him.

MOVING A CONSCIOUS PERSON
If the casualty is only slightly injured, and able to stand, this is a relatively simple operation.

MOVING AN UNCONSCIOUS PERSON
Sometimes such a casualty has to be moved quickly to prevent further injury occurring.

DRAGGING
A backwards drag is suitable for moving a light person, especially if you have to negotiate a flight or flights of stairs.

MOVING A CONSCIOUS PERSON/ACTION

Stand close to victim on the side on which she is injured, unless the wound is to the hand, arm or shoulder. In that case, support from the uninjured side. Put your arm around the casualty's waist and grip the clothing at the hip. Get her to put an arm around your neck. Grasp that hand unless she is bleeding heavily, when you should use your hand to staunch the blood. Take the casualty's weight with your body and move forward with slow, gentle steps. The same technique can be used with two helpers, one on either side of the casualty. Unless there is a hand, arm or shoulder injury, the helper on the injured side should take most of the weight.

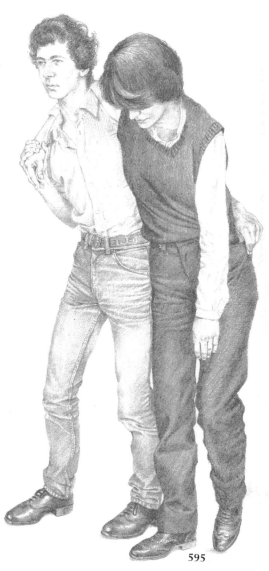

Moving an injured person/2

MOVING AN UNCONSCIOUS PERSON/*ACTION*

1

Clear the casualty's mouth of blood, mucus or vomit, and check breathing. Do not start artificial respiration until you are clear of danger. Turn the casualty face up and cross her arms at the wrists and rest them on the abdomen. If the casualty is very heavy, or there is a long way to go to safety, use a wrist-lash to help you take the strain.

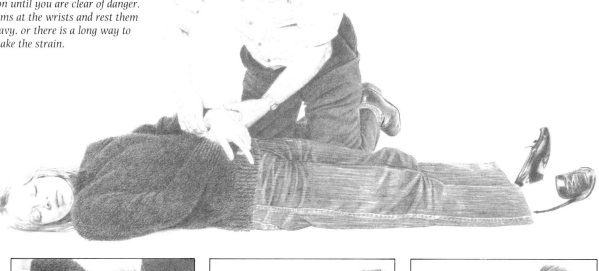

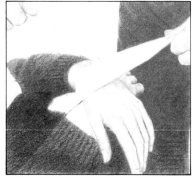

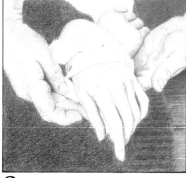

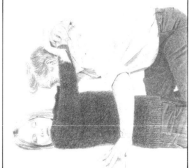

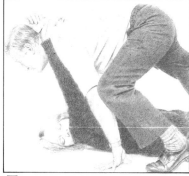

2

Use a belt, scarf, necktie or bandage to tie her wrists together. Wind the material around each wrist tightly, but not so tightly that the circulation is impeded.

3

Wind the material between the wrists to hold them together, and tie the ends with a reef knot. Check quickly with your fingers that the knot is fast and will not slip.

4

Kneel astride the casualty and slip your head through the tied wrists so that they are resting on your shoulders at the base of your neck. Push yourself up into a crouch.

5

Raise the casualty's head and upper body as far off the ground as you can comfortably manage, and work your way forward to safety. Use your arms to take the casualty's weight.

Nose-bleeds

Bleeding from the nose can be the result of a punch or blowing too hard and breaking the nasal blood vessels, or it may have no apparent cause. In elderly people, particularly, nose-bleeds may be a sign of high blood pressure.

If blood mixed with a straw-coloured fluid trickles from the nose of an unconscious person after a car accident, suspect a fracture of the skull. *See* HEAD AND FACIAL INJURIES *pages 591-3.*

NOSE-BLEEDS/*ACTION*

1

Sit the casualty down with his head leaning forwards so that the blood does not ooze down the back of his throat and possibly choke him. Loosen clothing about the neck.

2

Get the casualty to pinch the lower, soft part of the nose between his thumb and fingers for 10 minutes, and then to release the pressure slowly. If bleeding continues, get him to repeat the pressure for another 10 minutes.

3

When the bleeding has stopped, warn the casualty not to blow or pick his nose. If the bleeding does not stop, or if a broken nose or other injury is suspected, tell the victim to keep holding his nose and get medical aid.

DRAGGING A CASUALTY/*ACTION*

Stoop behind the casualty's head, so that you are looking down towards her feet. Pass your hands under the casualty's armpits. If she is very light—for example, a child—you can lift from there. Otherwise, grasp one of your wrists with the other hand across her chest and then lift. Do not lace your fingers together, as they may slip. Work your way backwards in a squatting or sliding position, letting the casualty's head rest on your upper arm. If you have to go down stairs or a steep slope, support the victim's head as much as possible on your thigh.

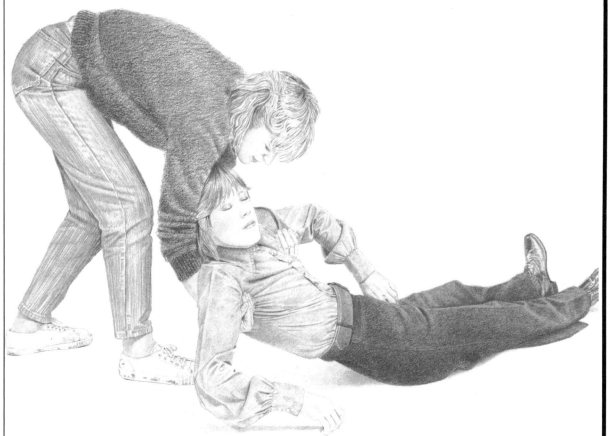

Overdose

Anyone who has taken an overdose of a drug needs immediate medical attention. Sufferers from asthma, hypersensitivity to certain medicines, or kidney disease often react more strongly to an overdose than would a more healthy person. Do *not* keep the casualty awake by giving him hot, black coffee and helping him to walk about. Wait until medical aid comes and his stomach can be pumped out.

Warning signs
• Depending on the size of the overdose and the drug concerned, the signs may vary from faintness to dizziness—sometimes with incoherent speech—to unconsciousness, absence of breath and heart stoppage.

OVERDOSE/*ACTION*

1
If breathing has stopped, start artificial respiration immediately, with chest compression if there is no pulse.

2
If the casualty is breathing but unconscious, treat for unconsciousness. If he is conscious, treat for poisoning.

3
Get medical aid immediately, even if casualty seems to have recovered. Keep any vomit, tablets, bottles or containers which will help identify the drug.

Poisoning

A poison can enter the body by being breathed in through the nose or mouth, as with gassing; or through the mouth alone, by being swallowed, as with a drug overdose.

Warning signs
• Anxiety, confusion or unconsciousness.
• Feelings of nausea, vomiting or sweating.

POISONING/*ACTION*

1
If the casualty is not breathing give artificial respiration with chest compression if necessary.

2
If the casualty is unconscious, but breathing, turn him on his stomach in the unconscious position. Check that his airway is clear and that his tongue has not fallen back.

3
If the casualty is conscious and has swallowed something caustic, get him to sip a pint of milk or water slowly to dilute the poison in his stomach. Do not *deliberately make him vomit.*

4
Get medical attention and prepare a full written report on the incident.

Pulse and respiration

In all but minor injuries, you should take the casualty's pulse and respiration rates as you are treating him—and regularly while you are waiting for medical assistance. You need a digital watch or one with a second hand. If you do not have one, get someone to count aloud for you (or count yourself), putting an 'and' between the numbers up to 12. Estimate roughly a second for the time it takes to say each number.

TWO AREAS TO TAKE A PULSE
The two usual areas for taking the pulse-rate (which coincides with the beat of the heart) are on the inside of the wrist and on the carotid area on the outer side of the neck, by the windpipe and slightly more than halfway to the jaw-line.

PULSE AND RESPIRATION
The normal adult pulse-rate, at rest, is 60-80 beats a minute, with an average of 72. It is slower in old people and faster in children—between 90 and 100 beats a minute in young children and up to 140 in babies.

In respiration, one breath is a complete cycle of breathing in, a slight pause, and then exhaling. Count only the number of times the chest *rises*. The average adult breathes 16-18 times a minute when at rest. In infants and young children, the rate is 24-40 breaths a minute.

Many people unknowingly alter their breathing rate if they are aware it is being checked. So it is best to take it at the same time as you are feeling the pulse if the casualty is conscious.

TWO WAYS TO TAKE A PULSE

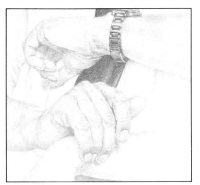

1
The wrist pulse can be felt about 1 in. (25 mm.) below the base of the thumb and ½ in. (13 mm.) from the edge of the arm. Place three fingers on the pulse and press slightly. Time the beats.

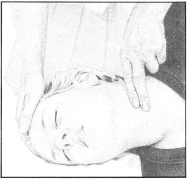

1
The carotid pulse can be felt on the outer side of the neck. Place two fingers on the pulse and press slightly. Time the beats. The pulse beats on both sides, but only feel on one.

Scalds

CHECKING PULSE AND RESPIRATION/*ACTION*

Bend the casualty's arm at the elbow so that it rests across the chest near the opposite shoulder, if that will not worsen injuries. Raise the wrist slightly and feel for the pulse with your fingertips—not your thumb. Count the beats for 30 seconds and remember the figure. Keep holding the wrist and count the number of times the casualty's chest rises in the next 30 seconds. Double the pulse and respiration figures you have obtained to express them per minute, and write them down, or have them noted by a helper.

The treatment for scalding is the same as for burns—cool the injured area with water and cover it with clean, non-fluffy material.
See BURNS AND SCALDS *pages 568-9.*

Severed limbs

Sometimes, if a limb, finger or toe has been severed, quick action can preserve the amputated part and it can be re-stitched later by micro-surgery. But the priority is to save the casualty, so do not waste time dealing with the severed limb until you have looked after him.

Never try to restore a severed limb yourself—for example, by binding it in place with surgical tapes—as you will cause the casualty a great deal of pain and will damage the tissues, making surgery more difficult.

SEVERED LIMBS/*ACTION*

1

Lie the casualty down and, as you do so, stop the bleeding by pressing a large piece of gauze, clean linen or the clean side of a handkerchief on the stump or raw area. Raise the injured part, propping it with a pillow, folded coat or on your knee, while you are treating it.

2

Put a pad of gauze or one improvised from clean linen on to the raw area and fix it in place with a bandage. Place another dressing on the raw end of the severed limb. If the injury is to an arm, immobilise it by bandaging it to the casualty's chest. If it is a leg, bandage it to the other one.

3

Encourage the casualty to remain still and get medical attention immediately.

4

Once you are sure that the casualty is in no immediate danger, deal with the severed part. If you can find it, wrap it in clean linen, put it in a plastic bag and keep it as cool as possible by packing ice around the bag. Do not let the ice come into direct contact with the limb. Give it to the ambulance crew or doctor, to go to hospital with the casualty.

Shock

Clinical shock is brought on by a reduction of the blood supply to the body's vital organs following severe injuries, such as burns or bleeding, heart attacks or abdominal emergencies—for example, a burst appendix. It can also be caused by heavy fluid loss through vomiting or diarrhoea. It may develop slowly and range from a feeling of faintness to unconsciousness or even death.

Clinical shock is not the same as the emotional fear which comes on immediately after an injury or other unpleasant experience, from which the victim may recover quickly.

Warning signs
• Pallid or grey skin which is cold and moist to touch.
• Fast, shallow breathing and a rapid, weak and thin pulse.
• Dizziness or fainting, blurred vision, nausea or vomiting.
• The casualty may complain of thirst.
• Anxiety and restlessness, sometimes progressing into unconsciousness.

SHOCK/*ACTION*

1

Lay the casualty down and treat any obvious injury or underlying condition which has caused the shock. Reassure the casualty.

2

Loosen the casualty's clothing at the neck, chest and waist. Lightly cover him with a coat or single blanket. If possible, raise his legs to return the blood supply to the brain.

3

If a conscious casualty complains of thirst, moisten his lips with water, but do not give him anything to drink. Give hot, sweet tea only in cases of emotional fright. Do not move the casualty unnecessarily. Try to comfort and reassure him.

4

If the casualty is unconscious, put him on his stomach in the unconscious position.

5

Get medical aid immediately, if you can do so without leaving the casualty unattended.

Slings/1

Once an injury to the hand, arm or ribs has been treated, put a sling on the casualty to give added protection and support. The hand should be just above elbow level for upper arm injuries, and on the shoulder for hand injuries.

ARM SLINGS
Made with a standard triangular bandage, these support the forearm and arm in cases of injuries of the upper limb. They are only effective when the casualty is sitting or standing.

ELEVATION SLINGS
These keep the hand and forearm in a well-raised position in cases of hand and shoulder injury. They provide extra support if a rough journey has to be undertaken.

IMPROVISED SLINGS
These are used if the casualty does *not* have an injured wrist or forearm. They are made from a large square of fabric, or from a belt, tie or scarf. If none of those is available, tuck the wrist inside the casualty's buttoned jacket, waistcoat, shirt or blouse.

MAKING AN ARM SLING/*ACTION*

1

Get the casualty to support the injured arm with his hand. Place an open triangular bandage between the casualty's chest and forearm, its side point stretching well beyond the elbow. Take the upper end over the shoulder on the uninjured side, around the back of the neck to the front of the injured side.

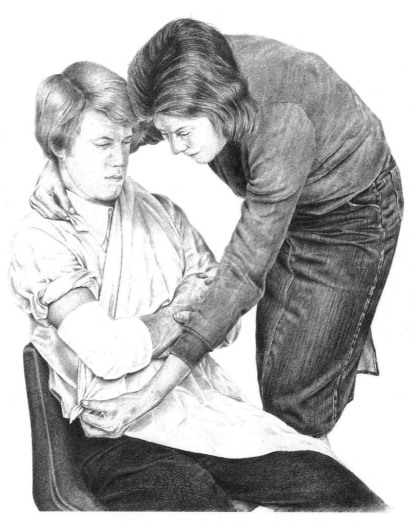

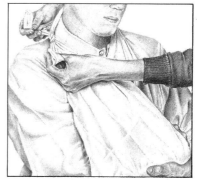

2

Take the lower end of the bandage up over the hand and forearm and tie it in the hollow just above the collar-bone. Use a reef bow or reef knot.

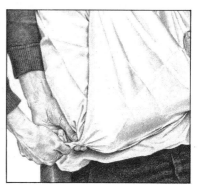

3

Pin the point of the sling near the elbow, or tuck it in. Check that the casualty's nail beds are not turning blue. If they are, the bandage is too tight and should be eased.

Slings/2

MAKING AN ELEVATION SLING/*ACTION*

1

If the hand or forearm is injured, raise the arm so that the hand rests on the opposite shoulder. Get the casualty to support it in place if possible.

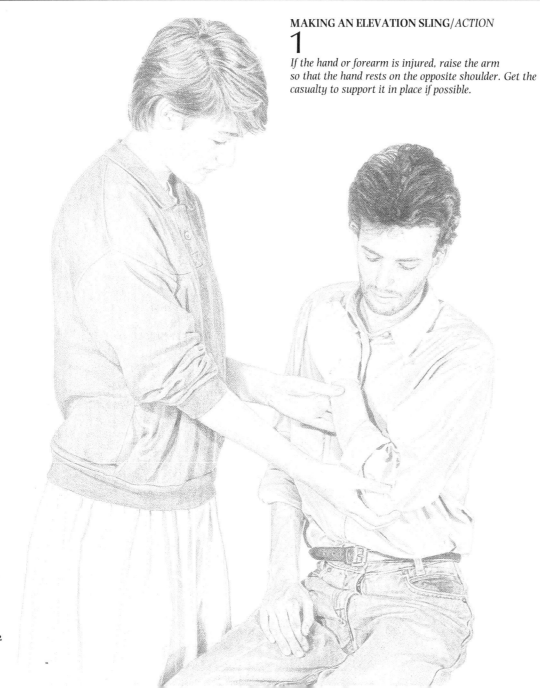

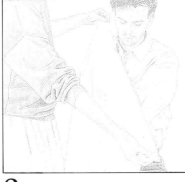

2

Put one point of the base of the sling over the casualty's shoulder on the uninjured side, with the point extended well beyond the elbow. The sling should then be hanging over the injured arm.

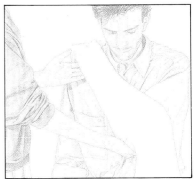

3

Gently push the base of the sling under the hand, forearm and elbow of the injured limb. Then bring the lower end of the base up and around the casualty's back on the injured side.

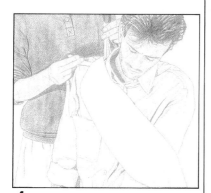

4

Bring the two ends of the sling together round the back of the casualty and on the uninjured side. Secure at the uninjured shoulder with a reef bow or reef knot.

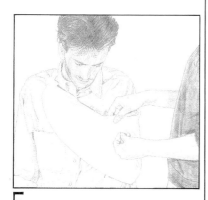

5

Fold the top of the sling at the elbow and fasten it with a pin or tape, or tuck it in. Check the nail beds to make sure they have not turned blue. If they have, ease the sling or bandage.

IMPROVISING A SLING/*ACTION*

1

If you do not have a triangular bandage or a square scarf, improvise a collar-and-cuff sling from a belt, tie, narrow scarf, or roller bandage.

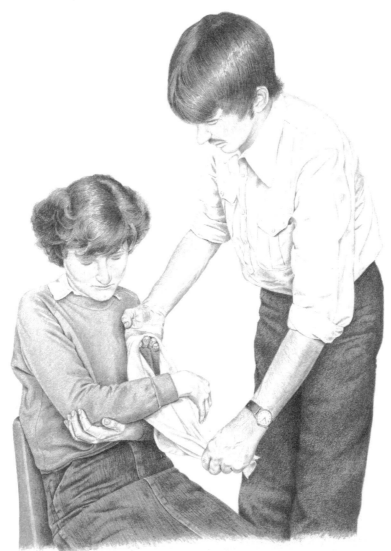

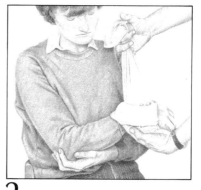

2

For an injured upper arm, wrap the improvised sling round the casualty's wrist on the injured side. Put one end of the sling over the casualty's shoulder on the injured side.

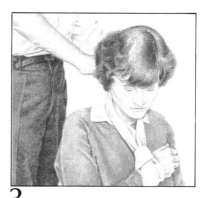

3

Bring the other end of the sling across the casualty's chest, round her back, and tie the ends in the hollow above the collar bone on the uninjured side.

Snow blindness Splinters

Skiers and others who spend long periods out in the snow risk snow-blindness if they do not protect their eyes with dark glasses. The ultra-violet rays from bright sunlight reflected on the snow inflame the cornea, causing loss of vision. With prompt treatment, the casualty usually recovers completely in a day or two.

Warning sign
• Vision begins to deteriorate three to five hours after the casualty is first exposed to bright sunlight on snow, and may be lost altogether.

SNOW BLINDNESS/*ACTION*

1

Cover the casualty's eyes with dressings or improvised pads. Do not allow him to remove them.

2

Get medical aid as quickly as possible.

Small pieces of wood or thorns embedded in the skin can cause infection if they are not carefully removed. Do not try to remove a large splinter, or one that does not protrude from the skin. In such cases seek medical aid.

SPLINTERS/*ACTION*

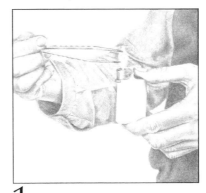

1

Sterilise a pair of tweezers—preferably with spade ends—by passing them through the flame from a lighter or gas stove (do not wipe any soot from them), or by boiling in water for ten minutes.

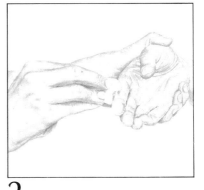

2

Wash the skin around the site of the injury carefully with warm, soapy water. Wipe downwards and outwards from the wound to avoid carrying dirt to it. Then dry the skin gently.

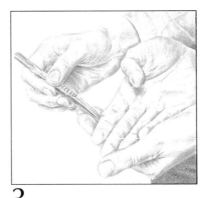

3

Using the tweezers, pull the splinter out. If it is a very small one, a magnifying glass may help you to see it. If the splinter does not come out, dress it lightly and get medical advice.

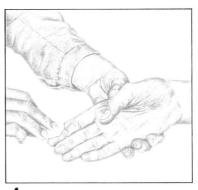

4

When the splinter has been removed, wash the wound with a mild antiseptic and dry gently. Cover it with a plaster or sterile dressing. If it swells or becomes painful get medical advice.

Splints/1

A bone which is broken, or suspected of being broken, should be immobilised. The best way to immobilise an arm is usually to bandage it against the chest, using a sling. A broken leg can be bandaged against the other leg, provided that plenty of padding is put between the ankles and knees to prevent chafing.

A splint for an arm or leg can be improvised from a tightly rolled blanket, provided it is long enough to go well beyond the joints above and below the break. Any rigid article, such as a walking-stick, umbrella or rolled cardboard, can also be used as a splint. Do not remove clothing to apply a splint and move the injured limb as little as possible.

If you expect an ambulance soon: Support the limb with the suspected fracture carefully, and ease it gently into its natural position. Steady and support it in this position until the ambulance arrives.
If you do not expect an ambulance soon, or if the casualty has to be moved: Take the action shown here.

SPLINTING WITH BANDAGES/*ACTION*

1

Whenever you do move the casualty, bear his comfort in mind. If one leg is injured, use the other as the splint. First place plenty of padding along the inside of the injured leg, especially at the ankle, knee and thigh. Then, supporting the injured leg constantly, gently move the uninjured leg across to it.
If a helper is available, he should support the injured leg at ankle and foot while bandaging is done. To show bandaging clearly, this support is omitted below.

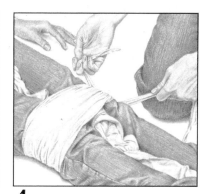

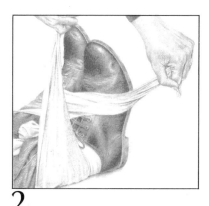

2

Tie the feet together in a figure of eight, using a narrow bandage. Pass the middle of the bandage under the ankles, cross the ends over the insteps and round to the soles.

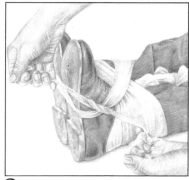

3

Tie the bandage ends together in a reef knot on the outer edge of the boot on the uninjured side.

4

Tie the knees together with a broad bandage knotted on the uninjured side. Tie extra bandages above and below the fracture site.

Splints/2

IMPROVISING A BLANKET SPLINT/*ACTION*

1

Roll a blanket lengthways as tightly as you can. Place one end between the casualty's legs, starting at the crotch. Bring the blanket around the foot of the injured leg and take the other end alongside the leg up to the thighs. Then tie the legs together with two bandages, unless the casualty needs to be taken on a rough or long journey to receive medical aid. In this case, use five bandages.

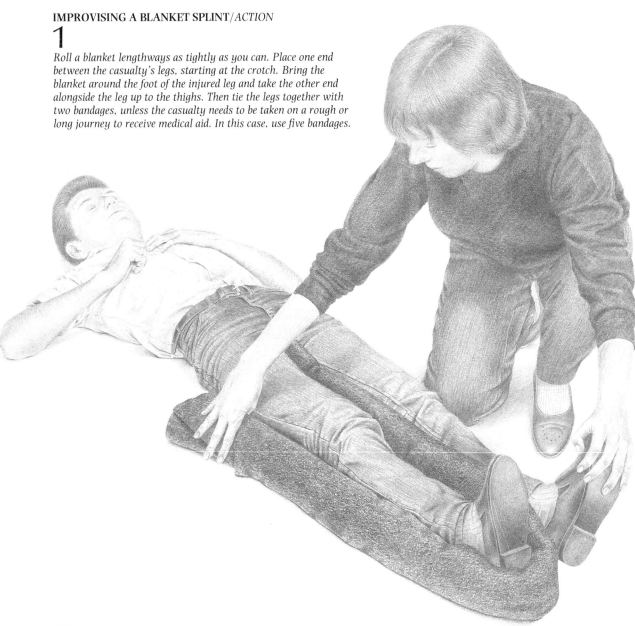

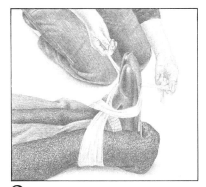

2

Tie the feet and ankles together with a bandage in a figure of eight. Then tie a broad fold bandage around the knees. Tie the knot on the uninjured leg.

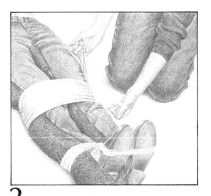

3

Tie the third and fourth bandages—if needed—above and below the fracture site. Use the fifth bandage to tie around the casualty's thigh or calf, depending on where the fracture is.

Sprains and strains

IMPROVISING ELBOW SPLINTS

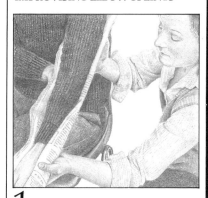

1

With a fractured elbow, sit the casualty in a chair and keep the injured arm straight. Roll up a newspaper and place it lengthways along the arm. Get the casualty to support the splint.

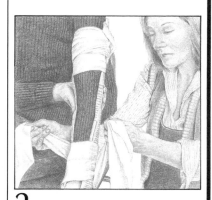

2

Make sure the casualty continues to support the improvised splint. Then secure the splint with two securing bandages—one at the top of the splint and the other at the bottom.

Sprains happen at joints, while strains involve muscles. Sprains occur when the ligaments connected with a joint are wrenched or torn. Strains occur when a muscle is over-stretched.

SPRAINS
The ankle joint is the joint most commonly affected by sprains, or the tearing of ligaments. But the wrist, elbow, knee, hip and shoulder can also suffer in this way. A severe sprain could mask a fractured ankle. If you suspect this, treat the injury as a fracture and get medical aid.

Warning signs
- Pain when moving the joint.
- Swelling of the joint and, sometimes, discoloration.
- The area over the torn ligament is tender.

STRAINS
Often muscles become strained by sudden or unaccustomed physical exertion, but they may result from an accident such as a fall.

Warning signs
- Pain over the muscle, which becomes rigid.
- There may be bruising or swelling and possible severe cramp.

SPRAINS/*ACTION*

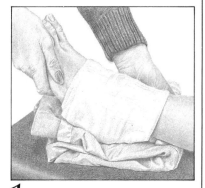

1

If indoors, remove the casualty's shoe and elevate the foot. Apply a cold compress to the injury. If outdoors, leave footwear on and apply a bandage in a figure of eight.

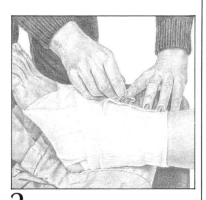

2

Place a bandage over the compress. Make one turn around the ankle, then go over the instep, under the foot, back across the instep, around the ankle again and pin. Bandage over footwear.

STRAINS/*ACTION*

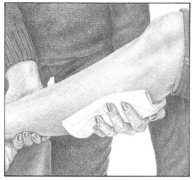

1

Place the casualty in the position most comfortable for him. Steady and support the injured part. Apply a cold compress to the area that is strained. Make sure you do not jolt the injured leg.

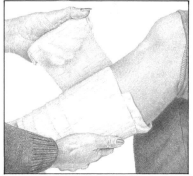

2

Keep the injured part steady and well supported and bandage firmly, but not too tightly as the muscles may swell, causing further discomfort. Then arrange for medical aid.

Stab wounds

An injury caused by stabbing or puncturing with a knife or other sharp object—for example, a bicycle spoke, steel knitting-needle, ice-pick or scissors—may appear trivial on the surface. But the skin tissues and internal organs can be severely damaged. Treat all stab or puncture wounds as serious and get medical attention immediately. *See* ABDOMINAL INJURIES *page 550*, CHEST INJURIES *page 570*.

Warning sign
• External bleeding.

STAB WOUNDS/*ACTION*

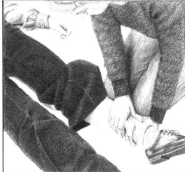

1

Stop any bleeding by pressing around the wound with clean material—such as a freshly laundered handkerchief—or your bare hands. Do not try to remove the object if it is still in the wound.

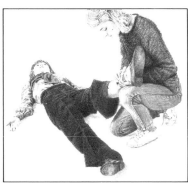

2

Rest the injured area on your knee to raise it above the level of the casualty's heart. This will help to stem the bleeding, but do not raise the area if an underlying fracture is suspected.

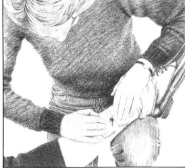

3

If a small object, such as a needle, is embedded apply a raised pad over the wound. If you do not have a raised pad, pack with matchboxes or other suitable objects.

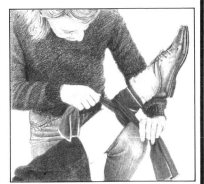

4

Put a clean dressing over the wound and bandage it lightly. If a raised pad or packing is used, apply the bandage diagonally to avoid pressure on the wound.

Stings

Treatment for stings varies according to their cause. Sometimes, antihistamine cream can help to relieve pain if applied immediately. But some people are allergic to the drug. *See* BITES AND STINGS *pages 562-3*.

Strangulation

If someone has been strangled, remove the pressure on the neck by cutting any rope, flex, scarf, tie or similar article.

Untie the knot if there is no way to cut the material, but otherwise try to preserve the knot as it may help in any police investigation to establish what happened.

If the victim has been hanged, support his body as you cut him free. Apply artificial respiration in case the casualty is still alive. *See* ASPHYXIATION *page 557.*

Stretchers

Someone who has been severely injured should be moved only if it is necessary to get urgent medical attention for him, and if it will not make his injuries worse.

If no stretcher is available, one can be improvised from coats and sticks, or from a flat, solid board such as a door. *See* MOVING AN INJURED PERSON *pages 595-7.*

There are several correct ways to load a stretcher, depending on the nature of the casualty's injuries and the number of helpers available.

With two helpers, one should roll the casualty gently on to his uninjured side, while the other pushes the open stretcher against and parallel to the casualty's back, if he is conscious, or his chest and stomach if he is unconscious.

Alternatively, the head of the open stretcher should be put at the casualty's feet. One helper supports his shoulders and the other his knees and thighs to lift him on.

IMPROVISING A STRETCHER

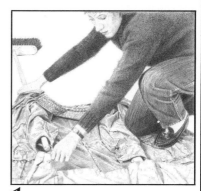

1

Turn the sleeves inside out of two or three unzipped or unbuttoned coats, and pass two strong poles through them— one on either side. With brooms, have one head at the top and one at the bottom.

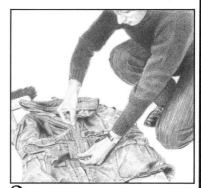

2

Secure the stretcher by zipping up or buttoning up the coats. If possible, get an uninjured person to lie on the stretcher and lift it to make sure it can take the weight.

Suffocation

In most cases of suffocation, the victim's mouth and nose have been blocked. Remove the object causing the blockage—if it is a polythene bag, by tearing it.

If the victim has been suffocated by smoke, protect yourself by tying a towel or thick piece of cloth— preferably wet—over your nose and mouth. Keep low to avoid the smoke and remove the victim as quickly as possible. Do not increase the fire risk by leaving windows and doors open. Treat the victim as for gassing. Apply artificial respiration. *See* GASSING *page 590.*

Sunburn

Sunstroke

Tooth injuries

Exposure to strong sunlight can produce skin reactions ranging from redness and itching to burns with blisters and swelling. Wind, salt water and reflected light—for example, from sea or snow—can increase the burning.

Excessive exposure to the heat of the sun can bring on headache, nausea and even death. Immediate medical treatment is needed. *See* HEAT STROKE *pages 593-4.*

All injuries to the teeth should be checked as soon as possible by a dentist or hospital dental department.

    In serious injuries to the mouth, the immediate aim is to ensure that the victim can breathe properly. Clear broken teeth and blood from his mouth with your fingers. If he is conscious, and has no other serious injuries, sit him in a chair with his head tilted forward over a bowl or basin. If he is unconscious, lie him on his stomach in the unconscious position. *See* UNCONSCIOUSNESS *page 612.*

    Never allow a casualty who is bleeding from the mouth to lie on his back, or he may choke on the blood. If bleeding continues for more than 30-40 minutes, take him to a hospital casualty department.

    Recurrent bleeding after tooth extraction may be due to over-frequent rinsing of the mouth. Tell the patient not to rinse his mouth for at least 12 hours.

SUNBURN/*ACTION*

1

Rest the casualty in the shade and give him plenty of liquids to drink. Do not allow him to go into the sun again without covering the affected areas with light, loose clothing.

2

Mild cases of sunburn can be soothed by applying calamine lotion, witch hazel or a proprietary lotion or cream, or by bathing in cool water.

3

If the sunburn is severe, get medical attention. Never deliberately burst blisters caused by sunburn.

TOOTH INJURIES/*ACTION*

1

If a tooth has been knocked completely out and is bleeding from the socket, make a pad slightly larger than the socket from sterile gauze. Get the casualty to put it on the affected area and bite firmly on it for 10 minutes. Tell him to spit out any blood that leaks through. If the bleeding does not stop, repeat the process for another 10 minutes. If the bleeding still does not stop, get medical or dental attention.

2

To try to save a whole tooth, the roots must be kept moist with saliva. Suck a piece of clean gauze until it is thoroughly damp, or get the casualty to do so. Wrap the tooth in the gauze and put it in a matchbox or other container, to take to the hospital or dentist.

Tourniquet

A tourniquet is a bandage tied above a wound and twisted tight with a stick to reduce bleeding. Although they are effective, they should *never* be applied, as they reduce the supply of oxygen in the blood and can permanently damage the tissues, leading to gangrene and possible loss of a limb.

Unconsciousness/1

An interruption in the normal activity of the brain causes unconsciousness. Anyone who has been unconscious, even for a short time, should receive immediate medical treatment.

There are three stages of unconsciousness to look for. A victim may quickly pass through all three, or remain in one. In each case, the test is the response to questions. The stages are:

Drowsiness, in which the victim is easily roused for a few moments, but then passes back into a sleep-like state. He may be able to answer questions about his condition.

Stupor, in which the victim does not react to questions easily or does so incoherently.

Coma, in which the victim cannot be roused at all, and is motionless and silent.

RECOVERY POSITION

All unconscious casualties who are breathing properly (except those with suspected fractures of the spine or neck) should be turned as quickly as possible on to their stomachs and arranged in the unconscious, or recovery, position.

The position prevents the casualty's tongue from falling into the back of his throat and choking him, and allows fluid—such as blood or vomit—to drain from his mouth.

Handle any serious wounds gently while arranging the casualty. But remember that the recovery position is a life-saver, and in most accidents involving a breathing, unconscious victim it has priority over other treatment.

UNCONSCIOUSNESS/*ACTION*

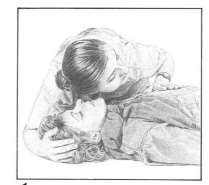

1

Check to see that the casualty is breathing. Put your ear to her nose or mouth and listen. Watch her chest to see if it rises and falls, or rest your hand lightly on it to feel for movement.

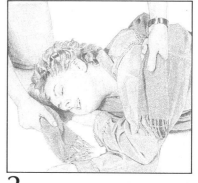

3

When breathing, loosen the casualty's clothing at the neck, chest and waist. Turn her to the recovery position. Try to ensure plenty of fresh air by opening windows and doors.

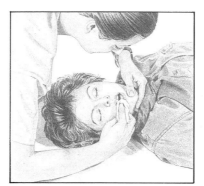

2

If she is breathing, clear her airway with your finger and clean up any blood. If she is not breathing, give artificial respiration, and if there is no pulse give chest compression.

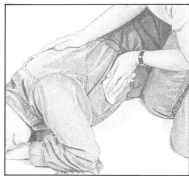

4

Check for any other injuries or bruises and stem any bleeding. Get medical aid as soon as possible. Then check to see if the victim is carrying a treatment card—say for diabetes.

Unconsciousness/2

Winding

RECOVERY POSITION/*ACTION*

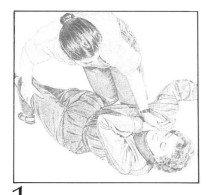

1
Kneel beside casualty. Tilt her head back and lift her chin to open her airway. Straighten both legs. Place nearer arm at right angles to body, elbow bent and palm of hand uppermost.

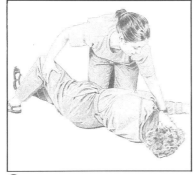

2
Bring the arm furthest from you over the casualty's chest, place the hand, with the palm outwards, against her nearer cheek, and hold it there.

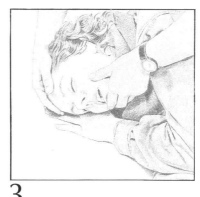

3
With your other hand, pull up her knee, keeping her foot flat on the ground. Roll her towards you, supporting her head and stopping her from rolling too far with your knees.

A hard blow in the upper part of the abdomen (the solar plexus) can cause a temporary collapse. The casualty usually gasps for air and doubles up, clutching his middle.

WINDING/*ACTION*

1
Let him curl up in a ball, or put him in the unconscious position.

2
Loosen tight clothing at the neck, chest and waist and gently massage the upper abdomen. Reassure the casualty that he is not seriously hurt and let him rest until he recovers.

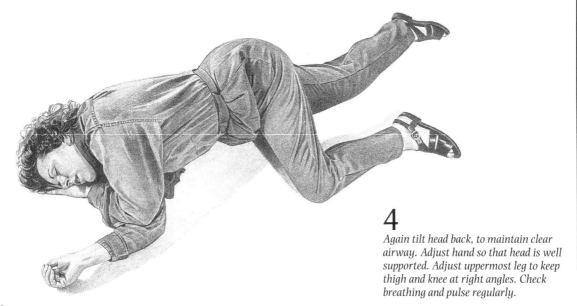

4
Again tilt head back, to maintain clear airway. Adjust hand so that head is well supported. Adjust uppermost leg to keep thigh and knee at right angles. Check breathing and pulse regularly.

INDEX

The page numbers in **black type** refer to main entries in the book. Numbers in *italic* refer to illustrations.

INDEX

INDEX

INDEX

INDEX

SELF-HELP AND VOLUNTARY ORGANISATIONS

The addresses of some of the many groups who provide support for patients, or parents of patients, with long-term health problems are given in the appropriate entries.

ACKNOWLEDGMENTS

Many members of the public
and of the medical profession
allowed themselves to be photographed
in their homes,
at their places of work
and in hospital
in order to provide reference
for many of the artists' drawings
which appear in this book.

The publishers thank them all,
together with the photographers
Ian Hooton and Andra Nelki,
and Mari Zipes Wallace
who researched the specialist photographs
used in the book.

Photographs and artwork in
FAMILY MEDICAL ADVISER
came from
the following people.

Credits read from left to right down the page. Work commissioned by Reader's Digest is shown in *italics*.

Pages 34–55 *Charles Raymond*; 81 Howard Sochurek/ John Hilleson Agency; Pages 84–85 *Charles Pickard*; 86– 87 *Jennifer Eachus*; 93 Emil Bernstein and Eila Kairinen, Gillette Research Institute/Science Magazine, August 27, 1971; 96–97 *Charles Pickard*; 98 Niels A. Lassen, MD, Bispebjerg Hospital, Denmark; 100–101 *Jennifer Eachus*; 102 John Watney; 116–117 *Keith Campbell, Howard Pemberton*; 118–125 *Howard Pemberton*; 126–127 *Keith Campbell, Howard Pemberton*; 130–139 *Howard Pemberton*; 140–141 *Keith Campbell, Howard Pemberton*; 142– 145 *Howard Pemberton*; 146–147 *Keith Campbell, Howard Pemberton*; 148 *Howard Pemberton*; 150–151 *Keith Camp- bell, Howard Pemberton*; 160–161 *Keith Campbell, Howard Pemberton*; 163 *Howard Pemberton*; 165 *Howard Pember- ton*; 166–169 *Howard Pemberton*; 174–175 Colour and vision tables from *Tests for Colour Blindness* by Dr Shinobu Ishihara, Kanehara Shuppan Co Ltd. This book should be used if an exact colour vision test is required; 180 *Andrew Aloof*, Medical Illustration Department, St Bartholomew's Hospital; 181 *Andrew Aloof*, Ron Boardman, Alltek Hospital Supplies Limited; 188–189 *Andrew Aloof*; 193 Howard Sochurek/John Hilleson Agency; 200 *Edward Williams*; 201 *Bill Prosser, Edward Williams*; 202 *Edward Williams, Bill Prosser*; 203 *Bill Prosser, Bill Prosser, Edward Williams*; 204 *Edward Williams*; 205 *Bill Prosser, Edward Williams*; 206 *Edward Williams*; 207 *Bill Prosser, Edward Williams*; 208 *Edward Williams, Bill Prosser*; 209 *Edward Williams*; 231 *Andrew Aloof*; 235–247 *Clive Arrowsmith*; 248–249 *Jennifer Eachus*; 258–261 *Jennifer Eachus*; 263 *Charles Pickard*; 265 *Charles Pickard*; 266 *Charles Pickard*; 276–285 *Jennifer Eachus*; 286–287 *Charles Pickard*; 289 E. H. Cook/Science Photo Library; 292–309 *Bill Prosser*; 310 A. R. Williams; 215 Petit Format/C. Edelmann, Petit Format/Guigoz; 316 Petit Format/Guigoz; 317 Petit Format/Guigoz; 326 Dr G. Paul Moore/Institute for the Advanced Study of Communication Processes, University of Florida; 332 Professor R. Damadian/Science Photo Library, *Andrew Aloof*; 333 *Andrew Aloof*; 334 A. R. Brody/ Science Photo Library, Dr A. Liepins/Science Photo Library; 335 Dr D. McLaren/Science Photo Library, Dr G. F. Lee- dale/Biofotos; 336 *Andrew Aloof*, Transparencies by William C. Nyberg and Alexander Tsiaras from Discover Magazine, March 1981 © Time Inc./Colorific!; 337 *Andrew Aloof*; 338 Dr R: P. Clark and Mervyn Goff/Science Photo Library; 341 Dr G. Bredberg/Science Photo Library; 356–357 *Andrew Aloof*; 363 CNRI/Vision International; 369 Dr G. Leedale/Biophotos/Science Photo Library; 370–371 *Andrew Aloof*; 392 Ray Ruddick/The London Hospital, Whitechapel, London; 393 David H. Trapnell/Queen Mary's Hospital, Roehampton, London; 398 Medtronic, Inc. Minneapolis; 414 Dr Mair, Northwick Park Hospital, Harrow, Middlesex; 415 *Andrew Aloof*; 416–417 *Charles Pickard*; 422–433 *Charles Pickard*; 434–435 *Andrew Aloof*; 443 *Image modification by Michael G. Gould, AIIP, FRSA, University of Warwick Photographic Department and Miss J. Silver, Moorfields Eye Hospital, London*; 445 Dr R. Dour- mashkin/Science Photo Library; 447 Howard Sochurek/ John Hilleson Agency; 454–459 *Jennifer Eachus*; 460 *Andrew Aloof*; Brookhaven National Laboratory and New York University Medical Centre; 461 Brookhaven National Laboratory and New York University Medical Centre; 472–475 *Jennifer Eachus*; 476 *Charles Pickard*; 488 John Watney; 496–499 *Jennifer Eachus*; 500 Gibbs Oral Hygiene Centre, CNRI/Vision International, Gibbs Oral Hygiene Centre, Gibbs Oral Hygiene Centre, Gibbs Oral Hygiene Centre; 501 *Jennifer Eachus*; 502 *Jennifer Eachus*; 503 Mr Alan Lynch; 528–537 *Clive Arrowsmith*; 541 *Gordon Lawson*; 542–549 *Andrew Aloof*; 550–551 *Gordon Lawson*; 552–557 *Andrew Aloof*; 558 *Bill Prosser*; 560–563 *Gordon Lawson*; 564–567 *Andrew Aloof*; 568–571 *Gordon Lawson*; 572–579 *Andrew Aloof*; 580 *Malcolm McGregor*; 581–585 *Andrew Aloof*; 586–589 *Malcolm McGregor*; 590 *Andrew Aloof*; 591 *Malcolm McGregor*; 592–593 Nicholas Hall; 594–595 *Malcolm McGregor*; 596–598 *Andrew Aloof*; 599 *Malcolm McGregor*; 600–607 *Stephen Pointer*; 608–612 *Andrew Aloof*.

A number of organisations
also gave assistance
and the publishers would like
to thank them.
They include:

Batricar Limited, Thrupp, Glos; British Dental Health Foundation, Milton Keynes, Bucks; S. Burvill & Son, Walton-on-Thames, Surrey; Classwood Limited, Per- shore, Worcestershire; Department of Helath and Social Security, Alexander Fleming House, London; M. Gilbert (Greenford) Limited, Greenford, Middlesex; Glemby Inter- national at Harvey Nichols, London; Habitat and Conran Associates, London; D. C. Hodge & Son Limited, Staines, Middlesex; Homecraft Supplies, London; Hozelock Limited, Haddenham, Bucks; Mecanaids Limited, Gloucester; Nicholls & Clarke Limited, London; Parker Bath Develop- ments Limited, New Milton, Hampshire; Tremorrah Indus- tries, Rentoul Works, Truro, Cornwall; Relax House- wares, Marlow, Bucks; Reselco Invalid Carriages Limited, London; Spear & Jackson (Tools) Limited, Wednesbury, West Midlands; The London Imaging Centre, London; Waves, Dorchester, Dorset; Wessex Medical Equipment Company Limited, Romsey, Hampshire; Wilkinson Sword Limited, High Wycombe, Bucks.

The table of weights on page 525 is reproduced by cour- tesy of Metropolitan Life Insurance Company, New York.

The publishers
also acknowledge their indebtedness
to the following books and journals
which were consulted
for reference:

Blakiston's Gould Medical Dictionary McGraw-Hill Inc.; *British National Formulary Number 1 1981*, British Medi- cal Association and The Pharmaceutical Society of Great Britain; Churchill Livingstone *Nurses Dictionary*, edited by Nancy Roper; *Common Diseases*, John Fry, MTP Press Limited; *Concise Medical Dictionary*, Elizabeth A. Martin, Oxford University Press; *Current Medical Diagnosis & Treat- ment 1981*, Marcus A. Krupp and Milton J. Chatton, Lange Medical Publications; *Emergency Care and Transpor- tation of the sick and injured*, The committee on injuries, American Academy of Orthopaedic Surgeons; *Family Health Guide*, The Reader's Digest Association Limited; The Royal Society of Medicine *Family Medical Guide*, edited by A. M. Cooke, Longman; *First Aid*, the authorised manual of British Red Cross Society; *Gray's Anatomy*, T. B. Johnston, D. V. Davies and F. Davies, Longman; *The Har- vard Medical School Health Letter*, Harvard Medical School; *Health and Personal Social Services for England*, HMSO; *Larousse Médical*, Librairie Larousse, Paris; *Martindale The Extra Pharmacopoeia*, edited by Ainley Wade, The Phar- maceutical Press; *The Medical Directory 1980*, Churchill Livingstone; *Medical Terminology in Hospital Practice*, Paul M. Davies, William Heinemann Medical Books Ltd; *The Merck Manual*, Robert Berkow, Merck, Sharp & Dohme Research Laboratories; *New Essential First Aid*, A. Ward and Peter J. Roylance, Pan Books Ltd; *Practice, A Handbook of Primary Medical Care*, edited by Jack Cormack, Marshall Marinker and David Morrell, Kluwer-Harrap Handbooks; Harrison's *Principles of Internal Medicine*, McGraw-Hill Inc.; *The Complete Medical Encyclopaedia, Symptoms*, edited by Sigmund Stephen Miller, Pan Books in association with Macmillan; *Scientific American*, Scientific American Inc.; *Towards Earlier Diagnosis in Primary Care*, Keith Hodgkin, Churchill Livingstone; *The Journal of Postgraduate Practice, Update*, Update Publications Ltd; *World Medicine*, New Medical Journals Ltd; *You and Your Rights*, The Reader's Digest Association Limited.

40-030-14